MW01203885

Handbook of Behavioral Medicine

Andrew Steptoe
Editor

Handbook of Behavioral Medicine

Methods and Applications

Editor

Andrew Steptoe
Department of Epidemiology and Public Health,
University College London, London, UK

Associate Editors

Kenneth E. Freedland
Department of Psychiatry, Washington University School of Medicine,
St. Louis, MO, USA

J. Richard Jennings
Department of Psychiatry, University of Pittsburgh, Pittsburgh, PA,
USA

Maria M. Llabre
Department of Psychology, University of Miami, Miami, FL, USA

Stephen B. Manuck
Department of Psychology, University of Pittsburgh, Pittsburgh, PA,
USA

Elizabeth J. Susman
Department of Biobehavioral Health, Pennsylvania State University,
University Park, PA, USA

Assistant Editor

Lydia Poole
Department of Epidemiology and Public Health,
University College London, London, UK

In association with the
Academy of Behavioral Medicine Research

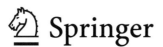 Springer

Editor

Andrew Steptoe
Department of Epidemiology
    and Public Health
University College London
London, UK
a.steptoe@ucl.ac.uk

Associate Editors

Kenneth E. Freedland
Department of Psychiatry
Washington University
    School of Medicine
St. Louis, MO, USA
freedlak@bmc.wustl.edu

J. Richard Jennings
Department of Psychiatry
University of Pittsburgh
Pittsburgh, PA, USA
jenningsjr@upmc.edu

Maria M. Llabre
Department of Psychology
University of Miami
Miami, FL, USA
mllabre@miami.edu

Stephen B. Manuck
Department of Psychology
University of Pittsburgh
Pittsburgh, PA, USA
manuck@imap.pitt.edu

Elizabeth J. Susman
Department of Biobehavioral Health
Pennsylvania State University
University Park, PA, USA
esusman@psu.edu

ISBN 978-0-387-09487-8   e-ISBN 978-0-387-09488-5
DOI 10.1007/978-0-387-09488-5
Springer New York Dordrecht Heidelberg London

Library of Congress Control Number: 2010933789

Printed on acid-free paper

Springer is part of Springer Science+Business Media (www.springer.com)

Preface

Behavioral medicine emerged in the 1970s as the interdisciplinary field concerned with the integration of behavioral, psychosocial, and biomedical science knowledge relevant to the understanding of health and illness, and the application of this knowledge to prevention, diagnosis, treatment, and rehabilitation. The Academy of Behavioral Medicine Research was founded in 1978 as a forum for established behavioral medicine researchers to exchange ideas in an informal atmosphere. The discipline has subsequently grown and evolved substantially. Recent years have witnessed an enormous diversification of behavioral medicine, with new sciences (e.g., genetics, life course epidemiology) and new technologies (e.g., neuroimaging) coming into play. New health problems have emerged, notably obesity and metabolic disorders, that present fresh challenges to the integration of behavioral sciences with public health. Traditional areas of behavioral medicine research such as the influence of psychological factors on physiological responses have been transformed with measures of intracellular processes, cell signaling molecules, cardiac morphology, and gene expression. Cardiovascular behavioral medicine and psychoneuroimmunology, the disciplines which underpin much of the pathophysiological research in behavioral medicine, have converged in the shared exploration of biobehavioral processes across a range of medical conditions. The field of psychological assessment has benefited from new techniques such as ecological momentary assessment and item response theory, while objective methods are being increasingly used in behavioral assessment. Interventional behavioral medicine has had a new lease on life with large clinical trials, the use of the Internet and other information technologies, and the introduction of the public health perspective into the individual-level behavioral change tradition. These developments have obliged practitioners to embrace new statistical and analytic approaches. Theoretical understanding has developed considerably, with concepts such as allostatic load, illness representations, and epigenetics enriching the diverse domains of behavioral medicine. The discipline has also become international, with learned societies in more than 20 countries, and high-quality research laboratories spread throughout the world.

There is a need to bring together these new developments in a compendium of methods and applications. This handbook aims to fill this need by providing an up to date survey of methods and applications drawn from the broad range of behavioral medicine research and practice. The handbook is divided into 10 sections that address key fields in behavioral medicine, ranging from basic biobehavioral processes, through individual developmental and socioemotional factors, to public health and clinical trials. Each section begins with one or two methodological or conceptual chapters, followed by contributions that address substantive topics within that field. There are very few disease-orientated chapters; rather, major health problems such as cardiovascular disease, cancer, HIV/AIDS, and obesity are explored from multiple perspectives. Our aim is to present behavioral medicine as an integrative discipline, involving diverse methodologies and research paradigms that converge on health and well-being.

As an editor, I should like to express my gratitude to the five associate editors who provided great expertise and support throughout the preparation of this book, to the assistant editor Lydia Poole for her unstinting work, and to the many contributors who have enabled the handbook to be completed in a timely fashion. The editorial team have also greatly benefited from the wisdom of an advisory group of distinguished members of the Academy of Behavioral Medicine Research, namely Ronald Glaser (Ohio State University), Kenneth E. Freedland (Washington University School of Medicine), Kathleen C. Light (University of Utah), Philip M. McCabe (University of Miami), and Andrew Baum (University of Texas, Arlington). Our thanks also go to the editorial and production groups at Springer for their efficiency and helpfulness during the production process.

London, UK   Andrew Steptoe
January 2010

Contents

Contributors

Pilvikki Absetz Adjunct Professor of Health Promotion, University of Tampere, School of Public Health and National Institute for Health and Welfare, P.O. Box 30, FI-00271 Helsinki, Finland, pilvikki.absetz@thl.fi

Sara Ahmed Assistant Professor, Faculty of Medicine, School of Physical and Occupational Therapy, McGill University, 3654 Prom Sir-William-Osler, Montréal, QC H3G 1Y5, Canada, sara.ahmed@mcgill.ca

Leona S. Aiken Professor of Psychology, Department of Psychology, Arizona State University, 950 S. McAllister Ave., P.O. Box 871104, Tempe, AZ 85287-1104, USA, leona.aiken@asu.edu

Michael H. Antoni Professor of Psychology, Department of Psychology, University of Miami, P.O. Box 248185, Coral Gables, FL 33124-0751, USA, mantoni@miami.edu

Michael A. Babyak Professor of Medical Psychology, Department of Psychiatry and Behavioral Sciences, Duke University Medical Center, Box 3119 DUMC, Durham, NC 27707, USA, babya001@mc.duke.edu

Stacy Cooper Bailey Clinical Research Associate and Program Director, Health Literacy and Learning Program, Center for Communication in Healthcare, Division of General Internal Medicine, and Institute for Healthcare Studies, Feinberg School of Medicine at Northwestern University, 750 N. Lake Shore Drive, 10th Floor, Chicago, IL 60611, USA, stacy-bailey@northwestern.edu

Michael T. Bailey Assistant Professor, Institute for Behavioral Medicine Research, The Ohio State University, 257 IBMR Building, 460 Medical Center Drive, Columbus, OH 43210, USA, michael.bailey@osu.edu

Kylie Ball Associate Professor, School of Exercise and Nutrition Sciences, Deakin University, 221 Burwood Highway, 3125 VIC, Australia, kylie.ball@deakin.edu.au

John C. Barefoot Research Professor, Department of Psychiatry and Behavioral Science, Duke University Medical Center, Box 2969, Durham, NC 27710, USA, john.barefoot@duke.edu

Silja Bellingrath Postdoctoral Fellow in Health Psychology, Jacobs Center on Lifelong Learning and Institutional Development, Jacobs University Bremen, Campus Ring 1, 28759 Bremen, Germany, s.bellingrath@jacobs-university.de

Yoav Ben-Shlomo Professor of Clinical Epidemiology, Department of Social Medicine, University of Bristol, Canynge Hall, 39 Whatley Road, Bristol BS8 2PS, UK, y.ben-shlomo@bristol.ac.uk

James A. Blumenthal Professor of Medical Psychology, Department of Psychiatry and Behavioral Sciences, Duke University Medical Center, Box 3119, Durham, NC 27710, USA, blume003@mc.duke.edu

Shawn D. Boykin Research fellow, Department of Epidemiology, Center for Integrative Approaches to Health Disparities, University of Michigan School of Public Health, 109 South Observatory St, Ann Arbor, MI 48109, USA, sdhb@umich.edu

Jessica Y. Breland Teaching Assistant, Department of Psychology, Institute for Health, Health Care Policy and Aging Research Rutgers, The State University of New Jersey, 30 College Ave., New Brunswick, NJ 08901-1293, USA, jbreland@eden.rutgers.edu

Michael P. Carey Director, Center for Health and Behavior, Syracuse University, 415-B Huntington Hall, Syracuse, NY 13244-2340, USA, mpcarey@syr.edu

Robert M. Carney Professor of Psychiatry, Behavioral Medicine Center, Washington University School of Medicine, 4320 Forest Park Avenue, Suite 301, St. Louis, MI 63108 USA, carneyr@wustl.edu

Charles S. Carver Professor of Psychology, Department of Psychology, University of Miami, 5665 Ponce de Leon Blvd., Coral Gables, FL 33124-0751, USA, ccarver@miami.edu

Carina K.Y. Chan Lecturer, Medicine and Health Sciences, Monash University (Sunway Campus), Building 3, Jalan Lagoon Selatan, Bandar Sunway, 46150 Selangor Darul Ehsan, Malaysia, carina.chan@med.monash.edu.my

Tarani Chandola Professor in Medical Sociology, CCSR, School of Social Sciences, Kantorovich Building, Humanities Bridgeford Street, University of Manchester, Manchester, M13 9PL, UK, tarani.chandola@manchester.ac.uk

Edith Chen Canada Research Chair in Health & Society, Associate Professor, Department of Psychology, University of British Columbia, 2136 West Mall, Vancouver, BC V6T 1Z4, BC, Canada, echen@psych.ubc.ca

Robert B. Cialdini Professor of Psychology and Marketing, Department of Psychology, Arizona State University, 950 S. McAllister Ave., P.O. Box 871104, Tempe, AZ 85287-1104, USA robert.cialdini@asu.edu

Cari J. Clark Research Associate, Department of Medicine, Program in Health Disparities Research, University of Minnesota Medical School, 717 Delaware Street SE, Suite 166, Minneapolis, MN 55414, USA, cjclark@umn.edu

Noreen M. Clark Myron E. Wegman Distinguished University Professor, Director, Center for Managing Chronic Disease, University of Michigan, 1415 Washington Heights, Ann Arbor, MI 48109, USA, nmclark@umich.edu

Verity J. Cleland Research Fellow, Centre for Physical Activity and Nutrition Research, Deakin University, 221 Burwood Highway, Burwood, VIC 3125, Australia, verity.cleland@utas.edu.au

Christopher L. Coe Professor of Psychology, Department of Psychology, Harlow Center for Biological Psychology, University of Wisconsin, 22 N. Charter Street, Madison, WI 53715, USA, ccoe@wisc.edu

Steve W. Cole Associate Professor, Department of Medicine, Division of Hematology-Oncology, UCLA School of Medicine, 11-934 Factor Building, Los Angeles, CA 90095-1678, USA, coles@ucla.edu

Mark Conner Professor of Applied Social Psychology, Institute of Psychological Sciences, University of Leeds, Leeds LS2 9JT, UK, m.t.conner@leeds.ac.uk

David Crawford Director, Centre for Physical Activity and Nutrition Research, Deakin University, 221 Burwood Highway, Burwood, VIC 3125, Australia, david.crawford@deakin.edu.au

Hugo D. Critchley Professor of Psychiatry, Clinical Imaging Sciences Centre, Brighton and Sussex Medical School, University of Sussex, Falmer, Brighton BN1 9RR, UK, h.critchley@bsms.ac.uk

Eco de Geus Professor of Psychology, Department of Biological Psychology, VU University, Van der Boechorststraat 1, 1081 BT, Amsterdam, The Netherlands, jcn.de.geus@psy.vu.nl

Ana V. Diez Roux Professor of Epidemiology, Department of Epidemiology, Center for Social Epidemiology and Population Health, University of Michigan School of Public Health, 109 Observatory St, Ann Arbor, MI 48109-2029, USA, adiezrou@umich.edu

Jenna Duffecy Assistant Professor, Department of Preventive Medicine, Northwestern University, Feinberg School of Medicine, 680 N. Lakeshore Drive, Suite 1220, Chicago, IL 60611, USA, j-duffecy@northwestern.edu

Jacqueline Dunbar-Jacob Professor and Dean of Nursing, University of Pittsburgh, 350 Victoria Building, 3500 Victoria St, Pittsburgh, PA 15261, USA, dunbar@pitt.edu

Victoria Egizio Graduate Student, Department of Psychiatry, University of Pittsburgh, Western Psychiatric Institute and Clinic, 3811 O'Hara St, Pittsburgh, PA 15213, USA, vbe1@pitt.edu

Susan E. Embretson Professor of Psychology, School of Psychology,
Georgia Institute of Technology, 654 Cherry St, Atlanta, GA 30332-0170,
USA, susan.embretson@psych.gatech.edu

Gina T. Eubanks Supervisor, Research Project Coordinator, Division of
Cardiovascular Medicine, Emory University, Atlanta, GA, USA; University
of South Florida, 1717 W Hills Ave Unit 3, Tampa, FL 33606, USA,
geubank@emory.edu

Susan A. Everson-Rose Associate Professor, Department of Medicine,
Program in Health Disparities Research, University of Minnesota Medical
School, 717 Delaware Street SE, Suite 166, Minneapolis, MN 55414, USA,
saer@umn.edu

Kenneth E. Freedland Professor of Psychiatry, Behavioral Medicine
Center, Department of Psychiatry, Washington University School of
Medicine, 4320 Forest Park Avenue, Suite 301, St. Louis, MI 63108, USA,
freedlak@bmc.wustl.edu

William Gerin Professor of Behavioral Health, Department of
Biobehavioral Health, College of Health and Human Development, The
Pennsylvania State University, 315 Health and Human Development East,
University Park, PA 16802, USA, wxg17@psu.ed

Peter J. Gianaros Assistant Professor of Psychiatry and Psychology,
Department of Psychiatry, University of Pittsburgh, Western Psychiatric
Institute and Clinic, 3811 O'Hara Street, Pittsburgh, PA 15213, USA,
gianarospj@upmc.edu

Andrea Gierens Director of the Biochemical Laboratories, Division of
Clinical and Physiological Psychology, University of Trier, Johanniterufer
15, D-54290 Trier, Germany, cortlab@uni_trier.de

Susan S. Girdler Professor and Director of the Stress and Health Research
Program, Department of Psychiatry, University of North Carolina at Chapel
Hill, Chapel Hill, NC 27599-7175, USA, susan_girdler@med.unc.edu

Ronald Glaser Professor of Molecular Virology, Immunology and
Medical Genetics, Director, Institute for Behavioral Medicine Research,
The Ohio State University, 120 IBMR Building, 460 Medical Center Drive,
Columbus, OH 43210, USA, ronald.glaser@osumc.edu, glaser.1@osu.edu

Ronald B. Goldberg Professor of Medicine, Division of Endocrinology,
Diabetes and Metabolism and Diabetes Research Institute, University of
Miami Miller School of Medicine, P.O. Box 016960, Miami, FL
33101-6960, USA, rgoldber@med.miami.edu

Marcus A. Gray Lecturer in Psychiatry and Neuroimaging, Trafford
Centre/Clinical Imaging Sciences Centre University of Sussex, Falmer,
Brighton, BN1 9PX, UK, m.gray@bsms.ac.uk

Tara L. Gruenewald Assistant Professor, Department of Medicine,
Division of Geriatrics, UCLA School of Medicine, 10945 Le Conte Avenue,

Suite 2339, Los Angeles, CA 90095-1687, USA,
tgruenewald@mednet.ucla.edu

Martica H. Hall Associate Professor of Psychiatry and Psychology,
Department of Psychiatry, University of Pittsburgh, Western Psychiatric
Institute and Clinic, 3811 O'Hara St, Pittsburgh, PA 15213, USA,
hallmh@upmc.edu

Anita L. Hansen Leader, Operational Psychology Research Group,
Department of Psychosocial Sciences, Faculty of Psychology, University of
Bergen, Christiesgate 12, N-5015 Bergen, Norway,
anita.hansen@psysp.uib.no

Mustafa Hassan Cardiology Fellow, Division of Cardiovascular Medicine,
University of Florida, 1600 SW Archer Rd., PO Box 100277, Gainesville,
FL 32610, USA, mustafa.mahmoudhassan@medicine.ufl.edu

Gerard Hastings Director, Institute for Social Marketing, University of
Stirling, Stirling FK9 4LA, Scotland, UK, gerard.hastings@stir.ac.uk

Larry V. Hedges Professor of Statistics and Policy Research, Professor in
the School of Education and social Policy, Department of Statistics,
Northwestern University, 2046 Sheridan Road, Evanston, IL 60208, USA,
l-hedges@northwestern.edu

Dirk H. Hellhammer Professor of Clinical and Physiological Psychology,
Division of Clinical and Physiological Psychology, University of Trier,
Johanniterufer 15, Trier, D-54290, Germany, hellhamm@uni-trier.de

Megan M. Hosey Graduate Student, Department of Psychology,
University of Maryland, Baltimore County, 1000 Hilltop Circle, Baltimore,
MD 21250, USA, mhosey1@umbc.edu

Christy R. Houle Postdoctoral Scholar, Center for Managing Chronic
Disease, University of Michigan, 1415 Washington Heights, Ann Arbor, MI
48109, USA, cmcd-info@umich.edu

Martin P. Houze Graduate Student, Center for Research and Evaluation,
School of Nursing, University of Pittsburgh, 350 Victoria Building, 3500
Victoria St, Pittsburgh, PA 15261, USA, houzem@pitt.edu

M. Bryant Howren Postdoctoral Fellow, VA Iowa City Healthcare System,
601 Hwy 6 west, Iowa City, IA 52240, USA, matthew.howren.va.gov

Ai Ikeda Research Fellow, Department of Society, Human Development
and Health, Harvard School of Public Health, 677 Huntington Avenue,
Kresge Building 7th Floor, Boston, MA 02115, USA, ai-ikeda@umin.ac.jp

Gail H. Ironson Professor of Psychology, Department of Psychology,
University of Miami, P.O. Box 248185, Coral Gables, FL 33124-0751,
USA, gironson@aol.com

J. Richard Jennings Professor of Psychiatry and Psychology, Department of Psychiatry, University of Pittsburgh, Western Psychiatric Institute and Clinic, 3811 O'Hara St, Pittsburgh, PA 15213, USA, jenningsjr@upmc.edu

Bjorn Helge Johnsen Professor of Personality Psychology, Faculty of Psychology, University of Bergen, Christiesgate 12, N-5015, Bergen, Norway, bjorn.johnsen@psysp.uib.no

Seth C. Kalichman Professor of Psychology, Department of Psychology, Center for Health, Intervention, and Prevention, University of Connecticut, 406 Babbidge Road, Storrs, CT 06269, USA, seth.k@uconn.edu

Ilia N. Karatsoreos Postdoctoral Fellow, Harold and Margaret Milliken Hatch Laboratory of Neuroendocrinology, The Rockefeller University, 1230 York Ave, New York, NY 10021, USA, ikaratsore@mail.rockefeller.edu

Ichiro Kawachi Professor of Social Epidemiology and Chair, Department of Society, Human Development and Health, Harvard School of Public Health, 677 Huntington Avenue, Kresge Building 7th Floor, Boston, MA 02115, USA, ikawachi@hsph.harvard.edu

Mee-Ae Kim-O Graduate Student, School of Psychology, Georgia Institute of Technology, 654 Cherry St, Atlanta, GA 30332-0170, USA, gth733b@mail.gatech.edu

Sarah W. Kinsinger Assistant Professor, Department of Medicine and Psychiatry, Division of Gastroenterology, Northwestern University, Feinberg School of Medicine, 680 N. St. Clair Street, Suite 1400, Chicago, IL 60611, USA, s-kinsinger@northwestern.edu

Helena Chmura Kraemer Professor of Biostatistics in Psychiatry (Emerita), Department of Psychiatry and Behavioral Sciences, Stanford University, 1116 Forest Avenue, Palo Alto, CA 94301, USA, hckhome@pacbell.net

Cameron Kramer Graduate Student, Department of Health and Community Systems, School of Nursing, University of Pittsburgh, 350 Victoria Building, 3500 Victoria St, Pittsburgh, PA 15261, USA, clkst32@pitt.edu

Diana Kuh Professor of Life Course Epidemiology, Director, 1MRC Unit for Lifelong Health and Ageing, Department of Epidemiology and Public Health, University College London, 33 Bedford Place, London WC1B 5JU, UK, d.kuh@nshd.mrc.ac.uk

Richard D. Lane Professor of Psychiatry, Psychology, and Neuroscience, Department of Psychiatry, University of Arizona, 1501 N. Campbell Ave., Tucson, AZ 85724-5002, USA, lane@email.arizona.edu

Caryn Lerman Mary W. Calkins Professor and Director, Tobacco Use Research Center, Department of Psychiatry, University of Pennsylvania, 3535 Market Street, Suite 4100, Philadelphia, PA 19104, USA, clerman@mail.med.upenn.edu

Elaine A. Leventhal Professor of Medicine, Department of Medicine, University of Medicine and Dentistry of New Jersey, UMDNJ-RWJ Medical School 125 Paterson Street - CAB 2310, New Brunswick, NJ 08903, USA, eleventh@umdnj.edu

Howard Leventhal Professor of Health Psychology, Department of Psychology, Institute for Health, Health Care Policy and Aging Research Rutgers, The State University of New Jersey, 30 College Ave., New Brunswick, NJ 08901-1293, USA, hleventhal@ifh.rutgers.edu

Kathleen C. Light Research Professor, Department of Anesthesiology, University of Utah, 615 Arapeen Drive, Suite 200, Salt Lake City, UT 84108, USA, kathleen.c.light@hsc.utah.edu

Maria Magdalena Llabre Professor of Psychology, Department of Psychology, University of Miami, P.O. Box 24-8185, Coral Gables, FL 33124, USA, mllabre@miami.edu

Ruth J.F. Loos Group Leader, Medical Research Council (MRC) Epidemiology Unit, Institute of Metabolic Science, Addenbrooke's Hospital – Box 285, Hills Road, Cambridge CB2 0QQ, UK, ruth.loos@mrc.epid.cam.ac.uk

Ray Lowry Senior Lecturer, Child Dental Health School of Dental Sciences, Newcastle University, Newcastle on Tyne, NE2 4BW, UK, r.j.lowry@ncl.ac.uk

Patrick J. Lustman Professor of Psychiatry, Department of Psychiatry, Washington University School of Medicine, 660 S. Euclid, Campus Box 8134, St. Louis, MI 63108, USA, lustmanp@wustl.edu

Faith Luyster Postdoctoral Scholar in Psychiatry, Department of Psychiatry, University of Pittsburgh, 350 Victoria Building, 3500 Victoria St., Pittsburgh, PA 15261, USA, fsl3@pitt.edu

Stephen B. Manuck Distinguished University Professor of Health Psychology and Behavioral Medicine, Behavioral Physiology Laboratory, Department of Psychology, University of Pittsburgh, 506 OEH, 4015 O'Hara Street, Pittsburgh, PA 15260, USA, manuck@imap.pitt.edu

Laura A.V. Marlow Research Associate, Department of Epidemiology & Public Health, Health Behaviour Research Centre, University College London, Gower Street, London WC1E 6BT, UK, l.marlow@ucl.ac.uk

Sir Michael G. Marmot Professor of Epidemiology, Department of Epidemiology and Public Health, University College London, London WC1E 6BT, UK, m.marmot@ucl.ac.uk

Scott C. Matthews Assistant Professor of Psychiatry, University of California San Diego, 3350 La Jolla Village Drive (Mail Code 116-A), San Diego, CA 92161, USA, scmatthews@ucsd.edu

Philip M. McCabe Professor, Associate Chairman, Department of
Psychology, University of Miami, P.O. Box 248185, Coral Gables, FL
33124, USA, pmccabe@miami.edu

Jeanne M. McCaffery Assistant Professor of Psychiatry and Human
Behavior, Weight Control and Diabetes Research Center, Brown Medical
School and The Miriam Hospital, 196 Richmond Street, Providence, RI
02903, USA, jeanne_mcCaffery@brown.edu

Kirsten J. McCaffery Senior Research Fellow, School of Public Health
and Centre for Medical Psychology and Evidence-Based Decision Making,
Edward Ford Building (A27), The University of Sydney, Sydney, NSW
2006, Australia, kirsten.mccaffery@sydney.edu.au

Maura McCall Graduate Student, Department of Health and Community
Systems, School of Nursing, University of Pittsburgh, 360 Victoria
Building, 3500 Victoria St, Pittsburgh, PA 15261, USA, mccallm@pitt.edu

Bruce S. McEwen Alfred E. Mirsky Professor, Head, Harold and Margaret
Milliken Hatch Laboratory of Neuroendocrinology, The Rockefeller
University, 1230 York Ave, New York, NY 10021, USA,
mcewen@mail.rockefeller.edu

Armando J. Mendez Assistant Professor of Medicine, Department of
Medicine, Division of Endocrinology, Diabetes and Metabolism and
Diabetes Research Institute, University of Miami Miller School of
Medicine, 1450 N.W. 10th Avenue, Miami, FL 33136, USA,
amendez2@med.miami.edu

Gregory E. Miller Associate Professor, Department of Psychology,
University of British Columbia, 2136 West Mall, Vancouver BC, Canada
V6T 1Z4, gemiller@psych.ubc.ca

Paul J. Mills Professor in Residence, Department of Psychiatry,
Behavioral Medicine Program, University of California at San Diego, 9500
Gilman Drive, La Jolla, CA 92093-0804, USA, pmills@ucsd.edu

Gita D. Mishra Programme leader, MRC Unit for Lifelong Health and
Ageing, Department of Epidemiology and Public Health, University
College London, 33 Bedford Place, London WC1B 5JU, UK,
g.mishra@nshd.mrc.ac.uk

David C. Mohr Professor of Preventive Medicine, Department of
Preventive Medicine, Northwestern University, Feinberg School of
Medicine, 680 N. Lakeshore Drive, Suite 1220, Chicago, IL 60611, USA,
d-mohr@northwestern.edu

Pablo A. Mora Assistant Professor of Psychology, Psychology
Department, University of Texas at Arlington, 501 S. Nedderman,
Arlington, TX 76019, USA, pmora@uta.edu

Mahasin S. Mujahid Assistant Professor of Epidemiology, Division of
Epidemiology, University of California Berkeley, School of Public Health,

50 University Hall, #7360, Berkeley, CA 94720-7360, USA,
mmujahid@berkeley.edu

Marian L. Neuhouser Associate Member, Cancer Prevention Program,
Fred Hutchinson Cancer Research Center, 1100 Fairview Avenue North,
M4-B402, Seattle, WA 98109-1024, USA, mneuhous@fhcrc.org

Ilja M. Nolte Statistical Geneticist, Unit of Genetic Epidemiology &
Bioinformatics, Department of Epidemiology, University Medical Center
Groningen, University of Groningen, Hanzeplein 1, PO Box 30.001, 9700
RB Groningen, The Netherlands, i.m.nolte@epi.umcg.nl

Judith K. Ockene Professor of Medicine, Division of Preventive and
Behavioral Medicine, University of Massachusetts Medical School, 55,
Lake Avenue North, Worcester, MA 01655-0214, USA,
judith.ockene@umassmed.edu

Brian Oldenburg Professor of International Public Health, Department of
Epidemiology and Preventive Medicine, Monash University, 89
Commercial Rd, Melbourne, VIC 3004, Australia,
brian.oldenburg@med.monash.edu.au

Lephuong Ong Clinical Associate, Department of Psychiatry and
Behavioral Sciences, Duke University Medical Center, Box 3119, Durham,
NC 27710, USA, lephuong.ong@duke.edu

Ikechukwu Onyewuenyi Graduate Student, Department of Psychiatry,
University of Pittsburgh, Western Psychiatric Institute and Clinic, 3811
O'Hara Street, Pittsburgh, PA 15213, USA, onyewuenyiic2@upmc.edu

C. Tracy Orleans Distinguished Fellow and Senior Scientist, Robert Wood
Johnson Foundation, Route 1 and College Road East, P.O. Box 2316,
Princeton, NJ 08543, USA, cto@rwjf.org

Frank J. Penedo Associate Professor of Psychology, Department of
Psychology & Psychiatry & Behavioral Sciences, University of Miami, P.O.
Box 248185, Coral Gables, FL 33124-0751, USA; Behavioral Medicine
Research Center, University of Miami, P.O. Box 248185, Coral Gables, FL
33124-0751, USA, fpenedo@miami.edu

Brenda W.J.H. Penninx Professor of Psychiatric Epidemiology,
Department of Psychiatry, VU University Medical Center, AJ Ernststraat
887, 1081 HL, Amsterdam, The Netherlands, b.penninx@vumc.nl

Lydia Poole Graduate Student, Psychobiology Group, Department of
Epidemiology and Public Health, University College London, 1-19
Torrington Place, London WC1E 6BT, UK, lydia.poole.09@ucl.ac.uk

Petra Puetz Research Associate, Department of Clinical and Physiological
Psychology, University of Trier, Johanniterufer 15, Trier, D-54290,
Germany, puet1301@uni-trier.de

Riju Ray Research Associate in Psychiatry, Department of Psychiatry, University of Pennsylvania, 3535 Market Street, Suite 4100, Philadelphia, PA 19104, USA, rijuray@mail.med.upenn.edu

Allecia E. Reid Graduate Research Associate, Department of Psychology, Arizona State University, 950 S. McAllister Ave., P.O. Box 871104, Tempe, AZ 85287-1104, USA, allecia.reid@asu.edu

Neil Schneiderman Professor of Psychology, Department of Psychology, University of Miami, P.O. Box 248185, Coral Gables, FL 33124-0751, USA, nschneid@miami.edu

Robert Schnoll Associate Professor, Department of Psychiatry, University of Pennsylvania, 3535 Market Street, Suite 4100, Philadelphia, PA 19104, USA, schnoll@mail.med.upenn.edu

Hannah M.C. Schreier Graduate Student, Department of Psychology, University of British Columbia, 2136 West Mall, Vancouver, BC V6T 1Z4, BC, Canada, hannahs@psych.ubc.ca

Carolyn Schwartz President and Chief Scientist, DeltaQuest Foundation Inc, 31 Mitchell Road, Concord, MA 01742, USA; Research Professor of Medicine and Orthopaedic Surgery, Tufts University School of Medicine, Boston, MA, USA, carolyn.schwartz@deltaquest.org

Lori A.J. Scott-Sheldon Research Assistant Professor of Psychology, Center for Health and Behavior, Syracuse University, 430 Huntington Hall, Syracuse, NY 13244-2340, USA, lajss@syr.edu

Teresa E. Seeman Professor of Medicine and Epidemiology, Department of Medicine, Division of Geriatrics, UCLA School of Medicine, 10945 Le Conte Avenue, Suite 2339, Los Angeles, CA 90095-1687, USA, tseeman@mednet.ucla.edu

David S. Sheps Professor of Medicine, Division of Cardiovascular Medicine, Emory University, EPICORE, 1256 Briarcliff Rd. NE, Building A, Suite 1N, Atlanta, GA 30306, USA, dsheps@emory.edu

Saul S. Shiffman Professor of Psychology, Department of Psychology, University of Pittsburgh, Sennott Square, 210 S. Bouquet Street, Pittsburgh, PA 15260, USA, shiffman@pitt.edu

Timothy W. Smith Professor of Psychology, Department of Psychology, University of Utah, 380 South 1530 East (Room 502), Salt Lake City, UT 84112-0251, USA, tim.smith@psych.utah.edu

Harold Snieder Professor, Unit of Genetic Epidemiology & Bioinformatics, Department of Epidemiology, University Medical Center Groningen, University of Groningen, Hanzeplein 1, PO Box 30.001, 9700 RB Groningen, The Netherlands, h.snieder@epi.umcg.nl

Andrew Steptoe British Heart Foundation Professor of Psychology, Department of Epidemiology and Public Health, University College

London, 1-19 Torrington Place, London WC1E 6BT, UK,
a.steptoe@ucl.ac.uk

Arthur A. Stone Distinguished Professor and Vice Chairman, Department
of Psychiatry and Behavioral Science, Stony Brook University, Stony
Brook, NY 11994-8790, USA, arthur.stone@sunysb.edu

Victor J. Strecher Professor and Director, Center for Health
Communications Research, Department of Health Behavior and Health
Education, Center for Health Communications Research, School of Public
Health, University of Michigan, 300 N. Ingalls – Room 5D-04 (0471), Ann
Arbor, MI 48109-0471, USA, strecher@umich.edu

S.V. Subramanian Associate Professor, Department of Society, Human
Development and Health, Harvard School of Public Health, 677 Huntington
Avenue, Kresge Building, 7th Floor, Boston MA 02115, USA,
svsubram@hsph.harvard.edu

Jerry Suls Professor of Psychology, Department of Psychology, Spence
Laboratories, University of Iowa, Iowa City, IA 52242, USA,
jerry-suls@uiowa.edu

Shelley E. Taylor Distinguished Professor of Psychology, Department of
Psychology, University of California, 1282A Franz Hall, Los Angeles, CA
90095, USA, taylors@psych.ucla.edu

Julian F. Thayer The Ohio Eminent Scholar Professor in Health
Psychology, Department of Psychology, The Ohio State University, 1835
Neil Avenue, Columbus, OH 43210, USA, thayer.39@osu.edu

Elizabeth Tipton Graduate Student, Department of Statistics,
Northwestern University, 2046 Sheridan Road, Evanston, IL 60208, USA,
e-tipton@u.northwestern.edu

Melissa A. Valerio Assistant Professor, Health Behavior and Health
Education, School of Public Health, University of Michigan, 1415
Washington Heights Street, Ann Arbor, MI 48109, USA,
mvalerio@umich.edu

Sara Vargas Graduate Student, Department of Psychology and Sylvester
Comprehensive Cancer Center, University of Miami, 5665 Ponce de Leon
Blvd., Coral Gables, FL 33124-0751, USA, s.vargas3@umiami.edu

Bas Verplanken Professor of Social Psychology, Department of
Psychology, University of Bath, Claverton Down, Bath, BA2 7AY, UK,
b.verplanken@bath.ac.uk

Karani S. Vimaleswaran Career Development Fellow, Medical Research
Council (MRC) Epidemiology Unit, Institute of Metabolic Science,
Addenbrooke's Hospital – Box 285, Hills Road, Cambridge, CB2 0QQ,
UK, vimaleswaran.karani-santhanakrishnan@mrc-epid.cam.ac.uk

Roland von Känel Professor of Medicine, Head, Psychosomatic Division, Department of General Internal Medicine, University Hospital/Inselspital, CH-3010 Bern, Switzerland, roland.vonkaenel@insel.ch

Nicole Vogelzangs Postdoctoral Researcher, Department of Psychiatry and EMGO Institute for Health and Care Research, VU University Medical Center, AJ Ernststraat 887, 1081 HL, Amsterdam, The Netherlands, n.vogelzangs@vumc.nl

Shari R. Waldstein Professor of Psychology, Department of Psychology; University of Maryland, Baltimore County, 1000 Hilltop Circle, Baltimore, MD 21250, USA, waldstei@umbc.edu

Jo Waller Senior Research Associate, Health Behaviour Research Centre, Department of Epidemiology & Public Health, University College London, Gower Street, London WC1E 6BT, UK, j.waller@ucl.ac.uk

Jane Wardle Professor of Clinical Psychology, Director, Health Behaviour Research Centre, Department of Epidemiology & Public Health, University College London, Gower Street, London WC1E 6BT, UK, j.wardle@ucl.ac.uk

Carrington Rice Wendell Graduate Student, Department of Psychology, University of Maryland, Baltimore County, 1000 Hilltop Circle, Baltimore, MD 21250, USA, rice3@umbc.edu

David R. Williams Professor of African and African American Studies and of Sociology, Department of Society, Human Development and Health, Harvard School of Public Health, 677 Huntington Ave, 6th Floor, Boston, MA 02115, USA, dwilliam@hsph.harvard.edu

Redford B. Williams Professor of Psychiatry & Behavioral Sciences, Director, Behavioral Medicine Research Center, Department of Psychiatry and Behavioral Sciences, Duke University Medical Center, Box 3926, Durham, NC 27710, USA, redfordw@duke.edu

Michael S. Wolf Associate Professor of Medicine and Learning Sciences, Division of General Internal Medicine, Feinberg School of Medicine, Northwestern University, 750 N. Lake Shore Drive, 10th Floor, Chicago, IL 60611, USA, mswolf@northwestern.edu

Ydwine Zanstra Postdoctoral Fellow, Department of Psychiatry, University of Pittsburgh, Western Psychiatric Institute and Clinic, 3811 O'Hara St, Pittsburgh, PA 15213, USA, zanstrayj@upmc.edu

Part I
Health Behaviors: Processes
and Measures

Chapter 1

Social and Environmental Determinants of Health Behaviors

Verity J. Cleland, Kylie Ball, and David Crawford

1 Introduction

Physical activity and healthy eating behaviors have an important role to play in the prevention of a range of adverse health outcomes. An extensive body of epidemiological evidence from large prospective cohort studies demonstrates that compared with those who are less physically active, those who are more active are at lower risk of all-cause mortality, cardiovascular diseases, stroke, type 2 diabetes, obesity, certain cancers (mainly breast and colon), musculoskeletal conditions, and poor mental health (US Department of Health and Human Services, 1996). Similarly, healthy eating behaviors have consistently been found to have positive health benefits: high fruit and vegetable consumption assists in the prevention of ischemic heart disease, obesity, certain cancers, and, to a lesser extent, stroke; fish and fish oil consumption is protective against coronary heart disease; and diets high in fiber protect against obesity and type 2 diabetes (World Cancer Research Fund and American Institute for Cancer Research, 2007; World Health Organization, 2002). Despite these well-documented health benefits, a large proportion of the population living in developed nations fail to meet physical activity and healthy eating recommendations.

Given the importance of physical activity and healthy eating behaviors for health, a number of countries have developed guidelines aimed at educating the public about optimal levels of physical activity and healthy eating patterns. Physical activity and healthy eating guidelines tend to be similar in countries such as the United States (US), Canada, Europe, the United Kingdom (UK), and Australia. Physical activity guidelines for adults generally recommend achieving at least 150 min per week of moderate-intensity activity, and that physical activity can be accumulated in 10-min bouts. Recent Physical Activity Guidelines for Americans suggest that physical activity can alternatively be accumulated through 75 min a week of vigorous-intensity aerobic physical activity, or an equivalent combination of moderate- and vigorous-intensity aerobic activity (US Department of Health and Human Services, 2008). The 2005 Dietary Guidelines for Americans suggest consuming a variety of nutrient-dense foods and beverages within and among the basic food groups, while choosing foods that limit the intake of saturated and trans fats, cholesterol, added sugars, salt, and alcohol (US Department of Health and Human Services, 2005). Dietary Guidelines for Australian Adults recommend enjoying a wide variety of nutritious foods (including plenty of vegetables, legumes, and fruits; wholegrain cereals; lean meat, fish, and poultry; reduced-fat milks, yoghurts, and cheeses; and drinking plenty of water) and taking care to limit saturated fat, moderate total

V.J. Cleland (✉)
Centre for Physical Activity and Nutrition Research,
Deakin University, 221 Burwood Highway, Burwood,
VIC 3125, Australia
e-mail: verity.cleland@utas.edu.au

A. Steptoe (ed.), *Handbook of Behavioral Medicine*, DOI 10.1007/978-0-387-09488-5_1,
© Springer Science+Business Media, LLC 2010

fat, choose low-salt foods, limit alcohol, and consume only moderate amounts of sugars and foods containing added sugars (National Health and Medical Research Council, 2003).

Despite these guidelines, in many developed countries, a significant proportion of the population eats poorly and is not physically active at levels recommended for good health. It is important to understand why so many people fail to meet physical activity and healthy eating recommendations, in order to inform the development of effective preventive strategies. A broad range of determinants of physical activity and healthy eating behaviors have been identified. Historically, much research examining determinants of health behavior, including physical activity and eating behaviors, has focused on individual and cognitive factors such as knowledge, motivation, and self-efficacy (described in Section 2). While selected individual factors have consistently been shown to be important in predicting physical activity and/or eating behaviors, more recently researchers have begun to examine the broader social and environmental contexts in which physical activity and eating behaviors occur. While research of this nature is new in its application to understanding physical activity and eating behaviors, it is not new in terms of its application to other public health issues. The classic example, where in 1854 John Snow removed the handle of the local public water pump on Broad Street, London, to end a cholera epidemic, highlights the importance of structural changes in influencing public health. A focus on understanding "upstream" determinants, such as social and environmental factors, of physical activity and eating behaviors may offer important opportunities for intervention. However, there are many challenges involved in the definition, conceptualization, and measurement of environments, which must be considered when attempting to understand the role of the environment as a determinant of health behavior.

While the challenges inherent in investigating environmental influences on health behavior have been discussed elsewhere (Ball et al, 2006c), their significance warrants mention here. Defining environments is difficult because people live and function in multiple contexts or settings (e.g., family, home, and work environments) and in multiple geographic areas (e.g., streets, neighborhoods, cities). Furthermore, there are different types of environmental influences, including factors within the built and natural environment, the social environment, the cultural environment, and the policy environment. Even defining a "neighborhood" environment, which has often been used as the unit of study in much of the research on environmental influences on health behavior, poses unique challenges. For instance, administratively classified definitions, such as postal (zip) codes or census block areas, may conflict with community perceptions of what constitutes a neighborhood. While defining neighborhoods with specificity to individuals (e.g., a 1 km radius of the home) may improve the ability to detect associations, studying environments at such a specific level can be time- and labor-intensive, and there is not yet agreement in defining appropriate geographical boundaries. For example, some studies have used a range of definitions including 400 m, 800 m, 1 km, 1 m, or 5 km. Another key issue is identifying which aspects of the environment to measure from thousands of potential exposure variables. Clear justification based on careful theoretical considerations must be provided in combination with thoughtful hypotheses, and consideration of the outcome being measured and the target group under investigation is recommended.

For the purposes of this chapter, social determinants are defined as the subjective social norms, support, and other social influences on physical activity and eating behaviors (Brug et al, 2008). Environments are defined here as the neighborhoods within which individuals, families, and communities exist, which in the health behavior literature has typically focused on aspects of the built environment. This chapter will focus primarily on the social and environmental determinants of physical activity and eating behaviors using evidence from systematic and narrative reviews and original research studies. It is acknowledged that other social and environmental influences are likely to be important in influencing physical activity and eating behaviors, but this chapter will focus on those determinants that have been most comprehensively examined in the scientific literature. Furthermore, because the social and environmental determinants of physical activity and eating behaviors are likely to be dramatically different in developing countries, this chapter is limited to research conducted in developed nations.

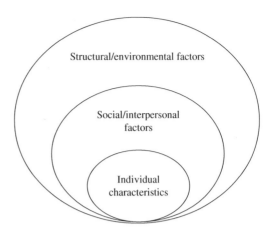

Fig. 1.1 Diagrammatic representation of the social–ecological model of influences on physical activity and eating behaviors

2 Theoretical Frameworks

In attempting to understand the determinants of physical activity and eating behaviors, theoretical frameworks offer a useful starting point to conceptualize the multitude of potential determinant factors. Many different theories have been developed in an attempt to explain behavior, and these can be broadly classified as intra-personal theories or inter-personal theories. Intra-personal theories, such as the health belief model (Becker and Maiman, 1975) and the theory of planned behavior (Ajzen, 1985), are primarily concerned with psychological factors and are based on the premise that behavior is largely choice-driven by individuals (see Chapter 2). In contrast, interpersonal theories, such as social cognitive theory (Bandura, 1986) and ecological models (Sallis and Owen, 2002; Stokols, 1992), posit that there are multiple layers of influence on behavior and emphasize the role of the broader environment in enabling or hindering individuals in their efforts to make healthy choices.

To date, much research on the determinants of physical activity and eating behavior has been atheoretical or has been largely driven by intra-personal theories (Baranowski et al, 1999; Cliska et al, 2000). This chapter will be based on social–ecological models because these give consideration to the broader social and environmental contexts in which physical activity and eating behaviors occur. Social–ecological models posit that there are multiple levels of influence, including individual factors, social factors, and environmental factors, and that these interact with each other to predict behavior (Fig. 1.1).

3 Social and Environmental Determinants of Physical Activity

Physical activity comprises a complex set of behaviors and as a result is difficult to measure. A detailed discussion of physical activity assessment is provided in Chapter 3, but is described briefly here. Physical activity can be classified by its type (e.g., swimming, walking, skiing, tennis, and basketball), intensity (e.g., light, moderate, vigorous), frequency (how many times per day/week/month/year), duration (how long per session), and the domain in which it occurs (e.g., leisure, transport, occupation, domestic). Self-reported (e.g., surveys and interviews) and objective (e.g., pedometers and accelerometers) measures of physical activity each have strengths and limitations, and a combination of both have been recommended for use. When considering the influence of social and environmental determinants of physical activity, it is important to measure context-specific physical activity behaviors (Brug et al, 2008; Giles-Corti et al, 2005). For instance, when trying to understand whether the presence of a walking trail influences physical activity, it may be more important to assess walking behaviors undertaken during leisure time, as opposed to a global measure of physical activity, since the latter may have been accumulated in other domains such as at work or in the home and is hence less likely to be related to the local presence of a walking trail.

3.1 Social Determinants of Physical Activity

There are a large number of potential social determinants of physical activity. This section focuses on four key social influences commonly examined in the literature: socioeconomic position, social support, personal safety/crime, and social capital/participation.

3.1.1 Socioeconomic Position

While there is some contention over the most appropriate indicator of socioeconomic position, there is relatively consistent evidence of a socioeconomic gradient in physical activity, whereby those experiencing the greatest socioeconomic disadvantage are least likely to report participating in physical activity during their leisure time. These findings tend to be independent of the measure of socioeconomic position used. A review of 57 studies examining relationships between socioeconomic position and physical activity found a socioeconomic gradient in physical activity in 90% of studies ($n = 10$) that used social class as the socioeconomic position indicator, 61% of studies ($n = 18$) that used income as the indicator, 71% that used education ($n = 24$), 50% that used an asset-based indicator ($n = 2$), and 100% that used an area-based indicator of socioeconomic position ($n = 3$) (Gidlow et al, 2006). In the United Kingdom, where social classification by employment grade is commonly used as an indicator of socioeconomic position, an examination of over 10,000 adults involved in the Whitehall II study found that men and women of low employment grade had significantly greater odds of no or low exercise compared with those

of high employment grade, independently of spousal social class (Bartley et al, 2004).

There is also some evidence of differences in the barriers to participation in physical activity according to socioeconomic position. For instance, a qualitative study conducted in Australia found that negative early life/family physical activity experiences and lack of time due to work commitments were consistent themes among women of lower socioeconomic position, but not among those of higher socioeconomic position (Ball et al, 2006b). A study in the United Kingdom of over 6000 adults found barriers such as lack of motivation, lack of time, lack of money, and lack of transport to be differentially distributed across different indicators of socioeconomic position (which included education, housing tenure, employment status, household social class, car ownership, and household income), with a higher proportion of adults of lower socioeconomic position identifying barriers to activity than those of higher socioeconomic position (Chinn et al, 1999).

3.1.2 Social Support

Social support is one of the strongest and most consistent predictors of physical activity behavior (Sallis and Owen, 1999; Trost et al, 2002). In their systematic review of articles published between 1998 and 2000, Trost and colleagues reported that a significant positive relationship was evident between social support and physical activity in each of the nine studies reviewed that included a measure of social support. Another review of studies published between 1980 and 2004 concluded that there was convincing evidence for a positive relationship between social support and general physical activity, vigorous physical activity/sports, moderate-to-vigorous physical activity, and walking (Wendel-Vos et al, 2007). Most evidence comes from cross-sectional studies, for example, an Australian study of 1803 adults aged 18–59 years found that perceptions of high social support for walking in the neighborhood were associated with an 80% increase in the odds of walking for recreation and a 50% increase in the odds of walking six times per week for at least 30 min each session (Giles-Corti and Donovan, 2002). Little evidence from prospective cohort studies is available. However, one Danish study examined changes in physical activity over 6 years among nearly 3000 adults aged 16 years and older and found in multivariable analyses that the only significant predictor of moving from the inactive category at baseline to the active category at follow-up was regularity of meeting with family, which may be an indirect indicator of social support (Zimmermann et al, 2008).

3.1.3 Personal Safety and Crime

The evidence surrounding the associations between personal safety, crime, and physical activity is equivocal, with inconsistencies in findings likely due to substantial differences in definitions, measures (perceived or objective), sampling, and the unit of analysis (individual, neighborhood, or state level) across studies. A lack of prospective and intervention studies also limits firm conclusions. A study of an ethnically diverse sample of 2338 urban and rural older women found no evidence of a relationship between perceived high levels of crime or lack of a safe place and participation in regular physical activity (Wilcox et al, 2000), while a smaller study of 291 adult women of low socioeconomic position identified no relationship between perceived neighborhood safety and meeting leisure time physical activity recommendations (Cleland et al, 2010; Epub ahead of print, Oct 29, DOI:10.1093/her/cyn054 Oct 29, DOI:10.1093/her/cyn054 #1861). In contrast, a study of 1659 adults aged 18 years and over found that lower perceived neighborhood crime was associated with leisure time physical activity, particularly activity conducted outdoors (McGinn et al, 2008). In a sub-sample of 303 participants from the same study, objective measures of low total crime and low criminal offences, but not incivilities or traffic offences, were associated with higher odds of meeting

leisure time physical activity recommendations, particularly outdoor physical activity.

3.1.4 Social Capital

Social capital has been defined as those features of social relationships, such as inter-personal trust, social participation, group membership, and norms of reciprocity, that facilitate collective action and cooperation for mutual benefit (Kawachi, 1999). While there is debate over whether social capital should be operationalized at the individual or community level (Putnam, 2000; Rose, 2000; Veenstra, 2000), it has been argued that a multilevel analytical approach is most appropriate because social capital may influence health at both levels (Kawachi et al, 2004). Although a number of studies have assessed relations between social capital and health outcomes, fewer have examined the association between social capital and physical activity.

Despite difficulties in conceptualizing and measuring social capital, of those studies that have examined relations with physical activity, findings have tended to suggest a positive association. For instance, a study of 11,837 Swedish adults found that those reporting lower levels of social participation had significantly higher odds of low leisure time physical activity, and social participation explained most of the association observed between socioeconomic position and leisure time physical activity (Lindstrom et al, 2001). A multilevel analysis of data from another Swedish survey found that an individual-level indicator of social capital (social participation), but not a neighborhood-level indicator of social capital (out-migration), was positively associated with leisure time physical activity (Lindstrom et al, 2003). A state- and county-level analysis of social capital and physical activity among 167,000 adults in 48 states in the United States identified positive associations between social capital and physical activity in multilevel, multivariable analyses (Kim et al, 2006).

3.2 Environmental Determinants of Physical Activity

There are a large number of potential determinants of physical activity in the physical environment, although research examining these is still relatively new. As discussed earlier, issues around definitions, measurement, and conceptualization of the environment and the infancy of this field make it difficult to draw firm conclusions about associations with physical activity. For instance, a recent review has highlighted an extensive range of issues associated with measuring the physical activity built environment and provides a useful summary of the many measurement tools currently available (Brownson et al, 2009). This section will focus on four key physical environment influences that have commonly been examined in the literature: availability and accessibility; aesthetics; infrastructure; and road safety.

3.2.1 Availability and Accessibility

Evidence from studies of the influence of the physical environment on physical activity suggests a positive association between availability of and access to facilities such as recreation centers, cycle paths, footpaths and swimming pools, and physical activity. While most studies examining this association have been cross-sectional in design, findings have been relatively consistent. For example, a population-based study of 1796 adults in the United States found that those who reported access to places to be physically active had more than twice the odds of doing any activity and of doing recommended amounts of activity, after adjusting for sociodemographic and other environmental factors (Huston et al, 2003). The same study also found that those reporting access to neighborhood trails had significantly higher odds of achieving recommended levels of leisure time physical activity, independent of other sociodemographic and environmental factors. A number of studies have also found positive associations

between physical activity and access to local parks (Booth et al, 2000; Foster et al, 2004; Nagel et al, 2008), residing in coastal areas (Ball et al, 2007; Bauman et al, 1999), convenience of physical activity facilities (De Bourdeaudhuij et al, 2003; Duncan et al, 2009; Humpel et al, 2004b), and negative associations between distance to cycle paths (Troped et al, 2001). A recent study of adults from 11 countries found the odds of being physically active were significantly higher among those who had access to low-cost recreational facilities, bicycle facilities, and sidewalks on most local streets (Sallis et al, 2009). Furthermore, the odds of being active improved with increasing number of favorable environmental characteristics, suggesting that "clusters" of activity friendly environmental features may be important for promoting physical activity.

3.2.2 Aesthetics

Consistent positive associations have been documented between aesthetic features of neighborhoods and participation in different types of physical activity (Humpel et al, 2002). Aesthetic features are often assessed through self-reported perceptions of the attractiveness of the environment, the amount of greenery or trees, the pleasantness of housing or the neighborhood, or the presence of enjoyable scenery. Cross-sectional evidence of a relationship between aesthetics and physical activity comes from a study of 3392 Australian adults which found those who reported less aesthetically pleasing environments had 28–39% lower odds of walking for exercise or recreation in the previous 2 weeks, compared with those reporting more aesthetically pleasing environments (Ball et al, 2001). Further longitudinal evidence of an association is provided by a 10-week prospective study of 512 Australian adults which found that men who reported positive changes in perceived aesthetics had twice the odds of increasing walking, although no relationship was observed among women (Humpel et al, 2004b), who are possibly more influenced by factors such as safety or accessibility.

3.2.3 Neighborhood Infrastructure

The evidence regarding the importance of neighborhood infrastructure in influencing physical activity is equivocal. However, this may be related to a lack of specificity in the assessment of physical activity. For example, Wilcox and colleagues found no relationship between the presence of sidewalks and total leisure time physical activity among urban and rural women (Wilcox et al, 2000), but the measure of physical activity used was overall leisure activity, which may include many different activity types, rather than walking per se. Plausibly, some of this leisure time physical activity could have been accumulated in recreational facilities or other places where the presence of sidewalks would not be expected to have an influence. Associations may have been observed if instead walking for leisure or walking for transport had been assessed, because these physical activity behaviors are more likely to be influenced by the presence of sidewalks. This was evident in an Australian study of mothers, where the presence of sidewalks and good street lighting at night were positively associated with walking for transport (Cleland et al, 2008). That study also found that limited public transport was inversely associated and having many alternative routes for getting from place to place was positively associated with both walking for leisure and walking for transport. Similarly, a study of Belgian adults found that a greater ease of the walk to a public transportation stop was associated with higher levels of walking, but only among women (De Bourdeaudhuij et al, 2003).

3.2.4 Road Safety

Road safety elements of the physical environment have been assessed objectively (for example, with a geographic information system) and subjectively (for example, self-reported perceptions), with contrasting findings observed. For instance, a North American study found that perceiving a busy street as a barrier was inversely associated with usage of a bikeway, but objective measurement of this same variable was not associated with bikeway usage among adults (Troped et al, 2001). Another North American study found perceptions of high-speed traffic were not associated with physical activity, but objectively measured low traffic speeds were positively associated with meeting leisure time physical activity guidelines among adults (McGinn et al, 2007). In contrast, a study in two North American cities found no relationship between self-reported perceptions of safety from traffic while riding or walking, or an objective audit of street safety and physical activity for transportation or for recreation (Hoehner et al, 2005). In one of the few longitudinal studies to examine the influence of road safety on physical activity, no relationship was observed between perceived road safety and walking for leisure, but participant reports of satisfaction with pedestrian crossings, the presence of traffic-slowing devices, and slow local traffic speed were positively associated with walking for transportation over 2 years (Cleland et al, 2008). The findings from this study further highlight the importance of examining physical activity behaviors specific to the environmental features being examined.

4 Social and Environmental Determinants of Eating Behaviors

Like physical activity, healthy eating comprises a complex set of behaviors that are challenging to measure. A detailed discussion of eating behavior assessment is provided in Chapter 4, but is described briefly here. A key consideration in dietary assessment is that there are many different elements of eating behavior that can be measured, including overall diet, patterns of food intake, consumption of specific foods, dietary habits, and nutrient intakes. It is therefore essential that a clear research question with a well-defined focus is established to assist in the selection of an appropriate assessment tool. Assessments of eating behaviors are generally conducted via self-report and involve either recording of intake (e.g., weekly food diary) or recalling intake, retrospectively (e.g., 24-h food recalls or recall of intake via food frequency questionnaires). Both methods have strengths and limitations, and there is currently no "gold standard" assessment tool.

4.1 Social Determinants of Healthy Eating Behaviors

There are many potential social determinants of healthy eating behaviors. This section will focus on three key social influences that have commonly been examined in the literature: socioeconomic position, social support, and family and household composition.

4.1.1 Socioeconomic Position

In general, those of lower socioeconomic position tend to consume poorer diets than those of higher socioeconomic position (Diez-Roux et al, 1999). For example, cross-sectional data from the Netherlands demonstrated that men and women in the lower socioeconomic groups (defined according to education, occupation, and occupational position) tended to have dietary patterns less conducive to good health, including greater intakes of sugars and sweets (Hulshof et al, 2003). Similarly, findings from the Australian National Nutrition Survey found men and women of higher socioeconomic status (defined according to occupation) more frequently consumed foods promotive of good health such as breakfast cereals and wholemeal bread (Mishra et al, 2002). A Swedish study found many differences in associations between dietary intake and socioeconomic position across two different measures of socioeconomic position, educational attainment, and occupational status (Galobardes et al, 2001). For instance, in that study fiber intake was significantly lower in men and women of lower socioeconomic position defined according to occupation, but

no significant differences were observed across educational categories. Similarly, meat intake was significantly higher among women of lower occupational status, but no significant difference across educational categories was evident. These findings highlight the importance of giving careful consideration to the measures of socioeconomic position and eating behavior employed.

4.1.2 Social Support

Social support from family and friends has demonstrated consistent positive associations with fruit and vegetable consumption in diverse populations (Kamphuis et al, 2006; Shaikh et al, 2008). A study of 271 adults from a low-income population found that increases over 12 months in fruit and vegetable intake associated with a brief behavioral intervention were predicted by baseline social support for dietary change (Steptoe et al, 1997). A study of 658 African-American adults found that social support was associated with overall fruit and vegetable intake, and with fruit intake among women (Watters et al, 2007), and an Australian study found a positive relationship between social support from family and friends and fruit and vegetable intake among women of varying socioeconomic position (Ball et al, 2006a). While studies assessing relationships with fat intake are less common, one study of 441 overweight and obese men found social support was significantly inversely associated with percentage of energy from fat intake after adjusting for demographic and other psychosocial factors (Hagler et al, 2007). An intervention study among older adults found correlations between a social support score and changes in fruit and vegetable consumption, but not changes in fat intake, over 1 year (Murphy et al, 2001).

4.1.3 Family and Household Composition

Given that many people spend much of their time in their home and that behavior is likely influenced by those who they are living with, household composition is likely to influence eating behavior. The available evidence suggests that being married is positively associated with fruit and vegetable intake (Kamphuis et al, 2006), but also positively associated with energy and total fat intake and inversely associated with saturated fat intake (Giskes et al, 2007a). Fewer studies have focused on associations with fruit and vegetable consumption than energy or fat intake, and those existing studies have tended to focus on women, limiting the ability to draw conclusions related to marital status and fruit and vegetable consumption among men. For instance, a UK study of more than 35,000 women found that married participants had 62% higher odds of having a high fruit and vegetable consumption compared with their single counterparts (Pollard et al, 2001). A Canadian study of older adults found that a significantly greater proportion of those who were married consumed fruit and vegetables at least five times per day compared with those who were single (Riediger and Moghadasian, 2008). Despite a larger number of studies having examined relationships between marital status and energy or fat intakes, evidence remains inconclusive. For instance, an Irish study of over 6500 adults found married men and women on average consumed more energy per day than single adults, and married women consumed more fat per day than single women, but these differences were not statistically significant (Friel et al, 2003).

Other features of the household that may impact on eating behavior are the presence and number of children. Women with children under the age of 16 years have been found to consume significantly more servings of fruit but significantly fewer servings of vegetables than women without children (Pollard et al, 2001). However, a Norwegian study found that those with children consumed fruits less often than participants without children (Wandel, 1995). One study found that, among white adults, those who had a young child, regardless of whether they were married or single, consumed significantly more fruit than did those who were married and had no children (Devine et al, 1999). Limited research has examined whether the presence and number

of children in the household is associated with energy or fat intake, making firm conclusions difficult to draw, and highlighting the need for further research in this area.

4.2 Environmental Determinants of Healthy Eating Behaviors

There are many potential environmental determinants of healthy eating behaviors. Much of the existing research on environmental influences on eating has focused on features of the built environment, in particular, the accessibility and availability of food outlets. However, a growing body of evidence has investigated the affordability of foods, and this research will also be summarized here.

4.2.1 Availability and Access

While a number of studies have investigated availability of different food stores, or of food items within food stores, across different neighborhoods, very few have linked these data with data on eating behaviors at the individual level. Consequently, evidence from empirical studies examining the relationship between availability of food and eating behaviors is relatively limited and remains equivocal. For instance, the presence of local grocery stores and the shelf space occupied by healthy foods in stores has been found to be negatively associated with fat intakes (Cheadle et al, 1991; Morland et al, 2002), but the presence of supermarkets, full-service restaurants, or fast-food restaurants has not (Morland et al, 2002). Two recent reviews of the relationship between the environment and fat and energy intake (Giskes et al, 2007a) and fruit and vegetable intake found that the limited available evidence made firm conclusions difficult (Kamphuis et al, 2006); however, there was some evidence to suggest that fruit and vegetable consumption is likely to be highest among those who have good local availability and accessibility of fruit and vegetables.

Associations between access and availability among different population groups may also differ. In one US study, the presence of a supermarket was positively associated with fruit and vegetable consumption among black but not white residents (Morland et al, 2002), and in another, proximity to a supermarket was associated with fruit consumption among low-income residents (Rose and Richards, 2004). Associations between access, availability, and eating behaviors may also be place-dependent. For example, in contrast to some US evidence, studies in Australia have found no relationship between the "objective" availability of recommended foods and food purchasing behavior (Giskes et al, 2007b), or between the density of supermarkets and fruit and vegetable stores in local neighborhoods and fruit and vegetable consumption among women (Ball et al, 2006a). These null findings may be partly attributable to ceiling effects in access to healthy foods, such that at least in urban areas of many developed countries, residents all have good access to food stores, and hence there may be insufficient variation in the availability of healthy foods to distinguish those with more healthy eating behaviors (Brug et al, 2008). It has also been suggested that findings of stronger or more consistent associations between access to healthy foods and eating behavior have been observed in countries such as the US, where there may be greater spatial segregation in availability of healthy food options (Brug et al, 2008).

4.2.2 Affordability

The perceived high cost or low affordability of healthy foods is one of the most frequently cited barriers to healthy eating, particularly among low-income individuals (Glanz et al, 1998; Inglis et al, 2005). A recent review of environmental correlates of fruit and vegetable consumption (Kamphuis et al, 2006) demonstrated that living in low-income households or neighborhoods, or being food insecure, was associated

with lower fruit and vegetable consumption. However, findings of studies examining economic factors and eating behaviors are equivocal. For example, another review found that low household income and neighborhood disadvantage were not strongly associated with energy or fat intakes (Giskes et al, 2007a). Similarly, while some studies have reported that healthy diets are more expensive than less healthy diets (Andrieu et al, 2006; Drewnowski et al, 2004; Jetter and Cassady, 2006), others have not – two studies in the US, for instance, showed that nutrient-dense diets are not more expensive than lower quality diets and may even cost less (Burney and Haughton, 2002; Raynor et al, 2002). It is possible that perceived costs may represent a greater barrier to healthy eating than actual costs, an argument supported by results of a recent Australian study which showed that perceived availability and price of healthy foods were more important than objective measures in predicting diet and mediating socioeconomic variations in diet (Giskes et al, 2007b).

Perhaps the strongest evidence for the impact of affordability on eating behaviors comes from experimental or intervention studies and several of these have suggested that cost is an important determinant of food consumption. For example, two community-based intervention studies demonstrated that price reduction strategies promote the choice of targeted foods. The Changing Individuals' Purchase of Snacks (CHIPS) study, based in 12 high schools and 12 worksites, found that lowering the prices of lower fat snacks increased the purchase of these snacks, with increases in direct proportion to the price reductions. Compared with usual price conditions, price reductions of 10, 25, and 50 on lower fat snacks resulted in an increase in sales of 9, 39, and 93%, respectively (French et al, 2001). The second study showed a fourfold increase in fresh fruit sales and a twofold increase in baby carrot sales resulting from a 50% price reduction in the costs of these items in two secondary school cafeterias (French et al, 1997).

While confirmation of these findings in settings other than schools and worksites is required, evidence from experimental studies such as those reviewed here suggests that cost appears a potent modifiable intervention level for strategies designed to promote healthy eating behaviors. This is particularly timely and important given that fiscal approaches to modifying eating behaviors (for instance, as a potential strategy to counter rising rates of obesity worldwide) are currently the topic of intense debate and increasing attention in research, public health, and policy circles internationally (e.g., McColl, 2009).

5 Conclusions

Physical activity and healthy eating are complex behaviors that are important predictors of a range of health outcomes and indicators. Despite recommendations that aim to promote these behaviors, a large proportion of the population fails to meet physical activity and eating guidelines. Given the importance of physical activity and healthy eating for good health, it is important to understand influences on these behaviors in order to develop effective interventions and strategies aimed at promoting health. While much past research has examined individual-level influences on physical activity and healthy eating, less is known about the influence of the broader social and physical environment on these behaviors. Social and physical environment influences offer significant public health prospects because of the opportunity to intervene "upstream". Despite the potential offered by these factors, there are many methodological issues that need to be resolved in order to advance our understanding of how social and environmental factors are related to physical activity and healthy eating.

Current evidence suggests that socioeconomic position and social support are consistently positively associated with physical activity, highlighting the importance of targeting those at risk of inactivity such as those facing socioeconomic disadvantage or who are socially isolated. Preliminary evidence also suggests that social capital, operationalized at either the individual or community level, is likely to have a positive relationship with physical activity. Evidence concerning the influence of personal safety and crime on physical activity is equivocal, and further research is required to better current understandings of these relationships. Access to and the availability and aesthetics of the physical environment appear to be positively associated with physical activity, while the evidence surrounding relationships between neighborhood infrastructure and road safety and physical activity remains inconclusive.

Evidence suggests a consistent positive association between socioeconomic position and social support and healthy eating, highlighting the importance of targeting those most at risk of social disadvantage or lack of support. While marital status and the presence and number of children in the household appear to be important influences on healthy eating, the lack of empirical studies makes strong conclusions and generalizations difficult to affirm. The evidence regarding access to and availability of healthy and unhealthy food choices is contentious, which is possibly related to conceptual and methodological issues. Limited intervention evidence suggests that food costs appear a potentially modifiable and effective intervention lever, although perceptions of affordability may also need to be addressed.

Despite the current evidence, further work is required in relation to the conceptualization, measurement, and definition of the social and particularly the environmental influences on physical activity and eating behaviors. Investigations based on theoretically driven research questions with consistent and comparable measures across studies are needed and specific research in at-risk populations such as those of lower socioeconomic position and minority groups will enhance understanding of how social and environmental factors relate to physical activity and eating behavior. The measurement of physical activity and eating behavior remains challenging despite technological advances, and different measures employed across studies make comparisons difficult. Consistent definitions and measures in future investigations will play a crucial role in helping to answer important research questions around determinants of physical activity and healthy eating behaviors.

Understanding the relative contribution of individual, social, and environmental factors and how these factors interact to influence physical activity and healthy eating behaviors within different population groups requires further investigation. Few studies have attempted to examine the independent contributions of these factors in multivariable models to determine which are the most important for physical activity and healthy eating behaviors. Disentangling these relationships will assist in the prioritization of factors to target in strategies aimed at promoting physical activity and healthy eating.

Most of the current evidence surrounding social and environmental influences on physical activity and healthy eating behaviors is cross-sectional. While cross-sectional study designs provide important information about the existence of associations, they do not allow for insights into the temporal nature of relationships, or about the influence of manipulations of, for example, features of the physical environment on behavior. Longitudinal and intervention studies are needed to help establish the sequential and ultimately causal nature of relationships between social and environmental factors and physical activity and healthy eating. Until these studies are conducted, it will be unknown whether those who are physically active and eat well are attracted to social and physical environments that are supportive of these behaviors or if supportive social and physical environments encourage physical activity and healthy eating behaviors.

Although there are gaps in the current scientific literature, the available evidence suggests that social and environmental factors have a role to play in influencing physical activity and healthy eating behaviors. Further development in the conceptualization, definition, and measurement of social and environmental determinants, as well as the examination of these determinants in longitudinal and intervention studies, will assist in our understanding of how these factors relate to physical activity and healthy eating behaviors. A better comprehension of these relations will enable the development of tailored programs and strategies to effectively promote physical activity and healthy eating behaviors, and consequently improve the health of the community.

References

Ajzen, I. (1985). From intentions to actions: a theory of planned behavior. In J. Kuhl & J. Beckman (Eds.), *Action-Control: From Cognition to Behavior* (pp. 11–39). Heidelberg: Springer.

Andrieu, E., Darmon, N., and Drewnowski, A. (2006). Low-cost diets: more energy, fewer nutrients. *Eur J Clin Nutr, 60*, 434–436.

Ball, K., Bauman, A., Leslie, E., and Owen, N. (2001). Perceived environmental aesthetics and convenience and company are associated with walking for exercise among Australian adults. *Prev Med, 33*, 434–440.

Ball, K., Crawford, D., and Mishra, G. (2006a). Socio-economic inequalities in women's fruit and vegetable intakes: a multilevel study of individual, social and environmental mediators. *Public Health Nutr, 9*, 623–630.

Ball, K., Salmon, J., Giles-Corti, B., and Crawford, D. (2006b). How can socio-economic differences in physical activity among women be explained? A qualitative study. *Women Health, 43*, 93–113.

Ball, K., Timperio, A., Salmon, J., Giles-Corti, B., Roberts, R. et al (2007). Personal, social and environmental determinants of educational inequalities in walking: a multilevel study. *J Epidemiol Community Health, 61*, 108–114.

Ball, K., Timperio, A. F., and Crawford, D. A. (2006c). Understanding environmental influences on nutrition and physical activity behaviors: where should we look and what should we count? *Int J Behav Nutr Phys Act, 3*, 33.

Bandura, A. (1986). *Social Foundations of Thought and Action: A Social Cognitive Theory*. Englewood Cliffs, NJ: Prentice Hall.

Baranowski, T., Cullen, K. W., and Baranowski, J. (1999). Psychosocial correlates of dietary intake: advancing dietary intervention. *Annu Rev Nutr, 19*, 17–40.

Bartley, M., Martikainen, P., Shipley, M., and Marmot, M. (2004). Gender differences in the relationship of partner's social class to behavioural risk factors and social support in the Whitehall II study. *Soc Sci Med, 59*, 1925–1936.

Bauman, A., Smith, B., Stoker, L., Bellew, B., and Booth, M. (1999). Geographical influences upon physical activity participation: evidence of a 'coastal effect'. *Aust N Z J Public Health, 23*, 322–324.

Becker, M. H., and Maiman, L. A. (1975). Sociobehavioral determinants of compliance with health and medical care recommendations. *Med Care, 13*, 10–24.

Booth, M. L., Owen, N., Bauman, A., Clavisi, O., and Leslie, E. (2000). Social-cognitive and perceived environment influences associated with physical activity in older Australians. *Prev Med, 31*, 15–22.

Brownson, R. C., Hoehner, C. M., Day, K., Forsyth, A., and Sallis, J. F. (2009). Measuring the built environment for physical activity: state of the science. *Am J Prev Med, 36*, S99–123 e12.

Brug, J., Kremers, S. P., Lenthe, F., Ball, K., and Crawford, D. (2008). Environmental determinants of healthy eating: in need of theory and evidence. *Proc Nutr Soc, 67*, 307–316.

Burney, J., and Haughton, B. (2002). EFNEP: a nutrition education program that demonstrates cost-benefit. *J Am Diet Assoc, 102*, 39–45.

Cheadle, A., Psaty, B. M., Curry, S., Wagner, E., Diehr, P. et al (1991). Community-level comparisons between the grocery store environment and individual dietary practices. *Prev Med, 20*, 250–261.

Chinn, D. J., White, M., Harland, J., Drinkwater, C., and Raybould, S. (1999). Barriers to physical activity and socioeconomic position: implications for health promotion. *J Epidemiol Community Health, 53*, 191–192.

Cleland, V. J., Ball, K., Salmon, J., Timperio, A. F., and Crawford, D. A. (2010). Personal, social and environmental correlates of resilience to physical inactivity among women from socio-economically disadvantaged backgrounds. *Health Educ Res, 25*(2), 268–281 (Epub ahead of print, Oct 29, DOI:10.1093/her/cyn054).

Cleland, V. J., Timperio, A., and Crawford, D. (2008). Are perceptions of the physical and social environment associated with mothers' walking for leisure and for transport? A longitudinal study. *Prev Med, 47*, 188–193 (Epub ahead of print, Oct 29, DOI:10.1093/her/cyn054 #1861).

Cliska, D., Miles, E., O'Brien, M. A., Turl, C., Tomasik, H. H. et al (2000). Effectiveness of community-based interventions to increase fruit and vegetable consumption. *J Nutr Educ, 32*, 241–252.

De Bourdeaudhuij, I., Sallis, J. F., and Saelens, B. E. (2003). Environmental correlates of physical activity in a sample of Belgian adults. *Am J Health Promot, 18*, 83–92.

Devine, C. M., Wolfe, W. S., Frongillo, E. A., Jr., and Bisogni, C. A. (1999). Life-course events and experiences: association with fruit and vegetable consumption in 3 ethnic groups. *J Am Diet Assoc, 99*, 309 314.

Diez-Roux, A. V., Nieto, F. J., Caulfield, L., Tyroler, H. A., Watson, R. L. et al (1999). Neighbourhood differences in diet: the Atherosclerosis Risk in Communities (ARIC) Study. *J Epidemiol Community Health, 53*, 55–63.

Drewnowski, A., Darmon, N., and Briend, A. (2004). Replacing fats and sweets with vegetables and fruits – a question of cost. *Am J Public Health, 94*, 1555–1559.

Duncan, M. J., Mummery, W. K., Steele, R. M., Caperchione, C., and Schofield, G. (2009). Geographic location, physical activity and perceptions of the environment in Queensland adults. *Health Place, 15*, 204–209.

Foster, C., Hillsdon, M., and Thorogood, M. (2004). Environmental perceptions and walking in English adults. *J Epidemiol Community Health, 58*, 924–928.

French, S. A., Jeffery, R. W., Story, M., Breitlow, K. K., Baxter, J. S. et al (2001). Pricing and promotion effects on low-fat vending snack purchases: the CHIPS Study. *Am J Public Health, 91*, 112–117.

French, S. A., Story, M., Jeffery, R. W., Snyder, P., Eisenberg, M. et al (1997). Pricing strategy to promote fruit and vegetable purchase in high school cafeterias. *J Am Diet Assoc, 97*, 1008–1010.

Friel, S., Kelleher, C. C., Nolan, G., and Harrington, J. (2003). Social diversity of Irish adults nutritional intake. *Eur J Clin Nutr, 57*, 865–875.

Galobardes, B., Morabia, A., and Bernstein, M. S. (2001). Diet and socioeconomic position: does the use of different indicators matter? *Int J Epidemiol, 30*, 334–340.

Gidlow, C., Johnston, L. H., Crone, D., Ellis, N., and James, D. (2006). A systematic review of the relationship between socio-economic position and physical activity. *Health Educ J, 65*, 338–367.

Giles-Corti, B., and Donovan, R. J. (2002). Socioeconomic status differences in recreational physical activity levels and real and perceived access to a supportive physical environment. *Prev Med, 35*, 601–611.

Giles-Corti, B., Timperio, A., Bull, F., and Pikora, T. (2005). Understanding physical activity environmental correlates: increased specificity for ecological models. *Exerc Sport Sci Rev, 33*, 175–181.

Giskes, K., Kamphuis, C. B., van Lenthe, F. J., Kremers, S., Droomers, M. et al (2007a). A systematic review of associations between environmental factors, energy and fat intakes among adults: is there evidence for environments that encourage obesogenic dietary intakes? *Public Health Nutr, 10*, 1005–1017.

Giskes, K., Van Lenthe, F. J., Brug, J., Mackenbach, J. P., and Turrell, G. (2007b). Socioeconomic inequalities in food purchasing: the contribution of respondent-perceived and actual (objectively measured) price and availability of foods. *Prev Med, 45*, 41–48.

Glanz, K., Basil, M., Maibach, E., Goldberg, J., and Snyder, D. (1998). Why Americans eat what they do: taste, nutrition, cost, convenience, and weight control concerns as influences on food consumption. *J Am Diet Assoc, 98*, 1118–1126.

Hagler, A. S., Norman, G. J., Zabinski, M. F., Sallis, J. F., Calfas, K. J. et al (2007). Psychosocial correlates of dietary intake among overweight and obese men. *Am J Health Behav, 31*, 3–12.

Hoehner, C. M., Brennan Ramirez, L. K., Elliott, M. B., Handy, S. L., and Brownson, R. C. (2005). Perceived and objective environmental measures and physical activity among urban adults. *Am J Prev Med, 28*, 105–116.

Hulshof, K. F., Brussaard, J. H., Kruizinga, A. G., Telman, J., and Lowik, M. R. (2003). Socio-economic status, dietary intake and 10 y trends: the Dutch National Food Consumption Survey. *Eur J Clin Nutr, 57*, 128–137.

Humpel, N., Marshall, A. L., Leslie, E., Bauman, A., and Owen, N. (2004a). Changes in neighborhood walking are related to changes in perceptions of environmental attributes. *Ann Behav Med, 27*, 60–67.

Humpel, N., Owen, N., and Leslie, E. (2002). Environmental factors associated with adults' participation in physical activity: a review. *Am J Prev Med, 22*, 188–199.

Humpel, N., Owen, N., Leslie, E., Marshall, A. L., Bauman, A. E. et al (2004b). Associations of location and perceived environmental attributes with walking in neighborhoods. *Am J Health Promot, 18*, 239–242.

Huston, S. L., Evenson, K. R., Bors, P., and Gizlice, Z. (2003). Neighborhood environment, access to places for activity, and leisure-time physical activity in a diverse North Carolina population. *Am J Health Promot, 18*, 58–69.

Inglis, V., Ball, K., and Crawford, D. (2005). Why do women of low socioeconomic status have poorer dietary behaviours than women of higher socioeconomic status? A qualitative exploration. *Appetite, 45*, 334–343.

Jetter, K. M., and Cassady, D. L. (2006). The availability and cost of healthier food alternatives. *Am J Prev Med, 30*, 38–44.

Kamphuis, C. B., Giskes, K., de Bruijn, G. J., Wendel-Vos, W., Brug, J. et al (2006). Environmental determinants of fruit and vegetable consumption among adults: a systematic review. *Br J Nutr, 96*, 620–635.

Kawachi, I. (1999). Social capital and community effects on population and individual health. *Ann N Y Acad Sci, 896*, 120–130.

Kawachi, I., Kim, D., Coutts, A., and Subramanian, S. V. (2004). Commentary: reconciling the three accounts of social capital. *Int J Epidemiol, 33*, 682–90; discussion 700–704.

Kim, D., Subramanian, S. V., Gortmaker, S. L., and Kawachi, I. (2006). US state- and county-level social capital in relation to obesity and physical inactivity: a multilevel, multivariable analysis. *Soc Sci Med, 63*, 1045–1059.

Lindstrom, M., Hanson, B. S., and Ostergren, P. O. (2001). Socioeconomic differences in leisure-time physical activity: the role of social participation and social capital in shaping health related behaviour. *Soc Sci Med, 52*, 441–451.

Lindstrom, M., Moghaddassi, M., and Merlo, J. (2003). Social capital and leisure time physical activity: a population based multilevel analysis in Malmo, Sweden. *J Epidemiol Community Health, 57*, 23–28.

McColl, K. (2009). "Fat taxes" and the financial crisis. *Lancet, 373*, 797–798.

McGinn, A. P., Evenson, K. R., Herring, A. H., Huston, S. L., and Rodriguez, D. A. (2007). Exploring associations between physical activity and perceived and objective measures of the built environment. *J Urban Health, 84*, 162–184.

McGinn, A. P., Evenson, K. R., Herring, A. H., Huston, S. L., and Rodriguez, D. A. (2008). The association of perceived and objectively measured crime with physical activity: a cross-sectional analysis. *J Phys Act Health, 5*, 117–131.

Mishra, G., Ball, K., Arbuckle, J., and Crawford, D. (2002). Dietary patterns of Australian adults and their association with socioeconomic status: results from the 1995 National Nutrition Survey. *Eur J Clin Nutr, 56*, 687–693.

Morland, K., Wing, S., and Diez Roux, A. (2002). The contextual effect of the local food environment on residents' diets: the atherosclerosis risk in communities study. *Am J Public Health, 92*, 1761–1767.

Murphy, P. A., Prewitt, T. E., Bote, E., West, B., and Iber, F. L. (2001). Internal locus of control and social support associated with some dietary changes by elderly participants in a diet intervention trial. *J Am Diet Assoc, 101*, 203–208.

Nagel, C. L., Carlson, N. E., Bosworth, M., and Michael, Y. L. (2008). The relation between neighborhood built environment and walking activity among older adults. *Am J Epidemiol, 168*, 461–468.

National Health and Medical Research Council (2003). *Dietary Guidelines for Australian Adults.* Canberra: National Health and Medical Research Council.

Pollard, J., Greenwood, D., Kirk, S., and Cade, J. (2001). Lifestyle factors affecting fruit and vegetable consumption in the UK Women's Cohort Study. *Appetite, 37*, 71–79.

Putnam, R. D. (2000). *Bowling Alone. The collapse and revival of American community.* New York, London: Simon & Schuster.

Raynor, H. A., Kilanowski, C. K., Esterlis, I., and Epstein, L. H. (2002). A cost-analysis of adopting a healthful diet in a family-based obesity treatment program. *J Am Diet Assoc, 102*, 645–656.

Riediger, N. D., and Moghadasian, M. H. (2008). Patterns of fruit and vegetable consumption and the influence of sex, age and socio-demographic factors among Canadian elderly. *J Am Coll Nutr, 27*, 306–313.

Rose, D., and Richards, R. (2004). Food store access and household fruit and vegetable use among participants in the US Food Stamp Program. *Public Health Nutr, 7*, 1081–1088.

Rose, R. (2000). How much does social capital add to individual health? A survey study of Russians. *Soc Sci Med, 51*, 1421–1435.

Sallis, J., and Owen, N. (1999). *Physical Activity and Behavioral Medicine*. California: Sage Publications.

Sallis, J., and Owen, N. (2002). Ecological models of health behavior. In K. Glanz, B. K. Rimer, & F. M. Lewis (Eds.), *Health Behavior and Health Education: Theory, Research & Practice, 3rd Ed* (pp. 462–484). San Francisco: Jossey-Bass.

Sallis, J. F., Bowles, H. R., Bauman, A., Ainsworth, B. E., Bull, F. C. et al (2009). Neighborhood environments and physical activity among adults in 11 countries. *Am J Prev Med, 36*, 484–490.

Shaikh, A. R., Yaroch, A. L., Nebeling, L., Yeh, M. C., and Resnicow, K. (2008). Psychosocial predictors of fruit and vegetable consumption in adults a review of the literature. *Am J Prev Med, 34*, 535–543.

Steptoe, A., Wardle, J., Fuller, R., Holte, A., Justo, J. et al (1997). Leisure-time physical exercise: prevalence, attitudinal correlates, and behavioral correlates among young Europeans from 21 countries. *Prev Med, 26*, 845–854.

Stokols, D. (1992). Establishing and maintaining healthy environments. Toward a social ecology of health promotion. *Am Psychol, 47*, 6–22.

Troped, P. J., Saunders, R. P., Pate, R. R., Reininger, B., Ureda, J. R. et al (2001). Associations between self-reported and objective physical environmental factors and use of a community rail-trail. *Prev Med, 32*, 191–200.

Trost, S. G., Owen, N., Bauman, A. E., Sallis, J. F., and Brown, W. (2002). Correlates of adults' participation in physical activity: review and update. *Med Sci Sports Exerc, 34*, 1996–2001.

US Department of Health and Human Services (1996). *Physical activity and health: a report of the Surgeon General*. Atlanta, GA: United States Department of Health and Human Services, Centers for Disease Control and Prevention, National Center for Chronic Disease Prevention and Health Promotion.

US Department of Health and Human Services (2005). *The Dietary Guidelines for Americans*. USA: US Department of Health and Human Services.

US Department of Health and Human Services (2008). *2008 Physical Activity Guidelines for Americans*. USA: US Department of Health and Human Services.

Veenstra, G. (2000). Social capital, SES and health: an individual-level analysis. *Soc Sci Med, 50*, 619–629.

Wandel, M. (1995). Dietary intake of fruits and vegetables in Norway: influence of life phase and socioeconomic factors. *Int J Food Sci Nutr, 46*, 291–301.

Watters, J. L., Satia, J. A., and Galanko, J. A. (2007). Associations of psychosocial factors with fruit and vegetable intake among African-Americans. *Public Health Nutr, 10*, 701–711.

Wendel-Vos, W., Droomers, M., Kremers, S., Brug, J., and van Lenthe, F. (2007). Potential environmental determinants of physical activity in adults: a systematic review. *Obes Rev, 8*, 425–440.

Wilcox, S., Castro, C., King, A. C., Housemann, R., and Brownson, R. C. (2000). Determinants of leisure time physical activity in rural compared with urban older and ethnically diverse women in the United States. *J Epidemiol Community Health, 54*, 667–672.

World Cancer Research Fund and American Institute for Cancer Research (2007). *Food, Nutrition, Physical Activity, and the Prevention of Cancer: A Global Perspective*. Washington, DC: American Institute for Cancer Research.

World Health Organization (2002). *Diet, Nutrition and the Prevention of Chronic Disease*. Report of a joint WHO/FAO Technical Expert Group. WHO Technical Report Series, 916. Geneva: World Health Organization.

Zimmermann, E., Ekholm, O., Gronbaek, M., and Curtis, T. (2008). Predictors of changes in physical activity in a prospective cohort study of the Danish adult population. *Scand J Public Health, 36*, 235–241.

Chapter 2

Cognitive Determinants of Health Behavior

Mark Conner

1 Introduction

The prevalence of health behaviors varies across social groups. For example, in the Western World smoking is generally more prevalent among those from economically disadvantaged backgrounds. This might suggest such socio-demographic factors as the focus of interventions to change health behaviors. However, such factors are frequently impossible to change or require political intervention at national or international levels (e.g., change in income distribution). This is one reason why a considerable body of research has focused on more modifiable factors assumed to mediate the relationship between socio-demographic factors and health-related behaviors. One important set of such factors is the thoughts and feelings the individual associates with the particular health-related behavior. These are often referred to as health cognitions and are the focus of this chapter. Although research does examine the role of individual health cognitions (e.g., outcome expectancies), most of the research in this area uses models that include sets of health cognitions that are assumed to combine in different ways to determine behavior. These models are collectively known as social cognition models (SCMs; Conner and Norman, 2005). They prominently include the Health Belief Model (HBM; e.g., Abraham and Sheeran, 2005; Janz and Becker, 1984), Protection Motivation Theory (PMT; e.g., Maddux and Rogers, 1983; Norman et al, 2005), Theory of Reasoned Action/Theory of Planned Behavior (TRA/TPB; e.g., Ajzen, 1991; Conner and Sparks, 2005), and Social Cognitive Theory (SCT; e.g., Bandura, 2000; Luszczynska and Schwarzer, 2005). Stage models represent a different form of SCM which does not assume behavior change to be linear, but rather to occur in discrete stages. Prochaska and DiClemente's (1984) Transtheoretical Model of Change (TTM) is the most commonly applied stage model. Below these SCMs are described and research using each is reviewed. There is considerable overlap between the models and the key health cognitions they identify. Building on this overlap some work has attempted to integrate SCMs into a unified theory of the determinants of health behaviors (Fishbein et al, 2001). This integrated model will also be described. Finally, this chapter overviews recent work in this area on intention stability as an important mediator of cognitive effects, affective expectancies as a highly predictive yet insufficiently considered variable, and implementation intentions as an important volitional technique to promote action.

2 Social Cognition Models

Social cognition models (SCMs) detail the important cognitions that distinguish between

M. Conner (✉)
Institute of Psychological Sciences, University of Leeds,
Leeds LS2 9JT, UK
e-mail: m.t.conner@leeds.ac.uk

A. Steptoe (ed.), *Handbook of Behavioral Medicine*, DOI 10.1007/978-0-387-09488-5_2,

those performing and not performing behaviors. The focus is on the cognitions or thought processes that intervene between observable stimuli and behavior in real-world situations (Fiske and Taylor, 1991). This approach is founded on the assumption that behavior is best understood as a function of people's perceptions of reality, rather than objective characterizations of the stimulus environment. SCMs can be seen as one part of *self-regulation* research. Self-regulation processes are defined as those "... mental and behavioral processes by which people enact their self-conceptions, revise their behavior, or alter the environment so as to bring about outcomes in it in line with their self-perceptions and personal goals" (Fiske and Taylor, 1991, p. 181). Self-regulation research has emerged from a clinical tradition in psychology which views the individual as striving to eliminate dysfunctional patterns of thinking or behavior and engage in adaptive patterns of thinking or behavior (Bandura, 1982; Turk and Salovey, 1986). Self-regulation involves cognitive re-evaluation of beliefs, goal setting, and ongoing monitoring and evaluating of goal-directed behavior. Two phases of self-regulation activities have been defined: motivational and volitional (Gollwitzer, 1990). In the motivational phase costs and benefits are considered in order to choose between goals and behaviors. This phase is assumed to conclude with a decision (or intention) concerning which goals and actions to pursue at a particular time. In the subsequent volitional phase, planning and action directed toward achieving the set goal predominate. The majority of SCMs focus on the motivational phase, although work with implementation intentions focuses on the volitional phase of action.

2.1 The Health Belief Model

The Health Belief Model (HBM) is the oldest and most widely used SCM (see Abraham and Sheeran, 2005, for a recent review). In one of the earliest studies, Hochbaum (1958) reported that perceived susceptibility to tuberculosis and

the belief that people with the disease could be asymptomatic (so that screening would be beneficial) distinguished between attendees and non-attendees for chest x-rays. Haefner and Kirscht (1970) extended this research by demonstrating that an intervention designed to increase participants' perceived susceptibility, perceived severity, and anticipated benefits resulted in a greater number of checkup visits to the doctor over an 8-month period compared to a control condition.

The HBM posits that health behavior is determined by two cognitions: perceptions of illness threat and evaluation of behaviors to counteract this threat (see Fig. 2.1). Threat perceptions are based on two beliefs: the perceived susceptibility of the individual to the illness ("How likely am I to get ill?") and the perceived severity of the consequences of the illness for the individual ("How serious would the illness be?"). Similarly, evaluation of possible responses involves consideration of both the potential benefits of and barriers/costs to action. Together these four beliefs are believed to determine the likelihood of the individual performing a health behavior. The specific action taken is determined by the evaluation of the available alternatives, focusing on the benefits or efficacy of the health behavior and the perceived costs or barriers of performing the behavior. Hence individuals are most likely to follow a particular health action if they believe themselves to be susceptible to a particular condition which they also consider to be serious and believe that the benefits outweigh the costs of the action taken to counteract the health threat.

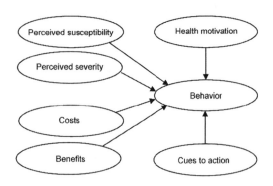

Fig. 2.1 The Health Belief Model

Two further cognitions usually included in the model are cues to action and health motivation. Cues to action are assumed to include a diverse range of triggers to the individual taking action which may be internal (e.g., physical symptom) or external (e.g., mass media campaign, advice from others) to the individual (Janz and Becker, 1984). An individual's perception of the presence of cues to action would be expected to prompt adoption of the health behavior if he/she already holds other key beliefs favoring action. Health motivation refers to more stable differences between individuals in the value they attach to their health and their propensity to be motivated to look after their health. Individuals with a high motivation to look after their health should be more likely to adopt relevant health behaviors.

The HBM has provided a useful framework for investigating health behaviors and has been widely used. It has been found to successfully predict a range of behaviors. For example, Janz and Becker (1984) found that across 18 prospective studies, the 4 core beliefs were nearly always significant predictors of health behavior (82, 65, 81, and 100% of studies report significant effects for susceptibility, severity, benefits, and barriers, respectively). Harrison et al (1992), in a review with more stringent inclusion criteria, reported that susceptibility and barriers were the strongest predictors of behavior. Some studies have found that these health beliefs mediate the effects of demographic correlates of health behavior. For example, Orbell et al (1995) reported perceived susceptibility and barriers to entirely mediate the effects of social class upon uptake of cervical screening. The HBM has also inspired a range of successful behavior change interventions (e.g., Jones et al, 1987).

The main strength of the HBM is the common-sense operationalization it uses including key beliefs related to decisions about health behaviors. However, further research has identified other cognitions that are stronger predictors of health behavior than those identified by the HBM, suggesting that the model is incomplete. This prompted a proposal to add self-efficacy and intention to the model to produce an "extended health belief model" (Rosenstock et al, 1988) which has generally improved the predictive power of the model (e.g., Hay et al, 2003).

2.2 Protection Motivation Theory

Protection Motivation Theory (PMT; Maddox and Rodgers, 1983; see Norman et al, 2005 for a review) is a revision and extension of the HBM which incorporates various appraisal processes identified by research into coping with stress. In PMT, the primary determinant of performing a health behavior is protection motivation or intention to perform a health behavior (see Fig. 2.2). Protection motivation is determined

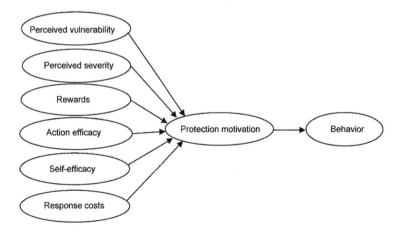

Fig. 2.2 Protection Motivation Theory

by two appraisal processes: threat appraisal and coping appraisal. Threat appraisal is based on a consideration of perceptions of susceptibility to the illness and severity of the health threat in a very similar way to the HBM. Coping appraisal involves the process of assessing the behavioral alternatives which might diminish the threat. This coping process is itself assumed to be based on two components: the individual's expectancy that carrying out a behavior can remove the threat (action-outcome efficacy) and a belief in one's capability to successfully execute the recommended courses of action (self-efficacy).

Together these two appraisal processes result in either adaptive or maladaptive responses. Adaptive responses are those in which the individual engages in behaviors likely to reduce the risk (e.g., adopting a health behavior) whereas maladaptive responses are those that do not directly tackle the threat (e.g., denial of the health threat). Adaptive responses are held to be more likely if the individual perceives himself or herself to be facing a health threat to which he/she is susceptible and which is perceived to be severe and where the individual perceives such responses to be effective in reducing the threat and believes that he/she can successfully perform the adaptive response. The PMT has been successfully applied to the prediction of a number of health behaviors (for a recent review see Norman et al, 2005). Meta-analytic reviews of PMT (Floyd et al, 2000; Milne et al, 2000) indicate protection motivation (i.e., intentions) and self-efficacy to be the most powerful predictors of behavior, while self-efficacy and response costs were most strongly associated with intentions.

2.3 Theory of Planned Behavior

The Theory of Planned Behavior (TPB; Ajzen, 1991) was developed by social psychologists and has been widely applied to understanding health behaviors (see Conner and Sparks, 2005, for a review). It specifies the factors that determine that individual's decision to perform a particular behavior (see Fig. 2.3). Importantly this theory added "perceived behavioral control" to the earlier Theory of Reasoned Action (TRA; Ajzen and Fishbein, 1980). The TPB proposes that the key determinants of behavior are intention to engage in that behavior and perceived behavioral control over that behavior. As in the PMT, intentions in the TPB represent a person's motivation or conscious plan or decision to exert effort to perform the behavior. Perceived behavioral control (PBC) is a person's expectancy that performance of the behavior is within his/her control and confidence that he/she can perform the behavior and is similar to Bandura's (1982) concept of self-efficacy.

In the TPB, intention is assumed to be determined by three factors: attitudes, subjective norms, and PBC. Attitudes are the overall evaluations of the behavior by the individual as positive or negative. Subjective norms are a person's

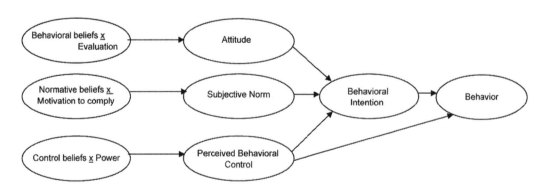

Fig. 2.3 Theory of Planned Behavior

beliefs about whether significant others think he/she should engage in the behavior. PBC is assumed to influence both intentions and behavior because we rarely intend to do things we know we cannot and because believing that we can succeed enhances effort and persistence and so makes successful performance more likely.

Attitudes are based on behavioral beliefs (or outcome expectancies), that is, beliefs about the perceived outcomes of a behavior. In particular, they are a function of the likelihood of the outcome occurring as a result of performing the behavior (e.g., "How likely is this outcome?") and the evaluation of that outcome (e.g., "How good or bad will this outcome be for me?"). It is assumed that an individual will have a limited number of consequences in mind when considering a behavior. This expectancy-value framework is based on Fishbein's (1967) earlier summative model of attitudes. Subjective norm is based on beliefs about salient others' approval or disapproval of whether one should engage in a behavior (e.g., "Would my best friend want me to do this?") weighted by the *motivation to comply* with each salient other on this issue (e.g., "Do I want to do what my best friend wants me to do?"). Again it is assumed that an individual will only have a limited number of referents in mind when considering a behavior. PBC is based on control beliefs concerning whether one has access to the necessary resources and opportunities to perform the behavior successfully (e.g., "How often does this facilitator/inhibitor occur?"), weighted by the perceived power, or importance, of each factor to facilitate or inhibit the action (e.g., "How much does this facilitator/inhibitor make it easier or more difficult to perform this behavior?"). These factors include both internal control factors (information, personal deficiencies, skills, abilities, emotions) and external control factors (opportunities, dependence on others, barriers). As for the other types of beliefs it is assumed that an individual will only consider a limited number of control factors when considering a behavior.

The TPB has been widely tested and successfully applied to the understanding of a variety of behaviors (for reviews see Ajzen, 1991; Conner and Sparks, 2005). For example, in a meta-analysis of the TPB, Armitage and Conner (2001) reported that across 154 applications, attitude, subjective norms, and PBC accounted for 39% of the variance in intention, while intentions and PBC accounted for 27% of the variance in behavior across 63 applications. Intentions emerged as the strongest predictors of behavior, while attitudes were the strongest predictors of intentions.

The TPB has also informed a number of interventions designed to change behavior. For example, Hill et al (2007) employed a randomized control trial to test the effectiveness of a TPB-based leaflet compared to a control condition in promoting physical exercise in a sample of school children. The leaflet condition compared to the control condition significantly increased not only reported exercise but also intentions, attitudes, subjective norms, and PBC. Additional analyses indicated that the impact on exercise was mediated by the increases the leaflet had produced (compared to the control group) in intentions and PBC.

2.4 Social Cognitive Theory

In Social Cognitive Theory (SCT; Bandura, 1982) behavior is held to be determined by three factors: goals, outcome expectancies, and self-efficacy (see Fig. 2.4). Goals are plans to act and can be conceived of as intentions to perform the behavior (see Luszczynska and Schwarzer, 2005). Outcome expectancies are similar to behavioral beliefs in the TPB but here are split into physical, social, and self-evaluative depending on the nature of the outcomes considered. Self-efficacy is the belief that a behavior is or is not within an individual's control and is usually assessed as the degree of confidence the individual has that he/she could still perform the behavior in the face of various obstacles (and is similar to PBC in the TPB). Bandura (2000) recently added socio-structural factors to

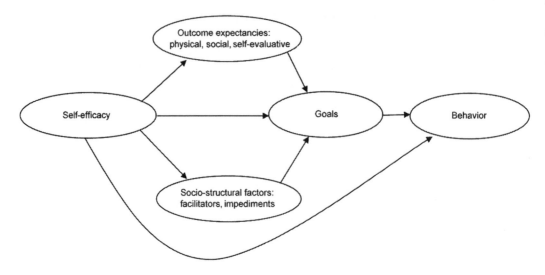

Fig. 2.4 Social Cognitive Theory

his theory. These are factors assumed to facilitate or inhibit the performance of a behavior and affect behavior via changing goals. Socio-structural factors refer to the impediments or opportunities associated with particular living conditions, health systems, political, economic, or environmental systems. They are assumed to inform goal setting and be influenced by self-efficacy. The latter relationship arises because self-efficacy influences the degree to which individuals pay attention to opportunities or impediments in their life circumstances. This component of the model incorporates perceptions of the environment as an important influence on health behaviors.

SCT has been successfully applied to predicting and changing various health behaviors. However, unlike a number of the other models considered above, many of the applications of SCT only assess one or two components of the model (usually self-efficacy) rather than all components. Self-efficacy and action-outcome expectancies along with intentions have been found to be the most important predictors of a range of health behaviors in a diverse range of studies (for reviews see Bandura, 2000; Luszczynska and Schwarzer, 2005).

2.5 Stage Models of Health Behavior

The SCMs considered above assume that the cognitive determinants of health behaviors act in a similar way during initiation (e.g., quitting smoking for the first time) and maintenance of action (e.g., trying to stay quit). In contrast, in stage models psychological determinants may change across such stages of behavior change (see Sutton, 2005, for a review). An important implication of the *stages* view is that different cognitions may be important determinants at different stages in promoting health behavior. The most widely used stage model is Prochaska and DiClemente's (1984) Transtheoretical Model of change (TTM). Their model has been widely applied to analyze the process of change in alcoholism treatment and smoking cessation. DiClemente et al (1991) identify five stages of change: pre-contemplation (not thinking about change), contemplation (aware of the need to change), preparation (intending to change in the near future and taking action in preparation for change), action (acting to change), and maintenance (of the new behavior). Individuals are seen to progress sequentially from one stage to the next, with maintenance the end stage of successful change. For example, in the case of smoking cessation, it is argued that in the pre-contemplation stage the smoker is unaware that his/her behavior constitutes a problem and has no intention to quit. In the contemplation stage, the smoker starts to think about changing his/her behavior, but is not committed to try to quit. In the preparation stage, the smoker has an intention to quit and starts to make plans to quit. The action stage is characterized by active attempts to quit, and after 6 months of successful abstinence the individual moves into the maintenance stage. This stage is characterized by attempts to prevent relapse and to consolidate the newly acquired non-smoking status.

Although widely applied, the evidence in support of stage models and different stages is modest (see Sutton, 2000, 2005). Sutton (2000) concludes that the distinctions between TTM stages are "logically flawed" and based on "arbitrary time periods." The sequential movement through stages has not generally been supported (Sutton, 2005). In addition, it has proved difficult to support the key prediction that there are different determinants of behavior change in different stages. Evidence from stage-matched versus stage-mismatched intervention studies does not generally provide support for the TTM (see Littell and Girvin, 2002, for a systematic review of the effectiveness of interventions applying the TTM to health-related behaviors). Thus, at present, research findings do not support the added complexity and increased cost of stage-tailored interventions compared to the linear approach advocated in other SCMs. West (2005) in reviewing stage models in relation to smoking has recently suggested that work on the TTM should be abandoned.

3 Integration of Social Cognition Models

The overlap between SCMs has prompted attempts to integrate them. This may be valuable, especially since they include some of the same cognitive determinants. For example, intention, self-efficacy, and outcome expectancies appear in several models. One important attempt to integrate these models was that by Bandura (SCT), Becker (HBM), Fishbein (TRA), Kaufen (self-regulation), and Triandis (Theory of Interpersonal Behavior) as part of a workshop organized by the US National Institute of Mental Health in response to the need to promote HIV-preventive behaviors. The workshop sought to "identify a finite set of variables to be considered in any behavioral analysis" (Fishbein et al, 2001, p. 3). They identified eight variables which, they argued, should account for most of the variance in any (deliberative) behavior. These were organized into two groups. First, those variables which were viewed as necessary and sufficient determinants of behavior. Thus, for behavior to occur an individual must (i) have a strong intention, (ii) have the necessary skills to perform the behavior, and (iii) experience an absence of environmental constraints that could prevent behavior. Second were those variables that were seen primarily to influence intention (although a direct effect on behavior was noted as possible). Thus, a strong intention is likely to occur when an individual (i) perceives the advantages (or benefits) of performing the behavior to outweigh the perceived disadvantages (or costs, i.e., outcome expectancies), (ii) perceives the social (normative) pressure to perform the behavior to be greater than that not to perform the behavior, (iii) believes that the behavior is consistent with his/her self-image, (iv) anticipates the emotional reaction to performing the behavior to be more positive than negative, and (v) has high levels of self-efficacy. Figure 2.5 illustrates this integrated model. This approach has been further developed by Fishbein (2008) in his integrative model (IM) of behavioral prediction although this has not, as yet, been widely tested.

4 Current Directions

A clear contribution of work with SCMs has been their ability to identify key correlates of health behavior that can be targeted

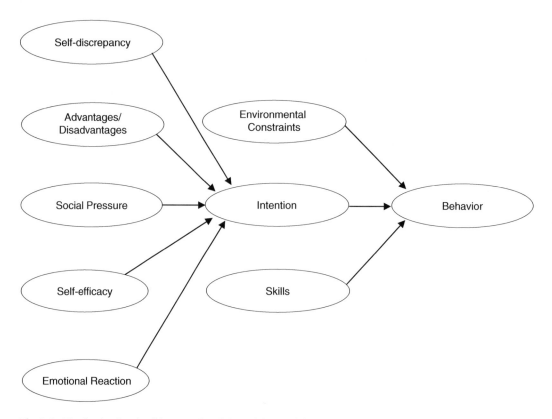

Fig. 2.5 The "major theorists" integrated social cognition model

in interventions to change behavior. Across studies the strongest relationships with behavior emerge for intentions, self-efficacy, and outcomes expectancies (Conner and Norman, 2005). However, in focusing on correlates of health behavior rather than examining causal relationships research may have overestimated the size of relationships. For example, while correlational research indicates intentions to have a strong effect size on behavior (Armitage and Conner, 2001), studies looking at manipulations of intentions indicate that a medium to large change in intentions is associated with only a small to medium effect sized change in behavior (Webb and Sheeran, 2006). A further important limitation with much work on SCMs is that while they usefully identify cognition change targets, they commonly do not specify the best means to change such cognitions (work on self-efficacy is an exception to this trend; Bandura, 2000). Recent work on classifying behavior change

interventions (e.g., Abraham and Michie, 2008) and the more widespread assessment of mediating cognitions in intervention studies may provide the basis for further insights into how best to change cognitions and assessing their causal impact on behavior change for health behaviors. In the remainder of this section three directions of current research on cognitive determinants of health behavior are briefly reviewed.

4.1 Intention Stability

In the vast majority of quality applications of SCMs to predicting health behavior, a prospective design is employed where the predictors of behavior are measured by questionnaire (at time 1) and then behavior is measured at a second time point (in stronger designs behavior change is the focus of interest). An important assumption of such a design is that the measured cognitions (e.g., attitudes) remain unchanged between their measurement and the opportunity to act. So, for example, the assumption is that intentions do not change in between when the (time 1) questionnaire is completed and the time points at which the respondent has the opportunity to act. This is an explicit limiting condition of the TRA/TPB (Ajzen and Fishbein, 1980). However, cognitions including intentions may indeed change in this time period and such change provides one important limitation on their power to predict behavior. Several studies have now demonstrated the power of intention stability to moderate the intention-behavior relationship (see Conner and Godin, 2007, for a review). For example, Conner et al (2002) found that intentions were strong predictors of healthy eating up to 6 years later, but only among those whose intentions had remained stable over an initial period of 6 months.

A number of factors have been found to influence the intention-behavior relationship. For example, anticipating feeling regret if one does not perform a behavior or perceiving a strong moral norm to act have both been found to significantly increase the intention-behavior relationship (see Cooke and Sheeran, 2004, for a review). Sheeran and Abraham (2003) showed intention stability to moderate the intention-behavior relationship for exercising and that intention stability mediated the effect of other moderators of the intention-behavior relationship (e.g., anticipated regret, certainty). This suggests that the mechanism by which a number of these other moderators may have their effect on intention-behavior relationships is through changing the temporal stability of intentions. Hence, factors that might be expected to make individual intentions more stable over time would be expected to increase the impact that these intentions have on behavior and so increase the intention-behavior relationship. Thus intention stability might be a useful focus of attention as a key mediating variable in intervention studies attempting to change health behavior.

4.2 Affective Influences

One criticism of work with SCMs has been the failure to explicitly consider affective influences on behavior (Conner and Armitage, 1998). Outcome expectancies included in PMT, TPB, and SCT do not preclude consideration of affective outcomes, although the outcomes typically considered do not focus on affective states. Over the last few years a number of studies have examined the impact of expectations of affect associated with performance of a behavior. For example, studies have examined anticipated regret as a determinant of behavior within the context of the TPB (see Sandberg and Conner, 2008, for a review). Regret is a negative affective state that can be anticipated pre-behaviorally and so influence subsequent behavior. Studies generally report that such anticipated affective states add significant variance to predictions of intentions but not behavior and may be particularly important in relation to certain *affective* behaviors (e.g., condom use; Glasman and Albarracin, 2006). Other studies have shown affective outcomes to be better predictors of behavior than more instrumental outcomes (e.g., Lawton et al, 2007). Work has also examined the affect that accompanies performance of the behavior (sometimes referred to as anticipatory affect or affective attitudes; Loewenstein, 1996) rather than following performance of the behavior. Such affective attitudes have been explicitly added to the TPB (Conner and Sparks, 2005) and been reported to be stronger predictors of intentions and behavior than instrumental attitudes (Ajzen, 2001; Lawton et al, 2009). In addition, some studies indicate affective attitudes to directly predict behavior independent of intentions (e.g., Lawton et al, 2009). Affective expectations and their influence on health behavior would appear to be an important and growing focus for research in this area.

4.3 Implementation Intentions

The majority of research reviewed thus far has focused on motivational influences of cognitive variables on behavior (i.e., impacting on intention formation). However, other research has begun to focus on the volitional phase of action (Bagozzi, 1993). One volitional variable that has been widely tested in relation to health behavior is implementation intentions. Gollwitzer (1993) makes the distinction between goal intentions and implementation intentions. While the former is concerned with intentions to perform a behavior or achieve a goal (i.e., "I intend to do x"), the latter is concerned with if-then plans which specify an environmental prompt or context that will determine when the action should be taken (i.e., "I intend to initiate the goal-directed behavior x when situation y is encountered"). Importantly, the if–then plan in an implementation intention commits the individual to a specific course of action when certain environmental conditions are met. Sheeran et al (2005) note that "to form an implementation intention, the person must first identify a response that will lead to goal attainment and, second, anticipate a suitable occasion to initiate that response. For example, the person might specify the behavior 'go jogging for 20 minutes' and specify a suitable opportunity 'tomorrow morning before work'" (p. 280). Gollwitzer (1993) argues that by forming implementation intentions individuals pass control of intention enactment to the environment. The specified environmental cue prompts the action so that the person does not have to remember the goal intention or decide when to act.

Sheeran et al (2005) provide an in-depth review of both basic and applied research with implementation intentions. For example, Milne et al (2002) found that an intervention using persuasive text based on PMT prompted positive pro-exercise cognition change but did not increase exercise. However, when this intervention was combined with encouragement to form implementation intentions, significant behavior change was observed (see Gollwitzer and Sheeran, 2006, for a meta-analysis of such studies). Thus implementation intention formation moderates the intention-behavior relationship demonstrating that two people with equally strong goal intentions may differ in their

volitional readiness depending on whether they have taken the additional step of forming an implementation intention. Implementation intention formation has been shown to increase the performance of a range of health behaviors with, on average, a medium effect size. Implementation intentions appear to be particularly effective for those with strong goal intentions and in overcoming forgetting that appears to be a common problem in enacting intentions. Provided effective cues are identified in the implementation intention (i.e., ones that will be commonly encountered and are sufficiently distinctive) forgetting appears to be much less likely.

5 Conclusions

A number of social cognition models have been developed to describe the key cognitive determinants and their relationship to behavior. These key cognitions include intentions, self-efficacy, and outcome expectancies. Recent research has sought to integrate such models (Fishbein et al, 2001). Current research has focused on intention stability as an important mediating variable explaining the impact of health cognitions on behavior. Other work is examining affective influences on health behaviors and how the formation of implementation intentions promotes the performance of behavior.

References

Abraham, C. and Michie, S. (2008). A taxonomy of behavior change techniques used in interventions. *Health Psychol, 27*, 379–387.

Abraham, C., and Sheeran, P. (2005). The health belief model. In M. Conner & P. Norman (Eds.), *Predicting Health Behaviour: Research and Practice with Social Cognition Models, 2nd Ed* (pp. 28–80). Maidenhead: Open University Press.

Ajzen, I. (1991). The theory of planned behavior. *Organiz Behav Hum Dec Proc, 50*, 179–211.

Ajzen, I. (2001). Nature and operation of attitudes. *Ann Rev Psychol, 52*, 27–58.

Ajzen, I., and Fishbein, M. (1980). *Understanding Attitudes and Predicting Social Behavior*. Englewood Cliff, NJ: Prentice Hall.

Armitage, C. J., and Conner, M. (2001). Efficacy of the theory of planned behaviour: a meta-analytic review. *Br J Soc Psychol, 40*, 471–499.

Bagozzi, R. P. (1993). On the neglect of volition in consumer research: a critique and proposal. *Psychol Marketing, 10*, 215–237.

Bandura, A. (1982). Self-efficacy mechanism in human agency. *Am Psychol, 37*, 122–147.

Bandura, A. (2000). Health promotion from the perspective of social cognitive theory. In P. Norman, C. Abraham, & M. Conner (Eds.), *Understanding and Changing Health Behaviour: From Health beliefs to Self-Regulation* (pp. 229–242). Switzerland: Harwood Academic.

Conner, M., and Armitage, C. J. (1998). Extending the theory of planned behavior: a review and avenues for further research. *J Appl Soc Psychol, 28*, 1430–1464.

Conner, M., and Godin, G. (2007). Temporal stability of behavioural intention as a moderator of intention-health behaviour relationships. *Psychol Health, 22*, 875–896.

Conner, M., and Norman, P. (Eds.) (2005). *Predicting Health Behaviour: Research and Practice with Social Cognition Models, 2nd Ed*. Maidenhead: Open University Press.

Conner, M., Norman, P., and Bell, R. (2002). The theory of planned behavior and healthy eating. *Health Psychol, 21*, 194–201.

Conner, M., and Sparks, P. (2005). The theory of planned behaviour and health behaviours. In M. Conner & P. Norman (Eds.), *Predicting Health Behaviour: Research and Practice with Social Cognition Models, 2nd Ed* (pp. 170–222). Maidenhead: Open University Press.

Cooke, R., and Sheeran, P. (2004). Moderation of cognition-intention and cognition-behaviour relations: a meta-analysis of properties of variables from the theory of planned behaviour. *Br J Soc Psychol, 43*, 159–186.

DiClemente, C. C., Prochaska, J. O., Fairhurst, S. K., Velicer, W. F., Velasquez, M. M., and Rossi, J. S. (1991). The process of smoking cessation: an analysis of precontemplation, contemplation, and preparation stages of change. *J Consult Clin Psychol, 59*, 295–304.

Fishbein, M. (1967). Attitude and the prediction of behavior. In M. Fishbein (Ed.), *Readings in Attitude Theory and Measurement* (pp. 477–492). New York: Wiley.

Fishbein, M. (2008). A reasoned action approach to health promotion. *Med Dec Making, 28*, 834–844.

Fishbein, M., Triandis, H. C., Kanfer, F. H., Becker M., Middlestadt, S. E., and Eichler, A. (2001). Factors influencing behavior and behavior change. In A. Baum, T. A. Revenson, & J. E. Singer (Eds.),

Handbook of Health Psychology (pp. 3–17). Mahwah, NJ: Lawrence Erlbaum Associates.

Fiske, S. T., and Taylor, S. E. (1991). *Social Cognition, 2nd Ed*. New York: McGraw-Hill.

Floyd, D. L., Prentice-Dunn, S., and Rogers, R. W. (2000). A meta-analysis of protection motivation theory. *J Appl Soc Psychol, 30*, 407–429.

Glasman, L. R., and Albarracin, D. (2006). Forming attitudes that predict future behavior: a meta-analysis of the attitude-behavior relation. *Psychol Bull, 132*, 778–822.

Gollwitzer, P. M. (1990). Action phases and mind-sets. In E. T. Higgins & R. M. Sorrentino (Eds.), *Handbook of Motivation and Cognition: Foundations of Social Behavior, Vol. 2* (pp. 53–92). New York: Guilford Press.

Gollwitzer, P. M. (1993). Goal achievement: the role of intentions. *Eur Rev Soc Psychol, 4*, 142–185.

Gollwitzer, P., and Sheeran, P. (2006). Implementation intentions and goal achievement: a meta analysis of effects and processes. *Adv Exp Soc Psychol, 38*, 69–119.

Haefner, D. P. and Kirscht, J. P. (1970). Motivational and behavioural effects of modifying health beliefs. *Public Health Rep, 85*, 478–484.

Harrison, J. A., Mullen, P. D., and Green, L. W. (1992). A meta-analysis of studies of the health belief model with adults. *Health Educ Res, 7*, 107–116.

Hay, J. L., Ford, J. S., Klein, D., Primavera, L. H., Buckley, T. R., Stein, T. R., Shike, M., and Ostroff, J. S. (2003). Adherence to colorectal cancer screening in mammography-adherent older women. *J Behav Med, 26*, 553–576.

Hill, C., Abraham, C., and Wright, D. (2007). Can theory-based messages in combination with cognitive prompts promote exercise in classroom settings? *Soc Sci Med, 65*, 1049–1058.

Hochbaum, G. M. (1958). *Public Participation in Medical Screening Programs: A Socio-psychological Study*. Public Health Service Publication No 572. Washington, DC: United States Government Printing Office.

Janz, N. K., and Becker, M. H. (1984). The health belief model: a decade later. *Health Educ Q, 11*, 1–47.

Jones, P. K., Jones, S. L., and Katz, J. (1987). Improving compliance for asthmatic patients visiting the emergency department using a health belief model intervention. *J Asthma, 24*, 199–206.

Lawton, R., Conner, M., and McEachan, R. (2009). Desire or reason: predicting health behaviors from affective and cognitive attitudes. *Health Psychol, 28*, 56–65.

Lawton, R., Conner, M., and Parker, D. (2007). Beyond cognition: predicting health risk behaviors from instrumental and affective beliefs. *Health Psychol, 26*, 259–267.

Loewenstein, G. (1996). Out of control: visceral influences on behavior. *Organiz Behav Hum Dec Proc, 65*, 272–292.

Littell, J. H., and Girvin, H. (2002). Stages of change. A critique. *Behav Modif, 26*, 223–273.

Luszczynska, A., and Schwarzer, R. (2005). Social cognitive theory. In M. Conner & P. Norman (Eds.), *Predicting Health Behaviour: Research and Practice with Social Cognition Models, 2nd Ed* (pp. 127–169). Maidenhead: Open University Press.

Maddux, J. E., and Rogers, R. W. (1983). Protection motivation and self-efficacy: a revised theory of fear appeals and attitude change. *J Exp Social Psychol, 19*, 469–479.

Milne, S., Sheeran, P., and Orbell, S. (2000). Prediction and intervention in health-related behavior: a meta-analytic review of protection motivation theory. *J Appl Soc Psychol, 30*, 106–143.

Milne, S., Orbell, S., and Sheeran, P. (2002). Combining motivational and volitional interventions to promote exercise participation: protection motivation theory and implementation intentions. *Br J Health Psychol, 7*, 163–184.

Norman, P., Boer, H., and Seydel, E. R. (2005). Protection motivation theory. In M. Conner & P. Norman (Eds.), *Predicting Health Behaviour: Research and Practice with Social Cognition Models, 2nd Ed* (pp. 81–126). Maidenhead: Open University Press.

Orbell, S., Crombie, I., and Johnston, G. (1995). Social cognition and social structure in the prediction of cervical screening uptake. *Br J Health Psychol, 1*, 35–50.

Prochaska, J. O., and DiClemente, C. C. (1984). *The Transtheoretical Approach: Crossing Traditional Boundaries of Therapy*. Homewood, IL: Dow Jones Irwin.

Rosenstock, I. M., Strecher, V. J., and Becker, M. H. (1988). Social learning theory and the health belief model. *Health Educ Q, 15*, 175–183.

Sandberg, T., and Conner, M. (2008). Anticipated regret as an additional predictor in the theory of planned behaviour: a meta-analysis. *Br J Soc Psychol, 47*, 589–606.

Sheeran, P., and Abraham, C. (2003). Mediator of moderators: temporal stability of intention and the intention-behavior relationship. *Pers Soc Psychol Bull, 29*, 205–215.

Sheeran, P., Milne, S., Webb, T. L., and Gollwitzer, P. M. (2005). Implementation intentions and health behaviours. In M. Conner & P. Norman (Eds.), *Predicting Health Behaviour: Research and Practice with Social Cognition Models, 2nd Ed* (pp. 276–323). Maidenhead: Open University Press.

Sutton, S. (2000). A critical review of the transtheoretical model applied to smoking cessation. In P. Norman, C. Abraham, & M. Conner (Eds.), *Understanding and Changing Health Behaviour: From Health Beliefs to Self-Regulation* (pp. 207–225). Reading, England: Harwood Academic Press.

Sutton, S. (2005). Stage models of health behaviour. In M. Conner & P. Norman (Eds.), *Predicting Health Behaviour: Research and Practice with Social Cognition Models, 2nd Ed* (pp. 223–275). Maidenhead: Open University Press.

Turk, D. C., and Salovey, P. (1986). Clinical information processing: bias inoculation. In R. E. Ingham (Ed.), *Information Processing Approaches to Clinical Psychology* (pp. 305–323). New York: Academic Press.

Webb, T. L., and Sheeran, P. (2006). Does changing behavioral intentions engender behavior change? A meta-analysis of the experimental evidence. *Psychol Bull, 132*, 249–268.

West, R. (2005). Time for a change: putting the transtheoretical (stages of change) model to rest. *Addiction, 100*, 1036–1039.

Chapter 3

Assessment of Physical Activity in Research and Clinical Practice

Lephuong Ong and James A. Blumenthal

1 Introduction

It is well established that physical activity is associated with significant physical and mental health benefits including increased longevity (Camacho et al, 1991; Leon et al, 1987; Paffenbarger et al, 1986; Powell et al, 1987). Physical inactivity, on the other hand, is associated with adverse health consequences and has been identified as a modifiable behavioral risk factor for mortality and diseases of lifestyle, such as cardiovascular disease, cancer, and diabetes mellitus (see Lee, 2003; Warburton et al, 2006). These data have prompted an increased interest in promoting physical activity, which requires accurate and objective quantification of activity. Because the validity of these associations rests upon the utilization of valid and reliable assessments of physical activity, precise measurements of physical activity are required to improve our understanding of the impact of physical activity on health outcomes and to provide a metric to evaluate the efficacy of clinical interventions designed to promote health and physical activity.

J.A. Blumenthal (✉)
Department of Psychiatry and Behavioral Sciences, Duke University Medical Center, Box 3119, Durham, NC 27710, USA
e-mail: blume003@mc.duke.edu

2 Physical Activity and Health Outcomes

2.1 All-Cause and CHD-Related Mortality

Epidemiologic studies have consistently identified an association between physical inactivity and a variety of poor health outcomes, ranging from cancer, heart disease, and osteoarthritis to all-cause mortality. In one of the earliest studies, Morris and colleagues (Morris and Heady, 1953; Morris et al, 1953) examined mortality data from the London Transport Executive between 1949 and 1952 and reported a lower total incidence of initial coronary episodes and cardiac-related deaths among middle-aged males engaged in more physically active occupations (e.g., postmen and bus conductors) compared to those in less active occupations (e.g., telephone operators and bus drivers; Morris et al, 1953). When cardiac-related mortality was examined for other occupations, a similar pattern of findings emerged, such that males performing "heavy" work (e.g., coal workers, laborers) had lower mortality rates relative to males performing "light" work (e.g., hairdressers, textile workers) (Morris et al, 1953). A trend for increased mortality due to lung cancers, appendicitis, prostate disease, duodenal ulcers, diabetes, and liver cirrhosis in middle-aged males performing light work as compared to heavy work was also found (Morris and Heady, 1953). This relationship between poorer health outcomes and lower physical activity was observed across the social classes.

In another large epidemiologic study in which 3686 San Francisco longshoremen between 35 and 74 years of age were followed for 22 years, Paffenbarger and colleagues reported that lower levels of energy expenditure (i.e., <8500 kcal/week), compared to high energy expenditure (i.e., >8500 kcal/week), were associated with a 1.46-fold increased risk of all-cause mortality after controlling for the effects of age, cigarette smoking, and high blood pressure (Paffenbarger et al, 1978a; Paffenbarger and Hale, 1975). Lower energy expenditure was also found to confer a 1.97-fold increased risk of heart attack and a 3.32-fold increased risk of sudden death (Paffenbarger and Hale, 1975; see Fig. 3.1). In a study of 12,138 healthy males, Leon et al (1987) found that after 7 years, middle-aged men in the top two tertiles of leisure time physical activity (mean minutes per day) had lower mortality rates compared to men in the lowest tertile. Relative to men in the lowest physical activity tertile, men in the highest tertile had 20% lower incidence of combined fatal and nonfatal coronary events.

There is evidence that the intensity of physical activity may moderate the relationship between physical activity and health outcomes. For example, in the Harvard Alumni Health Study, total physical activity was prospectively related to decreased risk of mortality in men who engaged in vigorous physical activities (i.e., ≥ 6 times the resting metabolic rate [MET]; Lee et al, 1995). In a follow-up study, Lee and Paffenbarger (2000) reported that vigorous physical activity conferred the greatest benefit in terms of reduced mortality, moderate physical activity was found to be somewhat beneficial, and light physical activity conferred no benefit.

Although there have been fewer studies in females, available data suggest a similar pattern. For example, in the Nurses' Health Study, in which 116,564 initially healthy, middle-aged women were followed for 24 years, physical inactivity (<1 h of exercise/week) was associated with a 52% increase in all-cause mortality, a twofold increase in cardiovascular mortality, and 29% increase in cancer-related mortality (Hu et al, 2004). Other investigators have also found that the relative risk of death due to all causes was reduced (RR, 0.77; 95% CI, 0.66–0.90) in a large cohort of postmenopausal women who reported regular physical activity compared with those who were sedentary (Kushi et al, 1997). With respect to frequency and intensity, the data indicate that engaging in moderate physical activity as infrequently as once per week appeared to have a protective effect on mortality (RR, 0.78; 95% CI, 0.64–0.96; Kushi et al,

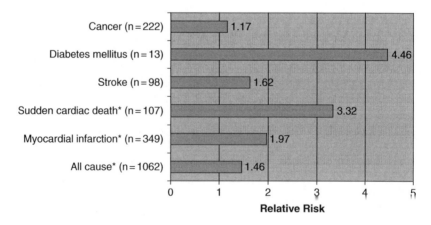

Fig. 3.1 Relative risk of death as related to work-related energy expenditure among 3686 San Francisco longshoremen (1951–1972). Data are adjusted for age, cigarette smoking, and systolic blood pressure. * $p<0.001$. Adapted from Paffenbarger, Brand et al (1978)

1997). Although data from women are less consistent and null findings have been reported (e.g., Blair et al, 1993; Kampert et al, 1996), studies generally show that physical activity has a beneficial effect on health and mortality in women as well as in men.

2.2 Incidence of Chronic Diseases

2.2.1 Coronary Heart Disease

Based on their review of 43 studies that examined the relationship between physical inactivity and CHD incidence, Powell and colleagues (1987) concluded that the risk of incident CHD due to physical inactivity ranges from 1.5 to 2.4 (median = 1.9). These values are similar in magnitude to other CHD risk factors, such as hypertension, hypercholesterolemia, and smoking. These data are consistent with recent evidence from the Nurses Health Study, in which physical inactivity (<1 h of exercise per week) was found to be associated with increased risk (RR = 1.58; 95% CI, 1.39–1.80) of incident coronary heart disease in 88,393 women followed for 20 years (Li et al, 2006). Data from the Womens' Health Study also indicate that the health benefits of physical activity are not limited to vigorous activity, such that participating in light to moderate physical activity, such as walking for at least 1 h per week, is associated with lower CHD risk (RR = 0.49; 95% CI, 0.28–0.86) (Lee et al, 2001).

Participation in physical activities also affects prognosis in patients with CHD. For instance, in older men with established CHD followed for 5 years ($N = 772$, mean age = 63), light to moderate physical activity conferred a reduction in risk for all-cause and cardiovascular mortality over a sedentary lifestyle after covariate adjustment (light, RR = 0.42; 95% CI, 0.25–0.71; moderate, RR = 0.47; 95% CI, 0.24–0.92; Wannamethee et al, 2000). These results are consistent with the findings of Taylor et al (2004), who conducted a systematic quantitative review of exercise-based cardiac rehabilitation programs and found

that, relative to usual care, cardiac rehabilitation was associated with reduced all-cause mortality (odds ratio [OR] = 0.80; 95% CI, 0.68–0.93) and fatal cardiac events (OR = 0.74; 95% CI: 0.61–0.96). Compared to usual care, cardiac rehabilitation was also associated with greater reductions in CHD-related risk factors, such as total cholesterol level, triglyceride level, and systolic blood pressure (Taylor et al, 2004).

2.2.2 Diabetes Mellitus

In a cohort of 87,253 of healthy females aged 34–59 years followed for 8 years, Manson et al (1991) reported that the age-adjusted relative risk of non-insulin-dependent diabetes mellitus in females who engaged in vigorous exercise at least once per week was 0.67. In another study of 21,271 initially healthy male physicians, Manson reported that vigorous exercise was found to be associated with reduced risk of non-insulin-dependent diabetes mellitus over a 5 year follow-up period (Manson et al, 1992). The age-adjusted relative risk of diabetes decreased with increasing frequency of physical activity (0.77 for once weekly, 0.62 for two to four times per week, and 0.58 for five or more times per week).

2.2.3 Cancer

Lee (2003) conducted a systematic review of epidemiologic studies that examined the relationship between physical activity and risk of developing cancer and found that physical activity is associated with reduced risk of certain, site-specific cancers, particularly colon and breast cancers. Specifically, physically active men and women showed a 30–40% reduction in risk of developing colon cancer compared to inactive persons. Relative to inactive women, physically active women exhibited a 20–30% decreased risk of developing breast cancer. The role of physical activity is less clear with prostate and lung cancers. Lee (2003) also concluded that moderate physical activity (>4.5 METs) had a greater protective effect compared to less intense activities. There also is evidence to suggest that regular, vigorous physical activity (i.e., participation in a sport >3 times/week) may reduce the risk of all-cause mortality (hazard ratio = 0.47; 95% CI, 0.23–0.96) in men and women following a cancer diagnosis (Hamer et al, 2008). Other data suggest that physical activity improves cardiorespiratory function and quality of life among cancer survivors (Courneya et al, 2003; McNeely et al, 2006; Schmitz et al, 2005).

2.2.4 Osteoporosis

In the Nurses Health Study, investigators followed 61,200 initially healthy postmenopausal women (aged 40–77 years) and found that walking for at least 4 h per week was associated with a 41% lower risk of hip fracture (RR, 0.59; 95% CI, 0.37–0.94) compared with walking less than 1 h per week (Feskanich et al, 2002). The reduced risk of hip fractures has also been observed in a prospective cohort study of men, such that men who engaged in vigorous physical activity (e.g., at least running or jogging) had a significantly lower risk of hip fracture (hazard ratio, 0.38; 95% CI, 0.16–0.91) relative to men who did not (Kujala et al, 2000). In addition, exercise may be an effective adjunctive treatment for individuals with osteoporosis, as it has been shown to relieve symptoms, improve quality of life, and maintain physical mobility (Sharkey et al, 2000).

2.2.5 Clinical Depression

In addition to the physical benefits of physical activity, regular exercise is also associated with significant mental health benefits, such as lower prevalence of mental disorders (Goodwin, 2003). There also are epidemiologic data that suggest that physical inactivity may be an independent risk factor for the development of depressive symptoms. For example, results from the National Health and Nutrition

Examination Survey Epidemiologic Follow-Up Study (NHANES I) suggest that females who engaged in little or no recreational physical activity are at a twofold increased risk of developing clinically elevated symptoms of depression over an 8 year follow-up period (OR, 1.9; 95% CI, 1.1–3.2) (Farmer et al, 1988). In males, however, physical inactivity predicted depressive symptoms over the follow-up period only if they reported clinically elevated symptoms at the baseline assessment (OR, 12.9; 95% CI, 1.7–98.9). In the Alameda County study, physical inactivity conferred an increased risk for depression in a population sample of non-depressed individuals of both genders (Camacho et al, 1991). Physical activity levels and depressive symptoms were assessed by self-report in 1965, 1974, and 1983. Compared to participants who reported high physical activity levels in 1965, men and women who reported low physical activity levels were at increased risk (males: OR, 1.76; 95% CI, 1.06–2.92; females: OR, 1.70; 95% CI, 1.06–2.70) of higher depressive symptoms in 1974. There is also evidence to suggest that maintaining high physical activity levels is important, as participants who decreased their activity levels from high to low between 1965 and 1974 were at increased risk for depressive symptoms in 1983. In addition to these epidemiological data, randomized trials of patients with major depression have shown that exercise is better than attention control and is comparable to psychotherapy (Lawlor and Hopker, 2001) and may be as effective as anti-depressant medication in reducing depressive symptoms (Babyak et al, 2000; Blumenthal et al, 2007; Blumenthal et al, 1999).

3 Defining Physical Activity

A discussion of assessment methods for physical activity cannot proceed without first defining physical activity and differentiating it from related constructs. Clear, operational definitions are essential for valid assessments and permit comparison across research studies.

Constructs related to physical activity relevant to researchers and clinicians in behavioral medicine are *exercise*, *physical fitness*, *exercise capacity*, and *functional capacity*.

The terms *physical activity* and *exercise* are frequently used interchangeably. Although physical activity and exercise share a number of common features such as energy expenditure and bodily movement of skeletal muscles, physical activity and exercise are distinct constructs (Caspersen et al, 1985). Caspersen et al (1985) define physical activity as "any bodily movement produced by skeletal muscles that results in energy expenditure" (p. 126). Physical activity thus defined is broad in scope and is performed in the contexts of leisure, household, and occupational domains of living. Alternatively, exercise is conceptualized as a subcategory of physical activity that is planned, structured, repetitive, and purposeful. Exercise is considered purposeful in that its aim is to maintain or improve physical fitness (Caspersen et al, 1985).

Physical fitness, exercise capacity, and *functional capacity* similarly refer to an individual's *ability* to perform physical activities. Physical fitness refers to "a set of attributes that people have or achieve that relates to the ability to perform physical activity" (Caspersen et al, 1985, p. 129). Physical fitness is positively correlated with physical activity and exercise. Markers of physical fitness include cardiorespiratory endurance, muscular strength, body composition, and flexibility. Exercise capacity specifically refers to the ability to perform aerobic exercise, while functional capacity specifically refers to an individual's ability to perform the physical demands associated with activities of daily living (Guyatt et al, 1985).

4 Dimensions of Assessment

With respect to the assessment of physical activity, the key dimensions of interest are *frequency*, *duration*, and *intensity*. *Frequency* refers to how often one engages in the physical activity of interest, within a specified interval of time (e.g., past week, past month). *Duration* is the total amount of time spent (e.g., in minutes, hours) performing the physical activity. *Intensity* reflects the amount of energy expended while performing the physical activity of interest and is typically expressed in metabolic equivalents (METs), a ratio of the metabolic rate during physical activity relative to the resting metabolic rate (3.5 ml O_2/kg/min). A MET value of 1.0 is roughly equivalent to the energy expenditure at rest; hence, if an individual engages in physical activity equivalent to a MET level of 10, they would expending 10 times the energy compared to their energy expenditure in a resting state. A compendium of physical activities and MET intensities can be used to estimate total energy expenditure (Ainsworth et al, 2000).

5 Laboratory Measures

5.1 Exercise Treadmill Testing

Exercise treadmill testing is the gold standard for the assessment of cardiorespiratory fitness or aerobic capacity. The results of exercise treadmill testing can be used to establish baseline cardiorespiratory fitness to facilitate the creation of a tailored exercise prescription. Exercise treadmill testing can also be utilized following exercise training as a post-treatment measure of change. In clinical cardiology, treadmill tests are routinely used to evaluate the presence and prognosis of ischemic heart disease.

Cardiorespiratory fitness is assessed directly by measuring maximum oxygen consumption, or $\dot{V}O_{2\,max}$, the rate of oxygen consumption during maximal aerobic activity (expressed in METs). To assess $\dot{V}O_{2\,max}$, individuals are instructed to exercise to exhaustion. Alternatively, the test may be discontinued when a maximum heart rate (calculated as $220 - $ age) is achieved.

Trained personnel are required to administer and supervise the graded exercise treadmill test and specialized equipment is necessary to assess $\dot{V}O_{2\,max}$. Typically, heart rate and electrocardiographic data are recorded during the treadmill test, which permits the monitoring of adverse events, such as cardiac arrhythmias and myocardial ischemia. Sphygmomanometry may also be employed to assess blood pressure. Expired air is collected to assess parameters such as maximum oxygen consumption, carbon dioxide production, minute ventilation, and respiratory exchange ratio.

A number of exercise treadmill testing protocols exist, such as the Bruce (Bruce et al, 1963), Naughton (Naughton et al, 1963), and Duke-Wake Forest (Blumenthal et al, 1988) protocols, which typically vary in the progression of the speed and incline of the treadmill, with optimal selection based on the clinical population and estimated duration of the test. The Bruce protocol (Bruce et al, 1963) is a routinely used and well-validated exercise treadmill test. There are seven stages in total, each lasting 3 min. There is a progressive increase in workload in terms of speed and incline with each successive stage. For instance, at stage 1, participants walk at a speed of 1.7 mph and an incline of 10%. At stages 2 and 3, the speed increases to 3.4 and 5.0 mph with inclines of 14 and 18%, respectively. A major disadvantage of the Bruce protocol is its high intensity, which limits its use to relatively healthy, physically fit individuals. Accordingly, the Bruce protocol has been modified for use with persons with diminished functional capacity. The modified Bruce is identical to the Bruce except that it features two initial, lower intensity stages (stage 1: 1.7 mph, 0% grade; stage 2: 1.7 mph, 5% grade). Stage 3 of the modified Bruce is equivalent to stage 1 of the regular Bruce protocol.

The Naughton protocol (Naughton et al, 1963) starts with a speed of 3.0–3.4 mph (0% grade), with 2 min increases in grade without increases in speed. The advantage of the Naughton is that it is a low intensity test that is suitable for patients with diminished functional capacity and low tolerance for aerobic exercise. The disadvantage of this protocol is that it may take a fair amount of time for healthier individuals to achieve heart rate targets or exercise to exhaustion.

In the Duke-Wake Forest protocol (Blumenthal et al, 1988), workloads are increased at the rate of 1 MET (3.5 ml O_2/kg/min) per minute: minute 1, 2.0 mph, 0% grade; minute 2, 2.5 mph, 0% grade; minute 3, 2.5 mph, 2.0% grade; and so on. The advantage of this protocol is that workload is increased in multiples of the resting metabolic rate, as opposed to more arbitrarily defined increments of speed and grade.

5.2 The 6-Minute Walk Test

The 6-minute walk test (6MWT; Butland et al, 1982) is a commonly performed test of functional capacity. The 6MWT is a self-paced, timed test of the total distance that a patient is able to walk in 6 min. Patients are instructed to walk as quickly as possible for the duration of the test, with voluntary rest permitted. Although other timed walk tests exist (e.g., 2-minute and 12-minute walk tests; Butland et al, 1982; McGavin et al, 1976), the 6MWT is the functional walk test of choice for clinical and research purposes as it is easy to administer, inexpensive, and considered to be reflective of activities of daily living (Lipkin et al, 1986). The 6MWT has been shown to be well-tolerated by patients with diminished functional capacity, thereby permitting the estimation of functional capacity in patients who are unable to achieve maximum treadmill tests (e.g., heart failure patients; Lipkin et al, 1986; Peeters and Mets, 1996).

Total distance walked on the 6MWT has been found to discriminate between normal subjects, New York Heart Association (NYHA) class II, and NYHA class III heart failure patients (Lipkin et al, 1986). Distance walked is also predictive of morbidity and mortality in patients with heart failure (Bittner et al, 1993; Cahalin et al, 1996), chronic obstructive pulmonary disease (Cote et al, 2007; Szekely et al, 1997), and end-stage lung disease awaiting transplantation

(Martinu et al, 2008). Reference values for distance and predictive equations for healthy adults are available (Camarri et al, 2006; Enright and Sherrill, 1998; Troosters et al, 1999). In healthy adults, walking distance ranges from 400 to 700 m and has been found to be predicted by age, gender, weight, and height (Chetta et al, 2006; Enright and Sherrill, 1998; Troosters et al, 1999). In patients with COPD, a change in walking distance of 54 m is considered clinically meaningful in that it is the difference in distance needed for patients to notice changes (i.e., improvement or worsening) in their functional capacity (Redelmeier et al, 1997).

5.3 The Step Test

The Step Test is a simple method for assessing cardiorespiratory fitness by evaluating heart rate response to stepping up and down a set of steps at a fixed rate (Whaley et al, 2006); post-exercise heart rate recovery may also be examined. Self-paced (Petrella et al, 2001) and fixed pace (Sykes, 1995) protocols are available. Depending on the protocol, step testing ends when a fixed number of steps at a given rate are complete or until a patient reaches the criterion heart rate (e.g., 80% of predicted maximum).

The Step Test has been found to be strongly correlated with $\dot{V}O_{2\,max}$ ($r = 0.92$; Sykes and Roberts, 2004) and is a sensitive index of change following exercise training (Petrella et al, 2001). Step testing is quick, inexpensive, and appropriate for the measurement of cardiorespiratory fitness in elderly subjects (Petrella et al, 2001).

6 Field Measures

6.1 Pedometers

A pedometer is a small, battery-operated electronic device worn at the waistband in the midline of the thigh that detects and records vertical pelvic displacements during ambulatory activities, such as walking and running (Berlin et al, 2006). The number of vertical displacements is stored as the number of steps taken and is presented on the pedometer's digital display (Berlin et al, 2006). The number of recorded steps need to be manually transcribed on either a daily or weekly basis and diaries may be provided so that participants may track the duration that the device is worn, type of activity, and the number of steps taken (Berlin et al, 2006). Some models allow the input of an individual's stride length in order to provide an estimate of the distance ambulated (Berlin et al, 2006).

Although step-counting accuracy has been found to vary between different pedometer brands and models, contemporary electronic pedometers are fairly accurate in counting steps in individuals with regular, steady, gait patterns (Bassett et al, 1996; Schneider et al, 2003). There is some evidence that pedometers may underestimate steps taken at slower speeds (e.g., 71% accuracy at speeds <2.0 mph) and that accuracy may reach 96% at speeds greater than 3.0 mph (Melanson et al, 2004). Pedometers have also been reported to be less reliable in individuals who have a body mass index >30 (Shepherd et al, 1999).

A major limitation associated with the use of the pedometer is that it does not record any information about the frequency, duration, or intensity of physical activity (Berlin et al, 2006). Hence, total energy expenditure cannot be reliably estimated with the pedometer. Another potential drawback of the pedometer is that its use is narrowly restricted to the assessment of walking and running, and that load-bearing, non-vertical movements, seated activities (e.g., cycling) cannot be validly monitored using the pedometer (Vanhees et al, 2005). Despite these limitations, the pedometer's relatively low cost, portability, and unobtrusiveness reduces participant and investigator burden, making it an attractive option for the assessment of physical activity in free living conditions.

6.2 Accelerometers

Routine daily physical activity can be assessed using an accelerometer, a compact, lightweight, noninvasive, and unobtrusive device that may be worn on the waist, ankle, or wrist (e.g., Actiwatch; Mini Mitter Co., Inc., Bend, Oregon). As the name implies, the accelerometer assesses physical activity in terms of acceleration (Chen and Bassett, 2005). Accelerometers measure and store frequency, pattern, duration, and intensity of movement through sensors that detect acceleration in one (uniaxial), two (biaxial), or three (triaxial) orthogonal planes (i.e., antero-posterior, mediolateral, and vertical; Berlin et al, 2006; Chen and Bassett, 2005). Raw data are expressed as "counts," a measure of the frequency and intensity of acceleration and deceleration (Berlin et al, 2006). Data are stored on the device and then uploaded to a PC for analysis. Accelerometers are also capable of recording the time of physical activity counts, permitting patterns of activity (time and duration) to be examined. Cumulative mean daily waking physical activity can be derived to provide an index of routine daily activity. If desired, sleep parameters, such as minutes of mobility during sleep,

total sleep time, and sleep efficiency (i.e., a ratio of actual sleep time to time in bed), also can be measured using accelerometry. Figures 3.2 and 3.3 display illustrative data obtained from the Lifecorder Plus (NEW-LIFESTYLES, Inc., Lee's Summit, Missouri) and the Actiwatch.

6.3 Questionnaires and Activity Rating Scales

Self-report measures in the form of questionnaires and activity rating scales are the most frequently used method to assess patterns of physical activity (see Table 3.1). Respondents may be asked to describe the type, frequency, intensity, and duration of their physical activities within a specific timeframe of interest (e.g., within the past day, week, month, or year). Questionnaires and activity rating scales can be self-administered (in person or by mail) or administered by trained personnel (in person or via telephone).

The primary advantages of self-report measures are that they are expedient, cost-effective, and associated with low participant

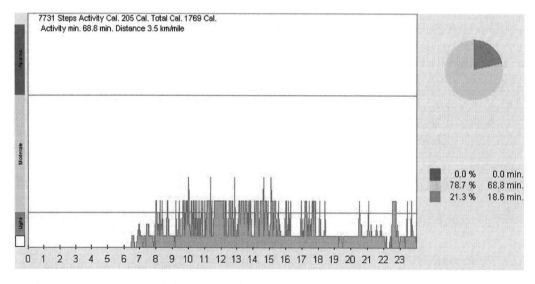

Fig. 3.2 Twenty-four hour physical activity data for a 73-year-old male using the Lifecorder Plus (NEW-LIFESTYLES, Inc., Lee's Summit, Missouri), a triaxial accelerometer. The subject ambulated 3.5 total miles and performed 68.8 min of moderate physical activity (defined as ≥ 2–5 METS)

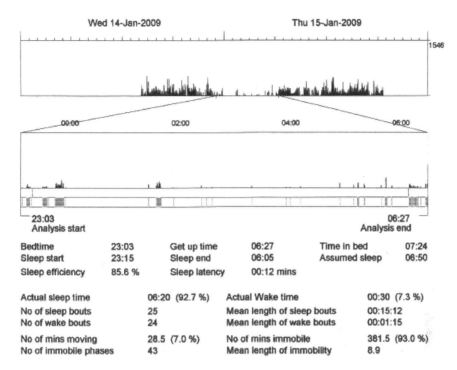

Bedtime	23:03	Get up time	06:27	Time in bed	07:24
Sleep start	23:15	Sleep end	06:05	Assumed sleep	06:50
Sleep efficiency	85.6 %	Sleep latency	00:12 mins		

Actual sleep time	06:20 (92.7 %)	Actual Wake time	00:30 (7.3 %)
No of sleep bouts	25	Mean length of sleep bouts	00:15:12
No of wake bouts	24	Mean length of wake bouts	00:01:15
No of mins moving	28.5 (7.0 %)	No of mins immobile	381.5 (93.0 %)
No of immobile phases	43	Mean length of immobility	8.9

Fig. 3.3 Sleep actigraphy data from a 48-year-old male using the Actiwatch (Mini Mitter Co., Inc., Bend, Oregon) showing activity distribution over a 24-h period and sleep parameters such as sleep time, sleep efficiency, and minutes of mobility during sleep

and investigator burden. Questionnaires can be administered to large groups of people with ease, making them an appropriate choice for large, epidemiologic studies. Notwithstanding these advantages, questionnaires and rating scales are associated with several important limitations. For instance, the reliance upon self-report measures creates the opportunity for study participants to respond in socially desirable ways to present themselves favorably or to answer in ways in which they think they are expected to answer. A potential solution to this problem would be to incorporate a social desirability scale, such as the Marlowe–Crowne Social Desirability Scale (Crowne and Marlowe, 1960), to detect potentially invalid questionnaires and either adjust their scores or exclude respondents who may for whatever reasons distort their reported activity levels. Another limitation associated with self-report measures is that the quality of the data is dependent on participant compliance, affected in turn by motivational and cognitive factors (e.g., memory).

6.3.1 Harvard Alumni Activity Survey

The Harvard Alumni Activity Survey is a brief, seven-item, expedient measure of physical activity (Paffenbarger et al, 1978b). It was constructed for use in the Harvard Alumni Health Study, which investigated the role of physical activity as a risk factor for myocardial infarction. This self-report questionnaire asks respondents to recall the types and duration of physical activities engaged in during the past week. The survey assesses the number of flights of stairs climbed, number of city blocks walked, and what sports were played (hours per week). A physical activity index representing total energy expenditure (expressed in kilocalories per week) is estimated based on values for each activity that is derived from the literature.

One year test–retest reliability is reported to be 0.73 and energy expenditure as measured using this scale has been shown to be inversely related to the risk of first heart attack (LaPorte et al, 1983).

Table 3.1 Characteristics of physical activity questionnaires

Measure	Format	Time frame	Activities assessed	Light intensity	Moderate/heavy intensity	Estimation of energy expenditure	Measures derived	Units
Harvard Alumni Activity Survey (Paffenbarger, Wing et al, 1978)	Self-report	Past week	Leisure	X	X	X	Physical activity index representing total energy expenditure	kcal/week
The Minnesota Leisure Time Physical Activity (Taylor et al, 1978)	Interview	Past 12 months	Leisure, household	X	X	X	Activity Metabolic Index for light, moderate, heavy, and total activities	MET*min/day
Seven-Day Physical Activity Recall (Sallis et al, 1985)	Interview or self-report	Past week	Leisure, household, work		X	X	Total energy expenditure	MET/week
Stages of Exercise Change Questionnaire (Marcus et al, 1992)	Self-report	Current exercise behavior	Exercise				Stage of change related to exercise	
CHAMPS (Stewart et al, 2001)	Self-report or interview	Typical week in past month	Leisure, work, household	X	X	X	Total caloric expenditure/week in moderate intensity or greater and in "all" physical activities; frequency of activity per week in moderate intensity or greater and in "all" physical activities	Kcal/week
Godin Leisure Time Exercise Questionnaire (Godin and Shephard, 1985)	Self-report	Typical 7-day period	Leisure	X	X	X	Activity score	MET/week
International Physical Activity Questionnaire (Craig et al, 2003)	Interview or self-report	Past week	Occupational, household, leisure, transport, rest	X	X	X	Total physical activity score	MET-minutes/week

6.3.2 Minnesota Leisure Time Physical Activity Questionnaire

The Minnesota Leisure Time Physical Activity Questionnaire (LTPA; Taylor et al, 1978) is designed to quantify energy expenditure during leisure time physical activities. It was originally created to assess the relationship between physical activity intensity and coronary heart disease risk. Respondents indicate which activities they have engaged in over the past 12 months and then a trained interviewer collects detailed information regarding activity type, duration, and frequency for each reported activity. Intensity codes in metabolic equivalents are available for 62 leisure activities. The product of each intensity code and duration of activity in minutes (MET*min) is summed for all activities to produce a total Activity Metabolic Index (AMI), expressed in MET*min/day. Light (sum of all activities with intensity codes $\leq$ 4.0 METs), moderate (sum of all activities with intensity codes between 4.5 and 5.5 METs), and heavy (sum of all activities with intensity codes $\geq$6.0 METs) AMIs may also be computed to examine the impact of physical activity intensity on health-related outcomes.

The LTPA has been shown to have satisfactory test–retest reliability at 5 weeks (r = .79–.88; Folsom et al, 1986) and at 1 year (r = .69; Jacobs et al, 1993; Richardson et al, 1994). Total AMI has been found to be moderately correlated with total exercise treadmill time (r = .45–.52; Taylor et al, 1978) and VO_{2peak} (r = .47; Richardson et al, 1994) but weakly correlated with 48-h Caltrac accelerometer readings (r = .23; Richardson et al, 1994). Findings from the Minnesota Heart survey and the Multiple Risk Factor Intervention Trial indicate that higher leisure time physical activity (assessed with the LTPA) is associated with fewer coronary risk factors (Folsom et al, 1985) and reduced risk of CHD morbidity and mortality (Leon et al, 1987).

6.3.3 Seven-Day Physical Activity Recall

Physical activity can be assessed with the 7-Day Physical Activity Recall (PAR; Blair et al, 1985; Sallis et al, 1985), a semi-structured interview designed to evaluate self-reported activity levels over a 7-day period. A self-report version of this questionnaire is also available. Respondents are asked to estimate the total time spent in sleep or engaged in occupational, household, or leisure activities of at least moderate intensity. Examples of moderate (e.g., brisk walking), hard (e.g., physical labor), and very hard (e.g., jogging) activities are provided. The energy expenditure for each activity is expressed in multiples of resting metabolic rate (MET; 1 MET = 1 kcal/kg/h). The MET for each activity is multiplied by hours spent in the activity, and the products are summed to provide an estimate of total energy expenditure.

The PAR is sensitive to changes in physical activity following exercise training (Blair et al, 1985) and is positively correlated with $VO_{2\,max}$ (r = .30; Jacobs et al, 1993). Acceptable inter-rater reliability coefficients have also been reported (r = 0.78–0.86) for PAR-estimated energy expenditure (Gross et al, 1990; Sallis et al, 1988), but 1 month test-retest reliability has been found to be low (r = .34; Jacobs et al, 1993).

6.3.4 Stages of Exercise Change Questionnaire

The Stages of Exercise Change Questionnaire (Marcus et al, 1992) was adapted from the smoking literature and is based on the Transtheoretical Model of Change (Prochaska and DiClemente, 1983). This scale is designed to assess respondents' stage of exercise change by asking them to choose the statement that best describes their current exercise behavior (e.g., precontemplation, *I currently do not exercise and I do not intend to start exercising in the next 6 months*). There is one statement for each of the five stages of readiness: precontemplation, contemplation, preparation, action, and maintenance. Two-week reliability is reported to be .78 (Marcus et al, 1992). Although it does not provide a measure of energy expenditure, exercise intensity, or exercise frequency, its stage-based approach facilitates the delivery of targeted interventions to promote physical activity at each stage of exercise change. It is not recommended as a reliable method for documenting the exact amount of activity in which a person regularly engages, but may be worthwhile for screening purposes.

6.3.5 Community Healthy Activities Model Program for Seniors Activities Questionnaire

The Community Healthy Activities Model Program for Seniors (CHAMPS) Activities Questionnaire (Stewart et al, 2001) is a comprehensive self-report measure of physical activity designed for use among sedentary older adults. It may be self- or interviewer administered to accommodate sensory deficits of elderly respondents. It assesses leisure, household, and work (e.g., volunteer) activities that are appropriate and relevant for older adults. Activity duration is multiplied by established metabolic equivalents for each activity and summed across all activities to yield an estimate of weekly caloric expenditure (kcal/week). The impact of activity intensity can be assessed by summing caloric expenditures only for activities of at least moderate intensity (MET $\geq$ 3.0).

The CHAMPS questionnaire has satisfactory 6-month test–retest reliability ($r = .62$–67) and is sensitive to change following an intervention designed to increase physical activity (Stewart et al, 2001). The CHAMPS questionnaire has also been found to significantly discriminate between groups with known differences in activity levels (e.g., sedentary, somewhat active, and active; Stewart et al, 2001). CHAMPS-derived estimates of total caloric expenditure has been shown to be positively correlated with 6-minute walk test performance ($r = .46$) and accelerometer data ($r = .36$–$.42$; Harada et al, 2001).

6.3.6 Godin Leisure Time Exercise Questionnaire

The Godin Leisure Time Exercise Questionnaire (Godin and Shephard, 1985) is a brief,

self-administered questionnaire that assesses leisure time physical activity. Respondents are asked to indicate the number of times during a typical week that they participate in mild (e.g., yoga, bowling), moderate (e.g., fast walking, baseball), or strenuous (e.g., running, jogging) exercise for at least 15 min. One additional item assesses how often during a typical week respondents engaged in sweat-inducing exercises. Each of the three exercise categories is assigned an intensity value, expressed as metabolic equivalents: strenuous, 9.0 METs; moderate, 5.0 METs; and mild, 3.0 METs. An activity score is computed by summing the products of the frequency of each of the three exercise categories and its corresponding METs value. One month test–retest reliability is reported to be 0.62 and the activity score is positively correlated with $\dot{V}O_{2\,max}(r = .56)$ and accelerometer ($r = .32$) data (Jacobs, 1993).

6.3.7 International Physical Activity Questionnaire

The International Physical Activity Questionnaire (IPAQ; Craig et al, 2003) is a set of four questionnaires designed for use in adults (15–69 years old) to derive internationally comparable data on physical activity during the last 7 days. Long and short versions of the IPAQ are available and are either interviewer- or self-administered. The 4-item, short version assesses the number of days per week the respondent has engaged in moderate or vigorous activity, as well as the time spent walking or sitting. The 27-item, long version assesses physical activity across five activity domains (e.g., occupational, transport, household, leisure, and time spent sitting). Data from the long and short forms are used to estimate total energy expenditure by weighting the reported minutes per week in each activity category by a MET energy expenditure estimate assigned to each activity category. The IPAQ has been found to have satisfactory test–retest reliability (long form: pooled Spearman's $\rho = 0.81$; short form: pooled Spearman's $\rho = 0.76$) and fair criterion validity (using accelerometers, pooled $\rho = 0.33$) in industrialized and developing nations (Craig et al, 2003).

7 Physiological Measures

7.1 Oxygen Uptake

Although not widely used, portable indirect calorimeters can be used to assess oxygen consumption ($\dot{V}O_2$) to estimate energy expenditure during physical activity (Duffield et al, 2004; Hausswirth et al, 1997). Although there is evidence to suggest that some models show good reliability and validity when compared to larger, traditional calorimeters (Hausswirth et al, 1997; Novitsky et al, 1995), issues related to cost and obtrusiveness have limited the use of these devices in larger population studies of physical activity.

7.2 Heart Rate Monitoring

Heart rate monitoring can be used as an objective measure of total energy expenditure in laboratory and free living conditions. Contemporary devices are small and unobtrusive, cost between $200 and $500, and consist of a chest strap transmitter and a receiver watch (Freedson and Miller, 2000). Its use is based on the premise that heart rate and oxygen consumption are linearly related, particularly between 110 and 150 bpm (Freedson and Miller, 2000; Livingstone, 1997). Using a regression equation, exercise heart rate can be used to estimate $\dot{V}O_2$. Monitors that provide minute-to-minute recordings of heart rate enable the evaluation of day-to-day variability of energy expenditure and provide information about the frequency, duration, and intensity of activity (Freedson and Miller, 2000).

Although there are several different methods to analyze heart rate data, a frequently used method is the FLEX heart rate method (Ceesay et al, 1989; Livingstone et al, 1990). In the FLEX

method, heart rate and oxygen consumption are monitored at different exercise intensities and different postures (i.e., sitting, supine, and standing). Basal metabolic rate is also estimated for each subject. These data are used to construct a calibration curve to estimate energy expenditure (Freedson and Miller, 2000). The FLEX heart rate is the threshold heart rate used to differentiate between resting and exercise heart rate (Livingstone, 1997). Satisfactory estimates of total energy expenditure have been reported using this method (Ceesay et al, 1989; Spurr et al, 1988).

There are several potential limitations associated with the use of heart rate monitors as a proxy for physical activity. First, extraneous factors other than physical activity can affect heart rate, which may lead to potentially biased estimates of energy expenditure. Factors such as temperature, humidity, emotional states, food intake, and body position may affect heart rate independent of physical activity (Livingstone, 1997). Second, the cost of heart rate monitors may be prohibitive for large, epidemiologic studies. Third, energy expenditure data derived from calibration curves may be invalid if heart rate data are not representative or poorly discriminate between resting and exercise heart rate (Livingstone, 1997).

8 Future Directions

8.1 Combination Devices

Combination devices that feature both physiological (e.g., heart rate, blood pressure) and activity (e.g., motion sensors) measures may improve physical activity assessment. Previous studies suggest that combining separately measured heart rate and accelerometry data yields more precise estimates of energy expenditure than estimates derived from accelerometry data alone (Brage et al, 2004; Strath et al, 2005).

One example of a combination device that simultaneously records physiological and actigraphy data is the Actiheart (Mini Mitter Co.,

Inc). The Actiheart features a heart rate monitor and uniaxial accelerometer and has been shown to reliably and accurately estimate walking and running intensity (Brage et al, 2005).

8.2 New Technologies

Technological advances have enabled computers and microprocessors to be lightweight and portable, leading to the development of wearable computers and sensors, incorporated into "smart clothing." Wearable computers, connected to cameras, microphones, and physiological sensors, may be utilized to continuously detect and record physical activity under free-living conditions (Healey, 2000). Audio, video, and physiological data may be used to verify self-reported activity data and to increase the accuracy of estimates of energy expenditure. Accelerometers and physiological sensors (e.g., heart rate, respiration, and skin conductance) may be sewn into clothing or disguised as jewelry (Healey, 2000). Activity and physiological data from the wearable unit may then be transmitted wirelessly to a personal digital assistant (i.e., PDA) or uploaded to a desktop computer for processing.

Several wearable units are currently available. The LifeShirt® System is a washable garment that contains embedded sensors to collect respiratory, ECG, postural, and activity data (VivoMetrics, Inc., Ventura, CA). An electronic diary can be used to record information about mood and activity. Data are encrypted and stored on a recorder, then uploaded to a personal computer for analysis. The SenseWear®, and its commercially available counterpart, the GoWear® fit ($160-350, Bodymedia, Pittsburgh, PA), are armbands that combine galvanic skin response, skin temperature, heat flux, and accelerometry data to assess activity intensity and duration, total energy expenditure, steps taken, and sleep duration. Data are uploaded to a personal computer or to the company's website for analysis.

These new technologies offer a continuous, automated approach to assessing and monitoring physical activity. Wearable computers and sensors reduce investigator and participant burden and offer a comprehensive assessment of activity and energy expenditure by combining physiological and activity data. This multidimensional approach requires greater sophistication in data modeling techniques, which may necessitate specialized personnel and equipment. Other factors affecting the widespread adoption of these devices include the high initial cost of wearable units and participant acceptability.

9 Conclusions

Depending on the physical activity parameter of interest (e.g., frequency, intensity, duration, energy expenditure), participant population, sample size, data sampling frequency, and study location and duration, researchers and clinicians have many assessment instruments to choose from. Laboratory, field, self-report, and physiological measures are each associated with unique costs and benefits; thus instrument selection should be tailored to the aims of the assessment. If appropriate, combined approaches, such as simultaneously utilizing questionnaire, accelerometer, and physiological data, may yield more and more comprehensive assessment of physical activity patterns than using a single instrument in isolation. The trend for the future may be the use of wearable devices that combine multiple types of data to improve the quantification of physical activity and to reduce participant and investigator burden.

References

Ainsworth, B. E., Haskell, W. L., Whitt, M. C., Irwin, M. L., Swartz, A. M. et al (2000). Compendium of physical activities: an update of activity codes and MET intensities. Med Sci Sports Exerc, 32, S498-501.

Babyak, M., Blumenthal, J. A., Herman, S., Khatri, P., Doraiswamy, M. et al (2000). Exercise treatment for major depression: maintenance of therapeutic benefit at 10 months. Psychosom Med, 62, 633-638.

Bassett, D. R., Jr., Ainsworth, B. E., Leggett, S. R., Mathien, C. A., Main, J. A. et al (1996). Accuracy of five electronic pedometers for measuring distance walked. *Med Sci Sports Exerc, 28*, 1071–1077.

Berlin, J. E., Storti, K. L., and Brach, J. S. (2006). Using activity monitors to measure physical activity in free-living conditions. *Phys Ther, 86*, 1137–1145.

Bittner, V., Weiner, D. H., Yusuf, S., Rogers, W. J., McIntyre, K. M. et al (1993). Prediction of mortality and morbidity with a 6-minute walk test in patients with left ventricular dysfunction. SOLVD investigators. *JAMA, 270*, 1702–1707.

Blair, S. N., Haskell, W. L., Ho, P., Paffenbarger, R. S., Jr., Vranizan, K. M. et al (1985). Assessment of habitual physical activity by a seven-day recall in a community survey and controlled experiments. *Am J Epidemiol, 122*, 794–804.

Blair, S. N., Kohl, H. W., and Barlow, C. E. (1993). Physical activity, physical fitness, and all-cause mortality in women: do women need to be active? *J Am Coll Nutr, 12*, 368–371.

Blumenthal, J. A., Babyak, M. A., Doraiswamy, P. M., Watkins, L., Hoffman, B. M. et al (2007). Exercise and pharmacotherapy in the treatment of major depressive disorder. *Psychosom Med, 69*, 587–596.

Blumenthal, J. A., Babyak, M. A., Moore, K. A., Craighead, W. E., Herman, S. et al (1999). Effects of exercise training on older patients with major depression. *Arch Intern Med, 159*, 2349–2356.

Blumenthal, J. A., Rejeski, W. J., Walsh-Riddle, M., Emery, C. F., Miller, H. et al (1988). Comparison of high- and low-intensity exercise training early after acute myocardial infarction. *Am J Cardiol, 61*, 26–30.

Brage, S., Brage, N., Franks, P. W., Ekelund, U., and Wareham, N. J. (2005). Reliability and validity of the combined heart rate and movement sensor Actiheart. *Eur J Clin Nutr, 59*, 561–570.

Brage, S., Brage, N., Franks, P. W., Ekelund, U., Wong, M. Y. et al (2004). Branched equation modeling of simultaneous accelerometry and heart rate monitoring improves estimate of directly measured physical activity energy expenditure. *J Appl Physiol, 96*, 343–351.

Bruce, R. A., Blackmon, J. R., Jones, J. W., and Strait, G. (1963). Exercising testing in adult normal subjects and cardiac patients *Pediatrics, 32*(Suppl) 742–756.

Butland, R. J., Pang, J., Gross, E. R., Woodcock, A. A., and Geddes, D. M. (1982). Two-, six-, and 12-minute walking tests in respiratory disease. *Br Med J, 284*, 1607–1608.

Cahalin, L. P., Mathier, M. A., Semigran, M. J., Dec, G. W., and DiSalvo, T. G. (1996). The six-minute walk test predicts peak oxygen uptake and survival in patients with advanced heart failure. *Chest, 110*, 325–332.

Camacho, T. C., Roberts, R. E., Lazarus, N. B., Kaplan, G. A., and Cohen, R. D. (1991). Physical activity and depression: evidence from the Alameda County Study. *Am J Epidemiol, 134*, 220–231.

Camarri, B., Eastwood, P. R., Cecins, N. M., Thompson, P. J., and Jenkins, S. (2006). Six minute walk distance in healthy subjects aged 55–75 years. *Respir Med, 100*, 658–665.

Caspersen, C. J., Powell, K. E., and Christenson, G. M. (1985). Physical activity, exercise, and physical fitness: definitions and distinctions for health-related research. *Public Health Rep, 100*, 126–131.

Ceesay, S. M., Prentice, A. M., Day, K. C., Murgatroyd, P. R., Goldberg, G. R. et al (1989). The use of heart rate monitoring in the estimation of energy expenditure: a validation study using indirect whole-body calorimetry. *Br J Nutr, 61*, 175–186.

Chen, K. Y., and Bassett, D. R., Jr. (2005). The technology of accelerometry-based activity monitors: current and future. *Med Sci Sports Exerc, 37*, S490–500.

Chetta, A., Zanini, A., Pisi, G., Aiello, M., Tzani, P. et al (2006). Reference values for the 6-min walk test in healthy subjects 20–50 years old. *Respir Med, 100*, 1573–1578.

Cote, C. G., Pinto-Plata, V., Kasprzyk, K., Dordelly, L. J., and Celli, B. R. (2007). The 6-min walk distance, peak oxygen uptake, and mortality in COPD. *Chest, 132*, 1778–1785.

Courneya, K. S., Mackey, J. R., Bell, G. J., Jones, L. W., Field, C. J. et al (2003). Randomized controlled trial of exercise training in postmenopausal breast cancer survivors: cardiopulmonary and quality of life outcomes. *J Clin Oncol, 21*, 1660–1668.

Craig, C. L., Marshall, A. L., Sjostrom, M., Bauman, A. E., Booth, M. L. et al (2003). International physical activity questionnaire: 12-country reliability and validity. *Med Sci Sports Exerc, 35*, 1381–1395.

Crowne, D., and Marlowe, D. (1960). A new scale of social desirability independent of psychopathology. *J Consult Clin Psychol, 24*, 329–354.

Duffield, R., Dawson, B., Pinnington, H. C., and Wong, P. (2004). Accuracy and reliability of a Cosmed K4b2 portable gas analysis system. *J Sci Med Sport, 7*, 11–22.

Enright, P. L., and Sherrill, D. L. (1998). Reference equations for the six-minute walk in healthy adults. *Am J Respir Crit Care Med, 158*, 1384–1387.

Farmer, M. E., Locke, B. Z., Moscicki, E. K., Dannenberg, A. L., Larson, D. B. et al (1988). Physical activity and depressive symptoms: the NHANES I Epidemiologic Follow-up Study. *Am J Epidemiol, 128*, 1340–1351.

Feskanich, D., Willett, W., and Colditz, G. (2002). Walking and leisure-time activity and risk of hip fracture in postmenopausal women. *JAMA, 288*, 2300–2306.

Folsom, A. R., Caspersen, C. J., Taylor, H. L., Jacobs, D. R., Jr., Luepker, R. V. et al (1985). Leisure time physical activity and its relationship to coronary risk factors in a population-based sample. The Minnesota Heart Survey. *Am J Epidemiol, 121*, 570–579.

Folsom, A. R., Jacobs, D. R., Jr., Caspersen, C. J., Gomez-Marin, O., and Knudsen, J. (1986). Test-retest reliability of the Minnesota Leisure Time Physical Activity Questionnaire. *J Chronic Dis, 39*, 505–511.

Freedson, P. S., and Miller, K. (2000). Objective monitoring of physical activity using motion sensors and heart rate. *Res Q Exerc Sport, 71*, S21–29.

Godin, G., and Shephard, R. J. (1985). A simple method to assess exercise behavior in the community. *Can J Appl Sport Sci, 10*, 141–146.

Goodwin, R. D. (2003). Association between physical activity and mental disorders among adults in the United States. *Prev Med, 36*, 698–703.

Gross, L. D., Sallis, J. F., Buono, M. J., Roby, J. J., and Nelson, J. A. (1990). Reliability of interviewers using the Seven-Day Physical Activity Recall. *Res Q Exerc Sport, 61*, 321–325.

Guyatt, G. H., Thompson, P. J., Berman, L. B., Sullivan, M. J., Townsend, M. et al (1985). How should we measure function in patients with chronic heart and lung disease? *J Chronic Dis, 38*, 517–524.

Hamer, M., Stamatakis, E., and Saxton, J. M. (2008). The impact of physical activity on all-cause mortality in men and women after a cancer diagnosis. *Cancer Causes Control*, Mar *20(2)*, 225–231.

Harada, N. D., Chiu, V., King, A. C., and Stewart, A. L. (2001). An evaluation of three self-report physical activity instruments for older adults. *Med Sci Sports Exerc, 33*, 962–970.

Hausswirth, C., Bigard, A. X., and Le Chevalier, J. M. (1997). The Cosmed K4 telemetry system as an accurate device for oxygen uptake measurements during exercise. *Int J Sports Med, 18*, 449–453.

Healey, J. (2000). Future possibilities in electronic monitoring of physical activity. *Res Q Exerc Sport, 71*, S137–145.

Hu, F. B., Willett, W. C., Li, T., Stampfer, M. J., Colditz, G. A. et al (2004). Adiposity as compared with physical activity in predicting mortality among women. *N Engl J Med, 351*, 2694–2703.

Jacobs, D. R., Jr., Ainsworth, B. E., Hartman, T. J., and Leon, A. S. (1993). A simultaneous evaluation of 10 commonly used physical activity questionnaires. *Med Sci Sports Exerc, 25*, 81–91.

Kampert, J. B., Blair, S. N., Barlow, C. E., and Kohl, H. W., 3rd. (1996). Physical activity, physical fitness, and all-cause and cancer mortality: a prospective study of men and women. *Ann Epidemiol, 6*, 452–457.

Kujala, U. M., Kaprio, J., Kannus, P., Sarna, S., and Koskenvuo, M. (2000). Physical activity and osteoporotic hip fracture risk in men. *Arch Intern Med, 160*, 705–708.

Kushi, L. H., Fee, R. M., Folsom, A. R., Mink, P. J., Anderson, K. E. et al (1997). Physical activity and mortality in postmenopausal women. *JAMA, 277*, 1287–1292.

LaPorte, R. E., Black-Sandler, R., Cauley, J. A., Link, M., Bayles, C. et al (1983). The assessment of physical activity in older women: analysis of the interrelationship and reliability of activity monitoring, activity surveys, and caloric intake. *J Gerontol, 38*, 394–397.

Lawlor, D. A., and Hopker, S. W. (2001). The effectiveness of exercise as an intervention in the management of depression: systematic review and meta-regression analysis of randomised controlled trials. *Br Med J, 322*, 763–767.

Lee, I. M. (2003). Physical activity and cancer prevention--data from epidemiologic studies. *Med Sci Sports Exerc, 35*, 1823–1827.

Lee, I. M., Hsieh, C. C., and Paffenbarger, R. S., Jr. (1995). Exercise intensity and longevity in men. The Harvard Alumni Health Study. *JAMA, 273*, 1179–1184.

Lee, I. M., and Paffenbarger, R. S., Jr. (2000). Associations of light, moderate, and vigorous intensity physical activity with longevity. The Harvard Alumni Health Study. *Am J Epidemiol, 151*, 293–299.

Lee, I. M., Rexrode, K. M., Cook, N. R., Manson, J. E., and Buring, J. E. (2001). Physical activity and coronary heart disease in women: is "no pain, no gain" passe? *JAMA, 285*, 1447–1454.

Leon, A. S., Connett, J., Jacobs, D. R., Jr., and Rauramaa, R. (1987). Leisure-time physical activity levels and risk of coronary heart disease and death. The Multiple Risk Factor Intervention Trial. *JAMA, 258*, 2388–2395.

Li, T. Y., Rana, J. S., Manson, J. E., Willett, W. C., Stampfer, M. J. et al (2006). Obesity as compared with physical activity in predicting risk of coronary heart disease in women. *Circulation, 113*, 499–506.

Lipkin, D. P., Scriven, A. J., Crake, T., and Poole-Wilson, P. A. (1986). Six minute walking test for assessing exercise capacity in chronic heart failure. *Br Med J (Clin Res Ed), 292*, 653–655.

Livingstone, M. B. E. (1997). Heart-rate monitoring: the answer for assessing energy expenditure and physical activity in population studies? *Br J Nutr, 78*, 869–871.

Livingstone, M. B. E., Prentice, A. M., Coward, A., Ceesay, S. M., Strain, J. J. et al (1990). Simultaneous measurement of free-living energy expenditure by the doubly labeled water method and heart-rate monitoring. *Am J Clin Nutr, 52*, 59–65.

Manson, J. E., Nathan, D. M., Krolewski, A. S., Stampfer, M. J., Willett, W. C. et al (1992). A prospective study of exercise and incidence of diabetes among US male physicians. *JAMA, 268*, 63–67.

Manson, J. E., Rimm, E. B., Stampfer, M. J., Colditz, G. A., Willett, W. C. et al (1991). Physical activity and incidence of non-insulin-dependent diabetes mellitus in women. *Lancet, 338*, 774–778.

Marcus, B. H., Rossi, J. S., Selby, V. C., Niaura, R. S., and Abrams, D. B. (1992). The stages and processes of exercise adoption and maintenance in a worksite sample. *Health Psychol, 11*, 386–395.

Martinu, T., Babyak, M. A., O'Connell, C. F., Carney, R. M., Trulock, E. P. et al (2008). Baseline 6-min walk distance predicts survival in lung transplant candidates. *Am J Transplant, 8*, 1498–1505.

McGavin, C. R., Gupta, S. P., and McHardy, G. J. (1976). Twelve-minute walking test for assessing disability in chronic bronchitis. *Br Med J, 1*, 822–823.

McNeely, M. L., Campbell, K. L., Rowe, B. H., Klassen, T. P., Mackey, J. R. et al (2006). Effects of exercise on breast cancer patients and survivors: a systematic review and meta-analysis. *CMAJ, 175*, 34–41.

Melanson, E. L., Knoll, J. R., Bell, M. L., Donahoo, W. T., Hill, J. O. et al (2004). Commercially available pedometers: considerations for accurate step counting. *Prev Med, 39*, 361–368.

Morris, J. N., and Heady, J. A. (1953). Mortality in relation to the physical activity of work: a preliminary note on experience in middle age. *Br J Ind Med, 10*, 245–254.

Morris, J. N., Heady, J. A., Raffle, P. A., Roberts, C. G., and Parks, J. W. (1953). Coronary heart-disease and physical activity of work. *Lancet, 262*, 1111–1120.

Naughton, J., Sevelius, G., and Balke, B. (1963). Physiological responses of normal and pathological subjects to a modified work capacity test *J Sports Med Phys Fitness, 44*, 201–207.

Novitsky, S., Segal, K. R., Chatr-Aryamontri, B., Guvakov, D., and Katch, V. L. (1995). Validity of a new portable indirect calorimeter: the AeroSport TEEM 100. *Eur J Appl Physiol Occup Physiol, 70*, 462–467.

Paffenbarger, R. S., Jr., Brand, R. J., Sholtz, R. I., and Jung, D. L. (1978a). Energy expenditure, cigarette smoking, and blood pressure level as related to death from specific diseases. *Am J Epidemiol, 108*, 12–18.

Paffenbarger, R. S., Jr., and Hale, W. E. (1975). Work activity and coronary heart mortality. *N Engl J Med, 292*, 545–550.

Paffenbarger, R. S., Jr., Hyde, R. T., Wing, A. L., and Hsieh, C. C. (1986). Physical activity, all-cause mortality, and longevity of college alumni. *N Engl J Med, 314*, 605–613.

Paffenbarger, R. S., Jr., Wing, A. L., and Hyde, R. T. (1978b). Physical activity as an index of heart attack risk in college alumni. *Am J Epidemiol, 108*, 161–175.

Peeters, P., and Mets, T. (1996). The 6-minute walk as an appropriate exercise test in elderly patients with chronic heart failure. *J Gerontol A Biol Sci Med Sci, 51*, M147–151.

Petrella, R. J., Koval, J. J., Cunningham, D. A., and Paterson, D. H. (2001). A self-paced step test to predict aerobic fitness in older adults in the primary care clinic. *J Am Geriatr Soc, 49*, 632–638.

Powell, K. E., Thompson, P. D., Caspersen, C. J., and Kendrick, J. S. (1987). Physical activity and the incidence of coronary heart disease. *Annu Rev Public Health, 8*, 253–287.

Prochaska, J. O., and DiClemente, C. C. (1983). Stages and processes of self-change of smoking: toward an integrative model of change. *J Consult Clin Psychol, 51*, 390–395.

Redelmeier, D. A., Bayoumi, A. M., Goldstein, R. S., and Guyatt, G. H. (1997). Interpreting small differences in functional status: the Six Minute Walk test in chronic lung disease patients. *Am J Respir Crit Care Med, 155*, 1278–1282.

Richardson, M. T., Leon, A. S., Jacobs, D. R., Jr., Ainsworth, B. E., and Serfass, R. (1994). Comprehensive evaluation of the Minnesota Leisure Time Physical Activity Questionnaire. *J Clin Epidemiol, 47*, 271–281.

Sallis, J. F., Haskell, W. L., Wood, P. D., Fortmann, S. P., Rogers, T. et al (1985). Physical activity assessment methodology in the Five-City Project. *Am J Epidemiol, 121*, 91–106.

Sallis, J. F., Patterson, T. L., Buono, M. J., and Nader, P. R. (1988). Relation of cardiovascular fitness and physical activity to cardiovascular disease risk factors in children and adults. *Am J Epidemiol, 127*, 933–941.

Schmitz, K. H., Holtzman, J., Courneya, K. S., Masse, L. C., Duval, S. et al (2005). Controlled physical activity trials in cancer survivors: a systematic review and meta-analysis. *Cancer Epidemiol Biomarkers Prev, 14*, 1588–1595.

Schneider, P. L., Crouter, S. E., Lukajic, O., and Bassett, D. R., Jr. (2003). Accuracy and reliability of 10 pedometers for measuring steps over a 400-m walk. *Med Sci Sports Exerc, 35*, 1779–1784.

Sharkey, N. A., Williams, N. I., and Guerin, J. B. (2000). The role of exercise in the prevention and treatment of osteoporosis and osteoarthritis. *Nurs Clin North Am, 35*, 209–221.

Shepherd, E. F., Toloza, E., McClung, C. D., and Schmalzried, T. P. (1999). Step activity monitor: increased accuracy in quantifying ambulatory activity. *J Orthop Res, 17*, 703–708.

Spurr, G. B., Prentice, A. M., Murgatroyd, P. R., Goldberg, G. R., Reina, J. C. et al (1988). Energy expenditure from minute-by-minute heart-rate recording: comparison with indirect calorimetry. *Am J Clin Nutr, 48*, 552–559.

Stewart, A. L., Mills, K. M., King, A. C., Haskell, W. L., Gillis, D. et al (2001). CHAMPS physical activity questionnaire for older adults: outcomes for interventions. *Med Sci Sports Exerc, 33*, 1126–1141.

Strath, S. J., Brage, S., and Ekelund, U. (2005). Integration of physiological and accelerometer data to improve physical activity assessment. *Med Sci Sports Exerc, 37*, S563–571.

Sykes, K. (1995). Capacity assessment in the workplace: a new step test. *J Occup Health, 1*, 20–22.

Sykes, K., and Roberts, A. (2004). The Chester step test: a simple yet effective tool for the prediction of aerobic capacity. *Physiotherapy, 90*, 183–188.

Szekely, L. A., Oelberg, D. A., Wright, C., Johnson, D. C., Wain, J. et al (1997). Preoperative predictors of operative morbidity and mortality in COPD patients undergoing bilateral lung volume reduction surgery. *Chest, 111*, 550–558.

Taylor, H. L., Jacobs, D. R., Jr., Schucker, B., Knudsen, J., Leon, A. S. et al (1978). A questionnaire for the assessment of leisure time physical activities. *J Chronic Dis, 31*, 741–755.

Taylor, R. S., Brown, A., Ebrahim, S., Jolliffe, J., Noorani, H. et al (2004). Exercise-based rehabilitation for patients with coronary heart disease: systematic review and meta-analysis of randomized controlled trials. *Am J Med, 116*, 682–692.

Troosters, T., Gosselink, R., and Decramer, M. (1999). Six minute walking distance in healthy elderly subjects. *Eur Respir J, 14*, 270–274.

Vanhees, L., Lefevre, J., Philippaerts, R., Martens, M., Huygens, W. et al (2005). How to assess physical activity? How to assess physical fitness? *Eur J Cardiovasc Prev Rehabil, 12*, 102–114.

Wannamethee, S. G., Shaper, A. G., and Walker, M. (2000). Physical activity and mortality in older men with diagnosed coronary heart disease. *Circulation, 102*, 1358–1363.

Warburton, D. E., Nicol, C. W., and Bredin, S. S. (2006). Health benefits of physical activity: the evidence. *CMAJ, 174*, 801–809.

Whaley, M. H., Brubaker, P. H., and Otto, R. M. (Eds.). (2006). *ACSM's Guidelines for Exercise Testing and Prescription, 7th Ed.* Philadelphia, PA: Lippincott, Williams & Wilkins.

Chapter 4

Dietary Assessment in Behavioral Medicine

Marian L. Neuhouser

1 Overview of Dietary Assessment in Behavioral Medicine

Nutritional status is one of the most important predictors of health risk. Research consistently demonstrates that diets rich in fruit, vegetables, whole grains, and lean meats from poultry and fish are inversely associated with risk of age-related chronic diseases such as cardiovascular disease, cancer, and diabetes (Kushi et al, 2006; Lampe, 1999; Neuhouser, 2004; Pool-Zobel et al, 1997; Prentice et al, 2004; World Cancer Research Fund/AICR, 2007). Conversely, diets high in refined grains and added sugars, but low in diverse plant foods, increase risk for obesity and obesity-related disorders including cardiovascular disease, cancer, and diabetes (Boynton et al, 2007; Kristal et al, 2000; National Research Council Committee on Diet and Health, 1989; Patterson et al, 2004). Despite the strong and consistent diet–disease associations and recommendations to the public to make healthy food choices and limit or avoid added fats, sodium, and empty calorie-type foods, consumers still, for the most part, select poor diets (Kant and Graubard, 2006). For example, only 11% of American adults obtain the recommended 5–9 servings of fruit and vegetables per day (Casagrande et al, 2007). Equally concerning is the high prevalence of daily consumption of sugar-laden empty calorie beverages, such as a soft drink; such high consumption is a common practice among young children, adolescents, and adults (Dubois et al, 2007; French et al, 2003; Rajeshwari et al, 2005; Rampersaud et al, 2003). This discrepancy between available knowledge of nutritional benefits and food intake patterns suggests a strong influence of culture and behavior on dietary practices.

Food choice is a complex behavior. Individuals and groups make dietary selections based on food familiarity, availability, cost, cultural norms, ease of preparation, individual taste, convenience, and many other factors (Drewnowski, 1997; Glanz et al, 1998a, b; Popkin et al, 2005). Therefore, assessment of diet, particularly for the purposes of promoting dietary change or improvement in dietary patterns, must include attention to the behavioral aspects of food intake (van Duyn et al, 2001). Dietary behaviors are extremely personal and efforts to promote healthful dietary changes that are based only on knowledge about foods are not likely to succeed.

Apart from behavioral predictors of food intake, measuring what people eat is particularly complicated for several reasons. To illustrate this point, we can compare the assessment challenges for two exposures: playing golf or tennis and diet. Playing golf or tennis is a single (yes/no) activity – people are either players or not, so individuals usually report with good accuracy whether or not they engage in these activities. Further, since for many people, these activities

M.L. Neuhouser (✉)
Fred Hutchinson Cancer Research Center,
1100 Fairview Avenue North, M4-B402, Seattle, WA
98109-1024, USA
e-mail: mneuhous@fhcrc.org

A. Steptoe (ed.), *Handbook of Behavioral Medicine*, DOI 10.1007/978-0-387-09488-5_4,
© Springer Science+Business Media, LLC 2010

occur on a weekly or monthly basis, most people would record with reasonable accuracy that they play golf or tennis once a week. In comparison, over the course of even 1 week, an individual can consume hundreds, even thousands of distinct food items in various combinations, making it cognitively challenging for respondents to accurately report on their intake. Meals can be prepared by others (e.g., in a restaurant, by a spouse, as prepackaged food) so that the respondent may not be cognizant of preparation details such as fat or salt used in cooking or portion size. Further, food choices often vary with seasons and other life activities (e.g., weekends, social engagements, holidays, vacations). In fact, in today's modern food environment with so many choices, particularly, myriad ready-to-eat choices available to consumers, the day-to-day variability in food intake can be so large that it is difficult to identify any underlying consistent pattern. Collectively, these issues make dietary assessment a very complex task for both researchers and clinicians.

2 Standard Dietary Assessment Tools for Use in Behavioral Medicine

Dietary assessment requires asking participants about their usual food habits. This process can take several forms, such as a structured interview, a self-administered questionnaire, or a diary. This section describes the more commonly used dietary assessment tools.

2.1 Food Records and Diaries

Multiple day food records or diaries require individuals to record all foods and beverages consumed over a specified period of time, often 3–7 days. Participants are typically asked to carry the paper record or diary with them and to record foods in real time as eaten. However, in reality,

many participants will record everything at the end of the day due to the burden of recording in real time. Some protocols require participants to weigh and/or measure foods before eating, while less stringent protocols use food models, photographs of food, measuring cups, and other aids to instruct respondents on estimating serving sizes. Often the food diary is carefully reviewed or documented by a trained dietitian to confirm food portion sizes, ingredients added in cooking and at the table (such as salt, oils, salad dressings, butter, and other condiments), and additional food details. However, this type of detailed review and documentation can add greatly to the participant burden since the minutiae required can seem overwhelming and time consuming to participants. In addition, this type of very detailed documentation adds to the overall cost of food record collection, but may not add significant or necessary food details. One study showed that when detailed, step-by-step instructions on food recording are provided to participants (including specific examples) prior to starting the diary, the detailed documentation by a dietitian may not be necessary (Kolar et al, 2005). Review by a dietitian can still occur during the data entry phase and follow-up queries can be made to the participants, as necessary, but the face-to-face questions and queries could be skipped when sufficient instruction is provided.

Regardless of the data collection protocol, ultimately the food consumption information from records/diaries must be coded and entered into a software program for calculation of nutrient intakes (Schakel et al, 1997). This data entry step is a time consuming task and requires trained data technicians or nutritionists. One reason these complex tasks are so time consuming is that the large food databases typically contain 15,000–20,000 individual food items, which represent only a fraction of the universe of food possibilities. Thus, the trained nutrition coder must make decisions about which foods to enter as substitutes. For example, an individual records "one 4-inch by 4-inch by 4-inch portion of 'Mama's' brand frozen lasagna." If "Mama's" is not listed among the various frozen lasagna choices in the database, the coder must make an informed decision about which brand is the closest match to "Mama's" in terms of total energy, protein, fat, and other nutrients. Some misclassification is unavoidable, but a well-trained and knowledgeable nutritionist should be able to select comparable substitutes.

Food records are somewhat burdensome for clients or study participants to complete. In fact, some studies have shown that individuals might change their food intake on recording days to consume more easy-to-prepare items that require less recording, but the ultimate influence of this practice is unknown (Craig et al, 2000; Rebro et al, 1998). Clients or study participants should always be reminded to eat as they normally do during the food-recording period. Advances in digital mobile devices (phones, cameras, PDAs) now make it possible to record and transmit food record data, which alleviates some of this participant burden and may provide more accurate data (Beasley et al, 2005; Kretsch and Fong, 1990; Wang et al, 2002). Digital devices are becoming such a routine part of people's lives that real-time digital recording of one's food and beverage intake may not feel as burdensome as a paper and pencil diary. Other disciplines in medicine, physical activity, and pain monitoring have been successfully using technological advances for quite sometime (Berg et al, 1998; Jamison et al, 2001). In addition, digital recording of food intake may alleviate problems with portion size estimation, which is a frequent source of error in dietary data collection (Williamson et al, 2003, 2004). In the future, pencil and paper food diaries are likely to disappear in favor of digital collection methods.

2.2 Dietary Recalls

A 24-h dietary recall is a structured interview in which detailed questions are asked about all foods and beverages consumed over the previous 24 h. Dietary recall interviews can be conducted in person or by telephone and typically last 20–30 min. Data from 24-h recalls have been used to characterize large populations in the United States via the survey, "What We

Eat in America" (Conway et al, 2004; Dwyer et al, 2003a). When conducted in large population groups, recalls provide a general "snapshot" of population dietary intake.

Regardless of whether 24-h dietary recalls are done in-person or over the telephone, the protocols work best when interviewer scripts are standardized on a computer screen with direct data entry into a software program. It is very important that the interviewer be well trained since tone of voice, body posture (when in-person), and reactions to participant descriptions of foods consumed can influence the quality of the data, including omissions or phantom food additions (Conway et al, 2004). Sometimes interviewers need to redirect the conversation back to the structured questions, should the respondent deviate off-topic, which can be a problem when assessing specific population subgroups, such as the elderly. As with food records, the use of portion size estimate aides, such as life-size food models, photographs, or dimensional aides including rulers and measuring cups, increases the ability to estimate portion size thereby improving the reliability of the recall data (Pietinen et al, 1988; Williamson et al, 2003).

Regarding the actual process of conducting the 24-h recall interviews, the currently most widely accepted methods follow the protocol established by the United States Department of Agriculture (USDA) and used in the "What We Eat in America" survey (Conway et al, 2003; Dwyer et al, 2003a, b). This five-step method includes the following sequence of queries:

1) *Quick list* – trained interviewers first ask participants to list all foods and beverages consumed during the previous 24 h.
2) *Forgotten food list* – interviewer asks detailed probes about foods or additions to foods that are frequently forgotten. Examples of foods that are often added to this list are milk on cereal, sugar in coffee, and between-meal snacks and beverages.
3) *Time and place* – the interviewer asks the participant to recall the time of day and the

location (e.g., home, school, restaurant) of the food consumption. This time and place memory probe frequently helps participants to better recall the foods consumed.

4) *Detail cycle* – the interviewer probes for details about each food named in the quick list and forgotten list, including cooking methods, portion size, brand names, type, and amount of fat added during cooking and at the table. The detail cycle includes the collection of information on mixed dishes and recipes. The questions in the detail cycle are highly standardized with computerized prompts to ensure uniform data collection.

5) *Final review* – the interviewer does a final review of the foods and beverages consumed and queries participants about any additional items that may have been omitted.

2.3 Food Frequency Questionnaires

Food frequency questionnaires (FFQ) are self-administered instruments that obtain data on frequency and portion size on anywhere from 60 to 150 foods or food groups. Respondents indicate on the form whether they eat a certain food and how often (i.e., once a month or several times a day). These instruments usually include various types of questions: (1) adjustment questions on food preparation or frequency of restaurant eating, (2) the food list, and (3) summary questions. The adjustment questions permit more refined analyses of fat intake by asking about food preparation practices (e.g., removing skin from chicken), types of added fats (e.g., use of butter vs. margarine on vegetables), or type of milk usually used (e.g., whole, skim, soy). Because details about food preparation are not obtained with FFQ in the same manner as food records and recalls, these adjustment questions can be useful approaches to fine-tune the food selections.

The main section of an FFQ consists of a food or food group list, with questions on usual frequency of intake and portion size. To allow for machine scanning of these forms, frequency responses are typically categorized from "never or less than once per month" to "2+ per day" for foods and "6+ per day" for beverages. Portion sizes are often assessed by asking respondents to mark "small," "medium," or "large" in comparison to a given medium portion size. However, some questionnaires only ask about the frequency of intake of a "usual" portion size (e.g., 3 ounces meat). Often a cartoon-type picture or very small photograph is provided as a "reference point" for the medium portion size. However, since the pictures must be small to fit onto the questionnaire, it is unclear how useful they may be in the long run.

FFQ food lists or line items are created to capture data on (1) major sources of energy and nutrients in the population of interest, (2) between-person variability in food intake, and (3) specific scientific hypotheses (Willett, 1998). Since the food list possibly cannot include the universe of all food and food combination possibilities, decisions must be made about which foods to include and which ones to omit. For example, one approach is to use national consumption data from 24-h dietary recalls to determine the most commonly eaten foods and major nutrient sources in the diet (Block et al, 1994, 1986; Willett, 1998). Details about nutrients are limited though for foods consumed in specific population groups (e.g., certain ethnic foods) and there are limited data on bioactive constituents of foods that are not considered nutrients but nonetheless have biological actions (e.g., isothiocyanates, polyphenols). Finally, to save space and reduce respondent burden, similar foods are often grouped into a single-line item (e.g., apples, peaches, plums). When grouping foods, important considerations include whether they are nutritionally similar enough to be grouped and whether the group will make cognitive sense to the respondent. For example, a food group composed of three types of fruit may have similar amounts of vitamin C, but be very different for other bioactive compounds such as flavonoids or carotenoids. These issues must be considered when selecting a dietary assessment instrument.

2.4 Advantages and Disadvantages of Standard Dietary Assessment Instruments

Dietary records and recalls provide similar types of data: detailed information on all foods and beverages consumed on specified days. While these methods are intended to capture data on actual foods consumed, there is a somewhat large respondent burden of recording (or recalling) food intake that can cause people to alter their food intake such that they consume less complex foods or they may avoid eating foods perceived to be less healthful (i.e., sweets, salty snacks). Further, even when participants record foods in real time, mistakes can still occur in food descriptions, portion size estimation, and lack of food composition data on various ethnic foods and complex mixtures. Theoretically, unannounced interviewer administered 24-h dietary recalls avoid the problem of changes in food intake since respondents cannot change what they ate retrospectively. However, a disadvantage of dietary recalls is that they rely on the respondent's memory and ability to estimate portion sizes, though the latter limitation can be alleviated by the use of portion size aides. An important advantage of recalls is that they are appropriate for low-literacy populations and children where use of diaries or records would not be appropriate (Sobo et al, 2000).

Today's modern diets give consumers a large amount of choice in food selection – both for home-prepared and ready-to-eat meals. As a result, there is quite high day-to-day variability in intake. In practice, for accurate dietary assessment, this means that several days of records/recalls are required to adequately assess "true" intake. Some foods may be consumed rather infrequently, but if they are an important contributor toward intake of specific nutrients, then many days of intake are needed to increase the probability of consumption of that food. For example, fatty fish, such as tuna, salmon, or mackerel, may be consumed only once a week or less, but these fish are very important sources of long-chain omega-3 fatty acids that are associated with reduced risk of cardiovascular disease and several other chronic health problems. A record or recall with insufficient days may not capture this fish intake. Unfortunately, research has also shown that reported energy intake, nutrient intake, and recorded numbers of foods decrease with increasing numbers of recorded days (Rebro et al, 1998). Thus, simply changing a protocol to increase the number of recorded days so as to capture this dietary variability may not be sufficient.

The major advantage of FFQs is that they attempt to assess usual, long-term diet, either current or in the past. In addition, they have relatively low respondent burden and are simple and inexpensive to analyze because they can be self-administered and are machine scannable. A disadvantage of these questionnaires is that respondents must estimate usual frequency of consumption of 100 or more foods and the associated usual portion sizes. These cognitive tasks can be exceedingly difficult for many respondents, and may contribute to the observed measurement error from FFQs (Neuhouser et al, 2008; Subar et al, 2003; Tooze et al, 2004). Another major disadvantage of these questionnaires is related to the close-ended nature of the form. For example, use of an FFQ with a typical American fixed-food list is not likely to be useful in some special populations or in places outside the United States. In addition, a questionnaire with appropriate foods and portion sizes for one population group (e.g., older African-American women) may be inappropriate for another subgroup (e.g., adolescent Hispanic females). Fortunately, some work has been completed to develop culturally appropriate FFQs. For example, FFQs have been developed for use in specialized populations, such as the elderly, rural residents, and various ethnic groups (Patterson et al, 1999; Resnicow et al, 2000; Yaroch et al, 2000). Finally, the fixed portion sizes on FFQs may make it extremely difficult to obtain accurate data. For example, most FFQs list a 12-ounce soft drink as a medium portion, when it is more likely a "small" using today's portion standards. Similarly, a medium hamburger from the 20th century was a 2-ounce patty, but in the 21st century, a medium hamburger is six ounces (Nielsen and Popkin, 2003; Nielsen et al, 2002). These fixed portion size issues do not occur with the open-ended records and recalls.

3 Non-traditional Dietary Assessment Instruments Used in Behavioral Medicine

Non-traditional assessment instruments have been a useful addition to the dietary assessment repertoire. For example, household food inventories, cash register receipts, and instruments focused more on behavioral aspects of eating, rather than absolute intake of nutrients have been useful.

3.1 Household Food Inventories

Household food inventories are ecological measures of diet. They cannot give information on an individual or even a family's absolute intake, but they provide a snapshot of eating behaviors or even "food culture." For example, households that have many high-fat, nutrient-poor foods (i.e., potato chips, candies, sweets, and other prepared snacks) and few fruits and vegetables may be more likely to have overall high-fat diets or be at risk for obesity. A common approach for family-level weight management programs is for the nutritionist to conduct a food inventory of the pantry and advise the family to discard items with excess energy and poor nutritional value. This point is illustrated in one study reporting that the presence (in the house) of 15 high-fat foods was found to correlate with household members' individual dietary fat intake at 0.42 ($p < 0.001$) (Patterson et al, 1997). Individuals with ≤ 4 high-fat foods in their house had a mean of 32% energy from fat compared to 37% for those with ≥ 8 high-fat foods. Household inventories can also provide information about

poverty and food availability. Poor household food availability may be associated with greater individual-level measures of food insecurity and is paradoxically associated with risk for obesity (Burdette and Whitaker, 2004; Mobley et al, 2006; Townsend, 2006). Appropriate referrals and interventions can be made when it is known that little food or poor nutrient quality food exists in the home. Finally, household inventories may be particularly good assessment tools to use with new immigrants where language or cultural barriers may preclude use of records, recalls, or FFQs (Satia et al, 2000, 2001a, b).

3.2 Targeted Instruments

Targeted instruments are those that are focused on a particular behavior or intake of a limited number of foods, such as fruit and vegetables, snacks, or sweets. While not useful for comprehensive dietary assessment, they are useful when evaluating or conducting an intervention on focused dietary behaviors. These types of targeted dietary assessment instruments are most useful when the target food/nutrient is not distributed throughout the food supply. For example, dietary fat is widely distributed in dairy foods, meats, added fats, desserts, prepared foods, etc. Therefore, short instruments that attempt to estimate fat intake tend to be imprecise since a short number of questions cannot capture this complex behavior (Neuhouser et al, 1999). A good example of a targeted instrument is one that was recently developed to assess soft drink and snack consumption among adolescents. Due to the tremendous and rapid increase in obesity among the entire population, including adolescents (French et al, 2003), many school districts are limiting the on-campus sale of sugar-laden beverages, such as soft drinks and other high-calorie drinks with few nutrients. To evaluate whether such policies are effective at reducing consumption of these beverages, researchers developed a short beverage and snack questionnaire. Similar to an FFQ in form, the questionnaire asks about frequency and location (at school or not at school) of soft drinks, sports-type drinks, fruit punch, and other sugar-sweetened beverages (Neuhouser et al, 2009). Other targeted instruments are those that assess fruit/vegetable, salty/savory snacks intake and food likes and dislikes (food propensity) (Neuhouser et al, 2000, 2001; Subar et al, 2006; Thompson et al, 2000, 2002). However, it is important to note that one disadvantage of these short checklists is that they may underestimate consumption of fruit and vegetables in particular. For example, "servings" of vegetables, such as a serving of green beans or green peas, is a relatively easy cognitive task. On the other hand, vegetables that are components of more complex dishes, such as vegetables on pizza or in casseroles, soups, and stews, are a bigger challenge for participants to deconstruct and record on a short questionnaire.

3.3 Eating Behavior Instruments

A class of dietary assessment instruments particularly well suited for behavioral medicine are those focused specifically on eating behaviors (in contrast to absolute intake measures in standard instruments). The development of these dietary behavior instruments was initially motivated by problems with assessing dietary intervention effectiveness, particularly low-fat interventions (Kristal et al, 1990). The fat-related diet habits questionnaire was based on an anthropologic model that described low-fat dietary change as four types: (1) avoiding high-fat foods (exclusion); (2) altering available foods to make them lower in fat (modification); (3) using new, specially formulated or processed, lower fat foods instead of their higher fat forms (substitution); and (4) using preparation techniques or food ingredients that replace the common higher fat alternative (replacement) (Shannon et al, 1997). A recently developed "mindful eating questionnaire" was designed as a cognitive approach for dietary assessment and intervention tool and incorporates a body awareness framework often used in the practice of yoga (Framson et al, 2009).

4 Summary and Conclusions

In conclusion, dietary assessment is a complex task. While it might seem intuitive to simply ask study participants or patients to recall foods eaten or complete a form on eating patterns, food intake behaviors are difficult to capture with reasonable accuracy due to the complex and varied items available to consumers, the burden that may be associated with asking participants to record foods and beverages and limitations in standard instruments that are currently available. In addition, underreporting of dietary intake has been identified as a significant problem in dietary assessment. Newer methods of dietary assessment that rely on PDAs, mobile phones, and other electronic technologies will likely be increasingly used in the future with the hope that more accurate data will be obtained. Nontraditional dietary assessment methods may be particularly useful. While not designed to measure absolute intake of foods or nutrients, they are intended to capture dietary behaviors, such as fat intake behaviors, food likes and dislikes (which may predict consumption), and intake of soft drinks and sweets. Despite the challenges in dietary assessment, efforts must continue to understand what people eat and offer dietary modification advice, as needed.

References

Beasley, J., Riley, W. T., and Jean-Mary, J. (2005). Accuracy of a PDA-based dietary assessment program. *Nutrition, 21*, 672–677.

Berg, J., Dunbar-Jacob, J., and Rohay, J. M. (1998). Compliance with inhaled medications: the relationship between diary and electronic monitor. *Ann Behav Med, 20*, 36–38.

Block, G., Coyle, L. M., Hartman, A. M., and Scoppa, S. M. (1994). Revision of dietary analysis software for the Health Habits and History Questionnaire. *Am J Epidemiol, 139*, 1190–1196.

Block, G., Hartman, A. M., Dresser, C. M., Carroll, M. D., Gannon, J. et al (1986). A data-based approach to diet questionnaire design and testing. *Am J Epidemiol, 124*, 453–469.

Boynton, A., Neuhouser, M. L., Wener, M. H., Wood, B., Sorensen, B. et al (2007). Associations between healthy eating patterns and immune function or inflammation in overweight or obese postmenopausal women. *Am J Clin Nutr, 86*, 1445–1455.

Burdette, H. L., and Whitaker, R. C. (2004). Neighborhood playgrounds, fast food restaurants, and crime: relationships to overweight in low-income preschool children. *Prev Med, 38*, 57–63.

Casagrande, S. S., Wang, Y., Anderson, C., and Gary, T. L. (2007). Have Americans increased their fruit and vegetable intake? The trends between 1988 and 2002. *Am J Prev Med, 32*, 257–263.

Conway, J. M., Ingwersen, L. A., and Moshfegh, A. J. (2004). Accuracy of dietary recall using the USDA five-step multiple-pass method in men: an observational validity study. *J Am Diet Assoc, 104*, 595–603.

Conway, J. M., Ingwersen, L. A., Vinyard, B. T., and Moshfegh, A. J. (2003). Effectiveness of the US Department of Agriculture 5-step multiple-pass method in assessing food intake in obese and nonobese women. *Am J Clin Nutr, 77*, 1171–1178.

Craig, M. R., Kristal, A. R., Cheney, C. L., and Shattuck, A. L. (2000). The prevalence and impact of 'atypical' days in 4-day food records. *J Am Diet Assoc, 100*, 421–427.

Drewnowski, A. (1997). Taste preferences and food intake. *Ann Rev Nutr, 17*, 237–253.

Dubois, L., Farmer, A., Girard, M., and Peterson, K. (2007). Regular sugar-sweetened beverage consumption between meals increases risk of overweight among preschool-aged children. *J Am Diet Assoc, 107*, 924–934.

Dwyer, J., Picciano, M. F., and Raiten, D. J. (2003a). Collection of food and dietary supplement intake data: What We Eat in America-NHANES. *J Nutr, 133*, 590–600.

Dwyer, J., Picciano, M. F., and Raiten, D. J. (2003b). Food and dietary supplement databases for What We Eat in America-NHANES. *J Nutr, 133*, 624S–634S.

Framson, C., Kristal, A. R., Schenk, J. M., Littman, A. J., Zeliadt, S. et al (2009). Development and validation of a mindful eating questionnaire. *J Am Diet Assoc, 109*, 1439–1444.

French, S. A., Lin, B. H., and Guthrie, J. F. (2003). National trends in soft drink consumption among children and adolescents age 6 to 17 years: prevalence, amounts, and sources, 1977/1978 to 1994/1998. *J Am Diet Assoc, 103*, 1326–1331.

Glanz, K., Basil, M., Maibach, E., Goldberg, J., and Snyder, D. (1998a). Why Americans eat what they do: taste, nutrition, cost, convenience, and weight control concerns are influences on food consumption. *J Am Diet Assoc, 98*, 1118–1126.

Glanz, K., Kristal, A. R., Tilley, B. C., and Hirst, K. (1998b). Psychosocial correlates of healthful diets among male auto workers. *Cancer Epidemiol Biomarkers Prev, 7*, 119–126.

Jamison, R. N., Raymond, S. A., Levine, J. G., Slawsby, E. A., Nedeljkovic, S. S. et al (2001). Electronic diaries for monitoring chronic pain: 1-year validation study. *Pain, 91*, 277–285.

Kant, A. K., and Graubard, B. I. (2006). Secular trends in patterns of self-reported food consumption of adult Americans: NHANES 1971–1975 to NHANES 1999–2002. *Am J Clin Nutr, 84*, 1215–1223.

Kolar, A. S., Patterson, R. E., White, E., Neuhouser, M. L., Frank, L. L. et al (2005). A practical method for collecting 3-day food records in a large cohort. *Epidemiology, 16*, 579–583.

Kretsch, M. J., and Fong, A. K. (1990). Validation of a new computerized technique for quantitating individual dietary intake: the Nutrition Evaluation Scale System (NESSy) vs the weighed food record. *Am J Clin Nutr, 51*, 477–484.

Kristal, A. R., Curry, S. J., Shattuck, A. L., Feng, Z., and Li, S. (2000). A randomized trial of a tailored, self-help dietary intervention: The Puget Sound Eating Patterns Study. *Prev Med, 31*, 380–389.

Kristal, A. R., Shattuck, A. L., Henry, H. J., and Fowler, A. (1990). Rapid assessment of dietary intake of fat, fiber, and saturated fat: validity of an instrument suitable for community intervention research and nutritional surveillance. *Am J Health Promot, 4*, 288–295.

Kushi, L. H., Byers, T., Doyle, C., Bandera, E. V., McCullough, M. et al (2006). American Cancer Society Guidelines on Nutrition and Physical Activity for Cancer Prevention: reducing the risk of cancer with healthy food choices and physical activity. *CA Cancer J Clin, 56*, 254–281.

Lampe, J. W. (1999). Health effects of vegetables and fruit: assessing mechanisms of action in human experimental studies. *Am J Clin Nutr, 70*, 475s–490s.

Mobley, L. R., Root, E. D., Finkelstein, E. A., Khavjou, O., Farris, R. P. et al (2006). Environment, obesity, and cardiovascular disease risk in low-income women. *Am J Prev Med, 30*, 327–332.

National Research Council Committee on Diet and Health. (1989). *Diet and Health: Implications for Reducing Chronic Disease Risk*. Washington, DC: National Academy Press.

Neuhouser, M. L. (2004). Dietary flavonoids and cancer risk: evidence from human population studies. *Nutr Cancer, 50*, 1–7.

Neuhouser, M. L., Kristal, A. R., McLerran, D., Patterson, R. E., and Atkinson, J. (1999). Validity of short food frequency questionnaires used in cancer chemoprevention trials: results from the Prostate Cancer Prevention Trial. *Cancer Epidemiol Biomarkers Prev, 8*, 721–725.

Neuhouser, M. L., Lelley, S., Lund, A., and Johnson, D. (2009). Development and validation of a beverage and snack questionnaire for use in evaluation of school nutrition policies. *J Am Diet Assoc, 109,* 1587–1592.

Neuhouser, M. L., Patterson, R. E., Kristal, A. R., Eldridge, A. L., and Vizenor, N. C. (2001). A brief dietary assessment instrument for assessing target foods, nutrients and eating patterns. *Public Health Nutr, 4,* 73–78.

Neuhouser, M. L., Patterson, R. E., Kristal, A. R., Rock, C. L., Neumark-Sztainer, D. et al (2000). Do consumers of savory snacks have poor quality diets? *J Am Diet Assoc, 100,* 576–579.

Neuhouser, M. L., Tinker, L., Shaw, P. A., Schoeller, D. A., Bingham, S. A. et al (2008). Use of recovery biomarkers to calibrate nutrient consumption self-reports in the Women's Health Initiative. *Am J Epidemiol, 167,* 1247–1259.

Nielsen, S. J., and Popkin, B. M. (2003). Patterns and trends in food portion sizes, 1977–1998. *JAMA, 289,* 450–453.

Nielsen, S. J., Siega-Riz, A. M., and Popkin, B. M. (2002). Trends in energy intake in US between 1977 and 1996: similar shifts seen across age groups. *Obese Res, 10,* 370–378.

Patterson, R. E., Frank, L. L., Kristal, A. R., and White, E. (2004). A comprehensive examination of health conditions associated with obesity in older adults. *Am J Prev Med, 27,* 385–390.

Patterson, R. E., Kristal, A. R., Shannon, J., Hunt, J. R., and White, E. (1997). Using a brief houschold food inventory as an environmental indicator of individual dietary practices. *Am J Public Health, 87,* 272–275.

Patterson, R. E., Kristal, A. R., Tinker, L. F., Carter, R. A., Bolton, M. P. et al (1999). Measurement characteristics of the Women's Health Initiative food frequency questionnaire. *Ann Epidemiol, 9,* 178–187.

Pietinen, P., Hartman, A. M., Haapa, E., Rasanen, L., Haapakoski, J. et al (1988). Reproducibility and validity of dietary assessment instruments: a self-administered food use questionnaire with a portion size picture booklet. *Am J Epidemiol, 123,* 655–666.

Pool-Zobel, B. L., Bub, A., Muller, H., Wollowski, I., and Rechkemmer, G. (1997). Consumption of vegetables reduces genetic damage in humans: first results of a human intervention trial with carotenoid-rich foods. *Carcinogenesis, 18,* 1847–1850.

Popkin, B. M., Duffey, K., and Gordon-Larsen, P. (2005). Environmental influences on food choice, physical activity and energy balance. *Physiol Behav, 86,* 603–613.

Prentice, R. L., Willett, W. C., Greenwald, P., Alberts, D., Bernstein, L. et al (2004). Nutrition and physical activity and chronic disease prevention: research strategies and recommendations. *J Natl Cancer Inst, 96,* 1276–1287.

Rajeshwari, R., Yang, S. J., Nicklas, T. A., and Berenson, G. S. (2005). Secular trends in children's sweetened-beverage consumption (1973 to 1994): The Bogalusa Heart Study. *J Am Diet Assoc, 105,* 208–214.

Rampersaud, G. C., Bailey, L. B., and Kauwell, G. P. A. (2003). National survey beverage consumption data for children and adolescents indicate the need to encourage a shift toward more nutritive beverages. *J Am Diet Assoc, 103,* 97–100.

Rebro, S., Patterson, R. E., Kristal, A. R., and Cheney, C. (1998). The effect of keeping food records on eating patterns. *J Am Diet Assoc, 98,* 1163–1165.

Resnicow, K., Odom, E., Wang, T., Dudley, W. N., Mitchell, D. et al (2000). Validation of three food frequency questionnaires and 24-hour recalls with serum carotenoid levels in a sample of African-American adults. *Am J Epidemiol, 152,* 1072–1080.

Satia, J. A., Patterson, R. E., Kristal, A. R., Hislop, E. G., and Pineda, M. (2001a). A household food inventory for North American Chinese. *Public Health Nutr, 4,* 241–247.

Satia, J. A., Patterson, R. E., Kristal, A. R., Hislop, T. G., Yasui, Y. et al (2001b). Development of scales to measure dietary acculturation among Chinese-Americans and Chinese-Canadians. *J Am Diet Assoc, 101,* 548–553.

Satia, J. A., Patterson, R. E., Taylor, V. M., Cheney, C. L., Shiu-Thornton, S. et al (2000). Use of qualitative methods to study diet, acculturation, and health in Chinese American women. *J Am Diet Assoc, 100,* 934–940.

Schakel, S. F., Buzzard, I. M., and Gebhardt, S. E. (1997). Procedures for estimating nutrient values for food composition databases. *J Food Comp Anal, 10,* 102–114.

Shannon, J., Kristal, A. R., Curry, S. J., and Beresford, S. A. (1997). Application of a behavioral approach to measuring dietary change: the fat- and fiber-related diet behavior questionnaire. *Cancer Epidemiol Biomarkers Prev, 6,* 355–361.

Sobo, E. J., Rock, C. L., Neuhouser, M. L., Maciel, T. L., and Neumark-Sztainer, D. (2000). Caretaker-child interaction during children's 24-hour dietary recalls: who contributes what to the recall record? *J Am Diet Assoc, 100,* 428–433.

Subar, A., Kipnis, V., Troiano, R. P., Midthune, D., Schoeller, D. A. et al (2003). Using intake biomarkers to evaluate the extent of dietary misreporting in a large sample of adults: The OPEN Study. *Am J Epidemiol, 158,* 1–13.

Subar, A. F., Dodd, K. W., Guenther, P. M., Kipnis, V., Midthune, D. et al (2006). The food propensity questionnaire: concept, development, and validation for use as a covariate in a model to estimate usual food intake. *J Am Diet Assoc, 106,* 1556–1563.

Thompson, F. E., Kipnis, V., Subar, A. F., Krebs-Smith, S. M., Kahle, L. L. et al (2000). Evaluation of 2 brief instruments and a food-frequency questionnaire to estimate daily number of servings of fruit and vegetables. *Am J Clin Nutr, 71,* 1503–1510.

Thompson, F. E., Subar, A. F., Smith, A. F., Midthune, D., Radimer, K. L. et al (2002). Fruit and vegetable assessment: performance of 2 new short instruments and a food frequency questionnaire. *J Am Diet Assoc,* *102,* 1764–1772.

Tooze, J. A., Subar, A. F., Thompson, F. E., Troiano, R., Schatzkin, A. et al (2004). Psychosocial predictors of energy underreporting in a large doubly labeled water study. *Am J Clin Nutr, 79,* 795–804.

Townsend, M. S. (2006). Obesity in low-income communities: prevalence, effects, a place to begin. *J Am Diet Assoc, 106,* 34–37.

Van Duyn, M. S., Kristal, A. R., Dodd, K., Campbell, M. K., Subar, A. F. et al (2001). Association of awareness, intrapersonal and interpersonal factors, and stage of dietary change with fruit and vegetable consumption: a national survey. *Am J Health Promot, 16,* 69–78.

Wang, D.-H., Kogashiwa, M., Ohta, S., and Kira, S. (2002). Validity and reliability of a dietary assessment method: the application of a digital camera with a mobile phone card attachment. *J Nutr Sci Vitaminol, 48,* 498–504.

Willett, W. (1998). *Nutritional Epidemiology, 2nd Ed.* New York: Oxford Universal Press.

Williamson, D. A., Allen, H. R., Martin, P. D., Alfonso, A. J., Gerald, B. et al (2003). Comparison of digital photography to weighed and visual estimation of portion size. *J Am Diet Assoc, 103,* 1139–1145.

Williamson, D. A., Martin, P. D., Alfonso, A., Gerald, B., and Hunt, A. (2004). Digital photography: a new method for estimating food intake in cafeteria settings. *Eat Weight Disord, 9,* 24–28.

World Cancer Research Fund/AICR. (2007). *Food, Nutrition, Physical Activity, and the Prevention of Cancer: A Global Perspective.* Washington, DC: AICR.

Yaroch, A. L., Resnicow, K., Davis, M., Davis, A., Smith, M. et al (2000). Development of a modified picture-sort food frequency questionnaire administered to low-income, overweight, African-American adolescent girls. *J Am Diet Assoc, 100,* 1050–1056.

Chapter 5

Assessment of Sexual Behavior

Lori A.J. Scott-Sheldon, Seth C. Kalichman, and Michael P. Carey

1 Assessment of Sexual Behavior

Sexuality is essential to human life, experienced through individual thoughts and desires, behaviors, relationships, and cultures (Robinson et al, 2002; WHO, 2006). A responsible, safe, and fulfilling sexual life experience requires a positive approach to sexuality and an understanding of the social, economic, and political factors (e.g., gender inequality and poverty) that may lead to sexual ill-health (WHO, 2006). Sexual well-being involves positive sexual expression, coupled with the possibility of satisfying and safe sexual experiences. To promote sexual health, public policy experts, health educators, physicians, and clinicians, benefit from extensive knowledge and understanding of sexual behavior including sexual aspects of relationships (e.g., sexual arousal and functioning).

Since the 1980s, research in sexual health has escalated due to the sexual revolution, advent of the HIV pandemic, and the pharmacological treatment of sexual problems. Advances in data collection methods and the assessment of sexual behavior have furthered our understanding of sexual behavior patterns and functioning. Although biological markers (e.g., incidence of sexually transmitted diseases or pregnancy) provide useful information about an individual's

behavior, these markers are incomplete because they convey little information about the frequency, number of sexual partners, and the co-occurrence of sexual behavior with other behaviors (e.g., alcohol or drug use). Because no objective indicators are available and sexual behavior cannot readily (or ethically) be measured through direct observation, researchers often rely on self-reports of sexual behavior. Obtaining detailed and accurate self-reports of sexual behavior are necessary to fully evaluate and further develop prevention programs, assess and treat sexual problems and trauma, and inform public policy and health care (Bogart et al, 2007; Catania et al, 1990; Cecil et al, 2005; Schroder et al, 2003b; Wincze and Carey, 2001).

Measurement of sexual behavior poses unique challenges to health researchers given (a) concerns about privacy, cultural taboos, and stigmatizing behaviors, (b) the nature of the behavior (i.e., dyadic rather than individual), and (c) motives for sexual behavior (Catania et al, 1990; Schroder et al, 2003a). Moreover, assessment of complex sexual behavior likely necessitates multiple types of assessment measures and methodology. In this chapter we address the importance of measuring sexual behaviors, measures and assessment methods, and challenges to sexual behavior measurement. We provide information about clinical interviewing and written assessments. Although we focus primarily on retrospective methods (e.g., questionnaires), we also present contemporaneous assessment methods (e.g., daily

L.A.J. Scott-Sheldon (✉)
Center for Health and Behavior, Syracuse University,
430 Huntington Hall, Syracuse, NY 13244-2340, USA
e-mail: lajss@syr.edu

A. Steptoe (ed.), *Handbook of Behavioral Medicine*, DOI 10.1007/978-0-387-09488-5_5,
© Springer Science+Business Media, LLC 2010

diary). We conclude by offering suggestions for improving sexual behavior assessments in future research.

2 Reasons for Measuring Sexual Behavior

Sexual expression is a fundamental aspect of human relationships. While most research has focused on the problems, risks, and dangers of sex, there are a number of physiological and psychological benefits of sexual expression (Whipple, 2006). For example, frequent sexual activity increases fertility (Cutler et al, 1985), the probability of conception (Wilcox et al, 1995), and improves sexual functioning and satisfaction (Laumann et al, 2006; Parish et al, 2007). Benefits aside, consequences related to sexual activity (e.g., sexual coercion, HIV) may threaten an individual's ability to have satisfying sexual experiences. Accurate, reliable, and valid self-reports of sexual behavior provide essential information to assist researchers and interventionists in developing efficacious programs to improve sexual health.

2.1 General Health Benefits

Studies examining the benefits of sexual activity on physical health have suggested sexual activity improves physical and psychological health in a number of domains. Sexual activity: (1) Increases longevity: Men with increased orgasmic frequency (i.e., had sex at least two times per week) had a 50% lower risk of mortality at a 10-year follow-up (Davey Smith et al, 1997); (2) Lowers the risk of chronic disease (e.g., heart disease and cancer): Among men, frequency of sex was associated with a lower risk of fatal coronary heart disease (Ebrahim et al, 2002). Furthermore, a national survey of US men found high ejaculation frequency (i.e., ≥ 21 ejaculations per month) was associated with decreased risk of total prostate cancer (Leitzmann et al,

2004); (3) Increases immunity: Increased levels of immunoglobulin A, an essential antibody used by the immune system to protect against viral infections, were found in college students reporting having sex at least three times per week (Charnetski and Brennan, 2004); (4) Associated with reduced stress: Participants who had vaginal sex in the last 2 weeks had lower blood pressure and stress response to stress-inducing tasks (Brody, 2006). Among medical residents, stress negatively affected desire, sexual arousal , and sexual satisfaction (Sangi-Haghpeykar et al, 2009); and (5) Increases physical fitness: Sexual intimacy was associated with physical fitness level among Fifty Plus Fitness Association members (Bortz and Wallace, 1999); frequency of sexual activity was higher among men enrolled in an intensive physical fitness program (White et al, 1990).

2.2 Sexual Health Outcomes

Prior research suggests sexual health and well-being are directly related to sexual behavior. Sexual experiences (e.g., frequency of sex or orgasm) have been associated with both positive and negative aspects of sexual and reproductive health.

2.2.1 Positive Sexual Health Outcomes

Among other benefits, fertility and conception are two ways by which sexual activity may have a positive effect on sexual health. Researchers have shown frequent vaginal sex (i.e., at least weekly) is associated with increased fertility (Cutler et al, 1985); women who have sex daily during their fertile period (i.e., five consecutive days in a woman's menstrual cycle culminating with a sixth day of ovulation) had a 37% chance of conceiving compare to a 15% chance among women having sex once during the same period (Wilcox et al, 1995). Moreover, frequent sexual activity, including sexual intercourse and orgasm, are positively associated with sexual and emotional satisfaction and relationship quality among both men and women (Costa and Brody, 2007; Laumann et al, 2006).

2.2.2 Negative Sexual Health Outcomes

Despite the benefits, sexual health is undermined by intimate partner violence (e.g., sexual coercion and rape) and by sexually transmitted infections (STIs). Recent US estimates of sexual coercion indicate that 1 in 59 adults have experienced unwanted sexual activity in the past year with 1 in 15 adults forced to have sex at least once in their lifetime (Basile et al, 2007). Among a diverse sample of women (adolescents, patients attending a STI clinic, homeless women, and college students), sexual coercion was consistently related to subsequent risky sexual behavior (Biglan et al, 1995). Risky sexual behavior (e.g., unprotected sex with infected partners) threatens sexual health and puts people at risk of contracting STIs. In the USA, an estimated 19 million new STIs are diagnosed each year, including 56,000 new cases of HIV/AIDS, over 1 million cases of chlamydia, 355,991 cases of gonorrhea, and 11,466 cases of syphilis (CDC, 2009; Hall et al, 2008).

3 Assessment of Sexual Behavior: How to Gather the Data

Biological outcomes (e.g., STI or pregnancy) can confirm sexual activity but provides limited information regarding the prevalence, frequency, or problems associated with sexual behavior. Both positive and negative effects of sexual expression vary depending on a number of highly complex contextual factors. Information regarding the prevalence of specific behaviors is contingent upon accurate, reliable, and valid self-reports of sexual behavior (Catania et al, 1990; Schroder et al, 2003b). Thus researchers need to make two fundamental decisions when they decide to assess sexual behavior: How to gather the data? What data to collect?

3.1 Modes of Assessment

The first question a researcher needs to answer involves the choice of data collection strategies or modes of assessment. In most clinical settings, it is customary to use a face-to-face interview, whereas in most public health and community settings, it is customary to use self-administered methods.

3.1.1 Interviews

In clinical settings, interviews are often preferred over self-administered assessments because interviewees are seeking treatment, have immediate questions and concerns that need to be addressed, and expect, and are often eager, to reveal sensitive information. In the clinical context, interviews are conducted by professionals (or trainees) who know how to establish rapport, elicit information efficiently, establish a diagnosis, formulate etiologic hypotheses, and suggest interventions. In the research context, by contrast, the goals of the interview are different but interviewers also need to be empathic, highly skilled, and efficient.

Several interviewer and process characteristics tend to increase the quality of sexual behavior data obtained. Assessment of behavior should occur after a respondent and interviewer have established rapport and the interviewer has assured the respondent of confidentiality. Sexual history interviews should always begin with an appropriate introduction for the respondent. During this time the reasons for asking questions about sexual and other socially sensitive behaviors should be provided. For example, one might explain the purpose of the research and how it will benefit the interviewee or the larger community. It can be helpful to contextualize sexual behavior as an important health behavior, just as one might discuss smoking, exercise, or stress management strategies. If biological specimens are to be collected, these can be likened to taking blood pressure or collecting serum for cholesterol levels (i.e., frame the assessment as a health inquiry, not an exploration of morality). Although sensitivity is essential, it is important to ask questions directly, without apology or hesitancy (Kinsey et al, 2003). If the interviewer appears embarrassed or unsure of the appropriateness of the questions, interviewees will detect this and may provide incomplete, ambiguous, or socially desirable responses.

After the introductory remarks, the respondent should be invited to ask any questions they might have. It is often important to "listen with the third ear" (Reik, 1983), that is, to use skills and intuition to sense what a respondent may be intending and to guide the interview accordingly. Careful listening serves as the cornerstone of the interview process. Some interviewees may freely offer information about their sexual behavior in response to direct questions. However, many interviewees will be embarrassed and perhaps confused by the range of questions and require patience and explanation. It is not uncommon for interviewees to have had distressing experiences in the past, for example, to report that they had tried previously to discuss sexual behavior with a health-care professional, but were met with avoidance, embarrassment, or apparent lack of interest; as a result, they did not pursue their concerns. So, interviewers need to be open to respondents' disclosures regarding sexual behavior and to be aware of subtle nonverbal cues that may discourage the disclosure of sensitive information.

When assessing sexual behavior, we have found it helpful to adopt assumptions in order to gather the most accurate information without wasting time and effort (Wincze and Carey, 2001). These assumptions reflect the preferred direction of error. Thus, for example, one might assume a low level of understanding on the part of the respondent so that language is directed to the respondent in a clear and concrete manner. Other useful assumptions include: respondents will (a) be embarrassed about and have difficulty discussing sexual matters; (b) not understand medical terminology; and (c) be misinformed about STIs. As the interviewer learns about the interviewees, these assumptions are adjusted.

Depending upon the interviewee and context, it may be useful to sequence the inquiry from the least to most threatening questions. Thus, questions about courtship, dating, or relationships might precede questions regarding sexual behavior, hookups, and casual sex. Experience in the assessment of sexual behavior also suggests that it can be helpful to place the "burden of denial" on the respondent (Kinsey et al, 2003). That is, rather than ask "if" a respondent has engaged in a particular sexual activity, the interviewer might ask "how many times have you ..." engaged in it. Use of this strategy will depend upon the nature of the relationship that has been established with the respondent and needs to be done sensitively.

Finally, it can often be helpful to follow a semi-structured format, so that information is gathered systematically, and no important areas are neglected. This, too, requires sensitivity because it is important to attend to interviewee responses and tailor the questions accordingly. Attention to the interview structure at the expense of the interpersonal dynamic can undermine rapport, which will jeopardize both the relationship and the quality of the data.

3.1.2 Self-Administered Questionnaires

The self-administered questionnaire (SAQ), an alternative approach to the in-person interview, is the most commonly used method of assessing self-report behavior. SAQs offer a number of advantages over in-person interviews such as providing a more private, less intrusive, and less threatening means of reporting sensitive behaviors, allowing participants to skip potentially embarrassing questions and administration to large numbers of people thus reducing costs (Catania et al, 1990; Durant and Carey, 2000; Schroder et al, 2003b). Despite these advantages, there are several disadvantages of SAQs. Self-administration precludes additional clarification of unclear questions or contingent questioning, increasing the chance for missing responses or inconsistent data reporting.

Several formats have been used for SAQs: paper-and-pencil, postal mail, electronic mail, or computer delivered. Studies examining differences between SAQ formats demonstrate that computer-administered self-interviews (CASI) may increase the reporting of sexual behaviors. Over a 3-month period, participants recalled their sexual behavior (e.g., frequency of unprotected sex) more accurately using the CASI compared with other types of self-report assessments (McAuliffe et al, 2007). College students completing CASI report more alcohol consumption and riskier sexual behaviors than those completing paper-based SAQ (Booth-Kewley et al, 2007). Finally, an increase in gynecological symptoms was reported among STI patients completing a CASI compared with those using a paper-based SAQ (Robinson and West, 1992). Higher self-reports of sensitive behavior among CASI users may be due to an increased a sense of privacy and credibility not provided by paper-and-pencil SAQs (Schroder et al, 2003b).

3.1.3 Internet Surveys

With the increasing popularity and availability of the Internet, researchers have begun using the Internet as a means to assess sexual behavior. Internet-based self-interviews (IBSI) share many of the advantages provided by CASI methods (e.g., increased sense of privacy, automated contingent questioning, eliminates data entry errors) but offer the potential to survey a wider range of participants and difficult-to-reach populations, allow completion at a time and place convenient for the participant, and participants are less vulnerable to coercion (Pequegnat et al, 2007; Rhodes et al, 2003). Limitations of using an IBSI include lack of Internet access among impoverished individuals (i.e., the digital divide), computer literacy issues, and concerns about data confidentiality or security (Baer et al, 2002; Pequegnat et al, 2007). Few studies have examined IBSI compared with other forms of self-assessments; to date, inconsistent results have been found between web- versus paper-based questionnaires (for a discussion, see Whittier et al, 2005).

3.1.4 Self-Monitoring and Diary Methods

Diaries have become an increasingly popular method of collecting health-related information almost contemporaneously to the actual event, thus avoiding recall bias and reducing measurement error (Bolger et al, 2003; Graham et al, 2005). Because diaries minimize memory demands and promise more accurate results, they are effective for eliciting highly detailed data on sensitive sexual behaviors (Graham et al, 2005; Schroder et al, 2003b). Compared with other SAQ formats, diaries allow for the assessment of events occurring in everyday situations as well as the contexts in which those events occur, assess behaviors closer in time to the actual event, increase privacy, credibility, and confidentiality, and require minimal reading and writing skills (Bolger et al, 2003; Schroder et al, 2003b). Moreover, diaries improve accuracy, have high completion rates over time, and can easily be used among participants with low literacy skills (Bolger et al, 2003; Schroder et al, 2003b).

Although there are several advantages to using daily diaries, researchers have begun to question the extent to which participants follow instructions regarding the date, time, and place of the diary entries (Bolger et al, 2003; Stone and Shiffman, 2002). The accuracy of written diaries (e.g., booklets, packets of questionnaires, postcards) is uncertain due to the lack of data monitoring (i.e., no time stamp), possibility of backfilling, retrospection errors, and incomplete data (Bolger et al, 2003; Green et al, 2006). Recent technological advances have enabled researchers to ascertain exactly when a report is completed and/or to impose a restricted time frame in which participants may complete those reports. Computers and other electronic devices (e.g., personal digital assistants, cell phones) allow researchers to not only record the date and time of each diary record but also provide the ability to signal participant responses at fixed or random intervals and send participants response reminders (Green et al, 2006). Similar rates of compliance between paper-and-pencil and electronic diaries have been found (Green et al, 2006).

Limited research has compared the accuracy of daily diaries with retrospective self-reports. After completing a written daily diary of their sexual activities, McAuliffe et al (2007) randomly assigned participants to complete one of the three types of retrospective measures (audio-CASI, CASI, or paper-based SAQ); these authors found substantially less sexual behavior reported retrospectively compared to the daily diaries. Although daily diaries yield more sexual behavior – and purportedly more accurate behaviors – diaries may not be appropriate in all contexts (e.g., among homeless persons) (Patterson and Strathdee, 2005). High demands on participants' need for adherence, likelihood of dropout rates, and increased likelihood of assessment reactivity may prevent researchers from using diaries in some public health contexts.

3.1.5 Virtual Reality

Virtual reality (VR), a computer-simulated environment in which an individual has the ability to control his/her actions, has recently been used to measure sexual behavior. Since sexual behavior cannot be readily or ethically measured via direct observation, VR has the ability to greatly enhance the ecological validity of sexual assessment by assessing behavior in a context similar to a real-life situation. Research examining the use of VR to measure sexual behavior is limited but there is some evidence that past sexual risk-taking behaviors predict VR risk taking and VR risk taking predicts future risk behaviors 3 months later (Godoy, 2007). Other research has shown VR to be an effective means of assessing sexual preferences (Renaud et al, 2002).

4 Measures of Sexual Behavior: What to Gather

Sexual behavior has been assessed using a wide range of measures (Noar et al, 2006; Schroder et al, 2003a; Sheeran and Abraham, 1994).

Although there has been a lack of consensus regarding the best method of assessing self-reports of sexual behaviors, some researchers have suggested focusing on using measures that are most appropriate for the specific context or goal of the research (e.g., risk screening, risk assessment, and risk event) (Noar et al, 2006; Patterson and Strathdee, 2005; Weinhardt et al, 1998b). For instance, if the goal is to assess the overall frequency of condom use among members of a specific community (e.g., among homeless adolescents), the researcher might ask global questions regarding the number of times a participant had sex and their overall frequency of condom use during a specific reporting period (e.g., past 3 months). Alternatively, if the goal is to assess the risk of HIV within the same community, a researcher might ask participants specific questions regarding the co-occurrence of sexual risk behavior (e.g., sex without a condom, alcohol and/or drug use prior to sex). Accurate measurement of sexual risk behavior is important not only in assessing the effectiveness of prevention programs, but also for ascertaining the prevalence of disease within a community, as well as informing policy decisions about how best to prevent STIs.

4.1 Question Types

4.1.1 Frequency of Sexual Behavior

Sexual behavior is most commonly assessed using frequencies. Reviews of the sexual behavior risk-reduction literature find 36–64% of studies measure the frequency of condom use (Noar et al, 2006; Schroder et al, 2003a; Sheeran and Abraham, 1994). Relative frequency measures of sexual behavior are often assessed using a single item such as "how often did you have sex in the past x months?" with a range of response options. Participants rate their frequency of sex using a Likert-type response with endpoints ranging from *never* to *always*; intermediate-scale points (e.g., *rarely*, *sometimes*, *almost always*) are inconsistently used.

Despite the popularity of relative frequency measures, research has shown the ability to accurately measure sexual behavior decreases as the frequency of the targeted behavior increases (Durant and Carey, 2000; Jaccard et al, 2002). Moreover, the accuracy of these ordinal measures of sexual behavior (specifically condom use) depends on shared definitions of labels both among participants and between the participants and researcher (Cecil et al, 2005). Research has shown category labels to be subject to individual interpretation. For example, nearly one-third of college students rate using condoms once or twice out of 20 events as "never" using condoms (Cecil and Zimet, 1998). Although most researchers would refer to "always using condoms" as 100% use, more than one-third of college students labeled using condoms 18 or 19 times out of 20 events as "always" using a condom. Cecil et al (2005) found similar results showing that "never" using condoms does not mean 0% of condom use, but could mean infrequent condom use (e.g., 1 time out of 20), and "always" using condoms docs not mean 100% condom use (i.e., 70% indicated always using condoms when condoms were used 19 out of 20 times).

4.1.2 Consistency of Sexual Behavior

Another question type focuses on the consistency of sexual behavior. Consistency of sexual behavior may be obtained directly or indirectly. For example, a direct measure of condom use would ask participants to respond to the question "over the past (time period), what proportion of the time did you use condoms when you had sex?" using an 11-point scale ranging from 0 to 100%. An indirect measure of consistent sexual behavior is calculated based on two separate questions representing the total number of sexual events in a specific time period and the total number of events in which, for example, a condom was used in that same time period; the proportion of time a participant used a condom is obtained by dividing the number of condom-protected events by the total number of

sexual events. Percentage ratings or proportions are problematic as both fail to capture variance in abstinence and/or reduced frequency rates. For instance, a value of zero using the indirect method may indicate a person abstained from sex *or* always used a condom for numerous sexual events, thus underestimating the risk of STI transmission among those with high frequencies of sexual events (Graham et al, 2005).

4.1.3 Dichotomies

Similar to ordinal measures of sexual behavior, dichotomies categorize individuals as low or high on a specified outcome measure. Participants are typically asked to respond *yes* or *no* regarding a particular sexual event (e.g., "Did you use a condom the last time you had sex?") but may also be asked about more general occurrences (e.g., "Have you ever used a condom?"). Dichotomies are useful when researchers are interested in examining differences between two groups (e.g., participants who have and have not had sex), but the use of dichotomies may be problematic because responses do not convey typical sexual activity patterns (i.e., may be restricted to a particular event). Dichotomies are descriptive and therefore reduce information available for analysis and interpretation (Graham et al, 2005).

4.1.4 Count Measures of Sexual Behavior

Instead of using *relative* measures (e.g., frequency of sex using assigned labels, percentage ratings, dichotomies), Schroder et al (2003a) suggest using *absolute* measures (i.e., count data) to assess sexual behavior because counts provide more specific data about a person's risk level. Count measures ask participants to provide the exact number of times they engaged in sexual behavior during a specific time period. For example, unprotected sex is assessed by asking participants the number of times they had vaginal sex in a specified period and the number of times they used a condom. An absolute measure of the number of unprotected sex events would be computed by subtracting the number of protected sex events from the number of times the participant had sex (not a ratio of unprotected sexual behavior). Absolute measures of sexual behavior can also be obtained using event-level data (e.g., daily diaries, timeline follow-back). For event-level data, researchers solicit information regarding condom use or other behaviors (e.g., drug and/or alcohol use) concurrent with a single or multiple sexual event(s); the number of sexual events are then summed.

Choice of sexual behavior measure depends upon the nature of the research question; however, count measures offer advantages not afforded by frequency or consistency data. Absolute measures of sexual behavior (1) reflect only the number of risk occurrences thus providing precise information regarding sexual behaviors and (2) are more versatile (i.e., can be converted to proportions) (Graham et al, 2005; Schroder et al, 2003a). Although count data yield both absolute and relative information useful in quantifying sexual behavior, count data have two primary disadvantages: (1) data collection is more time consuming and expensive especially if collecting event-level data (e.g., daily diaries) and (2) data analysis is more difficult because the data often deviate from the normal distribution (Schroder et al, 2003a).

4.1.5 Composite Measures of Sexual Behavior

Some researchers have suggested using composite measures (e.g., frequency and proportion items), safer sex algorithms, and risk indices to assess sexual behavior (Burkholder and Harlow, 1996; Miner et al, 2002a; Sheeran and Abraham, 1994). Sheeran and Abraham (Abraham and Sheeran, 1994; Sheeran and Abraham, 1994) measured condom use using a composite of frequency (*never* to *always*), temporal frequency (*never in the last year* to *most weeks in the last year*), and proportion of condom use (number of times participants used a condom divided by the total number of sex events). Miner et al

(2002b) developed a Safer Sex Algorithm consisting of decision rules for defining safe and unsafe sex as well as relationship variables and partner characteristics (i.e., length of relationship, partner type, HIV status, alcohol or drug use, and monogamy of individual and partner). Moderate correlations were found between measures taken 3 months apart ($r = 0.55$ for the number of unsafe sexual events and $r = 0.52$ for the number of unprotected anal and/or vaginal sex events).

4.2 Standardized (Published) Measures

Questionnaires used to assess sexual behavior and functioning can be accessed through professional journals or books devoted to self-report questionnaires. Although there are a limited number of reliable and valid scales of general sexual behavior, scales targeting specific populations are available. These scales include the *Coping and Change Sexual Behavior and Behavior Change Questionnaire* (Ostrow et al, 1995) for gay and bisexual men, the *HIV Risk-Taking Behavior Scale* (Darke et al, 1991) or the *Risk Behavior Assessment* (Needle et al, 1995) for drug users, and the *Adolescent Clinical Sexual Behavior Inventory* (Friedrich et al, 2004) targeting adolescents. An excellent resource containing measures of sexuality as well as the psychometric properties of each measure is the *Handbook of Sexuality-Related Measures* (Davis et al, 1998). As with any research, scales should be selected based on the psychometric properties (i.e., reliability and validity), research relevance (i.e., measure fits the intended purpose), and practicality (e.g., length of the questionnaire, culturally appropriate) (Weinhardt et al, 1998b).

5 Challenges to Sexual Assessment

Numerous factors can influence the accuracy of self-reports of sexual behavior. Cognitive, memory, and literacy challenges, social desirability, substance use, and level of assessment have all been associated with reporting bias (Catania et al, 1990; Graham et al, 2005; Schroder et al, 2003b; Weinhardt et al, 1998b). Recommendations for improving the assessment of sexual behavior include use terms that are clear and familiar to participants, pilot test with the target sample to facilitate measurement development, assess literacy skills, and evaluate whether an audio-administered version of the assessment is required (Weinhardt et al, 1998b). Understanding known problems associated with measuring sexual behavior will help increase the reliability and validity of self-reports.

5.1 Cognition and Memory Challenges

5.1.1 Length of Recall Period

Participants are typically asked questions about their behavior over a specific time period. To increase the accuracy of retrospective self-reports, researchers have recommended recall periods of 3 months or less. Research has shown sexual behaviors can be reliably assessed by self-report measures for intervals as long as 3 months but reliability decreases at longer intervals (Kauth et al, 1991). In a study comparing daily diaries to a SAQ 1, 2, and 3 months after diary completion, Graham et al (2003) found recall of condom use was stable across the 3-month period but participants reporting more frequent condom use had more errors. Jaccard et al (2002) compared weekly mailed self-report questionnaires with retrospective reports at 1, 3, 6, and 12 months finding no difference between type of method at the 3- and 12-month assessments, but not at the 1- or 6-month assessments. They concluded that retrospective SAQs accurately represent behavior for at least 3 months. Little evidence suggests that recall periods longer than 3 months provide accurate information (Schroder et al, 2003a; Sheeran and Abraham, 1994).

Reviews of the sexual risk behavior literature show that 28–49% of studies ask participants to recall condom use over a 3–6-month time frame whereas 15–18% provide no specific time frame (Noar et al, 2006; Sheeran and Abraham, 1994). Noar et al (2006) suggest that specific and brief recall periods should yield optimal responses but additional research is necessary to evaluate the reliability of various recall periods. Moreover, research shows high-frequency behaviors may be more difficult to recall over longer periods of time, whereas rarer behaviors may not occur over short recall periods. Since low-frequency behaviors are more salient, participants may be inclined to believe an event occurred more recently (i.e., telescoping) potentially leading participants to exaggerate sexual behaviors. Patterson and Strathdee (2005) recommended using absolute frequency counts for rare behaviors and relative frequency measures (e.g., proportion of time condom was used) for more frequent behaviors.

To enhance recall of retrospective self-reports, Weinhardt et al (1998) suggest using three strategies: (1) Provide anchor dates for recall periods, (2) Encourage participant to use calendars to aid the recall of memorable events, and (3) Prompt participant recall of extensive periods of sexual behavior (e.g., abstinence, consistent sexual activities). All three of the suggested strategies may be accomplished using the timeline follow-back (TFLB; Sobell and Sobell, 1996) procedure. The TLFB uses calendars marked with landmark events, personally meaningful dates, and other memory aides to facilitate accurate recall. Because of the interactive format used for the TLFB, memory is aided by the recalling of one event in reference to another event. Using the TLFB, behavioral patterns are recorded in greater detail and over multiple time points. Sexual risk information yielded by the TLFB include number of sexual partners, frequency of sexual events (vaginal, anal, oral), frequency of unprotected sexual events (vaginal, anal, oral), alcohol and/or drug use prior to sex, number of occasions and quantity of alcohol and/or drug use prior to sex, and STI history. Research has confirmed the stability of the 3-month retrospective self-reports using the

TLFB procedure (Carey et al, 2001; Weinhardt et al, 1998a).

5.1.2 Partner and Sexual Act Specificity

Failure to specify and/or define type of partner or sexual act may result in inaccurate self-reports of sexual behavior. Researchers recommend using measures that are specific to sexual partners and specific to sexual acts, rather than general measures (Fishbein and Pequegnat, 2000; Schroder et al, 2003b; Sheeran and Abraham, 1994). In Sheeran and Abraham's (1994) review of condom use measures, they found 79% of the measures did not specify type of partner and most (65%) did not specify the type of sexual act being assessed (i.e., vaginal, anal, or oral sex). An updated review of the literature examining 56 studies found 57% of measures did not specify partner type, 16% specified primary versus non-primary partners, and 16% were tailored to partner type (Noar et al, 2006); most studies reported the type of sexual activity (67%). Because different levels of risk are associated with various sexual practices, it is important for researchers to specify both sexual partner and sexual act to increase the accuracy of the data.

Research examining aggregate (i.e., summed across all sexual partners) versus partner-specific (i.e., questions specific for each sexual partner) formats has found partner-specific SAQs produce more accurate self-reports of sexual behavior than do aggregate question formats (McAuliffe et al, 2007). Thus, partner specificity (i.e., name of actual partner rather than primary versus non-primary labels) "may help cue the recall of sexual activities by providing both a context and a focus for past experiences and events" and improve the accuracy of self-reported sexual behavior (McAuliffe et al, 2007). Moreover, the use of multiple terms, without clear definitions, for partners (primary, steady, exclusive, regular versus secondary, casual, nonexclusive) makes comparisons between studies challenging.

5.2 Literacy Skills

Accuracy of self-reports hinges on the ability of people to read and comprehend questions. According to the 2003 National Assessment of Adult Literacy (Kutner et al, 2006, 2007), more than 30 million American adults had reading skills below basic level and 14% had below basic levels of health literacy (i.e., ability to read and understand health information). Moreover, illiteracy is more likely to occur in high-risk populations. Among adults living with HIV, Kalichman et al (2000) found 18% of participants had below basic levels of health literacy. Among people at risk for STIs, Al-Tayyib et al (2002) found a substantial proportion of adults scored at or below an eighth grade level (28%) including 12% scoring lower than a sixth grade level. Participants with lower literacy scores provided more logically inconsistent answers and had higher skip pattern errors when answering questions from a SAQ.

SAQs are particularly vulnerable to inaccurate estimates of sexual behavior caused by an inability to fully understand and comprehend the questions asked, failure to respond, and difficulty following complex question patterns. Both interviewer and audio-assisted methods (e.g., audio-CASI) allow individuals with low literacy to provide more meaningful responses. Interviewer-assisted questionnaires provide participants with additional instruction regarding unclear terms or skip patterns but reduce privacy and anonymity. Audio-CASI provides participants with an increased sense of anonymity whereby the participant listens to questions through headphones while keying in answers on a computer unassisted. Moreover, audio-CASI reduces cognitive demands and improves comprehension (Schroder et al, 2003b). Studies examining the effects of audio-CASI find fewer missing responses and "don't know" answers compared with participants assigned to complete written SAQs (Boekeloo et al, 1994; Turner et al, 1998). Thus, the various modes of assessment have different advantages and disadvantages, so selection of an optimal method depends upon the research question, sample, and context.

5.3 Social Desirability and Presentation Concerns

Because sexual behavior is typically a private activity, people may respond to sexual-related questions in ways designed to avoid embarrassment, reduce threat, or conform to social norms. Social desirability and impression management biases have been associated with refusal or failure to disclose sexual information and inaccurate reporting (Catania et al, 1990; Gibson et al, 1999; Schroder et al, 2003b). Whereas socially desirable behaviors tend to be over-reported, socially undesirable behaviors are more likely to be under-reported, because of this tendency, assessment strategies yielding higher self-reports of sexual risk behaviors are often assumed to be more accurate (Lau et al, 2000; Tourangeau and Smith, 1996). Accuracy is dependent upon participants' perceptions of anonymity, privacy, and credibility. The extent to which self-reports are biased by self-presentation concerns may impact our knowledge of the prevalence of sexual risk behavior and undermine efforts to measure the effects of prevention programs.

5.4 Cultural, Developmental, Sexual Orientation and Gender Matching

Assessments of sexual behavior should be appropriately matched to participants' culture, developmental status, and gender. Focus groups and pilot testing are needed to assist with the development and refinement of appropriate measures (Weinhardt et al, 1998b). Particular attention to language, specifically meanings and contexts of words, is critical in assessing sexual behavior among different ethnic groups. Conducting

separate focus groups with men and women may reveal cultural and contextual issues relevant for sexual behavior assessment (Carey et al, 1997). For example, the expression of machismo among Hispanic men is extremely important not only from a social standpoint but also for an individual's self-esteem; measures that fail to recognize cultural differences among Hispanic men and women may elicit inaccurate self-reports. Furthermore, emphasizing the personal and community benefits of the research is likely to increase participation and elicit more accurate reporting.

5.5 Individual Versus Dyadic Assessments

Even though sexual behavior occurs between people, it is typically measured at the individual rather than dyadic level. Since sexual behavior is intrinsically linked with other people, the strength of these linkages may be one of the most important research questions yet to be examined. Assessment of dyadic behaviors requires more resources and coordinated efforts to retain both partners. Because standard statistical methods assume independence, more complicated data analysis addressing the non-independence data issue is needed. Kenny et al (2006) provide an excellent resource on a variety of research designs to analyze dyadic data (e.g., structural equation modeling, longitudinal analyses).

6 Conclusions

Modalities and content of sexual behavior assessment best suited for a specific study will vary along several dimensions. The relative advantages of various methods require a careful weighing of administration approach (i.e., interviewer-, self-, or computer administered) as well as assessment targets (i.e., what behaviors to assess over what time frames using which response formats). Assessment decisions are decided optimally in the context of study populations and data collection context. The sensitive and private nature of sexual behavior places unique constraints on such assessments, including the absence of objective verifiable measures. New and improving technologies are increasing the assessment alternatives, suggesting that, in the future, our choices will be enhanced. It is likely that the expanded armamentarium of options will allow investigators to tailor their choices to the situation, resulting in improved reliability and validity of the data collected, and improved understanding of sexual behavior and its antecedents and consequences.

Acknowledgments Funding: The preparation of this chapter was supported by National Institute of Mental Health grants to Seth C. Kalichman (R01-MH71164) and Michael P. Carey (R01-MH068171).

References

Abraham, C., and Sheeran, P. (1994). Modelling and modifying young heterosexuals' HIV-preventive behaviour; a review of theories, findings and educational implications. *Patient Educ Couns, 23*, 173–186.

Al-Tayyib, A. A., Rogers, S. M., Gribble, J. N., Villarroel, M., and Turner, C. F. (2002). Effect of low medical literacy on health survey measurements. *Am J Public Health, 92*, 1478–1480.

Baer, A., Saroiu, S., and Koutsky, L. A. (2002). Obtaining sensitive data through the Web: an example of design and methods. *Epidemiology, 13*, 640–645.

Basile, K. C., Chen, J., Black, M. C., and Saltzman, L. E. (2007). Prevalence and characteristics of sexual violence victimization among U.S. adults, 2001–2003. *Violence Vict, 22*, 437–448.

Biglan, A., Noell, J., Ochs, L., Smolkowski, K., and Metzler, C. (1995). Does sexual coercion play a role in the high-risk sexual behavior of adolescent and young adult women? *J Behav Med, 18*, 549–568.

Boekeloo, B. O., Schiavo, L., Rabin, D. L., Conlon, R. T., Jordan, C. S. et al (1994). Self-reports of HIV risk factors by patients at a sexually transmitted disease clinic: audio vs. written questionnaires. *Am J Public Health, 84*, 754–760.

Bogart, L. M., Walt, L. C., Pavlovic, J. D., Ober, A. J., Brown, N. et al (2007). Cognitive strategies affecting recall of sexual behavior among high-risk men and women. *Health Psychol, 26*, 787–793.

Bolger, N., Davis, A., and Rafaeli, E. (2003). Diary methods: capturing life as it is lived. *Annu Rev Psychol, 54*, 579–616.

Booth-Kewley, S., Larson, G. E., and Miyoshi, D. K. (2007). Social desirability effects on computerized and paper-and-pencil questionnaires. *Comput Human Behav, 23*, 463–477.

Bortz, W. M., 2nd, and Wallace, D. H. (1999). Physical fitness, aging, and sexuality. *West J Med, 170*, 167–169.

Brody, S. (2006). Blood pressure reactivity to stress is better for people who recently had penile-vaginal intercourse than for people who had other or no sexual activity. *Biol Psychol, 71*, 214–222.

Burkholder, G. J., and Harlow, L. L. (1996). Using structural equation modeling techniques to evaluate HIV risk models. *Struct Eq Model, 3*, 348–368.

Carey, M. P., Carey, K. B., Maisto, S. A., Gordon, C. M., and Weinhardt, L. S. (2001). Assessing sexual risk behaviour with the Timeline Followback (TLFB) approach: continued development and psychometric evaluation with psychiatric outpatients. *Int J STD AIDS, 12*, 365–375.

Carey, M. P., Gordon, C. M., Morrison-Beedy, D., and McLean, D. A. (1997). Low-income women and HIV risk reduction: elaborations from qualitative research. *AIDS Behav, 1*, 163–168.

Catania, J. A., Gibson, D. R., Chitwood, D. D., and Coates, T. J. (1990). Methodological problems in AIDS behavioral research: influences on measurement error and participation bias in studies of sexual behavior. *Psychol Bull, 108*, 339–362.

Center for Disease Control and Prevention. (2009). Trends in reportable sexually transmitted diseases in the United States, 2007. http://www.cdc.gov/STD/stats07/trends.pdf.

Cecil, H., Pinkerton, S. D., Bogart, L. M., Pavlovic, J., and Kimball, A. M. (2005). An empirical study of ordinal condom use measures. *J Sex Res, 42*, 353–358.

Cecil, H., and Zimet, G. D. (1998). Meanings assigned by undergraduates to frequency statements of condom use. *Arch Sex Behav, 27*, 493–505.

Charnetski, C. J., and Brennan, F. X. (2004). Sexual frequency and salivary immunoglobulin A (IgA). *Psychol Rep, 94*, 839–844.

Costa, R. M., and Brody, S. (2007). Women's relationship quality is associated with specifically penile-vaginal intercourse orgasm and frequency. *J Sex Marital Ther, 33*, 319–327.

Cutler, W. B., Preti, G., Huggins, G. R., Erickson, B., and Garcia, C. R. (1985). Sexual behavior frequency and biphasic ovulatory type menstrual cycles. *Physiol Behav, 34*, 805–810.

Darke, S., Hall, W., Heather, N., Ward, J., and Wodak, A. (1991). The reliability and validity of a scale to measure HIV risk-taking behaviour among intravenous drug users. *AIDS, 5*, 181–185.

Davey Smith, G., Frankel, S., and Yarnell, J. (1997). Sex and death: are they related? Findings from the Caerphilly Cohort Study. *BMJ, 315,* 1641–1644.

Davis, C. M., Yarber, W. L., Bauserman, R., Schreer, G., and Davis, S. L. (Eds.). (1998). *Handbook of Sexuality-Related Measures.* Thousand Oaks, CA: Sage.

Durant, L. E., and Carey, M. P. (2000). Self-administered questionnaires versus face-to-face interviews in assessing sexual behavior in young women. *Arch Sex Behav, 29,* 309–322.

Ebrahim, S., May, M., Ben Shlomo, Y., McCarron, P., Frankel, S. et al (2002). Sexual intercourse and risk of ischaemic stroke and coronary heart disease: the Caerphilly study. *J Epidemiol Community Health, 56,* 99–102.

Fishbein, M., and Pequegnat, W. (2000). Evaluating AIDS prevention interventions using behavioral and biological outcome measures. *Sex Transm Dis, 27,* 101–110.

Friedrich, W. N., Lysne, M., Sim, L., and Shamos, S. (2004). Assessing sexual behavior in high-risk adolescents with the adolescent clinical sexual behavior inventory (ACSBI). *Child Maltreat, 9*(3), 239–250.

Gibson, D. R., Hudes, E. S., and Donovan, D. (1999). Estimating and correcting for response bias in self-reported HIV risk behavior. *J Sex Res, 36,* 96–101.

Godoy, C. G. (2007). *Using Virtual Environments to Unobtrusively Measure Real-Life Risk-Taking: Findings and Implications for Health Communication Interventions.* Unpublished Dissertation, University of Southern California.

Graham, C. A., Catania, J. A., Brand, R., Duong, T., and Canchola, J. A. (2003). Recalling sexual behavior: a methodological analysis of memory recall bias via interview using the diary as the gold standard. *J Sex Res, 40,* 325–332.

Graham, C. A., Crosby, R. A., Sanders, S. A., and Yarber, W. L. (2005). Assessment of condom use in men and women. *Annu Rev Sex Res, 16,* 20–52.

Green, A. S., Rafaeli, E., Bolger, N., Shrout, P. E., and Reis, H. T. (2006). Paper or plastic? Data equivalence in paper and electronic diaries. *Psychol Methods, 11,* 87–105.

Hall, H. I., Song, R., Rhodes, P., Prejean, J., An, Q. et al (2008). Estimation of HIV incidence in the United States. *JAMA, 300,* 520–529.

Jaccard, J., McDonald, R., Wan, C. K., Dittus, P. J., and Quinlan, S. (2002). The accuracy of self-reports of condom use and sexual behavior. *J Appl Soc Psychol, 32,* 1863–1905.

Kalichman, S. C., Benotsch, E., Suarez, T., Catz, S., Miller, J. et al (2000). Health literacy and health-related knowledge among persons living with HIV/AIDS. *Am J Prev Med, 18,* 325–331.

Kauth, M. R., St Lawrence, J. S., and Kelly, J. A. (1991). Reliability of retrospective assessments of sexual HIV risk behavior: a comparison of biweekly, three-month, and twelve-month self-reports. *AIDS Educ Prev, 3,* 207–214.

Kenny, D. A., Kashy, D. A., and Cook, W. L. (2006). *Dyadic Data Analysis.* New York: Guilford Press.

Kinsey, A. C., Pomeroy, W. R., and Martin, C. E. (2003). Sexual behavior in the human male. 1948. *Am J Public Health, 93,* 894–898.

Kutner, M., Greenberg, E., Jin, Y., Boyle, B., Hsu, Y. et al (2007). Literacy in everyday life: results from the 2003 National Assessment of Adult Literacy (NCES 2007480) (Vol. U.S. Department of Education). Washington, DC: National Center for Education.

Kutner, M., Greenberg, E., Jin, Y., and Paulsen, C. (2006). The Health Literacy of America's Adults: Results From the 2003 National Assessment of Adult Literacy (NCES 2006–483) (Vol. U.S. Department of Education). Washington, DC: National Center for Education.

Lau, J. T. F., Thomas, J., and Liu, J. L. Y. (2000). Mobile phone and interactive computer interviewing to measure HIV-related risk behaviours: the impacts of data collection methods on research results. *AIDS, 14,* 1277–1279.

Laumann, E. O., Paik, A., Glasser, D. B., Kang, J. H., Wang, T. et al (2006). A cross-national study of subjective sexual well-being among older women and men: findings from the Global Study of Sexual Attitudes and Behaviors. *Arch Sex Behav, 35,* 145–161.

Leitzmann, M. F., Platz, E. A., Stampfer, M. J., Willett, W. C., and Giovannucci, E. (2004). Ejaculation frequency and subsequent risk of prostate cancer. *JAMA, 291,* 1578–1586.

McAuliffe, T. L., DiFranceisco, W., and Reed, B. R. (2007). Effects of question format and collection mode on the accuracy of retrospective surveys of health risk behavior: a comparison with daily sexual activity diaries. *Health Psychol, 26,* 60–67.

Miner, M. H., Robinson, B. E., Hoffman, L., Albright, C. L., and Bockting, W. O. (2002a). Improving safer sex measures through the inclusion of relationship and partner characteristics. *AIDS Care, 14,* 827–837.

Miner, M. H., Robinson, B. E., Hoffman, L., Albright, C. L., and Bockting, W. O. (2002b). Improving safer sex measures through the inclusion of relationship and partner characteristics. *AIDS Care, 14,* 827–837.

Needle, R., Fisher, D. G., Weatherby, N., Chitwood, D., Brown, B. et al (1995). Reliability of self-reported HIV risk behaviors of drug users. *Psychol Addict Behav, 9,* 242–250.

Noar, S. M., Cole, C., and Carlyle, K. (2006). Condom Use Measurement in 56 studies of sexual risk behavior: review and recommendations. *Arch Sex Behav, 35,* 327–345.

Ostrow, D. G., DiFranceisco, W. J., Chmiel, J. S., Wagstaff, D. A., and Wesch, J. (1995). A case-control study of human immunodeficiency virus type 1 seroconversion and risk-related behaviors in the Chicago MACS/CCS Cohort, 1984–1992. Multicenter AIDS

Cohort Study. Coping and Change Study. *Am J Epidemiol, 142*, 875–883.

Parish, W. L., Luo, Y., Stolzenberg, R., Laumann, E. O., Farrer, G. et al (2007). Sexual practices and sexual satisfaction: a population based study of Chinese urban adults. *Arch Sex Behav, 36*, 5–20.

Patterson, T. L., and Strathdee, S. A. (2005). From Don Giovanni to Magic Johnson: methodological conundrums in the measurement of sexual risk behavior. *Ann Behav Med, 29*, 83–85.

Pequegnat, W., Rosser, B. R., Bowen, A. M., Bull, S. S., DiClemente, R. J. et al (2007). Conducting Internet-based HIV/STD prevention survey research: considerations in design and evaluation. *AIDS Behav, 11*, 505–521.

Reik, T. (1983). *Listening with the Third Ear*. New York: Farrar, Straus, and Giroux.

Renaud, P., Rouleau, J. L., Granger, L., Barsetti, I., and Bouchard, S. (2002). Measuring sexual preferences in virtual reality: a pilot study. *Cyberpsychol Behav, 5*, 1–9.

Rhodes, S. D., Bowie, D. A., and Hergenrather, K. C. (2003). Collecting behavioural data using the world wide web: considerations for researchers. *J Epidemiol Community Health, 57*, 68–73.

Robinson, B. B., Bockting, W. O., Rosser, B. R., Miner, M., and Coleman, E. (2002). The Sexual Health Model: application of a sexological approach to HIV prevention. *Health Educ Res, 17*, 43–57.

Robinson, R., and West, R. (1992). A comparison of computer and questionnaire methods of history-taking in a genito-urinary clinic. *Psychol Health, 6*, 77–84.

Sangi-Haghpeykar, H., Ambani, D. S., and Carson, S. A. (2009). Stress, workload, sexual well-being and quality of life among physician residents in training. *Int J Clin Pract, 63*(3), 462–467.

Schroder, K. E., Carey, M. P., and Vanable, P. A. (2003a). Methodological challenges in research on sexual risk behavior: I. Item content, scaling, and data analytical options. *Ann Behav Med, 26*, 76–103.

Schroder, K. E., Carey, M. P., and Vanable, P. A. (2003b). Methodological challenges in research on sexual risk behavior: II. Accuracy of self-reports. *Ann Behav Med, 26*, 104–123.

Sheeran, P., and Abraham, C. (1994). Measurement of condom use in 72 studies of HIV-preventive behaviour: a critical review. *Patient Educ Couns, 24*, 199–216.

Sobell, L. C., and Sobell, M. B. (1996). *Timeline Followback Users Guide*. Toronto, Canada: Alcohol Research Foundation.

Stone, A. A., and Shiffman, S. (2002). Capturing momentary, self-report data: a proposal for reporting guidelines. *Ann Behav Med, 24*, 236–243.

Tourangeau, R., and Smith, T. W. (1996). Asking sensitive questions: the impact of data collection mode, question format, and question context. *Public Opinion Quarterly, 60*, 275–304.

Turner, C. F., Ku, L., Rogers, S. M., Lindberg, L. D., Pleck, J. H. et al (1998). Adolescent sexual behavior, drug use, and violence: increased reporting with computer survey technology. *Science, 280*, 867–873.

Weinhardt, L. S., Carey, M. P., Maisto, S. A., Carey, K. B., Cohen, M. M. et al (1998a). Reliability of the timeline follow-back sexual behavior interview. *Ann Behav Med, 20*, 25–30.

Weinhardt, L. S., Forsyth, A. D., Carey, M. P., Jaworski, B. C., and Durant, L. E. (1998b). Reliability and validity of self-report measures of HIV-related sexual behavior: progress since 1990 and recommendations for research and practice. *Arch Sex Behav, 27*, 155–180.

Whipple, B. (2006). The health benefits of sexual expression. In M. S. Tepper & A. F. Owens (Eds.), *Sexual Health, Vol. 1* (pp. 17–42). Westport, CT: Greenwood.

White, J. R., Case, D. A., McWhirter, D., and Mattison, A. M. (1990). Enhanced sexual behavior in exercising men. *Arch Sex Behav, 19*, 193–209.

Whittier, D. K., Lawrence, J. S., and Seeley, S. (2005). Sexual risk behavior of men who have sex with men: comparison of behavior at home and at a gay resort. *Arch Sex Behav, 34*, 95–102.

World Health Organization (WHO). (2006). Defining sexual health: report of a technical consultation on sexual health. http://www.who.int/reproductive-health/publications/sexualhealth/index.html.

Wilcox, A. J., Weinberg, C. R., and Baird, D. D. (1995). Timing of sexual intercourse in relation to ovulation. Effects on the probability of conception, survival of the pregnancy, and sex of the baby. *N Engl J Med, 333*, 1517–1521.

Wincze, J. P., and Carey, M. P. (2001). *Sexual Dysfunction: A Guide for Assessment and Treatment, 2nd Ed*. New York, NY: Guilford Press.

Chapter 6

By Force of Habit

Bas Verplanken

1 By Force of Habit

Many behaviors of interest in behavioral medicine are highly repetitive. This holds of course for addictive behaviors, such as smoking and drinking alcohol, but also for many other behaviors that may have health consequences, such as eating, exercising, and hygiene-related behaviors. A number of popular socio-cognitive models in health psychology describe determinants of health behavior, such as the Health Belief Model (Janz and Becker, 1984), Protection Motivation Theory (e.g., Rogers and Mewborn, 1976), and the Theory of Planned Behavior (Ajzen, 1991). However, none of these models include constructs that represent the repetitive nature of behavior, such as an assessment of past behavior. The models implicitly suggest that past behavior influences future behavior through the model components. Yet, when past behavior is taken into the equation, it appears a powerful predictor of later behavior over and above the model variables (e.g., Albarracín et al, 2001).

Repetitive behaviors not only outperform the predictive power of socio-cognitive models, they also seem to pose limits on the validity of the models. In a meta-analysis of studies that included assessments of behavioral intentions, past behavior, and later behavior, Ouellette and Wood (1998) found that intentions, which are the most proximal predictors of behavior in the prevalent socio-cognitive models, predict behaviors fairly well when these are infrequently performed. However, when behaviors occur frequently, the predictive power of intentions attenuates, and past behavior becomes the strongest predictor (Triandis, 1980). A number of recent primary studies confirmed this notion (de Bruijn et al, 2007; Ferguson and Bibby, 2002; Ji and Wood, 2007; Verplanken et al, 1998). It thus seems that habitual behavior is no longer guided by conscious considerations or motivation, but is governed by other processes. This would of course have major implications for strategies to change habitual behaviors.

Why would such effects occur? As frequency of behavior in itself has no explanatory value (Ajzen, 2002), we need to focus in more detail on the concept of habit. In this chapter, I will thus first address the question what habits are and how they operate, and discuss variants of habits. I then address implications for interventions aimed at changing health behaviors. I will end the chapter by discussing the measurement of habit.

2 The Three Pillars of Habit

Three aspects are central to the nature of habits: a habit is behavior that is frequently performed, has acquired a high degree of automaticity, and is cued in stable contexts. These three pillars of habit will be elaborated in the following.

B. Verplanken (✉)
Department of Psychology, University of Bath,
Claverton Down, Bath, BA2 7AY, UK
e-mail: b.verplanken@bath.ac.uk

A. Steptoe (ed.), *Handbook of Behavioral Medicine*, DOI 10.1007/978-0-387-09488-5_6,
© Springer Science+Business Media, LLC 2010

2.1 Frequency

Psychologists have traditionally defined habit as frequency of past behavior. This conception stems from the behaviorist school, which focused primarily on overt behavior as the scientific object of interest (e.g., Hull, 1943). The behaviorist notion of what habits are (the number of repetitions of a behavior) and how they are formed (the impact of reinforcers) have remained relatively unchanged throughout the history of psychology, in spite of what has been known as the "cognitive revolution," which followed the decline of behaviorism. However, defining habit as frequency of past behavior is problematic for at least three reasons (Verplanken, 2006). The first is the question at which frequency we would designate a behavior as a habit. Ronis et al (1989) suggested that a behavior acquires habitual quality "...only if the behavior has been repeated both frequently (at least twice a month) and extensively (at least 10 times)" (p. 213). However, no rationale was given for this notion. A more serious concern is that frequent behavior does not necessarily imply a habit (Ajzen, 2002): "No matter how often we may have climbed the same mountain, it is difficult to believe that this behavior has become routine in the sense of constituting an automatic response sequence. Behaviors of this kind require conscious control, even after they have been performed many times" (p. 109). Frequency of behavior is thus a necessary but not sufficient feature to qualify a behavior as habitual. Indeed, a number of studies in which independent measures of habit were included in addition to measures of past behavior, demonstrated that the two constructs are not equivalent, and independently contribute to the prediction of intentions (Knussen and Yule, 2008), later behavior (Verplanken, 2006, Study 1), or habit strength measured at a later point in time (Verplanken and Melkevik, 2008).

2.2 Automaticity

Habits are characterized by automaticity (Aarts and Dijksterhuis, 2000; Aarts et al, 1998;

Sheeran et al, 2005; Verplanken and Aarts, 1999). The automaticity component, and not frequency per se, is likely to be responsible for why habits are experienced as natural elements of everyday life. We do not experience "making a travel mode decision" when commuting to work. Rather, we experience a sense of fluency and smoothness when taking the car.

Automaticity is not an all-or-none phenomenon. Bargh (1994) suggested to break down the concept into four features: lack of awareness, lack of conscious intent, the difficulty to control, and mental efficiency. A particular automatic process may thus include all or a combination of these features. For instance, lack of awareness and conscious intent may characterize habitual hand washing, while the difficulty to resist (lack of control) is a defining aspect of habitual snacking.

Habit automaticity is evident in minimal awareness, in the sense that people engage in shallow information processing when they perform a habit. Aarts et al (1997) demonstrated that habits were associated with using heuristic-based decision rules in making travel mode choices. Such decisions are based on using few attributes and thus require minimal mental effort. In another experiment, participants who had strong habits in one particular travel mode tended to ignore information about alternative options (Verplanken et al, 1997, Study 1), and needed less information about the nature of unknown travel mode choice situations before making choices (Verplanken et al, 1997, Study 2). Repeated exposure to stimuli also renders people insensitive to perceiving changes in the stimulus environment (Fazio et al, 2000). Taken together, strong habit individuals have a "tunnel vision" in that they are less interested in and attentive to information about available options and the context in which their habits are executed.

2.3 Context Cuing

The third pillar of habit relates to the context in which habits are performed and the process of eliciting a habitual response. Habits are intrinsically tied to the performance context. Behaviors such as snacking, exercising, hand washing, or purchasing food are typically performed at the same place and at the same time (Wood et al, 2002, 2005). In the behaviorist tradition a large body of knowledge has been built on how habits form. Paramount to habit formation is the systematic pairing of a cue, a response, and reinforcement. Operant conditioning forges the propensity to respond automatically to specific cues in a behavioral context. Habit formation and maintenance can thus only be expected to occur if performance contexts are stable, i.e., if the same cues reappear in the same fashion every time an individual is engaged in that context.

Wood and Neal (2007) suggested that habit cuing may occur in different fashions. A habitual response may be elicited by direct cuing. According to these authors, repeated coactivation of responses and contexts create associative links in memory. Context cues may activate those links and thus initiate the habitual response. Wood and Neal (2007) suggest a second, "hot," form of cuing in which the reward value of the response is conditioned into context cues. This was labeled motivated cuing. In this case the habitual response to a cue has a history of incentive conditioning, which empowers context cues with signaling reward.

It is important to note that cues may involve a wide spectrum of variants, including location, time, the presence of particular people, or internal states such as hunger or mood (e.g., Ji and Wood, 2007). Likewise, a wide range of reinforcers may be present, including physiological reinforcers such as satiation, social reinforcers such as approval, or efficiency such as time, money, or the absence of the need to deliberate. In order to understand particular habits it is extremely important to have insight into which contexts, cues, responses and reinforcers are at work.

Thisthird pillar of habit provides a bridge to a sociological analysis of habit as behavior that is part of wider socially and culturally defined social practices. For instance, Reckwitz (2002) describes a "practice" as unit of analysis. Practices are interconnected complexes of bodily and mental activities, objects, spaces as well as specific forms of knowledge (including emotions and desires), discourses, and language. For instance, "going out" may be defined as such a practice. In being socially or culturally defined, practices are routinized phenomena. Individuals are the agents that carry them out. Habits may be part of practices, which thus incorporate the context and cues that trigger habitual responses. The habit of binge drinking or eating junk food may thus be part of the practice of going out. Habits may thus be considered a wider and socially meaningful perspective.

3 Varieties of Habit

Although all habits share the features that were discussed as the three pillars of habit, i.e., frequent occurrence, automaticity, and context cuing, a wide variety of habits exist across the spectrum of health behaviors. In this section, I address the question where habits are located, levels of construal, and introduce mental habits.

3.1 The Location of a Habit

When we move away from simple habits such as nail biting or whistling to the behaviors that are of interest in behavioral medicine, we deal with complex, multi-layered, and multi-faceted behaviors. For instance, exercising includes decision-making and planning, preparation, and a sequence of behaviors when exercising is executed. Unhealthy snacking may start with purchasing unhealthy food items, may be embedded in other activities such as travelling or work, and may involve a mental component in the form of negative self-thinking or low self-esteem (Verplanken et al, 2005). It may thus often be difficult to locate where exactly the habit resides. In the case of exercising, the key habitual moment might be the moment of decision-making, whereas the exercising behaviors may be conducted and enjoyed mindfully (Verplanken and Melkevik, 2008). In the unhealthy snacking example it may be the impulsive purchasing of snacks which is crucial. In order to investigate a particular habit, it is thus necessary to analyze which part of the chain of events is the critical habitual part.

3.2 General Versus Specific Habits

Vallacher and Wegner (1987) contended that behaviors can be identified at various levels, ranging from a concrete and mechanistic level (e.g., eating a chocolate bar) to a more abstract and comprehensive level (e.g., high-calorie snacking). We thus may identify habits at different levels of construal. A particular habit may be innocent when it operates at a specific lower level, but harmful when it operates at higher levels. For example, suppose person A likes chocolate, frequently eats a chocolate bar, but has a perfectly healthy diet otherwise. Person B also frequently eats chocolate bars, but has a habit of eating sweet and fatty foods whenever he can. Person A simply likes chocolate. Person B's chocolate eating is thus part of a higher order habit, which designates an unhealthy and perhaps dangerous lifestyle. The level of construal is also important from a public health perspective, as higher order unhealthy habits add up to unhealthy populations.

3.3 Mental Habits

The habit concept may not have to be confined to overt behaviors, but is applicable to mental processes as well, in particular frequent recurrent thinking (Watkins, 2008). Thoughts that occur frequently and are elicited automatically in response to specific cues may thus qualify as a mental habit. In a comprehensive research program, Verplanken et al (2007) investigated negative self-thinking as mental habit. In these

studies, the habitual quality of negative self-thinking was pitted against the content of such thinking. Having negative self-thoughts every now and then is part of a healthy mental life, e.g., being self-critical at times, learning from past mistakes, or being aware of one's weaknesses. However, when negative self-thoughts occur frequently and automatically they may become dysfunctional. Verplanken et al (2007) indeed found that the mental habit component of negative self-thinking accounted for unique variance in explicit and implicit measures of self-esteem. Similar results were found in a longitudinal study over 9 months on anxiety and depression, even after controlling for traditional vulnerability measures such as previous symptoms, dysfunctional attitudes, and negative life events. Habitual negative thinking has also been found important in the more specific area of body image. Dissatisfied body image thinking is an increasing problem and is particularly associated with eating disturbances among young people in Western cultures (e.g., Thompson and Smolak, 2001). In a sample of 12–15 years old adolescents it was found that habitual negative thinking about appearance accounted for variance in self-esteem and eating disturbance propensity over and above the contributions of gender, age, and body dissatisfaction (Verplanken and Velsvik, 2008; see also Verplanken and Tangelder, 2010). In all, a mental habit seems a viable concept, which shows satisfactory construct and discriminant validity.

4 Breaking and Creating Habit

An important reason to study habit is the importance of the concept for behavior change. It is almost tautological to say that habits are difficult to change. However, this requires some more detailed scrutiny. I will briefly follow two strands of thought, on breaking old habits and creating new ones, respectively (see Verplanken and Wood, 2006, for a more detailed account), and bring these together by discussing the concept of habit discontinuity.

4.1 Breaking Habit

Frequency per se needs not be a barrier for behavioral change. What makes habits difficult to change is above all related to the other two pillars: automaticity and context cuing. This is particularly problematic when information-based interventions such as mass media campaigns are employed as a vehicle for change. As I explained in the beginning of this chapter, habit fosters conditions of minimal awareness and tunnel vision. Clearly, this does not bode well for the effectiveness of information campaigns. Even if campaigns change attitudes and intentions, the finding that habits attenuate the link between intentions and behavior suggests that investing in interventions that aim for attitude and motivation change is not an effective strategy. Another reason why informational campaigns may not easily affect habits is that these do not change the context cuing effect. The power of contextual cuing suggests that habituation shifts some control over behavior from an internal locus (e.g., an individual's willpower) to the external environment, and thus beyond the reach of information campaigns. Behavior change strategies that include modifications of the performance context, such as infrastructural changes, are thus deemed more effective.

4.2 Creating Habit

The features that make unhealthy habits resistant to change are the very features we would like healthy behaviors to acquire. Intervention planning often designates behavior change as the principle objective. However, although behavior change is of course an important milestone, habituation of the new behavior might be adopted as an intervention goal as well. Principles that govern habituation, such as reinforcement schedules, have been extensively investigated in the behaviorist tradition (e.g., Hull, 1943). These principles may thus be taken

into account when designing behavior change interventions. Lally et al (2010) demonstrated how habituation might be monitored. She asked participants to adopt a new, healthy, daily behavior, and obtained measures of habit strength every day over a period of 12 weeks. The habituation curves that resulted for each participant provided information on features such as the speed of habituation and degree of automaticity of the behavior.

4.3 Habit Discontinuities

Opportunities to break existing habits and build new ones may come together when people undergo naturally occurring changes that may, at least temporarily, disrupt existing routines (Verplanken and Wood, 2006). Such discontinuities may occur, for instance, because of moving house, starting a family, changing jobs, or retirement. Discontinuities may also arise from external changes, such as a period of economic downturn or new laws and regulations such as the smoking ban or congestion tax. In terms of our habit model, such discontinuities imply that habitual cue-response links are broken and the individual has to re-negotiate new solutions. During such windows of opportunity, individuals may be more open to information that assists or persuades them to find new solutions. Although this may seem an obvious suggestion, there has been little systematic empirical work to test this *habit discontinuity hypothesis* (Verplanken and Wood, 2006; Verplanken et al, 2008). Some studies provided circumstantial evidence in line with this hypothesis. Bamberg (2006) successfully delivered an intervention to promote the use of public transport after participants had moved residence. Verplanken et al (2008) found that university employees who had recently moved *and* were environmentally concerned commuted less frequently by car compared to those who were also environmentally concerned but had not recently moved. However, the habit discontinuity hypothesis awaits more rigorous testing.

5 The Measurement of Habit

In their seminal book *The Psychology of Attitudes*, Eagly and Chaiken (1993) wrote: "... the role of habit *per se* remains indeterminate (...) because of the difficulty of designing adequate measures of habit" (p. 181). The domain of habit seemed indeed to have stalled for a very long time. A major reason may be that habit has always been equated with behavioral frequency. As the measurement of a construct is intrinsically linked to the theory one has about the construct, the lack of progress in measuring habit strength can be traced back to the theoretical and conceptual problems that were inherited from the behaviorist school. However, to date a variety of measures are available, each of which has its strengths and weaknesses.

5.1 Frequency of Past Behavior

The most prevalent operationalization of habit is measures of self-reported frequency of past behavior. These may take the form of asking respondents how often they performed a particular behavior during some specified time frame. Responses are usually given on a bipolar response scale, for instance, a five-point scale ranging from *never* to *always*. The most obvious problem of this measure is that one-item measures are notoriously unreliable. There is of course an accuracy problem if one wants to assess objective frequency, rather than the experience of frequency. This particularly holds if such judgments rely on individuals' episodic memory, which is not likely to store traces of frequently occurring behavioral episodes. The most serious concern, however, is the conceptual problem that frequent behavior is not necessarily habitual. In other words, the measure only captures one of the three pillars of habit.

5.2 Past Behavioral Frequency and Habit Combined

Some authors assessed habit by adding statements such as "by force of habit" or "without awareness" (e.g., Mittal, 1988; Wittenbraker et al, 1983) to a self-reported frequency of past behavioral item (e.g. How often did you use your seatbelt during the past month by force of habit?). However, this measure should be disqualified due to its double-barreled nature: respondents are asked to provide one response to two different questions, i.e., on frequency and the degree to which they performed the behavior by force of habit.

5.3 Response Frequency Measure

The response frequency measure of habit was developed to assess habit strength in multiple choice contexts (e.g. Verplanken et al, 1994). Participants are presented with a series of situations and are asked to make a choice from multiple alternatives in each of these situations. For instance, in the context of travel mode choices participants were presented with situations such as going to the supermarket or visiting a friend in town, and a range of travel mode options as choice alternatives. The task is to be conducted under time pressure. The invariance of choices across situations (e.g., the number of times the car is chosen in a travel mode context) was then taken as an assessment of habit strength. The measure thus capitalizes on the automaticity component of habit, i.e., the assumption that under time pressure schematic or script-based responses will be elicited. Although the response frequency measure shows good test–retest reliability (Aarts, 1996) as well as construct and discriminant validity (e.g., Verplanken et al, 1998), it has some practical and conceptual limitations. For instance, new sets of situations need to be developed and tested in each new research context. The required time pressure prevents the measure to be used in self-paced questionnaires. Finally, the measure may be confounded with intentions or preferences.

5.4 Habit as a Reason for Behavior

Knussen and colleagues presented participants with lists of pre-tested reasons why one would recycle household waste (Knussen et al, 2004).

One of the alternatives was "because it is a habit." This measure rests on the assumption that people have insight into the reasons behind their behavior. Although this is not an unreasonable assumption in itself, it is questionable whether habit can qualify as a *reason* for behavior. In addition, the one-item format of the measure renders it potentially unreliable, and one may question whether people have unanimous interpretations of the concept of habit. For instance, habit may indeed be interpreted as repetitive and automatic behavior, but it is also used to refer to "bad" behaviors. This measure thus requires further testing and validation.

5.5 A Context-Focused Habit Measure

Wood and colleagues introduced a measure of habit strength that combines two pillars of habit: the frequency of past behavior and the stability of the context in which the habit occurs (e.g., Wood et al, 2005). The frequency aspect is measured as has traditionally been done by a one-item measure asking participants how often they performed the behavior. As an assessment of context stability participants are asked to indicate the extent to which they perform the behavior under similar circumstances. This may be operationalized by a single item (e.g. Danner et al, 2008) or by multiple items, such as items referring to location and time (e.g. Ji and Wood, 2007; Wood et al, 2005). The frequency item is then multiplied with the context item(s) to form (a) measure(s) of habit strength. By combining frequency with context stability, this measure is an improvement of the one-item frequency measure, although it still has potential reliability problems.

5.6 Self-Report Habit Index

Verplanken and Orbell (2003) developed the Self-Report Habit Index (SRHI). The SRHI is a generic 12-item instrument, which assesses

the experience of frequency and automaticity of behavior, i.e., two of the three pillars of habit. The experience of automaticity is broken down into a number of facets, i.e., the lack of awareness and conscious intent, mental efficiency, and difficulty to control (Bargh, 1994). In addition, the SRHI includes the experience of behavior being self-descriptive. The instrument is presented in Table 6.1. Verplanken and Orbell (2003) validated the SRHI in a number of studies and domains. For instance, the SRHI discriminates between repetitive behaviors that are executed weekly versus repetitive behaviors that are executed daily. Verplanken (2006, Study 3) showed that the measure discriminates between repetitive behavior that is executed in an automatic versus deliberative fashion (e.g., when behavior is easy versus difficult).

Table 6.1 The Self-Report Habit Index (Verplanken and Orbell, 2003)

Behavior X is something .....
1. I do frequently.
2. I do automatically.
3. I do without having to consciously remember.
4. That makes me feel weird if I do not do it.
5. I do without thinking.
6. That would require effort not to do it.
7. That belongs to my (daily, weekly, monthly) routine.
8. I start doing before I realize I am doing it.
9. I would find hard not to do.
10. I have no need to think about doing.
11. That is typically "me."
12. I have been doing for a long time.

Note: Five- or seven-point response scales anchored with "strongly disagree" and "strongly agree" may be used. From Verplanken and Orbell (2003, p. 1329). Copyright 2003 by John Wiley & Sons. Permission for reproduction should be sought.

To date the SRHI has been successfully used in a large variety of domains, such as food or snack consumption (Brug et al, 2006; Conner et al, 2007; de Bruijn et al, 2007; Honkanen et al, 2005; Verplanken et al, 2005), consumption of beverages (Kremers et al, 2007), food safety practices (Hinsz et al, 2007), physical activity (Chatzisarantis and Hagger, 2007; Verplanken and Melkevik, 2008), weight loss (Lally, 2007), Internet use (Lintvedt et al, 2008), and social behavior (Verplanken, 2004). The

12 items usually show high internal reliabilities (> 0.90), and satisfactory test–retest reliabilities of 0.71 over 1 week for unhealthy snacking (e.g., Verplanken, 2006) and 0.87 over 1 month for exercising (Verplanken and Melkevik, 2008) have been obtained. Importantly, Conner et al (2007) showed that the SRHI moderated the relationships between implicit measures of attitude and behavior, while no moderation was found in the relationship between explicit measures and behavior. These results validate the relationship between the SRHI and automaticity.

5.7 Conclusions

Which is the best measure? First, the availability of a set of different habit measures should be celebrated as an important step forward (Ajzen and Fishbein, 2005). The conceptual problem of the one-item self-reported past behavioral frequency measure (i.e., the fact that frequency is a necessary but not sufficient feature of habit), and potential reliability problems, renders this as an inadequate measure of habit. The combined one-item self-reported frequency and self-reported habit measure should not be used due to being double-barrelled. The habit-as-reason measure awaits further testing and validation. As for the other measures, each seems to capture some unique aspect of habit. Selecting the best alternative measure depends on the researcher's goal and the type of behavior under study. Different measures may also be used in conjunction with each other. The context-focused habit measure captures an important situational aspect of habitual behavior, i.e., context stability, in addition to past behavioral frequency. The response frequency measure (if properly applied) focuses on habits that are executed in multiple-choice contexts. The SRHI captures the experience of both frequency and automaticity and seems the most solid measure in terms of reliability and validity. In addition, this measure is generic and thus needs no adaptations or pilot testing for each new domain and can easily be used in questionnaires.

6 General Conclusions

Since the decline of behaviorism, habit has long been a forgotten concept in the social and behavioral sciences. This is the case in spite of the fact that many unhealthy behaviors are strongly habitual and that we would like to see healthy behaviors become habitual. The focus on deliberative thinking and motivated behavior such as represented by the prevalent socio-cognitive models may now be supplemented by the notion that these factors may wear off over time and be replaced by the more automatic and context-driven powers of habit (Dawes, 1998). The habit concept has much to offer to those who want to understand why people behave unhealthily, or why it remains such a challenge to establish healthier lifestyles. Researchers have now a choice of instruments at their disposal for measuring and monitoring habit strength. In all, habit theory seems a valuable contribution to the behavioral medicine field.

References

Aarts, H. (1996). *Habit and Decision Making: The Case of Travel Mode Choice*. Unpublished doctoral dissertation, University of Nijmegen, The Netherlands.

Aarts, H., and Dijksterhuis, A. (2000). Habits as knowledge structures: automaticity in goal-directed behavior. *J Pers Soc Psychol, 78*, 53–63.

Aarts, H., Verplanken, B., and van Knippenberg, A. (1997). Habit and information use in travel mode choices. *Acta Psychol, 96*, 1–14.

Aarts, H., Verplanken, B., and van Knippenberg, A. (1998). Predicting behavior from actions in the past: repeated decision-making or a matter of habit? *J Appl Soc Psychol, 28*, 1355–1374.

Ajzen, I. (1991). The theory of planned behavior. *Organ Behav Hum Decis Process, 50*, 179–211.

Ajzen, I. (2002). Residual effects of past on later behavior: habituation and reasoned action perspectives. *Pers Soc Psychol Rev, 6*, 107–122.

Ajzen, I., and Fishbein, M. (2005). The influence of attitudes on behavior. In D. Albarracín, B.T. Johnson, & M.P. Zanna (Eds.), *The Handbook of Attitudes* (pp. 173–221). Mahwah, NJ: Erlbaum.

Albarracín, D., Johnson, B. T., Fishbein, M., and Muellerleile, P. A. (2001). Theories of reasoned action and planned behavior as models of condom use: a meta-analysis. *Psychol Bull, 127*, 142–161.

Bamberg, S. (2006). Is a residential relocation a good opportunity to change people's travel behavior? Results from a theory-driven intervention study. *Environ Behav, 38*, 820–840.

Bargh, J. A. (1994). The four horsemen of automaticity: awareness, intention, efficiency, and control in social cognition. In: R. S. Wyer & T. K. Srull (Eds.), *Handbook of Social Cognition, vol. 1* (pp.1–40). Hillsdale, NJ: Erlbaum.

Brug, J., de Vet, E., Wind, M., de Nooijer, J., and Verplanken, B. (2006). Predicting fruit consumption: cognitions, intention, and habits. *J Nutr Educ Behav, 38*, 73–81.

Chatzisarantis, N. L., and Hagger, M. S. (2007). Mindfulness and the intention-behavior relationship within the theory of planned behavior. *Pers Soc Psychol Bull, 33*, 663–676.

Conner, M. T., Perugini, M., O'Gorman, R., Ayres, K., and Prestwich, A. (2007). Relations between implicit and explicit measures of attitude and behavior: evidence of moderation by individual difference variables. *Pers Soc Psychol Bull, 33*, 1727–1740.

Danner, U., Aarts, H., and de Vries, N. K. (2008). Habit vs. Intention in the prediction of future behaviour: the role of frequency, context stability and mental accessibility of past behaviour. *Br J Soc Psychol, 47*, 245–265.

Dawes, R. M. (1998). Behavioral decision making and judgment. In: D. T. Gilbert, S. T. Fiske, & G. Lindzey (Eds.), *The Handbook of Social Psychology, 4th Ed*, (pp. 497–548). Boston: McGraw-Hill.

de Bruijn, G.-J., Kremers, S., de Vet, E., de Nooijer, J., van Mechelen, W., and Brug, J. (2007). Does habit strength moderate the intention-behaviour relationship in the Theory of Planned Behaviour? The case of fruit consumption. *Psychol Health, 22*, 899–916.

Eagly, A. H., and Chaiken, S. (1993). *The Psychology of Attitudes*. Fort Worth, TX: Harcourt Brace Jovanovich.

Fazio, R. H., Ledbetter, J. E., and Towles-Schwen, T. (2000). On the costs of accessible attitudes: detecting that the attitude objects has changed. *J Pers Soc Psychol, 78*, 197–210.

Ferguson, E., and Bibby, P. A. (2002). Predicting future blood donor returns: past behavior, intentions, and observer effects. *Health Psychol, 21*, 513–518.

Hinsz, V. B., Nickell, G. S., and Park, E. S. (2007). The role of work habits in the motivation of food safety behaviors. *J Exp Psychol, 13*, 105–114.

Honkanen, P., Olsen, S. O., and Verplanken, B. (2005). Intention to consume seafood: the importance of habit strength. *Appetite, 45*, 161–168.

Hull, C. L. (1943). *Principles of Behaviour: An Introduction to Behaviour Theory*. New York: Appleton-Century Crofts.

Janz, N. K., and Becker, M. H. (1984). The health belief model: a decade later. *Health Educ Q, 11*, 1–47.

Ji, M. F., and Wood, W. (2007). Purchase and consumption habits: not necessarily what you intend. *J Consum Psychol, 17*, 261–276.

Knussen, C., and Yule, F. (2008). "I'm not in the habit of recycling": the role of habitual behavior in the disposal of household waste. *Environ Behav, 40*, 683–702.

Knussen, C., Yule, F., Mackenzie, J., and Wells, M. (2004). An analysis of intentions to recycle household waste: the roles of past behaviour, perceived habit, and perceived lack of facilities. *J Environ Psychol, 24*, 237–246.

Kremers, S. P., van der Horst, K., and Brug, J. (2007). Adolescent screen-viewing behaviour is associated with consumption of sugar-sweeted beverages: the role of habit strength and perceived parental norms. *Appetite, 48*, 345–350.

Lally, P. J. (2007). *Habitual Behavior and Weight Control*. Unpublished doctoral dissertation. University College London.

Lally, P., van Jaarsveld, C.H.M., Potts, H.W.W., and Wardle, J. (2010). How are habits formed: modelling habit formation in the real world. *Eur J Soc Psychol* (in press).

Lintvedt, O. K., Sørensen, K., Østvik, A. R., Verplanken, B., and Wang, C. E. (2008). The need for web-based cognitive behaviour therapy among university students. *J Tech Hum Serv, 26*, 239–258.

Mittal, B. (1988). Achieving higher seat belt usage: the role of habit in bridging the attitude-behavior gap. *J Appl Soc Psychol, 18*, 993–1016.

Ouellette, J. A., and Wood, W. (1998). Habit and intention in everyday life: the multiple processes by which past behavior predicts future behavior. *Psychol Bull, 124*, 54–74.

Reckwitz, A. (2002). Toward a theory of social practices. A development in culturalist theorizing. *Eur J Soc Theor, 5*, 243–263.

Rogers, R. W., and Mewborn, C. R. (1976). Fear appeals and attitude change: effects of anxiousness, probability of occurrence, and the efficiency of coping responses. *J Pers Soc Psychol, 34*, 54–61.

Ronis, D. L., Yates, J. F., and Kirscht, J. P. (1989). Attitudes, decisions, and habits as determinants of repeated behavior. In: A. R. Pratkanis, S. J. Breckler, & A. G. Greenwald (Eds.), *Attitude Structure and Function* (pp. 213–239). Hillsdale, NJ: Erlbaum.

Sheeran, P., Aarts, H., Custers, L., Rivis, A., Webb, T. L., and Cooke, R. (2005). The goal-dependent automaticity of drinking habits. *Br J Soc Psychol, 44*, 47–63.

Thompson, J. K., and Smolak, L. (Eds.) (2001). *Body Image, Eating Disorders, and Obesity in Youth: Assessment, Prevention, and Treatment*. Washington, DC: American Psychological Association.

Triandis, H. C. (1980). Values, attitudes, and interpersonal behavior. In: H. E. Howe, Jr. & M. M. Page

(Eds.), *Nebraska Symposium on Motivation, 1979* (pp. 195–259). Lincoln, NE: University of Nebraska Press.

Vallacher, R. R., and Wegner, D. M. (1987). What do people think they're doing? Action identification and human behavior. *Psychol Rev, 94*, 3–15.

Verplanken, B. (2004). Value congruence and job satisfaction among nurses: a human relations perspective. *Int J Nurs Stud*, 599–605.

Verplanken, B. (2006). Beyond frequency: habit as mental construct. *Br J Soc Psychol, 45*, 639–656.

Verplanken, B., and Aarts, H. (1999). Habit, attitude, and planned behaviour: is habit an empty construct or an interesting case of automaticity? *Eur Rev Soc Psychol, 10*, 101–134.

Verplanken, B., Aarts, H., and van Knippenberg, A. (1997). Habit, information acquisition, and the process of making travel mode choices. *Eur J Soc Psychol, 27*, 539–560.

Verplanken, B., Aarts, H., van Knippenberg, A., and Moonen, A. (1998). Habit versus planned behaviour: a field experiment. *Br J Soc Psychol, 37*, 111–128.

Verplanken, B., Aarts, H., van Knippenberg, A., and van Knippenberg, C. (1994). Attitude versus general habit: antecedents of travel mode choice. *J Appl Soc Psychol, 24*, 285–300.

Verplanken, B., Friborg, O., Wang, C. E., Trafimow, D., and Woolf, K. (2007). Mental habits: metacognitive reflection on negative self-thinking. *J Pers Soc Psychol, 92*, 526–541.

Verplanken, B., Herabadi, A. G., Perry, J. A., and Silvera, D. H. (2005). Consumer style and health: the role of impulsive buying in unhealthy eating. *Psychol Health, 20*, 429–441.

Verplanken, B., and Melkevik, O. (2008). Predicting habit: the case of physical exercise. *Psychol Sport Exerc, 9*, 15–26.

Verplanken, B., and Orbell, S. (2003). Reflections on past behavior: a self-report index of habit strength. *J Appl Soc Psychol, 33*, 1313–1330.

Verplanken, B., and Tangelder, Y. (2010). No body is perfect: The significance of habitual negative thinking about appearance for body dissatisfaction, eating disorder propensity, self-esteem, and suacking. *Psychology and Health,* in press.

Verplanken, B., and Velsvik, R. (2008). Habitual negative body image thinking as psychological risk factor in adolescents. *Body Image, 5*, 133–140.

Verplanken, B., Walker, I., Davis, A., and Jurasek, M. (2008). Context change and travel mode choice: combing the habit discontinuity and self-activation hypotheses. *J Environ Psychol, 9*, 15–26.

Verplanken, B., and Wood, W. (2006). Interventions to break and create consumer habits. *J Publ Pol Market, 25*, 90–103.

Watkins, E. R. (2008). Constructive and unconstructive repetitive thought. *Psychol Bull, 134*, 163–206.

Wittenbraker, J., Gibbs, B. L., and Kahle, L. R. (1983). Seat belt attitudes, habits, and behaviors: an adaptive amendment to the Fishbein model. *J Appl Soc Psychol, 13*, 406–421.

Wood, W., and Neal, D. T. (2007). A new look at habits and the habit-goal interface. *Psychol Rev, 114*, 843–863.

Wood, W., Quinn, J. M., and Kashy, D. A. (2002). Habits in everyday life: thought, emotion, and action. *J Pers Soc Psychol, 83*, 1281–1297.

Wood, W., Tam, L., and Guerrero Witt, M. (2005). Changing circumstances, disrupting habits. *J Pers Soc Psychol, 88*, 918–933.

Chapter 7

Adherence to Medical Advice: Processes and Measurement

Jacqueline Dunbar-Jacob, Martin P. Houze, Cameron Kramer, Faith Luyster, and Maura McCall

1 Introduction

Traditionally adherence has referred to the percent of a prescribed or recommended regimen that is carried out historically by patients and more recently by providers (Haynes, 1979). The definition is nonjudgmental and does not imply responsibility. The value of knowing adherence rates lies in the ability to assess the effectiveness of treatment, whether it be in the evaluation of new treatments or in the development of effective treatment for the individual.

A review of the research over the past 35 years suggests that adherence has been viewed in a global manner, with an emphasis on the identification of patient characteristics which may influence treatment behavior. Data have historically shown that adherence rates across regimen hover around 50% for both patients and providers (Baumhakel et al, 2009; Claxton et al, 2001; Dunbar-Jacob et al, 2000; Thier et al, 2008). Prediction has been difficult as the same characteristics examined in different studies show varying degrees of influence on the level of adherence, and many studies have focused on a limited number of characteristics (Baiardini et al, 2009; Stilley et al, 2004). Further confusing the picture is the fact that different studies both measure and define adherence in different ways. Thus, the behavioral processes underlying adherence and related measurement strategies become important considerations for the furtherance of an understanding of adherence and ultimately the prevention and remediation of poor adherence.

Any examination of adherence needs to consider the multiple steps from prescription to action and to consider these steps in refining the definition of adherence. First, of course, is the clarity and completeness of the prescription and related instruction. Second is the capability of the patient to carry out the instruction. Third is the availability of the resources needed to carry out the instruction. Fourth is the motivation to adhere to the prescription in part or in whole. And lastly is the system to support continued adherence, e.g., cues, self-monitoring, feedback, etc. Most commonly adherence studies have focused upon motivational factors with little attention to these other key elements.

Any examination of adherence also needs to consider the patient's decision making (Bieber et al, 2006; Loh et al, 2007). First the patient must decide whether to accept the recommended treatment. If treatment is accepted, then the patient must decide whether to initiate the treatment. If the patient decides to initiate the treatment, then she/he must determine whether the value of the treatment offsets any negative consequences to following it. If the patient decides to pursue the treatment, then the decision is whether to make it an integral part of daily habits. And finally the patient must decide whether to persist when problems occur.

J. Dunbar-Jacob (✉)
University of Pittsburgh, 350 Victoria Building, 3500 Victoria St, Pittsburgh, PA 15261, USA
e-mail: dunbar@pitt.edu

A. Steptoe (ed.), *Handbook of Behavioral Medicine*, DOI 10.1007/978-0-387-09488-5_7,
© Springer Science+Business Media, LLC 2010

A further consideration is whether the patient knows the state of their adherence. Considerable research suggests there is a poor relationship between patient self-report of adherence and adherence assessed through more direct mechanisms (Dunbar-Jacob et al, 2000; Wagner and Rabkin, 2000). While a portion of this may reflect a reluctance to report poor adherence to the provider (Sankar et al, 2007), it is likely that memory is a major factor in this discrepancy. To accurately report adherence, the patient must be able to recall and summarize their behavior over a period of time between provider visits, often as long as 6 months to a year. For the patient who has persisted with the regimen at some level over time, the regimen becomes habitual but not necessarily accurate. Such habitual behaviors become less salient and become part of a more general memory, making discrete events more difficult to recall (Barnhofer et al, 2005; McPherson, 2001; Warnecke et al, 1997). Cramer and colleagues (1990) showed that adherence improved 5 days prior to (88%) and after (86%) contact with the provider, in comparison to 1-month postvisit (67%). Hence it is reasonable to assume that many patients are recalling most recent behavior and not summarizing across time. Thus, measures may have different accuracy depending upon the variability of behavior and the length of time the patient is assessed.

Also of importance in the processes surrounding adherence is the quality of the communication that occurs within relationships (van Dulmen et al, 2008). Communication between the patient and the providers, communication between providers, communication within the interdisciplinary treatment team, and communication between inpatient and outpatient teams are all important to subsequent patient adherence. Problems in communication may further erode trust in the advice offered by the providers (Kerse et al, 2004; Thom et al, 2001). An assessment of conflicting recommendations or instruction may be important to the determination of whether adherence behavior represents poor adherence or selection among conflicting or suspect advice. This also appears in the adherence

of providers to guideline recommendations when multiple guidelines from different agencies are not consistent (Lewiecki, 2005).

2 Classification of Adherence

The multiple steps that the client or patient takes and the process through which the regimen is recommended leads to multiple points at which the patient may encounter errors or need to make decisions. At each of these points adherence may become a problem. Each point may suggest a different definition or method of assessment.

2.1 Acceptance of the Regimen

The first step is the period in which the regimen is initially presented, and the patient makes a decision about whether to follow it. One area of consideration is readiness to change. Studies examining readiness to adopt a regimen have varying results in predicting subsequent adherence (Aloia et al, 2005). Many factors may go into a patient's willingness to accept a regimen, such as the patient's preferences for type of treatment, the trust that the patient has in the provider, the level of burden imposed, the patient's beliefs about the illness or the treatment, the satisfaction with care, the consistency of the advice with previous advice or knowledge, and a host of other factors. It is at this step that negotiating a mutually satisfactory treatment may influence whether the patient adheres to the recommendation or not.

2.2 Adoption of the Regimen

Patients may agree to the regimen, or at least not object to it, but fail to initiate treatment. For example, between 66 and 84% of new antihypertensive prescription medicines were filled by persons with hypertension and who had at least two clinical encounters (Shah et al, 2009). In the same practice, 85% of new diabetes prescriptions were filled (Shah et al, 2008). For patients recently discharged from hospital after a myocardial infarction, 77% of discharge prescriptions were filled within 7 days (Jackevicius et al, 2006). In this situation, closed health-care systems may detect failure to fill through close monitoring of pharmacy fills. But for the open systems where patients may utilize any number of pharmacies, failure to adopt the regimen is unlikely to be detected until the next health-care visit, perhaps as long as 6–12 months after the prescription is written. It is unknown how many persons take the first step in behavioral interventions. Many factors may influence the patient's adoption of treatment including those noted above combined with a reluctance to question or challenge the provider. Other factors may include barriers to obtaining the prescription such as cost, accessibility, and availability.

2.3 Initiation of the Regimen

Even though the patient acquires the treatment or its resources, the regimen may not be initiated at all or may be discontinued after a brief exposure.

Indeed the first 6 months on treatment show a significant withdrawal from treatment (Perreault et al, 2005; Donnelly et al, 2008; Chapman et al, 2005). Data show as many as 50% or more of patients may terminate treatment by this point (Chapman et al, 2005; Rutledge et al, 1999; Newman et al, 2004). The factors which predict early termination of treatment are not clear. Hypotheses are directed toward the impact of side effects, financial concerns, or difficulty in carrying out the regimen.

2.4 Treatment Continuation

For those patients who continue treatment beyond the 6-month period, several adherence patterns emerge. This may constitute as many as 50% of this group. The series of figures below displays the variable patterns of adherence found in patients on medication for chronic disease who were monitored with the AARDEX Medication Event Monitoring System. Each of these patients had been on treatment for 1 year or longer before monitoring was initiated. For a portion of persons, adherence remains high and stable, though not necessarily perfect, over time (see Fig. 7.1).

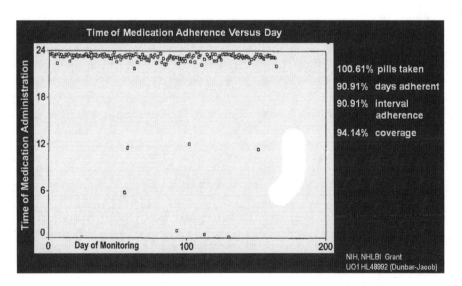

Fig. 7.1   Good adherer to once-a-day regimen

Other patients may demonstrate a persistently low adherence or a decline over time, as can be seen in Fig. 7.2.

The majority of the patients in this group, however, demonstrate variable levels of adherence over time showing a combination of missed doses (or episodes), double doses, and mistimed doses. These variable patterns are difficult to detect with the majority of measures of

adherence. See Fig. 7.3 for a visual view of a variable pattern of adherence for a twice-a-day medication.

Thus, adherence can be classified at several points, depending upon the outcome of interest, acceptance of the regimen (yes/no), initiation of the regimen (yes/no), and continuation or persistence with the regimen at varying levels of adherence.

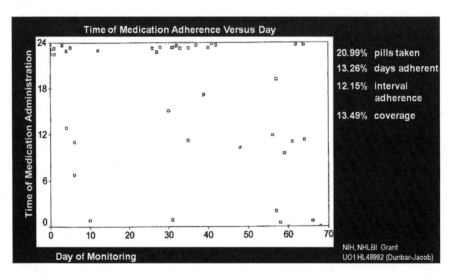

Fig. 7.2 Poor adherer to once-a-day regimen

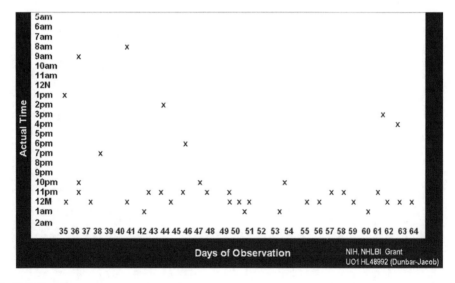

Fig. 7.3 Variable adherence to twice-a-day regimen

3 Defining Adherence

Before measuring adherence it is important to clearly define and specify just what adherence is and the step in the process that is of interest. Ideally, adherence would be defined as the proportion of the prescription or regimen required to create the desired clinical outcome. Haynes (1979) did so in the first adherence improvement randomized controlled trial (RCT) conducted. He examined adherence to antihypertensives and identified the average adherence (by home pill count) to obtain a diastolic blood pressure level of less than 90 mmHg (Haynes et al, 1976). Adherence was determined to be pill counts greater than 80%. Similarly, in the Lipid Research Clinics Coronary Primary Prevention Trial (LRC-CPPT) research subjects were prescribed six packets of cholestyramine per day designed to achieve a 20% reduction in low-density lipoprotein cholesterol (LDL). At the end of the trial, it was found that 70% adherence led to $\geq$20% reduction in LDL (Schaefer et al, 1994). Blagden and Chipperfield (2007) examined LDL cholesterol level changes with atorvastatin vs. atorvastatin plus ezetimibe. With 70% or greater adherence in their sample, monitored via pill counts, the LDL levels decreased by 36.5 and 50.5%, respectively. In contrast such levels of adherence are not effective in reducing viral load in HIV patients. Recommendations for effective treatment of HIV are to achieve adherence levels close to 100% (www.apha.org/ppp/hiv). Unfortunately, data are not readily available on other drugs to establish an optimal adherence level. Even less is known about optimal adherence for nonpharmacological interventions. For patients on multiple treatments, the common pattern for those with chronic disease, the picture of optimal adherence is even more confusing.

Further confounding the picture is the problem of medication which may have positive effects on one clinical parameter but negative effects on another. For example, Ames (1986) studied and reviewed studies of diuretics used in the treatment of hypertension to reduce high blood pressure levels and found that the hypertensive treatment may create a rise in various serum cholesterol measures by 4–56%; however, Ott and colleagues (2003) conducted an RCT in elderly that did not find such differences (Ott et al, 2003). Similarly, anti-hyperglycemic agents may lower blood glucose levels and glycated hemogloblin (HbA1c), but may lead to an increase in serum cholesterol (Gershberg et al, 1968). Thus, attempts to establish an optimal adherence to a cholesterol lowering regimen may potentially be confounded by adherence to the concurrent hypertension or diabetes regimen.

The answer to this dilemma has been to adopt a behavioral definition regarding the proportion of the regimen taken as the standard, typically about 80%. Alternatives to this have been to use unique definitions or qualitative definitions (good vs. poor with no numeric referent) or to fail to provide any definition at all. These variations in defining adherence impair the ability to perform adequate meta-analyses or systematic reviews of the magnitude of the problem or to evaluate the effectiveness of adherence interventions. At a minimum the provision of numeric definitions of adherence or cut points for classification is more informative. While it may not be clinically useful to set one behavioral standard across regimens or conditions, it is useful for comparison and summarization of adherence across populations.

4 Measurement of Adherence

4.1 Numeric Assessment of Adherence

The definition of adherence initially posed by Haynes and colleagues (1979), the percent or portion of the regimen carried out, suggests a numeric definition of adherence and the ability to count doses prescribed and taken. Four methods of assessment permit this, each with advantages and disadvantages. These include electronic monitoring, pill count, daily diary, and patient recall.

4.1.1 Electronic Monitoring

Electronic event monitoring (EEM) has been used increasingly over the past two decades for adherence to medication and to exercise regimens. In these cases the monitor itself is connected with the regimen and accepts passive participation on the part of the patient. The most commonly used EEM for medication consists of a microprocessor inserted in a medication bottle cap, which is activated by opening or closing of the cap (AARDEX MEMS). The date and time of opening (and subsequently closing) the cap are recorded on the microprocessor. Thus, it is possible to monitor the number of doses accessed, as well as the timing of doses. The interval between doses may be important for drug efficacy. Errors in timing (or intervals between doses) have been found to be the error of greatest magnitude in medication adherence (Claxton, 2001). Data may be monitored for short or long intervals.

Electronic technologies are also used in the assessment of adherence to lifestyle interventions, exercise, dietary behavior, and treatment of sleep apnea. Pedometers, accelerometers, and heart rate monitors allow freedom for the person exercising and are often used in research to measure physical activity (see Chapter 3). Studies have shown the reliability of these devices and often describe them as relatively inexpensive and simple to operate (Baker and Mautrie, 2005; Evangelista et al, 2005; Wilbur et al, 2001). Pedometers sense body motion and count footsteps. They are usually considered accurate if worn correctly and stride distance is predetermined. Pedometer readouts should be checked against known measurements like distance and time. Accelerometers are motion sensors that can detect changes in acceleration. Heart rate monitors usually strap a monitoring box with electrode on the chest and transmit the data to a watch-like receiver on the wrist that records heart rate over time. Dietary behavior also can be monitored through electronic diaries. Although current technologies such as personal digital assistants (PDAs) can provide dietary data in real time, all methods for collecting dietary data have inherent problems for monitoring adherence to diet recommendations (Glanz and Murphy, 2007). Similarly, in the management of sleep disorders, continuous positive airway pressure (CPAP) devices utilize smart cards, modem, or web-based methodology to convey data regarding the nightly duration of therapy at effective pressure and patterns of use. CPAP adherence typically is defined as ≥ 4 h of use for 70% of days. However, a standard definition of CPAP adherence has not been established.

With electronic monitoring, adherence itself is calculated by the number of presumptive events divided by the number of dosing events prescribed within the monitored time interval. The determination of what constitutes "good" adherence is left to the investigator or clinician. When gaps appear in dosing or a cessation of recorded events occurs, a concurrent interview is necessary to determine whether the patient utilized the monitor or whether the patient was hospitalized or otherwise had a change in either prescription or circumstances. The ultimate calculation of adherence permits the determination of the percent of doses or events, the percent of days on which the patient was adherent, as well as the percent of doses occurring within the scheduled interval. For exercise, intensity and duration can also be observed, and duration of CPAP use monitored. Additionally, information on "drug holidays," periods of time off, as well as patterns of adherence may be viewed. There is evidence that these monitors can stimulate behavior change itself (Baker and Mautrie, 2005; Deschamps et al, 2006).

There is evidence that the use of pedometers alone can increase reported motivation to exercise as well as increase self-reported physical activity, and actual physical activity as recorded by the pedometer, at least for the short term (Baker and Mutrie, 2005). In this particular study of intervention groups using the transtheoretical model to increase step count, significant reported increases in motivation and activity were only seen in the group using the pedometer.

4.1.2 Pill Counts

Pill counts, one of the common measures of adherence in pharmacological clinical studies, also permit a numeric estimate of adherence. Adherence is calculated as the number of pills taken divided by the number prescribed over the interval of interest, typically between periods of dispensing. It is important to note that the pill count does not identify patterns of adherence nor interdose intervals. Patients who miss a dose of medication and then compensate by taking an extra dose the next day, a pattern found with electronic monitoring, is not identifiable; nor is it possible to discriminate early cessation of treatment from low but relatively stable dosing, both resulting in low adherence estimates.

The pill count has been found to have a low but statistically significant correlation with EEM measures. For example, Hamilton (2003) reported correlation rates of 0.29–0.39, $p \leq 01$, for hypertensive patients. For AIDS patients, Bangsberg et al (2001) noted a correlation of $0.7, p < 0.001$, between unadjusted EEM and pill counts. Pill counts typically estimate a higher adherence than EEM (Bangsberg et al, 2001; Hamilton, 2003). Therefore the choice of methods of adherence depends upon what the clinician or investigator is interested in detecting. If one is interested in early changes in patterns of adherence, poor timing of medication, or information for the development of early intervention strategies, the EEM will most likely be useful. If an overall interest in adherence is of interest, then the pill count may give a reasonable estimate.

4.1.3 Pharmacy Refills

In a closed health system, where the provider of care and the dispensing pharmacy are fixed within the system, pharmacy refills may be used to estimate adherence. As with pill counts, the daily patterns of medication taking are not available. However a percent adherence can be calculated by examining the amount of medication dispensed divided by the number of tablets that should have been taken between refills. As long as the patient remains in the system it is possible to detect withdrawal from treatment.

Multiple methods of extracting data and estimating adherence are used, based on pharmacy fill rates and result in several measures. Hess and colleagues (2006) identified 11 measures in examination of pharmacy administration databases. These included "Continuous Measure of Medication Acquisition (CMA); Continuous Multiple Interval Measure of Oversupply (CMOS); Medication Possession Ratio (MPR); Medication Refill Adherence (MRA); Continuous Measure of Medication Gaps (CMG); Continuous, Single Interval Measure of Medication Aquisition (CSA); Proportion of Days Covered (PDC); Refill Compliance Rate (RCR); Medication Possession Ratio, modified (MPRm); Dates Between Fills Adherence Rate (DBR); and Compliance Rate (CR)" (Hess et al, 2006, p.280). Calculating rates of adherence to medication adherence by each mechanism for participants in a weight loss trial showed adherence rates ranging from 63 to 109.7%, depending on method of calculation. Thus, it is important to consider the procedure for calculating adherence over time from databases.

4.1.4 Daily Diaries

Daily diaries form a third method of evaluating event data. Diaries have been used for patient reporting of treatment-related behavior for several decades. Patients or research participants are instructed to record events near to the time of occurrence to minimize forgetting. Further detail around the events may be recorded either qualitatively or as a component of the structured diary. Thus, information can be learned about the circumstances that surround errors in regimen management or successful performance. Diaries have been particularly useful in monitoring food intake and exercise. However, there have been some examples of use in medication management.

Unfortunately, studies of the accuracy of self-report indicate that the data may be problematic. In a sample of women with sedentary lifestyles participating in a home-based walking program, self-report logs indicated that the women reported performing 64% of the prescribed walking exercises while the heart rate monitor data revealed that the women on average met 60% of the goal. This indicates a greater than 90% agreement (Wilbur et al, 2001). In a study comparing an instrumental paper and electronic diaries, however, 90% of events were reported on time but electronic assessment indicated that actual adherence was just 11%; in 32% of days with events entered, the diary had not been opened. Thus, false reporting was high (Stone et al, 2003). This also happens in the case of dietary diary entries. Patients may neglect to complete the diary as instructed and will consequently complete it prior to the clinic visit. The diary is dependent further upon the individual's recall of the foods and beverages consumed and, in some instances, the amount consumed and the nutritional and caloric content. Furthermore, the act of recording food consumption may influence the person's eating behavior resulting in an inaccurate representation of patient's dietary intake. Additionally, patients may censor the report of food consumption in order to be in accordance with known dietary recommendations.

4.1.5 Daily Recall

Recalls over a specific number of days may also be used to estimate percent adherence. If the patient can recall and is willing to report accurately, event data and timing can be assessed. Chesney and colleagues (2000) reported utility in 3 day recalls in identifying HIV patients with raised viral load. Studies have shown that physical activity recall questionnaires can provide a relatively accurate account of physical activity when compared with accelerometers with as much as 90% agreement. However, correlations between the subjective self-report data and the electronic data vary between gender, intensity of

the activity, and weight status of the individual (Timperio et al, 2003). Lu and colleagues (2008) reported that 1-month estimates were better than 3- or 7-day recalls when compared with EEM data. However, our own research has suggested that patients with rheumatoid arthritis may have difficulty in remembering the detail of medication taking beyond 3 days. In a 7-day recall of medication taking it was common for patients to begin to report "the same" beyond the third day (unpublished data). Lee et al, (2007) further reported that 24-h recalls were unrelated to pill counts and insensitive to temporal change. Thus, brief recalls may or may not correlate with concurrent clinical data. The question arises as to how much data can be reliably collected to build a picture of adherence over time.

5 Global Assessment of Adherence

Many adherence studies have used assessment strategies which lack a numeric estimate of the portion of the regimen carried out. Examples include a variety of self-report questionnaires, interviews, and clinician estimates. An examination of one measure may present the issues that arise when self-reported questionnaire assessment is used. The most commonly used generic adherence questionnaire is the Morisky Medication Adherence Questionnaire (MMAQ), a four-item (or eight-item version) self-report inventory used to screen for poor adherence (Morisky et al, 1986). An adherence percent is not obtained. The questionnaire yields a score of 0–4, with 0 reflecting good adherence. Studies reflect varying levels of sensitivity and usefulness. For example, Ruslami and colleagues (2008) reported that a combination of the self-report and clinical estimate detected all cases of nonadherence reported by the Medication Event Monitoring System. Yet Shalansky et al, (2004) noted a considerable difference in the detection of nonadherence between the MEMS (13%) and the MMAQ (3%). It has been noted that questionnaire data for adherence may not correlate with clinical data (Södergård et al, 2006) and that its utility may vary across settings (van de Steeg et al, 2009). As with patient recalls, the data rely upon the accuracy of the patient's memory. And, as noted, the questionnaire does not yield information on the level of adherence over time nor the pattern of adherence.

To be meaningful in assessing adherence the scoring and establishment of cut points would need to be considered carefully in conjunction with either more direct measures of adherence or established clinical cut points. It is also likely that the global measures will be most useful for recent periods when memory is most accurate. Analysis would only permit an estimation of the proportion of persons who recall and report problems related to adherence. It is unlikely to be useful in the assessment of adherence interventions as the sensitivity to change is unknown and unlikely to be sufficient to detect the modest changes seen in intervention studies (Arbuthnott and Sharpe, 2009; Conn et al, 2009; Kripalani et al, 2007).

6 Issues in Analysis of Adherence Data

Analysis is influenced by the method of measurement chosen within a study. For the use of electronic monitoring, where the most detailed information is collected, several issues arise. First is the length of time that data are collected and summarized. Current technology permits the capture of data for 1 day up to 1–2 years. Thus it is important to examine the length of time that data need to be collated to reach a stable estimate of adherence (Houze, Sereika, Dunbar-Jacob, unpublished). Deschamps and colleagues (2006) suggest that in HIV and in kidney transplant patients, an intervention effect of electronic monitoring can be found which decreased and stabilized over 35–50 days. Data can then be summarized over the relevant time period.

The next issue with electronic monitoring is the determination of what view of adherence

is important. For example, a simple count of adherence events can be determined, much like a pill count. This will provide a percent of actual events compared with the percent of prescribed events. The outcome can be influenced by over-adherent events, yielding rates greater than 100% or masking the extent of poor adherence. Summarizing across patients can inflate the level of group adherence if there are over-adherers within the group.

An alternative view is the proportion of days in which the events were accurate. This overcomes the problem of adherence above 100%. Individuals who miss a dose in the evening and make it up the next day will appear as adherent when the count of doses is performed but will have 2 days of poor adherence when the proportion of days adherent is calculated.

A third view is considering doses taken at the advised time, within a range. Adherence is likely to be lowest with this estimate. In cases where the timing of medication is important this assessment provides very useful data.

Thus, estimations of individual adherence and of group adherence need to consider the view of adherence that is important. Similar considerations can be given to daily diary adherence, although there is less likely to be reliable data gathered. These are the only two methods of assessment which require a decision of this nature before adherence can be estimated and ultimately analyzed.

Regardless of assessment method, the data for adherence over a group tend to be J-shaped (Dunbar-Jacob et al, 1998, see Fig. 7.4). Multiple strategies to transform the data have failed. Therefore non-parametric analyses are most useful. Newer strategies for analyzing J-shaped data are being examined and may yield more sensitive and accurate analytic strategies (Rohay, 2009).

Unfortunately, often the level of detail just noted is missing from studies of adherence. Further parametric analyses are often presented, typically in the absence of information about the nature of the distribution of the data. Attention to the nature of measurement, the definitions, and view of adherence, as well as the use of appropriate analytic strategies are important

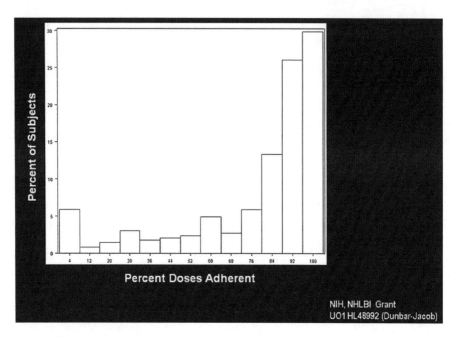

Fig. 7.4 Distribution of days adherent by EEM

to moving the field forward. Similarly meta-analyses need to consider not only intervention strategies, but also definitions and assessment strategies as well. Thus, the full picture of adherence, phase of adopting/managing the regimen, a prior definition of adherence, measurement method, and appropriate analytic strategy are crucial as we continue to develop an understanding of patient adherence.

7 Implications for Understanding Adherence

Numerous studies have been undertaken in an effort to understand who is likely to have adherence difficulties. The results of these studies have shown inconsistent relationships between predictors and adherence (Dunbar-Jacob et al, 2009). Few predictors have been found to be very robust within studies. It is not unreasonable to find inconsistency in the prediction of adherence when we note the variability in the phase of adhering to a treatment and the inconsistency in classification of a person's adherence given the varying methods of defining and assessing adherence. More careful description of the population and its stage of treatment (agreement with treatment, initiation of treatment, adjustment to new treatment, continuation of treatment) as well as clearer descriptions of the definition and assessment methodology will be required before we can begin to understand the predictors of adherence.

Similarly, numerous studies have examined strategies to improve adherence. A meta-analysis by Peterson et al (2003) showed that interventions increased adherence by 4–11%, a very small amount. Kripalani and colleagues (2007) reported that just 54% of studies reviewed reported improvements in adherence while just 30% showed clinical improvements, not always related to adherence. Looking within hypertension care, Schroeder et al (2004) found that 78% of adherence studies which simplified the regimen, 44% of those using complex interventions, and 42% of those using motivational strategies reported improvements in adherence. Adherence improvements ranged from 5 to 41%. However, the heterogeneity in measurement of adherence and methods of study prevented conduct of a pooled analysis. Thus, our knowledge of both intervention strategies and of predictors of adherence is hampered by the variability with which adherence is treated in studies.

8 Summary and Recommendations

As we examine the processes and measurement of patient adherence, we find considerable heterogeneity between studies in terms of definitions, measurement, analytic strategies, and the patient's phase of adopting and maintaining a new treatment regimen. This has resulted in difficulty in evaluating strategies for improving adherence as well as in identifying factors robustly and consistently associated with adherence. The processes required at the different phases of regimen behaviors are likely to be associated with different predictor variables and likely to be responsive to different strategies. However, future research is needed to evaluate more precisely the factors that impact the patient's behaviors during the various processes of accepting, initiating, implementing, and sustaining adherence to a new treatment. Similarly future research needs to examine intervention strategies designed for each phase. Both measurement and analysis strategies can influence the outcomes of studies. Measurement strategies should be chosen with care, selected with attention to the sensitivity to adherence itself and sensitivity to change. Similarly, analysis strategies need to be appropriate for the measurement strategy and the nature of the adherence distribution. While much has been learned about adherence over recent decades, our future understanding can be deepened with greater attention to processes and measures of adherence.

References

APHA (2004). Adherence to HIV treatment regimens: recommendations for best practices. www.apha.org/ppp/hiv June 2004. Accessed January 6, 2010.

Aloia, M. S., Arnedt, J. T., Stpenowsky, C., Hecht, J., and Borelli, B. (2005). Predicting treatment adherence in obstructive sleep apnea using principles of behavior change. *J Clin Sleep Med, 1*, 354–356.

Ames, R. P. (1986). The effects of antihypertensive drugs on serum lipids, I. diuretics. *Drugs, 32*, 260–278.

Arbuthnott, A., and Sharpe, D. (2009). The effect of physician-patient collaboration on patient adherence in non-psychiatric medicine. *Pat Educ Couns, 77*, 60–67.

Baiardini, I., Braido, F., Bonini, M., Compalati, E. and Canonica, G. W. (2009). Why do doctors and patients not follow guidelines? *Curr Opin Allergy Cl, 9*, 228–233.

Baker, G., and Mutrie, N. (2005). Are pedometers useful motivational tools for increasing walking in sedentary adults? Paper presented at Walk21-VI, 6th international conference on walking in the 21st century, Zurich, Switzerland.

Bangsberg, D. R., Hecht, F. M., Charlebois, E. D., Chesney, M., and Moss, A. (2001). Comparing objective measures of adherence to HIV antiretroviral therapy: electronic medication monitors and unannounced pill counts. *AIDS Behav, 5*, 275–281.

Barnhofer, T., Kuehn, E., and de Jong-Meyer, R. (2005). Specificity of autobiographical memory and basal cortisol levels in patients with major depression. *Psychoneuroendrocrinology, 30*, 403–411.

Baumhakel, M., Muller, U., and Bohm, M. (2009). Influence of gender of physicians and patients on guideline-recommended treatment of chronic heart failure in a cross-sectional study. *Eur J Heart Fail, 11*, 299–303.

Bieber, C., Muller, K. G., Blumenstiel, K., Schneider, A., Richter, A., et al (2006). Long-term effects of a shared decision-making intervention on physician-patient interaction and outcome in fibromyalgia: a qualitative and quantitative 1 year follow-up of a randomized controlled trial. *Patient Educ Couns, 63*(3), 357–366.

Blagden, M. D., and Chipperfield, R. (2007). Efficacy and safety of ezetimibe co-administered with atorvastatin in untreated patients with primary hypercholesterolaemia and coronary heart disease. *Curr Med Res Opin, 23*, 767–775.

Chapman, R. H., Benner, J. S., Petrilla, A. A., Tierce, J. C., Collins, S. R. et al (2005). Predictors of adherence with antihypertensive and lipid-lowering therapy. *Arch Intern Med, 165*, 1147–1152.

Chesney, M. A., Ickovics, J. R., Chambers, D. B., Gifford, A. L., Neidig, J. et al (2000). Self-reported adherence to antiretroviral medications among participants in HIV clinical trials: The AACTG Adherence Instruments. *AIDS Care, 12*, 255–266.

Claxton, A. J., Cramer, J. and Pierce, C. (2001). A systematic review of the associations between dose regimens and medication compliance. *Clin Ther, 23*, 1296–1310.

Conn, V. S., Hafdahl, A. R., Cooper, P. S., Ruppar, T. M., Mehr, D. R. et al (2009). Interventions to improve medication adherence among older adults: meta-analysis of adherence outcomes among randomized controlled trials. *Gerontologist, 49*, 447–462.

Cramer, J. A., Scheyer, R. D., and Mattson, R. H. (1990). Compliance declines between clinic visits. *Arch Intern Med 150*, 1509–1510.

Deschamps, A. E., van Wijngaerden, E., Denhaerynck, K., De Geest S., and Vandamme, A. M. (2006). Use of electronic monitoring induces a 40-day intervention effect in HIV patients. *J Acq Immun Def Synd, 43*, 247–248.

Donnelly, L. A., Doney, A. S. F., Morris, A. D., Palmer, C. N. A., and Donnan, P. T. (2008). Long-term adherence to statin treatment in diabetes. *Diabetes Med, 25*, 850–855.

Dunbar-Jacob, J., Erlen, J. A., Schlenk, E. A., Ryan, C. M., Sereika, S. M. et al (2000). Adherence in chronic disease. *Annu Rev Nurs Res, 18*, 48–90.

Dunbar-Jacob, J. Gemmell, l. A., and Schlenk, E. A., (2009). Predictors of patient adherence: patient characteristics. In J. K. Ockene & K. A. Riekert (Eds.). *The Handbook of Health Behavior Change, 3rd Ed* (pp. 397–410). New York: Springer.

Dunbar-Jacob, J., Sereika, S., Rohay, J., and Burke, L. (1998). Electronic methods in assessing adherence to medical regimens. In D. Krantz & A. Baum (Eds.). *Technology and Methods in Behavioral Medicine* (pp. 95–113). Mahwah, NJ, Lawrence Erlbaum Associates.

Evangelista, L. S., Dracup, K., Erickson, V., McCarthy, W. J., Hamilton, M. A. et al (2005). Validity of pedometers for measuring exercise adherence in heart failure patients. *J Cardiac Fail, 11*, 366–371.

Gershberg, H., Javier, Z., Hulse, M. and Hecht, A. (1968). Influence of hypoglycemic agents on blood lipids and body weight in ketoacidosis-resistant diabetics. *Ann New York Acad Sci, 148*, 914–924.

Glanz, K. and Murphy, S. (2007). Dietary assessment and monitoring in real time. In A. Stone, S. Shiffman, A. Atienza, & L. Nebeling (Eds.), *The Science of Real Time Data Capture: Self-Reports in Health Research* (pp. 151–168). New York: Oxford University

Hamilton, G. (2003). Measuring adherence in a hypertension clinical trial. *Eur J Cardiovasc Nurs, 2*, 219–228.

Haynes, R. B. (1979). Introduction. In R. B. Haynes, D. W. Taylor, & D. L. Sackett (Eds.), *Compliance in Health Care* (pp. i–xv). Baltimore: Johns Hopkins University Press.

Haynes, R. B., Sackett, D. L., Gibson, E. S., Taylor, D. W., Hackett, B. C. et al (1976). Improvement of medication compliance in uncontrolled hypertension. *Lancet, 1*, 1265–1268.

Hess, L. M., Raebel, M. A., Conner, D. A., and Malone, D. C. (2006). Measurement of adherence in pharmacy administrative databases: a proposal for standard definitions and preferred measures. *Ann Pharmacother, 40*, 1280–1288.

Houze, M., Sereika, S., and Dunbar-Jacob, J. (2009). Medication adherence: time to stability. Unpublished manuscript.

Rohay, J. (2009). Statistical assessment of medication adherence data: a technique to analyze the J-shaped curve. Doctoral Thesis, University of Pittsburgh.

Jackevicius, C. A., Paterson, J. M., and Naglie, G. (2006). Concordance between discharge prescriptions and insurance claims in post-myocardial infarction patients. *Pharmacoepidem Dr S,16*, 207–215.

Kerse, N., Buetow, S., Mainous, A. G., Young, G., Coster, G. et al (2004). Physician-patient relationship and medication compliance: a primary care investigation. *Ann Fam Med, 2*, 455–461.

Kripalani, S., Yao, X., and Haynes, R. B. (2007). Interventions to enhance medication adherence in chronic medical conditions: a systematic review. *Arch Intern Med, 167*, 540–549.

Lee, J. K., Grace, K. A., Foster, T. G., Crawley, M. J., Erowele, G. I. (2007). How should we measure medication adherence in clinical trials and practice? *Ther Clin Risk Manag, 3*, 685–690.

Lewiecki, E. M. (2005). Review of guidelines for bone mineral density testing and treatment of osteoporosis *Curr Osteo Rep, 3*, 75–83.

Loh, A., Simon, D., Wills, C. E., Kriston, L., Niebling, W. et al (2007). The effects of a shared decision-making intervention in primary care of depression: a cluster-randomized control trial. *Pat Educ Couns, 67*, 324–332.

Lu, M., Safren, S. A., Skolnik, P. R., Rogers, W. H., Coady, W. et al (2008). Optimal recall period and response task for self-reported HIV medication adherence. *AIDS Behav, 12*, 86–94.

McPherson, F. (2001). Autobiographical memory. http://www.memory-key.com/EverydayMemory/autobiographical.htm.

Morisky, D. E., Green, L. W., and Levine, D. M. (1986). Concurrent and predictive validity of a self-reported measure of medication adherence. *Med Care, 24*, 67–74.

Newman, S., Steed, L., and Mulligan, K. (2004). Self-management interventions for chronic illness. *Lancet, 364*, 1523–1537.

Ott, S. M., LaCroix, A. Z., Ichikawa, L. E., Scholes, D., and Barlow, W. E. (2003). Effect of low-dose thiazide diuretics on plasma lipids: results from a double-blind, randomized clinical trial in older men and women. *J Am Ger Soc, 5*, 340–347.

Perreault, S., Lamarre, D., Blais, L., Dragomir, A., Berbiche, D. et al (2005). Persistence with treatment in newly treated middle-aged patients with essential hypertension. *Ann Pharmacother, 39*, 1401–1408.

Peterson, A. M., Takiya, L., and Finley, R. (2003). Meta-analysis of trials of interventions to improve medication adherence. *Am J Health-Syst Pharm, 60*, 657–665.

Ruslami, R., Crevel, R. v., de, B. E. v., Alisjahbana, B., and Aarnouste, R. E. (2008). A step-wise approach to find a valid and feasible method to detect non-adherence to tuberculosis drugs. *SE Asian J Trop Med, 39*, 1083–1087.

Rutledge, J. C., Hyson, D. A., Garduno, D., Cort, D. A. et al (1999). Lifestyle modification program in management of patients with coronary artery disease: the clinical experience in a tertiary care hospital. *J Cardiopul Rehab Prev, 19*, 226–234.

Sankar, A. P., Nevendal, D. C., Neufeld, S., and Luborsky, M. R. (2007). What is a missed dose? Implications for construct validity and patient adherence. *AIDS Care, 19*, 775–780.

Schaefer, E. J., Lamon-Fava, S., Jenner, J. L., McNamara, J. R., Ordovas, J. M. et al (1994). Lipoprotein(a) levels and risk of coronary heart disease in men: The Lipid Research Clinics Coronary Primary Prevention Trial. *JAMA, 271*, 999–1003.

Schroeder, K., Fahey, T., and Ebrahim, S. (2004). How can we improve adherence to blood pressure-lowering medication in ambulatory care? *Arch Intern Med, 164*, 722–732.

Shah, N. R., Hirsch, A. G., Zacker, C., Taylor, S., Wood, G. C. et al (2008). Factors associated with first-filled adherence rates for diabetic medications: a cohort study. *J Gen Intern Med, 24*, 233.237.

Shah, N. R., Hirsch, A. G., Zacker, C., Wood, G. C., Schoenthaler, A. et al (2009). Predictors of first-fill adherence for patients with hypertension. *Am J Hypertension, 22*, 392–396.

Shalansky, S. J., Levy, A. R., and Ignaszewski, A. P. (2004). Self-reported Morisky score for identifying nonadherence with cardiovascular medications. *Ann Pharmacother, 38*, 1363–1368.

Södergård, B., Halvarsson, M., Brannstrom, J., Sonnerborg, A., and Tully, M. P. (2006). A comparison between AACTG adherence questionnaire and the 9-item Morisky medication adherence scale in HIV-patients. *Int Cong Drug Therapy HIV, 8*: Abstract No. P174.

Stilley, C. S., Sereika, S., Muldoon, M. F., Ryan, C. M., and Dunbar-Jacob, J. (2004). Psychological and cognitive function: predictors of adherence with cholesterol lowering treatment. *Ann Behav Med, 27*, 117–124.

Stone, A. A., Shiffman, S., Schwartz, J. E., Broderick, J. E., and Hufford, M. R. (2003). Compliance with paper and electronic diaries. *Comp Clin Trials 24*, 182–199.

Thier, S. L., Yu-Eisenberg, K. S., Leas, B. F., Cantrell, R., DeBussey, S., Goldfarb, N. I., and Nash, D. B. (2008). In chronic disease, nationwide data show poor adherence by patients to medication and by physicians to guidelines. *Managed Care, 17*, 48–52, 55–47.

Thom, D. H., and the Stanford Trust Study Physicians. (2001). Physician behaviors that predict patient trust. *J Fam Pract, 50*, 323–328.

Timperio, A., Salmon, J., and Crawford D. (2003). Validity and reliability of a physical activity recall instrument among overweight and non-overweight men and women. *J Sci Med Sport, 6*, 477–491.

Van Dulmen, S., Sluijs, E., van.Dijk, L., de.Ridder, D., Heerdink, R. et al (2008). Furthering patient adherence: a position paper of the international expert forum on patient adherence based on an internet forum discussion. *BMC Health Serv Res, 8*, 1–8.

Van de Steeg, N., Sielk, Pentzek, M., Bakx, C., and Altiner, A. (2009). Drug-adherence questionnaires not valid for patients taking blood-pressure-lowering drugs in a primary health care setting. *J Eval Clin Practice, 15*, 468–472.

Wagner, G., and Rabkin, J. G. (2000). Measuring medication adherence: are missing doses reported more accurately than perfect adherence?. *AIDS Care, 12*, 405–408.

Warnecke, R. B., Sudman, S., Johnson, T. P., O-Rourke, D., Davis, A. M. et al (1997). Cognitive aspects of recalling and reporting health-related events: Papanicolaou smears, clinical breast examinations, and mammograms. *Am J Epidemiol, 148*, 11, 982–992.

Wilbur, J., Chandler, P., and Miller, A. M. (2001). Measuring adherence to a women's walking program. *West J Nurs Res, 23*, 8–24.

Part II
Psychological Processes
and Measures

Chapter 8

Ecological Validity for Patient Reported Outcomes

Arthur A. Stone and Saul S. Shiffman

Asking people about their health, symptoms, attitudes, opinions, and behaviors is ubiquitous in the behavioral, social, and medical sciences (Stone et al, 2000). For many areas of inquiry in these fields, it is impossible to contemplate research programs without self-reports. Self-reports often serve as primary outcome measures, for instance, in assessing pain, fatigue, opinions, or attitudes; self-reports are the accepted standard for these constructs and "objective" alternative measures usually are not available. Even when objective measures are possible in principle, we often rely on self-report data (e.g., smoking behavior, asthma attacks, social interactions), because the costs of objective data collection (via behavioral observations, for example) are prohibitive.

Patient Reported Outcome (PRO) is a new term used to describe self-reports when they are used as outcome measures in trials (FDA Docket No. 2006D-0044; Rock et al, 2007). The importance of PROs to the behavioral and medical research enterprise has been highlighted

A.A. Stone (✉)
Department of Psychiatry and Behavioral Science, Stony Brook University, Stony Brook, NY 11994-8790, USA
e-mail: arthur.stone@sunysb.edu

AAS is the associate chair of the Scientific Advisory Board of invivodata, inc., a company that supplies electronic data capture services for clinical research and is a senior scientist at the Gallup Organization. SS is a founder of invivodata, inc. and the chair of its Scientific Advisory Board.

recently. The US Food and Drug Administration is in the process of setting standards for PROs used in clinical trials submitted in support of drug or device approvals and claims (FDA Docket No. 2006D-0044). The National Institutes of Health (NIH) has also devoted one of its Roadmap Projects, which are large-scale, high priority initiatives intended to advance health research, to the development of psychometrically sophisticated PROs for use with chronically ill individuals participating in clinical trials (www.nihpromis.org). There is also no doubt that PROs are essential for the delivery of medical care, where they provide essential information about patient functioning and satisfaction with services.

An important feature of PRO assessments, as they have traditionally been implemented, is that they have generally been obtained in relatively artificial or unusual settings, such as clinics and research laboratories, and by having participants recollect and/or reflect on their past experiences. The purpose of this article is to discuss the potential value of collecting PRO data in participants' natural environments and with minimal recourse to recall by systematically and repeatedly sampling self-reports in peoples' daily environments, offering the possibility of truly representative sampling. In the first section of the article, we review the concept of sampling everyday life, its implications for ecological validity, and how it could affect self-report information and PROs. We discuss studies from cognitive science, autobiographic memory, and survey design inform this discussion. In the second section, we review methodologies and technologies that enable collection of self-reports in peoples' typical environments, enhancing the representativeness of the resulting data.

1 Ecological Validity and Self-Reports

Today, when we think of the degree to which behavior observed in a research setting such as a research laboratory is generalizable to real-world behavior, we call this "ecological validity" (Hammond and Stewart, 2001). Over 70 years ago, ecological validity was first used in Brunswik's 1944 paper examining the perceptual phenomenon known as size constancy (Brunswik, 1944) – the ability of people to correctly judge the size of objects despite the fact that the projection of objects on the retina varies with viewing distance. Brunswik's interest was in how naturally occurring cues associated with objects, such as distance from object, were used by the individual to estimate size. In one study that presages the methods described later in this chapter, he recorded over several weeks randomly selected moments from a subject's daily routine and noted the retinal projection (via a photograph of the object), object size, and the subject's estimation of size.

The innovative feature of his design was the evaluation of the natural, ecological association of objects and their associated cues, in contrast to possibly artificial associations based on laboratory investigations, where the constellation of stimulus qualities bore little resemblance to those encountered by people in everyday life. "Representative design" was the term Brunswik coined to refer to the degree that a laboratory experiment corresponded with a particular set of environmental circumstances to which the results of the experiment were to be generalized – what we now call ecological validity. In keeping with contemporary parlance, we use the term ecological validity in its modern

meaning, while acknowledging its historical evolution.

2 Momentary, Retrospective, and Global Self-Report

For this discussion, we describe three types of self-reports defined by the cognitive tasks inherent in making the reports. We shall refer to these as *momentary states*, *retrospective summaries*, and *global reports*. Momentary state questions ask people to describe some aspect of their immediate state, for example, their current mood, symptoms, and circumstances. A question about immediate pain intensity could use, for example, the following wording: "Please indicate your *current* pain intensity."

Most assessment in medicine and behavioral science, however, does not focus on momentary assessment, but for practical reasons typically asks for a summary of experience over a period of time or about a past experience at a particular time. These are called retrospective self-reports, and the time frame for these questions can range from the last day to one's entire life. The important idea is that the intention of the question is to capture information outside of immediate experience, which is presumed to be available in memory. Examples of typical recall questions include "Please indicate your average pain intensity over the past month," which asks the respondent not only to recall but then to summarize (average) the retrieved results, and "When was the last time you stayed overnight in a hospital?" which asks for a specific fact relating to a particular occasion.

The third type of self-report, global report, does not have any time frame at all, but rather asks the respondent to generalize globally or universally. "Generally speaking, how happy a person are you?" and "Are you prone to anxiety?" are examples of global questions. These questions seek information about a person in general. They might be equivalent to retrospective summaries over a lifetime, but that is not clear.

3 Does Ecological Validity Matter for Self-Report?

Our focus is on the relevance of ecological validity in the three kinds of self-reports, and we believe this depends on two things. The first is whether or not the phenomenon to be captured by self-report varies over time and situation, and the second is whether or not individuals can accurately recall and summarize it without distortion. In brief, we believe that special procedures are needed to assure ecological validity when a phenomenon varies over time *and* when respondents are not able to accurately recall and/or summarize it. Under these conditions, asking respondents for their impression of experience over some finite time period will yield results that may not accurately reflect real-world experience.

3.1 Variability over Time and Situation

When the variable under study does not vary with time and circumstances (e.g., the respondent's gender), any method of self-report (your current state, your state yesterday, your state in general) will yield the same answer, making issues of recall and ecological validity moot. However, most of the phenomena we study do vary over time for several reasons. They may vary due to the impact of the immediate context (physical setting [work/home, outside/inside, and other physical qualities] or social setting [whom with, type of activity, and other interpersonal qualities]); due to maturation of the individual and associated change; or due to temporal effects such as time-of-day, day-of-week, season, etc. These factors create true variation, not just variation due to measurement error (noise), and investigators have an interest in that true variation. When such variation exists, and individuals are not capable of producing an unbiased summary of the variable experience (discussed

in next section), consideration of ecological validity is essential.

As an example of how environmental variability demands consideration in the design of studies to ensure ecological validity, consider an investigator who is trying to characterize participants' emotional state over a period of time. Now, affect is known to vary depending on the circumstances and setting. To achieve an accurate assessment of "average mood," which might serve as an investigator's outcome variable in trial, one would need to consider the full range of settings that the individual encountered – their mood may have been relaxed at home, but tense at work, or relaxed at work on Tuesday, but tense at work on Wednesday. In this case, it would be misleading to assess mood at work only or on Tuesdays only. The full range (or a representative range) of experiences and contexts would need to be taken into account, and properly weighted, to achieve an unbiased assessment of mood over the period. If one believes that individuals are capable of retrieving this information and weighting it appropriately, then recall summaries would be considered valid. If one concludes that we are not consistently capable of such cognitive feats, then one may need to actually sample and assess experiences across a range of time and settings (methods for doing so are discussed later).

3.2 Accuracy of Recall and Summary Processes

We have suggested that conclusions about respondents' ability to accurately recall and summarize the past are vital to determining how one collects data. Key to appreciating the limits of autobiographical memory is understanding the process of recording, retrieval, and summary of information about past experience. How, then, do we generate recall of and summarize our past states? Research indicates that the process of generating such "memories" is more accurately characterized as *reconstruction* (Menon and Yorkston, 2000; Schwarz and Strack, 1991) than simple retrieval.[1] Memories can be reconstructed using a variety of heuristic strategies to build plausible responses that usually serve adequately for memory's everyday adaptive uses. The use of heuristics is a critical point, because heuristic strategies can introduce significant bias. Ironically, for environmentally sensitive variables, the subject's state *at the time of the recall*, which is itself subject to the effects of the recall setting, can influence recall and summary processes. For example, several studies have shown that the pain levels experienced at the time of assessment biases the recall of past pain, such that respondents in current high levels of pain recall more pain (Eich et al, 1985; Linton and Melin, 1982; Smith and Safer, 1993).[2] In another example, Schwarz has shown that very small pleasures (finding a dime) just prior to assessment can have large impacts on responses to global well-being questions (Schwarz, 1996). Or, that bringing to mind remembrances of events that pertain, at least in part, to the broad question have the effect biasing responses toward the recently recalled experiences (Schwarz, 1996). Current states skew both what information we retrieve about the past (e.g., mood congruent recall; Clark and Teasdale, 1982) and how we interpret that information. In other words, our summaries of past experience are not built from objective, statistical summaries of the past, but are influenced by our present condition.

In a similar way, participants' recall of experience is overly influenced by the most intense and the most recent experiences during the target reporting period; this has been called the

"peak-end" effect (Fredrickson, 2000). Both the undue influence of our current state and that of recent and intense experiences are attributable to the influence of what is most "memorable" or salient, and the consequent under-weighting of routine experience – the fabric of everyday life – often resulting in systematic bias in recall (Kahneman et al, 1999). It should be noted that these heuristics operate rapidly and out of consciousness, as demonstrated by their impact in laboratory studies examining short-term recall (e.g., Redelmeier's colonscopy studies, Redelmeier and Kahneman, 1996). So, research participants, who are usually doing their best to provide accurate recall, are not aware that their recall reports are biased and have no ready way to avoid the bias. Not only do heuristics produce bias (that is, systematic errors) in contrast to merely injecting "noise" (random error) into recall, but the use of particular heuristics may vary between persons and across contexts, making it difficult to devise strategies that correct for heuristic bias and, more broadly, making the interpretation of recall reports exceedingly challenging.

Recall is also influenced by semantic memory, that is, generalized knowledge or belief (e.g., about myself, about work; Robinson and Clore, 2002; Ross, 1989). This may be especially prevalent when memories of an event, which may or may not be accurate, do not spring into mind. Memories constructed in this way are often "adjusted" to make them conform to logical scripts about events based on broader beliefs about behavior (in general or one's own) – they represent "what should have happened" or "what must have happened." Ross (1989) has shown that participants distort their recall to conform to their "personal theories" about behavior, for example, ideas about how stable or changeable their behavior is, beliefs about the influence of events on behavior, or their beliefs or ideals about themselves. These biases are particularly troubling, because they can generate "recall" that is psychologically coherent and consistent with theory (and thus easily accepted by scientists), but not based on fact. For example, participants who believe they have painful menstrual

---

[1]In fact, retrieval is not a simple process in that what is retrieved may be influenced by the individual's psychological state at the time of retrieval. For example, unpleasant memories are more accessible when an individual is in a negative affective state than when in positive affective state (Kihlstrom, et al 2000).

[2]A respondent's affective or pain state at the time of retrospection also influences the accessibility of certain memories and the heuristic processes used to summarize retrieved memories.

periods tend to "recall" such pain (and investigators may accept such reports), even when their own real-time reports showed they did not experience them (McFarland et al, 1989; see also Shiffman et al, 1997). Thus, cognitive science tells us that autobiographical memory is subject to substantial biases that can significantly distort self-reports. We next examine the implications of recall and summary processes for the different types of self-reports.

3.3 Implications for Global Reports

Evaluating the impact of accuracy and summary processes on global reports is difficult because it is not clear exactly how global assessment *should* line up with actual experience. If one assumes that global questions are meant to or are interpreted as reflecting experience – perhaps not an unreasonable assumption in many cases – then all of the troublesome processes associated with recall reports are applicable. Furthermore, there is evidence that ambiguity about what information is sought by a question and/or the inability to access that information from memory disposes respondents to answer on the basis of semantic memory (Robinson and Clore, 2002). Particularly when it is not clear what memories are relevant over what period, global questions will tend to pull for answers based on beliefs and attitudes. Although semantic memory has a connection to experience, that connection can be a loose one because other factors, such as beliefs, personality, and contextual cues. If it is actual experience that one seeks, then answers based on semantic memory are not ideal.

On the other hand, if one is interested in beliefs or opinions – and not actual experience – then global reports may be optimal. Beliefs and opinions can shape current and future behavior, so are of practical value and worthy of study in their own right, but care must be taken to distinguish between these beliefs and actual past behavior and experience, which may not be accurately reflected.

3.4 Implications for Retrospective Reports

The validity of retrospective self-reports depends on reporters' ability to accurately recall experience. As discussed above, cognitive research suggests that much of the information we seek about past behavior or experiences is not available in memory; we simply do not store such detailed and comprehensive information (Bradburn et al, 1987; Robinson and Clore, 2002; Schwarz and Oyserman, 2001; Schwarz et al, 1994; Thompson et al, 1996). Accuracy of recall and summary processes are, then, a major concern for interpreting recall reports. The extent of the concern, however, should be moderated by the nature of the recall content, as certain material (e.g., major, "unforgettable" events) may be less susceptible to memory failures, although still may be subject to the vagaries of summary processes.

It is also important to recognize that even "incorrect" or distorted recall can have substantial predictive validity. Some studies have shown that one's distorted memory or characterization of events can be a better predictor of future behavior than the actual experience. After all, it is this stored summary, however biased, that we later retrieve as a reference for future informing attitudes or directing our behavior (e.g., recalling how painful a previous colonoscopy was in order to decide whether to get another one; Redelmeier et al, 2003). Thus, there is value to the information held in retrospective reports, even when it does not faithfully reflect experience, but care must be taken not to interpret it as a true account of past events.

3.5 Implications for Momentary Reports

Assessments of current experience are not subject to recall bias, so the heuristics associated with memory processes are not much of a problem for these assessments. In contrast to the difficulty recovering accurate information about the past, Robinson and Clore (2002) and others have argued that we have good access to our current or very recent states; that is, questions about immediate state are answered by retrieval of experience and not by reference to beliefs. However, to say that momentary reports are immune to recall biases is not to say that such reports are entirely accurate and reliable, because self-reports are susceptible to other distortions that can influence the assessment (for example, the desire to present oneself in a favorable light; Schwarz, 2007), but at least the biases introduced by memory processes are minimized.

In summary, recall and global questions are prone to bias due to the limitations of memory capacity and to the ways that people reconstruct and summarize experiences over time. These biases threaten the validity of the resulting reports when those reports are meant to represent the actual experiences the individual had over the specified period recalled. Immediate reports can escape biases due to recall processes, but raise new challenges for achieving ecological validity.

4 Rationale for Taking Self-Report into Everyday Life

Despite the potential problems identified for recall and global questions, these types of questions have dominated the field of self-report assessment. First, recall is subjectively compelling: We trust our own memories unquestioningly most of the time, so it seems natural to trust our participants' memory as well, particularly when they don't seem to have a motive for dissembling. Yet research has shown that confidence in a particular memory is often unrelated to its accuracy (Busey et al, 2000; Wells and Bradfield, 1998). Additionally, the nature of memory and its tendency to bias is a relatively recent discovery and has not yet penetrated deeply into thinking about research methods.

Recall methods are also used because they are enormously convenient and efficient: In a relatively brief period, the researcher or clinician

is able to gather information on long periods of time, often up to years in duration, and on a wide variety of environments. If recall and global methods were capable of providing accurate information over such periods, there would be very little reason to consider alternatives. But, as the prior section of this chapter has shown, recall and recall self-reports may not be up to the task of providing truly accurate information about experience, at least some of the time.

If memory cannot be relied upon, then momentary assessments become essential. However, momentary assessments are limited by their very immediacy and narrow focus to what is happening *now*, at the moment of assessment, which is not often the investigator's focus. We earlier stated that many phenomena of interest vary across time and environmental context. It follows that momentary reports of those phenomena will vary by context. Thus, if momentary reports are to represent the person's overall experience, they would have to be collected in those contexts. No one momentary report could represent the subject's experience – there would have to be many. And, to achieve ecological validity, they would have to be collected in a wide range of real-world contexts, representatively sampling participants' momentary states across the range of settings they encounter.

These elements – real-time data collection about momentary states, repeated assessments, and sampling of real-world settings – form the core of the approach we have called Ecological Momentary Assessment (EMA; Stone et al, 1994, 2007; Shiffman et al, 2008).

Modern EMA methods have made use of innovations in data-collection technology, but EMA is not primarily a technological development. It more fundamentally addresses the design of data-collection protocols in relation to study objectives. Bolger and colleagues (2003) have enumerated three broad functions of EMA data collection: characterizing persons and individual differences (e.g., level of depressive symptoms); estimating within-person variability (e.g., standard deviation of pain intensity levels over a 1 month period); and estimating within-person associations among two or more variables (e.g., association between changes in sleep and gastrointestinal symptoms the following day or between time-of-day and fatigue levels). The reader is referred to Stone et al (2006) and Shiffman et al (2009) for examples demonstrating these uses of EMA data.

Aside from addressing issues of recall bias, EMA methods conceptually address other issues discussed in the psychological assessment literature. The first concerns the arbitrary nature of measurement often associated with psychological assessments, a topic recently reviewed by Blanton and Jaccard (2006). In essence, it is difficult to understand the meaning of scale scores on many instruments, because they are not linked to other referents. So, when an individual moves from an affect score of 50–60 on a 100-point scale, it is impossible to know exactly how their affect has changed. Because EMA protocols can representatively sample over time, it is possible to express the observations by estimating the proportion of time an individual has experienced some state (e.g., is angry, by some definition) or is in a particular environment (e.g., at work). Such "prevalence" metrics offer the advantage of being easily interpretable and, further, they possess ratio level measurement qualities. The clear labeling afforded by such measures enhances the opportunity to develop strong theories and interventions, which is not the case when there is less certainty about a measure's meaning (Blanton and Jaccard, 2006). Also consistent with recommendations of Blanton and Jaccard is the emphasis on the assessment of real-world occurrences.

A second conceptual issue concerns the place of EMA data in an assessment model, which is pertinent to considerations of its usefulness in theory development. Here we refer to the framework developed by McFall (2005) in an article on theory and utility in evidence-based assessment. In our view, self-report EMA data can be considered an instance of a "sample" approach versus the alternative "sign" approach to assessment. This is because EMA measures often directly assess the target experience or behavior, rather than some other construct that is simply

associated with the target. Signs, on the other hand, are indirect measures that simply have predictive utility (as in an actuarial prediction where any variable statistically associated with an outcome can be used to improve prediction, even if it has no conceptual overlap). Importantly, because there can be recall and summary problems with self-report data that can invalidate an assessment, EMA data may have unique value in providing proximal sample data for assessment. For example, one method for measuring coping with difficult events is based upon 1-month recall of the problem and the thoughts and behaviors used to cope with the problem. We compared real-time reports of these thoughts and behaviors with the recalled ones and found major discrepancies (Stone et al, 1998). Similarly, we compared global reports of smoking patterns to detailed real-time self-monitoring and found little correspondence (Shiffman, 1993); only the real-time data predicted subsequent relapse (Shiffman et al, 2007). In both cases, the real-time data might be considered a preferable sample.

The next issue concerns the isomorphism between recall measures of an outcome and EMA measures of an outcome. As mentioned above, using EMA to characterize overall levels of a self-report variable over a defined period of time is one of its primary uses. Little would be gained by using EMA methods if the resulting data were identical to those obtained by recall methods. Although there is a surfeit of information about *potential* reasons for achieving different results with the two methods, there is a paucity of empirical data documenting differences. In directly comparing data produced by the methods, two types of comparison emerge: (1) differences in levels (assuming the same measurement metric was used for both methods) and (2) differences in correspondence between rank-orderings of individuals by the methods (e.g., the correlation between the scores) (Stone et al, 2004; Shiffman et al, 2008).

Our own work on the assessment of pain intensity in patients with chronic pain disorders has partially addressed this question. Regarding differences in level of reporting, retrospective assessments produce higher levels of pain when compared to the average of momentary reports for the same period of time, and the discrepancy between the methods increases as the reporting period increases (Broderick et al, 2008). One possible explanation for these results is that the peak heuristic, which posits a particular focus on high levels of past pain, leads to an overemphasis of bouts of pain in the recalled reports (Stone et al, 2004). Others have also observed the higher level of reporting with recall measures (Linton and Gotestam, 1983; vandenBrink et al, 2001). On correspondence between the two methods, the situation is less clear because although there is a substantial correlation between the pain reports from the two methods (about 50% of the variance is shared), there is also a substantial proportion of variance that is unique to each method. This general finding led earlier researchers to call it a "half-empty or half-full" situation, depending upon one's perspective (Salovey et al, 1993).

Whether or not the magnitude of the association seems acceptable, there is evidence that recalled reports can be distorted in undesirable ways. For example, we found that how much pain a respondent experienced at the time of reporting their retrospective weekly level influenced the magnitude of retrospective report (Broderick et al, 2006). We have also reported that the degree of variability in EMA pain reports over a week is associated with recall of pain over the same week (Stone et al, 2005). The degree and direction of differences between recalled and actual immediate experience, and how these are affected by study conditions, needs further empirical exploration.

5 Conducting EMA Studies

Our purpose in this section of the chapter is to provide the reader with an overview of the many issues that confront the researcher endeavoring to collect self-reports from everyday life.

The presentation focuses on design considerations relating to ecological validity, but the reader is referred to many excellent comprehensive reviews (Affleck et al, 1999; Bolger et al, 2003; Delespaul, 1995; Shiffman et al, 2008; Stone et al, 2006). EMA is comprised of a variety of sampling designs that can be used singly or can be combined to meet the needs of investigators (Shiffman, 2006). A variety of schemes for scheduling assessments to ensure a representative sample of moments have been described (Delespaul, 1995; Shiffman, 2006).

The most commonly used schedules sample participants' experience through time-sampling; that is, they select a random sample of moments for assessment. The classic examples, from Experience Sampling Methodology (Csikszentmihalyi and Larsen, 1987; DeVries, 1987), are studies where participants are "beeped" at random times and prompted to complete an assessment of their momentary state. Random sampling of moments is seen as the key to representativeness, much as random sampling of individuals is seen as important for characterizing populations. As with sampling of individuals, any given sample of moments from a period of time will not yield a perfectly representative picture of a self-report variable; there will be an associated sampling error, just as there is when sampling people. Greater numbers of samples yield estimates with smaller sampling error.

Random time-sampling is not the only assessment schedule used in the EMA literature. An alternative is to schedule assessments at particular times of day, for example, every 2 h after 10 am, as a way to capture the day's experience. The limitations of this approach are discussed in Shiffman et al, (2008). Another alternative scheduling scheme is not based on time at all, but instead focuses on assessing particular events of interest. Thus, participants might be asked to complete an assessment every time they smoke a cigarette or engage in a social interaction. These event-based methods, which evolved from behavioral self-monitoring (Korotitsch and Nelson-Grey, 1999), are best suited to contexts where the phenomenon of interest is a discrete event (e.g., an asthma attack) or can be construed into episodes (e.g., exacerbations of pain).

A few examples can help characterize EMA methodology: In one study, patients with rheumatologic disorders rated their pain and mood up to 12 times a day when prompted at random times by a computer to complete an assessment (Stone et al, 2004). In another study, problem drinkers tracked each episode of drinking, recorded their level of intoxication and how they felt about their drinking (Muraven et al, 2005). A third study assessed the symptoms of people complaining of multiple chemical sensitivity several times per day, while simultaneously sampling the surrounding air for analysis of chemical exposures (Saito et al, 2005). In a study illustrating a combination of time-based and event-based sampling, Shiffman and Waters (2004) used time-sampled data to examine trends in affect in the days and hours preceding a focal event (smoking relapse). While the subject populations, assessments, and content focus differed, these EMA studies and others (Stone et al, 2006) share an approach involving multiple momentary assessments, collected near the time of experience, across a broad range of real-world settings the participants inhabit, and with attention to sampling of experience (e.g., random time-sampling). These are the core elements of EMA.

In another parallel with sampling of research participants, EMA researchers have been concerned about the loss of observations from the planned sample and accordingly have emphasized the importance of compliance with scheduled assessments and inclusion of all relevant moments in the sampling frame as key to representativeness (Hufford and Shields, 2002; Stone et al, 2002; Shiffman et al, 2008). Just as attrition from a sample of participants threatens the representativeness of the sample, so noncompliance with assessment prompts threatens the representativeness of the sample of moments. A variety of EMA sampling schemes, paralleling the variety of sampling designs for individuals in populations, have been described and used (stratified sampling, over-sampling, etc.) (Shiffman, 2006).

5.1 Implementation of EMA and Application of Technology

Advances in technology have enabled the conduct of efficient and imaginative EMA studies. Early diary studies had no reliable way of scheduling assessments or prompting participants to complete them, so assessments were often linked to standard events in participants' lives, such as meals or bedtime. However, these are hardly random moments in a person's day. An innovation was introduced by the developers of the Experience Sampling Method, who provided participants with electronic pagers and arranged to "beep" them to prompt them to complete a diary card (Csikszentmihalyi and Larsen, 1987). By providing a means of signaling the subject, beepers gave the investigator control over the intended schedule of assessments, which were typically recorded on traditional paper diary cards.

The use of electronic data capture for EMA has become increasingly common. Besides scheduling and issuing prompts, a palmtop can also collect and store the assessment data, while recording the exact time the assessment was completed. This is regarded as an important advantage, because of concerns about back-filling of data – that is, the completion of assessments after-the-fact, with falsification of the completion date and time, which negates the advantages of real-time data collection. There has been controversy about how often back-filling occurs, how it might be minimized, and what effects back-filling has on the resulting data (Green et al, 2006).

Nevertheless, several studies, with diverse populations and methods have demonstrated that participants do back-fill paper diary entries, even when they are electronically prompted for completion, and sometimes even when they are aware their entries are subject to verification (Hufford, 2007). This can be a serious concern, because participants who complete their diaries in retrospect reintroduce all of the problems of retrospective recall that the method was designed to avoid. Moreover, when participants choose when they complete the diaries, even if it's not long after the scheduled time, they can introduce additional bias because participants' choice of occasions can be biased (e.g., waiting until a symptom-free time to complete a diary or completing it when symptoms occur and serve as a reminder to do the diary). In essence, the sample of moments becomes like a convenience sample of volunteers, rather than like a random population sample. Accordingly, the ability of electronic data-collection methods to accurately record the time of diary completion is regarded by many investigators as an advantage over paper-and-pencil diaries.

Another advantage of many electronic data-collection systems is that they allow flexibility in the administration of questions, for example, item presentation can be contingent upon responses to prior items (e.g., skip patterns), greatly enhancing efficiency and reducing subject burden. Moreover, such electronic systems can also modify the sampling schedule based on algorithms applied to subject input, for instance, increasing the density of assessment when an event of interest has occurred or scheduling a series of assessments to follow up on a trigger event.

The most commonly used electronic devices for collecting self-report EMA data are palmtop computers and interactive voice response systems (IVRS). An advantage of palmtop computers is that they function independently and thus are not dependent on communication to a central center. They are also capable of presenting a variety of response options (Likert scales, Visual Analog Scale [VAS], Numeric Rating Scale, body diagrams) that are typically used in assessments. Since they present assessment content as text, the assessments resemble their paper ancestors, which probably accounts for the finding that such electronic assessments are psychometrically equivalent to parallel paper forms (Gwaltney et al, 2008).

In IVRS, assessment content is played to participants via recorded voice, and participants record their responses using the keypad ("press '1' if you are suicidal..."). While IVRS is most often used as a passive system requiring participants to call in, it can also be used to call participants on a schedule enabling time-sampling designs. With the advent of cell phones, the phone system can be used to reach participants in a wide variety of settings. An advantage is that IVRS uses the telephone – a technology familiar to participants. A disadvantage is that aural presentation of assessment and response options can limit the assessment (e.g., memory capacity limits the number of response options) and might change how participants respond.

As cell phones become more sophisticated, "smart phones" are increasingly able to function much like palmtop computers, displaying text-based assessments and sending assessment data to a central server. Desktop computer systems (web-based or otherwise), while not portable and thus not amenable to assessment in the full range of participants' settings, can be used to administer end-of-day or periodic assessments.

At the same time, these approaches are used to collect self-report data; a variety of specialized hardware can be used to assess participants' objective physiological states in a momentary way (e.g., ambulatory blood pressure, blood glucose, pulmonary function) (Kamarck et al, 1998). Other devices can objectively capture subject behavior (e.g., instrumented pill bottles, motion-detectors, audio or video recordings (Byerly et al, 2005)) or environmental conditions (e.g., noise, temperature, presence of chemical pollutants (e.g., Saito et al, 2005)). Collection of such objective data is often enriched by collecting concomitant self-report data, allowing these objective assessments to be linked to subjective states. Thus, technology has enabled a new age for collection of real-world data in real time (Kamarck et al, 1998).

5.2 Concerns About EMA

Nevertheless, there are issues that threaten the validity of these new methodologies. The frequency of EMA measurement and the fact that it takes place in participants' natural environments have raised concerns about reactivity – that is, the possibility that the act of measurement itself affects the phenomenon being measured. Evidence to date suggests that reactivity is minimal. One study randomized patients being assessed for pain to be assessed 3, 6, or 12 times daily, and it found no systematic change in their pain ratings (Stone et al, 2004), consistent with findings from an earlier study (Cruise et al, 1996). Other studies have found no effect on monitoring of behaviors such as drinking or smoking (Hufford et al, 2002). Empirical investigations have, then, reduced concern about reactivity, but further study may turn up contexts in which reactivity is a problem.

EMA studies can be demanding, often requiring participants to complete many assessments each day. This raises concerns about participants' ability or willingness to comply. Yet, across studies with diverse protocols and populations, a high degree of compliance is often achieved (Hufford and Shields, 2002). Some EMA studies make particularly high demands on participants, but what is striking is the degree of compliance observed even when the study demands might seem unrealistic on first blush. In that study where pain patients were randomized to complete 3, 6, or 12 assessments per day, compliance was excellent (averaging 94%) and was unaffected by the frequency of assessment (Stone et al, 2004). Even protocols with more than 20 prompts per day have achieved high compliance rates (Kamarck et al, 2007) Further, Freedman and colleagues (2006) showed that even homeless, crack cocaine addicts were able to complete an EMA study with multiple daily assessments with reasonable compliance. Thus, with proper management, participants seem able to bear the burden of intensive EMA sampling.

A related concern is whether the demands of EMA studies lead to bias in subject samples. We are not aware of any formal data on this, but some participants may not be willing or able to engage in these demanding protocols. In our experience, the demands of a subject's work are a common source of conflict; for example, neither surgeons nor waitresses can afford to be interrupted by unscheduled prompts. Such participant sampling bias should be evaluated and weighed in interpreting EMA data. Sometimes concerns are raised about whether older participants might have difficulty with technology such as palmtop computers. Analysis of compliance by age has demonstrated that older participants can be trained to operate the palmtops and actually demonstrate better compliance than younger participants.

There are, though, issues that may limit participants' participation. Deficits in eyesight (to see questions), hearing (to hear the phone or "beeps"), or manual dexterity (to manipulate a stylus or keypad) could certainly make some participants incapable of performing in an EMA study, though some of these deficits would also make traditional assessment difficult. More data on how EMA methods influence study participation and representativeness of subject samples would be useful.

6 Conclusion

We have argued that ecological validity is a critical component of self-report assessment for retrospective and global methods, one that is necessary for the validity of many content domains. Brunswik (1949) was correct in his assessment of the "formidable" nature of implementing representative designs to achieve what we now call "ecological validity," although he was not specifically referring to self-report data at that time. Recent developments in technology have made representative sampling of self-reports practical for most researchers, through the advent of sophisticated electronic diaries and interactive voice recording. There is no longer a need to personally shadow research participants as Brunswik did in order collect self-reports in a representative manner to achieve ecological validity. It is our hope that knowledge of these developments will hasten the adoption of methods for collecting real-time real-world data from research participants and overcome at least some aspects of the task envisioned by Brunswik over 50 years ago.

References

Affleck, G., Tennen, H., Keefe, F. J., Lefebvre, J. C., Kashikar-Zuck, S. et al (1999). Everyday life with osteoarthritis or rheumatoid arthritis: independent effects of disease and gender on daily pain, mood and coping. *Pain, 83*, 601–609.

Blanton, H., and Jaccard, J. (2006). Arbitrary metric in psychology. *Am Psychol, 61*, 27–41.

Bolger, N., Davis, A., and Rafaeli, E. (2003). Dairy methods: capturing life as it is lived. *Ann Rev Psychol, 54*, 579–616.

Bradburn, N., Rips, L., and Shevell, S. (1987). Answering autobiographical questions: the impact of memory and inference on surveys. *Science, 236*, 151–167.

Broderick, J., Schwartz, J., and Stone, A. (2006, 3–6 May). Context (pain and affect) influences recall pain ratings [Poster presented at the Annual Meeting of the American Pain Society]. San Antonio, TX.

Broderick, J., Schwartz, J., Vikingstad, G., Pribbernow, M., Grossman, S., and Stone, A. (2008). The accuracy of pain and fatigue items across different reporting periods. Pain, *139*, 146–157.

Brunswik, E. (1944). Distal focussing of perception: size constancy in a representative sample of situations. *Psychol Monogr, 56*, 1–49.

Brunswik, E. (1949). *Systematic and Representative Design of Psychological Experiments.* Berkeley and Los Angeles: University of California Press.

Busey, T., Tunnicliff, J., Loftus, G., and Loftus, E. (2000). Accounts of the confidence-accuracy relation in recognition memory. *Psychon Bull Rev, 7*, 26–48.

Byerly, M., Fisher, R., Whatley, K., Holland, R., Varghese, F. et al (2005). A comparison of electronic monitoring vs clinician rating of antipsychotic adherence in outpatients with schizophrenia. *Psychiat Res, 133*, 129–133.

Clark, D., and Teasdale, J. (1982). Diurnal variation in clinical depression and accessibility of memories of positive and negative experiences. *J Abnorm Psychol, 91*, 87–95.

Cruise, C., Porter, L., Broderick, J., Kaell, A., and Stone, A. (1996). Reactive effects of diary self-assessment in chronic pain patients. *Pain, 67*, 253–258.

Csikszentmihalyi, M., and Larsen, R. E. (1987). Validity and reliability of the experience sampling method. *J Nerv Med Dis, 175*, 526–536.

Delespaul, P. (1995). *Assessing Schizophrenia in Daily Life -- The Experience Sampling Method.* Maastricht: Maastricht University Press.

DeVries, M. (1987). Investigating mental disorders in their natural settings: introduction to the special issue. *J Nerv Men Dis, 175*, 509–513.

Eich, E., Reeves, J., Jaeger, B., and Graff-Radford, S. (1985). Memory for pain: relation between past and present pain intensity. *Pain, 223*, 375–379.

Fredrickson, B. (2000). Extracting meaning from past affective experiences: the importance of peaks, ends, and specific emotions. *Cogn Emot, 14*, 577–606.

Freedman, M., Lester, K., McNamara, C., Milby, J., and Schumacher, J. (2006). Cell phones for Ecological Momentary Assessment with cocaine-addicted homeless patients in treatment. *J Subst Abuse Treat, 30*, 105–111.

Green, A., Rafaeli, E., Bolger, N., Shrout, P., and Reis, H. (2006). Paper or plastic? Data equivalence in paper and electronic diaries. *Psychol Methods, 11*, 87–105.

Gwaltney, C., Shields, A., and Shiffman, S. (2008). Equivalence of electronic and paper-and-pencil administration of patient reported outcome measures. *Val Health , 11*, 322–333.

Hammond, K., and Stewart, T. (2001). *The Essential Brunswik: Beginnings, Explications, Applications.* New York, NY: Oxford University Press.

Hufford, M. (2007). Special methodological challenges and opportunities in Ecological Momentary Assessment. In A. Stone, S. Shiffman, A. Atienza, & L. Nebling (Eds.), *The Science of Real-Time Data Capture: Self-Reports in Health Research* (pp. 54–75). New York, NY: Oxford University Press.

Hufford, M., and Shields, A. (2002). Electronic diaries: an examination of applications and what works in the field. *Appl Clin Trials, 11*, 46–56.

Hufford, M., Shields, A., Shiffman, S., Paty, J., and Balabanis, M. (2002). Reactivity to ecological momentary assessment: an example using undergraduate problem drinkers. *Psychol Addict Behav, 16*, 205–211.

Kahneman, D., Diener, E., and Schwarz, N. (1999). *Well-Being: The Foundations of Hedonic Psychology.* New York: Russell Sage Foundation.

Kamarck, T., Shiffman, S., Smithline, L., Goodie, J., Paty, J. et al (1998). The effects of task strain, social conflict, and emotional activation on ambulatory cardiovascular activity: daily life consequences of "recurring stress" in a multiethnic sample. *Health Psychol, 17*, 17–29.

Kamarck, T., Shiffman, S., Muldoon, M., Sutton-Tyrell, K., Gwaltney, C. et al (2007). Ecological Momentary Assessment as a resource for social epidemiology. In A. Stone, S. Shiffman, A. Atienza, & L. Nebling (Eds.), *The Science of Real-Time Data Capture: Self-Reports in Health Research* (pp. 268–285). New York: Oxford University Press.

Kihlstrom, J., Eich, E., Sandbrand, D., and Tobias, B. (2000). Emotion and memory: implications for self-report. In A. Stone, J. Turkkan, C. Bachrach, J. Jobe, H. Kurtzman, & V. Cain (Eds.), *The Science of Self-Report: Implication for Research and Practice* (pp. 81–99). Mahwah, NJ: Erlbaum.

Korotitsch, W., and Nelson-Grey, R. (1999). An overview of self-monitoring research assessment and treatment. *Psychol Assess, 2*, 415–425.

Linton, S., and Gotestam, K. (1983). A clinical comparison of two pain scales: correlation, remembering chronic pain, and a measure of compliance. *Pain, 17*, 53–65.

Linton, S., and Melin, L. (1982). The accuracy of remembering chronic pain. *Pain, 13*, 281–285.

McFall, R. (2005). Theory and utility -- key themes in evidence-based assessment: comment on special section. *Am Psychol, 17*, 312–323.

McFarland, C., Ross, M., and DeCourville, N. (1989). Women's theories of menstruation and biases in recall of menstrual symptoms. *J Pers Soc Psychol, 57*, 522–531.

Menon, G., and Yorkston, E. (2000). The use of memory and contextual cues in the formation of behavioral frequency judgements. In A. Stone, J. Turkkan, C. Bachrach, J. Jobe, H. Kurtzman, & V. Cain (Eds.), *The Science of Self-Report: Implications for Research and Practice* (pp. 63–79). Mahwah, NJ: Lawrence Erlbaum Associates.

Muraven, M., Collins, R., Shiffman, S., and Paty, J. (2005). Daily fluctuations in self-control demands and alcohol intake. *Psychol Addict Behav, 19*, 140–147.

Redelmeier, D., and Kahneman, D. (1996). Patients' memories of pain medical treatments: real-time and retrospective evaluations of two minimally invasive procedures. *Pain, 66*, 3–8.

Redelmeier, D., Katz, J., and Kahneman, D. (2003). Memories of colonoscopy: a randomized trial. *Pain, 104*, 187–194.

Robinson, M., and Clore, G. (2002). Belief and feeling: evidence for an accessibility model of emotional self-report. *Psychol Bull, 128*, 934–960.

Rock, E., Scott, J., Kennedy, D., Sridhara, R., Pazdur, R., and Burke, L. (2007). Challenges to use of health-related quality of life for Food and Drug Administration Approval of anticancer products. *J Natl Cancer Inst Monogr, 25*, 27–30.

Ross, M. (1989). Relation of implicit theories to the construction of personal histories. *Psychol Rev, 96*, 341–357.

Saito, M., Kumano, H., Yoshiuchi, K., Kokubo, N., Ohashi, K., Yamamoto, Y. et al (2005). Symptom profile of multiple chemical sensitivity in actual life. *Psychosom Med, 67*, 318–325.

Salovey, P., Sieber, W., Jobe, J., and Willis, G. (1993). The recall of physical pain. In N. Schwarz & S. Sudman (Eds.), *Autobiographical Memory and the Validity of Retrospective Reports* (pp. 89–106). New York: Springer-Verlag.

Schwarz, N. (1996). *Cognition and Communication: Judgmental Biases, Research Methods, and the Logic of Conversation*. Hillsdale, NJ: Erlbaum.

Schwarz, N. (2007). Retrospective and concurrent self-report: the rationale for real-time data capture. In A. Stone, S. Shiffman, A. Atienza, & L. Nebling (Eds.), *The Science of Real-Time Data Capture: Self-Reports in Health Research* (pp. 11–26). New York: Oxford University Press.

Schwarz, N., and Oyserman, D. (2001). Asking questions about behavior: cognition, communication and questionnaire construction. *Am J Eval, 22*, 127–160.

Schwarz, N., Wanke, M., and Bless, H. (1994). Subjective assessments and evaluations of change: some lessons learned from social cognitive research. *Eeuro Rev Soc Psychol, 5*, 181–210.

Schwarz, N., and Strack, F. (1991). Evaluating one's life: a judgment model of subjective well-being. In F. Strack, M. Argyle, & N. Schwarz (Eds.), *Subjective Well-Being: An Interdisciplinary Approach* (pp. 27–47). Oxford: Pergamon Press.

Shiffman, S. (2006). Designing protocols for Ecological Momentary Assessment. In A. Stone, S. Shiffman, A. Atienza, & L. Nebling (Eds.), *The Science of Real-Time Data Capture: Self-Reports in Health Research*. New York: Oxford University Press.

Shiffman, S. (1993). Assessing smoking patterns and motives. *J Consult Clin Psychol, 61*, 732–742.

Shiffman, S., Balabanis, M., Gwaltney, C., Paty, J., Gnys, M. et al (2007). Prediction of lapse from associations between smoking and situational antecedents assessed by ecological momentary assessment. *Drug Alc Depend, 91*, 159–168.

Shiffman, S., Hufford, M., Hickcox, M., Paty, J. A., Gnys, M., and Kassel, J. D. (1997). Remember that? A comparison of real-time vs. retrospective recall of smoking lapses. *J Consult Clin Psychol, 65*, 292–300.

Shiffman, S., Hufford, M., and Stone, A. (2008). Ecological momentary assessment in clinical psychology. *Annu Rev Clin Psychol, 4*, 1–32.

Shiffman, S., and Waters, A. (2004). Negative affect and smoking lapses: a prospective analysis. *J Consult Clin Psychol, 72*, 1192–201.

Smith, W., and Safer, M. (1993). Effects of present pain level on recall of chronic pain and medication use. *Pain, 55*, 355–361.

Stone, A., Schwartz, J., Broderick, J., and Shiffman, S. (2005). Variability of momentary pain predicts recall of weekly pain: a consequence of the peak (or salience) memory heuristic. *Person Soc Psychol Bull 31*, 1340–1346.

Stone, A., Schwartz, J., Neale, J., Shiffman, S., Marco, C., Hickcox, M. et al (1998). How accurate are current coping assessments? A comparison of momentary versus end-of-day reports of coping efforts. *J Person Soc Psychol, 74*, 1670–1680.

Stone, A., Shiffman, S., Atienza, A., and Nebling, L. (2007). *The Science of Real-Time Data Capture: Self-Reports in Health Research.* New York: Oxford University.

Stone, A., Shiffman, S., Schwartz, J., Broderick, J., and Hufford, M. (2002). Patient non-compliance with paper diaries. *Br Med J, 324,* 1193–1194.

Stone, A., Turkkan, J., Jobe, J., Bachrach, C., Kurtzman, H., and Cain, V. (2000). *The science of self report.* Mahwah, NJ: Erlbaum.

Stone, A., Broderick, J., Shiffman, S., and Schwartz, J. (2004). Understanding recall of weekly pain from a momentary assessment perspective: absolute accuracy, between- and within-person consistency, and judged change in weekly pain. *Pain, 107,* 61–69.

Stone, A. A., and Shiffman, S. (1994). Ecological Momentary Assessment (EMA) in behavioral medicine. *Annals of Behavioral Medicine, 16,* 199–202.

Thompson, C., Skowronski, J., Larsen, S., and Betz, A. (1996). *Autobiographical Memory: Remembering What and Remembering When.* Mahwah, NJ: Erlbaum.

vandenBrink, M., Bandell-Hoekstra, F., and Abu-Saad, H. (2001). The occurrence of recall bias in pediatric headache: a comparison of questionnaire and diary data. *Headache, 41,* 11–20.

Wells, G., and Bradfield, A. (1998). "Good, you identified the suspect": feedback to eyewitnesses distorts their reports of the witnessing experience. *J Apply Psychol, 83,* 360–376.

Chapter 9

Item Response Theory and Its Application to Measurement in Behavioral Medicine

Mee-Ae Kim-O and Susan E. Embretson

1 Introduction

Item response theory (IRT) has become a mainstream approach for developing psychological measurement and standardized educational tests development in the 21st century. IRT is currently the mainstream method for measuring cognitive abilities and achievement. For the measurement in behavioral medicine, IRT models can be applied to personality traits (Reise and Waller, 1990), attitude measurements and behavioral ratings (Engelhard and Wilson, 1996), clinical testing issues (Santor et al, 1994), as well as to measures of psychopathology, moods, behavioral dispositions, and situational evaluations.

Applications of IRT models and associated methods can solve many practical problems in behavioral medicine. In the USA, the Patient-Reported Outcomes Measurement Information System (PROMIS) has been funded by the National Institute of Health to provide publically available computerized tests for many patient-reported outcomes of disease, such as depression, fatigue, and pain. IRT has been a major method for scaling and equating these tests because it solves many practical problems. For example, subsets of standardized self-report measures are often administered to reduce testing time in many clinical studies. IRT can be applied to equate item subsets to the original test. Further, IRT is the primary basis for adaptive testing to permit more reliable measurement of all levels of performance. This feature is particularly important in measuring change over time and treatment. Simulation studies have shown that treatment effects may not be adequately estimated if the test does not provide reliable measurement at the initial and later stages (Embretson, 1996).

This chapter will provide the overview of IRT and its models, as well as an example to illustrate applications. In Sections 2.1 and 2.2, the limitations of classical test theory will be reviewed and the contribution of IRT to overcome the limitations will be described. In Sections 3.1, 3.2, and 3.3, some fundamental IRT models will be reviewed in two categories (binary IRT models and polytomous IRT models). Then, in Sections 4.1 and 4.2, an application of IRT to questionnaires in behavioral medicine will be described.

2 Item Response Theory Versus Classical Test Theory

2.1 Limitations of Classical Test Theory

Psychometric theory can be divided into two categories: classical test theory (CTT) and item response theory (IRT). CTT was pioneered by Spearman (1904, 1907, 1913) and it has defined the standard for test development since the 1930s

M.-A. Kim-O (✉)
School of Psychology, Georgia Institute of Technology, 654 Cherry St, Atlanta, GA 30332-0170, USA
e-mail: gth733b@mail.gatech.edu

A. Steptoe (ed.), *Handbook of Behavioral Medicine*, DOI 10.1007/978-0-387-09488-5_9,
© Springer Science+Business Media, LLC 2010

(see Embretson and Reise, 2000). Allen and Yen (1979) characterize CTT as a simple model that describes how errors of measurement can influence observed scores. The CTT model can be expressed as

$$X_{ip} = T_{ip} + E_{ip}, \qquad (9.1)$$

where X_{ip} is an observed score for test i and person p, T_{ip} is a true score of test i and person p, and E_{ip} is an error score of test i and person p.

In the CTT model, estimates of examinees' true test scores are typically linear transformations of the raw test score, which are related to relevant normative populations by the transformation. Alternative test forms can be used to estimate true scores if the forms are parallel tests with the same expected true scores and error distributions. Psychometric indices for items in CTT are related to the properties of the test scores, particularly reliability and variance. That is, item difficulty is the proportion of persons passing or endorsing an item while item discrimination is the correlation of the item with the total test score.

However, CTT has three obvious limitations. First, an examinee's true score depends on the difficulty level of a test (test dependent). Scores will not be comparable between easy and hard tests. Second, the item characteristics depend on the ability of examinees (sample dependent). Item difficulty, for example, will vary substantially if the true score distributions vary between populations. Third, the parallel test assumption that two true test scores and two error variances are identical in the two tests is never fully met in practice. Therefore, it is difficult to compare examinees who take different tests and to contrast items whose characteristic indices are computed using different groups of examinees.

Because of these fundamental limitations of CTT, an alternative theory and model of mental measurement are desirable. Hambleton et al (1991) asserted that the desirable features of an alternative test theory would include (a) item characteristics that are not sample dependent, (b) examinees' true scores that are not test dependent, (c) a model that is expressed at the item level rather than at the test level, (d) a model that does not require the strictly parallel tests assumption, and (e) a model that provides a measure of precision for an individual's ability level.

2.2 Item Response Theory as Ideal Model

During the 1950s and 1960s, a revolutionary test theory, now known as IRT, was developed (Birnbaum, 1968; Lord, 1952; Lord and Novick, 1968; Rasch, 1960). IRT had the desirable features of an alternative test theory that were described above. That is, unlike CTT, the examinee's true score is not test dependent, the item parameters are not sample dependent, and the parallel test assumption is not necessary in IRT. In other words, if a given IRT model fits the test data of interest, ability estimates obtained from different sets of items will be comparable. Furthermore, item parameter estimates are also comparable regardless of the groups of examinees (Hambleton et al, 1991).

IRT also includes indices to discern the strength and weakness of each item in a test. In contrast, the CTT analyses are focused on the scale at the test level. For example, in IRT, we can distinguish good and bad items in terms of how accurately an item can measure examinees' at the different trait levels (i.e., *item information*). Also, IRT has provided solutions for many practical testing problems such as equating different test forms and examining measurement bias (Embretson and Reise, 2000).

There are two basic assumptions of IRT models about the data to which the models are applied: appropriate dimensionality and local independence. The first assumption means that the number of latent traits measured by the items corresponds to the number of trait parameters in the IRT model. For example, if test items depend on two or more latent traits, then IRT models with a single person trait parameter will not be appropriate. Factor analysis, among other methods, can be used to test the assumption. Models which assume the measurement of more than one trait for examinees' test scores are referred to as multidimensional models (Hambleton et al, 1991). Several multidimensional IRT (MIRT) models allow for more than one trait (θ) to be estimated, even though the most widely applied IRT models assume a unidimensional construct for which one θ estimate is sufficient to explain item responses (Reckase, 1997).

The unidimensionality assumption is closely related to the assumption of local independence. The local independence assumption means that when the abilities to influence test scores are controlled, examinees' responses to any of the items are statistically independent. Alternatively, within a given trait level, the probability of getting one item correct is independent of the probability of getting other items correct.

3 IRT Models

IRT models can be classified into two basic categories depending on how the items to analyze are scored: binary models and polytomous models. The binary IRT models are used for analyzing the items with dichotomously scored responses (e.g., yes/no or right/wrong), whereas the polytomous models can treat multiple category formats such as rating scales. IRT models were originally developed to handle binary response data. The polytomous IRT models were introduced later as generalized forms of the binary IRT models (e.g., Samejima, 1969). The polytomous IRT models can be divided into two categories depending on whether the test items have ordered response categories (e.g., Likert scale) or unordered response categories (e.g., unordered multiple choices). The models in each category will be described in detail.

3.1 Binary IRT Models

Binary response data may include ability tests (Right or Wrong), personality self-reports (True

or Not True), attitude endorsements (Agree or Disagree), and behavioral rating scales (Yes or No). Two separate lines of development lead to the currently available IRT models. Rasch (1960) developed a family of IRT models that fully met the properties of specific objectivity; that is, according to Rasch (1960) specific objectivity is met when item invariant person scores across items and person invariant item indices can be obtained. These models assume that the items are equally discriminating for the latent trait. In contrast, in the United States, families of models were developed that included item discrimination and other parameters. The normal ogive models (Lord, 1952) utilize the cumulative normal curve to model the relationship of item response probabilities to the latent trait. Birnbaum (1968) developed logistic models with multiple item parameters because they are mathematically and computationally simpler than the normal ogive models. There are three logistic models which are widely applied: the one-parameter logistic (1PL) model, the two-parameter logistic (2PL) model, and the three parameter logistic (3PL) model. The 1PL model may be written as follows:

$$P(X_{is} = 1|\theta_s, \beta_i) = \frac{\exp \alpha(\theta_s - \beta_i)}{1 + \exp \alpha(\theta_s - \beta_i)}, \quad (9.2)$$

where X_{is} = response of person s to item i (0, 1), θ_s = trait level for person s, α = a constant for item discrimination, and β_i = difficulty of item i.

The 1PL model is identical to the Rasch model if the value of the constant item discrimination is fixed to 1.

The 2PL model adds item discrimination parameter to the Rasch model as follows:

$$P(X_{is} = 1|\theta_s, \beta_i, \alpha_i) = \frac{\exp(\alpha_i(\theta_s - \beta_i))}{1 + \exp(\alpha_i(\theta_s - \beta_i))}, \quad (9.3)$$

where X_{is}, θ_s, and β_i are defined as above and α_i = discrimination for item i.

The 3PL model adds a lower-asymptote parameter to accommodate guessing possibility as follows:

$$P(X_{is} = 1|\theta_s, \beta_i, \alpha_i, \gamma_i) = \gamma_i$$
$$+ (1 - \gamma_i)\frac{\exp(\alpha_i(\theta_s - \beta_i))}{1 + \exp(\alpha_i(\theta_s - \beta_i))}, \quad (9.4)$$

where X_{is}, θ_s, β_i, and α_i are defined as above, and γ_i = lower asymptote (guessing) for item i.

The 1PL model is a special case of the 2PL model where all items have the a-parameter of a constant value, and the 2PL model is a special case of the 3PL model when the lower asymptote is 0. Which model is the best for the test development in behavioral medicine? The choice of a particular model depends on several considerations as follows: (a) the weights of items for scoring (equal vs. unequal), (b) the desired scale properties for the measure, (c) fit to the data, and (d) the purpose for estimating the parameters. If items are to be equally weighted and the strongest justification for scale properties is desired, then the 1PL or Rasch model is favored. For many tests, better fit is often obtained with the 2PL or 3PL models. However, a disadvantage of models with item discrimination parameters is that persons with the same total score may have different estimates of the latent trait, depending on which items they answer in the keyed direction.

3.2 Polytomous IRT Models

Several polytomous IRT models have been developed and they can be divided into two types: the indirect (or difference) models and the direct (or divided-by-total) models. The indirect (difference) models include the graded response model (GRM; Samejima, 1969) and the modified graded response model (M-GRM; Muraki, 1990). The direct (divided-by-total) models include the partial credit model (PCM; Masters, 1982), the generalized partial credit model (G-PCM; Muraki, 1992), the rating scale

model (RSM; Andrich, 1978a,b), and the nominal response model (NRM; Bock, 1972).

The GRM, M-GRM, PCM, and G-PCM are appropriate for responses with ordered multiple categories. Especially, the GRM and G-PCM models are appropriate for analyzing attitude or personality scale responses where subjects rate their beliefs or respond to statements on a multi-point scale (Embretson and Reise, 2000). The mathematical models and application of the GRM, G-PCM, and RSM will be introduced below. The NRM can be used when the response categories are not necessarily ordered along the persons' trait continuum.

The GRM was designed for a Likert-style survey questionnaire that was scored using more than two ordered categories such as "Strongly disagree (1)," "Disagree (2)," "Neutral (3)," "Agree (4)," and "Strongly agree (5)." The GRM is just an extension of the 2PL model for dichotomous data to polytomous data. Given the individual's trait level of θ, the probability that an individual responds to category x *or higher* is given as follows:

$$P_{ix}^*(\theta) = \frac{\exp[\alpha_i(\theta - \beta_{ij})]}{1 + \exp[\alpha_i(\theta - \beta_{ij})]}, \quad (9.5)$$

where x is the response category $j = 0, 1,\ldots, M$ score, α_i is common item slope parameter, and β_{ij} is a category threshold parameter.

The number of threshold parameters, β_{ij}, for each item is the number of response categories minus 1. Thus, the item operating characteristic curve (OCC) of the GRM includes $M-1$ separate curves, which represent the probabilities of responding in the lower category versus the successively higher categories.

The category response curve (CRC) of the GRM, the probability of responding to a specific category, can be expressed as

$$P_{ix}(\theta) = P_{ix}^*(\theta) - P_{i,x+1}^*(\theta), \quad (9.6)$$

where $P_{i,x+1}^*(\theta)$ is a cumulative probability of selecting a category score of $x+1$ or higher on item i given θ. Assuming five categories, the probability of responding in each of the five categories is as follows:

$$P_{i0}(\theta) = 1.0 - P_{i1}^{*}(\theta)$$
$$P_{i1}(\theta) = P_{i1}^{*}(\theta) - P_{i2}^{*}(\theta)$$
$$P_{i2}(\theta) = P_{i2}^{*}(\theta) - P_{i3}^{*}(\theta)$$
$$P_{i3}(\theta) = P_{i3}^{*}(\theta) - P_{i4}^{*}(\theta)$$
$$P_{i4}(\theta) = P_{i4}^{*}(\theta) - 0.$$

The PCM is an extension of the Rasch model using only item location parameters (b). The G-PCM is the extension of the PCM by substituting the 2PL model for the Rasch model (Dodd et al, 1995). Among several polytomous IRT models, G-PCM is widely used for ordered response categories. The G-PCM is expressed as follows:

$$P_{ix}(\theta) = \frac{\exp[\sum\limits_{j=0}^{x} \alpha_i(\theta - \delta_{ij})]}{\sum\limits_{r=0}^{m_i} [\exp \sum\limits_{j=0}^{r} \alpha_i(\theta - \delta_{ij})]}, \quad (9.7)$$

where $P_{ix}(\theta)$ is the probability of selecting a category score of x on item i given an individual's trait level of θ, $\sum\limits_{j=0}^{o}(\theta - \delta_{ij}) \equiv 0$ (when j is 0), j is the category score for item $i(j - 0, 1, \ldots m_i)$ is the discrimination parameter of item i and, δ_{ij} is the step difficulty parameter of item i with a category score of j.

Of the parameters above, the *item discrimination parameter,* α_i (also called slope), indicates how well an item uncovers the examinees' ability or trait. *Item information,* described earlier, depends partially on the item's discriminating power (Hambleton et al, 1991). Therefore, those two indices, *item discrimination parameter* and *item information,* play an important role to provide a basis for distinguishing good and bad items in IRT. The PCM can be regarded as a special case of the G-PCM in which item discriminations have a common value (usually constrained to 1.0).

The generalized rating scale model, G-RSM, can be expressed as

$$P_x(\theta) = \frac{\exp\left\{\sum\limits_{j=0}^{x} \alpha_i[\theta - (\lambda_i + \delta_j)]\right\}}{\sum\limits_{r=0}^{m_i} \exp\left\{\sum\limits_{j=0}^{x} \alpha_i[\theta - (\lambda_i + \delta_j)]\right\}},$$
(9.8)

where $\sum\limits_{j=0}^{o}(\theta - \delta_{ij}) \equiv 0$ (when j is 0), α_i is the item slope, λ_i is the item location, and δ_j is the category intersections.

The items vary in the item location and item discrimination in the RSM, but the relative distances of thresholds are uniform across items. Thus, the model often provides adequate fit to rating scale data with the same numerical format.

3.3 Evaluating Item Quality

Several indices are available to evaluate item quality; the item discrimination index, item information, and item fit. The item discrimination index is proportional to the slope of the ICC at the point β_i on the ability scale. Items with steeper slopes are more useful for separating examinees into different ability levels than are items with the less steep slopes. An item information value or function, $I_i(\theta)$, is a powerful method for describing and selecting items by displaying the accuracy of each item in measuring examinees' abilities or traits. The reciprocal of the sum of the $I_i(\theta)$ index is the standard error of measurement at each θ level. Thus, $I_i(\theta)$ index determines the contribution of an item to reducing measurement error and if it is not sufficiently high, the item can be deleted from the test. Finally, item fit indices are available. One widely used index is a goodness of fit test that compares the prediction of item probabilities from the model to the proportion of people responding to the item. All three indices are available in many computer programs, such as PARSCALE (Muraki and Bock, 1997).

4 Applying IRT to Questionnaires in Behavioral Medicine

A sample of 220 patients who were being treated for rheumatoid arthritis were surveyed with the Center for Epidemiologic Studies Depression Scale (CES-D). The mean age was 54.54 (*SD* =8.795) with a range between 38 and 70. Of the 220 subjects, 182 were females (82.7%) and 38 were males (17.3%). They were also composed of 187 (85%) Caucasians, 21 (9.5%) African Americans, 9 (4.1%) Hispanics, and 3 (1.4%) native Americans or Alaskan Natives.

4.1 Questionnaire and Analysis with Polytomous IRT

CES-D is a 20-item questionnaire which asks how subjects have felt and behaved during the last week for determining their depression level. A rating scale format with four categories is used

in the scales such as 0= rarely (<1 day), 1= some (1–2 days), 2= occasionally (3–4 days), and 3= all the time (5–7 days). Each item of the CES-D was analyzed with G-PCM because the model is widely used for analyzing attitude or personality scale responses where subjects rate their beliefs or respond to statements on a multi-point scale. The parameters of the G-PCM were estimated by the marginal maximum likelihood estimation (MMLE) method using the PARSCALE (Muraki and Bock, 1997) program.

4.2 Descriptive Statistics and Interpretation of IRT Results

Table 9.1 displays brief descriptions of the item content, the observed response frequencies within each category, and the item mean score when scored on a 0–3 scale for the CES-D. As shown in Table 9.1, the item means did not

Table 9.1 Content of the CES-D items, response frequencies, and item means (*N*=220)

Item	Content	Category 0	1	2	3	*M*
1	Bothered by things	134	65	17	4	1.51
2	Poor appetite	148	46	18	8	1.48
3	Unshakeable blues	155	45	14	6	1.41
4	Felt inferior	103	52	29	36	1.99
5	Trouble concentrating	104	80	33	3	1.71
6	Depression	122	66	27	5	1.61
7	Too much effort	74	91	39	16	1.99
8	Hopeful (reverse scored)	81	59	36	44	2.20
9	Feelings of failure	182	30	6	2	1.22
10	Fearful	155	53	11	1	1.36
11	Sleeplessness	64	71	59	26	2.21
12	Feeling happy (reverse scored)	84	93	29	14	1.88
13	Quiet	116	63	38	3	1.67
14	Feeling lonely	154	52	10	4	1.38
15	Unfriendly people	186	28	5	1	1.19
16	Joyful (reversed scored)	105	65	25	25	1.86
17	Crying	168	40	9	3	1.31
18	Sadness	128	40	9	3	1.54
19	Feeling disliked	194	20	5	1	1.15
20	Listless	70	89	47	14	2.62

Note: 0= rarely (<1 day); 1= some (1–2 days); 2= occasionally (3–4 days); 3= all the time (5–7 days)

demonstrate a wide spread, while within items the response frequencies across the categories were quite variable. Item 20 had the highest mean (2.62) with SD of 0.89 while item 19 had the lowest mean (1.15) with SD of 0.45. Subjects generally chose the response 2 (occasionally) or 3 (all the time) for item 20, while most of them selected the response 0 (rarely) or 1 (some) for item 19.

Table 9.2 displays the item discrimination parameters (slopes) and category intersection estimates. Since each item has four categories, three thresholds exist for each item. The last three columns in Table 9.2 present the fit index of each item (chi-square statistics). These statistics indicated that 6 of the 20 items were not well represented by the estimated G-PCM item parameters. These chi-square statistics were added across items and resulting in chi-square of 263.74 on 140 degrees of freedom ($p = 0.000$), which also indicated that overall model does not fit well. Table 9.3 presents item information at each point of seven "ability" levels ($\theta = -3$, $-2, -1, 0, 1, 2,$ and 3) along with the item discrimination parameters for each CES-D item. As

shown in Table 9.3, the amount of item information greatly depends on the item discriminating power.

As described above, good and bad items can be distinguished by the item discriminating power, item information, and item fit. Figures 9.1 and 9.2 show the CRC and the item information curve (IIC) for two items that had adequate fit to the model (see Table 9.2). Figure 9.1 shows that the CRC of item 6 has an ideal shape. The probability of each category is higher than the other categories within a certain range of the latent trait. Furthermore, the categories are very steep, which results from the high item discrimination estimate of 2.31. The IIC for item 6 shows generally high levels across the latent trait continuum, but is the highest value at around ability level of 1, which means that this item reduces measurement error the most within this range. Figure 9.2 shows the CRC and IIC of item 20 which has a more moderate item discrimination estimate of 0.56. The CRC are much flatter, which means that the category probabilities do not discriminate as well as item 20 between the various levels of the latent trait. The IIC for this item is

Table 9.2 Estimated item parameters for the generalized partial credit model and item fit statistics

	α_i	(SE)	$\delta 1$	$\delta 2$	$\delta 3$	χ^2	df	p
1	0.956	(0.13)	0.697	1.313	2.427	6.63	6	0.356
2	0.316	(0.06)	2.165	2.274	2.264	1.79	7	0.969
3	1.430	(0.20)	0.860	1.248	1.944	2.75	6	0.841
4	0.041	(0.01)	13.253	1.723	0.348	23.66	9	0.012
5	0.819	(0.10)	-0.069	1.583	2.761	4.64	6	0.592
6	2.308	(0.28)	0.239	1.096	1.950	3.40	5	0.641
7	0.751	(0.09)	-0.140	0.427	1.971	17.80	8	0.023
8	0.129	(0.03)	2.643	-0.343	0.676	38.22	9	0.000
9	0.425	(0.10)	2.860	2.570	2.823	12.55	6	0.050
10	0.831	(0.13)	0.931	2.070	3.152	6.62	7	0.470
11	0.238	(0.04)	0.773	1.110	2.188	10.55	9	0.307
12	0.511	(0.07)	6.385	0.344	2.400	45.03	8	0.000
13	0.412	(0.06)	-0.179	3.138	3.503	12.71	9	0.176
14	0.950	(0.14)	1.201	1.279	2.353	4.56	6	0.603
15	0.470	(0.11)	2.604	2.907	3.254	9.70	6	0.137
16	0.343	(0.05)	1.533	0.257	1.519	44.86	8	0.000
17	1.188	(0.18)	1.169	1.516	2.298	3.11	6	0.796
18	1.733	(0.21)	0.599	0.921	2.086	2.57	6	0.862
19	0.769	(0.15)	1.884	2.577	2.619	2.04	5	0.844
20	0.562	(0.07)	-0.401	0.694	2.256	10.51	8	0.230

Table 9.3 Item discrimination index and information at each theta (θ) value of the for the generalized partial credit model

Item no	α_i	Item information						
		$\theta = -3.0$	-2.0	-1.0	0	1.0	2.0	3.0
1	0.956	0.00847	0.04227	0.19711	0.69979	1.41373	1.65627	0.66798
2	0.316	0.01994	0.03701	0.07144	0.14056	0.25571	0.35185	0.31006
3	1.430	0.00064	0.00725	0.08104	0.77886	3.2106	2.75305	0.34424
4	0.041	0.00487	0.00524	0.00561	0.00595	0.00627	0.00653	0.00675
5	0.819	0.02585	0.09913	0.33315	0.77352	0.99499	0.84941	0.64768
6	2.308	0.00005	0.00235	0.11698	3.26809	4.81808	4.228	0.24304
7	0.751	0.06066	0.19027	0.46541	0.79663	1.11142	0.79088	0.27828
8	0.129	0.03242	0.04202	0.05209	0.06046	0.06453	0.06275	0.05575
9	0.425	0.00881	0.01861	0.04044	0.0928	0.22716	0.50691	0.64355
10	0.831	0.00747	0.03031	0.11821	0.39938	0.91518	1.18841	0.94659
11	0.238	0.06434	0.09298	0.12521	0.15038	0.15568	0.13844	0.10898
12	0.511	0.06485	0.1338	0.245	0.40401	0.60399	0.58926	0.31237
13	0.412	0.03622	0.07523	0.15187	0.26924	0.35589	0.32794	0.25191
14	0.950	0.00503	0.02505	0.11999	0.4876	1.35017	2.10951	0.63054
15	0.470	0.00741	0.01671	0.03835	0.09085	0.22339	0.50947	0.71499
16	0.343	0.04054	0.0759	0.14767	0.28046	0.41339	0.36451	0.20179
17	1.188	0.00121	0.00908	0.06724	0.44927	1.85309	2.89681	0.71557
18	1.733	0.00049	0.00936	0.17196	1.84155	2.78414	3.45956	0.25318
19	0.769	0.00217	0.00808	0.03054	0.12109	0.52057	1.61327	1.13995
20	0.562	0.07982	0.17943	0.34389	0.52878	0.63179	0.52597	0.29873

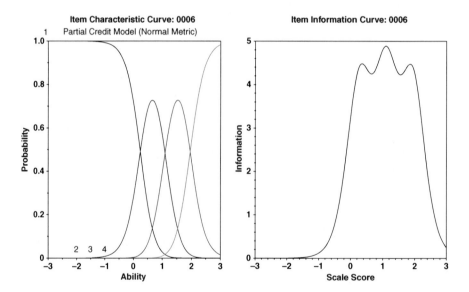

Fig. 9.1 Category response curves and item information curve for Item 6 under the generalized partial credit model

relatively flat and shows that the item does not reduce measurement error across all levels of the latent trait as compared to item 20.

Figures 9.3 and 9.4 illustrate two items of poor quality. Item 2 is shown in Fig. 9.3.

Although the fit of item 2 was adequate, it has a very low slope. Furthermore, Fig. 9.3 shows that three thresholds met very close together and do not discriminate well between levels of the latent trait. Further, the IIC show little contribution

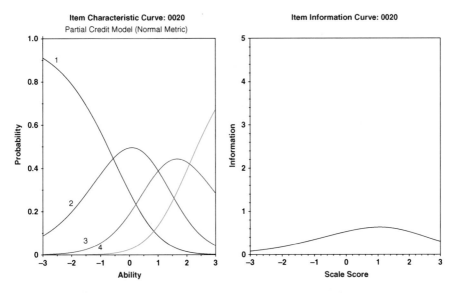

Fig. 9.2 Category response curves and item information curve for Item 20 under the generalized partial credit model

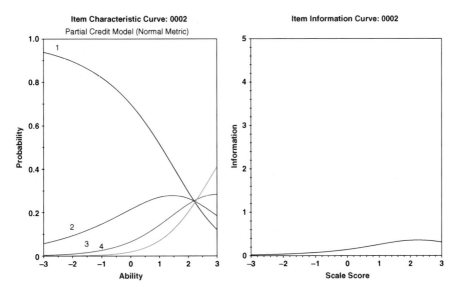

Fig. 9.3 Category response curves and item information curve for Item 2 under the generalized partial credit model

of this item to reducing measurement error. In Fig. 9.4, item 4 is shown. This item had poor fit to the model and very low discrimination. The CRC and IIC were almost flat. Figure 9.5 show the CRC for all 20 items.

To sum up, nine items of the CES-D were good or generally acceptable, but five items (2, 4, 8, 11, and 16) were unacceptable in terms

of the item discrimination parameter (less than 0.4) and item information. These results seemingly suggest that the CES-D should be revised for calibration with an IRT model. However, this conclusion would be premature. That is, the sample was somewhat limited; the sample size was somewhat small and had a limited range on the latent trait. The latter was indicated by

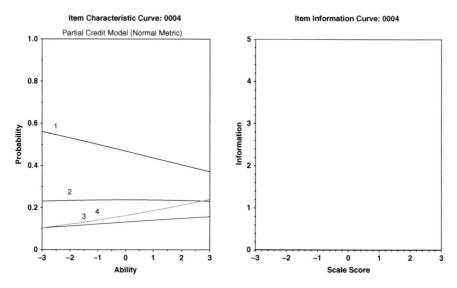

Fig. 9.4 Category response curves and item information curve for Item 4 under the generalized partial credit model

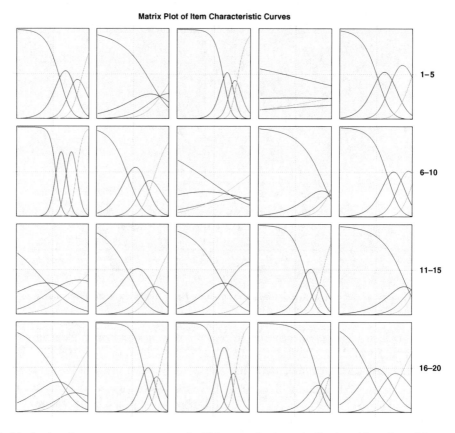

Fig. 9.5 Matrix plot of category response curves for 20 items under the generalized partial credit model

the relatively low means on many items, indicating low levels of depression. In this case, item discrimination parameters may be more poorly estimated, and it is possible that higher discriminations could be found in samples with greater degrees of depression. Nonetheless, more items and more discriminating items should be developed to measure depression, as the full advantages of IRT (i.e., adaptive testing) result from using item banks that have been calibrated with an appropriate model.

5 Summary

The purpose of this chapter was to present an overview of the development of item response theory as an alternative to classical test theory. Item response theory and the models that are relevant to applications in behavioral medicine were presented. An application to a self-reported patient outcome, depression, was also presented to illustrate the results from IRT modeling and to show how item quality could be assessed. Once an adequate item bank is established and the item parameters are estimated, IRT can be used to estimate trait levels from item subsets or from adaptive testing. Unlike classical test theory, the examinee's true score is not test dependent, and the item parameters are not sample dependent, therefore the parallel test assumption is not necessary in IRT.

References

Allen, M. J., and Yen, W. M. (1979). *Introduction to Measurement Theory*. Belmont, California: Wadsworth.

Andrich, D. (1978a). Application of a psychometric model to ordered categories which are scored with successive integers. *Appl Psychol Meas, 2*, 581–594.

Andrich, D. (1978b). A rating formulation for ordered response categories. *Psychometrika, 43*, 561–573.

Bock, R. D. (1972). Estimating item parameters and latent ability when responses are scored in two or more nominal categories. *Psychometrika, 37*, 29–51.

Birnbaum, A. (1968). Some latent trait models and their use in inferring an examinee's ability. In F.M. Lord & M. R. Novick, *Statistical Theories of Mental Test*

Scores (Chapters 17-20). Reading, MA: Addison-Wesley.

Dodd, B. G., De ayala, R. J., and Koch, W. R. (1995). Computerized adaptive testing with polytomous items. *Appl Psychol Meas, 19*, 5–22.

Embretson, S. E. (1996). Item response theory models and inferential bias in multiple group comparisons. *Appl Psychol Meas, 20*, 201–212.

Embretson, S. E., and Reise, S. P. (2000). *Item Response Theory for Psychologists*. Mahwah, NJ: Lawrence Erlbaum Associates.

Engelhard, G., and Wilson, M. (Eds). (1996). *Objective Measurement III: Theory into Practice*. Norwood, NJ: Ablex.

Hambleton, R. K., Swaminathan, H., and Rogers, H. J. (1991). *Fundamentals of Item Response Theory*. Newbury Park, CA: Sage Publications, Inc.

Lord, F. M. (1952). *A Theory of Test Scores (Psychometric Monograph No. 7)*. Iowa City, IA: Psychometric Society.

Lord, F. N., and Novick, M. R. (1968). *Statistical Theories of Mental Test Scores*. Reading, MA: Addison-Wesley.

Masters, G. N. (1982). A Rasch model for partial credit scoring. *Psychometrika, 47*, 149–174.

Muraki, E. (1990). Fitting a polytomous item response model to Likert-type data. *Appl Sychol Meas, 14*, 59–71.

Muraki, E. (1992). A generalized partial credit model: application of an EM algorithm. *Appl Psychol Meas, 16*, 159–176.

Muraki, E., and Bock, R. D. (1997). *PARSCALE 3: IRT Based Test Scoring and Item Analysis for Graded Items and Rating Scales*. Chicago: Scientific Software International, Inc.

Rasch, G. (1960). *Problabistic models for some intelligence and attainment tests*. Chicago: University of Chicago Press.

Reise, S. P., and Waller, N. G. (1990). Fitting the two-parameter model to personality data: the parameterization of the Multidimensional Personality Questionnaire. *Appl Psychol Meas, 14*, 45–58.

Reckase, M. (1997). The past and future of multidimensional item response theory. *Appl Psychol Meas, 21*, 25–36.

Samejima, F. (1969). *Estimation of Latent Ability Using a Response Pattern of Graded Scores*. Iowa City, IA: Psychometric Society.

Santor, D. A., Ramsay, J. O., and Zuroff, D. C. (1994). Nonparametric item analyses of the Beck depression inventory: evaluating gender item bias and response option weights. *Psychol Assess, 6*, 255–270.

Spearman, C. (1904). The proof and measurement of association between two things. *Am J Psychol, 15*, 72–101.

Spearman, C. (1907). Demonstration of formulae for true measurement of correlation. *Am J Psychol, 18*, 161–169.

Spearman, C. (1913). Correlations of sums and differences. *Br J Psychol, 5*, 417–426.

Chapter 10

Applications of Neurocognitive Assessment in Behavioral Medicine

Shari R. Waldstein, Carrington Rice Wendell, and Megan M. Hosey

1 Introduction

Neuropsychology is defined as the study of brain–behavior relations. Assessment of neurocognitive (or cognitive) function focuses more specifically on information processing abilities that can be grouped according to major domains of performance such as attention, learning and memory, executive functions, visuospatial and visuoconstructional skills, psychomotor abilities, perceptual skills, and language (see Lezak et al, 2004). These domains are assessed most thoroughly by a battery of neuropsychological tests, although under select circumstances such as initial dementia assessment, gross estimates can be derived from screening tests such as mental status exams.

Cognitive function is an important dimension of quality of life. Frank cognitive deficit, and even smaller decrements in cognitive performance, can be disruptive to well-being and daily functioning. A large literature has documented adverse effects of various chronic, non-neurological diseases and associated risk factors on cognitive function, and brain structure and function, across the life span (see Armstrong and Morrow, in press; Tarter et al, 2001; Waldstein, 2000; Waldstein and Elias, 2001). Interestingly, these are the very diseases and risk factors

commonly studied in the field of behavioral medicine. Inter-individual variability in cognitive performance has for decades been used as an important outcome variable in medical and behavioral medicine research. Indeed, the brain is increasingly recognized as a target organ of chronic disease. More recently, cognitive function has been examined as a predictor of other important endpoints in behavioral medicine such as quality of life, medical decision making, and treatment outcomes. Furthermore, recent data suggest that decreased cognitive function is a predictor of mortality in the context of clinical disease (e.g., Lee et al, 2006). Among older adults, chronic disease is known to increase risk for dementia, disability, and frailty.

In the present chapter, we will discuss several applications of cognitive assessment in behavioral medicine. We will first provide a brief overview of the major domains of cognitive function and provide select examples of commonly used tests. Next, we will briefly describe a spectrum of risk factors and chronic diseases with known relations to cognitive function. Lastly, we will examine use of cognitive performance to predict select outcomes in behavioral medicine research.

2 Neurocognition and Its Assessment

It is important to evaluate cognitive function in the behavioral medicine setting because such

S.R. Waldstein (✉)
Department of Psychology, University of Maryland, Baltimore County, 1000 Hilltop Circle, Baltimore, MD 21250, USA
e-mail: waldstei@umbc.edu

A. Steptoe (ed.), *Handbook of Behavioral Medicine*, DOI 10.1007/978-0-387-09488-5_10,
© Springer Science+Business Media, LLC 2010

function is apt to change in the face of medical illness or brain insult. Neurocognitive assessment is particularly complex in the field of behavioral medicine where patients can experience any number of health-related cognitive disruptions. Evaluation of cognitive function in patients or research participants in behavioral medicine is best accomplished by assessing each major domain of cognitive function.

Cognitive function can be categorized into multiple domains including (1) orientation, (2) perceptual processes, (3) attention and concentration, (4) executive function, (5) reasoning, (6) learning and memory, (7) visuospatial and visuoconstructional abilities, (8) psychomotor function, and (9) verbal or language function (Lezak et al, 2004). Making matters more complicated, tests rarely assess just one domain. In that regard, the nature of brain–behavior relations is such that several brain structures and functions are needed to complete even simple tasks. Furthermore, researchers and practitioners use differing terminology to describe similar constructs. Despite these challenges, neuropsychologists seek to accurately assess cognitive impairments in behavioral medicine populations and to make important recommendations to assist patients with these difficulties.

Patients who undergo neurocognitive testing may display a range of minor impairments across or even within any particular domain of function. Some patients may experience subtle decrements in cognitive function that are not of sufficient magnitude to qualify for diagnosis of a cognitive disorder. However, it is possible that these decrements remain noticeable or distressing to the patient. In contrast, other patients may experience declines that reach greater levels of clinical significance. For example, the diagnosis of mild cognitive impairment (MCI) is characterized as the presence of a significant deficit in one or more domains, though these impairments may not interfere with activities of daily living. However, more severe cognitive impairments, typically associated with pronounced functional limitations (e.g., caregiver dependence), may be indicative of a dementia

diagnosis such as Alzheimer's disease (AD). Varying levels of dementia and impairment exist along the continuum between MCI and AD, and MCI and AD are among a myriad of possible cognitive disturbances that patients may experience.

In the behavioral medicine setting, certain medical conditions are characterized by typical patterns of cognitive impairment, and neuropsychological batteries may be designed accordingly to target these patterns. For example, individuals with vascular disease often show decrements in the domains of attention and executive function (O'Brien, 2006). However, although it is important to emphasize patterns of impairment, individual findings from a neurocognitive assessment are rarely, if ever, pathognomonic for a particular diagnosis.

We next describe the major domains of cognitive function and several representative tests according to Lezak and colleagues (2004) who offer one of the most commonly used classification systems in neuropsychology. The interested reader is referred to her text for more detail. Further information about specific cognitive tests reflecting the different domains of function can also be found in Mitrushina et al (2005) and Strauss et al (2006).

2.1 Orientation

Prior to testing specific domains of function, an examiner may choose to include a general mental status measure that tests orientation, or the awareness of self relevant to time, place, and person. Screening measures such as the Mini-Mental State Examination accomplish this goal, or the investigator may simply ask questions regarding personal data and/or current events. Barring suspected dementia, particularly poor orientation may indicate the presence of a delirium. Postponement of neuropsychological testing is preferable until the delirium clears and the examinee is able to perform more optimally.

2.2 Perception

Performance on most cognitive tests is affected by perceptual processes, but certain tests better isolate basic perception by limiting physical interaction with test materials. As an example, the Judgment of Line Orientation (JLO) test is a commonly administered test of visual perception. The JLO is presented in flip-book style; two lines appear on the top page, and a standard fan-shaped array of 11 lines appears on the bottom page. Examinees must identify the lines from the bottom page that match the angles of the two lines at the top page. Depending on the examinee's presentation, tests are available for a variety of other basic perceptual processes, including visual neglect, color perception, auditory perception, tactile perception, and olfaction.

2.3 Attention and Concentration

Similar to perception, attentional processes are tapped by numerous neurocognitive tests, but select tests disproportionately target attention. Basic attention refers to the ability to focus on, or perceive, specific information. Complex attention (including working memory) tasks require the examinee to hold information in mind while manipulating it in some way. Concentration (or vigilance) refers to the ability to maintain basic or complex attention over a period of time. Attentional deficits may occur at one, some, or all of these levels, and neurocognitive testing helps to distinguish among these respective functions. For example, the Digits Forward portion of the Digit Span test of the Wechsler Adult Intelligence Scales (WAIS) assesses basic attention. Examinees are asked to immediately recall strings of digits spoken by the examiner at an approximate rate of one digit per second. The digit sequences increase in length until participants fail two trials of a particular length. In contrast, the Digits Backward portion of the test, which taps more complex attentional and

working memory processes, requires examinees to immediately recall additional strings of digits and repeat them to the examiner in reverse order.

2.4 Executive Functions

The executive functions are integral to the completion of the most complex human behaviors, particularly (a) adapting to novel situations, (b) engaging in social interactions, (c) abstract reasoning, and (d) regulating cognition and emotion. Executive functioning is a multi-component construct with dimensions that are generally defined as (a) volition, (b) purposive action, and (c) effective performance. Executive functions include the ability to sustain or flexibly redirect attention, the inhibition of inappropriate behavioral or emotional responses, the planning of strategies for future behavior, the initiation and execution of these strategies, and the ability to switch among problem-solving strategies. There are several multi-step tests designed to assess select executive functions. For example, the Trail Making Test Part B is a test easily administered in a behavioral medicine setting. To complete the test, patients draw lines connecting alternating numbers and letters in sequence (i.e., 1 to A, A to 2, 2 to B). The number of errors and task completion time are recorded and used to evaluate performance. There are also longer, more complex tests, such as the Wisconsin Card Sorting Test, that have the potential to yield more detailed information.

2.5 Reasoning

Like executive function, reasoning is usually characterized by a person's ability to integrate multiple facts or stimuli. Reasoning is distinguished from executive function in that an examinee must make a conscious effort to make rational judgments or to reach a conclusion about related stimuli. Tests intended to assess this domain usually involve reasoning about verbal or visually presented stimuli. An example of such a test is Comprehension, a subtest of the various versions of the WAIS. This test presents the examinee with increasingly difficult open-ended questions that assess social competence and practical reasoning.

2.6 Learning and Memory

Learning refers to the process of acquiring new information, whereas memory involves the encoding, retention, and later retrieval of that information. Tests of learning and memory are classified according to the modality of adminis-tration (e.g., verbal versus visual). Verbal learn-ing and memory tests frequently take one of two forms: (a) list recall or (b) story recall. The California Verbal Learning Test is an exam-ple of the former. Examinees are asked to recall a 16-item list across five learning trials after a short delay and a longer 20-min delay. The Logical Memory subtest of the Wechsler Memory Scales is an example of story recall. Examinees hear simple stories of a few lines and are asked to repeat as much information as possible from each story. In contrast, the Benton Visual Retention Test assesses visual memory; examiners show examinees 10 con-secutive cards, each containing three geometric figures of varying sizes and shapes. Following a 10-s exposure period, examiners remove the card from view, and examinees immediately repro-duce the figures from memory on a blank sheet of paper.

2.7 Visuospatial and Visuoconstructional Abilities

Tests of visuospatial and visuoconstructional abilities go beyond tests of simple perception to assess an individual's ability to organize visual information, orient objects in two- or three-dimensional space, and perform construc-tion via drawing, building, or assembling test materials. In the Hooper Visual Organization Test examinees are presented with line drawings of objects that have been divided into multi-ple "puzzle" pieces. The examinee must cor-rectly identify the object presented by men-tally rotating the pieces to form a coherent picture. Commonly used examples of construc-tional tasks include the Copy trial of the Rey Complex Figure Test and the Block Design subtest of the WAIS. In the Rey Complex Figure Test, examinees are presented with a two-dimensional complex drawing and are asked to copy the figure. Copies are then systematically scored for accuracy using a 36-point scale. For Block Design, examinees are presented with red and white blocks, each with two red sides, two white sides, and two half-red half-white sides. Examinees must assemble the blocks to repli-cate a two-dimensional target stimulus within a specified amount of time. The number of blocks utilized increases with increasing item difficulty.

2.8 Psychomotor Function

In neuropsychology, two facets of psychomo-tor function are typically assessed – speed and strength. The examiner is typically interested in centrally mediated deficit, rather than fatigue or damage to the extremities. The Finger Tapping Test is an example of a test of psychomotor speed. Examinees are asked to use their index finger to tap a key that is connected to a counter as quickly as they can for a specified period of time. Several trials are typically completed and then averaged. Higher counts are associated with better performance. The Grip Strength Test (or Hand Dynamometer) is designed to test hand strength. Examinees are instructed to squeeze the device as hard as they can. Performance is measured in the amount of pressure the exami-nee is able to apply to the device. Two trials per hand are completed, usually alternating hands between trials, and the trials are averaged by hand.

2.9 Verbal and Language Function

Neurocognitive assessment of verbal and language function is aimed at assessing (a) verbal production (e.g., articulation and sound sequence), (b) fluency (e.g., the ability to produce spontaneous speech or to name objects), and (c) reading and writing abilities. The Boston Naming Test is a common test of naming abilities. Examinees are presented with ink drawings that range in familiarity and are asked to name the object in the picture. Verbal fluency, another facet of verbal and language function, is commonly assessed with the Controlled Oral Word Association Test. In this test, examinees are given 1 min to name as many words as they can that begin with a particular letter of the alphabet. The first (and still most common) set of letters used is F-A-S. Importantly, verbal fluency also assesses aspects of executive function, so conclusions regarding performance on this test should take into account this overlap of assessed domains.

2.10 General Assessment Issues

It is apparent that cognitive function is not a unitary construct and cannot be assessed as such. Indeed, adequate assessment of cognitive performance typically depends on at least brief evaluation of all or almost all major domains of performance (or a hypothesis-driven focus on fewer domains). Use of composite scores is discouraged because they can mask understanding of specific cognitive processes. Importantly, cognitive screening measures such as the Mini-Mental State Examination are grossly inadequate to evaluate cognitive abilities, their prospective change, or response to treatment (Tombaugh and

McIntyre, 1992). Concerns about floor or ceiling effects must be considered when working with those of considerably low or high levels of cognitive ability. In research and clinical contexts, it is necessary to consider known sociodemographic influences on performance such as age, sex, education, race/ethnicity, and socioeconomic status. Emotional status (e.g., symptoms of anxiety or depression), psychiatric disorders, sleep, and acute ingestive behaviors (e.g., smoking, caffeine, alcohol) are also highly relevant. Testers must be sure to make participants feel comfortable and promote motivation. For more detailed discussion see Lezak et al (2004). As we discuss below, a host of chronic diseases and their risk factors also influence cognitive performance.

3 Chronic Diseases, Risk Factors, and Neurocognition

An increasingly broad spectrum of chronic diseases and their risk factors have been associated with decrements in cognitive function across the life span (Armstrong and Morrow, in press; Tarter et al, 2001; Waldstein and Elias, 2001; Waldstein et al, in press). Here we will briefly overview a sample of relevant areas of investigation, beginning with several known and putative risk factors for chronic diseases, followed by select diseases and their treatments. Space limitations preclude us from describing specific patterns of cognitive difficulties associated with any particular risk factor or disease. However, data suggest that almost all major domains of function are affected, with measures of attention, executive functions, learning and memory, and psychomotor abilities showing particular vulnerability to various conditions. The interested reader is referred to the above reviews for further detail and for reference to the extensive and growing literature documenting potential underlying neurobiological mediators of risk factor/disease – neurocognition associations.

3.1 Risk Factors and Neurocognition

A host of behavioral, biomedical, psychosocial, and psychophysiological risk factors can influence cognitive performance. Importantly, relations of these risk factors (and diseases) to cognitive outcomes may be moderated by select genotypes. For example, the apolipoprotein E (APOE) ε4 allele is associated with AD, cognitive decline (Farrer et al, 1997), cardiovascular disease, and stroke (Eichner et al, 2002). Haan and colleagues (1999) noted that among individuals with cardiovascular and metabolic diseases, those who had an APOE ε4 allele experienced a significantly greater rate of cognitive decline than those without.

Numerous lifestyle factors that promote or reduce risk for chronic disease have known a impact on cognitive function and its decline. Various health-compromising behaviors exert a negative influence on cognitive function, whereas health-enhancing behaviors are associated with higher levels of performance or potential improvement with intervention. Lifestyle factors can influence cognitive performance by impacting the brain directly or by promoting or reducing the development of chronic diseases that in turn affect the brain. Examples of health-compromising behaviors that are associated with lower levels of cognitive function include smoking (Swan and Lessov-Schlaggar, 2007), heavy alcohol consumption (Oscar-Berman and Marinkovic, 2007), dietary insufficiencies (Gillette et al, 2007), and physical inactivity (Colcombe et al, 2004). Health-enhancing behaviors such as greater intake of antioxidants including omega-3 fatty acids, and vitamins C and E have been associated with higher levels of cognitive performance (Del Parigi et al, 2006; Morris et al, 2004), although results of randomized clinical trials have been mixed. Greater levels of fitness or physical activity have also been related to better cognitive performance (Colcombe et al, 2004). Further, aerobic exercise has demonstrated exciting associations with cognitive improvements and even neuroplasticity in both animal models and humans (Dishman et al, 2006; Lautenschlager et al, 2008).

Various traditional biomedical risk factors for disease and newer biomarkers are associated with lower levels of cognitive function and decline. Examples include high levels of blood pressure (or hypertension; Waldstein and Katzel, 2001), cholesterol (Muldoon et al, 2001), glucose (even in a non-diabetic range; Taylor and MacQueen, 2007), insulin (Stolk et al, 1997), homocysteine (Elias et al, 2005), obesity (Gunstad et al, 2007), pro-inflammatory markers (e.g., interleukin-6; Yaffe et al, 2003), and indices of oxidative stress (Berr et al, 2000). Interestingly, both high and low levels of several of these risk factors (e.g. blood pressure, cholesterol, body mass index, alcohol consumption) have been related to poorer cognitive outcomes (see Waldstein et al, in press).

Various hormones are known to have a direct biological influence on the brain while potentially promoting diseases that affect cognitive function. In that regard, low levels of estrogen and androgens (Sherwin, 2003, 2006) and both low and high levels of thyroid hormones (Smith et al, 2002) have been related to poorer cognitive function. Hormone therapy in postmenopausal women may help prevent cognitive decline (Sherwin, 2003). Numerous studies have revealed associations between higher resting cortisol levels and lowered levels of cognitive performance, particularly on tests of learning and memory (Lupien et al, 2005). It has also been noted that stress-induced cortisol elevations are associated with decreased cognitive performance (Kirschbaum et al, 1996).

The latter findings reflect a larger literature on the negative relations of stress to cognitive performance and brain structure and function, at least in part via aberrations in cortisol (Sapolsky, 1999; McEwen, 2002). Stress-induced blood pressure responses have also been related to lower levels of cognitive function (Waldstein and Katzel, 2005). In addition to stress-related constructs, it is increasingly recognized that a number of psychosocial factors that may confer risk for chronic disease are related to cognitive function (see Waldstein et al, in press). Depression is such a factor that has long been known to have negative relations to brain and cognition. Other psychosocial factors such as hostility and anxiety may confer a negative influence on cognitive function whereas social support – a factor usually associated with better health outcomes – may have a protective relation to cognitive function.

A number of the aforementioned risk factors such as less healthy lifestyles, psychosocial stressors, and an accumulation of biomedical risk factors may, in part, explain associations of low levels of education or socioeconomic status (SES) and race/ethnicity (e.g., African American) to cognitive performance (Waldstein, 2000). Those of lower SES may also be more likely to experience neurotoxic exposures that impact the brain and cognitive function negatively (Morrow et al, 2001) and are less likely to have access to adequate treatment of their medical conditions.

3.2 Chronic Diseases and Neurocognition

Disease of any physiological system can negatively impact the brain and cognitive function (see Armstrong and Morrow, in press; Tarter et al, 2001; Waldstein and Elias, 2001). Cardiovascular diseases have been studied fairly extensively, and a range of conditions are associated with cognitive decrements. These include cardiac arrythmias (Mead and Keir, 2001), clinical coronary disease or myocardial infarction (Vingerhoets et al, 1997), heart failure (Vogels et al, 2007), and peripheral arterial disease (Waldstein et al, 2003). Various indices of subclinical vascular disease such as carotid intimal-medial thickening (Wendell et al, 2009), pulse wave velocity (Waldstein et al, 2008), brachial flow-mediated dilation (Cohen et al, 2009), and left ventricular hypertrophy (Elias et al, 2007) are similarly associated with poor cognitive outcomes.

Negative cognitive outcomes are also associated with type I and type II diabetes mellitus, pulmonary diseases such as chronic obstructive pulmonary disease and asthma, hepatic diseases such as cirrhosis, kidney diseases, autoimmune diseases such as systemic lupus erythematosus, various cancers, sleep disorders such as obstructive sleep apnea, and the human immunodeficiency virus (HIV) and the acquired immunodeficiency syndrome (AIDS) (see Bellia et al, 2007; Biessels et al, 2008; Borson et al, 2008; Kurella et al, 2005; Tarter et al, 2001; Zhang et al, 2007).

Medical and surgical treatments for disease affect cognitive function though in inconsistent directions. For example, prospective investigations generally indicate better cognitive outcomes for those taking antihypertensive medication than untreated hypertensives (Murray et al, 2002). Yet, results of double-blind, placebo controlled trials of antihypertensive have yielded complex and conflicting findings. Statin use may also be related to lesser prospective decline in cognitive performance (Szwast et al, 2007), although results of investigations of statin administration are mixed. Treatments for asthma (e.g., corticosteroid, theophylline) have yielded similarly mixed findings. Acute improvements in cognitive function have been associated with oxygen-related treatments for chronic obstructive pulmonary disease and obstructive sleep apnea syndrome and with hemodialysis (see Tarter et al, 2001). Coronary artery bypass surgery – a major surgical intervention – has been associated with both short- and long-term cognitive difficulties, although long-term alterations in performance may be attributable to the underlying disease (Royter et al, 2005).

3.3 Summary

Identifying future needs for research, Waldstein (2000) has suggested a need for increased multidisciplinary collaboration to address research questions related to associations between health/disease and cognitive function such as (a) understanding what domains of cognitive function are most affected by risk factors and diseases; (b) determining relevant effect modification variables (e.g., age, education, race/ethnicity, genetic polymorphisms, comorbidities) in order to identify vulnerability and resilience factors; (c) understanding the biological and/or psychological mechanisms intervening between health and cognition relations; (d) determining whether medical, surgical, or lifestyle interventions improve or further compromise cognitive performance; and (e) identifying whether changes in cognitive function associated with health status have an influence on quality of life, daily functioning, medical adherence, medical decision making, or treatment outcomes. Below we briefly consider aim (e).

4 Applications of Neuropsychology in Behavioral Medicine

Use of neurocognitive measures to predict outcomes in behavioral medicine research is, to date, less common than examining cognitive functions as outcome variables. Here we provide examples of several ways in which investigators are using cognitive performance measures in behavioral medicine research contexts.

4.1 Medical Decision Making

A primary application of neurocognitive assessment in behavioral medicine involves the role of certain cognitive functions in a patient's medical decision making. Here we conceptualize medical decision making broadly, including health behaviors and health behavior changes relevant to diet, exercise, substance use, and medical treatment adherence. We also focus on executive function, as this domain has been linked most often to patients' medical decision making.

By definition, all health behaviors and health behavior changes involve executive functions (Williams and Thayer, 2009), as they require the

planning of strategies for future behavior, the initiation and execution of these strategies, and the ability to troubleshoot ineffective strategies and implement new ones. Emotion regulation is also relevant to the maintenance of health behaviors and implementation of behavior changes. As an example, an obese individual interested in losing weight must initiate, execute, and maintain a weight loss plan in order to successfully achieve his or her goal. Furthermore, good problem-solving strategies and effective regulation of emotional reactions to this process may increase chances of success.

In their review of executive functions and changing substance use behavior, Blume and Marlatt (2009) point out that the conceptual relation between executive function and substance use behavior is reciprocal. That is, poor executive function contributes to poor substance-related decisions, such as excessive or illegal substance use. In turn, substance use behavior may result in further decrements in executive function through temporary or permanent damage to relevant brain circuits. Such deficits in executive function then become significant barriers to successful behavior change. Importantly, this cycle may be easily applied to the range of health behaviors described above, including diet and fitness. In fact, Sabia and colleagues (2009) show evidence of an association between a number of unhealthy behaviors (including smoking, alcohol abstinence, low physical activity, and low fruit and vegetable consumption) and likelihood of poor executive functioning. Specifically, individuals with three to four unhealthy behaviors were more likely to have poor executive function, and this association grew stronger with increasing age.

Similarly, executive functioning deserves consideration in the context of management of chronic illness and adherence to medical treatment regimens. As noted above, on average, individuals with obesity, diabetes, hypertension, peripheral vascular disease, renal dysfunction, pulmonary disease, HIV/AIDS, and other illnesses demonstrate poorer executive function than individuals without these diseases. Deficits in executive function may result directly from disease or indirectly through treatments of disease (via mechanisms such as hypoperfusion of the brain or systemic inflammation). Moreover, these decrements in executive function are associated with poor treatment adherence, which may serve to perpetuate or exacerbate the disease processes. For example, executive function has been associated with poor adherence to medication regimens for cholesterol lowering (Stilley et al, 2004) and HIV/AIDS (Hinkin et al, 2003). Other cognitive functions, such as attention, prospective memory, and visuospatial-constructional ability, are also implicated in poor adherence to medication regimens (Hinkin et al, 2003; Stilley et al, 2004; Woods et al, 2008). Decisions to adhere poorly to prescribed treatments should therefore be understood as potential end-products of decrements in various cognitive functions.

Chronic pain, a common treatment target for behavioral medicine practitioners, provides a final example of the relevance of the neurocognitive examination to medical decision making. In their review of executive functions, self-regulation, and chronic pain, Solberg et al (2009) propose a model in which executive functions and associated decrements in self-regulation cause and maintain chronic pain disorders. Specifically, the cognitive, emotional, social, behavioral, and physiological challenges associated with chronic pain are more poorly managed in the context of poor executive function. Optimally designed chronic pain interventions may therefore require components aimed at improving executive functions and self-regulatory capacity, such as cognitive techniques and physical activity.

4.2 Quality of Life

Although the literature is limited, diminished cognitive function has been associated with decreases in health-related quality of life (HRQoL) in those with chronic disease. For example, patients with peripheral vascular disease and lower scores on measures of cognitive function exhibited diminished everyday adaptive functioning (Phillips, 2001) – itself a major predictor of HRQoL (Andersen et al, 2004). Cognitive difficulties have also been associated with lower levels of HRQoL in persons with chronic obstructive pulmonary disease (McSweeney and Labuhn, 1996), HIV (Tozzi et al, 2003), or those undergoing cancer treatments (O'Shaughnessy, 2002). Cognitive difficulties may also, in part, explain lower levels of HRQoL among those with hypertension (Thyrum and Blumenthal, 1995) or diabetes (Kuo et al, 2005).

5 Summary and Conclusions

Cognitive function has a long and extensive history as an important outcome variable in behavioral medicine research. There is a large available literature indicating that a multitude of chronic diseases and their risk factors can exert a negative impact on cognitive function. Despite an already impressive knowledge base, there remain as many questions as answers in terms of identifying the specific neurocognitive tests that are most sensitive to particular diseases and risk factors, understanding of relevant vulnerability and resilience factors, and study of underlying neurobiological mechanisms. Furthermore, there is a relative paucity of research on the daily life impact of cognitive difficulties related to chronic diseases and their risk factors, although work to date suggests associations with medical decision making, quality of life, physical and daily function, disability, and frailty. Improvements in our understanding of these areas will only strengthen the existing relevance of neurocognitive assessment to the practice of behavioral medicine.

References

Andersen, C. K., Wittrup-Jensen, K. U., Lolk, A., Andersen, K., and Kragh-Sørensen, P. (2004). Ability to perform activities of daily living is the main factor affecting quality of life in patients with dementia. *Health Qual Life Outcomes, 2,* 1–7.

Armstrong, C., and Morrow, L. A. (in press) *Handbook of Medical Neuropsychology: Applications of Cognitive Neuroscience.* New York: Springer.

Bellia V, Pedone C, Catalano F, Zito A, Davì E et al (2007). Asthma in the elderly: mortality rate and associated risk factors for mortality. *Chest, 132,* 1175–1182.

Berr, C., Balansard, B., Arnaud, J. et al (2000). Cognitive decline is associated with systemic oxidative stress: the EVA study. *J Am Geriatr Soc, 48,* 1285–1291.

Biessels, G. J., Deary, I. J., and Ryan, C. M. (2008). Cognition and diabetes: a lifespan perspective. *Lancet Neurol, 7,* 184–190.

Blume, A. W., and Marlatt, G. A. (2009). The role of executive cognitive functions in changing substance use: what we know and what we need to know. *Ann Behav Med, 37,* 117–125.

Borson S, Scanlan J, Friedman S, Zuhr E, Fields J et al (2008). Modeling the impact of COPD on the brain. *Int J Chron Obstruct Pulmon Dis, 3,* 429–434.

Cohen, R. A., Poppas, A., Forman, D. E. et al (2009). Vascular and cognitive functions associated with cardiovascular disease in the elderly. *J Clin Exp Neuropsychol, 31,* 96–110.

Colcombe, S. J., Kramer, A. F., Erickson, K. I., Scalf P, McAuley E et al (2004). Cardiovascular fitness, cortical plasticity, and aging. *Proc Natl Acad Sc, 101,* 3316–3321.

Del Parigi, A., Panza, F., Capurso, C., and Solfrizzi, V. (2006). Nutritional factors, cognitive decline, and dementia. *Brain Res Bull, 69,* 1–19.

Dishman, R. K., Berthoud, H. R., Booth, F. W. et al (2006) Neurobiology of exercise. *Obesity, 14,* 345–356.

Eichner, J. E., Dunn, S. T., Perveen, G., Thompson, D. M., Stewart K. E. et al (2002). Apolipoprotein E polymorphism and cardiovascular disease: a HuGE review. *Am J Epidemiol, 155,* 487–495.

Elias, M. F., Sullivan, L. M., Elias, P. K., D'Agostino, R. B., Wolf, P. A. et al (2007). Left ventricular mass, blood pressure, and lowered cognitive performance in the Framingham offspring. *Hypertension, 49,* 439–445.

Elias, M. F., Sullivan, L. M., D'Agostino, R. B., Elias, P. K., Jacques, P. F. et al (2005). Homocysteine and cognitive performance in the Framingham Offspring Study: age is important. *Am J Epidemiol 162,* 644–653.

Farrer, L. A., Cupples, L. A., Haines, J. L., Hyman, B., Kukull, W. A. et al (1997). Effects of age, sex, and ethnicity on the association between apolipoprotein E genotype and Alzheimer disease. A meta-analysis. APOE and Alzheimer Disease Meta Analysis Consortium. *JAMA, 278,* 1349–1356.

Gillette, G. S., Abellan, V. K. G., Andrieu, S., Barberger, G. P., Berr, C. et al (2007). IANA task force on nutrition and cognitive decline with aging. *J Nutr Health Aging, 11,* 132–152.

Gunstad, J., Paul, R. H., Cohen, R. A., Tate, D. F., Spitznagel, M. B. et al (2007). Elevated body mass index is associated with executive dysfunction in otherwise healthy adults. *Compr Psychiatry, 48,* 57–61.

Haan, M. N., Shemanski, L., Jagust, W. J., Manolio, T. A., and Kuller, L. (1999). The role of APOE epsilon4 in modulating effects of other risk factors for cognitive decline in elderly persons. *JAMA, 282,* 40–46.

Hinkin, C. H., Castellon, S. A., Durvasula, R. S., Hardy, D. J., Lam, M. N. et al (2003) Medication adherence among HIV+ adults: effects of cognitive dysfunction and regimen complexity. *Neurology, 59,* 1944–1950.

Kirschbaum, C., Wolf, O. T., May, M., Wippich, W., and Helhammer, D. H. (1996). Stress- and treatment-induced elevations of cortisol levels associated with impaired declarative memory in healthy adults. *Life Sci, 58,* 1475–83.

Kuo, H. K., Jones, R. N., Milberg, W. P., Tennstedt, S., Talbot, L. et al (2005). Effect of blood pressure and diabetes mellitus on cognitive and physical functions in older adults: a longitudinal analysis of the advanced cognitive training for independent and vital elderly cohort. *J Am Geriatr Soc, 53,* 1154–61.

Kurella, M., Chertow, G. M., Fried, L. F., Cummings, S. R., Harris, T. et al (2005). Chronic kidney disease and cognitive impairment in the elderly: the health, aging, and body composition study. *J Am Soc Nephrol, 16,* 2127–2133.

Lautenschlager, N. T., Cox, K. L., Flicker, L., Foster, J. K., van Bockxmeer, F. M. et al (2008). Effect of physical activity on cognitive function in older adults at risk for Alzheimer's disease: a randomized trial. *JAMA, 309.* 1027–1037.

Lee, H. B., Kasper, J. D., Shore, A. D., Yokley, J. L., Black, B. S. et al (2006). Level of cognitive impairment predicts mortality in high-risk community samples: The Memory and Medical Care Study. *J Neuropsychiatry Clin Neurosci, 18,* 543–545.

Lezak, M., Howieson, D. B., and Loring, D. W. (2004). *Neuropsychological Assessment, 4th Ed.* New York: Oxford University Press.

Lupien, S. J., Fiocco, A., Wan, N., Maheu, F., Lord, C. et al (2005). Stress hormones and human memory function across the lifespan. *Psychoneuroendocrinology, 30,* 225–242.

McEwen, B. S. (2002). Sex, stress and the hippocampus: allostasis, allostatic load and the aging process. *Neurobiol Aging, 23,* 921–939.

McSweeney, A. J., and Labuhn, K. T. (1996). The relationship of neuropsychological functioning to health related quality of life in systemic medical disease: the example of chronic pulmonary artery disease. In I. Grant & K. M. Adams (Eds.), *Neuropsychological Assessment of Neuropsychiatric Disorders* (pp. 3–30). New York: Oxford University Press.

Mead, G. E., and Keir, S. (2001). Association between cognitive impairment and atrial fibrillation: a systematic review. *J Stroke Cerebrovasc Dis, 10,* 35–43.

Mitrushina, M., Boone, K. B., Razani, J., and D'Elia, L. F. (2005). *Handbook of Normative Data for Neuropsychological Assessment, 2nd Ed.* New York: Oxford.

Morris, M. C., Evans, D. A., Bienias, J. L., Tangney, C. C., Wilson, R. S. (2004) Dietary fat intake and 6-year cognitive change in an older biracial community population. *Neurology, 62,* 1573–1579.

Morrow, L. A., Muldoon, S. B., and Sandstrom, D. J. (2001). Neuropsychological sequelae associated with occupational and environmental exposure to chemicals. In R. E. Tarter, M. A. Butters, & S. R. Beers (Eds.), *Medical neuropsychology* (2nd ed.). New York: Plenum Press.

Muldoon, M. F., Flory, J. D., and Ryan, C. M. (2001). Serum cholesterol, the brain and cognition. In, S. R. Waldstein & M. F. Elias (Eds.) *Neuropsychology of Cardiovascular Disease* (pp. 37–59). Mahwah, NJ: Erlbaum.

Murray, M. D., Lane, K. A., Gao, S., Evans, R. M., Unverzagt, F. W. et al (2002). Preservation of cognitive function with anithypertensive medications. *Arch Intern Med, 162,* 2090–2096.

O'Brien, J. T. (2006). Vascular cognitive impairment. *Am J Geriatr Psychiatry, 14,* 724–733.

O'Shaughnessy, J. A. (2002). Effects of epoetin alfa on cognitive function, mood, asthenia, and quality of life in women with breast cancer undergoing adjuvant chemotherapy, *Clin Breast Cancer, 3,* S116–S120.

Oscar-Berman. M., and Marinkovic, K. (2007). Alcohol: effects on neurobehavioral functions and the brain. *Neuropsychol Rev, 17,* 239–257.

Phillips, N. A. (2001). Thinking on your feet: A neuropsychological review of peripheral vascular disease. In S. R. Waldstein & M. F. Elias (Eds.), *Neuropsychology of cardiovascular Disease.* Florence, KY: Erlbaum.

Royter, V., Bornstein, N. M., and Russell, D. (2005). Coronary artery bypass grafting (CABG) and cognitive decline: a review. *J Neurol Sci, 230,* 65–67.

Sabia, S., Nabi, H., Kivimaki, M., Shipley, M. J., Marmot, M. G. et al (2009). Health behaviors from early to late midlife as predictors of cognitive function: The Whitehall II study. *Am J Epidemiol, 170,* 428–437.

Sapolsky, R. M. (1999). Glucocorticoids, stress, and their adverse neurological effects: relevance to aging. *Exp Gerontol, 34,* 721–32.

Sherwin, B. B. (2003). Steroid hormones and cognitive functioning in aging men: a mini-review. *J Mol Neurosci, 20,* 385–393.

Sherwin, B. B. (2006). Estrogen and cognitive aging in women. *Neuroscience, 138,* 1021–1026.

Smith, J. W., Evans, A. T., Costall, B., and Smythe, J. W. (2002). Thyroid hormones, brain function, and cognition: a brief review. *Neurosci Biobehav Rev, 26,* 45–60.

Solberg Nes, L., Roach, A. R., and Segerstrom, S. C. (2009). Executive functions, self-regulation, and chronic pain: a review. *Ann Behav Med, 37,* 173–182.

Strauss, E., Sherman, E. M. S., and Spreen, O. (2006). *A Compendium of Neuropsychological Tests: Administration, Norms, and Commentary, 3rd Ed.* Oxford: Oxford University Press.

Stilley, C. S., Sereika, S., Muldoon, M. F., Ryan, C. M., and Dunbar-Jacob, J. (2004). Psychological and cognitive function: predictors of adherence with cholesterol lowering treatment. *Ann Behav Med, 27,* 117–124.

Stolk, R. P., Breteler, M. M., Ott, A., Pols, H. A., Lamberts, S. W. et al (1997). Insulin and cognitive function in an elderly population. The Rotterdam Study. *Diabetes Care, 20,* 792–795.

Swan, G. E., and Lessov-Schlaggar, C. N. (2007). The effects of tobacco smoke and nicotine on cognition and the brain. *Neuropsychol Rev,17,* 259–273.

Szwast, S. J., Hendrie, H. C., Lane, K. A., Gao, S., Taylor, S. E. et al (2007). Association of statin use with cognitive decline in elderly African Americans. *Neurology, 69,* 1873–1880.

Tarter, R. E., Butters, M. A., and Beers, S. R. (Eds). (2001). *Medical Neuropsychology, 2nd Ed.* New York: Plenum Press.

Taylor, V. H., and MacQueen, G. M. (2007). Cognitive dysfunction associated with metabolic syndrome. *Obes Rev, 8,* 409–418.

Thyrum Towner, E., and Blumenthal, J. A. (1995). The effects of hypertension on neurobehavioral functioning. In J. E. Dimsdale & A. Baum (Eds.) *Quality of Life in Behavioral Medicine Research* (pp. 161–170). Florence, KY: Erlbaum.

Tombaugh, T. N., and McIntyre, N. J. (1992). The Mini-Mental State Examination: a comprehensive review. *J Am Geriatr Soc, 40,* 22–935.

Tozzi, V., Balestra, P., Galgani, S., Murri, R., Bellagamba, R. et al (2003). Neurocognitive performance and quality of life in patients with HIV infection. *AIDS Res Hum Retroviruses, 19,* 643–52.

Vingerhoets, G., Van Nooten, G., and Jannes, C. (1997). Neuropsychological impairment in candidates for cardiac surgery. *J Int Neuropsychol Soc, 3,* 480–484.

Vogels, R. L., Scheltens, P., Schroeder-Tanka, J. M., and Weinstein, H. C. (2007). Cognitive impairment in heart failure: a systematic review of the literature. *Eur J Heart Fail, 9,* 440–449.

Waldstein, S. R. (2000). Health effects on cognitive aging. In P. C. Stern & L. L. Carstensen (Eds.), *The Aging Mind: Opportunities in Cognitive Research* (pp. 189–217). Committee on Future Directions for Cognitive Research on Aging. Commission on Behavioral and Social Sciences and Education. Washington, DC: National Academy Press.

Waldstein, S. R., and Elias, M. F. (2001). *Neuropsychology of Cardiovascular Disease.* Mahwah, NJ: Lawrence Erlbaum Associates.

Waldstein, S. R., and Katzel LI. (2001) Hypertension and cognitive function. In S. R. Waldstein & M. F. Elias (Eds.) *Neuropsychology of Cardiovascular Disease* (pp. 15–36). Mahwah, NJ: Erlbaum.

Waldstein, S. R., Katzel, L. I. (2005). Stress-induced blood pressure reactivity and cognitive function. *Neurology, 64*, 1750–1755.

Waldstein, S. R. Rice, S. C., Hosey, M. M., Seliger, S. L., and Katzel, L. I. (in press). Cardiovascular disease and neurocognitive function. In C. Armstrong & L. A. Morrow (Eds.), *Handbook of Medical Neuropsychology: Applications of Cognitive Neuroscience.* New York: Springer.

Waldstein, S. R., Rice, S. C., Thayer, J. F., Najjar, S. S., Scuteri, A. et al (2008). Pulse pressure and pulse wave velocity are related to cognitive decline in the Baltimore Longitudinal Study of Aging. *Hypertension, 51*, 99–104.

Waldstein, S. R., Tankard, C. F., Maier, K. J., Pelletier, J. R., Snow, J. et al (2003). Peripheral arterial disease and cognitive function. *Psychosom. Med, 65*, 757–763.

Wendell, C. R., Zonderman, A. B., Metter, E. J., Najjar, S. S., and Waldstein, S. R. (2009). Carotid intimal medial thickness predicts cognitive decline among adults without clinical vascular disease. *Stroke, 40*, 3180–3185.

Williams, P. G., and Thayer, J. F. (2009). Executive functioning and health: introduction to the special series. *Ann Behav Med, 37*, 101–105.

Woods, S. P., Moran, L. M., Carey, C. L., Dawson, M. S., Iudicello, J. E. et al (2008). Prospective memory in HIV infection: is "remembering to remember" a unique predictor of self-reported medication management? *Arch Clin Neuropsychol, 23*, 257–270.

Yaffe, K., Lindquist, K., Penninx, B. W. et al (2003). Inflammatory markers and cognition in well-functioning African-American and white elders. *Neurology, 61*, 76–80.

Zhang, L. J., Yang, G., Yin, J., Liu, Y., Qi, J. (2007). Neural mechanism of cognitive control impairment in patients with hepatic cirrhosis: a functional magnetic resonance imaging study. *Acta Radiol, 48*, 577–587.

Chapter 11

Lay Representations of Illness and Treatment: A Framework for Action

Howard Leventhal, Jessica Y. Breland, Pablo A. Mora, and Elaine A. Leventhal

1 What Are Lay Representations?

There is a lengthy history to the idea that a "common-sense" framework derived from culture and life experience (for a history see Cameron and Leventhal, 2003; Skelton and Croyle, 1991) shapes people's actions (i.e., goals, selection, and evaluation of actions for goal attainment). While philosophers (Stich, 1992), sociologists (Angel and Thoits, 1987), and anthropologists (Garro, 2000; Kleinman et al, 1978) agree on the nature of lay representations, there is no consensus on the processes underlying the content and function of representations (i.e., what representations are, how they come into play, and how they shape behavior). To transform the notion of lay representations from idle chatter to a legitimate area of cognitive and behavioral science that contributes to practice, it is necessary to specify the variables or domains of representations and the processes involved in their operation and suggest ways of implementing specific variables, i.e., issues of measurement and procedures for intervention.

H. Leventhal (✉)
Department of Psychology, Institute for Health, Health Care Policy and Aging Research Rutgers, The State University of New Jersey, 30 College Ave., New Brunswick, NJ 08901-1293, USA
e-mail: hleventhal@ifh.rutgers.edu

1.1 The Domains of Common-Sense Representations

As is the case with the other chapters in this handbook, our emphasis is on methods, that is, how to assess and use Common-Sense Model (CSM) concepts in empirical research. However, we will begin by describing the processes underlying the domains and functions of lay representations that make up the fundamental properties of the CSM. Indeed, this step is essential to the development of methods for measuring representations to understand and predict behavior as well as the use of lay representations in different types of investigations.

1.1.1 Common-Sense Representations as Central Components in Feedback and Feedforward Control Systems

The CSM was developed to describe the processes underlying health (i.e., prevention) and illness behaviors (i.e., secondary and tertiary prevention). As with all feedback and feedforward models, it divides the behavioral process into (1) a *perceptual stage,* in which a discrepancy between a perceived input and a reference value is detected (*the representation of a potential threat to health*); (2) a *response stage* in which an action is sought and performed to remove the discrepancy (*removal of the threat*); and (3) an *appraisal stage,* in which the results of an action to control the threat are evaluated (Fig. 11.1). Therefore, the initial focus is on the

A. Steptoe (ed.), *Handbook of Behavioral Medicine*, DOI 10.1007/978-0-387-09488-5_11,
© Springer Science+Business Media, LLC 2010

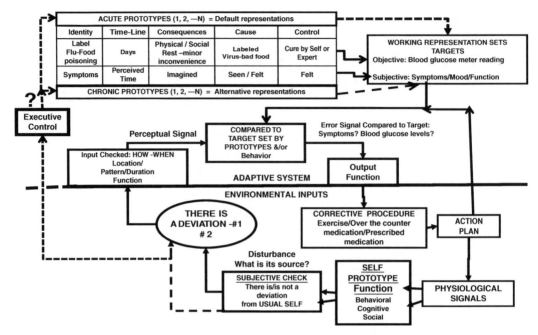

Fig. 11.1 Physiological signals are compared to prototypes of self (*lower right*). If evaluated as deviant from the usual self, they are processed (location, pattern/duration, function, etc.) and compared to targets set by underlying prototypes (familiar acute models are "safe" defaults). If match to default is ambiguous and/or suggestive of an unsafe alternative, action is considered (output function leading to corrective action) and performed once an action plan is in place. A key question is whether the output from the action is evaluated against the target for the prototype (my diabetes is still out of control) or the corrective behavior (my blood glucose went down after walking, or went up after eating). Executive controls (far left) are aware of the ongoing test process and can shift the prototype, the response for management, and the responses and targets for appraisal. Executive control is closer to focal awareness, more deliberative and effortful than the processes elicited by the automatic system

specific content of the threats that create targets for action, the specific features of the action to ameliorate the threat, and the targets used to appraise outcomes. Specificity is essential to convert a general feedback model into a set of tools and principles for the creation of measures to predict behavioral outcomes and to develop interventions to influence behavioral processes.

Lay representations specify five sets of domains that define health threats: (1) *identity*: what the threat is called, a conceptual or propositional statement representing the threat, and how it is experienced including the symptoms and/or functional changes observed in oneself or another person that are concrete features of the threat; (2) *temporal features*: its rate of onset, duration, and temporal trajectory; each of which is assessed subjectively and can be assessed objectively, with clocks and calendars;

(3) *consequence:* physical, psychological, social, economic, etc.; (4) *causes:* perceived contact with pathogens, age, stress, etc.; and (5) *controllability*: whether the threat is understood and perceived to be susceptible to control, as distinct from the efficacy of the responses to control it. These five domains apply to the procedures that are available and used to deal with health threats, that is, to reduce the gap between the targets (symptoms or objective values) defined by the illness representation and the outcomes appraised after acting.

1.1.2 Representations Are Multi-level

Representations involve both concrete experiences (e.g., symptoms, experienced time, and/or disruption of work) and abstract or propositional cognitive processes (e.g., disease labels or chronological time). The meaning (semantics) of propositional statements is anchored in experience (Andrews et al, 2009; Shanon, 1988). Because representations are multi-level, the targets for action based on representations are also multi-level. Thus, patients may use concrete experiences (i.e., symptoms) to decide when they are hypertensive (Meyer et al, 1985) or believe that they have asthma only when they are symptomatic (Halm et al, 2006). The experiential base of concepts are often targets for management and may differ from patients' statements that people "can't tell when their blood pressure is high," and "will have asthma for the rest of their lives."

1.2 Prototypes: Creating Representations of Illness and Targets for Management

Representations are dynamic; a "sore/blemish" on the skin may transform from an infection to a skin cancer, and the type of cancer (basal cell versus melanoma) may change the meaning of the prognosis from life threatening to curable. Feedback from self-examination, social comparisons, and care-seeking can reshape illness and treatment representations. Representations are unstable and the instability of a dynamic process poses challenges for descriptive studies and interventions.

The schemata and/or prototypes in declarative and procedural memory that underlie representations and shape behavioral strategies and the prototype checks (PCs) that activate and connect schemata to ongoing experiences are likely more stable and therefore better targets for assessment. Numerous studies have assessed and demonstrated the importance of the check mechanisms in predicting care-seeking. However, the empirical literature for assessing prototypes is less robust and not well integrated with findings regarding representations and the check process.

1.2.1 The Formation of Prototypes and the Activation of Representations

Representations of illness, treatments, and outcomes are dynamic, and both their experiential base and abstract features can be implicit (active and below awareness) (Henderson et al, 2007; Williams et al, 2003) or in conscious awareness. In this regard, they are similar to other everyday experiences. For example, when we enter the waiting room of a medical office, we scan the behavioral environment, occupied and unoccupied seats, and walk to sit in one of the unoccupied chairs. The rug and floor are likely implicit (unnoticed unless one slips), while selected features of the chairs and seated patients are represented in consciousness at different levels of salience. The representations guiding movement (the affordances perceived in the environment) are activated by perceptual features that activate underlying schemata of rooms, floors, chairs, and people.

The CSM provides a detailed description of the processes involved in the activation of prototypes, the process that elaborates the meaning of implicit and explicit observations of somatic and functional cues. The core of the process is an ongoing scanning, checking, and comparing of somatic sensations, as well as physical and mental function, to the underlying prototype and schemata of the physical and functional self. A representation of illness is activated when the scanning or *check process* detects a deviation in somatic sensations and/or physical and mental function that exceeds normally expected variability in the self and matches an underlying *illness prototype*. The representation formed at that moment is an operating hypothesis about the nature and meaning of the experienced deviations. For example, the deviations may reflect one of several acute conditions such as a migraine headache, common cold, heartburn, and/or stomach ache from bad food, or a potentially chronic condition such as an ulcer, hypertension, diabetes, a cancer, or something more benign such as psychological stress or normal aging. The checks connecting experience to prototypes address these questions by evaluating the *sensory properties* (e.g., sharp, dull, or throbbing), *location* (e.g., head, belly, legs, or heart), *duration* (e.g., felt and clock time), *rates of change* (e.g., sudden onset, gradual increase, steady), *consequences* (e.g., disrupted breathing or impaired walking), *causes* (e.g., bad tasting food or little sleep), and the effects of behavior or, *control of,* the experience (e.g., used alcohol or salve, rested and it cleared). The "primary prototype checks" built into the nervous system match the specific attributes of experience to "slots" in the underlying prototype (Gobet, 1998). The representation that emerges and changes from this ongoing process of matching experience to prototypes generates motivation for action, and the feedback from these actions confirms or disconfirms the meaning of the somatic experience.

1.2.2 Prototype Checking Is a Social Process

Prototype checks are not only at the core of the intra-personal processes that give meaning to experience but also central for interpersonal communication. Once the opening niceties are completed ("How are you?"), a medical practitioner will address the presenting complaint with the same checks the patient uses: "What is bothering you?" "Where is it?" "How does it feel?" "How long has it been going on?" "Has it been getting worse?" "What were you doing when it started?" "Have you done anything to self-treat it?" "What happened?" This exchange reinforces the check process and may or may not provide an alternative explanation for the presenting symptoms and physical and cognitive dysfunctions. An additional set of PCs emerge from social comparison processes. We assign meaning to symptoms and functional changes by checking for common exposure (e.g., exposure to someone with SARS), familial linkage (e.g., family member had breast cancer), similarities in physiognomy, temperament, and response to aging (e.g., parental dementia a sign of risk to self). These processes are less well explored in the CSM (Leventhal et al, 2007).

1.3 Representations Create a Context for Management

1.3.1 Relating Treatment and Action Plans to Illness Representations

The activation of a representation of a condition such as asthma, cancer, diabetes, or hypertension creates a framework within which individuals engage in a common-sense selection and appraisal of procedures to prevent, detect, control, and cure potential threats to health. These specific procedures can be selected from culturally prescribed nostrums, the shelf of family remedies, or be medically prescribed. Procedures are highly valued if they are perceived and believed to attack the disease at its location, address its mode of action, and/or affect a perceptible target (e.g., a subjective symptom or objective reading), and do so quickly. The match between the procedure representations and the illness representation determines the relevance of the procedure for illness control: if "heart burn" is the problem, ingesting an anti-acid makes good "common sense"; if cancer is a growth or lump, then surgical removal makes good "common sense" (radiation less so as it leaves something in the body). If asthmatic patients perceive that they have asthma only when they experience symptoms and that asthma has few negative consequences, they will doubt the necessity and will not take their inhaled corticosteroid as prescribed (i.e., Halm et al, 2006; Horne and Weinman, 2002). It is more difficult to sustain a procedure that fits this formula less well and has less distinctive and/or delayed feedback. For example, feedback will be less rapid and clear for attempts to control diabetic blood glucose levels with diet and physical activity than with medication. On the other hand, behavioral practices sustained by widely held, culturally supported beliefs could support possibly risky actions that are of little benefit biologically (e.g., the belief that natural foods enhance the body's immune system). It is important to note that in each of these examples the combination of an illness and treatment representation created the context for management, but the actual performance required the creation of an action plan.

In summary, the system is dynamic and the representations and actions are fluid. The underlying prototypes can vary from highly stable (e.g., the self) to moderately stable (e.g., lifetime experience with colds and migraine), to vague and readily changeable (e.g., SARS). Given its complexity and flexibility, the model speaks to a wide range of situations and poses challenges to our ingenuity in creating interventions and measures to test specific hypotheses.

1.3.2 The "Executive Self" and Strategies for Management

So far, our focus has been on the "nitty gritty" of the CSM – the details involved in creating structures for performance in a specific place and time. The CSM postulates a second, executive level of strategies involved in evaluating and protecting the self-system, testing and choosing among illness representations, screening and selecting procedures for management, and selecting targets for evaluating outcomes. The model mirrors gerontological views of age-related change (Baltes and Baltes, 1990) and overlaps with psychological models focusing on properties of the self, such as self-efficacy (Bandura, 1998), coping and stress management (Carver et al, 1989; Lazarus, 1993), and procedures involved in cognitive behavioral therapy (e.g., Friedman et al, 2003). The CSM has examined, in detail, the procedures involved in global self-assessments of health (e.g., Mora et al, 2008) and the "executive level" coping strategies for protecting and enhancing the self, conservation of resources (i.e., the belief that one will live longer by conserving energy) and "use it or lose it" (i.e., using competencies to avoid loss) approaches to self-management frequently expressed by older patients (Leventhal and Crouch, 1997). A longitudinal study examining the impact of a major health event on giving up activities and the factors associated with later replacement used a 3 item scale to assess belief

in the need to conserve resources and found the expected negative association (high scores interfered with action) with finding a replacement (Duke et al, 2002). The CSM has not yet advanced hypotheses as to how strategies for regulating functional resources will relate to specific approaches to problem solving (i.e., the sequence in which risks and action plans are identified and put in place).

2 The Empirical Challenges

The CSM can serve as a powerful conceptual tool for addressing the methodological issues in qualitative and quantitative studies describing and explaining behavioral processes in cross-sectional and longitudinal investigations. The CSM can also be a tool in experiments and clinical trials designed to reshape behavior and improve objective outcomes. No model as comprehensive as the CSM can be used effectively, however, without careful attention to its implementation.

2.1 Contextual Factors Critical for the Implementation of the CSM

Contextual factors alter the relevance of different aspects of lay representations whether they are used in descriptive studies to predict specific behavioral outcomes or in interventions to influence behavioral processes. For example, the participants, the disease, and the treatment all affect prototype checks and representations. The CSM also assumes that there are multiples routes to a goal and recognizes the role of contextual factors in determining which routes will be used and by whom. Although the use of "common sense" elements is essential for implementing any conceptual model, including the CSM, we recommend researchers and practitioners use the following elements to guide their work.

2.1.1 Are Participants Well or Ill?

Different CSM variables are relevant when predicting and/or intervening to alter the behavior of individuals who are "physically well" versus those with one or more medical diagnoses. Predicting or intervening to encourage the use of screening or preventive care for undiagnosed patients will require a more intensive focus on the processes involved in making appraisals of the future self. This would include factors such as how individuals come to perceive themselves at risk, the proximity and evolution of risk, and how to create action plans for integrating screening or care into daily routines. On the other hand, studies examining treatment adherence among patients with a diagnosed chronic illness will need to focus more intensely on the perception of specific treatments; for example, how the effects of treatment are experienced and understood in relation to the experience and understanding of the disease.

Context will also affect the salience of the various aspects of illness representations to patients diagnosed with a specific condition. For example, patients hospitalized for uncontrolled attacks of asthma or a myocardial infarction will likely be focused on the disease, how it was experienced prior to and during hospitalization, and why they were unable to avoid the episode. Patients who have avoided uncontrolled attacks and hospitalization are more likely to focus on treatment and how they experience maintaining safety. However, these examples are not "fixed" and it is essential to consider the specific properties of the context, disease, and behavior. The perceived properties of a recommended behavior for adjusting treatment (e.g. the aversive nature of using a peak flow meter every day) may be as important as the perceived properties of a recommended treatment.

2.1.2 Multiple Routes to Goal

The CSM identifies multiple routes to a goal for patients managing chronic conditions. For example, consistent with the CSM emphasis on the effects of monitoring and interpretation of symptoms, few of the 19 patients in a qualitative study of congestive heart failure (CHF) used medication to treat symptoms, like swollen legs or breathlessness while lying down, as they failed to perceive a relationship between those symptoms and "heart" conditions such as CHF (Horowitz et al, 2004). One participant, however, was in excellent control despite the fact that she was cognitively compromised and unaware of any relationship between symptoms and CHF. She maintained control because her son-in-law, a cardiologist, called every day and told her, "Mom, you have to take your medication now." In this case, social control of the behavior was the pathway to treatment adherence, as social control was able to override a biologically incorrect illness representation.

Along the same lines, multiple pathways are likely responsible for the contrasting results of clinical trials (e.g., assessing the efficacy of blood glucose monitoring among type 2 diabetics). The carefully controlled trials by Farmer and colleagues (2007) showed significant and equivalent improvement in HbA1c levels in the non-monitoring control arm and the two intervention arms. The composition of the sample provides a clue as to why control and intervention patients may have been equally successful in managing blood glucose. Slightly more than half of the participants in each of the three arms were professional, managerial, or clerically trained (53–56%) and the majority of the remainder were skilled manual and/or manually employed (44–45%). Thus, virtually all participants (98–99% in each arm) were accustomed to operating in a conceptual framework. Therefore, it is likely that most participants managed food intake and physical activity by creating and adhering to a daily action plan without monitoring. By contrast, in a multinational study with a diverse array of participants, the monitoring arm showed significant improvements in HbA1c levels relative to the non-monitoring controls (Barnett et al, 2008). We will return to this issue when discussing interventions.

2.1.3 Disease and Procedures for Control

Different components of the CSM will play a critical role in initiating and maintaining behavior for the management of different diseases and treatments. While acute and chronic conditions may share some "common-sense" attributes, representations of acute and chronic conditions differ sharply with respect to time-line and perceived likelihood of complete resolution. Within chronic conditions, a major division occurs between symptomatic and asymptomatic conditions. Diseases like osteoarthritis are highly symptomatic (or "noisy") conditions that provide cues for monitoring, the need for treatment and treatment efficacy. Diseases like hypertension and hyperglycemia are relatively "silent," or asymptomatic, creating an opening for self-generated symptoms, possibly due to situation-specific factors, that elicit worry and psychological stress. For example, blood pressure is elevated in clinical settings among individuals who have labeled themselves as hypertensive (white coat hypertension) whether or not their blood pressure is elevated during 24-h ambulatory monitoring (Spruill et al, 2007). Continually "noisy" and "silent" conditions differ from asthma, a chronic condition whose symptoms appear episodically and is therefore both noisy and silent. Patients are likely to only manage symptoms when their asthma is noisy even though it requires treatment when both noisy and silent (Halm et al, 2006). The risks entailed with symptom-focused treatment are present for other chronic conditions, like myocardial infarction (Akincigil et al, 2008).

Finally, interventions, whether for primary, secondary, or tertiary prevention, vary along multiple features of commonsense representations. Treatments vary in generating distressing side effects (e.g., identity), time-line (e.g., time to perceived benefits), method for detecting benefit (e.g., alleviation of symptoms or objective readings), and possible discrepancies between onset of side effects and perceived benefits. For example, side effects of anti-depressant medications occur soon after treatment initiation, while benefits in mood are delayed.

2.1.4 Co-morbidities

Although CSM is ideally suited to the examination of the mechanisms involved in the behavioral management for patients with co-morbid conditions, the specific properties of the conditions are still extremely important. For example, patients with two or more physical disorders may attribute symptoms incorrectly and use inappropriate targets for monitoring treatment efficacy. Depressive symptoms, frequently reported in conjunction with cardiovascular disease and diabetes, provide an example of the intricacies involved in patients' perception of the separateness and causal relationship among symptoms and physical conditions. While the depressive symptoms may be perceived as separate from, or as symptoms of, the physical illness, the perceived direction of cause may differ among patients and between patients and providers. The relationship between depression and physical illness also highlights the impact of depressive symptoms on generating action plans due to perceptions of inconsistencies between behaviors for managing depression (e.g., go out with friends and have fun) and the physical disease (e.g., if diabetic, avoid party foods) (Detweiler-Bedell et al, 2008).

2.1.5 Defining Goals by Action or by Target

Different features of CSM will be relevant for assessment depending upon the participant's goals. Therefore, investigations examining the relationship of common-sense factors to the use of health care must distinguish the purpose of patient visits. Visits scheduled for annual examinations or flu shots depend on a different set of variables than visits generated by the appearance of unexpected symptoms or novel changes in function. Prior studies have distinguished between spontaneous and scheduled visits (Cameron et al, 1995). Once again, however, multiple pathways exist to the same goal. Thus, patients with new unexplained symptoms may decide to seek care because the symptoms are painful, painless but feared as signs of a life threatening illness, or as a routine approach to any deviations from somatic norm (Mora et al, 2002).

The CSM suggests that interventionists must identify cues for monitoring efficacy and timing as well as clarify the meaning of these cues. For example, diabetics monitoring blood glucose need to know how and when to monitor as well as what they are monitoring. Diabetic patients must recognize that blood glucose readings monitor the effects of various behaviors on their blood sugar levels NOT their diabetes in general, which is measured by their doctor with HbA1c levels. Misinterpreting individual blood glucose readings as measuring diabetes control unnecessarily raises threat, emotional fears and disrupts management.

2.1.6 Gender and Age

The prototype of the self and an individual's illness history are shaped by the person's gender and age. Some of these effects are pronounced, while others are subtle. Women's pubertal history generates a wide array of somatic experiences, interests, and skills in managing health events (Verbrugge, 1985). Since studies show that women are more likely to share somatic experiences, the CSM check process can be seen as a focus for communication and sharing interpretations of changes in symptoms and function for women (Gijsbers Van Wijk and Kolk, 1997). Age introduces two factors for use with the CSM. First, the aging prototype, a factor encouraging the interpretation of gradual and chronic somatic and functional changes as being due to age. Second, strategies for managing resources, such as the previously discussed conservation strategy (Duke et al, 2002; Leventhal et al, 1993, 1995) and use it or lose it (Leventhal and Crouch, 1997).

3 Methods for Implementation of the CSM

The difference between concepts when assessed and when implemented in an experimental framework was commented upon decades ago with respect to test anxiety (Mandler and Kremen, 1958). As this is the case for the concepts in the CSM, our presentation is divided into two sections, the first describing the instruments available for cross-sectional and longitudinal descriptive studies.

3.1 Description and Prediction in Cross-Sectional and Longitudinal Studies

Six sets of factors have proven critical for the prediction of behavioral and bio-medical measures in both cross-sectional and longitudinal studies using the CSM: (1) properties of the self; (2) checks for comparing experience to prototypes of self and prototypes of illness; (3) representations of illness; (4) representations of treatment; (5) the prototypes underlying illness and treatment representations; and (6) action plans. The availability of standardized methods for assessment in these areas differs widely. The three areas with the strongest empirical base are representations of illness, representations of treatment, and the checks involved in self-appraisal.

3.1.1 Illness Representations

The Illness Perception Questionnaire (IPQ) provides both long and short forms for the assessment of an individual's representations of illness, i.e., the active and dynamic perceptions and beliefs about illness (Broadbent et al, 2006; Moss-Morris et al, 2002; Weinman et al, 1996). The instruments assess the five domains of CSM illness representations: identity, time-line, consequences, causes, and controllability (Weinman et al, 1996). Recent versions have included a factor to assess the respondent's belief that his or her representation makes sense, that it is "coherent" (Moss-Morris et al, 2002). The instrument has been used in a wide range of studies predicting treatment adherence and health outcomes for multiple chronic conditions such as asthma (Horne and Weinman, 2002), diabetes (Searle et al, 2007), cardiovascular disease (Horne et al, 2000), rheumatic conditions (Moss-Morris and Chalder, 2003), and emotional disorders (Fortune et al, 2004). As one would expect, the five domains also define the properties of the prototypes underlying the representation of illness that an individual is actively managing. Although there may be exceptions (Bishop et al, 1987), the few studies that have assessed prototypes used scaling methods (e.g., multidimensional scaling) to identify groups or subsets of illnesses and have not focused on identifying the specific features of disease prototypes and whether they match the domains of illness representations.

The following four advantages and disadvantages of the IPQ are worth noting. First, the IPQ is flexible. Investigators are encouraged to add items to specific scales to match the disease and population being studied. This makes excellent sense given the variability of experiences and management routines across diseases and individuals. Second, as is the case with many "survey"-oriented instruments, the IPQ relies upon the respondents' verbal responses. This may give insufficient attention to the hard, perceptual-behavioral level of representations the experiential level that provides the concrete affordances that cue and guide behavior and are at best only partially captured by verbal descriptions. Third, the IPQ represents only one component of the CSM and it has not been used to examine specific procedures and action plans. Investigators have had little or no success in describing pathways for self-management by combining the IPQ with measures of coping styles to test the hypotheses that coping mediates the relationship of the IPQ to behavior. This is not surprising as representations of specific actions or procedures, not styles, are connected to representations of illness. Finally, it is important to note there are differences between the assessment of illness representations using the IPQ and how illness representations need to be treated when implementing interventions.

3.1.2 Prototype Checks

Prototype checks are also involved in the formation of prototypes, though we know of no studies in this area. Given their function in matching experience to prototypes, it is not surprising that the PCs fit within the domains of representations: *symptom pattern and location* (identity); *duration* and *rates of onset and change* (timelines); *injury, ingested food, stress, etc.* (cause); *stress, fatigue, pain, dysfunctions, etc.* (consequences); and *response to intervention* (control). Studies examining medical care-seeking report extremely robust effects for duration, novelty ("How long has it been going on?") (Mora et al, 2002), labeling and consequences (Cameron et al, 1993), and response to self-management (i.e., control: Easterling and Leventhal, 1989).

That the sensory properties, severity and location of symptoms define a self-checking process was recognized long before prototype checks were assigned a formal role in the CSM; national organizations have and continue to list them as warning signs of cancer and heart attack. A recent study examining the delay from symptom onset to care-seeking for patients subsequently diagnosed with myocardial infarction makes an unusually strong case for the independent contribution of each check to care-seeking. The beta weights in the regression model relating delay in care-seeking to reports of specific prototype checks (location, novelty, sensory properties) are essentially identical to the bivariate correlations (Bunde and Martin, 2006). Studies are needed to examine whether prototype checks are truly independent of one another or operate in clusters within a domain of illness representations such as identity or time-line.

3.1.3 Prototype Checks Connect Representations to Context

Finally, prototype checks play a critical role in social communication. It has long been known that people describe the properties of symptom and functional experience when sharing information about health (Brody and Kleban, 1981), and do so in clinical visits when describing presenting complaints and responding to a review of systems. Thus, prototype checks define a key component of the mechanism involved in linking and allowing the social context to share and shape individual cognition (Greeno, 1998; Newell and Simon, 1972). In the final section we will address the critical role of prototype checks in the implementation of interventions.

3.1.4 Treatment Representations

Our preference is to conceptualize treatment representations using the same framework as illness representations and adapting instruments such as the IPQ for assessment. A treatment would have an identity (e.g., label, how to use/take it), time-lines (e.g., when and for how long to take), causal factors (e.g., works by removing, killing, neutralizing pathogenic material), control (e.g., cure and control of symptoms and objective indicators of disease), and consequences or costs (e.g., symptoms or side effects, physical damage, addiction, financial costs, etc.) and benefits (e.g., life extension, improved quality of life). Some of the factors assess the initiation of the treatment, others its expected and/or experienced outcomes. Although the experiential base of representations is more readily specified for the treatment of ongoing, symptomatic conditions than for asymptomatic conditions or prevention, people may "find" or create symptoms to provide a match between a condition and an experience and use the symptoms as evidence of treatment efficacy (Meyer et al, 1985).

To develop an instrument useful for clinical practice, Horne and colleagues (Horne et al, 1999) approached the assessment of perception and beliefs about medication by factor analyzing the responses to a large pool of items by patients with different chronic conditions. The result was two scales addressing the necessity of medication (medication in general and one's own specific medications) and two scales assessing concerns about medication (medication in general and one's own specific medications) (Horne et al, 2004). These scales have been used to predict medication adherence for several chronic conditions (Horne and Weinman, 1999), and can be modeled as mediators between representations of illness and secondary and tertiary prevention behaviors. Although the scales generated by Horne and colleagues do not carry the labels associated with the five domains of illness representations, many of the items can be classified within one of the five. Their approach also has the advantage of providing treatment (medication)-specific scales that are easy to use and meet the criteria for reliability and predictive validity (i.e., prediction of medication adherence) (Horne et al, unpublished).

Although the assessment of "necessities and concerns" regarding specific treatment behaviors is useful for predicting behavior and identifying adherence problems in clinical settings (Horne, 2003), intervening to enhance adherence requires understanding the representation underlying a treatment behavior, the cues for initiating and evaluating action (symptoms versus objective reading), the time for observing effects, and the coherence of this representation with that of the illness. For example, symptoms reinforce treatment necessity beliefs if they are attributed to the illness (Baumann and Leventhal, 1985; Meyer et al, 1985), but symptoms can enhance treatment concerns if they are attributed to the medication (Cooper et al, 2009). Similarly, patients who perceive their condition to be episodic rather than chronic are less likely to be convinced of the need for regular maintenance treatment if they perceive the purpose of treatment to be palliative (symptom relief) (Halm et al, 2006; Horne et al, 2009; Horne and Weinman, 2002). Representations of the risks (and benefits) of treatment will comprise beliefs about the timeline for onset of effects (both positive and negative), their duration and consequences, and the potential for control (e.g., over side effects). Moreover, the expectation of medication side effects may promote a search for confirmatory symptoms as predicated by the CSM (Meyer et al, 1985; Nestoriuc et al, 2010). Necessity beliefs and concerns are also influenced by prototypic beliefs about the properties of specific medicines (e.g., effect of symptoms, time-line for action, consequences and potential for control of beneficial and adverse effects). They are also influenced by more general beliefs about pharmaceuticals as a class of treatment (i.e., social representations) (Gonzalez et al, 2007; Horne et al, 2009).

4 The CSM: A Conceptual Tool for Generating Interventions

Four issues must be considered when using the CSM to design interventions. First, there are many ways to get from an educational/behavioral input to behavioral outcomes that impact objective biological markers. Second, clinical trials differ from experiments: experiments target specific pathways. On the other hand, the typical trial involves a complex "package" that differentiates the intervention arm from the control arm. Even when a single agent is involved (e.g., a drug or blood glucose monitor), there is typically more than one pathway in the system from input to output. Third, the essential ingredient for success will differ across individuals. Some participants may need to revise their illness representations (e.g., revising their view of the cause of their disease), others may need to change their behavior for controlling outcomes (e.g., learning to use an inhaler), still others may need to change the targets for assessing outcomes (e.g., using a glucometer). We would not compare the efficacy of antibiotics between patients with bacterial or viral conditions. Nor should we compare the efficacy of behavioral interventions for individuals for whom they are irrelevant. Fourth, and perhaps most importantly, interventions often face the challenging and intriguing task of reframing recipients' perceptions. Reframing involves the following steps: (1) identifying the experiences (symptoms – presence or absence; functional and/or affective changes; observed similarities to others) that match an underlying prototype that support the individual's active representation

of a threat (perceived vulnerability, current condition or absence of a prior condition); (2) connecting these experiences to a plausible, alternative prototype. Failure to connect with an alternative, biologically valid prototype risks re-activation of the dysfunctional representation. With these issues clearly in mind, how would the CSM enhance the design of clinical trials?

4.1 Many Paths to Outcomes: Focusing Clinical Experiments and Trials

Feinstein (1984) describes two divergent approaches to trials, the fastidious and the pragmatic. The fastidious trial is highly focused, recruiting a well-defined set of participants of a specific age and gender who are suffering from a specific disease for a specific period of time. These participants are then randomized to either a specific treatment or an appropriate control, either an alternative treatment or usual care, with the goal of altering or remediating a specific target (e.g., a symptom or measure). By contrast, the pragmatic trial randomizes participants varying in age, gender, ethnic background and, over a lengthy timeframe, compares usual care to a new treatment to prevent the occurrence or progression of a specific disease or set of diseases presumed to respond to that treatment. Pragmatic trials are preferred by clinicians who seek answers to questions respecting how to treat the typical patient in their practice. The following issues can be raised when looking at the contrast between fastidious and pragmatic trails from a CSM point of view.

4.1.1 "Needs" Assessment

The catchment (i.e., where participants are recruited), whether they are sick and with what, their educational level, and the physical and social structure of their home environments determines what participants bring to clinical settings and intervention trials. Within the CSM framework, these factors will shape measures, procedures, media, and content used to create an intervention.

4.1.2 Participant Selection

A clinical trial focused on prevention or disease management may be carefully designed and meet many criteria for fastidiousness, but fail to test its key hypothesis by ignoring factors specified by the CSM. For example, trials comparing the efficacy of blood glucose monitoring to usual care have produced mixed results (see McAndrew et al, 2007). As discussed above, despite high standards of fidelity to treatment implementation, the three-arm trial conducted by Farmer and colleagues (2007) showed no differences in HbA1c values among the intervention and control arms. This trial ignored a basic premise of the CSM, that there are multiple pathways to adherence, which limited the possibility of detecting benefits from monitoring. In fact, care in selecting participants increased the probability of including individuals who could manage their behavior at a conceptual level (i.e., without monitoring blood glucose). Good problem solvers can alter their life styles (e.g., food intake and activity) and use their physician's feedback on HbA1c levels as evidence for the success of their changed life styles, thereby having no need for monitoring.

4.1.3 Identifying Moderators and Mediators

In addition to individual differences in conceptual skills and environmental contexts, patients bring specific problems related to their perceptions and beliefs about their condition, possibilities for treatment and control, and the outcomes they expect to feel and observe with treatment. As it is assumed that outcomes reflect the impact of the intervention on patients' experience-based belief systems, baseline and repeat assessments of representations of illness and treatment provide critical data for identifying moderators of effects and pathways responsible for treatment outcomes (Kraemer et al, 2002).

4.1.4 Identifying Gaps and/or Targets for Change

Neither assessments nor interventions need to cover every aspect of disease and treatment representations for each participant. For example, in settings where all participants are diagnosed with and are knowledgeable about a common disease, studies will focus on treatment representations and criteria for evaluating outcomes. Although illness representations are probably less important in such settings, it will be important to address illness model features that are key to initiating and maintaining treatment (Baldwin et al, 2006). For example, whether a chronic disease is understood and perceived as chronic, acute, or episodic, whether perceptions and beliefs about symptoms drive self-management, or whether the disappearance and/or absence of symptoms is perceived as a cure negating the continuation of treatment.

4.2 Implementing Interventions

Because the CSM was generated by the integration of clinical experience and cognitive-behavioral theory and data, the conceptual framework is suitable for generating tailored interventions and developing step-wise approaches for representations of illness, treatment, and action plans. As limited space precludes addressing each of these approaches, we will discuss the general issues involved in the implementation of interventions in each of these areas. Implementation of such interventions involves specification and agreement between study participant and interventionist regarding the abstract and concrete features of representations and action plans, and, most importantly, the prototype checks used in checking experience against underlying illness schemata. Interventions need to address and create a valid match between patients' perceptions and procedural knowledge, the cognitive affective structures that underlie behavior, and the words describing the disease and treatment protocol (Phillips, 2008). Neither the traditional "medical" nor the current "patient-centered psychosocial" approach to communication address this requirement.

4.2.1 Implementing Illness Representations

To ensure that patients are working with an illness representation that is biologically valid, it is critical to ascertain the prototype that appears to underlie the representation. The checks play a critical role in this process. An intervention for "silent" diseases must provide a simple and convincing illustration that the disease is present when the patient is asymptomatic. For example, to illustrate the inadequacy of symptoms to predict hypertensive status, patients could take their blood pressure upon arising from a good night sleep. In this situation the context (post-sleep) and check for a prototype of wellness (feeling rested) would be inconsistent with the elevated reading they are sure to get if they are hypertensive. For asthma, a chronic condition that manifests episodically, a simple, vivid analogy of inflammation would be valuable for explaining the episodic nature of a chronic condition (you may not feel a sore on your arm till I touch you: when dust touches your lungs, you feel it). Finding a familiar, alternative prototype is critical for reframing both the meaning of symptoms (disease is chronic) and behavioral control. Alternatively, prototypes can be found to re-map symptoms for multiple conditions (e.g., chest pain can be reframed from heart diseases to chondritis).

Reframing is most successful when symptoms are connected to an explicit and plausible alternative prototype using the prototype checks that created the initial, biologically invalid representation (Rubin et al, 2005). However, not every patient will require concrete evidence, which may be difficult or impossible to generate for some disorders. Creating alternative prototypes where none currently exist is a challenge that has yet to be addressed empirically. Incorporating concrete evidence into an intervention ensures that patients and interventionists are using the same cues (e.g., symptom by location, pattern, and/or meter readings) and the same explicit time frames (e.g., onset and/or duration). Measurement of prototypes at baseline can be used in analyses as moderators and changes in illness prototypes as mediators.

4.2.2 Implementing Treatment Representations

The steps involved in the implementation of interventions that target treatment representations overlap with many of the steps in cognitive behavioral therapy. The response in a treatment protocol needs to be defined and practiced. Implementation guided by the CSM makes use of feedback and feedforward principles: it requires defining and experiencing the sensations involved in performance of the response, anticipated sensations or benefits, and the time frames for experiencing them. For example, a patient with asthma needs to know how to hold the inhaler, to breathe deeply, and to feel sensations deep in the chest when inhaling. The same patient also needs to know how often to engage in this process and when she/he is likely to notice benefits (e.g., what to feel when climbing steps or to observe in peak flow readings, and how many days it will take before observing change). Musculoskeletal treatments have similar properties. The steps in the exercise regimen must be defined and practiced, the sensory properties associated with appropriate performance must be kept in mind, the anticipated outcomes and time frames before benefits must be clear. The implementation is defined by the prototype checks that link experience to abstractions, that is, sensations in locations and time frames in response to intervention.

Causal features and consequences will be critical for specific interventions. For example, asthmatics may be concerned about causal features and consequences of corticosteroid use because the term steroids evokes consequences seen in athletes' drug use, and inhaling is perceived as similar to using other substances, eliciting fears of addiction. Similarly, conceptualizing cancer as caused by either gene mutations (e.g., BRCA1) or behaviors (e.g., smoking) may result in very different post-treatment monitoring and management behaviors. As behaviors can be altered, a belief in behavioral causes could encourage patients to quit smoking, engage in regular exercise, and/or follow a healthy diet. On the other hand, genes are associated with immutability, which could lead to inaction.

4.2.3 Implementing Action Plans

Implementation of action plans involves translating the words in a guideline for screening or treatment into specific actions that occur at specific places and times in the patient's environment (Leventhal et al, 1965, 1967). The checks, location, time, and sensory/perceptual events experienced during performance and experienced outcomes are central to the translation process. Adherence to daily medication for blood pressure control requires translating each component of the protocol into the environment where the patient is expected to act. For example, "take the pill" means keeping the pill where you have a glass of water handy (i.e., location). Similarly, "take it in the morning" (i.e., time-line) means eliciting the patient's morning routine (e.g., does the patient have breakfast every morning?) and fitting the pill into that routine (e.g., if a patient always has juice before leaving home, the medication should be placed adjacent to it). Actions are performed in the physical environment; the words used by executive processes can serve to review and improve the relationship between the environment and the action (e.g., make sure the pills are where you will see them so you do not have to think about it).

The sensory properties of pill taking are innocuous and unlikely to need explaining; that is not the case for the sensory properties of the outcomes! Knowing what to look for and when to experience it (i.e., time-line for results) will enhance experiencing benefits and detection of risks (i.e., consequences). Detecting optimal locations and time for performance to generate action plans for the management of musculoskeletal problems is more complex than taking a pill. In these cases, the environmental matching (location; time to perform; duration of performance) needs to be matched to the sensory properties of the action at both sides (input and output) of the control process. The location, timing, and duration of the action can facilitate or pose barriers to detecting the sensory patterns essential for effective performance. For example, if a patient is instructed to walk everyday, it is important to consider whether the patient has the space and time to safely carry out the intervention. If the patient works and lives in an unsafe neighborhood, he or she cannot implement a walking-based treatment in the same way as a non-working patient living in an affluent neighborhood (King et al, 2008).

4.3 Practitioner Participant Relationships: Executive Function and Expert Performance

Although we have focused on the details of assessing and intervening in the realm of experience and behavior (affordances) for illness management by patients and practitioners, the CSM does not ignore the role of executive functioning in this process. The most important area in which the CSM addresses executive function concerns its suggestions about how the roles and relationships among practitioners and patients will affect the possibility of achieving expertise in management. These suggestions are based on the assumption that practitioners and patients are striving to develop shared models of an illness threat and an agreed upon approach to threat reduction. We have stressed the role of prototype checks in the process of information sharing. Prototype checks are important from the clinic visit through the health promotion message to conversations with family members and friends. Questions about prototypes help clinicians and family members generate hypotheses about the nature of the problem and treatment. When the interlocutor is a physician, the information exchanged sets the stage for a bio-medical appraisal of the presenting problem, the conduct of the physical examination, and ordering objective tests if necessary. When the interlocutor is a layperson, the information is appraised in a common-sense framework, absent actual experience accompanying the reports of the problems' features. The prototype checks involved in this process extend beyond those involved in appraising deviations from the "normal self"; they include an array of checks specific to the social comparison process. Specifically, how does the self compare to a parent, sibling, or other relative similar in physical properties (e.g., weight, breast size) and emotional temperament (e.g., sanguine, anxious). The appraisal process includes checks on similarity between relatives and self regarding physical and emotional properties perceived as disease-relevant (Leventhal et al, 2007).

4.3.1 Executive Function

Both the CSM and current trends in clinical practice and medical education (de Ridder et al, 2007; Michie et al, 2003) recognize that openness and listening (Baron, 1985) in a trusting and respectful relationship is essential for communication and developing shared models. Mutual respect and trust provide a context within which the clinician and patient share essential details for linking experience to credible illness and treatment prototypes, and forming action plans relevant to the patient's environment. Respect and trust can be gained through working and communicating within the patient's common-sense framework. However, respect and trust are not sufficient to produce the content essential for behavioral change and favorable health outcomes. To maintain trust and shared perspectives, practitioners and patients must recognize that the fit between diagnoses, treatments, and expected outcomes leads to questions about the nature of the diagnoses as well as questions regarding the appropriateness of treatment and its outcomes. Questioning involves executive function, that is, the deliberative and/or automatic consideration and testing of alternatives. For patients, this means the evaluation of the fit of experience to alternative prototypes, considering and trying alternative self-selected "treatments" to evaluate alternatives. Failure to recognize and share these processes can disrupt the trust essential to the treatment relationship.

The CSM points to at least four areas in which failure to recognize the operation of executive function can create difficulties for management disrupting adherence and trust. First, it takes time to develop expertise. The time frame set for avoidance and control of health threats by a patient's executive function is often extremely unrealistic. The history of management of acute diseases teaches that satisfactory outcomes, including cure and alleviation of symptoms and risk, should be achieved in days or hours. Patients need to understand that it may take weeks, months, or even years to become expert and move from conscious and deliberate disease management to operation on an automatic, perceptual basis. Unless the threat to life is immediate, clinicians and interventionists need to provide long-term, realistic time frames with sequential goals.

Second, it is critical to address the perceptual space in which action occurs! Verbally oriented patients and practitioners expect words to automatically transfer to performance. However, words do not fully, and often not even partially, define performance. This disconnect can lead to a breakdown in trust and shared goals. The perceptual space includes internal somatic representations. For some diseases (e.g., arthritis), recognition and readiness to respond to the internal perceptual framework may be more important than developing a view of the environment for performance. Third, executive function, skillful though it may be, often focuses on limited features of the problem-solving process. Many current theoretical models focus on skills (i.e., the physical action) with insufficient attention to the context in which action takes place. Expert performance in soccer requires not only knowing how to dribble or shoot the ball but also how to perceive the position of opponents (disease) and team members (treatments) and judge when to shoot (self treat) and when to pass (ask questions and get advice). Behavioral skills are not sufficient. The executive self, conscious that it doesn't know what to do, may be unaware that expertise in self-management requires perceptual and cognitive skills involved in identifying cues and time frames for action and cues and time frames for evaluating feedback. This must be shared.

Finally, a patient and family will need input from multiple sources (e.g., primary and specialty care, dietician, and exercise specialists) and the inclusion of the family and/or social network to become expert in managing chronic illnesses like asthma, congestive heart failure, and diabetes. To create shared management, the CSM raises the challenge of creating an efficient and effective "language" that is intelligible to all parties, free of jargon and that addresses the internal and external environments for performance. In short, the language must integrate words and sentences (the abstract level) with perceptions and/or images (the concrete level) of how, where, and when to act, as well as what to expect following action and when and how to see and recognize benefit and/or risk. Health literacy, whether for primary, secondary or tertiary prevention, is a multi-person affair; it requires literacy by providers for patients and families and literacy by patients and families for providers.

Acknowledgments We would like to thank Drs. Linda Cameron, Michael Diefenbach, and Robert Horne for helpful comments. We recommend readers contact them if they have special interest in dynamic visual models (Dr. Cameron), risk perception (Dr. Diefenbach), and treatment representations (Dr. Horne). Preparation was supported by grant R24 AG023958 from the NIH.

References

Akincigil, A., Bowblis, J. R., Levin, C., Jan, S., Patel, M. et al (2008). Long-term adherence to evidence based secondary prevention therapies after acute myocardial infarction. *J Gen Intern Med, 23*, 115–121.

Andrews, M., Vigliocco, G., and Vinson, D. (2009). Integrating experiential and distributional data to learn semantic representations. *Psychol Rev, 116*, 463–498.

Angel, R., and Thoits, P. (1987). The impact of culture on the cognitive structure of illness. *Cult Med Psychiatry, 11*, 465–494.

Baldwin, A. S., Rothman, A. J., Hertel, A. W., Linde, J. A., Jeffery, R. W. et al (2006). Specifying the determinants of the initiation and maintenance of behavior change: an examination of self-efficacy, satisfaction, and smoking cessation. *Health Psychol, 25*, 626–634.

Baltes, P. B., and Baltes, M. M. (1990). Psychological perspectives on successful aging: the model of selective optimization with compensation. In P. B. Baltes & M. M. Baltes (Eds.), *Successful Aging: Perspectives from the Behavioral Sciences* (pp. 1–34). Cambridge, MA: Cambridge University Press.

Bandura, A. (1998). Health promotion from the perspective of social cognitive theory. *Psychol Health, 13*, 623–649.

Barnett, A. H., Krentz, A. J., Strojek, K., Sieradzki, J., Azizi, F. et al (2008). The efficacy of self-monitoring of blood glucose in the management of patients with type 2 diabetes treated with a gliclazide modified release-based regimen. A multicentre, randomized, parallel-group, 6-month evaluation (DINAMIC 1 study). *Diabetes Obes Metab, 10*, 1239–1247.

Baron, R. J. (1985). An introduction to medical phenomenology: I Can't Hear You While I'm Listening. *Ann Intern Med, 103*, 606–611.

Baumann, L. J., and Leventhal, H. (1985). "I can tell when my blood pressure is up, can't I?" *Health Psychol, 4*, 203–218.

Bishop, G. D., Briede, C., Cavazos, L., Grotzinger, R. et al (1987). Processing illness information: the role of disease prototypes. *Basic Appl Soc Psyc, 8*, 21–43.

Broadbent, E., Petrie, K. J., Main, J., and Weinman, J. (2006). The Brief Illness Perception Questionnaire (BIPQ). *J Psychosom Res, 60*, 631–637.

Brody, E. M., and Kleban, M. H. (1981). Physical and mental health symptoms of older people: who do they tell? *J Am Geriatr Soc, 29*, 442–449.

Bunde, J., and Martin, R. (2006). Depression and prehospital delay in the context of myocardial infarction. *Psychosom Med, 68*, 51–57.

Cameron, L., Leventhal, E. A., and Leventhal, H. (1993). Symptom representations and affect as determinants of care seeking in a community-dwelling, adult sample population. *Health Psychol, 12*, 171–179.

Cameron, L., Leventhal, E. A., and Leventhal, H. (1995). Seeking medical care in response to symptoms and life stress. *Psychosom Med, 57*, 37–47.

Cameron, L. D., and Leventhal, H. (2003). *The Self-Regulation of Health and Illness Behaviour*. London; New York: Routledge.

Carver, C. S., Scheier, M. F., and Weintraub, J. K. (1989). Assessing coping strategies: a theoretically based approach. *J Pers Soc Psychol, 56*, 267–283.

Cooper, V., Gellaitry, G., Hankins, M., Fisher, M., and Horne, R. (2009). The influence of symptom experiences and attributions on adherence to highly active anti-retroviral therapy (HAART): a six-month prospective, follow-up study. *AIDS Care, 21*, 520–528.

de Ridder, D. T., Theunissen, N. C., and van Dulmen, S. M. (2007). Does training general practitioners to elicit patients' illness representations and action plans influence their communication as a whole? *Patient Educ Couns, 66*, 327–336.

Detweiler-Bedell, J. B., Friedman, M. A., Leventhal, H., Leventhal, E. A., and Miller, I. W. (2008). Integrating co-morbid depression and chronic physical disease management: identifying and resolving failures in self-regulation. *Clin Psychol Rev, 28*, 1426–1446.

Duke, J., Leventhal, H., Brownlee, S., and Leventhal, E. A. (2002). Giving up and replacing activities in response to illness. *J Gerontol B Psychol Sci Soc Sci, 57*, P367–376.

Easterling, D. V., and Leventhal, H. (1989). Contribution of concrete cognition to emotion: neutral symptoms as elicitors of worry about cancer. *J Appl Psychol, 74*, 787–796.

Farmer, A., Wade, A., Goyder, E., Yudkin, P., French, D. et al (2007). Impact of self monitoring of blood glucose in the management of patients with non-insulin treated diabetes: open parallel group randomised trial. *BMJ 335*, 132–132.

Feinstein, A. R. (1984). Current problems and future challenges in randomized clinical trials. *Circulation, 70*, 767–774.

Fortune, G., Barrowclough, C., and Lobban, F. (2004). Illness representations in depression, *Br J Clin Psychol, 43*, 347–364.

Friedman, M. A., Cardemil, E. V., Gollan, J., Uebelacker, L. A., and Miller, I. W. (2003). The GIFT program for major depression. *Cogn Behav Pract, 10*, 157–168.

Garro, L. C. (2000). Remembering what one knows and the construction of the past: a comparison of cultural consensus theory and cultural schema theory. *Ethos, 28*, 275–319.

Gibson, J. J. (1977). The theory of affordances. In R. Shaw & J. Bransford (Eds.), *Perceiving, Acting and Knowing: Toward an Ecological Psychology* (pp. 67–82). Hillsdale, NJ: Lawrence Erlbaum Associates.

Gijsbers Van Wijk, C. M. T., and Kolk, A. M. (1997). Sex differences in physical symptoms: the contribution of symptom perception theory. *Soc Sci Med, 45*, 231–246.

Gobet, F. (1998). Expert memory: a comparison of four theories. *Cognition, 66*, 115–152.

Gonzalez, J., Penedo, F., Llabre, M., Durán, R., Antoni, M. et al (2007). Physical symptoms, beliefs about medications, negative mood, and long-term HIV medication adherence. *Ann Behav Med, 34*, 46–55.

Greeno, J. G. (1998). The situativity of knowing, learning, and research. *Am Psychol, 53*, 5–26.

Halm, E. A., Mora, P., and Leventhal, H. (2006). No symptoms, no asthma: the acute episodic disease belief is associated with poor self-management among inner city adults with persistent asthma. *Chest, 129*, 573–580.

Henderson, C. J., Hagger, M. S., and Orbell, S. (2007). Does priming a specific illness schema result in an attentional information-processing bias for specific illnesses? *Health Psychol, 26*, 165–173.

Horne, R., Buick, D., Fisher, M., Leake, H., Cooper, V. et al (2004). Doubts about necessity and concerns about adverse effects: identifying the types of beliefs that are associated with non-adherence to HAART. *Int J STD AIDS, 15*, 38–44.

Horne, R. (2003). Treatment perceptions and self-regulation. In L. D. Cameron & H. Leventhal (Eds.), *The Self-Regulation of Health and Illness Behaviour* (pp. 138–153). New York, NY: Routledge.

Horne, R., James, D., Petrie, K., Weinman, J., and Vincent, R. (2000). Patients' interpretation of symptoms as a cause of delay in reaching hospital during acute myocardial infarction. *Heart, 83*, 388–393.

Horne, R., Parham, R., Driscoll, R., and Robinson, A. (2009). Patients' attitudes to medicines and adherence to maintenance treatment in inflammatory bowel disease. *Inflamm Bowel Dis, 15*, 837–844.

Horne, R., Parham, R., Freemantle, N., and Cooper, V. (unpublished). The utility of the Necessity-Concerns Framework for conceptualising salient beliefs for understanding adherence to medication in chronic illness: a meta-analysis.

Horne, R., and Weinman, J. (1999). Patients' beliefs about prescribed medicines and their role in adherence to treatment in chronic physical illness. *J Psychosom Res, 47*, 555–567.

Horne, R., and Weinman, J. (2002). Self-regulation and self-management in asthma: exploring the role of illness perceptions and treatment beliefs in explaining non-adherence to preventer medication. *Psychol Health, 17*, 17–32.

Horne, R., Weinman, J., and Hankins, M. (1999). The Beliefs About Medicines Questionnaire: the development and evaluation of a new method for assessing the cognitive representation of medication. *Psychol Health, 14*, 1–24.

Horowitz, C. R., Rein, S. B., and Leventhal, H. (2004). A story of maladies, misconceptions and mishaps: effective management of heart failure. *Soc Sci Med, 58*, 631–643.

King, A. C., Satariano, W. A., Marti, J., and Zhu, W. (2008). Multilevel modeling of walking behavior:

advances in understanding the interactions of people, place, and time. *Med Sci Sports Exerc, 40*, S584–593.

Kleinman, A., Eisenberg, L., and Good, B. (1978). Culture, illness, and care: clinical lessons from anthropologic and cross-cultural research. *Ann Intern Med, 88*, 251–258.

Kraemer, H. C., Wilson, G. T., Fairburn, C. G., and Agras, W. S. (2002). Mediators and moderators of treatment effects in randomized clinical trials. *Arch Gen Psychiatry, 59*, 877–884.

Lazarus, R. S. (1993). From psychological stress to the emotions: a history of changing outlooks. *Annu Rev Psychol, 44*, 1–21.

Leventhal, E. A., and Crouch, M. (1997). Are there differences in perceptions of illness across the lifespan? In K. J. Petrie & J. A. Weinman (Eds.), *Perceptions of Health and Illness: Current Research and Applications* (pp. 77–102). Singapore: Harwood Academic Publishers.

Leventhal, E. A., Easterling, D., Leventhal, H., and Cameron, L. (1995). Conservation of energy, uncertainty reduction, and swift utilization of medical care among the elderly: II. *Med Care, 33*, 988–1000.

Leventhal, E. A., Leventhal, H., Schaefer, P., and Easterling, D. (1993). Conservation of energy, uncertainty reduction, and swift utilization of medical care among the elderly. *J Gerontol, 48*, 78.

Leventhal, H., Forster, R., and Leventhal, E. (2007). Self-regulation of health threats, affect, and the self: lessons from older adults. . In C. M. Aldwin, C. L. Park, & A. Spiro, III (Eds.), *Handbook of Health Psychology and Aging* (pp. 341–366). New York, NY: Guilford Press.

Leventhal, H., Singer, R., and Jones, S. (1965). Effects of fear and specificity of recommendation upon attitudes and behavior. *J Pers Soc Psychol, 2*, 20–29.

Leventhal, H., Watts, J. C., and Pagano, F. (1967). Effects of fear and instructions on how to cope with danger. *J Pers Soc Psychol, 6*, 313–321.

Mandler, G., and Kremen, I. (1958). Autonomic feedback: a correlational study. *J Pers, 26*, 388–399.

McAndrew, L., Schneider, S. H., Burns, E., and Leventhal, H. (2007). Does patient blood glucose monitoring improve diabetes control? A systematic review of the literature. *Diabetes Educ, 33*, 991–1010.

Meyer, D., Leventhal, H., and Gutmann, M. (1985). Common-sense models of illness: the example of hypertension. *Health Psychol, 4*, 115–135.

Michie, S., Miles, J., and Weinman, J. (2003). Patient-centredness in chronic illness: what is it and does it matter? *Patient Educ Couns, 51*, 197–206.

Mora, P. A., DiBonaventura, M. D., Idler, E., Leventhal, E. A., and Leventhal, H. (2008). Psychological factors influencing self-assessments of health: towards an understanding of the mechanisms underlying how people rate their own health *Ann Behav Med, 36*, 292–303.

Mora, P. A., Robitaille, C., Leventhal, H., Swigar, M., and Leventhal, E. A. (2002). Trait negative affect relates to prior week symptoms, but not to reports of illness episodes, illness symptoms and care seeking among older people. *Psychosom Med, 64*, 436–449.

Moss-Morris, R., and Chalder, T. (2003). Illness perceptions and levels of disability in patients with chronic fatigue syndrome and rheumatoid arthritis. *J Psychosom Res, 55*, 305–308.

Moss-Morris, R., Weinman, J., Petrie, K. J., Horne, R., Cameron, L. D. et al (2002). The revised illness perception questionnaire (IPQ-R). *Psychol Health, 17*, 1–16.

Nestoriuc, Y., Orav, E. J., Liang, M. H., Horne, R., and Barsky, A. J. (2010). Prediction of non-specific side-effects in rheumatoid arthritis patients by beliefs about medicines. *Arthritis Care & Res, 62*, 791–799.

Newell, A., and Simon, H. A. (1972). *Human Problem Solving.* Englewood Cliffs, NJ: Prentice-Hall.

Phillips, L. A. (2008). Construct validation of the doctor expertise scale in a primary care setting Unpublished Thesis (MS), Rutgers University.

Rubin, J., Wunsche, B. C., Cameron, L., and Stevens, C. (2005). Animation and modelling of cardiac performance for patient monitoring. In B. McCane (Ed.), *Proceedings of Images and Vision Computing New Zealand. Otago, New Zealand* (pp. 476–481). Otago, New Zealand: University of Otago.

Searle, A., Norman, P., Thompson, R., and Vedhara, K. (2007). Illness representations among patients with type 2 diabetes and their partners: relationships with self-management behaviors. *J Psychosom Res, 63*, 175–184.

Shanon, B. (1988). Semantic representation of meaning: a critique. *Psychol Bull, 104*, 70–83.

Skelton, J. A., and Croyle, R. T. (1991). *Mental Representation in Health and Illness.* New York: Springer-Verlag.

Spruill, T., Pickering, T., Schwartz, J., Mostofsky, E., Ogedegbe, G. et al (2007). The impact of perceived hypertension status on anxiety and the white coat effect. *Ann Behav Med, 34*, 1–9.

Stich, S. (1992). What is a theory of mental representation? *Mind, 101*, 243–261.

Verbrugge, L. M. (1985). Gender and health: an update on hypotheses and evidence. *J Health Soc Behav, 26*, 156–182.

Weinman, J., Petrie, K. J., Moss-Morris, R., and Horne, R. (1996). The Illness Perception Questionnaire: a new method for assessing the cognitive representation of illness. *Psychol Health, 11*, 431–445.

Williams, P. G., Wasserman, M. S., and Lotto, A. J. (2003). Individual differences in self-assessed health: an information-processing investigation of health and illness cognition. *Health Psychol, 22*, 3–11

Chapter 12

Conceptualization, Measurement, and Analysis of Negative Affective Risk Factors

Timothy W. Smith

Since long before the inception of behavioral medicine as a scientific field, negative emotions have been described as contributing to the development and course of serious physical illness. A substantial and growing body of research now supports this hypothesis (Smith and MacKenzie, 2006; Steptoe, 2007a; Suls and Bunde, 2005). Among the specific negative affects studied, anger and related constructs (e.g., hostility) have the longest history of research, especially in cardiovascular disease (Chida and Steptoe, 2009; see Chapter 13). More recently, depression has emerged as a major research focus as a risk factor for the development and adverse course of physical illness (Nicholson et al, 2006; Steptoe, 2007b). Anxiety and related constructs (e.g., worry) are increasingly documented as having similar effects (Roy-Byrne et al, 2008; Suls and Bunde, 2005). Whether studied as symptoms of emotional distress, diagnosed mood or anxiety disorders, or related personality traits, it is increasingly clear that these affective characteristics pose significant health risks.

Yet, inconsistencies in this literature underscore the need for additional research (c.f., Nicholson et al, 2006), especially since some intervention trials based on these associations have not demonstrated expected health benefits (e.g., ENRICHD Investigators, 2003).

Nonetheless, management of negative emotions and stress can potentially improve health outcomes (e.g., Linden et al, 2007). As a guide to future research, this chapter reviews implications of the fact that these negative affective characteristics are often closely related, despite distinct labels and clear conceptual differences. Until recently studies have typically examined only one such characteristic at a time. As a result, observed associations could reflect the individual risk factor studied, a closely related but unmeasured affective trait, or a broader individual difference in propensity to negative affect (Suls and Bunde, 2005).

Studies of the overlapping versus independent nature of associations between multiple negative affective characteristics and health outcomes are important not only in providing more precise answers to age-old questions about negative affect and physical health, but also for the design of interventions. In order to select or develop maximally useful treatments, it is important to determine if one of the individual negative affects is the predominant influence on health, if multiple specific affects are important, or if the observed associations reflect the role of a broader disposition to experience negative affect generally. The present chapter reviews the conceptual, measurement, and data analytic challenges in producing this more refined understanding.

T.W. Smith (✉)
Department of Psychology, University of Utah,
380 South 1530 East (Room 502), Salt Lake City, UT
84112-0251, USA
e-mail: tim.smith@psych.utah.edu

A. Steptoe (ed.), *Handbook of Behavioral Medicine*, DOI 10.1007/978-0-387-09488-5_12,
© Springer Science+Business Media, LLC 2010

1 Overview of Recent Research

As in much of the literature on the health consequences of negative affect, the endpoints examined in studies of anger have predominantly
included not only cardiovascular diseases such
as coronary heart disease (CHD) and stroke but
also other specific illnesses and all-cause mortality. A recent quantitative review found a significant association between initial levels of anger,
hostility, and related traits and the subsequent
development of CHD in initially healthy populations, as well as with negative outcomes (e.g.,
cardiac death, recurrent events) among patients
with pre-existing CHD (Chida and Steptoe,
2009). Similar conclusions have been reached in
quantitative (Nicholson et al, 2006) and qualitative reviews (Lett et al, 2007; Steptoe, 2007b)
of the association of depression and CHD. The
smaller and less conclusive literature on anxiety
suggests similar effects (Roy-Byrne et al, 2008;
Suls and Bunde, 2005).

The few studies addressing the overlapping
versus independent nature of these associations
have produced mixed results. Frasure-Smith
and Lesperance (2003) found that symptoms
of depression predicted recurrent cardiac events
among post-myocardial infarction patients, but
anxiety and anger did not. A measure of general
negative affectivity identified via factor analysis of the depression, anxiety, and anger scales
also predicted cardiac events. When considered simultaneously, depressive symptoms and
the negative affectivity factor were both significant predictors. In patients with coronary
artery disease, Frasure-Smith and Lesperance
(2008) found that diagnosed major depressive
disorder (MDD) and generalized anxiety disorder (GAD) were both independent predictors of
subsequent cardiac events. Further, co-morbid
MDD and GAD did not increase risk beyond
either condition occurring in isolation. Although
self-reported symptoms of anxiety and depression also predicted coronary events, most of
the risk associated with elevated symptoms was
accounted for by diagnosed MDD or GAD.
Other studies of CHD patients have found that

both anxiety and depressive symptoms predict
outcomes such as re-hospitalization (Tully et al,
2008a) or that only anxiety had significant
effects (Tully et al, 2008b).

Studies of pre-clinical coronary disease (i.e.,
atherosclerosis) and the initial onset of CHD are
similarly mixed. For example, Stewart and colleagues (2007) found that depressive symptoms
predicted progression of carotid atherosclerosis,
whereas anxiety and anger did not. In contrast,
Smith et al (2008) found that individual differences in anxiety and anger were independently
associated with asymptomatic coronary artery
disease in outwardly healthy adults, but depression was not. In a study of initially healthy men,
Kubzansky and colleagues (2006) derived scales
from the Minnesota Multiphasic Personality
Inventory – 2 to assess specific symptoms of
anxiety, depression, and anger, attempting to
minimize their overlap. Using these novel scales,
they found that self-reported anxiety, depression,
and anger each predicted CHD when considered
individually, as did a measure of general emotional distress that contained items reflecting all
three of these negative affects and general emotional distress. When the four scales were considered simultaneously, only anxiety and general distress predicted CHD. In another report
from this study sample, a self-report measure
of general anxiety predicted incident myocardial
infarction when controlling several other negative affective risk factors (e.g., depression, anger,
hostility), whereas these other traits did not have
significant effects when anxiety was controlled
(Shen et al, 2008). In a sample of male veterans,
Boyle and colleagues (2006) found that anxiety, anger, and depression individually predicted
CHD onset, but none of these characteristics
predicted CHD when considered simultaneously.
Further, a composite measure of general negative
affect was the strongest predictor.

Grossardt et al (2009) found that higher
scores on MMPI-based scales assessing anxiety,
depression, and pessimism were each associated with increased risk of all-cause mortality
when considered separately, as was a general distress scale that combined these individual predictors. When anxiety, depression,

and pessimism were considered simultaneously, depression and pessimism independently predicted increased risk of death, whereas anxiety was *inversely* associated with mortality. Finally, Phillips et al (2009) found that both diagnosed MDD and GAD predicted all-cause mortality and co-morbid MDD/GAD was associated with particularly increased risk.

Clearly, additional research is needed on the initial development of disease and mortality among initially healthy samples. As in the case of the course of established disease, the relative importance and overlapping versus specific nature of the associations between negative affective characteristics and the initial development of disease are presently not clear. There is intriguing, albeit preliminary evidence that general emotional distress may be an important predictor of later disease.

2 Conceptual Foundations

Effective measurement and analysis of negative affective risk factors must be based on a clear and empirically supported conceptual model of this domain (McFall, 2005). Without a sound conceptual structure describing these risk factors, the process of measurement is likely to be flawed and quantitative analysis often ill informed. Terms reflecting these negative affective traits and related constructs are often used without careful reference to such conceptual matters. Yet, useful conceptual distinctions are available from theory and research on emotion, personality, and psychopathology.

2.1 Essential Distinctions

2.1.1 Distinctions Among Negative Affects

Virtually all descriptions of basic emotions distinguish among anxiety and related emotions (e.g., fear), depression and related emotions (e.g., sadness), and anger (e.g., Beck, 1976;

Izard, 1991; Lazarus, 1991). In contrast to a state of calm relaxation, anxiety reflects nervousness, tension, apprehension, and at the extreme is characterized by dread. In contrast, depression involves sadness, sorrow, unhappiness, and at the extreme includes despair. Anger varies from mild irritation and annoyance to rage. These emotional constructs are also distinguished in terms of the cognitive content that accompanies them. Threat and perceived vulnerability to harm are associated with anxiety; loss, deprivation, separation, hopelessness, and failure are associated with depression; and frustrated goals, interpersonal transgression, and victimization are associated with anger (Beck, 1976; Lazarus, 1991).

2.1.2 Distinctions Among Types of Affective Phenomena

These affective characteristics can also be distinguished in terms of the forms they take, ranging from brief experiences well within normal emotional experience to more enduring and dysfunctional conditions. Episodes of specific emotion (e.g., anxiety, anger) can be relatively brief, and are often studied as precipitants of negative health outcomes such as acute coronary events (Bhattacharyya and Steptoe, 2007). Such episodic emotions can be distinguished from moods, in that emotions are briefer, more intense, and more strongly related to both behavioral response tendencies and physiological changes (Watson, 2000).

There are stable individual differences in the experience of negative affect and most comprehensive conceptual models or taxonomies of personality traits include related dimensions labeled *neuroticism* (Costa and McCrae, 1992; Eysenck, 1952) or *negative affectivity* (Watson and Clark, 1984). These traits contrast individuals who are generally calm and emotionally stable with those who are prone to frequent, pronounced, and prolonged episodes of negative affect – often in response to lower levels of situational precipitants. Neuroticism also includes non-affective aspects such as self-consciousness and feelings of vulnerability, inferiority, or insecurity, whereas trait negative affectivity does not. Related conceptual models focus on more specific emotional dispositions, such as trait anxiety or trait anger. These more specific affective individual differences are seen as lower order components or "facets" of the broader trait of neuroticism (Costa and McCrae, 1992) or negative affectivity (Watson and Clark, 1984).

In psychopathology research, a distinction is made between emotional distress and diagnosable emotional disorders. Individuals can report elevated levels of emotional distress, without meeting the criteria for an emotional disorder. Elevated symptoms are also presumed to be less enduring than those seen in related personality traits and diagnosable disorders are typically seen as related to but distinct from personality traits in their severity, related symptoms, and associated levels of dysfunction or impairment.

2.2 Empirical Challenges to Conceptual Distinctions

Although anxiety, depression, and anger can be clearly distinguished at a conceptual level, as can their various forms (i.e., symptoms, personality traits, and diagnosable disorders), these distinctions are difficult to support empirically (Suls and Bunde, 2005). Hence, research faces a difficult task in parsing what has been labeled a "big mush" of negative affective risk factors (Ketterer et al, 2002).

2.2.1 Specific Symptoms Scales Are Often Indistinguishable

This issue is illustrated by the high correlation between self-report inventories intended to measure symptoms of depression and those intended to assess symptoms of anxiety. In the parlance of construct validation (Campbell and Fiske, 1959), correlations between measures of anxiety and depression (i.e., hetero-trait correlations)

often equal the correlations between multiple measures of either of these constructs considered alone (i.e., mono-trait correlations). This indicates a troublesome lack of discriminant validity, a key component of construct validity. Multiple studies across a variety of populations and measures suggest that despite their distinct labels, measures of anxiety and depressive symptoms are more accurately interpreted as assessing a single dimension of emotional distress or negative affectivity (Feldman, 1993; Watson, 2009a). This problem has been acknowledged in psychopathology research for many years, but researchers in behavioral medicine often still interpret measures of depressive symptoms or anxiety as if they assessed the specific characteristic indicated by the scale label. Block (1995) refers to this interpretive error as the "jangle fallacy" in which distinct scale labels are accepted as evidence that distinct constructs are measured, when in fact it is an unrecognized instance of imprecisely labeled scales assessing highly overlapping if not equivalent constructs.

Some anxiety, depression, and anger scales demonstrate the expected structure of three distinct but closely correlated components, including expected patterns of convergent and discriminant validity (i.e., mono-trait correlations significantly larger than hetero-trait correlations) (e.g., Costa and McCrae, 1992; Watson et al, 2008). However, these measures of negative affective traits are still closely related, suggesting that associations of health outcomes with one might reflect the others.

In analyses of convergent and discriminant validity, anger is often more easily distinguished from anxiety and depression than the latter are from each other. Although a strong case can be made for anger as a component of neuroticism and negative affectivity (Costa and McCrae, 1992; Watson, 2009b), there is also mounting evidence that it has distinct motivational underpinnings relative to anxiety and depression (Carver and Harmon-Jones, 2009). Although anger may be easier to distinguish conceptually and psychometrically, this affective characteristic is consistently related to both anxiety and depression. Hence, its associations with health could easily overlap with the other two aspects of negative affect (Suls and Bunde, 2005).

The overlap among anxiety, depression, and anger is also seen in their cognitive correlates. Each of these negative affects is associated with the hypothesized cognitive aspects of anxiety (i.e., threat, vulnerability to harm), depression (e.g., loss, failure), and anger (e.g., transgression by others, victimization). However, in some cases associations with the hypothesized specific cognitive content are detectably larger than the non-specific associations (Beck and Perkins, 2001; Smith and Mumma, 2008).

2.2.2 Symptoms of Emotional Distress Overlap with Personality Traits

Inventories assessing symptoms of emotional distress typically ask respondents to rate symptoms during the past 1 or 2 weeks. This presumably increases the likelihood of capturing symptoms of distress and disorder and decreases the likelihood that scores will reflect more stable characteristics (i.e., personality traits). Researchers sometimes place undue confidence in this distinction, as scores on such symptom measures include substantial levels of stable variance as well as the intended, fluctuating states (Kenny and Zautra, 1995). This has been well documented in studies of anxiety, depression, and their co-occurrence (Cole et al, 1998; Dumenci and Windle, 1996). Hence, interpretation of symptom measures as assessing something clearly distinct from personality traits represents another example of the jangle fallacy.

Interestingly, although measures of trait neuroticism or negative affectivity demonstrate high levels of temporal stability (i.e., test–retest reliability) from during to after an episode of depression, mean scores are significantly elevated during the episode (Costa et al, 2005; De Fruyt et al, 2006). Hence, measures intended to capture only stable individual differences in negative affect (i.e., personality traits) also reflect at least to some extent fluctuating symptoms of emotional distress. Here again, uncritical acceptance that these trait measures assess the intended category

of affective phenomenon – and *only* that phenomenon – are not entirely warranted.

2.2.3 Emotional Disorders and Personality Traits Overlap

Associations between personality traits related to negative affect and diagnosable psychopathology (i.e., mood and anxiety disorders) are not surprising. Elevated neuroticism is a common feature in depression and anxiety disorders (Weinstock and Whisman, 2006). This association can reflect a causal influence of neuroticism on subsequent risk for these disorders, the effect of the disorders on fluctuations in neuroticism scores as described above, or the fact that personality traits and forms of psychopathology involving negative affect may fall on a common spectrum (Widiger and Smith, 2008). Although most research of this type involves anxiety and depression, preliminary evidence suggests that clinically diagnosable anger disorders (i.e., intermittent explosive disorder) are associated with personality traits involving anger and aggressive behavior (McClosky et al, 2008).

This overlap between personality and diagnosable psychopathology suggests that associations of one type of affective characteristic with health outcomes might easily overlap with – or perhaps even largely reflect – the other. For example, given that MDD and GAD are common in medical populations (Benton et al, 2007; Goodwin et al, 2009), some of the variance in trait neuroticism scores in studies of the course of disease could reflect psychopathology rather than normal personality, per se. Similarly, associations of diagnosed emotional disorders with health outcomes could also reflect related personality traits (i.e., neuroticism, negative affectivity).

2.2.4 Diagnosed Emotional Disorders Are Not Discrete Categories

An underlying assumption of diagnostic systems such as the DSM-IV (American Psychiatric

Association, 1994) is that these disorders are discrete entities that are qualitatively distinct from sub-threshold levels of related symptoms. In this view, for example, elevated levels of depressive symptoms below the threshold for MDD or even dysthymic disorder are qualitatively distinct from the diagnosable conditions. That is, taxonomies of discrete categorical diagnoses suggest that these disorders exist as natural types, rather than simply more severe levels of otherwise continuous distributions of symptoms.

Recent quantitative taxometric analyses of anxiety and mood disorders have produced conflicting results regarding this issue. Some studies suggest that MDD exists as a discrete category or taxon (Ruscio et al, 2009), whereas others suggest that depressive symptoms are a continuous dimension with no "natural breaks" indicative of discrete categories (Prisciandaro and Roberts, 2005). Similarly, there is evidence for both the discrete category of anxiety disorders (Kotov et al, 2005) and the continuous dimensions of anxiety severity (Broman-Fulks et al, 2006). Presently, the view of anxiety and mood disorders as discrete categories as opposed to the extreme of continuous distributions of symptoms is open to question (Haslam, 2007). It is possible that such categories reflect professional conventions more than natural types. Hence, studies of diagnosed categorical disorders as risk factors might mask continuous effects of symptoms severity, perhaps artificially dichotomizing that risk dimension.

Studies of diagnosable disorders as risk factors are also complicated by the high degree of co-morbidity. Depressive disorders are quite commonly co-morbid with GAD (Kessler et al, 2008; Moffitt et al, 2007). Depressive disorders are also often co-morbid with other anxiety disorders (e.g., post-traumatic stress disorder), though less so than with GAD (Watson, 2009a). Anger and closely related emotional symptoms such as irritability are common in depressive disorders, and their co-occurrence with depression is further associated with increased likelihood of co-morbid anxiety disorders (Fava et al, 2009). The DSM-IV diagnosis most specifically related to anger and aggressive behavior

(i.e., intermittent explosive disorder) is also quite commonly co-morbid with MDD and anxiety disorders (Kessler et al, 2006). Hence, associations of one of these diagnosed disorders with health outcomes might overlap with one or both of the others.

The close association between anxiety and depression in general, and between MDD and GAD in particular, has prompted efforts to revise the related conceptual models and diagnostic frameworks. In one influential alternative, Clark and Watson (1991) suggested that anxiety and depression share a common core of general negative affect. Depression combines this core with low levels of positive emotionality (i.e., anhedonia). In contrast, anxiety combines negative emotionality with high levels of physiological hyperarousal. This overlap has prompted calls for reorganization in the classification of the mood and anxiety disorders. Specifically, Watson (2005) has argued that the mood and anxiety disorders should be collapsed into a broad category of emotional disorders, with three subclasses: bipolar disorders, distress disorders (i.e., MDD, dysthymic disorder, GAD, post-traumatic stress disorder), and fear disorders (i.e., panic disorder, agoraphobia, social phobia, specific phobia). The extensive evidence regarding the overlap of anxiety and depressive disorders suggests that studying these risk factors individually implies an unjustified level of specificity and efforts to test their independent associations with health likely involve a forced separation of naturally co-occurring phenomena rather than an easily justified effort to carve nature at its joints.

2.3 Implications

This brief review demonstrates two types of confounding that complicate research on negative affective risk factors. First, when anxiety, depression, or anger is studied separately, observed results may overlap with the other, unstudied risk factors. Second, when symptoms of emotional distress, affective personality traits, or diagnosable disorders are studied separately, observed results may overlap with the other types of affective constructs. As noted above, this complicates translation of research on these risk factors into interventions, as specific emotional targets and optimal populations are not yet well defined. Hence, future research must go beyond the single-risk factor approach.

3 Measurement

In this future research, measurement of the affective risk factors will be a critical consideration. As noted above, measurement must be founded on a well specified and empirically supported model of these constructs (McFall, 2005; Smith, 2007).

3.1 Models of the Domain

The simplest model that accommodates the evidence described above is presented in Fig. 12.1a. Anxiety, depression, and anger should be considered, as well as the various forms they take. Comprehensive assessment of all of the resulting constructs might not be feasible in any given study, but the matrix depicted in Fig. 12.1a at a minimum serves to illustrate the range of alternative interpretations for any given set of measures. Figure 12.1b presents an alternative based on the more recent models of the overlapping and specific features of anxiety,

depression, and anger. The common core of negative affective symptoms, traits, or even re-conceptualized disorders could be measured, along with more specific distinguishing characteristics (e.g., anhedonia, physiologic hyperarousal).

3.2 Evaluating Measures

As discussed above, associations among anxiety, depression, and anger are to be expected, as are associations among symptoms, traits, and disorders. Therefore, even large associations between such measures do not by themselves challenge their construct validity; specifically, it is not necessarily evidence of poor discriminant validity. Rather, such associations are problematic only if they are as large as those between multiple measures of a single construct. That is, correlations among measures of anxiety, depression, and anger are expected, but they should be smaller than correlations among multiple measures of any individual affective construct if those measures are intended to support inferences about specific affective constructs.

Theory-based predictions about the relative magnitude of associations among measured variables provide the basis of strong, a priori tests of measurement models using structural equation modeling and related techniques. Valid inferences about the relative importance or independence of effects involving any specific affective construct require evidence that those constructs are, in fact, measured with at least

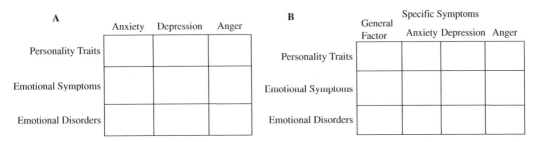

Fig. 12.1 (a) Conceptual framework for overlapping negative affective risk factors. (b) Alternative framework including general and specific aspects of negative affect

some degree of specificity. Other theory-based tests of measurement models should also include specific a priori hypotheses, such as the greater temporal stability of personality measures as compared to symptom measures, or the discontinuous nature of diagnostic categories. The strength of the evidence regarding associations between affective risk factors and health outcomes hinges on this often overlooked step of careful testing of well-articulated measurement models, and the ability to measure overlapping constructs with adequate specificity is essential in the eventual development of optimally focused interventions.

Symptoms of emotional distress include not only affective phenomenon but also physical symptoms, such as the fatigue associated with depression and the racing heart associated with anxiety. Some evidence suggests that such somatic symptoms of emotional distress are better predictors of health outcomes than are cognitive or affective symptoms (e.g., Linke et al, 2009; Stewart et al, 2007). It is possible that this pattern indicates that somatic symptoms of emotional distress actually reflect the presence or severity of underlying medical illness or co-occurring inflammation (Dantzer et al, 2007), rather than emotional distress per se. Analyses of the relative importance of somatic and non-somatic symptoms of distress will be more informative if the meaning of somatic symptom measures is carefully established in measurement research.

patterns. Multiple measurement occasions can also help disentangle transitory symptoms and personality traits. Further, prior histories of emotional disorder can provide incremental predictive utility over current assessments of symptoms and disorders in studies of health risks (Agatisa et al, 2005; Rutledge et al, 2006). Many if not most episodes of MDD are recurrent episodes (Coyne et al, 1999), but reports of prior episodes are often unreliable (Coyne et al, 2001).

3.4 Methods of Measurement

The vast majority of studies of negative emotions as risk factors for poor health outcomes rely on self-reports of anxiety, depression, or anger. This approach assumes that participants are willing and able to provide generally accurate descriptions of their emotional functioning. Even interview-based assessments (e.g., structured diagnostic interviews) rely heavily on what participants are willing and able to report. A small but growing literature suggests that self-reports of these risk factors have less predictive utility than do other methods, such as ratings provided by significant others (c.f., Smith et al, 2008). Hence, reliance on self-reports could produce an underestimate of the importance of negative affective risk factors. Here again, design and implementation of optimal interventions would be facilitated by attention to basic issues in measurement.

3.3 Considering Temporal Factors in the Measurement Strategy

Most studies in this area assess negative affective risk factors only at one point in time, yet temporal aspects of these risk factors may be important. For example, using multiple waves of personality assessment, Mrocek and Spiro (2007) found that high initial levels of neuroticism accompanied by further increases was a stronger predictor of mortality than other

4 Analysis

Clear conceptual models of negative affective characteristics are also essential as guides to statistical analyses, as future research must disentangle associations involving inherently interrelated or confounded influences on health. There are many procedural and interpretive challenges in using statistical control to address such confounds (Christenfeld et al, 2004), some of which stem from limitations in measurement.

For example, limited reliability or validity of measures of confounding factors can result in their "under-correction" and residual confounding. However, even when measurement limitations are minimized, major challenges remain.

4.1 Approaches to Confounding and Statistical Control

As noted above, analysis of a single affective risk factor creates obvious alternative interpretations; observed associations could involve not only the measured risk factor but also an unmeasured but correlated affective characteristic or a general affective characteristic. Further, these alternative risk factors could involve symptoms, traits, or disorders. These interpretive ambiguities inherent in the "one-at-a-time" approach are a clear impediment to progress. Inclusion of multiple affective risk factors raises the issue of optimal approaches to statistical analysis. Automated step-wise procedures in which predictors (e.g., symptoms of anxiety, depression, or anger) are entered into the analysis in order of magnitude of their association with the outcome (e.g., incident CHD) have severe limitations (see Chapter 54). When predictors are closely correlated, trivial differences in effect sizes across samples can result in highly unstable results. Selection as the first predictor included can vary across studies as the result of meaningless sample-specific differences in the magnitude of associations with the outcome. Once the first predictor is included for this essentially arbitrary reason, high levels of overlap among predictors are likely to produce misleading results regarding the importance of the remaining predictors.

Simultaneous analyses in which multiple affective risk factors are included concurrently has some advantages. The instability of results inherent in automated step-wise procedures is avoided and the significance of the independent associations for each predictor controlling the others is tested. However, the results may be misleading in another respect, one that has been described as the "perils of partialling" (Lynam et al, 2006). Specifically, the variance in a measured variable that is independent of a closely related variable might not reflect the construct of original interest in the way it did before partialling. For example, variance in a measure of anxiety might not reflect the construct of anxiety to the same extent once it is shorn of overlapping variance with depressive symptoms. This is especially true in instances where large correlations between the predictors reflect substantive overlap (Lynam et al, 2006). Given the well-established substantive reasons for overlap among anxiety, depression, and anger described above, as well as among related symptoms, traits, and disorders, the perils of partialling are a serious challenge to valid interpretations of related statistical analyses.

The results of Grossardt and colleagues (2009) described previously provide an example. When considered individually, anxiety predicted increased risk of death. However, when forced to be independent of depression and pessimism via simultaneous analysis, the anxiety scale was *inversely* related to mortality risk. The uncorrected anxiety measure suggested a risk factor, whereas anxiety shorn of its overlap with depression and pessimism was somehow protective. The two versions of the anxiety measure apparently assess distinct constructs. As construct validation studies are rarely repeated across the original and "corrected" or "independent" versions of such scales, it is often virtually impossible to know with confidence what the modified versions actually assess.

To address the confounding among negative affects, Kubzansky and colleagues (2006) developed research scales where the overlap across anxiety, depression, and anger was minimized. However, if these affective characteristics are naturally correlated, then scales that successfully minimize their overlap are virtually by definition not fully representative of the constructs of interest. At a minimum, construct validation research would be required to establish the extent to which the atypical scales are valid measures. Kubzansky et al (2006), Boyle et al (2006), and Frasure-Smith and Lesperance (2003) did examine whether a general negative affectivity factor predicted health outcomes. This useful analysis addresses an important question, but it is incomplete in that it does not test the importance of individual affective risk factors and their independent effects.

4.2 Recommendations

Each individual analytic strategy described above has important limitations and it is essential that these be stated explicitly when interpreting statistical results. However, when used in combination and with careful attention to the specific conceptual question tested in each option, these approaches can be much more informative. For example, a composite or general negative affectivity risk factor could be tested initially. Regardless of the significance of this general factor, separate affective risk factors within that general factor could be tested individually. Finally, the individual negative affective risk factors could be tested in a simultaneous analysis, with appropriate interpretive caution regarding the constructs assessed by the partialled predictors. If the partialled, independent effects of individual predictors are quite different from those for the same predictors considered separately, then the partialled predictors should interpreted with still greater caution. This sequence of analyses tests (a) the significance of the broader affective characteristic, (b) the individual (and potentially overlapping) affective characteristics within that broader domain, and (c) the unique or independent role of these individual risk factors. The pattern of results across these analyses can provide valuable information about the role of general negative emotionality versus specific components. It is important to note that these conceptual considerations can guide a variety of specific types of analyses. The optimal quantitative technique will depend on several factors, such as the scaling of the outcome variable and the consideration of time (e.g., survival analysis). Some approaches, such as structural equation modeling, permit tests the general negative affectivity factor and independent effects of its components in a single analysis.

This multi-part analytic approach to disentangling the role of anxiety, depression, anger, and general negative affectivity could be used to distinguish the effects of symptoms, personality traits, and diagnosable emotional disorders. Distinguishing among these types of affective characteristics similarly requires a multi-part approach. As noted above, the assumption that diagnosed mood or anxiety disorders reflect discrete categories rather than simply the extremes of continuous distributions of symptomatology has been challenged in recent taxometric research (Haslam, 2007). Comparing diagnostic groups could result in an unnecessary loss of statistical power similar to that occurring when continuous predictors are arbitrarily dichotomized. The prediction that diagnosed disorders have a qualitatively distinct association with health outcomes could be tested as higher order effects (i.e., curvilinear, quadratic) beyond linear associations with health outcomes of a continuous measure of the symptoms contributing to the diagnosis.

Ideally, the measurement strategy for these risk factors in a given study should be designed in advance to support testing the specific question(s) of interest. Those questions, in turn, should be tied to a specific a priori analysis plan. For reasons discussed above, such measurement strategies should also consider the temporal course of these risk factors. Analysis of such temporal patterns in the affective risk factors can be accomplished in a variety of ways (e.g., growth curve modeling, latent trajectory models), depending on the specific question and sampling frame for the risk factors.

The recommendation to utilize multiple analyses to address specific conceptual questions regarding correlated affective risk factors might seem to conflict with generally sound advice to keep the number of analyses to a minimum. Further, emphasizing the importance of clear ties between statistical analysis and conceptual models regarding the nature of overlapping predictors might clash with an occasionally expressed skepticism in the biomedical research community regarding the seemingly speculative nature of psychological theory. Nonetheless, a conceptually based, a priori analysis plan with these multiple components can maximize the information gleaned from any given study.

5 Conclusions and Implications

Various measures and categorizations of negative affective characteristics have predictive utility in epidemiological and clinical studies of serious physical illness. Because anxiety, depression, and anger have typically been examined separately, as have related symptoms, personality traits, and diagnosed emotional disorders, several questions remain before this literature can optimally guide intervention research. The overlapping versus specific nature of these effects must be clarified to guide the focus of interventions. Similarly, clarification of the role of symptoms, traits, and disorders, as well as related temporal patterns, will be critical in the selection of individuals for treatment. Empirically supported theoretical models of this affective domain are invaluable as a guide to the measurement and analysis issues in this needed research.

The conceptual models emphasized here are based on structural accounts of the negative affects, related personality traits, and psychopathology. There are other theoretical frameworks that could prove useful, such as developmental approaches that focus on the emergence of these affective risk factors from common and specific pathways. The negative affective risk factors are correlated with other psychological risk factors for disease (Kubzanski et al, 2005), suggesting that the approach described here could be applied to other individual differences. Further, the negative affective risk factors are also associated with risk factors that are traditionally construed as aspects of the social environment, such as interpersonal conflict and low levels of social support. Other conceptual frameworks can guide an integrative approach to overlap among intrapersonal and social–environmental risk factors (Smith et al, 2010).

Over time, such research can provide incrementally specific answers to essential questions;

among the multiple kinds and forms of negative affective risk factors, is there a principle "bad actor" that takes the form of a specific or general emotional characteristic? Further, is there a level of severity or temporal pattern that would help to identify those individuals most likely to profit from related interventions? This more refined understanding of affective risks for physical illness could help maximize the benefits – and minimize the costs – of the next generation of psychosocial interventions.

References

Agatisa, P. K., Matthews, K. A., Bromberger, J. T., Edmundowicz, D., Chang, Y. F. et al (2005). Coronary and aortic calcification in women with a history of major depression. *Arch Intern Med, 165,* 1229–1236.

American Psychiatric Association (1994). *Diagnostic and Statistical Manual of Mental Disorders, 4th Ed.* Washington, DC: American Psychiatric Association.

Beck, A. T. (1976). *Cognitive Therapy and the Emotional Disorders.* New York: International Universities Press.

Beck, R., & Perkins, T. S. (2001). Cognitive content-specificity for anxiety and depression: A meta-analysis. *Cognitive Therapy Research, 25,* 651–663.

Benton, T., Staab, J., and Evans, D. L. (2007). Medical co-morbidity in depressive disorders *Ann Clin Psychiatry, 19,* 289–303.

Bhattacharyya, M. R., and Steptoe, A. (2007). Emotional triggers of acute coronary syndromes: strength of evidence, biological processes, and clinical implications. *Prog Cardiovascular Dis, 49,* 353–365.

Block, J. (1995). A contrarian view of the five-factor approach to personality description. *Psychol Bull, 117,* 187–215.

Boyle, S. H., Michalek, J. E., and Suarez, E. C. (2006). Covariation of psychological attributes and incident coronary heart disease in U.S. Air Force veterans of the Vietnam War. *Psychosom Med, 68,* 844–850.

Broman-Fulks, J. J., Ruggerio, K. J., Green, B. A., Kilpatric, D. G., Danielson, C. K. et al (2006). Taxometric investigation of PTSD: data from two nationally representative samples. *Behav Ther, 37,* 364–380.

Campbell, D. T., and Fiske, D. W. (1959). Convergent and discriminant validation by the multitrait-multimethod matrix. *Psychol Bull, 56,* 81–105.

Carver, C. S., and Harmon-Jones, E. (2009). Anger is an approach-related affect: evidence and implications. *Psycho Bull, 135,* 183–204

Chida, Y., and Steptoe, A. (2009). The association of anger and hostility with future coronary heart disease:

a meta-analytic review of prospective evidence. *J Am Coll Cardiol, 53*, 774–778.

Christenfeld, N. J. S., Sloan, R. P., Carroll, D., and Greenland, S. (2004). Risk factors, confounding, and the illusion of statistical control. *Psychosom Med, 66*, 868–875.

Clark, L. A., and Watson, D. (1991). Tripartite model of anxiety and depression: psychometric evidence taxonomic implications. *J Abnorm Psychol, 100*, 316–336.

Cole, D. A., Peek, L. G., Martin, J. N., Truglio, R., and Seroczynski, A. D. (1998). A longitudinal look at the relation between depression and anxiety in children and adolescents. *J Consult Clin Psychol, 66*, 451–460.

Costa, P. T., Jr., Bagby, R. M., Herbst, J. H., and McCrae, R. R. (2005). Personality self-reports are concurrently reliable and valid during acute depressive episodes. *J Affect Dis*, 89, 45–55.

Costa, P. T., Jr., and McCrae, R. R. (1992). *NEO-PI-R Professional Manual*. Lutz, FL: Psychological Assessment Resources.

Coyne, J. C., Pepper, C. M., and Flynn, H. (1999). Significance of prior episodes of depression in two patient populations. *J Consult Clin Psychol, 67*, 76–81.

Coyne, J. C., Thompson, R., & Racioppo, M. W. (2001). Validity and efficiency of screening for history of depression by self-report. *Psychological Assessment, 13*, 163–170.

Dantzer, R, Castanon, N., Lestage, J., Moreau, M., and Capuron, L. (2007). Inflammation, sickness behaviour and depression. In A. Steptoe (Ed.), *Depression and Physical Illness* (pp. 265–279). Cambridge, UK: Cambridge University Press.

De Fruyt, F., Van Leeuwen, K., Bagby, R. M., Rolland, J. P., and Rouillon, F. (2006). Assessing and interpreting personality change and continuity in patients treated for major depression. *Psychol Assess*, 18, 71–80.

Dumenci, L., and Windle, M. (1996). A latent trait-state model of adolescent depression using the Center for Epidemiologic Studies Depression Scale. *Multivariate Beh Res, 31*, 313–330.

ENRICHD Investigators. (2003). Effects of treating depression and low perceived social support on clinical events after myocardial infarction. *JAMA, 289*: 3106–3116.

Eysenck, H. J. (1952). *The scientific study of personality*. New York: Praeger.

Fava, M., Hwang, I., Rush, A. J., Sampson, N., Walters, E. E., and Kessler, R. C. (2009). The importance of irritability as a symptom of major depressive disorder: results from the National Comorbidity Survey replication. *Mol Psychiatry*. doi: 10.1038/mp.2009.20

Feldman, L. A. (1993). Distinguishing depression and anxiety in self-report: evidence from confirmatory factor analysis on nonclinical and clinical samples. *J Consul Clin Psychol, 61*, 631–638.

Frasure-Smith, N., and Lesperance, F. (2003). Depression and other psychological risks following myocardial infarction. *Arch Gen Psychiatry, 60*, 627–636.

Frasure-Smith, N., and Lespérance, F. (2008). Depression and anxiety as predictors of 2-year cardiac events in patients with stable coronary artery disease. *Arch Gen Psychiatry, 65*, 62–71.

Goodwin, R. D., Davidson, K. W., and Keyes, K. (2009). Mental disorders and cardiovascular disease among adults in the United States. *J Psychiatric Res, 43*, 239–246.

Grossardt, B. R., Bower, J. H., Geda, Y. E., Colligan, R. C., and Rocca, W. A. (2009). Pessimistic, anxious, and depressive personality traits predict all-cause mortality: The Mayo Clinic Cohort Study of personality and aging. *Psychosom Med*, 71, 491–500.

Haslam, N. (2007). The latent structure of mental disorders: a taxometric update on the categorical vs. dimensional debate. *Curr Psychiatry Rev, 3*, 172–177.

Izard, C. E. (1991). *The Psychology of Emotions*. New York: Plenum Press.

Kenny, D., and Zautra, A. (1995). The trait-state-error model for multi-wave data. *J Consult Clin Psychol, 63*, 52–59.

Kessler, R. C., Cocarro, E. F., Favia, M., Jaeger, S., Jin, R. et al (2006). The prevalence and correlates of DSM-IV intermittent explosive disorder in the National Comorbidity Survey replication. *Arch Gen Psychiatry, 63*, 669–678.

Kessler, R. C., Gruber, M., Hettema, J. M., Hwang, I., Sempson, N. et al (2008). Co-morbid major depression and generalized anxiety disorders in the National Comorbidity Survey follow-up. *Psychol Med, 38*, 365–374.

Ketterer, M. W., Denollet, J., Goldberg, A. D., McCullough, P. A., John, S. et al (2002). The big mush: psychometric measures are confounded and non-independent in their association with age at initial diagnosis of ischaemic coronary heart disease. *J Cardiov Risk, 9*, 41–48.

Kotov, R., Schmidt, N., Lerew, D., Joiner, T., and Ialongo, N. (2005). Latent structure of anxiety: taxometric exploration. *Psychol Assess, 17*, 369–374.

Kubzansky, L. D., Cole, S. R., Kawachi, I., Volonas, P., and Sparrow, D. (2006). Shared and unique contributions of anger, anxiety, and depression to coronary heart disease: a prospective study in the normative aging study. *AnnBehav Med, 31*, 21–29.

Kubzanski, L. D., Davidson, K. W., and Rozanski, A. (2005). The clinical impact of negative psychological states: expanding the spectrum of risk for coronary artery disease. *Psychosom Med, 67*, S10–S14.

Lazarus, R. S. (1991). *Emotion and Adaptation*. New York: Oxford University Press.

Lett, H. S., Sherwood, A., Watkins, L, and Blumenthal, J. A. (2007). Depression and prognosis in cardiac patients. In A. Steptoe (Ed.), *Depression and Physical Illness* (pp. 87–108). Cambridge, UK: Cambridge University Press.

Linden, W., Phillips, M. J., and Leclerc, J. (2007). Psychological treatment of cardiac patients: a meta-analysis. *Eur Heart J*, 28, 24, 2964–6.

Linke, S., Rutledge, T., Johnson, B., Vaccarino, V., Bittner, V., Cornell, C. et al (2009). Depressive symptom dimensions and cardiovascular prognosis among women with suspected myocardial ischemia. *Arch Gen Psychiatry, 66*, 499–507.

Lynam, D. R., Hoyle, R. H., and Newman, J. P. (2006). The perils of partialling: cautionary tales from aggression and psychopathy. *Assessment, 12*, 328–341.

McClosky, M. S., Lee, R., Berman, M. E., Noblett, K. L., and Coccaro, E. F. (2008). The relationship between impulsive verbal aggression and intermittent explosive disorder. *Aggress Behav, 35*, 51–60.

McFall, R. M. (2005). Theory and utility—key themes in evidence-based assessment: comment on the special section. *Psychol Assess, 17*, 312–333.

Moffitt, T. D., Harrington, H., Caspi, A., Kim-Cohen, J., Goldberg, D. et al (2007). Depression and generalized anxiety disorder: cumulative and sequential comorbidity in a birth cohort followed prospectively to age 32 years. *Arch Gen Psychiatry, 64*, 651–660.

Mrocek, D., and Spiro, A. (2007). Personality change influences mortality in older men. *Psychol Sci, 18*, 371–376.

Nicholson, A., Kuper, H., and Hemingway, H. (2006). Depression as an aetiologic and prognostic factor in coronary heart disease: a meta-analysis of 6362 events among 146,538 participants in 54 observational studies. *Eur Heart J, 27*, 2763–2774.

Phillips, A. C., Batty, G. D., Gale, C. R., Deary, I. J., Osborn, D. et al (2009). Generalized anxiety disorder, major depressive disorder and their comorbidity as predictors of all-cause and cardiovascular mortality: The Vietnam Experience Study. *Psychosom Med, 71*, 395–403.

Prisciandaro, J., and Roberts, J. (2005). A taxometric investigation of unipolar depression in the National Comorbidity Survey. *J Abnormal Psychol, 114*, 718–728.

Roy-Byrne, P. P., Davidson, K. W., Kessler, R. C., Asmundson, G. J. G., Psych, R. D., Goodwin, R. D. et al (2008). Anxiety disorders and comorbid mental illness. *Gen Hosp Psychiatry, 30*, 208–225.

Ruscio, J. Brown, T. A., and Ruscio, A. M. (2009). A taxometric investigation of DSM-IV major depression in a large outpatient sample. *Assessment, 16*, 127–144.

Rutledge, T., Reis, S. E., Olson, M. B., Owens, J., Kelsey, S. F. et al (2006). Depression symptom severity and reported treatment history in the prediction of cardiac risk in women with suspected myocardial ischemia: the NHLBI-sponsored WISE study. *Arch Gen Psychiatry,63*, 874–80.

Shen, B. -J., Avivi, Y. E., Todaro, J. F., Spiro, A., Laurenceau, J., Ward, K. D., and Niaura, R. (2008). Anxiety characteristics independently and prospectively predict myocardial infarction in men. *J Am Coll Cardiol, 51*, 113–119.

Smith, P. N., & Mumma, G. H. (2008). A multiwave web-based evaluation of cognitive content specificity for depression, anxiety, and anger. *Cognitive Therapy Research, 32*, 50–65.

Smith, T. W. (2007). Measurement in health psychology research. In R. Silver & H. S. Friedman (Eds.), *Foundations of Health Psychology* (pp. 19–51). Oxford, UK: Oxford Press.

Smith, T. W., Traupman, E., Uchino, B. N., and Berg, C. A. (2010). Interpersonal circumplex descriptions of psychosocial risk factors for physical illness: application to hostility, neuroticism, and marital adjustment. *J Personal, 78*, 1011–1036.

Smith, T. W., and MacKenzie, J. (2006). Personality and risk of physical illness. *Ann Rev Clin Psychol, 2*, 435–467.

Smith, T. W., Uchino, B. N., Berg, C. A., Florsheim, P., Pearce, G. et al (2008). Self-reports and spouse ratings of negative affectivity, dominance and affiliation in coronary artery disease: where should we look and who should we ask when studying personality and health? *Health Psychol, 27*, 676–684.

Steptoe, A. (Ed.). (2007a). *Depression and Physical Illness.* Cambridge, UK: Cambridge University Press.

Steptoe, A. (2007b). Depression and specific health problems. In A. Steptoe (Ed.), *Depression and Physical Illness* (pp. 53–86). Cambridge, UK: Cambridge University Press.

Stewart, J. C., Janicki, D. L., Muldoon, M. F. Sutton-Tyrell, K. and Kamarch, T. W. (2007). Negative emotions and 3-year progression of subclinical atherosclerosis. *Arch Gen Psychiatry, 64*, 225–233.

Suls, J. and Bunde, J. (2005). Anger, anxiety, and depression as risk factors for cardiovascular disease: the problems and implications of overlapping affective dispositions. *Psychol Bull, 131*, 260–300.

Tully, P. J., Baker, R. A. and Knight, J. L. (2008a). Anxiety and depression as risk factors for mortality after coronary artery bypass surgery. *J Psychosom Res, 64*, 285–290.

Tully, P. J., Baker, R. A., Turnbull, D., and Winefield, H. (2008b). The role of depression and anxiety symptoms in hospital readmissions after cardiac surgery. *J Beh Med, 31*, 281–290.

Watson, D. (2000). *Mood and Temperament.* New York: Guilford Press.

Watson, D. (2005). Rethinking the mood and anxiety disorders: a quantitative hierarchical model for DSM-V. *J Abnormal Psychol, 114*, 522–536.

Watson, D. (2009a). Differentiating the mood and anxiety disorders: a quadripartite model. *Ann Rev Clin Psychol, 5*, 221–247.

Watson, D. (2009b). Locating anger in the hierarchical structure of affect: comment on Carver and Harmon-Jones (2009). *Psychol Bull, 135*, 205–208.

Watson, D., and Clark, L. A. (1984). Negative affectivity: the disposition to experience aversive emotional states. *Psychol Bull, 96*, 465–490.

Watson, D., O'Hara, M. W., and Stuart, S. (2008). Hierarchical structures of affect and psychopathology and their implications for the classification of emotional disorders. *Depress Anxiety, 25*, 282–288.

Weinstock, L. M., and Whisman, M. A. (2006). Neuroticism as a common feature of the depressive and anxiety disorders: a test of the revised integrative hierarchical model in a national sample. *J Abnormal Psychol, 115*, 68–74.

Widiger, T. A., and Smith, G. T. (2008). Personality and psychopathology. In O. P. John, R. W. Robbins, & L. A. Pervin (Eds.) *Handbook of Personality: Theory and Research, 3rd Ed.* (pp. 743–769). New York: Guilford Press.

Chapter 13

Hostility and Health

John C. Barefoot and Redford B. Williams

The idea that interpersonal animosity can have adverse health consequences is centuries old and has been part of multiple cultures. Inquiry into the phenomenon using scientific methodology also has a long history, with one of the most prominent examples being the popularity of the concept of Type A Behavior in the 1970s and 1980s. Hostility was one component of the Type A complex and eventually emerged as the focus of a great deal of behavioral medicine research (Williams and Barefoot, 1988). That work has resulted in a clearer delineation of the concept, documentation of its health effects, and description of several mechanisms that can account for those effects. This progress has set the stage for interventions to alleviate those effects.

1 Components and Definitions

As with many other terms whose origin is from common parlance, the word "hostility" is used to refer to a number of different, but highly

related phenomena. For example distrust, anger, and aggression are part of the overall hostility complex even though they are clearly distinct phenomena. Further complications in the definition arise because some authors use the term to refer only to hostile beliefs about others.

One useful conceptual principle is to rely on the well-known distinction between cognitive, affective, and behavioral components of experience (Barefoot and Lipkus, 1994). Hostile beliefs, including cynicism and suspicion, are cognitive phenomena that characterize a hostile way of thinking about others. The affective component contains emotions such as anger and contempt, while the behavioral component includes various forms of aggression and interpersonal challenge, although these can be expressed in subtle ways. These various manifestations of hostility are clearly interrelated, with suspicion and hostile beliefs often resulting in a proneness to see others as threatening, leading to anger-related emotions that may then be expressed as antagonistic behavior.

While the cognitive, affective, and behavioral components of hostility are interrelated, they can influence health through different pathways and each can be subdivided into more complex phenomena. An example is the process of anger regulation (John and Gross, 2004). Once anger has been aroused there are many pathways for its expression or, if it is not expressed, there are multiple ways of dealing with it more covertly. For example, one can express anger through aggression or discussion, and nonexpression strategies may take forms such as rumination, distraction, or reflection.

J.C. Barefoot (✉)
Department of Psychiatry and Behavioral Science, Duke University Medical Center, Box 2969, Durham, NC 27710, USA
e-mail: john.barefoot@duke.edu

Disclosure: Redford Williams is a founder and major stockholder in Williams LifeSkills, Inc., a company that develops, tests, and markets behavioral interventions that target psychosocial risk factors. Redford Williams holds a U.S. patent on the use of the 5HTTLPR L allele as a marker of increased CVD risk in persons exposed to chronic stress.

A great deal of research has been devoted to identifying the differential health consequences of anger coping styles, illustrating that the connections between hostility and health are far less clear-cut than straightforward main effects.

This recognition of distinct components of hostility and their potentially different psychological and physiological effects results in the need to be aware of the particular aspects of hostility that a measure is assessing when interpreting the literature. Factor analyses of multiple hostility measures reveal that they differentially tap the cognitive, affective, and behavioral factors (Barefoot et al, 1993; Martin et al, 2000). For example, the widely used Cook Medley scale (1954) primarily reflects cognitive predispositions, while the Trait Anger scale (Spielberger, 1983) and Expression subscales of the Buss-Durkee Inventory (Buss and Durkee, 1957) obviously reflect quite different psychological phenomena.

Another definitional issue that is important for behavioral medicine stems from the fact that measures of hostility are usually correlated with other health-related negative psychosocial factors such as depression, anxiety, and low social support (see Chapter 12). In addition, these psychosocial risk factors tend to co-occur in socially disadvantaged groups (Gallo and Matthews, 2003). This co-variation has prompted some researchers to focus on the variance that is shared among these constructs and search for genetic and physiological explanations that might account for this phenomenon (Raynor et al, 2002; Williams et al, 2003a). It has been suggested that a single underlying psychological tendency might account for the most important health effects (Suls and Bunde, 2005). We feel that this is a useful strategy with a great deal of potential, but we also recognize that much of the variance among these measures is not shared and that psychosocial factors like hostility may also have health effects that are different from those associated with other psychosocial factors (e.g., Yan et al, 2003).

For example, hostility is also inversely associated with positive psychosocial factors such as an optimistic outlook on life and positive

expectations for recovery, which have been found to be associated with adverse cardiac heart disease (CHD) outcomes, ranging from rehospitalization after coronary bypass surgery (Scheier et al, 1999) to both cardiac and all-cause mortality in CHD patients (Barefoot et al, APS, 2008). A recent study involving 97,253 women participants in the Women's Health Initiative (Tindle et al, 2009) provides a particularly strong demonstration that positive and negative psychosocial factors like cynical hostility and optimism co-occur in the same persons, yet still have independent effects on health and disease. In this large, diverse sample of American women, the correlation between optimism and hostility was -0.27 ($P<0.001$). In multivariable analyses adjusting for a broad range of potential confounders, however, *both* hostility – adjusted HR 1.16 (95% CI, 1.07–1.27) – and optimism – adjusted HR 0.86 (0.79–0.93) – were independently associated with all-cause mortality. Furthermore, individual components of the complex may interact in ways that have an important impact on health outcomes (Gallo and Matthews, 2003). Therefore, the present chapter will address both approaches to the studies of the health consequences of hostility.

2 Origins of Hostile Predispositions

There are two general approaches to the question of the sources of hostility: one derived from developmental psychology and the other from the perspective of genetics and physiology. These research strategies are not competing, but should be viewed as complementary.

2.1 Developmental Influences

Hostile attribution tendencies are the basis of cynical and mistrusting attitudes that can foster anger and subsequent antagonistic behavior. One prominent theory that deals with the development of such thought patterns has been proposed by Dodge (2006), who argues that suspicion and wariness to threat are natural reactions and it is the task of socialization to train children to become open to more trusting and positive approaches to interactions. This is done through modeling, positive family experiences, and belonging to a culture that values cooperative interactions. The developmental psychology literature is consistent with this approach, documenting that those who report that their family backgrounds were abusive or characterized by conflict are themselves more likely to be hostile and have interpersonal conflicts. A convincing demonstration of this was provided by Matthews et al (1996), who conducted a longitudinal study of fathers and sons, coding their interaction on a conflict arousing laboratory task at baseline. The more hostile the father's interactions with the son during the task, the higher the son's hostility score was when measured 3 years later.

Of course, opposite effects would be expected in families with supportive atmospheres that encourage a more benign attributional style. The results of Luecken (2000) and Simons and colleagues (2006) illustrate this by showing that those from positive family backgrounds are less likely to become hostile in the face of stressful environments.

2.2 Effects of Adult Adversity

Suspicious attitudes can also be viewed as a rational response to environments that are truly threatening and combative behavior can be adaptive under those conditions. Therefore, it is not surprising that cynicism and mistrust are more prevalent in those faced with harsh life circumstances. This may help explain the high levels of hostility typically reported by members of lower socioeconomic status and minority groups (e.g., Barefoot et al, 1991). It is also consistent with the hostile attitudes present in those who have suffered trauma. Anger proneness is one of the hallmark symptoms of Post Traumatic Stress Disorder (PTSD; Orth and Wieland, 2006;

Jakupcak et al, 2007). Although hostile tendencies are elevated in all types of trauma victims, they are especially prevalent in men whose exposure was related to military experiences. The prevalence of PTSD in women is high as well and is most often associated with sexual trauma. The presence of anger proneness can partially explain the high levels of cardiovascular reactivity that have been observed in studies of PTSD patients (Beckham et al, 1996).

2.3 Genetic and Physiological Influences

Based on the extensive evidence relating central nervous system (CNS) serotonin function to the expression of psychosocial factors like hostility and the potentially pathogenic biobehavioral characteristics that are found in persons with high hostility, Williams (1994) proposed that reduced CNS serotonin function is one brain mechanism that could account for the clustering of hostility and biobehavioral factors that increase disease risk. Using the prolactin response to fenfluramine/citalopram challenge as an index of CNS serotonin function, Manuck's research group has provided extensive evidence supporting this hypothesis, showing that lower CNS serotonin function is associated with increased aggressiveness (Manuck et al, 1998, 2002), increased expression of the metabolic syndrome (Muldoon et al, 2006), and even increased carotid arteriosclerosis (Muldoon et al, 2007). They have also used cerebrospinal fluid (CSF) levels of the major serotonin metabolite 5HIAA to index CNS serotonin function in cynomolgus macaques and found that males with lower CSF 5HIAA levels exhibit increased dominance behaviors (Kaplan et al, 2002).

It is not surprising, given these findings linking CNS serotonin function with hostility and associated biobehavioral characteristics that could mediate the effects of hostility on pathogenesis, that considerable research attention has been devoted to evaluating the effects of genes that influence serotonin function on these psychosocial and biobehavioral characteristics. In a seminal early study, Lesch and colleagues (1996) found that persons carrying the less active short (S) allele of a functional polymorphism of the serotonin transporter promoter (5HTTLPR) have higher levels of neuroticism (including the angry hostility facet) and lower levels of agreeableness – a profile that is characteristic of high hostility – than those homozygous for the more active long (L) allele. Manuck and colleagues (2000) found that the less active alleles of a functional polymorphism in another gene that influences CNS serotonin function, monoamine oxidase A (MAOA-uVNTR), are associated with increased aggressiveness in men.

While these studies finding main effects of serotonin gene variants on hostility and related psychosocial characteristics are informative, it has become clear that any attempts to identify gene variants that influence the expression of psychological and biobehavioral phenotypes involved in disease etiology and/or course must include consideration of environmental exposures that can modify the influence of the genes on these characteristics (Moffitt et al, 2005). In a study employing this strategy that provides one example of a gene × environment interaction influencing the development of hostility, Caspi et al (2002) showed that in men who had been abused during childhood those with the less active alleles of the MAOA-uVNTR polymorphism were more likely than those with the more active alleles to engage in violent behaviors during adulthood.

Further evidence linking CNS serotonin function with hostility and other negative and positive psychological characteristics comes from a study by Siegler and colleagues (2008) in which high brain serotonin levels – indexed by high CSF 5HIAA in men with less active MAOA-uVNTR alleles – were found to be associated with lower levels of hostility and depression and higher levels of conscientiousness, altruism, and perceived social support. In addition to providing evidence that low CNS serotonin function is associated with high hostility, this study also provides evidence that CNS serotonin function could account

for the clustering of hostility with other negative and positive psychosocial characteristics.

While the examples cited thus far may appear fairly straightforward, it is important to understand that this work has only recently begun, that the mechanisms being studied are far from simple, and that much additional research will be required before the final story has been told. This complexity can be illustrated with a few additional examples. Williams et al (2003) found that CSF 5HIAA levels are associated with 5HTTLPR genotypes, but in ways that vary as a function of both race and sex. In men and whites, the SS genotype is associated with lower CSF 5HIAA levels, but in women and blacks those with the SS genotype have higher 5HIAA levels than carriers of the L allele of both races and sexes. This finding suggests that both race and sex need to be tested in any attempts to relate 5HTTLPR genotypes to phenotypes whose expression may be influenced by CNS serotonin function. The importance of this approach is illustrated by recent findings in a study by Brummett and colleagues (2008a) in which the 5HTTLPR S allele was associated with increased depressive symptom levels in women exposed to chronic stress during both childhood and adulthood, while in men it was the L allele that was associated with increased depressive symptoms. Brummett et al (2008b) documented this sex moderation of 5HTTLPR genotype effects on negative affects in an experimental study in which the increase in negative affects induced by intravenous infusion of the amino acid precursor of serotonin, tryptophan, was larger in men with the 5HTTLPR LL genotype, but larger in women with the SS genotype. In contrast to these moderations of 5HTTLPR effects on CSF 5HIAA and negative affects by race and sex, the 5HTTLPR L allele has been found associated with larger cardiovascular responses to acute mental stress in the lab in both men and women, blacks and whites (Williams et al, 2008). Support for the pathogenic effects of the 5HTTLPR L allele comes from three independent case–control studies, one in Japan (Arinami et al, 1999) and two from Europe (Coto et al, 2003; Fumeron et al, 2002) in which the 5HTTLPR LL genotype was found associated with increased risk of myocardial infarction (MI).

The foregoing indicates that the strategy of evaluating CNS serotonin function – and genes that influence it whether as main effects or via gene × environment interactions – has enabled us to make good progress towards understanding the origins of hostility and associated potentially pathogenic biobehavioral factors. But it is also clear that there is much more work to be done, both with respect to serotonin and related genes. This work will also need to focus on a broad range of other biologically plausible candidate genes, including those that influence the sympathetic nervous system (SNS) and hypothalamic–pituitary–adrenal (HPA) axis as well as the metabolic, cardiovascular, hemostatic, and inflammatory functions whose expression is influenced by the SNS and HPA axis.

2.4 Social Environment

It is important to also be aware of the magnitude of social influences on a person's psychological outlook and disease risk. One approach to this task has been through the concept of social capital (Kawachi and Berkman, 2000), which is based on the notion that group-level atmospheres and characteristics have important influences on individual well-being. Thus, cohesive groups with constructive attitudes can result in more productive and healthier atmospheres. One important component of social capital is the level of interpersonal trust, which can foster or hinder cooperative behavior and foster the achievement of goals. The impact of group level trust can be seen in the work of Kopp and colleagues (2006), who compared subregions of Hungary on a variety of psychosocial characteristics based on a large-scale survey. Death rate differences across regions were predicted by a variety of psychosocial characteristics including hostility and attributes such as supportive social

conditions that are both a cause and a product of individual level trust.

Social networks constitute another important influence on a person's attitudes and behavior. Friends help set examples and provide conditions conducive to health-related behaviors and attitudes. Studies of the patterns of the distribution of health habits, obesity, and psychological characteristics such as happiness in the population have documented their similarity to patterns of social connections (Christakis and Fowler, 2008; Fowler and Christakis, 2008).

3 Hostility and Health Outcomes

3.1 Coronary Disease Development

The most frequently studied disease outcome in the hostility literature is coronary heart disease. Multiple reviews (e.g., Chida and Steptoe, 2009; Everson-Rose and Lewis, 2005; Smith et al, 2004) have concluded that ample evidence exists to establish a link between hostility and coronary heart disease incidence even though not all studies are positive and there are questions about issues such as the equality of the effect for both sexes. These studies have used a variety of hostility measures as predictors. For example, instruments that have predicted cardiac events include those designed to assess cynicism and mistrust (e.g., Barefoot et al, 1995; Niaura et al, 2002) as well as anger proneness (e.g., Williams et al, 2001) and ratings of hostile behavior during an interview (Matthews et al, 2004). The variety and quality of the various studies boost confidence in the overall conclusion that antagonistic personal characteristics lead to an elevated incidence of coronary events.

Another valuable research strategy is the examination of atherosclerosis levels in asymptomatic samples with noninvasive procedures that quantify the amount of plaque present in important arteries. This strategy provides more detail about the course of the disease by separating plaque generation from other components of the disease process such as event triggering and by examining the early stages of CHD development. These studies also avoid potential confounding psychological factors such as individual differences in health care seeking and sensitivity to symptoms (Barefoot et al, 1992; Mechanic, 1972). Studies of coronary artery calcification have found associations between hostility and atherosclerosis in both cross-sectional comparisons (e.g. Everson-Rose et al, 2006) and prospective studies of plaque growth (e.g., Julkunen et al, 1994). These investigations have included both women and men and subjects of a variety of age groups (e.g., Iribarren et al, 2000; Knox et al, 2004). Not all studies have had positive findings (e.g., Stewart et al, 2007), but the bulk of the evidence favors an association of hostility with subclinical disease progression.

Another aspect of the coronary heart disease process is the actual triggering of coronary events, a process that has been frequently hypothesized to be linked to the influence of both physical and psychological stressors (Strike and Steptoe, 2005). Anger is an obvious candidate for one such category of triggers, and studies that inquire about a patient's activities prior to the coronary episode find a high prevalence of anger episodes (Mittleman et al, 1995; Möller et al, 1999). The presence of anger prior to an event is more common in younger patients and those of lower socioeconomic status, a different pattern than the one characterizing those with apparent physical exertion triggers (Strike et al, 2006). Of course, such studies face the problems of possible recall bias. However, there are physiological mechanisms that make the anger triggering effect plausible and potential methods for identifying those at risk (Burg et al, 2009).

3.2 Prognosis in Those with Established Coronary Disease

The case for elevated risk of recurrent events in hostile patients is not as clear-cut as it is for disease incidence, partially because fewer studies have addressed the issue. Chaput and colleagues (2002) found that scores on the Cook Medley scale were an independent risk factor for recurrent events in postmenopausal women. Denollet and Brutsaert (1998) found that anger was one of several negative emotions conferring excess risk in MI patients. There have been some negative studies, however (e.g., Frasure-Smith and Lesperance, 2003), other researchers have observed the effect only under certain conditions. For example, two studies (Angerer et al, 2000; Boyle et al, 2004) found some hostility measures to be predictive while others were not, and Boyle and colleagues (2005) observed a stronger effect in younger patients. Although the picture painted by the literature is not completely clear, it is highly probable that hostility does convey increased risk of future coronary events in those with established disease. The exact conditions and aspects of hostility that maximize that risk are yet to be established.

The incidences of other cardiovascular disease have also been linked to various aspects of hostility. For example, Williams and colleagues (2002) found that trait anger predicted stroke incidence among participants in a large national study who were aged 60 or older, and Yan and colleagues (2003) observed a link between Cook Medley scores and the development of hypertension in the Coronary Artery Risk Development in Young Adults (CARDIA) study.

3.3 Total Mortality and Other Diseases

The impact of hostility on specific diseases that are not cardiovascular in nature has not been very extensively documented although there are investigations linking it to cancer incidence (Tindle et al, 2009) and to various indicators of general health (e.g., Adams, 1994; Kivimaki et al, 1998). Many studies have demonstrated the ability of hostility measures to predict mortality from all causes. Most studies of coronary disease incidence find that the prediction of total mortality is as strong, or stronger, than the effects obtained for the cardiac mortality outcome.

3.4 Demographic Factors, Hostility, and Health Risks

Findings that age may moderate the risks of hostility (e.g., Boyle et al, 2005; Williams et al, 2002) serve as a reminder that we should consider the role that age might play in the association between hostility and health. There are substantial age trends in the levels of hostility in the population (Barefoot et al, 1991), with higher scores in young adults and somewhat higher scores in older adults compared to middle-aged adults. However, not all of the hostility components show the same trends. Comparisons among middle-aged and older adults found higher levels of the cognitive aspects of hostility such as cynicism in the older group, but lower levels of overt anger expression and no differences in the affective component (Barefoot et al, 1993). These factors become especially relevant in light of the general trends for hostility to be a less potent risk factor for cardiovascular disease among older adults, a phenomenon observed for several other risk indicators as well (Williams, 2000). However, the potential role of hostility in healthy aging is a topic that deserves more attention. Experiences of anger and conflict in a laboratory setting have been found to lead to increases in proinflammatory cytokine production and slower wound healing (Kiecolt-Glaser et al, 2005). Chronic reactions of this type can lead to a variety of illnesses associated with aging such as osteoporosis, arthritis, and diabetes, in addition to cardiovascular disease. Similar effects were observed in a longitudinal study of older adults in which Cook and Medley hostility scores were associated with elevated levels of C-reactive protein, suggesting that disease processes might be accelerated for those individuals (Graham et al, 2006). Another suggestion of the role of hostility in the aging process comes from the observation that high hostility in older men was associated with poorer lung function at baseline and a more rapid decline in pulmonary function over an 8-year study period (Kubzansky et al, 2006). These findings suggest that aging processes may be a fruitful topic for more extensive study.

Strong trends have also been observed for socio-economic status, with the poorer and less educated members of the population expressing much higher levels of cynicism and distrust (Barefoot et al, 1993). Despite this, those with less education score lower on measures of anger expression (Haukkala, 2002).

Cultural differences in hostility should also be taken into account. These are not only associated with the level of hostility in a population as documented in the study of social networks and social capital (see above), but the manifestations of hostility components as well. For example, norms regarding emotional expressivity differ between Asian and American cultures (Butler et al, 2007). Cross-cultural studies in Singapore have also documented significant blood pressure differences in response to stress and in daily life between hostile subjects of Chinese and Indian ethnicity despite the similarity of their environments (Bishop and Robinson, 2000; Enkleman et al, 2005).

Gender is another factor that has strong influence on hostility scores, with women scoring lower on many measures (e.g. Barefoot et al, 1993). As with socio-economic status, this difference is not seen for all hostility components. Women are most likely to have lower scores on cognitive and behavioral measures, but not necessarily on measures of anger, indicating they may employ different modes of dealing with and expressing their negative reactions. Men appear to be more likely to engage in aggressive behavior, but women are more likely to communicate their angry feelings (Stoney and Engebretson, 1994).

4 Mechanisms

4.1 Social Stressors

One of the major ideas in research on hostility is that those with antagonistic cognitive, emotional, and behavioral predispositions tend to lead more stressful lives. The underlying behavioral mechanisms can be outlined using

Smith's transactional model (Smith et al, 2004). The transactional account of the process begins with a cognitive predisposition to be cynical and suspicious, leading to a tendency to perceive threat or hostile intent on the part of others; a bias that has been demonstrated in the laboratory by having high and low hostile subjects report their reactions to standardized social stimuli (Allred and Smith, 1991; Larkin et al, 2002). These attributions can lead to anger with its many physiological and behavioral consequences. They can also lead to another outcome likely to have an impact on stress: the failure to recognize or make use of potential sources of social support, consistent with the finding that those with high hostility scores tend to report lower levels of social support and more negative relationships (Benotsch et al, 1997; McCann et al, 1997). This lack of support can reduce a resource for dealing with stressors, an important component in the reserve capacity model that outlines the sources of resilience that promote coping with adversity (Gallo and Matthews, 2003).

Yet another part of the transactional model is based on the high likelihood that people will act in accordance with their expectations and emotions, leading to antagonistic behavior in hostile individuals. Of course, such actions are likely to elicit negative or antagonistic behavior from others, producing an environment that is more stressful from both objective and subjective perspectives.

The most convincing illustrations of the consequences of these transactional processes can be seen in studies that monitor the experiences of high and low hostile individuals during their daily lives. For example, Brissette and Cohen (2002) interviewed subjects on seven consecutive days about their experiences and interactions. Those with high hostility scores who had conflicts reported more negative affects and poorer sleep on those days. This is consistent with recent studies showing disturbed sleeping patterns among hostile individuals and those with high negative affect (Grano et al, 2008; Stoia-Caraballo et al, 2008). This is a particularly noteworthy set of findings in light of the importance of sleep for physical health.

Ambulatory blood pressure monitoring has been used by another set of investigators to assess differences in the daily experiences of high and low hostile individuals. This method samples the subject's blood pressure at frequent intervals during the day and gets a record of his/her activities and feelings at the time. Although there are some differences in the findings across studies, the general pattern is for high hostile persons to report more negative affect, especially during social interactions or potentially stressful encounters, and these subjective experiences were generally accompanied by elevated blood pressure readings (Benotsch et al, 1997; Brondolo et al, 2003; Guyll and Contrada, 1998; Jamner et al, 1991).

5 Physiological Links Between Social Stress and Disease Processes

A large body of evidence points to both biological and behavioral accompaniments of hostility that could account for increased disease risk. Beginning with biological studies, Suarez and colleagues (1998) found that while physiological functions did not differ in high and low hostile men while solving anagrams, when harassment was added to the experiment, high hostiles showed larger blood pressure, heart rate, and forearm blood flow responses during the task as well as slower recovery in blood levels of norepinephrine and cortisol. Sloan et al (1994) found decreased vagal tone as indexed by heart rate variability in younger men with high hostility levels. Using T-wave amplitude responses to isoproterenol, with and without atropine pretreatment, to index vagal antagonism of SNS effects on myocardial function, Fukudo et al (1992) found weaker vagal antagonism among high hostile Type A men. Markowitz (1998) and Shimbo and colleagues (2009) have observed increased platelet activation in both CHD patients and healthy persons.

Following an earlier study that found hostility associated with increased fasting glucose, insulin, and insulin resistance (HOMA) in a mixed sample (Surwit et al, 2002), it has recently been found that this association of hostility with fasting glucose and insulin resistance is present only in African American women (Georgiades et al, 2009). It now appears, moreover, that increased CNS serotonin function, as indexed by CSF levels of the tryptophan pathway metabolites 5OH-tryptophan (5HTP) and 5HIAA, is responsible for this association between hostility and fasting glucose and insulin resistance in African American women (Boyle et al, 2009).

6 Health Behaviors

There is also considerable evidence that hostility is associated with a broad range of risky health behaviors (Bunde and Suls, 2006). In a prospective study of over 4000 college graduates who had taken the MMPI as freshmen, Siegler and colleagues (1992) found that when followed up 25 years later, those with higher hostility at age 18 had higher lipid ratios, body mass index, smoking rates (and lower quit rates), and alcohol consumption as well as lower exercise rates. In a cross-sectional evaluation of hostility–risk factor associations in the CARDIA study, Scherwitz et al (1992) found high hostility associated with increased waist/hip ratio, caloric intake (600 more calories/day in high hostiles), smoking rates, marijuana use, and alcohol consumption.

Associations of smoking and alcohol use with hostility scores have been reported in a number of studies. These associations are present in adolescence (e.g., Pulkki et al, 2003) and in highly educated samples (e.g., Siegler et al, 1992) as well as the general population (Whiteman et al, 1997). These differences extend to usage patterns as well as the incidence and prevalence of these behaviors. For example, Boyle and colleagues (2008) found that hostility was not significantly associated with the frequency of alcohol drinking, but it was associated with heavy episodic drinking, a pattern that accounted for a good deal of the hostility's prediction of higher mortality. The effect of hostility applies not only

to the prevalence of these behaviors, but the ability to change these habits as well (Kahler et al, 2004). There may be a set of physiological underpinnings for these phenomena because it has been shown that physiological reactions to nicotine, alcohol, and their withdrawal differ according to hostility level (al' Absi et al, 2007; Fallon et al, 2004; Jamner et al, 1999; Zeichner et al, 1995).

7 Interventions

Ultimately, the reason we do research to identify psychosocial factors that predict increased disease risk, as well as the biobehavioral mechanisms responsible for the effects of the psychosocial factors on etiology and course of disease, is to guide translational research that will enable us to develop interventions that can prevent disease from developing in healthy persons and improve prognosis in those who already have disease. Most of the work on such interventions thus far has been conducted in clinical populations, in which any benefits on disease outcomes will be easier to demonstrate than would primary prevention effects in healthy samples.

To our knowledge the first such attempt to reduce hostility in a clinical sample was carried out by Gidron and colleagues (1999), using an adaptation of a behavioral intervention developed by Williams and Williams (1993). In a small sample of post-MI men with high hostility levels, those randomized to receive a hostility reduction workshop showed significantly larger decreases than those randomized to usual care in both self-report and observer ratings of hostility both at the end of training and at 2-months follow-up. Those in the active treatment arm also showed significantly larger decreases in depression and diastolic blood pressure at the end of training that became larger at 2-months follow-up. A follow-up study found that, despite the small sample size, those randomized to the hostility reduction group incurred significantly lower medical care costs over the ensuing 6 months than the usual care group. (Davidson et al, 2007).

Bishop et al (2005) conducted a randomized clinical trial in 58 male patients who had undergone coronary bypass surgery in which patients were randomized to either a six-session cognitive-behavioral stress-coping skills intervention using the Williams LifeSkills Workshop (Williams and Williams, 1998) or a 1-h lecture on stress and the heart with "tips" on how to manage stress better. It is important to note that there were no selection criteria for this study – all patients were eligible and asked to participate in a study to determine whether stress coping skills training (in short or long formats) helps patients do better after coronary bypass surgery. Compared to those receiving only the 1-h lecture on stress, the patients randomized to the LifeSkills workshop showed significantly larger improvements in trait anger, depression, satisfaction with social support, satisfaction with life, resting systolic blood pressure and heart rate, as well as systolic blood pressure and heart rate responses to an anger recall task. These improvements were present at the end of training and were even more pronounced at 3-months follow-up. In contrast to the improvements observed in the active treatment arm patients in this trial, those randomized to the placebo condition showed moderate deterioration in all measures at the end of the training period as well as at 3-months follow-up. Their scores on the CES-D depression scale rose from the subclinical range prior to randomization to levels that were in the clinical range (>16) at the end of the training period and at 3-months follow-up.

There are several aspects of this trial that are worth noting. First, not only did negative psychosocial factors like depression and trait anger improve with the training, but positive factors like satisfaction with social support and satisfaction with life also improved, suggesting that this form of stress-coping skills training has broad effects, that both reduce negative psychosocial factors and increase positive factors. In addition to the psychosocial improvements, there were also marked improvements in cardiovascular function, with patients in the active treatment arm showing a decrease in the systolic blood pressure response to anger recall from +26 mmHg prior to randomization to +16 mmHg at the end of training to +11 mmHg at 3-months follow-up.

It is worth emphasizing that there were no selection criteria for this trial. Patients were eligible to participate regardless of depression or trait anger or social support levels; and while the active treatment arm showed marked improvements at the end of training and 3-months follow-up, those patients randomized to the attention-placebo control condition showed further deterioration in all measures, with the mean depression score for the group being in the clinical range at follow-up. This suggests that rather than selecting – and potentially stigmatizing – patients for this sort of intervention on the basis of elevated hostility/anger, depression and/or social isolation levels, it may be better to train (rather than "treat") all patients in stress-coping skills, much the same as all CHD patients are seen as needing training in good nutrition and exercise habits.

The relevance of this point for clinical practice is highlighted by the results of the ENRICHD study – a large randomized clinical trial of cognitive behavior therapy for post-MI patients who met criteria for depression and/or social isolation. Despite high hopes that this ambitious trial of a behavioral intervention known to be effective in treating depression would be effective in also reducing the incidence of mortality and non-fatal MI over a 3-year follow-up period, there was no difference in the survival curves of the active treatment and usual care arms (Berkman et al, 2003). Post-hoc analyses in the (non-random) subset of 30% of the patients in the active treatment arm who were able to participate in a group-based coping skills workshop revealed that they did experience a reduction in mortality and non-fatal MI that was significant at the trend level even after control for all potential confounders, including the survival time required to make it into a group (Saab et al, 2009).

The evidence regarding stress-coping skills training to reduce hostility (and other psychosocial risk factors) and effects of such interventions on prognosis in CHD patients is clearly too limited at present to recommend such training for use in clinical settings. The evidence that is available does provide some encouragement, however, that properly conducted randomized trials of such training – perhaps in all CHD patients, rather than those selected because of depression or high hostility levels – have real potential to document improvements not only in a broad range of psychosocial factors and potential biological mechanisms (i.e., blood pressure at rest and in response to mental challenge) but also in morbidity and mortality in this high-risk patient population.

Acknowledgement This work was supported by National Heart, Lung, and Blood Institute grant P01HL36587 (RBW), Clinical Research Unit grant M01RR30, RO1 HL54780 and the Duke University Behavioral Medicine Research Center.

References

Adams, S. H. (1994). The role of hostility in women's health during midlife: a longitudinal study. *Health Psychol, 13*, 488–495.

Allred, K. D., and Smith, T. W. (1991). Social cognition in cynical hostility. *Cog Ther Res, 15*, 399–412.

al' Absi, M., Carr, S. B., and Bongard, S. (2007). Anger and psychobiological changes during smoking abstinence and in response to acute stress: prediction of smoking relapse. *Int J Psychophys, 66*, 109–115.

Angerer, P., Siebert, U., Kothny, W., Muhlbauer, D., Mudra, H. et al (2000). Impact of social support, cynical hostility and anger expression on progression of coronary atherosclerosis. *J Am Coll Card 36*, 1781–1788.

Arinami, T., Ohtsuki, T., Yamakawa-Kobayashi, J. R., Amemiya, H., Fujiwara, H. et al (1999). A synergistic effect of serotonin transporter gene polymorphism and smoking in association with CHD. *Thromb Haemost, 81*, 853–856.

Barefoot, J. C., Beckham, J. C., Peterson, B. L., Haney, T. L., and Williams, R. B. (1992). Measures of neuroticism and disease status in coronary angiography patients. *J Consult Clin Psycho, 60*, 127–132.

Barefoot, J. C., Beckham, J. C., Haney, T. L., Siegler, I. C., and Lipkus, I. M. (1993). Age differences in hostility among middle-aged and older adults. *Psych Aging, 8*, 3–9.

Barefoot, J. C., Brummett, B. H., Clapp-Channing, N., Williams, R. B., Siegler, I. C. et al (2008). Recovery expectations of cardiac patients as predictors of survival. *APS Meeting Abstract 2008, 70, Number 3, A-117.*

Barefoot, J. C., Larsen, S., von der Lieth, L., and Schroll, M. (1995). Hostility, incidence of acute myocardial infarction, and mortality in a sample of older Danish men and women. *Am J Epid, 142*, 477–484.

Barefoot, J. C., and Lipkus, I. M. (1994). Assessment of anger-hostility. In A. W. Siegman & T. W. Smith (Eds.), *Anger, Hostility and the Heart.* Hillside, NJ: Lawrence Erlbaum.

Barefoot, J. C., Peterson, B. L., Dahlstrom, W. G., Siegler, I. C., Anderson, N. B. et al (1991). Hostility patterns and health implications: correlates of Cook-Medley scores in a national survey. *Health Psych, 10*, 18–24.

Beckham, J. C., Roodman, A. A., Barefoot, J. C., Haney, T. L., Helms, M. J. et al (1996). Interpersonal and self-reported hostility among combat veterans with and without Posttraumatic Stress Disorder. *J Traumatic Stress, 9*, 335–340.

Benotsch, E. G., Christensen, A. J., and McKelvey, L. (1997). Hostility, social support, and ambulatory cardiovascular activity. *J Behav Med, 20*, 163–176.

Bishop, G. D., Kaur, D. J., Tan, V. L. M., Chua, Y. L., Liew, S. M. et al (2005). Effect of a psychosocial skills training workshop on psychophysiological and psychosocial risk in patients undergoing coronary artery bypass grafting. *Am Heart J, 150*, 602–609.

Bishop, G. D., and Robinson, G. (2000). Anger, harassment, and cardiovascular reactivity among Chinese and Indian men in Singapore. *Psychosom Med, 62*, 684–692.

Boyle, S. H., Mortensen, L., Grønbæk, M., and Barefoot, J. C. (2007). Hostility, drinking pattern, and mortality. *Addiction, 163*, 54–59.

Boyle, S. H., Williams, R. B., Mark, D. B., Brummett, B. H., Siegler, I. C., and Barefoot, J. C. (2004). Hostility as a predictor of survival in patients with coronary artery disease. *Psychosom Med, 66*, 629–632.

Boyle, S. H., Williams, R. B., Mark, D. B., Brummett, B. H., Siegler, I. C. et al (2005). Hostility, age, and mortality in a sample of cardiac patients. *Am J Card, 96*, 64–66.

Boyle, S. H., Wang, L., Surwit, R. S., Zeng, Z., Holden, W. et al (2009). Central nervous system serotonin, hostility and glucose metabolism in African American women. *APS Meeting Abstract 2009, 71, Number 3, A-26.*

Brissette, I., and Cohen, S. (2002). The contribution of individual differences in hostility to the associations between daily interpersonal conflict, affect, and sleep. *Pers Soc Psychol Bull 28*, 1265–1274.

Brondolo, E., Rieppi, R., Erickson, S. A., Bagiella, E., Shapiro, P. A. et al (2003). Hostility, interpersonal interactions, and ambulatory blood pressure. *Psychosom Med, 65*, 1003–1011.

Brummett, B. H., Boyle, S. H., Siegler, I. C., Kuhn, C. M., Ashley-Koch, A. et al (2008a). Effects of environmental stress and gender on associations among symptoms of depression and the serotonin transporter gene linked polymorphic region (5-HTTLPR). *Behav Genet 38*, 34–43.

Brummett, B. H., Muller, C. L., Collins, A. L., Boyle, S. H., Kuhn, C. M. et al (2008b). 5-HTTLPR and gender moderate changes in negative affect responses to tryptophan infusion. *Behav Genet, 38*, 476–483.

Bunde, J., and Suls, J. (2006). A quantitative analysis of the relationship between the Cook-Medley Hostility Scale and traditional coronary artery disease risk factors. *Health Psychol, 25*, 493–500.

Burg, M. M., Graeber, B., Vashist, A., Collins, A., Earley, C. et al (2009). Noninvasive detection of risk for emotion provoked myocardial ischemia. *Psychosom Med, 71*, 14–21.

Buss, A. H., and Durkee, A. (1957). An inventory for assessing different kinds of hostility. *J Consult Psychol, 21*, 343–349.

Butler, E. A., Lee, T. L., and Gross, J. J. (2007). Emotion regulation and culture: are the social consequences of emotion suppression culture specific? *Emotion, 7*, 30–48.

Caspi, A., McClay, J., Moffitt, T. E., Mill, J., Martin, J. et al (2002). Role of genotype in the cycle of violence in maltreated children. *Science, 297*, 851–854.

Chaput, L. A., Adams, S. H., Simon, J. A., Blumenthal, R. S., and Vittinghoff, E. et al (2002). Hostility predicts recurrent events among postmenopausal women with coronary heart disease. *Am J Epid, 156*, 1092–1099.

Chida, Y., and Steptoe, A. (2009). The association of anger and hostility with future coronary heart disease: a meta-analytic review of prospective evidence. *J Am Coll Card, 53*, 936–946.

Christakis, N. A., and Fowler, J. H. (2008). The collective dynamics of smoking in a large social network. *NEJM, 358*, 2249–2258.

Cook, W. W., and Medley, D. M. (1954). Proposed hostility and pharisaic virtue scales for the MMPI. *J Applied Psychol, 38*: 414–418.

Coto, E., Reguero, J. R., Alvarez, V., Morales, B., Batalia, A. et al (2003). 5-Hytroxytrptamine 5-HT_{2A} receptor and 5-hydroxytryptamine transporter polymorphisms in acute myocardial infarction. *Clin Sci, 104*, 241–245.

Denollet, J., and Brutsaert, D. L. (1998). Personality, disease severity, and the risk of long-term cardiac events in patients with a decreased ejection fraction after myocardial infarction. *Circulation, 97*, 167–173.

Dodge, K. A. (2006). Translational science in action: hostile attributional style and the development of aggressive behavior problems. *Devel Psychopathol, 18*, 791–814.

Davidson, K. W., Gidron, Y., Mostofsky, E. et al (2007). Hospitalization cost offset of a hostility intervention for coronary heart disease patients. *J Consult Clin Psychol, 75*, 657–672.

Enkleman, H. C., Bishop, G. D., Tong, E. M. W., Diong, S. M., Why, Y. P. et al (2005). The relationship of hostility, negative affect, and ethnicity to cardiovascular responses: an ambulatory study in Singapore. *Int J Psychophys, 56*, 185–197.

Berkman, L. F., Blumenthal, J., Burg, M., Carney, R. M., Catellier, D. et al (2003). Effects of treating depression and low perceived social support on clinical events after myocardial infarction: the Enhancing Recovery in Coronary Heart Disease Patients (ENRICHD) Randomized Trial. *JAMA, 289*, 3106–3116.

Everson-Rose, S. A., and Lewis, T. T. (2005). Psychosocial factors and cardiovascular disease. *Ann Rev Pub Health, 26*, 469–500.

Everson-Rose, S. A., Lewis, T. T., Karavolos, K., Matthews, K. A., and Sutton-Tyrrell, K. (2006). Cynical hostility and carotid atherosclerosis in African American and white women: The Study of Women's Health Across the Nation (SWAN) Heart Study. *Am Heart J, 152*, 982.e7–13.

Fallon, J. H., Keator, D. B., Mbogori, J., Turner, J., and Potkin, S. G. (2004). Hostility differentiates the brain metabolic effects of nicotine. *Cog Brain Res, 18*, 142–148.

Fowler, J. H., and Christakis, N. A. (2008). Dynamic spread of happiness in a large social network: longitudinal analysis over 20 years in the Framingham Heart Study. *BMJ, 337*, a2338.

Frasure-Smith, N., and Lesperance, F. (2003). Depression and other psychological risks following myocardial infarction. *Arch Gen Psychiatry, 60*, 627–636.

Fukudo, S., Lane, J. D., Anderson, N. B., Kuhn, C. M., Schanberg, S. M. et al (1992). Accentuated vagal antagonism of beta-adrenergic effects on ventricular repolarization: differential responses between Type A and Type B men. *Circulation, 85*, 2045–2053.

Fumeron, F., Betoulle, D., Nicaud, V., Evans, A., Kee, F. et al (2002). Serotonin transporter gene polymorphism and myocardial infarction. *Circulation, 105*, 2943–2945.

Gallo, L. C., and Matthews, K. A. (2003). Understanding the association between socioeconomic status and health: do negative emotions play a role? *Psych Bull, 129*, 10–51.

Georgiades, A., Lane, J. D., Boyle, S. H., Brummett, B. H., Barefoot, J. C. et al (2009). Hostility and fasting glucose in African American women. *Psychosom Med, 71*, 642–645.

Gidron, Y., Davidson, K., and Bata, I. (1999). The short-term effects of a hostility-reduction intervention in CHD patients. *Health Psychol, 18*, 416–420.

Graham, J. E., Robles, T. F., Kiecolt-Glaser, J. K., Malarkey, W. B., Bissell, M. G. et al (2006). Hostility and pain are related to inflammation in older adults. *Brain Behav Immun, 20*, 389–400.

Grano, N., Vahtera, J., Virtanen, M., Keltikangas-Jarvinen, L., and Kivimaki, M. (2008). Association of hostility with sleep duration and sleep disturbances in an employee population. *Int J Behav Med, 15*, 73–80.

Guyll, M., and Contrada, R. (1998). Trait hostility and ambulatory cardiovascular activity: responses to social interaction. *Health Psychol, 17*, 30–39.

Haukkala, A. (2002). Socio-economic differences in hostility measures – a population based study. *Psychol Health, 17*, 191–202.

Iribarren, C., Sidney, S., Bild, D. E., Liu, K., Markowitz, J. H. et al (2000). Association of hostility with coronary artery calcification in young adults: The CARDIA Coronary Artery Risk Development in Young Adults study. *JAMA, 283*, 2546–2551.

Jakupcak, M., Conybeare, D., Phelps, L., Hunt, S., Holmes, H. A. et al (2007). Anger, hostility, and aggression among Iraq and Afghanistan War veterans reporting PTSD and subthreshold PTSD. *J Traum Stress, 20*, 945–954.

Jamner, L. D., Shapiro, D., Goldstein, I. B., and Hug, R. (1991). Ambulatory blood pressure and heart rate in paramedics: effects of cynical hostility and defensiveness. *Psychosom Med, 53*, 393–406.

Jamner, L. D., Shapiro, D., and Jarvik, M. E. (1999). Nicotine reduces the frequency of anger reports in smokers and nonsmokers with high but not low hostility: an ambulatory study. *Exp Clin Psychopharm, 7*, 454–463.

John, O. P., and Gross, J. J. (2004). Healthy and unhealthy emotional regulation: personality processes, individual differences, and life span development. *J Personality, 72*, 1301–1333.

Julkunen, J., Salonen, R., Kaplan, G. A., Chesney, M. A., and Salonen, J. T. (1994). Hostility and the progression of carotid atherosclerosis. *Psychosom Med, 56*, 519–525.

Kahler, C. W., Strong, D. R., Niaura, R., and Brown, R. A. (2004). Hostility in smokers with past major depressive disorder: relation to smoking patterns, reasons for quitting, and cessation outcomes. *Nicot Tobac Res, 6*, 809–818.

Kaplan, J. R., Manuck, S. B., Fontenot, M. B. et al (2002). Central nervous system monoamine correlates of social dominance in cynomolgus monkeys (Macaca fascicularis). *Neuropsychopharmacology, 26*, 431–443.

Kawachi, I., and Berkman, L. (2000). Social cohesion, social capital, and health. In L. F. Berkman & I. Kawachi (Eds.), *Social Epidemiology*. New York: Oxford University Press.

Kiecolt-Glaser, J. K., Loving, T. J., Stowell, J. R., Malarkey, W. B., Lemeshow, S. et al (2005). Hostile marital interactions, proinflammatory cytokine production, and wound healing. *Arch Gen Psychiatry, 62*, 1377–1384.

Kivimaki, M., Vahtera, J., Koskenvuo, M., Uutela, A., and Pentti, J. (1998). Response of hostile individuals to stressful changes in their working lives: test of a psychosocial vulnerability model. *Psychol Med, 28*, 903–913.

Knox, S. S., Weidner, G., Adelman, A., Stoney, C. M., and Ellison, R. C. (2004). Hostility and physiological risk in the National Heart, Lung, and Blood Institute Family Heart Study. *Arch Int Med, 164*, 2442–2448.

Kopp, M., Skrabski, A., Szántó, Z., and Siegrist, J. (2006). Psychosocial determinants of premature cardiovascular mortality differences within Hungary. *J Epid Commun Health, 60*, 782–788.

Kubzansky, L. D., Sparrow, D., Jackson, B., Cohen, S., Weiss, S. T. et al (2006). Angry breathing: a prospective study of hostility and lung function in the Normative Aging Study. *Thorax, 61*, 833–834.

Larkin, K. T., Martin, R. R., and McClain, S. E. (2002). Cynical hostility and the accuracy of decoding facial expressions of emotions. *J Behav Med, 25*, 286–292.

Lesch, K. P., Bengel, D., Heils, A., Sbol, S. Z., Greenberg, B. P. et al (1996). Association of anxiety-related traits with a polymorphism in the serotonin transporter gene regulatory region. *Science, 274*, 1527–1531.

Luecken, L. J. (2000). Attachment and loss experiences during childhood are associated with adult hostility, depression, and social support. *J Psychosom Res, 49*, 85–91.

Manuck, S. B., Flory, J. D., Ferrell, R. E., Mann, J., and Muldoon, M. F. (2000). A regulatory polymorphism of the monoamine oxidase-A gene may be associated with variability in aggression, impulsivity, and central nervous system serotonergic responsivity. *Psychiat Res, 95*, 9–23.

Manuck, S. B., Flory, J. D., McCaffery, J. M., Matthews, K. A., Mann, J. J. et al (1998). Aggression, impulsivity, and central nervous system serotonergic responsivity in a nonpatient sample. *Neuropsychopharmacology, 19*, 287–299.

Manuck, S. B., Flory, J. D., Muldoon, M. F., and Ferrell, R. E. (2002). Central nervous system serotonergic responsivity and aggressive disposition in men. *Physiol Behav, 77*, 705–709.

Markowitz, J. H. (1998). Hostility is associated with increased platelet activation in coronary heart disease. *Psychosom Med, 60*, 586–591.

Martin, R., Watson, D., and Wan, C. (2000). A three-factor model of trait anger: dimensions of affect, behavior, and cognition. *J Personality, 68*, 869–897.

Matthews, K. A., Gump, B. B., Harris, K. F., Haney, T. L., and Barefoot, J. C. (2004). Hostile behaviors predict cardiovascular mortality among men enrolled in the Multiple Risk Factor Intervention Trial. *Circulation, 109*, 66–70.

Matthews, K. A., Woodall, K. L., Kenyon, K., and Jacob, T. (1996). Negative family environment as a predictor of boys' future status on measures of hostile attitudes, interview behavior, and anger expression. *Health Psych, 15*, 30–37.

McCann, B. S., Russo, J., Benjamin, G., and Andrew, H. (1997). Hostility, social support, and perceptions of work. *J Occup Health Psychol, 2*, 175–185.

Mechanic, D. (1972). Social psychologic factors affecting the presentation of bodily complaints *New Eng J Med, 286*, 1132–1139.

Mittleman, M. A., Maclure, M., Sherwood, J. B., Mulry, R. P., Tofler, G. H. et al (1995). Triggering of acute myocardial infarction onset by episodes of anger. Determinants of Myocardial Infarction Onset Study Investigators. *Circulation, 9*, 1720–1725.

Moffitt, T. E., Caspi, A., and Rutter, M. (2005). Strategy for investigating interactions between measured genes and measured environments. *Arch Gen Psychiatry, 62*, 473–481.

Muldoon, M. F., Mackey, R. H., Korytkowski, M. T., Flory, J. D., Pollock, B. G. et al (2006). The metabolic syndrome is associated with reduced central serotonergic responsivity in healthy community volunteers. *J Clin Endocrinol Metab, 91*, 718–721.

Muldoon, M. F., Mackey, R. H., Sutton-Tyrrell, K., Flory, J. D., Pollock, B. G. et al (2007). Lower central serotonergic responsivity is associated with preclinical carotid artery atherosclerosis. *Stroke, 38*, 2228–2233.

Möller, J., Hallqvist, J., Diderichsen, F., Theorell, T., Reuterwall, C. et al (1999). Do episodes of anger trigger myocardial infarction? A case-crossover analysis in the Stockholm Heart Epidemiology Program (SHEEP). *Psychosom Med, 61*, 842–849.

Niaura, R., Todaro, J. F., Stroud, L., Spiro, A., III, Ward, K. D. et al (2002). Hostility, the metabolic syndrome, and incident coronary heart disease. *Health Psychol, 21*, 588–593.

Orth, U., and Wieland, E. (2006). Anger, hostility, and posttraumatic stress disorder in trauma-exposed adults: a meta-analysis. *J Consult Clin Psych, 74*: 698–706.

Pulkki, L,. Kivimaki, M., Elovainio, M., Viikari, J., and Keltikangas-Jarvinen, L. (2003). Contribution of socioeconomic status to the association between hostility and cardiovascular risk behaviors: a prospective cohort study. *Am J Epid, 158*, 736–742.

Raynor, D. A., Pogue-Geile, M. F., Kamarck, T. W., McCaffery, J. M., and Manuck, S. B. (2002). Covariation of psychosocial characteristics associated with cardiovascular disease. *Psychosom Med, 64*, 191–203.

Saab, P. G., Bang, H., Williams, R. B., Powell, L. H., Schneiderman, N. et al (2009). The impact of cognitive behavioral group training on event-free survival in patients with myocardial infarction: the ENRICHD experience. *J Psychosom Res, 67*, 45–56.

Scheier, M. F., Matthews, K. A., Owens, J. F., Schultz, R., Bridges, M. W. et al (1999). Optimism and rehospitalization after coronary artery bypass surgery. *Arch Intern Med, 159*, 829–835.

Scherwitz, L. W., Perkins, L. L., Chesney, M. A., Hughes, G. H., Sidney, S. et al (1992). Hostility and health

behaviors in young adults: The CARDIA study. *Am J Epidemiol, 136*, 136–145.

Shimbo, D., Chaplin, W., Kuruvilla, S., Wasson, L. T., Abraham, D. et al (2009). Hostility and platelet reactivity in individuals without a history of cardiovascular disease events. *Psychosom Med, 71*, 741–747.

Siegler, I. C., Peterson, B. L., Barefoot, J. C., and Williams, R. B. (1992). Hostility during late adolescence predicts coronary risk factors at mid-life. *Am J Epidemiol, 136*, 146–154.

Siegler, I. C., Helms, M. J., Kuhn, C. M., Surwit, R. S., James, S. A. et al (2008). Personality associations of high brain serotonin in men. *APS Meeting Abstract 2008, 70, Number 3, A79.*

Simons, R. L., Simons, L. G., Burt, C. H., Drummund, H., Stewart, E. et al (2006). Supportive parenting moderates the effect of discrimination upon anger, hostile view of relationships, and violence among African American boys. *J Health Soc Behav, 47*, 373–389.

Sloan, R. P., Shapiro, P. A., Bigger, J. T., Bagiella, E., Steinman, R. C. et al (1994). Cardiac autonomic control and hostility in healthy subjects. *Am J Cardiol, 74*, 298–300.

Smith, T. W., Glazer, K., Ruiz, J. M., and Gallo, L. C. (2004). Hostility, anger, aggressiveness, and coronary heart disease: an interpersonal perspective on personality, emotion, and health. *J Personality, 72*, 1217–1270.

Spielberger, C. D., Jacobs, G., Russell, S. F., and Crane, R. J. (1983). Assessment of anger: The State-Trait Anger Scale. In J. N. Butcher & C. D. Spielberger (Eds.), *Advances in personality assessment, vol 2*. Hillsdale, NJ: Lawrence Erlbaum.

Stewart, J. C., Janicki, D. L., Muldoon, M. F., Sutton-Tyrrell, K., and Kamarck, T. W. (2007). Negative emotions and 3-year progression of subclinical atherosclerosis. *Arch Gen Psychiat, 64*, 225–233.

Stoia-Caraballo, R., Rye, M. S., Pan, W., Brown-Kirschman, K. J., Lutz-Zois, C. et al (2008). Negative affect and anger rumination as mediators between forgiveness and sleep quality. *J Behav Med, 31*, 478–488.

Stoney, C. M., and Engebretson, T. O. (1994). Anger and hostility: Potential mediators of the gender difference in cardiovascular disease. In A. W. Siegman & T. W. Smith (Eds.), *Anger, hostility and the heart* (pp. 215–238). Hillsdale, NJ: Erlbaum.

Strike, P. C., Perkins-Porras, L., Whitehead, D. L., McEwan, J., and Steptoe, A. (2006). Triggering of acute coronary syndromes by physical exertion and anger: clinical and sociodemographic characteristics. *Heart, 92*, 1035–1040.

Strike, P. C., and Steptoe, A. (2005). Behavioral and emotional triggers of acute coronary syndromes: a systematic review and critique. *Psychosom Med, 67*, 179–186.

Suarez, E. C., Kuhn, C. M., Schanberg, S. M., Williams, R. B., and Zimmerman, E. A. (1998).

Neuroendocrine, cardiovascular, and emotional responses of hostile men: the role of interpersonal challenge. *Psychosom Med, 60,* 78–88.

Suls, J., and Bunde, J. (2005). Anger, anxiety, and depression as risk factors for cardiovascular disease: the problems and implications of overlapping affective dispositions. *Psych Bull, 131,* 260–300.

Surwit, R. S., Williams, R. B., Siegler, I. C., Lane, J. D., Helms, M. J. et al (2002). Hostility, race, and glucose metabolism in non-diabetic individuals. *Diabetes Care, 25,* 835–839.

Tindle, H. A., Chang, Y. F., Kuller, L. H., Manson, J. E., Robinson, J. G. et al (2009). Optimism, cynical hostility, and incident coronary heart disease and mortality in the Women's Health Initiative. *Circulation, 20,* 656–662.

Whiteman, M. C., Fowkes, F. G., Deary, I. J., and Lee, A. J. (1997). Hostility, cigarette smoking and alcohol consumption in the general population. *Soc Sci Med, 44,* 1089–1096.

Williams, J. E., Nieto, F. J., Sanford, C. P., and Tyroler, H. A. (2001). Effects of an angry temperament of coronary heart disease risk. *Am J Epidemiol, 154,* 230–235.

Williams, J. E., Nieto, F. J., Sanford, C. P., Couper, D. J., and Tyroler, H. A. (2002). The association between trait anger and incident stroke risk: the Atherosclerosis Risk in Communities (ARIC) Study. *Stroke, 33:* 13–19.

Williams, R. B. (2000). Psychological factors, health, and disease: the impact of aging and the life cycle. In: S. B. Manuck, R. Jennings, B. S. Rabin, & A. Baum (Eds.), *Behavior, Health, and Aging.* Hillsdale, NJ: Lawrence Erlbaum Associates.

Williams, R. B. (1994). Neurobiology, cellular and molecular biology, and psychosomatic medicine. *Psychosom Med, 56,* 308–315.

Williams, R. B., and Barefoot, J. C. (1988). Coronary-prone behavior: the emerging role of the hostility complex. In B. K. Houston, & C. R. Snyder (Eds.), *Type A Behavior Pattern: Research, Theory, and Intervention.* New York: Wiley.

Williams, R. B., Barefoot, J. C., and Schneiderman, N. (2003a). Psychosocial risk factors for cardiovascular disease: more than one culprit at work. *JAMA, 290,* 2190–2192.

Williams, R. B., Marchuk, D. A., Gadde, K. M., Barefoot, J. C., Grichnik, K. et al (2003b). Serotonin-Related gene polymorphisms and central nervous system serotonin function. *Neuropsychopharmacology, 28,* 533–541.

Williams, R. B., Marchuk, D. A., Siegler, I. C., Barefoot, J. C., Helms, M. J. et al (2008). Childhood socioeconomic status and serotonin transporter gene polymorphism enhance cardiovascular reactivity to mental stress. *Psychosom Med, 70,* 32–39.

Williams, R. B., and Williams, V. P. (1993). *Anger Kills: Seventeen Strategies for Controlling the Hostility That Can Harm Your Health.* New York: Times Books. Trade paperback edition published by Harper-Collins, Spring, 1994.

Williams, V. P., and Williams, R. B. (1998). *LifeSkills: 8 Simple Ways to Build Stronger Relationships, Communicate More Clearly, Improve Your Health, and Even the Health of Those Around You.* New York: Times Books/Random House.

Williams, V. P., Brenner, S. L., Helms, M. J., and Williams, R. B. (2009). Coping skills training to reduce psychosocial risk factors for medical disorders: a field trial evaluating effectiveness in multiple worksites. *J Occup Health, 51,* 437–442.

Yan, L. L., Liu, K., Matthews, K. A., Daviglus, M. L., Ferguson, T. F. et al (2003). Psychosocial factors and risk of hypertension: The Coronary Artery Disease Risk Development in Young Adults (CARDIA) study. *JAMA, 290,* 2138–2148.

Zeichner, A., Giancola, P. R., and Allen, J. D. (1995). Effects of hostility on alcohol stress-response-dampening. *Alcoholism: Clin Exper Res, 19,* 977–983.

Chapter 14

Positive Well-Being and Health

Andrew Steptoe

1 Introduction

Positive well-being can be defined as optimal psychological experience and functioning. It has an important relationship with health. Illness often leads to reduced well-being and to unhappiness, while there is mounting evidence that positive well-being has health-protective effects and may even foster longevity. This chapter outlines the nature and determinants of psychological well-being, its relationship with health and the central nervous system, other physiological and behavioral pathways through which well-being may influence health status.

1.1 The Nature of Positive Well-Being

There are two broad perspectives on positive well-being that have been delineated in the research literature over the past 20 years. The first focuses on subjective well-being or the experience of high positive affect, low negative affect, and satisfaction with life (Diener, 1984). This affective experience has also been described as happiness, hedonic well-being, pleasure, and enjoyment of life. The second construct has come to be called eudaimonic well-being, and

emphasizes the actualization of human potential and the sense of meaning and fulfillment in life, determined by perceptions of autonomy, and the ability to determine one's own path in life (Ryan and Deci, 2001). This latter concept derives from the humanistic psychological tradition and has been characterized by Ryff as comprising of six dimensions, namely feeling of self-acceptance, personal growth, relationships with others, autonomy, environmental mastery, and purpose in life (Ryff and Keyes, 1995). A third concept derives from the international development and economic literature, and defines well-being through the possession of capabilities or freedoms such as bodily integrity, affiliation, and control over the environment (Nussbaum and Sen, 1993); this has had less impact in the behavioral medicine and psychological literature, though it has been highly influential in government and policy circles.

There has been considerable debate about the importance of these differences in the concept of positive well-being, and the extent to which they reflect coherent measurable entities or relate differentially to other life outcomes such as health and success in relationships (Kashdan et al, 2008). From the perspective of research in health, perhaps the most important issue is whether the current interest in positive well-being reflects a meaningful agenda for investigation, or is a passing fashion. It is well established in psychiatry and behavioral medicine that negative psychological states such as depression, anxiety, and hostility are associated with adverse effects on physical health (see Chapters 12 and 13). If positive psychological states and traits are

A. Steptoe (✉)
Department of Epidemiology and Public Health,
University College London, 1-19 Torrington Place,
London WC1E 6BT, UK
e-mail: a.steptoe@ucl.ac.uk

A. Steptoe (ed.), *Handbook of Behavioral Medicine*, DOI 10.1007/978-0-387-09488-5_14,
© Springer Science+Business Media, LLC 2010

nothing more than the absence of emotional distress, research in this field is likely to have little substantive to contribute. This chapter will argue that the impact of positive well-being on health, biology, and behavior is in part independent of negative affect, suggesting that it does make an important independent contribution.

1.2 The Determinants of Positive Well-Being

Positive well-being has multiple determinants at the individual, social, and ecological levels, and these have been extensively studied by a variety of social scientists ranging from personality psychologists to economists (Diener et al, 1999; Dolan et al, 2008). There is good evidence that positive affect is moderately heritable (Lykken and Tellegen, 1996), and this association may be mediated through temperamental dispositions such as high extraversion, low neuroticism, and optimism. Positive well-being is strongly related to satisfying social relationships and social engagement, though the causal sequence can be difficult to disentangle (Lyubomirsky et al, 2005). The issues of causation and reverse causation also bedevil analyses of the relationship between positive well-being and income or wealth. There is evidence, on one hand, that changes in income stimulate changes in well-being and, on the other hand, that high positive well-being predicts future increases in income and wealth. It would appear in developed countries that relative income is more influential on well-being than absolute income (Clark et al, 2008). Across the population, positive well-being tends to be greater in younger and older people, with the lowest levels in the middle years of adult life (Dolan et al, 2008). The experience of stressful life events leads to a deterioration in well-being, while positive events have the reverse effect, but there is controversy over the extent which longer-term adaptation takes place (Diener et al, 2006). Happiness appears to be transmitted through social networks (Fowler and Christakis, 2008),

while interpersonal interactions such as generosity and giving also promote positive affect (Dunn et al, 2008). Many of the diverse findings in the literature are a result of differences in measurement, including whether the measure is immediate (e.g. "how do you feel right now?") or reflective (e.g. "if you were to consider your life in general these days, how happy or unhappy would you say you are?"). Studies in which psychological states are measured repeatedly over time using ecological momentary assessment (EMA) or the day reconstruction method may generate different results from those that involve questionnaires that require integration of subjective states over days or weeks (Kahneman and Krueger, 2006).

2 Positive Well-Being and Health-Protective Characteristics

One of the difficulties in evaluating the contribution of positive well-being to health is that it does not occur in isolation, but tends to be associated with a range of other psychosocial characteristics that may themselves have health benefits. This is illustrated in Table 14.1 with data from around 700 men and women aged 60.7 years on average, who were members of the Whitehall II epidemiological cohort (see Steptoe et al, 2008b for further details). Positive affect was assessed using EMA ratings of happiness obtained four times over a single day, while eudaimonic well-being was associated with the autonomy, self-realization, and control scales from the CASP-19 questionnaire (Hyde et al, 2003). The table summarizes the associations between these two dimensions of positive well-being and a series of psychosocial factors relevant to health. All analyses were adjusted for age, gender, socioeconomic status, employment status, and self-rated health. It can be seen that both positive affect and eudaimonic well-being were associated with protective psychosocial factors (number of friends, low social isolation, emotional and practical support), and with psychological factors that may reflect more effective

Table 14.1 Psychosocial correlates of positive well-being

	Positive affect		Eudaimonic well-being	
	Standardized β (S.E.)	P	Standardized β (S.E.)	P
Social factors				
Number of close friends	0.095(0.037)	0.01	0.165(0.035)	0.001
Social isolation	−0.144(0.037)	0.001	−0.188(0.035)	0.001
Emotional support	0.172(0.030)	0.001	0.219(0.034)	0.001
Practical support	0.121(0.037)	0.001	0.140(0.035)	0.001
Psychological factors				
Optimism	0.217(0.043)	0.001	0.436(0.038)	0.001
Coping by problem engagement	0.084(0.042)	0.048	0.179(0.040)	0.001
Coping by eliciting social support	0.108(0.042)	0.01	0.209(0.039)	0.001
Avoidant coping	0.001(0.042)	0.99	−0.156(0.040)	0.001

Regression coefficients adjusted for age, gender, socioeconomic status, employment status, and self-rated health. $N = 690$–702 for different analyses. Based on Steptoe et al (2008b)

adaptation including optimism and actively oriented coping. Other research indicates that psychological well-being is associated with trust and social capital (Helliwell and Putnam, 2004), and with good marital relationships and high self-esteem (Lyubomirsky et al, 2005).

In many ways, these associations are not surprising. Positive affect serves to engage and attract other people, so may bolster social resources. Ong et al (2009) have argued that the effects of resilience are also mediated through positive affect, and that positive emotions lead to a broadening of activities, helping to build enduring physical, intellectual, and social resources, and to enhance cognitive flexibility. Similarly, in the broaden-and-build theory, Fredrickson (2004) has argued that positive emotions broaden repertoires of thought and action that in turn increase wider functional resources, improving the chances of effective coping. However, it is also the case that many of these psychosocial factors such as coping and social support have been independently related to health outcomes in other research (see Chapters 15, 17 and 18), so defining a distinct role for positive well-being requires care.

3 Positive Well-Being and Physical Health

The research literature relating positive well-being with physical health is growing

(Pressman and Cohen, 2005; Veenhoven, 2008). Theoretically, the strongest research design for establishing causality is the experimental study, in which participants are assigned at random to different levels of positive well-being and tracked for health outcomes. Although several controlled positive psychological intervention studies have now been conducted, the emphasis to date has been on subjective well-being and the alleviation of depression rather than on physical health and biological outcomes (Sin and Lyubomirsky, 2009).

One of the stronger population-based research designs for studying predictors of the development of physical illness is the prospective epidemiological cohort study. This involves recruiting a sample of initially healthy individuals, assessing positive well-being (along with traditional risk factors for disease), then tracking the cohort over several years. The relationship between positive psychological factors and future illness can then be investigated. It is essential in such a study to have as complete a follow-up of participants as possible, since loss to follow-up may distort the results. It is also important to assess potential confounders. This has been a limitation in some studies of positive well-being. For example, Danner and coworkers (2001) published a well-known study of elderly Catholic nuns, showing that those whose writings in early life contained high levels of positive emotional content had a reduced risk of mortality when the participants were aged over 75 years.

Interesting though this association is, it supplies weak evidence for a protective role for positive emotions; no health assessments were performed at baseline, so it is possible that the nuns whose writings had less positive content had clinical or subclinical health problems before the writing task was carried out; only women who survived to age 75 were included, so it is conceivable that a different association between well-being and survival was present earlier in life; and apart from age and education, no other factors that might potentially influence either positive emotion or future mortality were controlled.

Fortunately, other studies provide stronger evidence. A good example is Kubzansky and Thurston's (2007) study of emotional vitality and coronary heart disease (CHD). A cohort of 6025 men and women aged 25–75 years who were initially free of CHD were followed for an average of 15 years, during which time 1141 developed CHD. Emotional vitality, a combination of vitality (sense of energy and pep), positive well-being (happiness and life satisfaction), and emotional self-control (feeling emotionally stable and secure), was assessed at baseline. Participants with greater emotional vitality were at markedly reduced risk for CHD, and this effect remained significant after accounting statistically for age, gender, ethnicity, marital status, educational attainment, blood pressure, cholesterol, body mass index (BMI), smoking, alcohol use, physical activity level, diabetes, hypertension, and psychological illness. All three components of emotional vitality appeared to contribute to the health outcomes in this study. In the model adjusting for risk factors, the relative risk of CHD in the highest compared with lowest tertile of emotional vitality was 0.74 (95% confidence intervals 0.64–0.85), indicating a 26% reduction in relative risk.

These effects are not only observed in Western populations. An analysis was conducted of 88,175 Japanese men and women aged 40–69 years at baseline who were followed up for an average of 12 years (Shirai et al, 2009). A simple rating of enjoyment of life that correlates well with more elaborate measures of happiness was administered. Over the follow-up period, 3523 had newly diagnosed cardiovascular disease, and there were 1860 fatalities. Low enjoyment of life was associated with increased risk of cardiovascular disease incidence (hazard ratio 1.23, C.I. 1.05–1.44) and mortality (1.61, C.I. 1.32–1.96) in men, after adjustment for age, occupation, BMI, smoking, physical activity, alcohol consumption, diabetes, hypertension, and participation in health screening. Interestingly, effects were maintained when the deaths within the first 6 years were excluded, arguing against the possibility that some participants were already sick with the early stages of cardiovascular disease (and therefore unhappy) at the start of the study. It is not clear why there were no significant associations among women, but their low disease rates may have been responsible.

We published a meta-analysis of prospective studies relating psychological well-being with mortality in 2008 (Chida and Steptoe, 2008). Twenty-six articles involving initially healthy populations and 28 articles studying people with an established illness such as head and neck cancer or HIV/AIDS were identified. The follow-up periods ranged between 2 and 44 years in the healthy population studies and 1–20 years in studies of illness groups. We found that positive affect and positive traits such as optimism and hopefulness were associated with reduced mortality, with stronger effects in healthy populations (adjusted hazard ratio 0.82, 95% C.I. 0.76–0.89, $p < 0.001$) than in those with existing illnesses (hazard ratio 0.98, C.I. 0.95–1.00, $p = 0.03$). These associations persisted when negative affect was controlled, and were also strong in studies that were judged to be of high quality on the basis of criteria such as the measurement of covariates and the rigor of outcome ascertainment. However, there were indications of publication bias, implying that studies finding a positive association were more likely to be published than those which did not. It is also possible that, despite controlling for standard risk factors such as age, socioeconomic position, gender, and marital status, other unmeasured factors were responsible for the apparent protective effects.

Positive affect is related to other severe health outcomes as well. For example, Ostir and colleagues (2001) have reported that positive affect was associated with a reduced risk of stroke in a population of older men and women after controlling for relevant covariates, and in another analysis with lower blood pressure and less hypertension (Ostir et al, 2006). A study of older patients with coronary artery disease demonstrated that functional decline was reduced in those reporting high levels of positive emotion (Brummett et al, 2009b). Cohen and colleagues (2003, 2006) have used experimental exposure to infectious respiratory pathogens such as influenza virus, in order to analyze the role of emotional states under relatively controlled conditions. In these studies, volunteers were administered standard doses of virus and were then quarantined for a number of days to assess the development of objective illness. It was found that participants with a more positive emotional style (those with high levels of positive affect over several days) had reduced risk of developing upper respiratory illness. Interestingly, these effects were independent of optimism, extraversion, self-esteem, purpose in life, and other covariates, suggesting rather specific associations between positive affect and health outcome.

Not all studies of positive affect or happiness have shown health protective effects (Eaker et al, 2007; Lampert et al, 2002). Nevertheless, from this brief review it can be seen that much of the evidence to date does suggest that there are important associations between positive well-being and health outcomes, and that these are not merely the mirror image of the effects of depression and distress.

4 Pathways Linking Positive Well-Being with Health

If the effects of positive well-being on health are robust, a crucial issue is to increase the understanding of what mechanisms are involved. There are at least four possibilities. The first

is that there is a common genetic substrate. As noted in Section 1.2, positive affect is moderately heritable and genetic factors also contribute to risk of common diseases such as type 2 diabetes and CHD. Theoretically, there might be genetic factors common to positive affect and health risk. These genetic factors could be functional, reflecting perhaps the role of central neurotransmitters both in mood regulation and physiological dysfunction, or might be due to co-aggregation of alleles. There is no direct evidence for such pathways at present. However, it has been argued that there are common genetic contributions to negative affective states such as depression, and to biological factors relevant to common diseases such as inflammatory responses and heart rate variability, so it is conceivable that similar processes could relate positive affective states with health (Su et al, 2009; Vaccarino et al, 2008).

The second possibility is that positive well-being is a marker of the broader set of psychosocial factors discussed in Section 2, which are themselves related to health, and has no direct functional role. This possibility has not been investigated very thoroughly to date, since although studies of positive well-being and health have controlled for factors such as socioeconomic status, age, and negative affect, they have seldom included the wide range of potential social and psychological mediators. However, in one investigation we studied the associations between sleep problems and both positive affect and eudaimonic well-being in a population of middle-aged men and women (Steptoe et al, 2008c). Poor sleep was related both to low positive affect and impaired eudaimonic well-being, and both effects remained significant after controlling for socioeconomic position, stress factors (financial strain and neighborhood crime), psychological distress, and social factors (social isolation, emotional support, and negative social interactions). Findings like this suggest that the relationship between positive well-being and health is distinct from more general psychosocial resources, at least in some cases.

The third possibility is that lifestyle factors are responsible, with happy individuals having more favorable health habits and making healthier behavioral choices than less happy people. Numerous lifestyle factors, including smoking, alcohol consumption, regular physical exercise, dietary choice, and sexual risk behavior are potentially associated with positive affect. The fourth possibility is that differential psychobiological activation is involved, implicating differences in neuroendocrine, autonomic, immune, and inflammatory responses. Both these pathways are discussed in further detail below.

5 Psychological Well-Being and Health Behaviors

Studies of the relationship between positive well-being and healthy behavior choices have generated rather variable results. Although positive affect and more enduring traits such as life satisfaction have been associated with greater physical activity, not smoking and moderate alcohol consumption in some studies (Dear et al, 2002; Patterson et al, 2004; Schnohr et al, 2005), other investigations have generated null or even reverse results (Diener and Seligman, 2002; Graham et al, 2004; Murphy et al, 2005). Rather less is known about the associations between well-being and other health behaviors such as dietary choice. We carried out an analysis of the relationship between life satisfaction and seven health behaviors using data on more than 17,000 young adults in 21 countries (Grant et al, 2009). Greater life satisfaction was consistently associated with a reduced likelihood of smoking and with an increased rate of regular exercise in all the regions of the world that were tested, independently of age, gender, and clustering within countries. Less consistent associations were recorded for daily fruit consumption and for the use of sunscreen to protect against skin cancer, since relationships were positive in some regions of the world but not in others.

Many of the relationships between positive well-being and health behavior are bidirectional.

For example, exercise training studies have shown that increasing physical activity has beneficial effects on mood, while depressed people are typically sedentary but become more physically active when their depression lifts (Steptoe, 2006). The current evidence is therefore consistent with the hypothesis that lifestyle factors partly mediate the associations between positive psychological states and health outcomes. However, it is notable that several studies of positive affect, mortality, and morbidity discussed in Section 3 controlled statistically for health behaviors such as smoking and physical activity, and that associations nevertheless persisted (Chida and Steptoe, 2008). More direct psychobiological pathways may therefore be involved.

6 Biological Processes Linking Positive Well-Being and Health

Activation of cardiovascular and neuroendocrine processes is regulated by corticolimbic brain circuitry involving divisions of the cingulate gyrus, the insula and the amygdala (see Chapter 51). Gianaros et al (2008) have demonstrated that blood pressure stress reactivity is associated with stronger positive functional connectivity between the amygdala and the perigenual anterior cingulate cortex, while connections between the ventromedial prefrontal cortex and the midbrain structures are implicated in cardiac responses to social stress (Wager et al, 2009). It is now evident that these same brain regions are involved in emotion regulation. Furthermore, the circuitry involved in physical pain and pleasure appears to be activated by positive and negative socially induced emotion (Takahashi et al, 2009). The possibility therefore arises that positive well-being may be embodied in the activation of neural circuitry in a reciprocal fashion to negative emotional states such as depression and distress.

There are three broad approaches to studying the peripheral biological correlates of positive well-being. The first is to obtain a single reading or a few measures of biological state, for example, a measure of plasma interleukin (IL-6) or blood pressure, and relate this to positive well-being. This technique is used in epidemiological studies (often in large samples) and in smaller studies of convenience, with measures of heart rate, blood pressure, cortisol output, and immune parameters such as natural killer cells cytotoxicity or IL-6 concentration. The results of such studies have been varied, due in part to the range of measures of positive well-being applied, but also because of small samples sizes and failure to control for covariates (Pressman and Cohen, 2005). Many of the biological variables assessed are affected by age, gender, smoking, adiposity, socioeconomic status, and other factors, so failure to control for these variables may generate spurious findings.

The cross-sectional single measure approach has demonstrated some important associations between the activation of health-related biological pathways and positive well-being. For instance, we carried out a study of 2873 healthy men and women in which in an inverse relationship between the positive affect and the inflammatory markers, C-reactive protein and IL-6, was observed. These affects were independent of age, ethnicity, socioeconomic position, body mass, smoking, and depressed mood (Steptoe et al, 2008a). However, they were found in women only and not in men. Interestingly, low IL-6 was also related to high ratings on measures of eudaimonic well-being in a sample of older women in Wisconsin (Friedman et al, 2007). Positive affect has also been linked with functional immune measures such as heightened antibody responses following vaccination for hepatitis B, independently of age, gender, health behavior, and negative affect (Marsland et al, 2006).

The evidence for associations between positive well-being and biology can be strengthened by the use of two other more dynamic approaches to measuring of biological responses: namely experimental studies and naturalistic ambulatory monitoring.

6.1 Experimental Studies of Biology and Well-Being

Experimental studies of biology and well-being are typically involved of the assessment of cardiovascular, neuroendocrine, or immunological responses under controlled laboratory conditions. Two types of experimental studies have been reported. The first has evaluated the biological effects of short-term manipulation of mood state. Pressman and Cohen's (2005) systematic review identified 16 studies with strong methodology that assessed the cardiovascular effects of mood manipulations using procedures such as listening to cheerful music or watching amusing videos. In the majority of studies, positive mood inductions stimulated increased blood pressure (BP) and heart rate compared with neutral conditions, probably because of general activation effects. Nonetheless, Vlachopoulos et al (2009) recently showed that a positive mood induction (amusing movie) led to decreases in arterial stiffness, while the reverse was found for stress induction. Arterial stiffness is an indicator of vascular health that is positively related to coronary artery disease. The impact of positive affect experimental manipulations on cortisol and immunological parameters has been mixed.

However, all these studies involved very short-term changes in mood. More relevant for the investigation of potential health effect is the comparison of people high and low in trait measures of positive affect. For example, Tugade and Fredrickson (2004) tested cardiovascular recovery following challenging tasks, and found that individuals high in resilience showed more rapid post-stress recovery. This association was accentuated in people high in positive affect. We have carried out two studies assessing these phenomena. The first involved 216 middle aged men and women from the Whitehall II epidemiological cohort who were monitored during and after the administration of two standardized tasks: color/word interference and mirror tracing (Steptoe et al, 2005). Positive affect was assessed by aggregating EMA assessments of happiness obtained every 20 min over a working day. Blood pressure and heart rate reactivity and recovery were not related to positive affect. However, stress-induced fibrinogen responses were inversely associated with positive affect after adjusting for age, gender, socioeconomic status, BMI, smoking, baseline fibrinogen, and negative affect. Fibrinogen is a mark of inflammation, and is also a precursor of fibrin, one of the main constituents of vascular thrombi, and is an important independent risk factor for coronary heart disease (Danesh et al, 1998, see chapter 45).

It is possible that an explanation for our failure to observe effects on cardiovascular stress recovery was that recovery measures were taken 45 min post-stress, and effects might have emerged earlier in the adaptation process. In the second study carried out with 72 healthy working men, we monitored BP and heart rate during tasks and then for a period 5–10 min after task completion (Steptoe et al, 2007). Positive affect was assessed both with aggregated EMA scores obtained over two working days and with standard questionnaire measures, the positive and negative affect schedule (PANAS). Positive affect assessed with EMA was associated with significantly improved diastolic BP recovery after task, controlling for age, BMI, work stress, and negative affect. Notably, we found no relationship between stress recovery and positive affect assessed with the PANAS, suggesting that effects are more prominent when affect is recorded using an immediate rather than reflective measure. However, another recent study using a reflective questionnaire assessment has shown that positive affect is inversely related to systolic and diastolic BP reaction to a sadness recall task, independently of gender, age, socioeconomic status, race, BMI level, smoking, and negative affect (Brummett et al, 2009a).

6.2 Naturalistic Physiological Monitoring Studies

The third strategy for investigating the biological correlates of positive well-being involves monitoring physiological function in everyday life. Naturalistic monitoring has the advantage of assessing effects in ecologically valid real-life situations as people go about their normal activities, rather than in the rarified atmosphere of the laboratory. Naturalistic studies are limited to a few biological variables by technology, but key measures such as cortisol can be assessed from saliva, while ambulatory BP, heart rate, and heart rate variability (HRV) can be assessed relatively unobtrusively.

We recorded salivary cortisol eight times over a working day and eight times over a leisure day in the study of 216 Whitehall participants mentioned earlier. We found that salivary cortisol averaged over the day was inversely related to positive affect after controlling for other relevant factors such as age, grade of employment, BMI, and smoking. The effect also remained significant after adjusting for psychological distress, indicating that the potentially beneficial effect of positive affect is distinct from the absence of distress. Associations were observed both on working and on nonworking days, and persisted in a second assessment of the same participants carried out 3 years later (Steptoe and Wardle, 2005). We also found that at the 3-year follow-up, ambulatory systolic BP was inversely related to positive affect after controlling for relevant covariates including psychological distress.

The relationship between positive affect and reduced cortisol in everyday life has been observed by other groups as well, albeit with some variation between men and women and in the time of day most sensitive to affective state (Ice, 2005; Lai et al, 2005; Polk et al, 2005). For example, Brummett et al (2009) found that positive affect was inversely related to the cortisol awakening response after controlling for several relevant covariates. Pressman et al (2009) assessed participation in enjoyable leisure activities in 1399 participants from four studies. Participation (which was strongly linked with positive affect) was inversely related to cortisol monitored over the day, independently of covariates including age, gender, income, education, race, BMI, and health status.

A relatively under-researched variable in this context has been HRV. As detailed in Chapter 47,

HRV is an indicator of autonomic cardiac regulation, and greater high frequency (HF-HRV) power in the HRV spectrum is suggestive of greater parasympathetic activation. Reduced HF-HRV is commonly found in depression (Rottenberg, 2007), but the impact of positive affect has not yet been extensively studied. Our group recently carried out a study of patients with suspected coronary artery disease, measuring HRV for 24 h while people went about their everyday lives (Bhattacharyya et al, 2008). Positive affect was assessed retrospectively using the day reconstruction method, the technique of reconstructing the events of the day and their associated affect devised by Kahneman and colleagues (2004). Greater positive affect over the monitoring period was associated with higher HF-HRV, and this difference remained significant after controlling for age, gender, cardiovascular disease status, and the use of medication. This result suggests that positive affect is linked with healthier cardiac autonomic control processes.

7 Interventions and Implications for Health

There are as yet no large-scale studies that have convincingly demonstrated that improving positive affect results in favorable changes in objectively assessed physical health outcomes or biological responses. Several intervention methods have been proposed for enhancing happiness and resilience, using treatments such as Fordyce's happiness program, and gratitude and mindfulness interventions. These interventions may not only augment happiness but also build resilience resources that enhance effective coping with trauma (Cohn et al, 2009). It is important to investigate the impact of interventions on potential biological and behavioral mediators, and ultimately disease etiology and prognosis, in order to establish the true importance of positive affect in health. It is even possible that some of the benefits of cognitive-behavioral

interventions result not from their effects on negative affective states directly but also from changes in positive well-being. But such notions will remain speculations rather than scientifically founded observations until the necessary research is completed.

8 Conclusions

Growing interest in potentially health protective factors in the psychological and social environment has stimulated research linking positive affect with health. There is now some evidence that positive affect is an independent predictor of health outcomes, although findings are mixed. It may also be associated with positive health behaviors, and with health-protective biological responses. Many studies of behavioral and biological mediators have been cross-sectional, so causal sequences have not been documented. Interventions to enhance positive affect have not yet been shown directly to reduce risk of health deterioration or biological and behavioral correlates. Nonetheless, this is an exciting field of behavioral medicine research that promises to increase the understanding of connections between the mind and body, to relieve suffering, and to postpone ill health.

References

Bhattacharyya, M. R., Whitehead, D. L., Rakhit, R., and Steptoe, A. (2008). Depressed mood, positive affect, and heart rate variability in patients with suspected coronary artery disease. *Psychosom Med, 70,* 1020–1027.

Brummett, B. H., Boyle, S. H., Kuhn, C. M., Siegler, I. C., and Williams, R. B. (2009a). Positive affect is associated with cardiovascular reactivity, norepinephrine level, and morning rise in salivary cortisol. *Psychophysiology, 46,* 862–869.

Brummett, B. H., Morey, M. C., Boyle, S. H., and Mark, D. B. (2009b). Prospective study of associations among positive emotion and functional status in older patients with coronary artery disease. *J Gerontol B Psychol Sci Soc Sci, 64,* 461–469.

Chida, Y., and Steptoe, A. (2008). Positive psychological well-being and mortality: a quantitative review of prospective observational studies. *Psychosom Med, 70*, 741–756.

Clark, A. E., Frijters, P., and Shields, M. A. (2008). Relative income, happiness, and utility: an explanation for the Easterlin paradox and other puzzles. *J Econ Lit, 46*, 95–144.

Cohen, S., Alper, C. M., Doyle, W. J., Treanor, J. J., and Turner, R. B. (2006). Positive emotional style predicts resistance to illness after experimental exposure to rhinovirus or influenza a virus. *Psychosom Med, 68*, 809–815.

Cohen, S., Doyle, W. J., Turner, R. B., Alper, C. M., and Skoner, D. P. (2003). Emotional style and susceptibility to the common cold. *Psychosom Med, 65*, 652–657.

Cohn, M. A., Fredrickson, B. L., Brown, S. L., Mikels, J. A., and Conway, A. M. (2009). Happiness unpacked: positive emotions increase life satisfaction by building resilience. *Emotion, 9*, 361–368.

Danesh, J., Collins, R., Appleby, P., and Peto, R. (1998). Association of fibrinogen, C-reactive protein, albumin, or leukocyte count with coronary heart disease: meta-analyses of prospective studies. *JAMA, 279*, 1477–1482.

Danner, D. D., Snowdon, D. A., and Friesen, W. V. (2001). Positive emotions in early life and longevity: findings from the nun study. *J Pers Soc Psychol, 80*, 804–813.

Dear, K., Henderson, S., and Korten, A. (2002). Well-being in Australia--findings from the National Survey of Mental Health and Well-being. *Soc Psychiatry Psychiatr Epidemiol, 37*, 503–509.

Diener, E. (1984). Subjective well-being. *Psychol Bull, 95*, 542–575.

Diener, E., Lucas, R. E., and Scollon, C. N. (2006). Beyond the hedonic treadmill: revising the adaptation theory of well-being. *Am Psychol, 61*, 305–314.

Diener, E., and Seligman, M. E. (2002). Very happy people. *Psychol Sci, 13*, 81–84.

Diener, E., Suh, E. M., Lucas, R. E., and Smith, H. L. (1999). Subjective well-being: three decades of progress. *Psychol Bull, 125*, 276–302.

Dolan, P., Peasgood, T., and White, M. (2008). Do we really know what makes us happy? A review of the economic literature on the factors associated with subjective well-being. *J Econ Psychol, 29*, 94–122.

Dunn, E. W., Aknin, L. B., and Norton, M. I. (2008). Spending money on others promotes happiness. *Science, 319*, 1687–1688.

Eaker, E. D., Sullivan, L. M., Kelly-Hayes, M., D'Agostino, R. B., Sr., and Benjamin, E. J. (2007). Marital status, marital strain, and risk of coronary heart disease or total mortality: the Framingham Offspring Study. *Psychosom Med, 69*, 509–513.

Fowler, J. H., and Christakis, N. A. (2008). Dynamic spread of happiness in a large social network:

longitudinal analysis over 20 years in the Framingham Heart Study. *Br Med J, 337*, a2338.

Fredrickson, B. L. (2004). The broaden-and-build theory of positive emotions. *Philos Trans R Soc Lond B Biol Sci, 359*, 1367–1378.

Friedman, E. M., Hayney, M., Love, G. D., Singer, B. H., and Ryff, C. D. (2007). Plasma interleukin-6 and soluble IL-6 receptors are associated with psychological well-being in aging women. *Health Psychol, 26*, 305–313.

Gianaros, P. J., Sheu, L. K., Matthews, K. A., Jennings, J. R., Manuck, S. B. et al (2008). Individual differences in stressor-evoked blood pressure reactivity vary with activation, volume, and functional connectivity of the amygdala. *J Neurosci, 28*, 990–999.

Graham, C., Eggers, A., and Sukhtankar, S. (2004). Does happiness pay? An exploration based on panel data from Russia. *J Econ Behav Org, 55*, 319–342.

Grant, N., Wardle, J., and Steptoe, A. (2009). The relationship between life satisfaction and health behavior: a cross-cultural analysis of young adults. *Int J Behav Med, 16*, 259–268.

Helliwell, J. F., and Putnam, R. D. (2004). The social context of well-being. *Philos Trans R Soc Lond B Biol Sci, 359*, 1435–1446.

Hyde, M., Wiggins, R. D., Higgs, P., and Blane, D. B. (2003). A measure of quality of life in early old age: the theory, development and properties of a needs satisfaction model (CASP-19). *Aging Ment Health, 7*, 186–194.

Ice, G. H. (2005). Factors influencing cortisol level and slope among community dwelling older adults in Minnesota. *J Cross Cult Gerontol, 20*, 91–108.

Kahneman, D., and Krueger, A. B. (2006). Developments in the measurement of subjective well-being. *J Econ Perspect, 20*, 3–24.

Kahneman, D., Krueger, A. B., Schkade, D. A., Schwarz, N., and Stone, A. A. (2004). A survey method for characterizing daily life experience: the day reconstruction method. *Science, 306*, 1776–1780.

Kashdan, T. B., Biswas-Diener, R., and King, L. A. (2008). Reconsidering happiness: the costs of distinguishing between hedonics and eudaimonia. *J Posit Psychol, 3*, 219–233.

Kubzansky, L. D., and Thurston, R. C. (2007). Emotional vitality and incident coronary heart disease: benefits of healthy psychological functioning. *Arch Gen Psychiatry, 64*, 1393–1401.

Lai, J. C., Evans, P. D., Ng, S. H., Chong, A. M., Siu, O. T., et al (2005). Optimism, positive affectivity, and salivary cortisol. *Br J Health Psychol, 10*, 467–484.

Lampert, R., Joska, T., Burg, M. M., Batsford, W. P., McPherson, C. A. et al (2002). Emotional and physical precipitants of ventricular arrhythmia. *Circulation, 106*, 1800–1805.

Lykken, D., and Tellegen, A. (1996). Happiness is a stochastic phenomenon. *Psychol Science, 7*, 186–189.

Lyubomirsky, S., King, L., and Diener, E. (2005). The benefits of frequent positive affect: does happiness lead to success? *Psychol Bull, 131*, 803–855.

Marsland, A. L., Cohen, S., Rabin, B. S., and Manuck, S. B. (2006). Trait positive affect and antibody response to hepatitis B vaccination. *Brain Behav Immun, 20*, 261–269.

Murphy, J. G., McDevitt-Murphy, M. E., and Barnett, N. P. (2005). Drink and be merry? Gender, life satisfaction, and alcohol consumption among college students. *Psychol Addict Behav, 19*, 184–191.

Nussbaum, M. C., and Sen, A. (1993). *The Quality of Life*. Oxford: Clarendon Press.

Ong, A. D., Bergeman, C. S., and Boker, S. M. (2009). Resilience comes of age: defining features in later adulthood. *J Pers, 77*, 1777–1804.

Ostir, G. V., Berges, I. M., Markides, K. S., and Ottenbacher, K. J. (2006). Hypertension in older adults and the role of positive emotions. *Psychosom Med, 68*, 727–733.

Ostir, G. V., Markides, K. S., Peek, M. K., and Goodwin, J. S. (2001). The association between emotional well-being and the incidence of stroke in older adults. *Psychosom Med, 63*, 210–215.

Patterson, F., Lerman, C., Kaufmann, V. G., Neuner, G. A., and Audrain-McGovern, J. (2004). Cigarette smoking practices among American college students: review and future directions. *J Am Coll Health, 52*, 203–210.

Polk, D. E., Cohen, S., Doyle, W. J., Skoner, D. P., and Kirschbaum, C. (2005). State and trait affect as predictors of salivary cortisol in healthy adults. *Psychoneuroendocrinology, 30*, 261–272.

Pressman, S. D., and Cohen, S. (2005). Does positive affect influence health? *Psychol Bull, 131*, 925–971.

Pressman, S. D., Matthews, K. A., Cohen, S., Martire, L. M., Scheier, M. et al (2009). Association of enjoyable leisure activities with psychological and physical well-being. *Psychosom Med, 71*, 725–732.

Rottenberg, J. (2007). Cardiac vagal control in depression: a critical analysis. *Biol Psychol, 74*, 200–211.

Ryan, R. M., and Deci, E. L. (2001). On happiness and human potentials: a review of research on hedonic and eudaimonic well-being. *Annu Rev Psychol, 52*, 141–166.

Ryff, C. D., and Keyes, C. L. (1995). The structure of psychological well-being revisited. *J Pers Soc Psychol, 69*, 719–727.

Schnohr, P., Kristensen, T. S., Prescott, E., and Scharling, H. (2005). Stress and life dissatisfaction are inversely associated with jogging and other types of physical activity in leisure time--The Copenhagen City Heart Study. *Scand J Med Sci Sports, 15*, 107–112.

Shirai, K., Iso, H., Ohira, T., Ikeda, A., Noda, H. et al (2009). Perceived level of life enjoyment and risks of cardiovascular disease incidence and mortality: the Japan public health center-based study. *Circulation, 120*, 956–963.

Sin, N. L., and Lyubomirsky, S. (2009). Enhancing well-being and alleviating depressive symptoms with positive psychology interventions: a practice-friendly meta-analysis. *J Clin Psychol Sess, 65*, 467–487.

Steptoe, A. (2006). Depression and physical activity. In A. Steptoe (Ed.), *Depression and Physical Illness* (pp. 348–368). Cambridge: Cambridge University Press.

Steptoe, A., Gibson, E. L., Hamer, M., and Wardle, J. (2007). Neuroendocrine and cardiovascular correlates of positive affect measured by ecological momentary assessment and by questionnaire. *Psychoneuroendocrinology, 32*, 56–64.

Steptoe, A., O'Donnell, K., Badrick, E., Kumari, M., and Marmot, M. G. (2008a). Neuroendocrine and inflammatory factors associated with positive affect in healthy men and women: Whitehall II study. *Am J Epidemiol, 167*, 96–102.

Steptoe, A., O'Donnell, K., Marmot, M., and Wardle, J. (2008b). Positive affect and psychosocial processes related to health. *Br J Psychol, 99*, 211–217.

Steptoe, A., O'Donnell, K., Marmot, M., and Wardle, J. (2008c). Positive affect, psychological well-being, and good sleep. *J Psychosom Res, 64*, 409–415.

Steptoe, A., and Wardle, J. (2005). Positive affect and biological function in everyday life. *Neurobiol Aging, 26 Suppl 1*, 108–112.

Steptoe, A., Wardle, J., and Marmot, M. (2005). Positive affect and health-related neuroendocrine, cardiovascular, and inflammatory processes. *Proc Natl Acad Sci U S A, 102*, 6508–6512.

Su, S., Miller, A. H., Snieder, H., Bremner, J. D., Ritchie, J. et al (2009). Common genetic contributions to depressive symptoms and inflammatory markers in middle-aged men: the twins heart study. *Psychosom Med, 71*, 152–158.

Takahashi, H., Kato, M., Matsuura, M., Mobbs, D., Suhara, T. et al (2009). When your gain is my pain and your pain is my gain: neural correlates of envy and schadenfreude. *Science, 323*, 937–939.

Tugade, M. M., and Fredrickson, B. L. (2004). Resilient individuals use positive emotions to bounce back from negative emotional experiences. *J Pers Soc Psychol, 86*, 320–333.

Vaccarino, V., Lampert, R., Bremner, J. D., Lee, F., Su, S., et al (2008). Depressive symptoms and heart rate variability: evidence for a shared genetic substrate in a study of twins. *Psychosom Med, 70*, 628–636.

Veenhoven, R. (2008). Healthy happiness: effects of happiness on physical health and the consequences for preventive health care. *J Happiness Studies, 9*, 449–469.

Vlachopoulos, C., Xaplanteris, P., Alexopoulos, N., Aznaouridis, K., Vasiliadou, C. et al (2009). Divergent effects of laughter and mental stress on arterial stiffness and central hemodynamics. *Psychosom Med, 71*, 446–453.

Wager, T. D., van Ast, V. A., Hughes, B. L., Davidson, M. L., Lindquist, M. A. et al (2009). Brain mediators of cardiovascular responses to social threat, part II: prefrontal-subcortical pathways and relationship with anxiety. *Neuroimage, 47*, 836–851.

Chapter 15

Coping and Health

Charles S. Carver and Sara Vargas

1 Stress

Over the years, a number of models of stress have been proposed. Though they vary in emphasis, nearly all recent statements relate back in one way or another to the work of Richard Lazarus and Susan Folkman (e.g., Lazarus, 1966, 1999; Lazarus and Folkman, 1984). The Lazarus and Folkman model conceptualizes stress as a transaction between person and context. Stress exists when a person confronts a circumstance that taxes or exceeds his or her ability to manage it. The circumstance itself is termed a stressor.

1.1 Appraisals and Psychological Stress

Lazarus (1966) was the first to emphasize that people's *appraisal* of the circumstance often matters more in the transaction than does the objective circumstance itself. Appraisals are cognitive processes that incorporate not only information from the stressor but also information from inside the person. Being approached by a small dog is not alarming for most people, but for people with phobias pertaining to dogs the circumstance is appraised quite differently.

A student who is actively and thoughtfully engaged in a course will appraise the announcement of a surprise quiz very differently than will a student who uses that class hour mostly to text friends.

Also important is the person's appraisal of whether he or she will be able to handle the circumstance being confronted. A person who can readily bring to mind effective ways to avoid or minimize potential bad outcomes will experience less stress than a person who can think of nothing to do. The appraisal that an aversive outcome is looming or is at hand is termed primary appraisal; the appraisal of whether there are ways to respond to it is termed secondary appraisal. Obviously these appraisals influence one another. The more confident the person is about having useful strategies, the less problematic the circumstance is likely to seem.

Several further labels have been applied to different appraisals of stressors. *Threat* appraisal means that one views the stressor as an impending event that may have bad or harmful consequences. *Harm* appraisal implies that something bad has already happened. *Loss* appraisal is a specific kind of harm appraisal in which a desired end becomes inaccessible. That is, although harm can mean either occurrence of pain and punishment or removal of something desirable, loss tends to be restricted to the latter.

Another appraisal is also commonly mentioned in this context. *Challenge* appraisal means viewing the circumstance as difficult and demanding, but also as something the person can benefit from. Challenge constitutes an "optimal" obstacle – one that appears surmountable (with

C.S. Carver (✉)
Department of Psychology, University of Miami, 5665 Ponce de Leon Blvd., Coral Gables, FL 33124-0751, USA
e-mail: ccarver@miami.edu

A. Steptoe (ed.), *Handbook of Behavioral Medicine*, DOI 10.1007/978-0-387-09488-5_15,
© Springer Science+Business Media, LLC 2010

effort), the removal of which will promote a better state of affairs. Challenge also implies expectation of good outcomes. The characteristics (and consequences) of challenge are different enough from those of threat and loss as to cast doubt on the position that challenge should be viewed as a form of stress (Blascovich, 2008; Tomaka et al, 1993).

Another popular analysis of stress uses an economic metaphor (Hobfoll, 1989, 1998), starting with the idea that people have resources that they try to protect, defend, and conserve. Resources are anything the person values. They can be physical (e.g., house, car), conditions of life (e.g., having friends and relatives, stable employment), personal qualities (e.g., a positive world view, work skills), or other assets (e.g., money or knowledge). From this view, stress occurs when resources are threatened or lost. Though this view emphasizes the utility of the resources as critical to stress, confrontation with threat and loss remains the crux of the issue.

1.1.1 Physiological Responses

Confronting threat and loss produces emotional distress. Distress emotions incorporate a variety of involuntary physiological changes within the body: cardiovascular, neuroendocrine, and immune. Many kinds of emotional arousal (e.g., fear or anger) prepare the body for sudden or sustained action. Thus, the physiological changes that occur are those that make energy available to muscles and direct resources away from other functions such as digestion or self-repair (Miller et al, 2002). Fear prepares the body for escape, anger for attack. Some kinds of emotions associated with stress, however – particularly those related to loss – have a different character. Dejection or sadness is not about preparing for action, but about giving up the effort to attain desired ends (Nesse, 2000).

These responses are functional for the purposes to which they evolved. In the short term, it is more important to devote resources to escape an imminent threat than (for example) to quell an infection. However, even adaptive processes

can result in problems if they are engaged too frequently or for too long. Several sorts of problems may occur. As one example, extensive and repeated cardiovascular stress responses place an abnormally high burden on arteries. Over time, this creates small tears in the artery and the depositing of protective plaques. This is normal. Too much depositing of plaques, however, eventually results in atherosclerosis, a clogging of the artery (e.g., Krantz and McCeney, 2002; Rozanski et al, 1999; Smith and Ruiz, 2002). This example represents an acceleration of a normal function, so that it reaches a maladaptive endpoint sooner than it otherwise would.

As another example, the processes by which blood pressure is regulated cause increases from baseline levels in response to situational demands. If those increases occur too frequently or are too sustained, the regulatory process begins to adjust the baseline upward. Now when the stressor ends, blood pressure returns not to its preexisting resting level, but to a higher level. Over iterations of adjustment, the resting level becomes elevated, becoming hypertension (cf. Fredrikson and Matthews, 1990). A gradual shift in resting level to a value that is too extreme for the well-being of the overall system has been termed allostasis (McEwen, 2000, see Chapter 42). Consistent with this line of reasoning, chronic stress has been linked to hypertension (Sparrenberger et al, 2009).

Another focal point in stress-related physiological responding is the hypothalamic–pituitary–adrenocortical (HPA) axis. This set of structures plays a major role in the body's stress response (McEwen, 2006, 2008). HPA activation is reflected in increases in levels of several hormones, including the catecholamines (epinephrine and norepinephrine) and cortisol. Cortisol is considered a particularly important stress hormone because of its links to other processes in the overall stress response. For example, elevation of cortisol can suppress diverse aspects of immune functioning (e.g., Choi et al, 2008; Kronfol et al, 1997). That is, as noted earlier, when strong demands are made on behavior (fight-or-flight), immune surveillance takes a lower priority and is suppressed (Miller et al, 2002).

Indeed, the immune system itself is another target of analyses of stress-related physiological responding (Segerstrom and Miller, 2004). The immune system obviously has important implications for health. The immune system is the body's main line of defense against disease agents, ranging from bacteria to cancer cells. If immune functioning is impaired over a sustained period, rather than just temporarily, the person thereby becomes more vulnerable both to opportunistic infectious agents and to agents of disease that had already been at work in the body. The result may be either disease promotion or disease progression (Glaser and Kiecolt-Glaser, 1994). The immune system is far more complicated than was assumed two decades ago, and there are several ways in which stress can influence immune function (Kiecolt-Glaser et al, 2002; Robles et al, 2005).

One last point should be made here about the nature of psychophysiological response patterns. Stress can be acute (relatively short-term) or chronic (existing over sometimes extended periods of time). Short-term stress responses are generally adaptive, unless previous damage has primed the body for a system failure. However, chronic activation of the body's stress response itself can have damaging effects on the body. When you bring to mind an example of stress, it may be easiest to think of an acute and time-limited situation. Many of the stressors that people confront in today's world, however, are relatively chronic and long-lasting.

2 Coping

Coping is generally defined in terms such as this: efforts to deal in some manner with a threatening or harmful situation, either to remove the threat or to diminish the ways in which it can have an adverse impact on the person. This definition is very broad. Not surprisingly, many distinctions have been made within the coping concept (see also Compas et al, 2001; Folkman and Moskowitz, 2004; Skinner et al, 2003).

2.1 Emotion-Focused and Problem-Focused Coping

A distinction made early on by Lazarus and Folkman (1984) and their colleagues was between problem-focused coping and emotion-focused coping. Problem-focused coping is aimed at the stressor itself. It may involve taking steps to remove or evade the stressor's arrival, or to reduce its physical impact. Emotion-focused coping stems from the fact that stress experiences typically incorporate distress emotions. Emotion-focused coping is aimed at reducing distress in one fashion or other. Because there are many ways to try to reduce distress, emotion-focused coping includes a very wide range of responses.

This distinction between problem- and emotion-focused coping raises a number of points. First, although the distinction is useful, it is imperfect. There are some coping responses that do not fit neatly into either category. For example, self-blame does not appear to be an attempt to remove the stressor; it may be an effort to dampen distress by assigning responsibility, but it often has the opposite effect. In contrast, some responses can fit into either category, depending on the intended effect. For example, one can seek social support for problem-focused efforts or for emotion regulation.

Second, it is generally believed that the controllability of the stressor that one is encountering influences the relative usefulness of problem-versus emotion-focused coping (certainly it seems to affect the likelihood of deploying these types of coping). Problem-focused coping strategies are well-suited to stressors that seem to have controllable aspects; emotion-focused strategies are better-suited to stressors that the person sees as uncontrollable (Park et al, 2004).

Third, although the two classes of responses can be distinguished by their goals, they often facilitate one another. For example, when people engage in effective problem-solving strategies, they indirectly reduce their emotional distress. When people engage in effective emotion-focused coping strategies, they may therefore be able to face a problem more calmly and generate more effective problem-focused strategies.

2.2 Approach and Avoidance Coping

Another very important distinction among coping responses is between approach and avoidance, or engagement and disengagement responses (Roth and Cohen, 1986; Skinner et al, 2003). Approach coping strategies are efforts to deal with the stressor or related emotions (as described in the preceding paragraphs). Avoidance strategies are attempts to escape from having to deal with the stressor.

Disengagement coping is often emotion-focused, because it involves an attempt to escape from feelings of distress. Sometimes disengagement coping is almost literally an effort to act as though the stressor does not exist, so that it does not have to be reacted to. Wishful thinking and fantasy distance the person from the stressor, at least temporarily, and denial creates a boundary between reality and the person's experience.

Avoidance coping can be useful in the short term, but it is generally ineffective when confronting a stressor that poses a real threat, that is, something that will have to be dealt with eventually. If you go out partying to avoid a stressor, it is likely to still be there the next day. Indeed, for many stressors, the longer you avoid dealing with it, the more difficult and urgent the problem becomes. Finally, some kinds of disengagement coping create problems of their own. Excessive use of alcohol or drugs can create social and health problems, and shopping or gambling as an escape can create financial problems.

2.3 Positive, Meaning-Focused, and Spiritual Coping

Researchers who study coping have increasingly become aware that positive as well as negative experiences occur during periods of stress.

For example, people report both negative emotions and positive emotions during stressful periods (e.g., Andrykowski et al, 1993; Norekvål et al, 2008). There is some basis for holding that positive emotions per se can have beneficial effects on health (Folkman and Moskowitz, 2000, 2004; Frederickson et al, 2000), though evidence is mixed (Pressman and Cohen, 2005, see Chapter 14).

Another positive experience that sometimes occurs with stress is finding meaning or experiencing positive life changes in response to the stressor (e.g., Jim and Jacobsen, 2008; Park et al, 2009; Tomich and Helgeson, 2004). Such experiences are variously called *stress-related growth* (Park et al, 1996), *post-traumatic growth* (Tedeschi and Calhoun, 2004), or *benefit finding* (Tomich and Helgeson, 2004). Such positive experiences have been associated with other positive psychosocial outcomes (Carver and Antoni, 2004; Helgeson et al, 2006). Though these responses are often treated as equivalent, these category labels appear to capture several phenomena that are distinguishable from each other (Sears et al, 2003; Weaver et al, 2008).

Another sort of coping that has elicited widespread interest in recent years is coping through spirituality or religiosity. Spirituality and religiosity are distinct concepts (Zinnbauer and Pargament, 2005), but they are often considered together, and we will do so here. Use of spiritual or religious coping can mean many different things. It may mean attending religious services and activities; it may mean frequent prayer; it may mean taking strength in one's faith; it may mean turning oneself over to a higher power.

The obvious focus for this class of coping response is on distress emotions. Religious or spiritual coping is generally aimed at least in part at producing a psychological sense of peace. In some circumstances, however, it can be thought of as indirect problem-focused coping, to the extent the coping means praying to change a stressful situation. Spiritual/religious coping is common among people with chronic illnesses, such as HIV/AIDS (Cotton et al, 2006), cancer (Vachon, 2008), and chronic pain (Büssing et al,

2009). This type of coping may be appealing to people with these diseases because the diseases have an uncontrollable nature that may be amenable to spiritual/religious coping strategies (Baldacchino and Draper, 2001).

2.4 Conclusions and Methodological Issues

Even this brief review of distinctions among types of coping, which is far from exhaustive (Compas et al, 2001; Skinner et al, 2003), makes clear that there are many ways to group coping responses. No single distinction fully represents the structure of coping. Factor analyses clearly indicate that coping is organized in a multidimensional way (Skinner et al, 2003). Nor, unfortunately, do the various distinctions represent a neat matrix into which coping responses can be sorted. In the grand scheme, the distinction that may matter most is between approach (engagement) versus avoidance (disengagement) coping. In general, approach coping keeps the person engaged in the effort to deal with the stressor; avoidance coping amounts to a tacit admission of defeat.

As researchers address the question of how coping influences well-being, a large number of methodological issues arise (Carver, 2006). Perhaps the most difficult issue is how, and how often, to assess coping. Coping is viewed conceptually as an ever-changing response to evolving situational demands, but the procedures of most coping studies do not reflect this view very well. Even many of the studies that would be regarded as good representatives of research on this topic assess coping only once a week, or once a month, across the span of adapting to some stressor. Usually, the measure asks the extent to which the person has engaged in various responses over the past day (or week). Unfortunately, those studies can tell us little about how the timing, order, combination, or duration of coping influences the outcome under study. These factors may in fact be quite important.

For example, Tennen et al (2000) have proposed that people typically use emotion-focused coping mostly after they have tried problem-focused coping and found it ineffective. This suggests an approach to research in which the question is whether the person changes from one sort of coping to another across successive assessments as a function of ineffectiveness of the first response. Tennen et al (2000) argued convincingly that, if we are to be able to understand these more subtle issues, coping must be assessed on-line and repeatedly. Unfortunately, not much work of that sort has yet been done.

3 Stress, Coping, and Health

The field of behavioral medicine is interested in coping largely insofar as coping has some measurable influence on health. Much of the existing research on coping has focused on psychosocial outcomes such as emotional well-being and quality of life, or on physiological responses that occur quite early in the pathway towards illness. Thus, what can be said about how coping affects health per se remains relatively limited. On the other hand, some of the effects of stress on health are much clearer.

3.1 What Is Health?

For our purposes, health is the presence or absence of a diagnosable, verifiable illness or disorder. Even within this definition, there is a great deal of diversity. Health-related outcomes include disease initiation (who develops the disease and who does not), disease progression (how quickly an early form of a disease evolves into a more advanced form), recurrence of disease, side effects of treatment, and mortality rates or survival time.

This diversity raises further issues. For example, it may be that stress and coping affects some health outcomes but not others (e.g., disease initiation but not progression). It may be that stress and coping affects some diseases but not others (e.g., cardiovascular disease but not cancer). It is necessary, therefore, to investigate effects of stress and coping on diverse outcomes separately, and be cautious about making broad statements about the impact of stress or specific coping strategies on "health" or "disease" in general.

Nonetheless, some broad hypotheses can be posed in principle. As suggested earlier, the typical view of the relationships among stress, coping, and health begins with adverse events leading to negative emotions, with physiological components or concomitants. If the distress is intense, prolonged, or repeated, disruption of one or more physiological systems may develop. The disruption then affects disease outcomes, directly or indirectly. From this view, effective coping acts largely to minimize initial stress arousal and to influence how intense and prolonged the negative emotions are. Coping that is ineffective or maladaptive can worsen the response, resulting in sustained distress and accompanying physiological responses.

3.2 Coping and Health: Behavioral Pathways

Before we turn to literature bearing on those hypotheses, one side point. Although much of the discussion of coping and health emphasized the physiological reactivity that comes along with distress and disease pathways that follow from that reactivity, there are also simpler and more direct ways in which maladaptive coping can produce health problems. Specifically, people sometimes cope via behaviors that themselves are inimical to health. We begin our discussion of coping and health with a brief discussion of that pathway to illness.

As noted earlier, in the context of the distinction between problem-focused and emotion-focused coping, there is great diversity among responses that bear the label emotion-focused. As we said there, virtually anything a person does with the intent of diminishing distress can legitimately be called emotion-focused coping. Some of these responses themselves have effects other than the desired one. Indeed, some can promote health problems.

For example, smoking, alcohol and drug use, and casual sex are common ways to self-sooth, or regulate emotions, when under stress (cf. Cohen et al, 1991; Holahan et al, 2003; Horowitz and White, 1991). Such activities may reduce negative feelings over the short term, thereby serving as emotion-focused coping. However, they ultimately can have adverse effects on health.

Maladaptive coping is partly doing behaviors that are inimical to health. It is partly abandoning behaviors that are beneficial to health. For example, maintaining an exercise regimen and a well-balanced diet is important to maintaining good health. Yet exercise and proper eating are often the first things to be disregarded when stress arises. Abandoning these health-promoting activities prevents the person from gaining incremental benefits he or she would otherwise experience (Smith and Leon, 1992). Abandoning those beneficial behaviors thus can be considered maladaptive coping.

3.3 Psychophysiological Pathways

Despite these direct behavioral pathways to health, most discussions of adaptive and maladaptive coping refer to the creation or reduction of physiological changes over extended periods of time (Ursin and Olff, 1993). In addressing such effects of stress and coping, one might focus at several levels of abstraction. The focus could be on episodic change in some endocrine or immune parameter, emergence of an intermediate disease state such as atherosclerosis, or eventual emergence of full-blown clinical events such as heart attacks. Outcomes at all these levels have been examined. Here we provide just a few relevant examples at several levels.

One set of physiological parameters that has received attention concerns the stress hormone cortisol. In general, problem-focused and approach coping styles are related to lower overall levels of cortisol, more favorable diurnal cortisol rhythms, and faster recovery to normal patterns after a stressor (Mikolajczak et al, 2007; Nicolson, 1992; O'Donnell et al, 2008; Sjogren et al, 2006). A number of qualities that reflect social integration and support have also been linked to favorable cortisol profiles. Use of social support relates to lower daily cortisol levels (O'Donnell et al, 2008). Social isolation (living alone and little contact with friends and family) predicts a greater cortisol response at awakening and greater cortisol output over the day (Grant et al, 2009). Higher levels of religiosity have also been associated with favorable cortisol patterns in women with fibromyalgia, even after controlling for social support (Dedert et al, 2004).

Coping responses have also been linked to variations in immune system functioning. For example, among HIV patients, those who showed difficulty in recognizing and expressing their emotions had higher levels of an immune marker related to HIV disease progression (Temoshok et al, 2008). Also among HIV patients, those expressing disengagement tendencies had higher viral loads and lower immune cell counts (Wald et al, 2006). In a non-patient sample, instrumental coping was linked to better immune system functioning, along with lower HPA activation (Olff et al, 1995).

Another intermediate physiological condition that has received a good deal of attention is atherosclerosis. A good deal is known about stress and atherosclerosis, though less about coping. Even mild chronic stress promotes atherosclerosis in laboratory animals, a process that seems to be mediated by HPA activation, reflected in elevated stress hormones (Kumari et al, 2003). Inflammatory immune responses, which are induced by stress, are central to development of atherosclerosis (Libby, 2006), acting as a mediator between stress and atherosclerosis (Black, 2006; see Grippo and Johnson, 2009, for review).

Chronic occupational stress consistently predicts hypertension and atherosclerosis (Everson-Rose and Lewis, 2005; Sparrenberger et al, 2009), but social disruptions can also create chronic stress, with similar results. For example, both social isolation and crowding promote atherosclerosis in monkeys (Shively et al, 1989). Similar relationships have been found between social disruption (social isolation and lack of perceived social support) and atherosclerosis in humans (Everson-Rose and Lewis, 2005; Smith and Ruiz, 2002).

Another body of work examines disease progression. Studies have shown that denial coping and lower satisfaction with social support relate to the progression from HIV to AIDS (Leserman et al, 2000). Optimism, active coping, and spirituality show some evidence of predicting slower disease progression (Ironson and Hayward, 2008). A meta-analysis of coping among men with prostate cancer found that approach coping (both problem-focused and emotion-focused) improved physical outcomes such as self-reported fatigue and physical well-being, and that avoidance coping was associated with lower self-reported physical functioning (Roesch et al, 2005).

Cardiovascular disease is unusual in that there are both gradually developing outcomes (e.g., atherosclerosis) and also more abrupt outcomes (e.g., heart attacks). Negative emotional states have been linked to atherosclerosis (Everson-Rose and Lewis, 2005; Suls and Bunde, 2005) and also to triggering of acute cardiac events (Steptoe and Brydon, 2009). The latter effect is not limited to high arousal emotions such as anger. Acute depressed mood is also a trigger of cardiac events (Steptoe et al, 2006). Fitting this, bereavement is an acute stressor that has been long associated with elevated rates of cardiac events (Parkes, 1964). The acute stressor need not be death, disaster, or war, however. A recent study showed that watching a stressful soccer match more than doubled the risk of cardiac events for men in Germany (Wilbert-Lampen et al, 2008).

Enough research has examined coping and health-related outcomes in nonclinical samples to warrant a meta-analysis (Penley et al, 2002). This analysis found that certain kinds of problem-focused coping (self-control and use of social support) related positively to diverse kinds of good health outcomes (ranging from self-reports of symptoms to objective illness-related measures), while other types of coping (e.g., confrontive coping and wishful thinking) related to poorer health outcomes. There were also cases in which the controllability of the stressor and whether the stressor was acute or chronic moderated the relationship between coping and outcomes. For example, distancing was related to poorer health outcomes when the stressor was chronic and controllable; taking responsibility was related to poorer outcomes when the stressor was acute and uncontrollable.

Another meta-analysis was reported even more recently, on a more focused set of studies (Moskowitz et al, 2009). All of these studies examined persons with HIV. Outcomes were categorized as emotional, health-related behavior, and physical. Coping that involved direct action and positive reappraisal had consistently positive relations to better results across all categories of outcome. Disengagement coping was consistently associated with poorer outcomes.

3.4 Cautions and Qualifications

Before leaving this discussion of coping and health, we should say a bit more about what the literature does and does not show. As noted earlier, in some cases much more is known about effects of stress than about effects of coping. A good deal of research on coping, even research that bears on health, has other limitations. For one, some of these studies rely on self-reported health outcomes. These are much less reliable as indicators of health than are objective outcomes, and must be interpreted much more cautiously.

Further, a good deal of this research assesses coping tendencies in general rather than coping with a specific problem, or assesses at a single time how people coped with a specific problem over an extended period. This research may be

telling us about coping and health. However, it may be telling us about something slightly different: personality and health. That is, an important determinant of how a given person copes with a given stressor at a given moment is that person's personality (Carver and Connor-Smith, 2010).

As an example of how the line between these concepts can be blurred, consider the literature on optimism. Optimism is a personality trait, but its essence has much in common with certain ways of coping (positive reframing, looking on the best side of things, moving forward with a positive outcome in mind). To the extent that optimism predicts favorable health-related outcomes (Chida and Steptoe, 2008; Ironson and Hayward, 2008; Segerstrom, 2005), an unanswered question remains. Are better outcomes a product of differences in coping, or are they a product of something else embedded in personality? This question actually pertains to a good deal of the literature on coping and health.

4 Coping Interventions for Disease Populations

We close the chapter by looking briefly at the possibility of changing in ways that may foster better health. The emergence of a literature, limited though it may be, which suggests that health benefits may follow from certain coping strategies, has helped to encourage creation of a number of interventions for people who already are suffering from various kinds of disease. Here are two examples (for a more thorough review see de Ridder and Schreurs, 2001).

Antoni and his colleagues developed a 10-week cognitive behavioral stress management intervention involving relaxation, cognitive restructuring, and coping skills training for women being treated for non-metastatic breast cancer. This intervention led to improved psychosocial outcomes (Antoni et al, 2006a, b). It also led to greater reductions in cortisol levels through a 12-month follow-up, compared with a control group (Phillips et al, 2008), and to greater cytokine production through 6-month follow-up (Antoni et al, 2009).

Another research team tested a year-long intervention (4 months of weekly sessions and 8 monthly sessions), which trained breast cancer patients strategies to reduce stress, improve mood, and maintain treatment adherence. This intervention improved symptoms and functional status, compared to a control group (Andersen et al, 2007). A recent report indicated that it even increased survival rates (Andersen et al, 2008). This is a particularly encouraging result, given the considerable controversy about whether such interventions can influence survival.

A number of other coping-based interventions have been developed for other health populations. Examples include dyadic interventions for enhancing communication skills for persons with HIV and their partners (Fife et al, 2008) and pain-specific coping skills for persons suffering from sickle cell anemia (Gil et al, 2000). It seems likely that further exploration of such coping-based interventions will be an important agenda for the future in behavioral medicine.

Acknowledgments Preparation of this chapter was facilitated by grants from the National Cancer Institute (CA64710) and the National Science Foundation (BCS0544617).

References

Andersen, B. L., Farrar, W. B., Golden-Kreutz, D., Emery, C. F., Glaser, R. et al (2007). Distress reduction from a psychological intervention contributes to improved health for cancer patients. *Brain Behav Immun, 21*, 953–961.

Andersen, B. L., Yang, H. C., Farrar, W. B., Golden-Kreutz, D. M., Emery, C. F. et al (2008). Psychologic intervention improves survival for breast cancer patients: a randomized clinical trial. *Cancer, 113*, 3450–3458.

Andrykowski, M. A., Brady, M. J., and Hunt, J. W. (1993). Positive psychosocial adjustment in potential bone marrow transplant recipients: cancer as a psychosocial transition. *Psychooncology, 2*, 261–276.

Antoni, M. H., Lechner, S., Diaz, A., Vargas, S., Holley, H. et al (2009). Cognitive behavioral stress management effects on psychosocial and physiological

adaptation in women undergoing treatment for breast cancer. *Brain Behav Immun, 23*, 580–591.

Antoni, M. H., Lechner, S. C., Kazi, A., Wimberly, S. R., Sifre, T. et al (2006a). How stress management improves quality of life after treatment for breast cancer. *J Consult Clin Psychol, 74*, 1143–1152.

Antoni, M. H., Wimberly, S. R., Lechner, S. C., Kazi, A., Sifre, T. et al (2006b). Reduction of cancer-specific thought intrusions and anxiety symptoms with a stress management intervention among women undergoing treatment for breast cancer. *Am J Psychiatry, 163*, 1791–1797.

Baldacchino, D., and Draper, P. (2001). Spiritual coping strategies: a review of the nursing research literature. *J Adv Nurs, 34*, 833–841.

Black, P. H. (2006). The inflammatory consequences of psychologic stress: relationship to insulin resistance, obesity, atherosclerosis and diabetes mellitus, type II. *Med Hypotheses, 67*, 879–891.

Büssing, A., Michalsen, A., Balzat, H. J., Grünther, R. A., Ostermann, T. et al (2009). Are spirituality and religiosity resources for patients with chronic pain conditions? *Pain Med, 10*, 327–339.

Blascovich, J. (2008). Challenge and threat. In A. J. Elliot (Ed.), *Handbook of Approach and Avoidance Motivation* (pp. 431–445). New York: Psychology Press.

Carver, C. S. (2006). Stress, coping, and health. In H. S. Friedman & R. C. Silver (Eds.), *Foundations of Health Psychology* (pp. 117–144). New York: Oxford Press.

Carver, C. S., and Antoni, M. H. (2004). Finding benefit in breast cancer during the year after diagnosis predicts better adjustment 5 to 8 years after diagnosis. *Health Psychol, 23*, 595–598.

Carver, C. S., and Connor-Smith, J. (2010). Personality and coping. *Annu Rev Psychol, 61*, 679–704.

Chida, Y., and Steptoe, A. (2008). Positive psychological well-being and mortality: a quantitative review of prospective observational studies. *Psychosom Med, 70*, 741–756.

Choi, J., Fauce, S. R., and Effros, R. B. (2008). Reduced telomerase activity in human T lymphocytes exposed to cortisol. *Brain Behav Immun, 22*, 600–605.

Cohen, S., Schwartz, J. E., Bromet, E. J., and Parkinson, D. K. (1991). Mental health, stress, and poor health behaviors in two community samples. *Prev Med, 20*, 306–315.

Compas, B. E., Connor-Smith, J. K., Saltzman, H., Thomsen, A. H., and Wadsworth, M. E. (2001). Coping with stress during childhood and adolescence: problems, progress, and potential in theory in research. *Psychol Bull, 127*, 87–127.

Cotton, S., Puchalski, C. M., Sherman, S. N., Mrus, J. M., Peterman, A. H. et al (2006). Spirituality and religion in patients with HIV/AIDS. *J Gen Intern Med, 21*, S5–S13.

Dedert, E. A., Studts, J. L., Weissbecker, I., Salmon, P. G., Banis, P. L., and Sephton, S. E. (2004). Religiosity may help preserve the cortisol rhythm in women with stress-related illness. *Int J Psychiatry Med, 34,* 61–77.

de Ridder, D., and Schreurs, K. (2001). Developing interventions for chronically ill patients: is coping a helpful concept? *Clin Psychol Rev, 21,* 205–240.

Everson-Rose, S. A., and Lewis, T. T. (2005). Psychosocial factors and cardiovascular disease. *Annu Rev Public Health, 26,* 469–500.

Fife, B. L., Scott, L. L., Fineberg, N. S., and Zwickl, B. E. (2008). Promoting adaptive coping by persons with HIV disease: evaluation of a patient/partner intervention model. *J Assoc Nurses AIDS Care, 19,* 75–84.

Folkman, S., and Moskowitz, J. T. (2000). Positive affect and the other side of coping. *Am Psychol, 55,* 647–654.

Folkman, S., and Moskowitz, J. T. (2004). Coping: pitfalls and promise. *Annu Rev Psychol, 55,* 745–774.

Frederickson, B. L., Mancuso, R. A., Branigan, C., and Tugade, M. M. (2000). The undoing effect of positive emotions. *Motiv Emot, 24,* 237–258.

Fredrikson, M., and Matthews, K. A. (1990). Cardiovascular responses to behavioral stress and hypertension: a meta-analytic review. *Ann Behav Med,* 12, 30–39.

Gil, K. M., Carson, J. W., Sedway, J. A., Porter, L. S., Schaeffer, J. J. et al (2000). Follow-up of coping skills training in adults with sickle cell disease: analysis of daily pain and coping practice diaries. *Health Psychol, 19,* 85–90.

Glaser, R., and Kiecolt-Glaser, J. K. (Eds.). (1994). *Handbook of Human Stress and Immunity.* San Diego, CA: Academic Press.

Grant, N., Hamer, M., and Steptoe, A. (2009). Social isolation and stress-related cardiovascular, lipid, and cortisol responses. *Ann Behav Med,* 37, 29–37.

Grippo, A. J., and Johnson, A. K. (2009). Stress, depression, and cardiovascular dysregulation: a review of neurobiological mechanisms and the integration of research from preclinical disease models. *Stress, 12,* 1–21.

Helgeson, V. S., Reynolds, K. A., and Tomich, P. L. (2006). A meta-analytic review of benefit finding and growth. *J Consult Clin Psychol, 74,* 797–816.

Hobfoll, S. E. (1989). Conservation of resources: a new attempt at conceptualizing stress. *Am Psychol, 44,* 513–524.

Hobfoll, S. E. (1998). *Stress, Culture, and Community.* New York: Plenum.

Holahan, C. J., Moos, R. H., Holahan, C. K., Cronkite, R. C., and Randall, P. K. (2003). Drinking to cope and alcohol use and abuse in unipolar depression: a 10-year model. *J Abnorm Psychol, 112,* 159–165.

Horowitz, A. V., and White, H. R. (1991). Becoming married, depression, and alcohol problems among young adults. *J Health Soc Behav, 32,* 221–237.

Ironson, G., and Hayward, H. (2008). Do positive psychosocial factors predict disease progression in HIV-1? A review of the evidence. *Psychosom Med, 70,* 546–554.

Jim, H. S., and Jacobsen, P. B. (2008). Posttraumatic stress and posttraumatic growth in cancer survivorship: a review. *Cancer J, 14,* 414–419.

Kiecolt-Glaser, J. K., McGuire, L., Robles, T. F., and Glaser, R. (2002). Emotions, morbidity, and mortality: new perspectives from psychoneuroimmunology. *Annu Rev Psychol, 53,* 83–107.

Krantz, D. S., and McCeney, M. K. (2002). Effects of psychological and social factors on organic disease: a critical assessment of research on coronary heart disease. *Annu Rev Psychol, 53,* 341–369.

Kronfol, Z., Madhavan, N., Zhang, Q., Hill, E. E., and Brown, M. B. (1997). Circadian immune measures in healthy volunteers: relationship to hypothalamic-pituitary-adrenal axis hormones and sympathetic neurotransmitters. *Psychosom Med, 59,* 42–50.

Kumari, M., Grahame-Clarke, C., Shanks, N., Marmot, M., Lightman, S. et al (2003). Chronic stress accelerates atherosclerosis in the apolipoprotein E deficient mouse. *Stress, 6,* 297–299.

Lazarus, R. S. (1966). *Psychological Stress and the Coping Process.* New York: McGraw-Hill.

Lazarus, R. S. (1999). *Stress and Emotion: A New Synthesis.* New York: Springer.

Lazarus, R. S., and Folkman, S. (1984). *Stress, Appraisal, and Coping.* New York: Springer.

Leserman, J., Petitto, J. M., Golden, R. N., Gaynes, B. N., Gu, H. et al (2000). Impact of stressful life events, depression, social support, coping, and cortisol on progression to AIDS. *Am J Psychiatry, 157,* 1221–1228.

Libby, P. (2006). Inflammation and cardiovascular disease mechanisms. *Am J Clin Nutr, 83,* 456S–460S.

McEwen, B. S. (2000). Allostasis and allostatic load: Implications for neuropsychopharmacology. *Neuropsychopharmacology, 22,* 108–124.

McEwen, B. S. (2006). Protective and damaging effects of stress mediators: central role of the brain. *Dialogues Clin Neurosci, 8,* 367–381.

McEwen, B. S. (2008). Central effects of stress hormones in health and disease: understanding the protective and damaging effects of stress and stress mediators. *Eur J Pharmacol, 538,* 174–185.

Mikolajczak, M., Roy, E., Luminet, O., Fillée, C., and de Timary, P. (2007). The moderating impact of emotional intelligence on free cortisol responses to stress. *Psychoneuroendocrinology, 32,* 1000–1012.

Miller, G. E., Cohen, S., and Ritchey, A. K. (2002). Chronic psychological stress and the regulation of pro-inflammatory cytokines: a glucocorticoid-resistance model. *Health Psychol, 21,* 531–541.

Moskowitz, J. T., Hult, J. R., Bussolari, C., and Acree, M. (2009). What works in coping with HIV? A meta-analysis with implications for coping with serious illness. *Psychol Bull, 135,* 121–141.

Nesse, R. M. (2000). Is depression an adaptation? *Arch Gen Psychiatry, 57,* 14–20.

Nicolson, N. A. (1992). Stress, coping and cortisol dynamics in daily life. In M. W. De Vries (Ed.), *The Experience of Psychopathology*. Cambridge: Cambridge University Press.

Norekvål, T. M., Moons, P., Hanestad, B. R., Nordrehaug, J. E., Wentzel-Larsen, T. et al (2008). The other side of the coin: perceived positive effects of illness in women following acute myocardial infarction. *Eur J Cardiovasc Nurs, 7*, 80–87.

O'Donnell, K., Badrick, E., Kumari, M., and Steptoe, A. (2008). Psychological coping styles and cortisol over the day in healthy older adults. *Psychoneuroendocrinology, 33*, 601–611.

Olff, M., Brosschot, J. F., Godeart, G., Benschop, R. J., Ballieux, R. E. et al (1995). Modulatory effects of defense and coping on stress-induced changes in endocrine and immune parameters. *Int J Behav Med, 2*, 85–103.

Park, C. L., Armeli, S., and Tennen, H. (2004). Appraisal-coping goodness of fit: a daily internet study. *Pers Soc Psychol Bull, 30*, 558–569.

Park, C. L., Cohen, L. H., and Murch, R. L. (1996). Assessment and prediction of stress-related growth. *J Pers, 64*, 71–105.

Park, C. L., Lechner, S. C., Antoni, M. H., and Stanton, A. L. (Eds.). (2009). *Medical Illness and Positive Life Change: Can Crisis Lead to Personal Transformation?* Washington, DC: American Psychological Association.

Parkes, C. M. (1964). Effects of bereavement on physical and mental health: a study of the medical records of widows. *BMJ, 2*, 274–279.

Penley, J. A., Tomaka, J., and Wiebe, J. S. (2002). The association of coping to physical and psychological health outcomes: a meta-analytic review. *J Behav Med, 25*, 551–603.

Phillips, K. M., Antoni, M. H., Lechner, S. C., Blomberg, B. B., Llabre, M. M., Avisar, E. et al (2008). Stress management intervention reduces serum cortisol and increases relaxation training during treatment for nonmetastatic breast cancer. *Psychosom Med, 70*, 1044–1049.

Pressman, S. D., and Cohen, S. (2005). Does positive affect influence health? *Psychol Bull, 131*, 925–971.

Robles, T. F., Glaser, R., and Kiecolt-Glaser, J. K. (2005). Out of balance: a new look at chronic stress, depression, and immunity. *Curr Dir Psychol Sci, 14*, 111–115.

Roesch, S. C., Adams, L., Hines, A., Palmorse, A., Vyas, P. et al (2005). Coping with prostate cancer: a meta-analytic review. *J Behav Med, 28*, 281–293.

Roth, S., and Cohen, L. J. (1986). Approach, avoidance, and coping with stress. *Am Psychol, 41*, 813–819.

Rozanski, A., Blumenthal, J. A., and Kaplan, J. (1999). Impact of psychological factors on the pathogenesis of cardiovascular disease and implications for therapy. *Circulation, 99*, 2192–2217.

Sears, S. R., Stanton, A. L., and Danoff-Burg, S. (2003). The yellow brick road and the emerald city: benefit finding, positive reappraisal coping, and posttraumatic growth in women with early-stage breast cancer. *Health Psychol, 22*, 487–497.

Segerstrom, S. C. (2005). Optimism and immunity: do positive thoughts always leave to positive effects? *Brain Behav Immun, 19*, 195–200.

Segerstrom, S. C., and Miller, G. E. (2004). Psychological stress and the human immune system: a meta-analytic study of 30 years of inquiry. *Psychol Bull, 130*, 601–630.

Shively, C. A., Clarkson, T. B., and Kaplan, J. R. (1989). Social deprivation and coronary artery atherosclerosis in female cynomolgus monkeys. *Atherosclerosis, 77*, 69–76.

Sjogren, E., Leanderson, P., and Kristenson, M. (2006). Diurnal saliva cortisol levels and relations to psychosocial factors in a population sample of middle-aged Swedish men and women. *Int J Behav Med, 13*, 193–200.

Skinner, E. A., Edge, K., Altman, J., and Sherwood, H. (2003). Searching for the structure of coping: a review and critique of category systems for classifying ways of coping. *Psychol Bull, 129*, 216–269.

Smith, T. W., and Leon, A. S. (1992). *Coronary Heart Disease: A Behavioral Perspective*. Chapaign-Urbana, IL: Research Press.

Smith, T. W., and Ruiz, J. M. (2002). Psychosocial influences on the development and course of coronary heart disease: current status and implications for research and practice. *J Consult Clin Psychol, 70*, 548–568.

Sparrenberger, F., Cichelero, F. T., Ascoli, A. M., Fonseca, F. P., Wiess, G. et al (2009). Does psychosocial stress cause hypertension? A systematic review of observational studies. *J Hum Hypertens, 23*, 12–19.

Steptoe, A., and Brydon, L. (2009). Emotional triggering of cardiac events. *Neurosci Biobehav Rev, 33*, 63–70.

Steptoe, A., Strike, P. C., Perkins-Porras, L., McEwan, J. R., and Whitehead, D. L. (2006). Acute depressed mood as a trigger of acute coronary syndromes. *Biol Psychiatry, 60*, 837–842.

Suls, J, and Bunde, J. (2005). Anger, anxiety, and depression as risk factors for cardiovascular disease: the problems and implications of overlapping affective dispositions. *Psychol Bull, 131*, 260–300.

Tedeschi, R. G., and Calhoun, L. G. (2004). Posttraumatic growth: conceptual foundations and empirical evidence. *Psychological Inquiry, 15*, 1–18.

Temoshok, L. R., Waldstein, S. R., Wald, R. L., Garzino-Demo, A., Synowski, S. J. et al (2008). Type C coping, alexithymia, and heart rate reactivity are associated independently and differentially with specific immune mechanisms linked to HIV progression. *Brain Behav Immun, 22*, 781–792.

Tennen, H., Affleck, G., Armeli, S., and Carney, M. A. (2000). A daily process approach to coping. Linking theory, research, and practice. *Am Psychol, 55*, 626–636.

Tomaka, J., Blascovich, J., Kelsey, R. M., and Leitten, C. L. (1993). Subjective, physiological, and behavioral effects of threat and challenge appraisal. *J Pers Soc Psychol, 65*, 248–260.

Tomich, P. L., and Helgeson, V. S. (2004). Is finding something good in the bad always good? Benefit finding among women with breast cancer. *Health Psychol, 23*, 16–23.

Ursin, H., and Olff, M. (1993). Psychobiology of coping and defence strategies. *Neuropsychobiology, 28*, 66–71.

Vachon, M. L. (2008). Meaning, spirituality, and wellness in cancer survivors. *Semin Oncol Nurs, 24*, 218–225.

Wald, R. L., Dowling, G. C., and Temoshok, L. R. (2006). Coping styles predict immune system parameters and clinical outcomes in patients with HIV. *Retrovirology, 3*, P65.

Weaver, K. E., Llabre, M. M., Lechner, S. C., Penedo, F., and Antoni, M. H. (2008). Comparing unidimensional and multidimensional models of benefit finding in breast and prostate cancer. *Qual Life Res, 17*, 771–781.

Wilbert-Lampen, U., Leistner, D., Greven, S., Pohl, T., Sper, S. et al (2008). Cardiovascular events during World Cup Soccer. *N Engl J Med, 358*, 475–483.

Zinnbauer, B. J., and Pargament, K. I. (2005). Religiousness and spirituality. In R. F. Paloutzian & C. L. Park (Eds.), *Handbook of the Psychology of Religion and Spirituality* (pp. 21–42). New York: Guilford Press.

Part III
Social and Interpersonal Processes

Chapter 16

Experimental Approaches to Social Interaction for the Behavioral Medicine Toolbox

Jerry Suls and M. Bryant Howren

Why should health psychologists conduct laboratory experiments to understand the role that social behavior plays in physical health? Lab experiments, by their very nature, are artificial and rarely can recruit representative samples. Would not it be far better to study the influence of social factors on health in real-life situations? These questions and complaints represent a misunderstanding of the purposes of laboratory experimentation. Festinger (1953), one of the foremost social psychologists of the 20th century, provided a succinct answer:

> The laboratory experiment should be an attempt to create a situation in which the operation of variables will be clearly seen under special identified and defined conditions. It matters not whether such a situation would ever be encountered in real life. In most laboratory experiments, such a situation would certainly "never" be encountered in real life. In a laboratory, however, we can find out exactly how a certain variable affects behavior or attitudes under special, or "pure," conditions (p. 139).

In other words, if researchers want to learn whether certain variables lead to a particular outcome, then the constraints of the laboratory provide the arena in which systematic variation of different variables is possible and confounding factors can be minimized. The opportunity afforded by laboratory experiments to assess how combinations of manipulated variables may interact is a distinct advantage. Only rarely does a real-life situation allow for this option. Moreover, knowledge regarding relationships between or among variables resulting from laboratory experiments can provide the basis for predictions about real-life situations.

One difficulty associated with the laboratory experiment is that rarely is the strength of independent variables likely to be comparable to the strength these variables exert in real-life situations; thus, the power to detect effects may be very small. This can be compensated for, to some extent, by the increased control the researcher has in the laboratory setting. In the case of social-psychological variables, the use of cover-stories or deception is often important to increase the power of the manipulations. It is here the term "experimental realism" applies. This refers to the extent to which experimental procedures have an impact on the participants or the extent to which events in the experimental setting are credible, involving, and taken seriously (Carlsmith et al, 1976).

To illustrate how experimental approaches to social interaction have been conducted regarding questions in health psychology/behavioral medicine, five research paradigms will be briefly described in this chapter. These five were chosen to reflect the breadth of problems studied in laboratory research, which have broad-ranging implications for understanding the etiology, prevention, experience, and/or treatment of physical disease. Some approaches, which were seminal for the growth of behavioral medicine, such as Schachter's research on obesity and smoking or Glass's (1977) research on Type

J. Suls (✉)
Department of Psychology, Spence Laboratories,
University of Iowa, Iowa City, IA 52242, USA
e-mail: jerry-suls@uiowa.edu

A. Steptoe (ed.), *Handbook of Behavioral Medicine*, DOI 10.1007/978-0-387-09488-5_16,
© Springer Science+Business Media, LLC 2010

A behavior were not chosen simply because they have received extensive coverage in other sources (Glass, 1977; Schachter, 1971a, b). As each approach is described, we also will explain what assets the psychological laboratory offered to advance each topic domain.

1 Thioamine Acetylase Paradigm for Studying Illness Cognition

The study of symptom and illness cognition is an important topic because the ways in which individuals think about physical symptoms partly determines whether they decide they are ill and, further, perceive the need to seek medical care. For some time, those interested in illness cognition relied on questionnaire, interview, or ethnographic methods (Croog et al, 1971; Mechanic, 1972; Taylor et al, 1984; Zola, 1966). Such non-experimental approaches yielded rich insights, but third-variable explanations were often plausible. However, at the time, these methods seemed to be the only viable options; health researchers had not yet developed methods to experimentally (and ethically) manipulate the experience of physical illness.

Jemmott et al (1986), who were trained as experimental social psychologists, developed the thioamine acetylase (TAA) saliva reaction test, a fictitious medical test for an enzymatic deficiency, in order to experimentally test hypotheses about illness cognition. They hypothesized that people perceive medical deficiencies which are prevalent as less serious than those that are rare. In other words, if a condition is perceived to be common, people do not believe it is serious and, therefore, there is no need for them to take corrective action.

In order to increase experimental realism and maximize external validity, Jemmott and colleagues conducted their experiment in a psychology laboratory outfitted with items typically seen in a medical clinic, such as stethoscopes, blood pressure gauges, and health posters. Additionally, the experimenters wore white lab coats. Participants were recruited by telephone

under the guise that they would be taking part in a study conducted by the "Health Awareness Project," which required completion of some health-related questionnaires, several standard medical tests, and some "recently developed" tests, including the TAA test and a hearing test. Participants also were administered a short hypochondriasis scale as a screening device. Those who were high in hypochondrical tendencies were excluded from participation to minimize potential risk due to deception.

Upon arrival, participants' blood pressure and pulse were taken as part of the cover-story and they were seated in individual soundproof booths in preparation for the hearing test. Although groups were limited to two or three individuals, participants were led to believe that they were part of a group of five individuals. Once seated, the experimenter explained (via an intercom system) that the hearing test would be postponed due to technical difficulties and that the next test would be the TAA saliva reaction test, which was described in a booklet that was read aloud by the experimenter.

Participants were told that an enzyme found in saliva, thioamine acetylase (TAA), was a marker of pancreatic function and that some individuals have the enzyme while others do not. Further, participants were led to believe that individuals *lacking* the TAA enzyme were at increased risk for several "mild, but irritating pancreatic disorders." All of this information was actually fictitious; however, it was necessary to create the experimental conditions.

The booklet included detailed instructions on how to self-administer the TAA test using a strip of chemically coated paper. Participants were asked to rinse with mouthwash (under the pretense of removing potential test contaminants such as food residue) before expectorating into a cup and placing the strip of TAA test paper in the saliva. The strip of test paper, however, was actually glucose-sensitive and the mouthwash used prior to the "test" contained a trace amount of the substance. Consequently, each participant's test paper turned from yellow to green.

The supposed meaning of this reaction was manipulated as a function of the experimental condition. Prior to the test, one group of randomly assigned participants was told the color change indicated that TAA was *absent* from their saliva while another group was told the change denoted that TAA was *present*. The prevalence of the deficiency was also manipulated; that is, some participants were led to believe either one or four individuals per group lacked the TAA enzyme. After the test, a battery of health-related questionnaires was completed including the main dependent measures – items assessing how serious the participants believed the enzyme deficiency to be.

Jemmott et al found that participants assigned to the low-prevalence condition perceived the deficiency to be more serious than those in the high-prevalence condition. Moreover, individuals with the supposed TAA deficiency not only rated it as less serious but were also more likely to question the validity of the test itself than those who were led to believe they did not have the deficiency. In sum, both prevalence and personal relevance influenced appraisal of the supposed health threat.

In other experiments using the TAA paradigm, Ditto and Jemmott (1989) demonstrated that perceived prevalence influenced judgments of both positive and negative health characteristics. In a pair of studies, participants were led to believe that the lack of TAA was either a *benefit* or a *detriment* to health (i.e., the deficiency made a person more/less susceptible to disease). The prevalence of the deficiency was manipulated in a manner similar to that described above. Results indicated that, as the scarcity of the condition increased, the more positive or negative the subsequent appraisals of this characteristic tended to be. Rather than simply leading to more negative appraisals of a medical condition, scarcity information had an *extremetizing* effect on appraisals. Also, participants were more likely to take informational pamphlets and sign-up for detailed medical evaluations as a function of the scarcity of the condition.

This paradigm has been used to investigate a number of other phenomena in illness cognition, including the relationships between diagnostic

status, symptom perception, and risk behaviors (see Croyle and Ditto, 1990 for a review). For example, using a similar procedure, Croyle and Sande (1988) manipulated subjects' diagnostic status. Consistent with prior results, participants who were led to believe that their test indicated a TAA deficiency rated the disorder as less serious and the test as less valid than individuals who were without the fictitious deficiency.[1,2] These results indicated that the participants were using minimization, a kind of denial of the potentially threatening diagnosis.

In the same experiment, participants also were asked to report whether they had recently experienced several common symptoms (e.g., headache, backache) or engaged in certain "risk behaviors" (e.g., use of aspirin, getting less than 7 h of sleep per night) that were purportedly related to the deficiency. Those participants who were led to believe that they lacked the TAA enzyme, and thus were supposedly at greater risk of pancreatic disorder, reported more diagnostic-consistent symptoms and behaviors than those without the deficiency. Similar results have been reported by individuals who were led to believe that they had elevated blood pressure (Baumann et al, 1989). Hence, believing that they were at risk prompted individuals to mislabel ambiguous, common sensations as signs of illness and to recall otherwise ordinary or innocuous behaviors that they believed might have placed them at risk.

The TAA paradigm permits the use of experimental manipulations to study questions about illness cognition and to draw causal inferences,

---

[1]Of note, Croyle and Sande's (1988) study took place in the exam room of a student health clinic—a conventional medical setting. Additionally, participants did not self-administer the TAA test; instead, a research assistant posing as a nurse performed the test. The fact that previous results were replicated in the context of these alterations served to underscore the validity of this experimental paradigm.

[2]Comparable procedures have been used to demonstrate that individuals likewise discount the seriousness of *actual* health disorders, namely hypertension (Croyle, 1990).

thereby improving upon descriptive, correlational methodologies. Of course, for ethical reasons it was important to disabuse participants regarding the fictitious information and feedback. To reduce potential aversiveness, the TAA deficiency was not depicted as an extremely serious condition, but described as a risk factor rather than a disease. The investigators also used a careful debriefing process (Ross et al, 1975) in which participants were first asked whether they had any questions about the study. They were then told that TAA was fictitious and the saliva test had been engineered so the test strip always changed color. Of note, only 3–5% of subjects had any suspicions about the procedure (Croyle and Ditto, 1990). Further, they were told the test actually had no bearing on their susceptibility to pancreatic disease and that the interpretation they had been given depended only on the experimental condition to which they had been randomly assigned. Only after all questions were answered and concerns were addressed were the participants permitted to leave.

2 Trier Social Stress Test (TSST) Paradigm

Both epidemiological and animal research documents the role of acute and chronic life stressors in physical illness risk (e.g., Holmes and Rahe, 1967; Lazarus and Folkman, 1984; Lovallo, 2005). A major premise of this research is that stress induces arousal of the sympathetic and hypothalamic–adrenal–pituitary axes resulting in increased neuroendocrine activity, which in turn elicits bodily changes that may have deleterious effects (e.g., Lovallo, 2005). In particular, the *reactivity hypothesis* posits that certain individuals exhibit exaggerated psychophysiological reactivity to stressors, which produces pathogenic processes that increase the risk of subsequent physical illness over time (Krantz and Manuck, 1984).

Although advances in biomedical technology have made it possible to measure ambulatory physiological reactivity such as blood pressure, heart rate, and neuroendocrine markers (Kamarck et al, 2002), uncontrolled factors routinely encountered in daily life introduce many possible sources of confounding. The study of psychophysiological responses to stress in the laboratory, where confounding variables can be minimized, has assumed a major role in identifying potential pathogenic processes that place persons at risk (Matthews et al, 1986).

In particular, psychological stress, or challenge, tests have been frequently used to assess hypothalamic–pituitary–adrenal (HPA) reactivity (e.g., salivary cortisol) in laboratory settings (see Chapter 43). Many hormones may be reliably measured in saliva and such techniques have been used extensively in psychobiological research (Kirschbaum and Hellhammer, 2000). Previous research aimed at elucidating the factors responsible for individual differences in HPA reactivity obtained mixed results (e.g., Berger et al, 1987) due, in part, to use of stressors that yielded unreliable stimulation of the HPA axis. Consequently, the Trier social stress test (TSST; Kirschbaum et al, 1993) was developed to allow for reliable stimulation of the HPA axis and subsequent measure of both physiological and psychological responses to stress in a controlled laboratory setting. The TSST has now become the "...standard protocol for the experimental induction of psychological stress in healthy participants, as well as clinical populations," (Kudielka et al, 2007, p. 57). Since numerous studies have demonstrated the reliability of the TSST to elicit physiological reactivity in healthy samples (e.g., Kirschbaum et al, 1992, 1995; Kudielka et al, 2004b), the TSST has also been used extensively in clinical populations in order to study stress-response profiles for various disorders and diseases (e.g., Bower et al, 2005; Gaab et al, 2005; Heim et al, 2000; Young et al, 2004).[3]

---

[3]For an extensive review of research in both nominally healthy and clinical samples related to the TSST paradigm, see Kudielka et al (2007).

Developed at the University of Trier, the TSST protocol induces moderate stress via a combination of psychological and social stressors. Specifically, upon arrival, each participant answers a series of questions regarding physical health and is led to a room in which a baseline saliva sample will be obtained. The participant is first asked to rest for 10 min in order to avoid potential activation of the HPA axis. After 10 min, a saliva sample is taken.

Next, the participant is escorted to another experiment room in which a 20-min period of psychosocial stress follows. The participant is told that she/he will be asked to play the role of a job applicant and deliver a speech (which will be videotaped) before a selection committee of three individuals, for which she/he will have 10 min to prepare in an adjacent room. In an effort to increase anticipatory stress, the participant is told that she/he will be evaluated on both content and style and that the committee members are trained in public speaking analysis. Further, the participant is told that any written notes generated during the preparation phase will not be allowed during the speech. After the preparation phase is over, an additional saliva sample is obtained. The participant is then led back before the committee and asked to give the speech for 5 min. Prior to the initiation of the speaking task, the participant is also informed that another unrelated task will follow the speech, but details are withheld until the completion of the speech. During the speech itself, certain nonverbal cues are presented or withheld by the committee in an effort to further increase stress, such as withholding encouraging smiles or nods and only presenting the time remaining if the participant stops before 5 min have elapsed.

Finally, upon completion of the speech, the participant is informed that she/he must complete a serial subtraction task. The task requires the participant to continuously subtract 13 from 1022 as quickly as possible.[4] To increase stress,

the participant is told that each error will result in the task starting over from 1022. After 5 min of this task, the participant is led to an adjacent room in order to obtain post-test assessments (i.e., additional saliva samples, a battery of questionnaires) and debriefing information. In essence, the TSST is an experimental social stress procedure.

Many experiments in behavioral medicine have utilized the TSST paradigm over the past decade. For example, the TSST has been used to evaluate stress reactivity in breast cancer patients and survivors. Giese-Davis and colleagues (2006) investigated the role of depression on stress reactivity in patients with metastatic breast cancer, finding that in response to challenge, depressed (vs. non-depressed) women reported increased levels of negative affect in addition to reduced high-frequency heart rate variability, a risk factor for cardiovascular disease. Both groups, however, demonstrated blunted HPA responses to challenge, suggesting that the HPA axis may be hyporesponsive in patients suffering from breast cancer.

Bower and colleagues (2005) evaluated cortisol responses to the TSST in fatigued and non-fatigued early-stage breast cancer survivors. The researchers found that women with persistent fatigue showed blunted cortisol responses after adjustment for depression and other covariates. Non-fatigued survivors, however, showed a significant increase in salivary cortisol comparable to that found in healthy individuals exposed to the TSST.

Other research has evaluated patients suffering from chronic fatigue syndrome (CFS), type I diabetes, atopic dermatitis, and individuals with elevated cardiovascular disease risk. For example, Gaab and colleagues (2005) compared cortisol and proinflammatory cytokine responses in patients with CFS versus healthy controls. They found that both groups demonstrated increased cortisol response to the TSST, but cytokine levels in those with CFS were significantly attenuated compared with controls. In type I diabetic patients, a significant delay in the decrease of glucose levels after food intake was observed post-challenge (Wiesli et al, 2005). Additionally,

---

[4]Actual numbers may vary, but primes are recommended to maximize difficulty.

adults with atopic dermatitis have been found to exhibit attenuated cortisol and ACTH responses to psychosocial stress (Buske-Kirschbaum et al, 2002a, b). Similarly, depressed adults at risk for cardiovascular disease showed a hypocortisol response to the TSST (Taylor et al, 2006).

Given the robust pattern of HPA hyperreactivity observed in response to the TSST in healthy individuals, the findings detailed above suggest that the response profiles of various patient populations may have a markedly different pattern – potentially indicating a depletion of physiological resources. Further study may help elucidate mechanisms that contribute to the relationship between stress and disease.

3 Mental Harassment in the Context of Hostility and Cardiovascular Risk

Cynical hostility, measured with various self-report measures (e.g., Cook-Medley Hostility Scale, Ho Scale; Cook and Medley, 1954), has been identified as a behavioral risk factor for the development and progression of cardiovascular disease (e.g., Chida and Steptoe, 2009; Smith, 1992), but the ways in which this psychological characteristic contribute to atherogenesis and subsequent coronary events are not well understood. The reactivity hypothesis described in the preceding section has been considered as one plausible explanation for the risk conferred by cynical hostility (e.g., Williams et al, 1985). The idea is that cynically hostile persons may respond with exaggerated cardiovascular physiological responses to provocation. If this is a common phenomenon, then heightened neuroendocrine responses may increase the risk of atherogenesis (see Chapter 13).

Although evidence from research with animal models supports this general idea (Manuck et al, 1989), cynical hostility has no direct analog in animals. Suarez and Williams (1989) developed a paradigm to test the cardiovascular effects of behavioral stress on individuals

high and low in hostility. Consequently, Suarez and colleagues (1989, 1990, 1993, 1998) initiated a series of studies using mental harassment in an attempt to isolate physiological responses directly attributable to behavioral stress.

Specifically, the paradigm involved preliminary screening of potential participants to identify individuals with high and low hostility scores (as measured using the Ho Scale). Once identified, participants were randomly assigned to harassment and non-harassment conditions involving an elaborate cover-story and deceptions. Upon arrival to the laboratory, all participants were told that the purpose of the study was to evaluate physiological responses to a mental stressor and then were asked to read and sign informed consent documents. In the harassment condition, the procedural script required that the experimenter receive a phone call during the consent process from his/her supposed supervisor, indicating that the supervisor would be unable to attend to experiment. The experimenter conveyed this information to the participants and let them know that a technician would substitute for the remainder of the protocol. Participants were then led to the experimental room and introduced to the technician, who had just been informed that she/he would have to run the experiment. Using a condescending tone, the technician then responded that she/he would "not be responsible for any problems" and that she/he would "stop the experiment if any problems occurred." The non-harassment condition utilized the same scenario except that there was no confrontation between the technician and experimenter. Participants were then led to the experiment room where they were fitted with a blood pressure cuff, electrodes, and/or a venous catheter.

After physiological data were collected over two 5-min baseline periods, participants were given instructions for the mental task, which comprised a series of five-letter anagrams presented during $3\frac{1}{2}$ min intervals. Participants were instructed to solve these anagrams after viewing them on a large projector screen and that each of the anagrams had but one correct answer. During the trials, the technician reported the time remaining every 30 seconds. As an incentive, participants were told that the individual with the highest score would receive a $25 cash prize.

This standard protocol was used in both conditions. In the harassment condition, however, participants were subjected to harassing statements during the completion of the anagram task. Specifically, the technician delivered these statements when reporting the time remaining. Statements included, "I told you these are five letter words!" "Stop mumbling, I can't understand your answers!," and "You are getting paid to be in this experiment!" Any response from the participant was ignored unless she/he requested to cease participation. Physiological data were again collected at the conclusion of the anagram task.

The studies conducted by Suarez and colleagues (1989, 1990, 1993, 1998) yielded several, consistent findings. In studies of both men and women, those who scored high in hostility and also experienced mental harassment during the anagram task consistently exhibited increased cardiovascular and/or neuroendocrine responses. For example, Suarez and colleagues (1998) demonstrated that increased (and protracted) blood pressure, heart rate, forearm blood flow, forearm vascular resistance, norepinephrine, testosterone, and cortisol responses resulted from harassment of those high in hostility. In addition, throughout the series of studies conducted by Suarez and colleagues, these same individuals also reported increased levels of negative affect including anger, anxiety, and depression. In contrast, individuals who were not harassed during the anagram task showed no increases in physiological or emotional arousal. Excessive cardiovascular reactivity has also been demonstrated in studies using similar behavioral stress paradigms such as a conflict discussion task or unsolvable anagrams, which participants were led to believe were "fairly easy" (Hardy and Smith, 1988; Smith and Allred, 1989; Weidner et al, 1989; cf. Suls and Wan, 1993).

It is noteworthy that heightened reactivity is not exhibited by hostile persons in response to stressors that do not involve interpersonal conflict. Both hostile and non-hostile persons demonstrate similar responses to mental stressors, suggesting that provocation is the key element distinguishing them.

4 Social Support in the Context of Behavioral Stress

Epidemiological studies consistently find that individuals without adequate social support are at increased risk of all-cause and cardiovascular morbidity and mortality (e.g., Berkman, 1985; Cohen, 1988; Kaplan et al, 1988; Orth-Gomer and Johnson, 1987; see Chapter 17). In contrast, individuals who are socially integrated have improved health (House et al, 1988) and, in particular, a reduced incidence or prevalence of cardiovascular disease (e.g., Medalie and Goldbourt, 1976; Seeman and Syme, 1987). Even population studies that are prospective in design, however, can only be suggestive with respect to the mechanisms by which social support confers such benefits (Uchino et al, 1996).

Laboratory experiments can be informative regarding some of the potential mechanisms, however. It has been hypothesized that social support reduces physiological responses to stress and thereby improves cardiovascular health (e.g., Cohen et al, 1994; House, 1981). Given this, several researchers have experimentally investigated the influence of social support on physiological reactivity while exposed to various laboratory stress tasks.

In this area of research, the general procedures involve the random assignment of participants to conditions in which a stressful task is completed either alone or in the presence of a partner, usually a close friend. The behavioral stressors used in this category of studies have varied with some using a combination of tasks, such as mental arithmetic, vocabulary, or concept formation tasks (Kamarck et al, 1990), and others utilizing public speaking to induce reactivity (Lepore et al, 1993). The support conditions also have varied, with some studies manipulating the effects of a close friend's presence during stress, others comparing the influence of friends versus strangers, and still others manipulating the behavior of the experimenter to further increase the level of stress. Before and after the completion of these tasks, measures of physiological reactivity (e.g., blood pressure, heart rate, impedance cardiography) were taken and questionnaires completed.

Kamarck et al (1990) initiated one of the first studies to experimentally investigate the effects of social support on cardiovascular reactivity. Their study randomly assigned participants to "friend" and "alone" conditions. After a series of baseline assessments, participants were asked to complete mental arithmetic and concept formation tasks, either alone or in the presence of a close, same-sex friend. The friend was given specific instructions to silently support the partner, touch the partner's wrist throughout the testing period, and take care not to interrupt or distract the partner. Additionally, the friend was given a set of questionnaires to complete during the tasks in order to control the interaction between the individuals. Kamarck and colleagues found that individuals in the presence of a supportive friend exhibited lower heart rate and blood pressure reactions to the stressors.

Lepore and colleagues (1993) conducted a similar study using a speech task as the behavioral stressor. However, these researchers used slightly different support conditions. In addition to the "alone" condition, participants were randomly assigned to give a speech in the presence of a same-sex *supportive* or *non-supportive* confederate. Support behaviors included reassuring comments ("Remember, it will all be over in a few minutes.") and compliments ("You did fine."), in addition to non-verbal gestures such as smiles and an open-body posture. The non-supportive condition included neutral behaviors and actual interaction was minimal. Lepore et al found that participants who delivered a speech in the presence of a supportive partner had significantly less reactivity (as measured via systolic and diastolic blood pressure) than those who gave a speech in the presence of a non-supportive partner. The same was true when supported participants were compared with those

in the alone condition. A study by Christenfeld and colleagues (1997) also found that individuals delivering a speech in the presence of a friend or supportive stranger exhibited significantly less cardiovascular reactivity when compared with those giving a speech in the presence of a neutral stranger.

Kamarck et al (1995) went a step further by manipulating the behavior of the experimenter, adding an aspect of social threat during the completion of the tasks. Specifically, in the high-threat condition, the experimenter was formally dressed, introduced himself using his title, and gave instructions in a loud, inpatient manner. Additionally, participants were explicitly reminded of the experimenter's presence during the mental stressors. In the low-threat condition, the experimenter was informally dressed, introduced himself using his first name, and gave instructions using a normal tone. Kamarck et al found that, under conditions of high social threat, the presence of a close friend resulted in lower cardiovascular reactivity in response to mental challenge. Similarly, Kors et al (1997) manipulated social threat by assigning participants to conditions in which a close friend was more or less evaluative of the participant's performance. Results indicated attenuated reactivity during a mental arithmetic task, but only for participants whose friend was non-evaluative.[5]

By manipulating stress and type of support while measuring physiological parameters, it was possible to detect stress-buffering effects. Only lab experiments allow for this kind of control of theory-driven factors and extraneous variables in order to identify the social support effects suggested by descriptive epidemiological research studies.

---

[5]Although the studies summarized here primarily demonstrated the protective effects of social support, the evidence is somewhat mixed as others have reported that the presence of a friend or supportive other can increase reactivity and hinder performance (e.g., Allen et al, 1991) or does not differ from those tested alone (Sheffield and Carroll, 1994). See Uchino et al, 1996 for a more detailed review.

5 Experimental Research on Advanced Directives

Experimental methods have also helped to increase understanding of the use of advanced directives, or living wills, for end-of-life care. As advocated by the American Medical Association (Orentlicher, 1990) and other prominent health-related organizations (e.g., American Geriatrics Society, 1991), advanced directives (AD) – which are legally recognized in all 50 states and the District of Columbia (The Patient Self-Determination Act, 1990) – allow individuals to make explicit their preferences for treatment and care given the event of serious illness and, therefore, provide some control if situations arise in which the individual is otherwise incapable of making such preferences known.

The use of such instruments assumes, however, that ADs improve the ability of a surrogate decision-maker to substitute judgment on behalf of the patient. Indeed, numerous studies have reported that, without ADs, the ability of family members and healthcare providers to accurately predict treatment-related preferences is very poor (e.g., Ouslander et al, 1989; Seckler et al, 1991). But research had not evaluated whether discussion of ADs between patients and proxies improves the accuracy of substituted judgment. Ditto and colleagues (2001) developed an experimental paradigm to study the agreement between patients and surrogates for different illness scenarios.

Specifically, a randomized clinical trial (The Advance Directives, Values Assessment, and Communication Enhancement project, ADVANCE) was undertaken. The distinctive feature of ADVANCE was that it manipulated the nature of discussion between the relevant parties. Previous work on ADs has tended to be descriptive and correlational, so it was not possible to draw causal inferences about what factors influence the accuracy or effects of ADs. The trial recruited patients who were 65 years or older from primary care facilities. Potential participants were randomly selected to receive a letter from their healthcare provider inviting

them to participate. The study entailed three 1–2 h interviews over 24 months and the participation of a surrogate decision-maker; if the patient was hospitalized, additional interviews were required.

Participants and their surrogates were randomized to one of five experimental conditions. In the control condition, patients and surrogates had no contact beyond the informed consent process, nor were any AD documents completed. There were two "no-discussion" conditions in which the patients and surrogates were separated after consent, but the patient completed a series of AD documents. Finally, two "discussion" conditions required that patients complete the AD documents in the presence of the surrogate. A trained interviewer then facilitated questions and discussion between the two parties via a series of structured prompts. The primary outcome, accuracy of substituted judgment, was measured using the Life-Support Preferences/Predictions Questionnaire (LSPQ; Coppola et al, 1999), which presents nine different illness scenarios intended to capture a range of potential conditions of varying severity such as coma, stroke, and cancer scenarios.

Surprisingly, none of the intervention conditions improved accuracy between patients and their surrogates, but the discussion conditions did increase perceived understanding and comfort for those without a previous AD. Ditto and colleagues have also used similar, quasi-experimental designs to further investigate judgments related to end-of-life care (e.g., Coppola et al, 2001).

Thus, even surrogates provided with an instructional AD completed by a patient were no more accurate in their predictions of that patient's life-sustaining preferences than surrogates making predictions without a patient-completed directive. This was the case even when the surrogate discussed the directive with the patient prior to the prediction task.

Fagerlin and colleagues (2001) conducted research to further investigate such inaccuracies. Based on social psychological research on interpersonal perception, they measured surrogates' own treatment preferences and compared them to their predictions of patients' preferences. In one study, a sample of older adult patients was asked to designate the individual that they would want to make medical decisions on their behalf – most often spouses or adult children – and this person was also recruited to participate. Next, all patient participants were asked to complete treatment preferences for themselves. Surrogate participants were asked to also complete treatment preferences for themselves and then make predictions regarding the patient's preferences.

In addition to finding an "overtreatment" bias (i.e., surrogates overpredicted the patient's desire for treatment in several illness scenarios), surrogates' decisions about life-sustaining medical treatments were strongly associated with their personal treatment wishes and this helped to account for inaccuracy between the parties. Although these results may seem surprising, they actually are quite consistent with a standard social normative bias, the false consensus effect, whereby people overestimate the extent to which their own opinions and behavioral choices are shared by others (Ross et al, 1977; Krueger and Clement, 1997).

Medical ethicists, policy makers, and the medical community maintain that when patients do not have decisional capacity, medical decisions should be based on the standard of substituted judgment (Baergen, 1995). The research of Ditto, Fagerlin, and their associates demonstrate that this policy is uninformed by basic social psychological research on interpersonal perception. In other words, this means that the surrogate decision maker will encounter difficulties in trying to honor the wishes of the incapacitated patient. There is cause for optimism, however, because there are psychological strategies that increase the accuracy of social judgments (Funder, 1995). It remains for researchers to test the effects of these manipulations on the accuracy of ADs.

6 Conclusions

As described in this chapter, experimental approaches to social interaction in health psychology and behavioral medicine typically involve elaborate cover stories, scripts, and sometimes deception. At its best, it takes the form of experimental theater in which researchers adopt the roles of producer, director, and actor. With such methods, social factors can be manipulated under controlled circumstances to identify and elucidate causal relationships as well as develop and test theories. In many cases, results based on experimental methods may help to explain findings from epidemiological and intervention research where mechanisms can only be inferred. Further, these approaches may identify novel relationships and explore speculative causal directions, which may not be feasible to test in patients or the broader medical setting without preliminary supportive evidence. The strengths of such methods are a major reason why the subdiscipline of social-health psychology has been growing steadily over the past several years (e.g., Suls and Wallston, 2003).

Of course, these methods comprise only a few of the tools available to the behavioral medicine researcher. The biopsychosocial model requires the collaboration of biological, psychological, and other social scientists and practitioners (Suls and Rothman, 2004), with all parties bringing their respective methods of inquiry to the table. As such, the experimental methods discussed here should be considered as much a part of the behavioral medicine toolbox as clinical assessments, medical indices, advanced biostatistical procedures, and behavioral interventions.

References

Allen, K. M., Blascovich, J., Tomaka, J., and Kelsey, R. M. (1991). Presence of human friends and pet dogs as moderators of autonomic responses to stress in women. *J Pers Soc Psychol, 61*, 582–589.

American Geriatrics Society Public Policy Committee (1991). *AGS Position Statement: Medical Treatment Decisions Concerning Elderly Persons*. New York: American Geriatrics Society.

Baergen, R. (1995). Revising the substituted judgment standard. *J Clin Ethics, 6*, 30–38.

Baumann, L. J., Cameron, L. D., Zimmerman, R. S., and Leventhal, H. (1989). Illness representations and matching labels with symptoms. *Health Psychol, 8,* 449–469.

Berger, M., Bossert, S., Krieg, J. C., Dirlich, G., Ettmeier, W., Schreiber, W. et al (1987). Interindividual differences in the susceptibility of the cortisol system: an important factor for the degree of hypercortisolism in stress situations? *Biol Psychiatry, 22,* 1327–1339.

Berkman, L. F. (1985). The relationship of social networks and social support to morbidity and mortality. In S. Cohen & S. L. Syme (Eds.), *Social Support and Health* (pp. 241–262). Orlando, FL: Academic Press.

Bower, J. E., Ganz, P. A., and Aziz, N. (2005). Altered cortisol response to psychologic stress in breast cancer survivors with persistent fatigue. *Psychosom Med, 67,* 277–280.

Buske-Kirschbaum, A., Geiben, A., Hollig, H., Morschhauser, E., and Hellhammer, D. (2002a). Altered responsiveness of the hypothalamus-pituitary-adrenal axis and the sympathetic adrenomedullary system to stress in patients with atopic dermatitis. *J Clin Endocrinol Metab, 87,* 4245–4251.

Buske-Kirschbaum, A., Gierens, A., Hollig, H., and Hellhammer, D. H. (2002b). Stress-induced immunomodulation is altered in patients with atopic dermatitis. *J Neuroimmunol, 129,* 161–167.

Carlsmith, J. M., Ellsworth, P. C., and Aronson, E. (1976). *Methods of Research in Social Psychology.* Reading, MA: Addison-Wesley.

Chida, Y., and Steptoe, A. (2009). The association of anger and hostility with future coronary heart disease: a meta-analytic review of prospective evidence. *J Am Coll Cardiol, 53,* 936–946.

Christenfeld, N., Gerin, W., Linden, W., Sanders, M., Mathur, J. et al (1997). Social support effects on cardiovascular reactivity: is a stranger as effective as a friend? *Psychosom Med, 59,* 388–398.

Cohen, S. (1988). Psychosocial models of the role of social support in the etiology of physical disease. *Health Psychol, 7,* 269–297.

Cohen, S., Kaplan, J. R., and Manuck, S. B. (1994). Social support and coronary heart disease: underlying psychologic & biologic mechanisms. In S. A. Shumaker & S. M. Czajkowski (Eds.), *Social Support and Cardiovascular Disease.* New York: Plenum.

Coppola, K. M., Bookwala, J., Ditto, P. H., Lockhart, L. K., Danks, J. H. et al (1999). Elderly adults' preferences for life-sustaining treatments: the role of impairment, prognosis, and pain. *Death Stud, 23,* 617–634.

Coppola, K. M., Ditto, P. H., Danks, J. H., and Smucker, W. D. (2001). Accuracy of primary care and hospital-based physicians' predictions of elderly outpatients' treatment preferences with and without advance directives. *Arch Intern Med, 161,* 431–440.

Cook, W. W., and Medley, D. M. (1954). Proposed hostility and pharisaic-virtue for the MMPI. *J Appl Psychol, 38,* 414–418.

Croog, S. H., Shapiro, D. S., and Levine, S. (1971). Denial among heart patients. *Psychosom Med, 33,* 385–397.

Croyle, R. T. (1990). Biased appraisal of high blood pressure. *Prev Med, 19,* 40–44.

Croyle, R. T., and Ditto, P. H. (1990). Illness cognition and behavior: an experimental approach. *J Behav Med, 13,* 31–52.

Croyle, R. T., and Sande, G. N. (1988). Denial and confirmatory search: paradoxical consequences of medical diagnosis. *J Appl Soc Psychol, 18,* 473–490.

Ditto, P. H., Danks, J. H., Smucker, W. D., Bookwala, J., Coppola, K. M. et al (2001). Advanced directives as acts of communication. *Arch Intern Med, 161,* 421–430.

Ditto, P. H., and Jemmott, J. B. (1989). From rarity to evaluative extremity: effects of prevalence information on the evaluation of positive and negative characteristics. *J Pers Soc Psychol, 57,* 16–26.

Fagerlin, A., Ditto, P. H., Danks, J. H., Houts, R. M., and Smucker, W. M. (2001). Projection in surrogate decisions about life-sustaining medical treatments. *Health Psychol, 20,* 166–175.

Festinger, L. (1953). Laboratory experiments. In L. Festinger & D. Katz (Eds.), *Research Methods in the Behavioral Sciences* (pp. 136–172). New York: Dryden Press.

Funder, D. C. (1995). On the accuracy of personality judgment: a realistic approach. *Psychol Rev, 102,* 652–670.

Gaab, J., Rohleder, N., Heitz, V., Engert, V., Schad, T. et al (2005). Stress-induced changes in LPS-induced pro-inflammatory cytokine production in chronic fatigue syndrome. *Psychoneuroendocrinology, 30,* 188–98.

Giese-Davis, J., Wilhelm, F. H., Conrad, A., Abercrombie, H. C., Sephton, S. et al (2006). Depression and stress reactivity in metastatic breast cancer. *Psychosom Med, 68,* 675–683.

Glass, D. (1977). *Behavior Patterns, Stress, and Coronary Disease.* Hillsdale, NJ: Erlbaum.

Hardy, J. H., and Smith, T. W. (1988). Cynical hostility and vulnerability to disease: social support, life stress, and physiological response to conflict. *Health Psychol, 7,* 447–459.

Heim, C., Newport, D. J., Heit, S., Graham, Y. P., Wilcox, M. et al (2000). Pituitary-adrenal and autonomic responses to stress in women after sexual and physical abuse in childhood. *JAMA, 284,* 592–597.

Holmes, T. H., and Rahe, R. H. (1967). The Social Readjustment Rating Scale. *J Psychosom Res, 11,* 213–218.

House, J. S. (1981). *Work Stress and Social Support.* Reading, MA: Addison-Wesley.

House, J. S., Landis, K. R., and Umberson, D. (1988). Social relationships and health. *Science, 241,* 540–545.

Jemmott, J. B., Ditto, P. H., and Croyle, R. T. (1986). Judging health status: effects of perceived prevalence and personal relevance. *J Pers Soc Psychol, 50*, 899–905.

Kamarck, T., Annunziato, B., and Amateau, L. M. (1995). Affiliation moderates the effects of social threat on stress-related cardiovascular responses: boundary conditions for a laboratory model of social support. *Psychosom Med, 57*, 183–194.

Kamarck, T. W., Janicki, D. L.; Shiffman, S., Polk, D., Muldoon, M. F. et al (2002). Psychosocial demands and ambulatory blood pressure: a field assessment approach. *Physiol Behav, 77*, 699–704.

Kamarck, T. W., Manuck, S. B., and Jennings, J. R. (1990). Social support reduces cardiovascular reactivity to psychological challenge: a laboratory model. *Psychosom Med, 52*, 42–58.

Kaplan, G., Salonen, J., Cohen, R., Brand, R., Syme, L. et al (1988). Social connections and mortality from all causes and from cardiovascular disease: prospective evidence from Eastern Finland. *Am J Epidemiol, 128*, 370–380.

Kirschbaum, C., and Hellhammer, D. (2000). *The John D. and Catherine T. MacArthur Research Network on Socioeconomic Status and Health: Salivary Cortisol and Challenge Tests*. Retrieved April 1st, 2009, from http://www.macses.ucsf.edu/Research/Allostatic/notebook/challenge.html.

Kirschbaum, C., Pirke, K. M., and Hellhammer, D. H. (1993). The 'Trier Social Stress Test'—a tool for investigating psychobiological stress responses in a laboratory setting. *Neuropsychobiology, 28*, 76–81.

Kirschbaum, C., Prüssner, J., Gaab, J., Schommer, N., Lintz, D. et al (1995). Persistent high cortisol responses to repeated psychological stress in a subpopulation of healthy men. *Psychosom Med, 57*, 468–474.

Kirschbaum, C., Wüst, S., and Hellhammer, D. H. (1992). Consistent sex differences in cortisol responses to psychological stress. *Psychosom Med, 54*, 648–657.

Kors, D. J., Linden, W., and Gerin, W. (1997). Evaluation interferes with social support: effects on cardiovascular stress reactivity in women. *J Soc Clin Psychol, 16*, 1–23.

Krantz, D. S., and Manuck, S. B. (1984). Acute psychophysiological reactivity and risk of cardiovascular disease: A review and methodologic critique. *Psychological Bulletin, 96*, 435–464.

Krueger, J., and Clement, R. W. (1997). Estimates of social consensus by majorities and minorities: the case of social perception. *Pers Soc Psychol Rev, 1*, 299–313.

Kudielka, B. M., Buske-Kirschbaum, A., Hellhammer, D. H., and Kirschbaum, C. (2004b). HPA axis responses to laboratory psychosocial stress in healthy elderly adults, younger adults, and children: impact of age and gender. *Psychoneuroendocrinology, 29*, 83–98.

Kudielka, B. M., Hellhammer, D. H., Kirschbaum, C. (2007). Ten years of research with the Trier Social Tress Test-revisited. In E. Harmon-Jones & P. Winkielman (Eds.), *Social neuroscience: Integrating biological and psychological explanations of social behavior* (pp. 56–83). New York: Guilford Press.

Lazarus, R. S., and Folkman, S. (1984). *Stress, Appraisal, and Coping*. New York: Springer.

Lepore, S. J., Mata, K. A., and Evans, G. W. (1993). Social support lowers cardiovascular reactivity to an acute stressor. *Psychosom Med, 55*, 518–524.

Lovallo, W. R. (2005). *Stress and Health: Biological and Psychological Interactions, 2nd Ed*. Thousand Oaks, CA: Sage Publications.

Manuck, S. B., Muldoon, M. F., Kaplan, J. R., Adams, M. R., and Polefrone, J. M. (1989). Coronary artery atherosclerosis and cardiac response to stress in cynomolgus monkeys. In A. W. Siegman & T. M. Dembroski (Eds.), *In Search of Coronary-Prone Behavior* (pp. 207–228). Hillsdale, NJ: Erlbaum.

Matthews, K. A. et al (Eds.). (1986). *Handbook of Stress, Reactivity and Cardiovascular Disease*. New York: Wiley.

Mechanic, D. (1972). Social psychologic factors affecting the presentation of bodily complaints. *N Engl J Med, 286*, 1132–1139.

Medalie, J. H., and Goldbourt, U. (1976). Angina pectoris among 10,000 men: II. Psychosocial and other risk factors as evidenced by multivariate analysis of a five-year incidence study. *Am J Med, 60*, 910–919.

Orentlicher, D. (1990). Advance medical directives. *JAMA, 263*, 2365–2367.

Orth-Gomer, K., and Johnson, J. (1987). Social network interaction and mortality: a six-year follow-up study of a random sample of the Swedish population. *J Chronic Dis, 40*, 949–957.

Ouslander, J. G., Tymchuk, A. J., and Rahbar, B. (1989). Health care decisions among elderly long-term residents and their potential proxies. *Arch Intern Med, 149*, 1367–1372.

Ross, L., Greene, D., and House, P. (1977). The "false consensus effect": an egocentric bias in social perception and attribution processes. *J Exp Soc Psychol, 13*, 279–301.

Ross, L., Lepper, M., and Hubbard, M. (1975). Perseverance in self perception and social perception: biased attributional processes in the debriefing paradigm. *J Pers Soc Psychol, 32*, 880–892.

Schachter, S. (1971a). *Emotion, Obesity, and Crime*. New York: Academic Press.

Schachter, S. (1971b). Some extraordinary facts about obese humans and rats. *Am Psychol, 26*, 129–144.

Seckler, A. B., Meier, D. E., Mulvihill, M., and Cammer-Paris, B. E. (1991). Substituted judgment: how accurate are proxy predictors? *Ann Intern Med, 115*, 92–98.

Seeman, T. E., and Syme, S. L. (1987). Social networks and coronary artery disease: a comparison of the structure and function of social relations as predictors of disease. *Psychosom Med, 49*, 341–354.

Sheffield, D., and Carroll, D. (1994). Social support and cardiovascular reactions to active laboratory stressors. *Psychol Health, 9*, 305–316.

Smith, T. W. (1992). Hostility and health: current status of a psychosomatic hypothesis. *Health Psychol, 11*, 139–150.

Smith, T. W., and Allred, K. D. (1989). Blood pressure reactivity during social interaction in high and low cynical hostile men. *J Behav Med, 11*, 135–143.

Suarez, E. C., Harlan, E., Peoples, M. C., and Williams, R. B. (1993). Cardiovascular and emotional responses in women: the role of hostility and harassment. *Health Psychol, 12*, 459–468.

Suarez, E. C., Kuhn, C. M., Schanberg, S. M., Williams, R. B., and Zimmerman, E. A. (1998). Neuroendocrine, cardiovascular, and emotional responses of hostile men: the role of interpersonal challenge. *Psychosom Med, 60*, 78–88.

Suarez, E. C., and Williams, R. B. (1989). Situational determinants of cardiovascular and emotional reactivity in high and low hostile men. *Psychosom Med, 51*, 404–418.

Suarez, E. C., and Williams, R. B. (1990). The relationships between dimensions of hostility and cardiovascular reactivity as a function of task characteristics. *Psychosom Med, 52*, 558–570.

Suls, J., and Rothman, A. (2004). Evolution of the biopsychosocial model: prospects and challenges. *Health Psychol, 23*, 119–125.

Suls, J., and Wallston, K. A. (Eds.). (2003). *Social Psychological Foundations of Health and Illness*. Malden, MA: Blackwell Publishing.

Suls, J., and Wan, C. K. (1993). The relationship between trait hostility and cardiovascular reactivity: a quantitative review and analysis. *Psychophysiology, 30*, 615–626.

Taylor, C. B., Conrad, A., Wilhelm, F. H., Neri, E., DeLorenzo, A. et al (2006). Psychophysiological and cortisol responses to psychological stress in depressed and nondepressed older men and women with elevated cardiovascular disease risk. *Psychosom Med, 68*, 538–546.

Taylor, S. E., Lichtman, R. R., and Wood, J. V. (1984). Attributions, beliefs about control, and adjustment to breast cancer. *J Pers Soc Psychol, 46*, 489–502.

Uchino, B. N., Cacioppo, J. T., and Kiecolt-Glaser, J. K. (1996). The relationship between social support and physiological processes. A review with emphasis on underlying mechanisms and implications for health. *Psychol Bull, 119*, 488–531.

Weidner, G., Friend, R., Ficarrotto, T. J., and Mendell, N. R. (1989). Hostility and cardiovascular reactivity to stress in women and men. *Psychosom Med, 51*, 36–45.

Wiesli, P., Schmid, C., Kerwer, O., Nigg-Koch, C., Klaghofer, R. et al (2005). Acute psychological stress affects glucose concentrations in patients with type 1 diabetes following food intake but not in the fasting state. *Diabetes Care, 28*, 1910–1915.

Williams, R. B., Barefoot, J. C., and Shekelle, R. B. (1985). The health consequences of hostility. In M. A. Chesney & R. H. Rosenman (Eds.), *Anger and Hostility in Cardiovascular and Behavioral Disorders* (pp. 173–186). Washington, DC: Hemishpere.

Young, E. A., Abelson, J. L., and Cameron, O. G. (2004). Effect of comorbid anxiety disorders on the hypothalamic-pituitary-adrenal axis response to a social stressor in major depression. *Biol Psychiatry, 56*, 113–120.

Zola, I. K. (1966). Culture and symptoms—an analysis of patients' presenting complaints. *Am Sociol Rev, 31*, 615–630.

Chapter 17

Social Support and Physical Health: Links and Mechanisms

Tara L. Gruenewald and Teresa E. Seeman

1 Social Support and Health

For centuries, theorists and philosophers have postulated that social relationships are important determinants of health and well-being. Widespread scientific interest in the role of social relationships and health was kindled in the latter part of the 20th century by epidemiological investigations which documented that level of social integration, measured as number of social relationships and connections to social groups, prospectively predicted morbidity and mortality outcomes (see House et al, 1988, for review; see also Ikeda and Kawachi, this volume). Interest in social relationships as determinants of health was further flamed by the fact that the magnitude of the relationship between social integration and mortality was comparable to standard risk factors, such as smoking and a sedentary lifestyle. As epidemiological evidence mounted that greater social integration was associated with better health outcomes, attention shifted toward understanding the mechanisms through which the social environment affects physical health. In two early reviews, Cobb (1976) and Cassell (1976) argued that *supportive* aspects of social ties were important components of the salubrious impact of social integration and activity. As we review below, a large and growing body of evidence supports the hypothesis that not only the existence of social connections but also the *supportive qualities* of social relationships are linked to physical health outcomes, such as disease morbidity and mortality, and considerable effort is being devoted to understanding the behavioral, psychosocial, and biological pathways that underlie these links.

2 Social Support: Definitions and Measurement

The supportive functions of social ties, typically referred to as *social support*, can be differentiated from structural aspects of social relationships, such as number and type of social ties. The term social support is sometimes used to refer to both structural and functional characteristics; however, as our focus is on the potential health benefits of *supportive functions* of social relationships, we will use the term social support to refer to specific functions performed by network ties and will examine the health correlates of such functions in this review. Relationships can provide a wide array of support functions, but a common formulation divides support functions into three main types: *emotional support*, which is the perceived availability or receipt of indications of caring and acceptance from a support target or the sharing of thoughts and emotions with a support target; *informational support*, which includes perceived availability or receipt of knowledge or information from a

T.L. Gruenewald (✉)
Department of Medicine, Division of Geriatrics, UCLA School of Medicine, 10945 Le Conte Avenue, Suite 2339, Los Angeles, CA 90095-1687, USA
e-mail: tgruenewald@mednet.ucla.edu

A. Steptoe (ed.), *Handbook of Behavioral Medicine*, DOI 10.1007/978-0-387-09488-5_17,
© Springer Science+Business Media, LLC 2010

support target; and *instrumental/tangible support*, which includes perceived availability or receipt of goods, resources, and practical help in addressing a need/problem. Other forms of support that have been defined in the literature include support functions that provide companionship or a feeling of intimacy, enhance self-esteem, provide validation or reassurance of worth, or provide opportunities for nurturance. A number of self-report instruments are available which measure one or more of these support functions (see Wills and Shinar, 2000).

In addition to differentiating among types of support functions, a distinction can also be made between perceptions of support availability and actual receipt of support from social targets, what is often referred to as a distinction between *perceived* and *received* or *enacted* support (Barrera, 1986). Dunkel-Schetter and Bennett (1990) have argued that this difference can also be conceptualized as the *cognitive* versus *behavioral* components of social support, that is, a distinction between individuals' cognitions about support availability and the actual interpersonal transactions and exchanges that occur in the giving and receiving of support. Interestingly, only a moderate correspondence between perceived and received support has been found in studies that have measured both forms (Haber et al, 2007). The weight of the evidence suggests that *perceptions* of support may be more important for well-being than actual support receipt, but support receipt is less often measured in health research, perhaps due to the challenge of measuring specific support transactions. Thus, it may be premature to conclude that perceived support is more strongly linked to physical well-being than received support.

The scientific literature on social support and health has predominantly focused on the perceived availability or receipt of support *from* others; relatively little attention has been given to the potential health benefits of providing support *to* others. However, as we review below, evidence is accumulating that giving support may be as beneficial to health as receiving support. Of course, there exist potential negative

aspects of support provision; support expectations or expenditures can be sources of felt demands and burdens, chronic stress can take a toll on support networks, and relationship conflicts may arise when mismatches occur between expected and enacted support among support targets and providers (see Dunkel-Schetter and Bennett, 1990, for a review). The importance of attending to the interpersonal nature of social support, including exchange transactions and the relationship context within which support occurs, has also been noted (e.g., Shumaker and Brownell, 1984), but there is little research on the health correlates of such characteristics.

Another aspect to consider in the measurement of social support is the *source* of supportive functions. Social support measures vary in the degree of detail collected regarding level and type of support provided by different sources (e.g., intimate partner, family members, friends, co-workers), but often global or average scores that ignore specific sources or divide sources into broad categories (e.g., family versus friends) are used in health research. Although differential health benefits have been found for the *presence* of different types of social ties (e.g., marital, friends, group membership; e.g., Giles et al, 2005), less information is available on the health impact of support from different sources. We should also note that support from paid professionals (e.g., therapists, physicians) may be conducive to health, but we focus solely on support from targets within individuals' natural social networks in this review.

3 Social Support: Links to Physical Health Outcomes

A sizable body of research documents that perceived availability of, as well as actual receipt of, support from others is positively associated with psychological well-being (see Cohen and Wills, 1985; Kawachi and Berkman, 2001, for reviews). The literature on links to physical health outcomes is considerably smaller, but a solid evidence base which supports connections between social support and morbidity and mortality outcomes is emerging. Similar to research findings for social integration, greater social support, particularly greater perceived availability of emotional support, is related to lower risk for mortality in both community samples (e.g., Berkman et al, 1992; Blazer, 1982; Hanson et al, 1989; Lyyra and Heikkinen, 2006; Orth-Gomer et al, 1993) and specific patient populations (e.g., Brummett et al, 2005). However, such links are not always observed (Walter-Ginzburg et al, 2002) and inverse associations have also been documented (e.g., Birditt and Antonucci, 2008).

Social support has also been examined as a predictor of disease onset and/or progression. Within the domain of heart disease, greater emotional and instrumental support have been linked to more favorable cardiovascular outcomes, including slower progression of coronary atherosclerosis and lower likelihood of fatal and non-fatal cardiovascular events (e.g., Angerer et al, 2000; Krumholz et al, 1998; Seeman and Syme, 1987; Wang et al, 2005; Woloshin et al, 1997), with some evidence of stronger associations for functional as compared to structural relationship measures in studies assessing both forms (e.g., Seeman and Syme,1987). Greater perceived support, especially perceived availability of emotional support, has also been found to predict lower mortality risk among women with breast cancer in some studies (see Falagas et al, 2007, for review). During pregnancy, greater perceived and received social support are linked to fewer labor complications and better birth outcomes in newborns, such as higher birth weight (Collins et al, 1993; Feldman et al, 2000). At the other end of the lifespan, higher levels of emotional support predict better cognitive and physical functioning in older adults (Seeman et al, 1995; 2001), but greater levels of instrumental support are often associated with higher levels of disability cross-sectionally and prospectively (e.g., Mendes de Leon et al, 2001; Seeman et al, 1996), which may indicate greater need for assistance, or negative impact of receipt assistance on feelings of self-efficacy and

control, constructs thought to affect functional ability over time.

One neglected aspect of the study of social support in relation to health is the study of potential health benefits of *support provision*. Brown and colleagues (2003) found that the provision of instrumental and emotional support was associated with lower mortality risk over a 5-year period in a sample of community-dwelling older adults. Interestingly, associations between support receipt and mortality risk were no longer significant when taking into account support provision. Sato and colleagues (2008) also found that the provision of instrumental support was associated with lower mortality risk in older men over a 12-year follow-up, although this association was not observed in women. A growing body of research also indicates that feeling useful to others is associated with lower risk of disability and mortality in older adulthood (e.g., Gruenewald et al, 2007; Okamoto and Tanaka, 2004). Such findings indicate that the salubrious impact of helping and providing for others may be an important target for future health research, especially in older adult populations.

The other qualitative aspects of social relationships that have not received much attention in the study of health are the health impacts of negative relationship characteristics, such as relationships characterized by conflicts, demands, criticism, and rejection. A number of theorists have suggested that negative aspects of relationships may be as or even more influential to health and well-being as compared to the positive, supportive qualities of relationships (e.g., Coyne and Bolger, 1990; Rook, 1984). A growing body of research provides support for this hypothesis in the study of psychological distress (e.g., Ingersoll-Dayton et al, 1997; Newsom et al, 2005) and research is emerging that links negative relationship qualities to physical health, as well. A study by Krause (2005) indicated that greater perceived frequency of criticism, prying, demands, and being taken advantage of by network members, was associated with greater risk of heart disease in older adults of low, but not high, socioeconomic status. Birditt and Antonucci (2008) found that increases in negativity in relationships with spouses and children over a 3-year period predicted greater mortality risk over a 16-year follow-up. Consistent with previous research, these authors also found that consistently low levels of support were associated with greater mortality risk, but associations between positive relationship qualities (e.g., increased love from spouse, consistently high love from friends/relatives) and mortality hazard were also observed, highlighting the complex nature of associations between support and health that may emerge when considering both positive and negative relationship qualities, different support sources, and change in these characteristics over time. An interesting topic for future research is the health consequences of the relative balance of positive and negative relationship characteristics.

3.1 Direct Versus Buffering Effects of Social Support on Health

There are two dominant hypotheses regarding how social support may act to benefit health. The direct effects model asserts that perceived availability or receipt of social support has a direct effect on health, while the stress-buffering model posits that support is salutogenic within the context of stressor experience. In both conceptualizations, social support is thought to affect psychological, behavioral, or biological processes that, in turn, render one more or less susceptible to disease and illness. However, the stress-buffering model suggests that social support will have an impact on health primarily by reducing ("buffering" against) the negative effects of life stress, while the direct effects model suggests that social support is beneficial even outside of stressor experience (see Cohen and Wills, 1985, for review).

A significant research effort has been devoted to understanding whether social support benefits mental and physical well-being through a direct or buffering process. A comprehensive review of investigations comparing the two models in studies of psychological distress by Cohen and Wills (1985) indicated that perceived availability of

social support primarily played a buffering role, while structural aspects, such as level of social integration, had a direct association with psychological symptomatology (see also Kawachi and Berkman, 2001). There are few studies that have carefully compared whether supportive qualities of relationships work through direct or buffering routes to affect physical health. A small number of studies that have assessed both direct and buffering roles support both pathways; mortality risk is greater in individuals experiencing life stress who also suffer from low levels of social support, but impoverished levels of support also predict mortality risk directly (Falk et al, 1992; Rosengren et al, 1993). Additional research comparing buffering and direct effects of both functional and structural aspects of social ties in the prediction of physical health outcomes is needed.

4 Social Support and Health: Pathways

Armed with a burgeoning body of evidence linking social support to physical health outcomes, researchers have turned to understanding the pathways through which supportive functions of social relationships may influence health. Most conceptual models identify psychological, behavioral, and physiological processes as underlying pathways through which supportive qualities of relationships affect physical well-being (e.g., Cohen, 2004; House et al, 1988; Uchino et al, 1996). Although each of these pathways may operate independently to link social support to physical health, it is also likely that these processes are influenced by, and interact with, each other to mediate associations between social support and health.

4.1 Psychological Pathways

Social support may impact psychological states and perceptions in both a direct and a stress-buffering fashion. The perceived availability or enacted experience of support and companion-ship from others in one's network is thought to promote general feelings of esteem, inti-macy, belongingness, self-efficacy, control, and a sense of life meaning and purpose (Cohen and Wills, 1985; Uchino, 2006). These psycho-logical states, in turn, are thought to promote better mental and physical well-being directly or indirectly via positive influences on engage-ment in health-promoting behaviors and more positive physiological states. The belief that oth-ers would provide support when needed is also thought to play a key role in stress appraisal pro-cesses, such that an individual will be less likely to appraise a stimulus as a potential threat alto-gether, or will perceive a lower overall level of threat, to the extent that perceptions of avail-able support bolster an individual's perceptions of being able to cope with, or minimize the harm of, a stressor (Cohen and Wills, 1985). Over time, less adverse psychological, behavioral, and physiological responses to potential stressors as a result of such appraisals are thought to limit risks for disease development. As previously noted, a large body of evidence suggests that social support can buffer against the adverse psy-chological impacts of stress (Cohen and Wills, 1985), as well as enable more positive adjust-ment to chronic illness (Helgeson and Cohen, 1996).

4.2 Behavioral Pathways

The importance of social support in the adoption and maintenance of health-promoting behaviors and the avoidance of health-damaging behaviors have long been noted (see Burg and Seeman, 1994; Campbell, 2003). Social support may be especially beneficial to successful management of chronic disease conditions. A meta-analytic review of over 100 studies by DiMatteo (2004) indicated that instrumental, emotional, and uni-dimensional (i.e., aggregate measure) support are associated with better adherence to medical regimens with instrumental support exhibiting the strongest association; the risk of nonad-herence is twice as great in those not receiv-ing instrumental support as compared to those

receiving such support. Adherence is also better in patients from cohesive families and worse in patients from families characterized by conflict, highlighting the important influence of both pos-itive and negative relationship qualities on health behavior. Although structural characteristics of relationships are correlated with adherence, social support characteristics are more strongly associated with adherence behavior (DiMatteo, 2004), indicating that the supportive qualities of relationships may be especially important for engagement in health-promoting behavior. Of course, social relationships can also encourage engagement in health-damaging behaviors, such as smoking and poor diet, through modeling and peer influence mechanisms (Burg and Seeman, 1994).

4.3 Biological Pathways

A major thrust of research efforts in recent decades has been the identification of biolog-ical mechanisms which may explain observed links between social support and physical health outcomes, including cardiovascular, endocrine, and immune pathways, which play a role in disease and disability. An impressive body of evidence is accumulating that greater social sup-port is associated with more positive profiles of physiological functioning, as well as more positive patterns of physiological reactivity to stressor experience (see Uchino, 2006; Uchino et al, 1996). Consistent with a focus on car-diovascular health outcomes in the social sup-port literature, the majority of studies examining physiological correlates of social support have examined indicators of cardiovascular function-ing. In a comprehensive review, Uchino and colleagues (1996) documented that structural and functional social relationship measures show similar associations with indicators of cardiovas-cular functioning, including lower basal levels of blood pressure and heart rate. Studies of buffer-ing effects of social support on cardiovascular reactivity during acute exposure to stressful sit-uations in laboratory settings indicate that both experimentally manipulated exposure to social support (e.g., expressions of encouragement during task performance) and perceived level of support from natural network members that an individual brings to the stressful situation can dampen cardiovascular reactivity.

Studies have also documented associations between greater social support and lower levels of ambulatory cardiovascular activity in individual's naturalistic environments (see Uchino, 2006, for review). Support for a stress-buffering role of social support was documented in an investigation by Steptoe (2000) who found that only individuals low in perceived social support exhibited increased ambulatory cardiovascular activity under periods of high stress throughout the day. Consistent with the potential health benefits of support provision, Piferi and Lawler (2006) found that the tendency to provide support to others was also associated with lower blood pressure throughout the day. Although ambulatory cardiovascular activity is believed to have prognostic value for cardiovascular health outcomes, to date, the more favorable profiles of ambulatory cardiovascular activity in those with greater social support have not been directly linked to better cardiovascular health outcomes within the same participants.

Social support is also linked to functioning of hormonal (endocrine) stress regulatory systems, such as the sympathetic–adrenal–medullary (SAM) and hypothalamic–pituitary–adrenal (HPA) systems, which regulate blood levels of catecholamines (epinephrine, norepinephrine) and the glucocorticoid hormone, cortisol, respectively, in humans. Catecholamines and cortisol modulate cardiovascular and immune function, as well as a variety of other physiological processes (e.g., metabolism, growth, reproduction), and thus play important roles in functioning and disease. A study of female breast cancer patients found that those with higher reported levels of social support had lower mean levels of cortisol across the day, a physiological state which may confer favorable outcomes in terms of cancer progression (Turner-Cobb et al, 2000). Seeman and colleagues (1994, 2002) have found associations between greater levels of social support and lower levels of urinary

catecholamines and cortisol, as well as lower levels of physiological dysregulation on a composite "allostatic load" index of cardiovascular, metabolic, and endocrine functioning in older men, but not older women. In this cohort, higher levels of relationship demands and conflicts are also linked to these physiological variables in older men. Such findings might suggest that endocrine activity is more sensitive to qualitative relationship characteristics in older men, but a recent study found that salivary cortisol levels were associated with behavior patterns during spousal conflict in older women, but not in older men (Heffner et al, 2006). Methodological and sample characteristics vary greatly across the small number of studies examining endocrine correlates of social support and conflict, thus more research will be needed to delineate the positive and negative relationship characteristics and the characteristics of individuals for whom hormone activity is linked to social support.

Social support has also been examined as a buffer of stress-induced cortisol increases in laboratory stress paradigms. As with studies of cardiovascular reactivity, both experimentally manipulated provision of social support within the laboratory (see Thorsteinsson and James, 1999, for review) and greater experience of support in the natural environment that individuals bring with them to the laboratory (Eisenberger et al, 2007) are associated with lower cortisol reactivity. Another important biological factor that may be involved in HPA downregulation, especially under conditions of support experience, is oxytocin, a neuropeptide involved in parental behavior, bonding, and other prosocial behavior. In a novel paradigm in which oxytocin or a placebo was administered to participants before participation in a set of challenging stressor tasks, Heinrichs and colleagues (2003) demonstrated that either oxytocin or social support from a friend was associated with smaller task-induced increases in cortisol levels, but the lowest levels of reactivity were observed in those who received both oxytocin and support. Experimentally administered oxytocin also increased positive behaviors during a conflict discussion and reduced cortisol responses to the conflict in a recent study of heterosexual couples (Ditzen et al, 2009).

Supportive characteristics of relationships are also linked to disease-relevant aspects of immunity. Greater levels of social support are generally linked to more positive profiles of immunologic functioning (e.g., greater proliferation of immune cells to antigenic stimulation, greater killing activity of natural killer cells, more robust immune response to vaccine), in both healthy and disease-afflicted individuals, under both stress and non-stress conditions (see Uchino et al, 1996, 2006, for reviews). An interesting study demonstrated that perceptions of support may be related to immune functioning relatively early in the life course; young asthmatic children who perceived low levels of parental support had higher levels of eosinophil activation, an immune cell involved in asthma symptoms, and were also more likely to have immune cells that were resistant to the inhibitory effects of glucocorticoids, suggesting a possible impairment in endocrine systems that downregulate inflammatory immune activity (Miller et al, 2009).

5 Modifying Factors

Links between functional aspects of social relationships and health may be moderated by individual difference factors, such as individual beliefs, coping styles, and personality factors, which influence perception and behavior within interpersonal relationships. For example, associations between social support and health or psychological and physiological states thought to play a role in support–health associations have been found to vary by individual difference factors such as attachment style (Collins and Feeney, 2004; Davila and Kashy, 2009) and hostility (Holt-Lunstad et al, 2008), as well as the presence of other psychological states, like depression (e.g., Frasure-Smith et al, 2000; Lett et al, 2007).

Associations between social support and health may also vary by sociodemographic factors, such as gender, age, and socioeconomic status. Whether social support has a greater impact on health at different stages of the life course is unclear. Krause (1999) observed substantial individual variability in change in frequency of social contact and level of perceived, received and provided support in older adults over time; the physical health correlates of such patterns are an interesting topic for future research. Interestingly, older adults have been found to report more positive perceptions of social support than younger adults (Schnittker, 2007), but the association between support characteristics and mental well-being has been found to weaken with age (Segrin, 2003). However, support needs may increase with age due to greater level of disease and functional limitation, thus creating greater potential for well-being to be impacted by the positive and negative aspects of support transactions. Across the lifespan, women report giving and receiving more support than men and females are often identified as support sources for both men and women (Shumaker and Hill, 1991). Early epidemiologic studies suggested that the association between social integration/support and disease might be stronger in men than in women, but such differences have not always been found and some studies suggest that women may actually be more sensitive to both the positive and the negative qualities of relationships (see Lett et al, 2005, for review). A number of investigations also suggest stronger associations between both positive and negative relationship qualities and health in those of lower socioeconomic status (Krause, 2005; Strogatz and James, 1986; Vitaliano et al, 2001), suggesting that those with low resources may experience a greater boost from support but may also be more vulnerable to the negative impacts of conflict, as compared to those with greater resources.

6 Intervention Research

The sizable body of evidence linking supportive aspects of relationships to physical health outcomes calls into question whether interventions to improve social support might benefit health. A review of 100 interventions of either group- or individual-level formats designed to modify perceptions of support availability and/or skills related to seeking and receiving social support documented that a majority of interventions were successful in improving psychosocial (e.g., psychological well-being, perceptions of support availability, or receipt) and behavioral outcomes (e.g., adherence to medical treatments, maintenance of adopted health behaviors; Hogan et al, 2002). However, a much smaller body of research has examined physical health impacts of social support interventions. Campbell (2003) noted that interventions for physical health conditions that involve family members, such as interventions which educate families about the target health condition and provide social support skills training, generally support the salutary benefits of family intervention for a number of health conditions (e.g., better glycemic control in diabetics, better asthma control, lower blood pressure in hypertensive patients; see also Martire et al, 2004).

Given the large body of evidence suggesting that low levels of social integration/social support are predictive of cardiovascular disease outcomes, the Enhancing Recovery in Coronary Heart Disease (ENRICHD) trial was designed to provide psychosocial treatment to individuals who had recently suffered an MI and also perceived low social support availability (Berkman et al, 2003). Over 2000 individuals with low levels of perceived social support, high levels of depressive symptoms, or both, were randomized to either usual care (with private physician) or psychosocial treatment, which consisted of both individual cognitive behavioral therapy and group therapy. A tailored therapy program was designed for each participant that addressed social skill deficits, cognitive factors contributing to dissatisfaction with social support in one's network, network development, support needs and preferences, and individual factors (e.g., anxiety) that might be contributing to deficiencies with support processes. For those with depressive symptomatology, cogni-

tive behavioral therapy also addressed depression. The intervention was successful in decreasing depressive symptoms and increasing perceptions of social support to a greater degree in intervention subjects, although both intervention and control groups actually experienced improvements in these parameters. The crushing blow, however, was a failure of greater improvements in these psychosocial outcomes in the intervention group to translate into better cardiovascular outcomes. Post hoc analyses did indicate that perceptions of low levels of perceived support at study entry predicted risk of recurrent MI or mortality, consistent with observational research linking low perceived support to greater risk of poor cardiovascular outcomes; however, change in social support in trial participants did not alter mortality outcome. Other post hoc analyses indicated greater treatment effects for social support in those without as compared to those with a partner, suggesting that such interventions might be particularly beneficial in those without an intimate support source (Burg et al, 2005), or alternatively that efforts to modify support transactions through therapy with support recipients may be at odds with the preferences of established support providers, or redundant with already available support. Another possibility is that the critical period for support intervention in terms of effecting change in cardiovascular disease outcomes may be earlier in the disease process; there may be less of an opportunity for improvements in social support to effect change at a physiological level late in the progression of the disease.

7 Future Directions

As we have reviewed, there is considerable support for the hypothesis that the supportive qualities of our social relationships are linked to our physical well-being. Epidemiological research establishes links between support characteristics and disease morbidity and mortality, as well as the psychosocial, behavioral, and biological pathways through which social support may get under the skin to affect health. Experimental research also highlights social support as a buffer against the adverse physiological effects of stressor experience, which when experienced over a lifetime may explain the better health outcomes of those with more supportive networks.

Despite incredible advances in our understanding of connections between social support and health, we still have much to learn. Although research clearly establishes a link between greater perceived availability of emotional support and better physical health, the salubrious impact of other forms of support still needs clarification and greater attention needs to be paid to the potential health benefits of actual support receipt. A focus on the other side of the support equation, that of the health benefits of giving, may also be a fruitful area for future research. Accumulating evidence that negative aspects of social relationships, such as demands and conflicts, are associated with risk of poor health highlights the need to consider both positive and negative relationship qualities, and their relative balance, in the study of physical health.

A number of methodological developments may help advance our knowledge of how social support influences physical well-being. Advances in the measurement and analysis of daily measures of both physiological activity and psychosocial and behavioral processes, especially in real-life settings, have the potential to yield important discoveries regarding complex interactions between actual support transactions and individual-level characteristics and responses that have importance for health. The field has also established an impressive array of social support measurements; the time is ripe for comparative analyses of those dimensions of social support most strongly linked to physical health, under what conditions, and for whom. The mixed record of success with interventions designed to affect physical disease outcomes by modifying social support factors should not discourage future intervention efforts. Much success has been recognized for the modification of psychosocial and behavioral factors associated with disease progression (e.g., self-efficacy, adherence). Longer term follow-up of disease

outcomes in such interventions may demonstrate the tremendous physical health benefits of social support interventions that occur at earlier stages in the disease process. In short, an impressive body of research demonstrates that the supportive qualities of our relationships are linked to physical well-being. Our objective for the future is to more clearly delineate specific support characteristics, mediating mechanisms, and moderating factors involved in these links with the aim of developing more effective interventions for improving social and physical well-being.

References

Angerer, P., Siebert, U., Kothny, W., Muhlbauer, D., Mudra, H. et al (2000). Impact of social support, cynical hostility and anger expression on progression of coronary atherosclerosis. *J Am Coll Cardiol, 36,* 1781–1788.

Barrera, M. (1986). Distinctions between social support concepts, measures, and models. *Am J Community Psychol, 14,* 413–445.

Berkman, L. F., Blumenthal, J., Burg, M., Carney, R. M., Catellier, D. et al (2003). Effects of treating depression and low perceived social support on clinical events after myocardial infarction: the Enhancing Recovery in Coronary Heart Disease Patients (ENRICHD) Randomized Trial. *J Am Med Assoc, 289,* 3106–3116

Berkman, L. F., Leo-Summers, L., and Horwitz, R. I. (1992). Emotional support and survival after myocardial-infarction: a prospective, population-based study of the elderly. *Ann Intern Med, 117,* 1003–1009.

Birditt, K., and Antonucci, T. C. (2008). Life sustaining irritations? Relationship quality and mortality in the context of chronic illness. *Soc Sci Med, 67,* 1291–1299.

Blazer, D. G. (1982). Social support and mortality in an elderly community population. *Am J Epidemiol, 115,* 684–694.

Brown, S. L., Nesse, R. M., Vinokur, A. D., and Smith, D. M. (2003). Providing social support may be more beneficial than receiving it: results from a prospective study of mortality. *Psychol Sci, 14,* 320–327.

Brummett, B. H., Mark, D. B., Siegler, I. C., Williams, R. B., Babyak, M. A. et al (2005). Perceived social support as a predictor of mortality in coronary patients: effects of smoking, sedentary behavior, and depressive symptoms. *Psychosom Med, 67,* 40–45.

Burg, M. M., Barefoot, J., Berkman, L., Catellier, D. J., Czajkowski, S. et al (2005). Low perceived social support and post-myocardial infarction prognosis in the enhancing recovery in coronary heart disease clinical trial: the effects of treatment. *Psychosom Med, 67*, 879–888.

Burg, M. M. and Seeman, T. E. (1994). Families and health: the negative side of social ties. *Ann Beh Med, 16*, 109–115.

Campbell, T. L. (2003). The effectiveness of family interventions for physical disorders. *J Marital Fam Ther, 29*, 263–281.

Cassell, J. (1976). The contribution of the social environment to host resistance. *Am J Epidemiol, 104*, 107–123,

Cobb, S. (1976). Social support as a moderator of life stress. *Psychom Med, 38*, 300–314.

Cohen, S. (2004). Social relationships and health. *Am Psychol, 59*, 676–684.

Cohen, S., and Wills, T. A. (1985). Stress, social support, and the buffering hypothesis. *Psychol Bull, 98*, 310–357.

Collins, N. L., Dunkel-Schetter, C., Lobel, M., and Scrimshaw, S. C. (1993). Social support in pregnancy: psychosocial correlates of birth outcomes and postpartum depression. *J Pers Soc Psychol, 65*, 1243–1258.

Collins, N. L., and Feeney, B. C. (2004). Working models of attachment shape perceptions of social support: evidence from experimental and observational studies. *J Pers Soc Psychol, 87*, 363–383.

Coyne, J. C., and Bolger, N. (1990). Doing without social support as an explanatory concept. *J Soc Clin Psychol, 9*, 148–158.

Davila, J., and Kashy, D. A. (2009). Secure base processes in couples: daily associations between support experiences and attachment security. *J Fam Psychol, 23*, 76–88.

DiMatteo, M. R. (2004). Social support and patient adherence to medical treatment: a meta-analysis. *Health Psychol, 23*, 207–18

Ditzen, B., Schaer, M., Gabriel, B., Bodenmann, G., Ehlert, U. et al (2009). Intranasal oxytocin increases positive communication and reduces cortisol levels during couple conflict. *Biol Psychiatry, 65*, 728–731.

Dunkel-Schetter, C. and Bennett, T. L. (1990). Differentiating the cognitive and behavioral aspects of social support. In B. R. Sarason, I. G. Sarason, & G. R. Pierce (Eds.), *Social Support: An Interactional View* (pp. 267–296). New York: Wiley.

Eisenberger, N. I., Taylor, S. E., Gable, S. L., Hilmert, C. J., and Lieberman, M. D. (2007). Neural pathways link social support to attenuated neuroendocrine stress responses. *Neuroimage, 35*, 1601–12

Falagas, M. E., Zarkadoulia, E. A., Ioannidou, E. N., Peppas, G., Christodoulou, C. et al (2007). The effect of psychosocial factors on breast cancer outcome: a systematic review. *Breast Cancer Res, 9*, 23.

Falk, A., Hanson, B. S., Isacsson, S. O., and Ostergren, P. O. (1992). Job strain and mortality in elderly men: social network, support and influence as buffers. *Am J Public Health, 82*, 1136–1139.

Feldman, P. J., Dunkel-Schetter, C., Sandman, C. A., and Wadhwa, P. D. (2000). Maternal social support predicts birth weight and fetal growth in human pregnancy. *PsychosomMed, 62*, 715–725.

Frasure-Smith, N., Lesperance, F., Gravel, G., Masson, A., Juneau, M. et al (2000). Social support, depression, and mortality during the first year after myocardial infarction. *Circulation, 101*, 1919–1924.

Giles, L. C., Glonek, G. F. V., Luszcz, M. A., and Andrews, G. R. (2005). Effect of social networks on 10 year survival in very old Australians: the Australian longitudinal study of aging. *J Epidemiol Community Health, 59*, 574–579.

Gruenewald, T. L., Karlamangla, A. S., Greendale, G. A., Singer, B. H., and Seeman, T. E. (2007). Feelings of usefulness to others, disability, and mortality in older adults: The MacArthur study of successful aging. *J Gerontol Psychol Sci Soc Sci, 62*, P28–P37.

Haber, M. G., Cohen, J. L., Lucas, T., and Baltes, B. B. (2007). The relationship between self-reported received and perceived social support: a meta-analytic review. *Am J Community Psychol, 39*, 133–144.

Hanson, B. S., Isacsson, S. O., Janzon, L., and Lindell, S. E. (1989). Social network and social support influence mortality in elderly men: the prospective population study of men born in 1914, Malmo, Sweden. *Am J Epidemiol, 130*, 100–111.

Heffner, K. L., Loving, T. J., Kiecolt-Glaser, J. K., Himawan, L. K., Glaser, R. et al (2006). Older spouses' cortisol responses to marital conflict: associations with demand/withdraw communication patterns. *J Behav Med, 29*, 317–25.

Heinrichs, M., Baumgartner, T., Kirschbaum, C., and Ehlert, U. (2003). Social support and oxytocin interact to suppress cortisol and subjective responses to psychosocial stress. *Biol Psychiatry, 54*, 1389–1398.

Helgeson, V. S., and Cohen, S. (1996). Social support and adjustment to cancer: reconciling descriptive, correlational, and intervention research. *Health Psychol, 15*, 135–148.

Hogan, B. E., Linden, W., and Najarian, B. (2002). Social support – do they interventions work? *Clin Psychol Rev, 22*, 381–440.

Holt-Lunstad, J., Smith, T. W., and Uchino, B. N. (2008). Can hostility interfere with the health benefits of giving and receiving social support? The impact of cynical hostility on cardiovascular reactivity during social support interactions among friends. *Ann Beh Med, 35*, 319–330.

House, J. S., Landis, K. R., and Umberson, D. (1988). Social relationships and health. *Science, 241*, 540–545.

Ingersoll-Dayton, B., Morgan, D., and Antonucci, T. (1997). The effects of positive and negative social exchanges on aging adults. *J Gerontol Psychol Sci Soc Sci, 52*, S190–S199.

Kawachi, I., and Berkman, L. F. (2001). Social ties and mental health. *J Urban Health, 78*, 458–467.

Krause, N. (1999). Assessing change in social support during late life. *Res Aging, 21*, 539-569.

Krause, N. (2005). Negative interaction and heart disease in late life: exploring variations by socioeconomic status. *J Aging Health, 17*, 28–55.

Krumholz, H. M., Butler, J., Miller, J., Vaccarino, V., Williams, C. S. et al (1998). Prognostic importance of emotional support for elderly patients hospitalized with heart failure. *Circulation, 97*, 958–964.

Lett, H. S., Blumenthal, J. A., Babyak, M. A., Catellier, D. J., Carney, R. M. et al (2007). Social support and prognosis in patients at increased psychosocial risk recovering from myocardial infarction. *Health Psychol, 26*, 418–427.

Lett, H. S., Blumenthal, J. A., Babyak, M. A., Strauman, T. J., Robins, C. et al (2005). Social support and coronary heart disease: epidemiologic evidence and implications for treatment. *Psychosom Med, 67*, 869–878.

Lyyra, T. M., and Heikkinen, R. L. (2006). Perceived social support and mortality in older people. *J Gerontol Psychol Sci Soc Sci, 61*, S147–S152.

Martire, L. M., Lustig, A. P., Schulz, R., Miller, G. E., and Helgeson, V. S. (2004). Is it beneficial to involve a family member? A meta-analysis of psychosocial interventions for chronic illness. *Health Psychol, 23*, 599–611.

Mendes de Leon, C. F., Gold, D. T., Glass, T. A., Kaplan, L., and George, L. K. (2001). Disability as a function of social networks and support in elderly African Americans and Whites: The Duke EPESE 1986–1992. *J Gerontol Psychol Sci Soc Sci, 56*, S179–S190.

Miller, G. E., Gaudin, A., Zysk, E., and Chen, E. (2009). Parental support and cytokine activity in childhood asthma: the role of glucocorticoid sensitivity. *J Allergy Clin Immunol, 123*, 824–830.

Newsom, J. T., Rook, K. S., Nishishiba, M., Sorkin, D. H., and Mahan, T. L. (2005). Understanding the relative importance of positive and negative social exchanges: examining specific domains and appraisals. *J Gerontol Psychol Sci Soc Sci, 60*, P304–P312.

Okamoto, K., and Tanaka, Y. (2004). Subjective usefulness and 6-year mortality risks among elderly persons in Japan. *J Gerontol Psychol Sci Soc Sci, 59*, P246–249.

Orth-Gomer, K., Rosengren, A., and Wilhelmsen, L. (1993). Lack of social support and incidence of coronary heart disease in middle-aged Swedish men. *Psychosom Med, 55*, 37–43.

Piferi, R. L., and Lawler, K. A. (2006). Social support and ambulatory blood pressure: an examination of both receiving and giving. *Int J Psychophysiol, 62*, 328–336.

Rook, K. S. (1984). The negative side of social interaction: impact on psychological well-being. *J Pers Soc Psychol, 46*, 1097–1108.

Rosengren, A., Orth-gomer, K., Wedel, H., and Wilhelmsen, L. (1993). Stressful life events, social support and mortality in men born in 1933. *Br Med J, 307*, 1102–1105.

Sato, T., Kishi, R., Suzukawa, A., Horikawa, N., Saijo, Y. et al (2008). Effects of social relationships on mortality of the elderly: how do the influences change with the passage of time? *Arch Gerontol Geriatr, 47*, 327–339.

Schnittker, J. (2007). Look closely at all the lonely people: age and the social psychology of social support. *J Aging Health, 19*, 659–682.

Seeman, T. E., Berkman, L. F., Blazer, D., and Rowe, J. W. (1994). Social ties and support and neuroendocrine function: The MacArthur studies of successful aging. *Ann Beh Med, 16*, 95–106.

Seeman, T. E., Berkman, L. F., Charpentier, P. A., Blazer, D. G., Albert, M. S. et al (1995). Behavioral and psychosocial predictors of physical performance: MacArthur Studies of Successful Aging. *J Gerontol Biol Sci Med Sci, 50*, M177–M183.

Seeman, T. E., Bruce, M. L., and McAvay, G. J. (1996). Social network characteristics and onset of ADL disability: MacArthur studies of successful aging. *J Gerontol Psychol Sci Soc Sci, 51*, S191–S200.

Seeman, T. E., Lusignolo, T. M., Albert, M., and Berkman, L. (2001). Social relationships, social support, and patterns of cognitive aging in healthy, high-functioning older adults: MacArthur studies of successful aging. *Health Psychol, 20*, 243–255.

Seeman, T. E., Singer, B. H., Ryff, C. D., Love, G. D., and Levy-Storms, L. (2002). Social relationships, gender, and allostatic load across two age cohorts. *Psychosom Med, 64*, 395–406.

Seeman, T. E., and Syme, S. L. (1987). Social networks and coronary artery disease: a comparison of the structure and function of social relations as predictors of disease. *Psychosom Med, 49*, 341–354.

Segrin, C. (2003). Age moderates the relationship between social support and psychosocial problems. *Hum Commun Res, 29*, 317–342.

Shumaker, S. A., and Brownell, A. (1984). Toward a theory of social support: closing conceptual gaps. *J Soc Issues, 40*, 11–36.

Shumaker, S. A., and Hill, D. R. (1991). Gender differences in social support and physical health. *Health Psychol, 10*, 102–111.

Steptoe, A. (2000). Stress, social support and cardiovascular activity over the working day. *Int J Psychophysiol, 37*, 299–308.

Strogatz, D. S., and James, S. A. (1986). Social support and hypertension among blacks and whites in a rural, southern community. *Am J Epidemiol, 124*, 949–956.

Thorsteinsson, E. B., and James, J. E. (1999). A meta-analysis of the effects of experimental manipulations of social support during laboratory stress. *Psychol Health, 14*, 869–886.

Turner-Cobb, J. M., Sephton, S. E., Koopman, C., Blake-Mortimer, J., and Spiegel, D. (2000). Social support and salivary cortisol in women with metastatic breast cancer. *Psychosom Med*, 62, 337–45

Uchino, B. N. (2006). Social support and health: a review of physiological processes potentially underlying links to disease outcomes. *J Beh Med, 29*, 377–387.

Uchino, B. N., Cacioppo, J. T., and Kiecolt-Glaser, J. K. (1996). The relationship between social support and physiological processes: a review with emphasis on underlying mechanisms and implications for health. *Psychol Bull, 119*, 488–531.

Vitaliano, P. P., Scanlan, J. M., Zhang, J., Savage, M. V., Brummett, B. et al (2001). Are the salutogenic effects of social supports modified by income? A test of an "added value hypothesis". *Health Psychol, 20*, 155–165.

Walter-Ginzburg, A., Blumstein, T., Chetrit, A., and Modan, B. (2002). Social factors and mortality in the old-old in Israel: The CALAS study. *J Gerontol Psychol Sci Soc Sci, 57*, S308–S318.

Wang, H. X., Mittleman, M. A., and Orth-Gomer, K. (2005). Influence of social support on progression of coronary artery disease in women. *Soc Sci Med, 60*, 599–607.

Wills, T. A. and Shinar, T. A. (2000). Measuring perceived and received social support. In S. Cohen, B. H. Gottlieb, & L. G. Underwood (Eds.), *Social Support Measurement and Intervention: A Guide for Health and Social Scientists*. New York: Oxford University Press.

Woloshin, S., Schwartz, L. M., Tosteson, A. N. A., Chang, C. H., Wright, B., Plohman, J. et al (1997). Perceived adequacy of tangible social support and health outcomes in patients with coronary artery disease. *J Gen Intern Med, 12*, 613–618.

Chapter 18

Social Networks and Health

Ai Ikeda and Ichiro Kawachi

1 Definitions and Measurement

Social network is defined as "the web of social relationships that surround an individual" (Berkman and Glass, 2000). An important distinction that is drawn between the concepts of social networks versus social support is while that the former term refers to the *structure* of social ties, the latter refers to their *functional* aspects (such as the exchange of information, instrumental aid, and affection).[1] Social networks can be further characterized according to their size (number of members connected to the index individual), frequency of contact, and the diversity of domains in which the individual maintains social relations (e.g., marital ties, friendships, voluntary groups, and church membership).

Broadly speaking, two approaches exist by which to measure social networks: (a) the *egocentric* network assessment approach, which inquires about the extent of an individual's (the ego's) social ties (e.g., "Are *you* married?", and "How many close friends do *you* have?") and (b) the *sociometric* (or whole social network) approach which attempts to measure the totality of social connections within a structure. For reasons of practicality, most epidemiologic research has focused on the egocentric network approach. In large-scale epidemiological studies, the typically adopted approach has been to include a few brief items on a survey inquiring about a respondent's social ties (size, frequency, and diversity of domains), and then following the individuals over time to observe the incidence of health outcomes (morbidity and mortality). For example, the widely used Berkman-Syme Social Network Index (1979) consists of just seven items inquiring about marital status, number and frequency of contact with children, number and frequency of contact with close friends, and membership in voluntary organizations and church groups. The virtues of this approach consist of its brevity as well as proven ability to predict future health outcomes.

By contrast, the sociometric approach is far more demanding, since the method requires that every person nominated by the ego as a personal contact (the *alters*) must in turn be approached in order to map the entire social network. Sociometric approaches are most useful when examining network structures with clearly defined *boundaries*, and for that reason they tend to be used in examining phenomena such as the spread of high-risk behaviors in networks of injection drug users (Friedman and Aral, 2001) or the spread of suicidal ideation in school settings (Bearman and Moody, 2004).

A. Ikeda (✉)
Department of Society, Human Development and Health, Harvard School of Public Health, 677 Huntington Avenue, Kresge Building 7th Floor, Boston, MA 02115, USA
e-mail: ai-ikeda@umin.ac.jp

---

[1] Medical students are familiar with the distinction between structure and function. For example, the structure of the cardiovascular system consists of a central pump (the heart) and some pipes (arteries, veins), while the function of the system is to convey oxygen to tissues.

2 Mechanisms Linking Social Networks to Health Outcomes

Cohen and Wills (1985) distinguished between two models to explain the mechanisms by which social relationships influence health outcomes: (a) the *main effects* model and (b) the *stress-buffering* model. According to the stress-buffering model, social ties influence health outcomes only for individuals who happen to be experiencing stress – in other words, social resources *buffer* the individual against the deleterious effects of stress – whereas the main effects model posits that social relationships are beneficial regardless of the presence of stress. While these two models are not mutually exclusive, the emerging consensus in the field is that social networks operate via the main effects model, whereas social support is mobilized (and is most effective in promoting well-being) under stressful circumstances.

Berkman and Glass (2000) have gone further to identify a set of four distinct processes and mechanisms by which social networks exert their main effects on health outcomes. They are: (a) social influence over health-related behaviors, (b) social engagement, (c) exchange of social support, and (d) access to material resources. *Social influence* refers to the notion that our behaviors are influenced and regulated by others – an idea that harks back to Durkheim (1897). Socially more well-connected individuals tend to exhibit healthier profiles of lifestyle behaviors compared to socially isolated individuals, e.g., less smoking, better quality diet, more physical activity (Berkman and Syme, 1979; Eng et al, 2002; Kawachi et al, 1996). Social influence is particularly salient in marriage, which is for many people the most intimate of social ties. Longitudinal studies of marital transitions demonstrate the influence of marriage on health behaviors within spousal dyads. For example, when men become widowed or divorced, their alcohol consumption increases relative to men who stay married. Conversely, when widowed or divorced men become remarried, their alco-

hol consumption declines (Eng et al, 2005).[2] Just the opposite is observed among women – that is, their level of drinking decreases when they become widowed or divorced, but rises when they re-marry (Lee et al, 2005). From the foregoing examples, it is evident that social influence does not uniformly promote healthier behaviors, and the intriguing gender differences may partly explain why the health benefits of marital ties have been reported to be stronger for men than for women (House et al, 1988).

A separate pathway linking social networks to health is through *social engagement*, which refers to participation in social activities through one's social relationships. Participation in turn defines and reinforces an individual's social roles, identity, meaning, and sense of belongingness. Lifelong engagement in social activities has additionally been linked to maintenance of cognitive ability at older ages (Bassuk et al, 1999) through what appears to be a "use it or lose it" mechanism.

Thirdly, social networks are the conduits through which the transfer and exchange of *social support* take place. Social support is further classified into several subtypes, ranging from emotional support (love and affection) to the exchange of information and advice, and instrumental support (cash loans, labor in kind). Of these different types, particular attention has been paid to emotional support because of its direct influence in producing positive affective states, which are in turn believed to dampen neuroendocrine responses to stress (the stress-buffering mechanism referred to earlier). We emphasize again that social networks and social support are distinct constructs. Hence, it is possible to receive emotional support from others who are not part of one's social network (e.g., a crisis interventionist volunteering on a suicide hotline). Conversely, social networks may produce differences in immune, inflammatory, or

---

[2]In popular parlance, this effect may be dubbed "nagging", but we will stick to the term "social influence".

neuroendocrine responses even in the absence of mobilizing emotional support. For example, in Sheldon Cohen's experiments exposing volunteers to an intranasal dose of the cold virus, individuals reporting high social network diversity (i.e., the presence of social ties in many domains including the work-place, community groups, churches) experienced roughly half the risk of succumbing to a symptomatic cold compared to more isolated individuals, *even though the experiments did not involve any manipulation of social support in the laboratory* (1997). Presumably, this finding is explained by some as-yet unaccounted for the effect of social network integration on immune functioning (i.e., the ability to fend off the cold virus). Furthermore, longitudinal data from the Framingham Study (Loucks et al, 2006) as well as the MacArthur Successful Aging Study (Loucks et al, 2006) have reported associations between higher levels of social networks and lower levels of inflammatory markers such as interleukin-6 and C-reactive protein, even after controlling for depressive symptoms, SES, smoking, body mass index, and physical activity.

The fourth distinct mechanism through which social networks may affect well-being is through improving *access to material resources*. This mechanism is distinct from the mobilization of instrumental social support (e.g. cash loans) during times of crisis. The idea here is that people with wider social networks are able to access more opportunities (e.g., job openings) by virtue of their connections.[3] Crucially, the connections need not be particularly strong or intimate. As Granovetter (1973) demonstrated in his classic study of job seekers, most successful job hunters found their work not through their closest contacts, but through "friends of friends" – i.e., their so-called "weak ties". The explanation for this seemingly paradoxical finding is that close

friends tend to share access to the same information, whereas novel information is likely to originate from more remote sources. In other words, social networks do not represent an undifferentiated source of "host resistance" to illness. Different aspects of social network promote health through distinct mechanisms. Thus, when a person is in need of emotional support, having strong social network contacts (e.g., confidants) matters the most, but when one is unemployed and seeking work, having a far-flung network of weak ties matters more.

3 The Empirical Evidence Based Linking Social Networks to Health

We reviewed the epidemiological evidence linking social networks to selected health outcomes, focusing on studies examining four broad sets of endpoints: (a) all-cause mortality, (b) cardiovascular disease incidence and survival, (c) cancer incidence and survival, and (d) maintenance of cognitive function. Our reviews are restricted to prospective cohort studies, given that evidence from cross-sectional studies are too numerous to summarize. We have also not summarized the studies focusing exclusively on marital status and health outcomes, of which there are a huge number – for more detailed reviews of marital status and health, readers are referred to Ross et al (1990), Waite (1995), Rogers et al (2000), Kiecolt-Glaser and Newton (2001), and Wilson and Oswald (2005).

Causal inference poses a challenge in observational studies of social networks and health outcomes. Broadly speaking, the two sets of challenges to inferring causality are: (a) reverse causation, i.e., the onset of illness resulting in a change in social networks, rather than the other way round, and (b) omitted variable bias, or confounding by unobserved characteristics which predict both an individual's level of integration within a social network as well as his/her risk of disease. Reverse causation can be

---

[3]Sometimes, this concept has been referred to by the term "individual social capital" (see van der Gaag and Webber, 2008).

theoretically overcome with prospective observational studies with careful restriction of the study sample at entry to individuals without symptomatic illness (hence, our focus on cohort data in this review). Omitted variable bias is trickier to deal with since there are a number of potential variables – such as personality traits (e.g., hostility, general orneriness) – that could simultaneously account for social isolation and subsequent risk of major disease (e.g., cardiovascular disease). Large-scale prospective studies have seldom controlled for a comprehensive set of potential confounding variables. An additional level of complexity is introduced when the health outcome is in the realm of mental health, where negative affectivity could influence the reporting of social networks and be associated with increased risk of the outcomes of interest (Kawachi and Berkman, 2001). Novel methods for causal inference – such as instrumental variable analysis or propensity score matching – could be attempted, but it is hard to think of clever instruments for social networks.[4] Last but not least, it is difficult to conceive of randomized trials that directly manipulate people's social networks. This is in contrast to social support, which can and has been directly subjected to experimental manipulation, e.g., through cognitive behavioral therapy, family systems therapy, and social support groups, albeit with mixed results on the health outcomes of interest, i.e., survival after myocardial infarction (Berkman et al, 2003) and functional recovery following a cerebral stroke (Glass et al, 2004). In short, prospective observational studies are likely to remain the main source of evidence linking social networks to health outcomes.

3.1 All-Cause Mortality

Following the seminal study by Berkman and Syme in Alameda County, California (1979), no fewer than 28 prospective studies have sought to document the relationship between social networks and all-cause mortality (Table 18.1). As Table 18.1 indicates, the preponderance of evidence suggests that social networks are related to risk of subsequent all-cause mortality, i.e., individuals with the lowest level of social connectedness (e.g., not being married, having few close friends, not belonging to groups) experience roughly a doubling of all-cause mortality compared to those with the highest level of social integration. This finding is robust with respect to control for a range of potential confounding variables (such as co-existing morbidity) as well as even variables that may be considered to be on the pathway between social networks and mortality (such as smoking status).

Two additional observations from the table are that: (a) social networks are more consistently associated with mortality risk among men compared to women (more on this later); and (b) the association between social networks and mortality is characterized by a "dose response" relation between the degree of social connectedness (e.g., greater size and frequency of social contacts, greater network diversity across different social domains) as opposed to a "threshold effect" of social isolation compared to everyone else. In other words, more is better. The benefits of social networks extend beyond having just one strong social bond (e.g., being married). Moreover, one type of bond may substitute for another – for example, having a close friend/confidante may be just as beneficial as being married.[5]

One of the limitations of using all-cause mortality as the outcome is that the endpoint conflates disease incidence with prognosis. While deaths are convenient to count and they provide

[4]A notable exception is the case of marital ties and risk of mortality, which has been instrumented using U.S. state-level variation in the strictness of divorce laws (Lillard and Panis, 1996). The authors found evidence of causation in both directions, i.e. from marriage to health, as well as from health to marriage.

[5]Or in some cases, even better if you happen to be hitched to an uncaring, emotionally distant spouse.

Table 18.1 Prospective studies of social network and all-cause mortality

Country, published year study population	Sample size	Age at entry	Follow-up years	Social network measures	Relative risk
Berkman and Syme (1979). Residents of Alameda County, USA	2,229 (men)	30–69	9	Marital status, friends and relatives, church and group membership	RR=2.3[†] of all-cause mortality for low *vs.* high social network index
	2,496 (women)				RR=2.8[†] of all-cause mortality for low *vs.* high social network index
Blazer (1982). Elderly residents of Durham County, USA	331 (men and women)	65+	3	Social interaction with relatives and friends (phone calls and visits)	RR=1.88[†] of all-cause mortality for frequency of social interaction
House et al (1982). Residents of Tecumseh, USA	2,754 (men and women)	35–69	12	Social relationships (marital status, visit friends and relatives), social activity (church, group membership, social leisure activity)	Social relationships and activity was associated with all-cause mortality in men ($\beta = -0.410$[†], by mean social relationships and activity index)
Welin et al (1985). Random sample of residents in Gothenburg, Sweden	989 (men)	50, 60	9	Social activities (visiting friends and relatives, participating group activities)	RR=3.4[†] of all-cause mortality for low *vs.* high social activity group
Schoenbach et al (1986). Residents of Evans County, USA	2,059 (men and women)	15+	12	Marital status, friends and relatives, church membership	No association with all-cause mortality
Seeman et al (1987). Residents of Alameda County, USA	4,174 (men and women)	38–94	17	Marital status, friends and relatives, church and group membership.	HR=2.00[†] of all-cause mortality for low *vs.* high social network index in 38–49 years old and HR=1.49[†] in 70+ years old
Orth-Gomer and Johnson (1987). Random sample of population, Sweden.	17,433 (men and women)	29–74	6	Marital status, children and relatives, contacts with neighbors and co-workers	RR=1.34[†] of all-cause mortality for the lowest compared with upper two tertiles of social network interaction index
Kaplan et al (1988). Residents of Kuopio and North Karelia, Finland.	13,301 (men and women)	39–59	5	Marital status, friends and relatives, group membership	OR=1.54[†] of all-cause mortality for the first and second lowest *vs.* highest quintile of social connections index in men

Table 18.1 (continued)

Country, published year study population	Sample size	Age at entry	Follow-up years	Social network measures	Relative risk
Hanson et al (1989). Elderly residents of Malmo, Sweden	621 (men)	68	5	Social anchorage, contact with children, relatives, friends, neighbors and co-workers, participation in social activities	HR=2.2[†] of all-cause mortality for low vs. high social participation
Astrand et al (1989). Pulp and paper company employees, Sweden	391 (men)	35–65	22	Group membership, contact with relatives, friends, neighbors, and co-workers, participation in social activity	No association of social network with all-cause mortality
Olsen et al (1991). Random sample of elderly residents in Odense, Denmark	715 (men)	70–100	15–16	Contact with siblings, children, friends, grandchildren, and other relatives	No association with all-cause mortality
	1,037 (women)				No association with all-cause mortality
Ho (1991). Stratified sample of elderly residents in Hong Kong	1,054 (men and women)	70+	2	Size and frequency of contact with children, relatives and friends, social integration (neighbors and group membership), participation in social and family activity	OR=1.9[†] for low vs. high social integration, OR=1.8[†] for contact/network, OR=1.5[†] for participation in social and family activity
Vogt et al (1992). Random sample of HMO members, USA	2,603 (men and women)	18+	15	Scope, size and frequency of contact within and across family, friends, and community	HR=2.7[†] of all-cause mortality for low vs. high tertiles of network scope, HR=1.5[†] for network frequency, HR=1.4[†] for network size
Falk et al (1992). Elderly residents of Malmo, Sweden	621 (men)	68	7	Social anchorage, contact with children, relatives, friends, neighbors and co-workers, participation in social activities and its adequacy	RR=1.6[†] of all-cause mortality for low vs. high social anchorage score, RR=1.9[†] for adequacy of social participation
Seeman et al (1993). Elderly residents of New Haven, East Boston, and Iowa, USA	2,812 (men and women)	65+	5	Marital status, contact with close friends and relatives, church and groups membership	HR=2.40[†] of all-cause mortality for social tie in men and HR=1.78[†] in women of New Heaven, HR=1.89[†] in women of Iowa

Table 18.1 (continued)

Country, published year study population	Sample size	Age at entry	Follow-up years	Social network measures	Relative risk
Sugisawa et al (1994). A national probability sample of elderly Japanese	2,200 (men and women)	60+	3	Contact with children, relatives, and friends, participation in organization	Social participation was associated with all-cause mortality ($\beta = -0.384^{\dagger}$, the risk of dying for persons who had no social participation)
Shye et al (1995). Random sample of HMC elderly members, USA	209 (men)	65+	15	Size and frequency of contact within and across family, friends, co-worker, and community	HR=1.49* of all-cause mortality for low social network size
	246 (women)				HR=1.62* of all-cause mortality for low social network size
Kawachi et al (1996). Dentists, veterinarians, pharmacists, optometrists, osteopathic physicians, podiatrists, USA	32,624 (men)	42–77	4	Marital status, friends and relatives, church and group membership	RR=1.38* of all-cause mortality for low vs. high social network index (P for trend=0.06)
Yasuda et al (1997). Elderly residents of northeast Baltimore, USA	806 (women)	65+	5	Size and frequency of contact within children, relatives, friends, group membership, participation in organization	HR=3.1† for no contact with children, HR=2.2† for no contact with friends, HR=2.4† for no group membership, HR=2.8† for no participation in organization in =75 years old
Cerhan and Wallace (1997). Elderly residents of Iowa and Washington counties, USA	903 (men)	65–102	11	Marital status, friends and relatives, church, group membership	HR=1.8† of all-cause mortality for lower vs. higher level of social tie index at 1982, HR=2.0† at 1985. HR=1.8† for a decrease to a lower level compared with higher levels at both times, HR=2.2† for lower levels at both time
	1,672 (women)				HR=1.6† of all-cause mortality for lower vs. higher level of social tie index at 1982, HR=2.3† at 1985. HR=2.1† for a decrease to a lower level compared with higher levels at both times, HR=2.2† for lower levels at both time

Table 18.1 (continued)

Country, published year study population	Sample size	Age at entry	Follow-up years	Social network measures	Relative risk
Penninx et al (1997). Stratified/random sample of elderly residents of Amsterdam, the Netherlands	2,829 (men and women)	55–85	2	Partner status, contact with children, relatives, neighbors, co-workers, organization, other contacts	No association of social network size with all-cause mortality
Fuhrer et al (1999). Random sample of elderly residents in southwest France	1,576 (men) 2,201 (women)	65+	5	Marital status, children, relatives, friends, group membership	HR=1.82[†] for few or no connections compared with many connections in social network index No association between social network index and all-cause mortality
Eng et al (2002).Dentists, veterinarians, pharmacists, optometrists, osteopathic physicians, podiatrists, USA	28,369 (men)	42–77	10	Marital status, friends and relatives, church and group membership	HR=1.19[†] of all-cause mortality for the two most isolated levels of social network index combined compared with highest (p for trend =0.009)
Iwasaki et al (2002). Residents of Komochi Village and Isesaki City, Japan	11,565 (men and women)	40–65	7	Contact with relative and friends, participation in religious and other group activity	HR=1.50[†] of all-cause mortality for not participating in hobbies, club activities and community groups in men, HR=1.78[†] for those who rarely/never met close relatives in women
Rutledge et al (2003). Elderly residents of Baltimore, Minneapolis, Portland, Monongahela Valley, USA	7,524 (women)	65+	6	Size and frequency of contact with family and friends, interdependent relationships	HR=0.92[†] of all-cause mortality for high vs. low social network scale

Table 18.1 (continued)

Country, published year study population	Sample size	Age at entry	Follow-up years	Social network measures	Relative risk
Berkman et al (2004). French employees of Electricity of France-Gas, France	12,347 (men)	40–50	10	Marital status, friends and family, voluntary group membership	HR=2.70† of all-cause mortality for the least vs. most socially integrated men (P for trend=0.0006)
	4,352 (women)	35–50			HR=3.64 of all-cause mortality for the least vs. most socially integrated women (P for trend=0.012)
Giles et al (2005). Stratified/Random sample of elderly residents of Adelaide, Australia	1,477 (men and women)	70+	10	Contact with children, relatives, friends and confidants (phone calls and visits)	HR=0.78† of all-cause mortality for highest vs. lowest tertile of friends networks, HR=0.83† for confidants networks
Barefoot et al (2005). Random sample of residents of Copenhagen, Denmark	9,573 (men and women)	21–93	6	Marital status, children and relatives, contacts with neighbors and co-workers	HR=0.83† of all-cause mortality for =3 types of contacts compared with <3 types

HMO, health maintenance organization; OR, odds ratio; HR, hazard ratio; RR, relative risk; *, borderline; †, $p<0.05$

a combined summary measure of the effects of social networks on health, they fail to distinguish between potential differences in the impact of social networks on disease incidence versus survival following established diagnosis. The distinction is important from the point of view of identifying potential entry points for intervention. To obtain a more fine-grained view of the impacts of social networks on health, we turn to studies of cardiovascular disease and cancer incidence versus survival.

3.2 Cardiovascular Disease

Table 18.2 summarizes the studies linking social networks to cardiovascular disease (myocardial infarction and stroke) incidence, mortality, and survival. The distinction between mortality versus survival is that prospective studies using the former endpoint typically used death register linkage for follow-up, i.e., they did not have information on disease incidence (for example, using medical record review). These studies share the same limitation as studies of all-cause mortality, i.e., they are unable to distinguish between the effects of social networks on disease incidence versus disease prognosis. By contrast, studies using survival as the endpoint typically begin with a sample of incident cases of cardiovascular disease and proceed to follow them within a Kaplan-Meier survival analysis framework.

As Table 18.2 illustrates, studies are fairly consistent in indicating a protective effect of social networks on coronary heart disease incidence. In the U.S. Health Professional Follow-up Study – to date the largest prospective study on this topic – stronger social networks were associated with lower incidence of both stroke as well as fatal coronary heart disease (defined as death within 48 h of the onset of symptoms) (Eng et al, 2002; Kawachi et al, 1996). Studies using survival as the endpoint are also broadly consistent in suggesting improved prognosis following established cardiovascular disease among more socially integrated individuals. Taken together, these studies suggest that social networks are

protective for both cardiovascular incidence as well as survival following the onset of disease.[6]

3.3 Cancer

To our knowledge, only two prospective studies to date (based on the Alameda County Study and a study of a health maintenance organization's members in the USA) have examined the association between social isolation (paucity of social networks) and overall cancer incidence. The Alameda County Study found elevated risks of cancer incidence and mortality in socially isolated women, but not in men. The study also found elevated risk of cancer mortality, particularly for tobacco-related cancers in socially isolated women. On the other hand, social connections were not associated with incidence or mortality in men, though the socially isolated had a significantly lower risk of cancer survival. The study of health maintenance organization members did not find an elevated risk of cancer incidence, but poorer cancer survival in persons with fewer social networks. When we turn to studies of cancer mortality, however, the evidence is quite mixed, with three of five studies indicating no association with social networks. Once again, cancer mortality may not be the optimal endpoint to test the potential influence of social networks because of the inability to distinguish incidence from prognosis, and the very long latency period between exposure and the outcome (typically a decade or longer for cancer outcomes). Moreover, cancers represent a heterogeneous mix of tumors with different levels of prognosis. Thus there is little reason to believe that social networks would exert a similar influence on the course of metastatic breast cancer or lung cancer (median survival about 9 months) compared to, say, a more indolent tumor such

---

[6]We should note here that randomized trials of social *support* provision have not found improved prognosis following myocardial infarction (Berkman et al, 2003) or stroke (Glass et al, 2004).

Table 18.2 Prospective studies of social network and cardiovascular disease

Author, published year study population, country	Sample size	Age at entry	Follow-up years	Social network measures	Relative risk
Incidence					
Reed et al (1983). Residents of Hawaii, USA	4,653 (men)	52–71	8	Marital status, contact with relatives, co-workers, religious and social organizations	No association with CHD incidence
Vogt et al (1992). Random sample of HMO members, USA.	2,603 (men and women)	18+	15	Scope, size and frequency of contact within and across family, friends, and community	HR=1.5† of CHD incidence for network scope HR=0.72† of survival for high vs. low tertiles of network scope, HR=0.73† for network frequency, HR=0.76† for network size in CHD incidence cases. HR=0.73† for network scope in stroke incidence cases
Orth-Gomer et al (1993). Random sample of residents in Goteborg, Sweden	736 (men)	50	6	Relatives, friends and confidants	OR=3.8† of CHD incidence for lower vs. upper quartile of social integration score (*P* for trend=0.04)
Kawachi et al (1996). Dentists, veterinarians, pharmacists, optometrists, osteopathic physicians, podiatrists, USA	32,624 (men)	42–77	4	Marital status, friends and relatives, church and group membership	HR=2.02† of stroke incidence for low vs. high social network index (P for trend=0.03), and HR=1.86 (NA) of non-fatal stroke incidence (*P* for trend=0.03) HR=1.76 (NA) of cardiovascular disease (stroke and coronary heart disease) mortality for low vs. high social network index (*P* for trend=0.02)
Eng et al (2002). Dentists, veterinarians, pharmacists, optometrists, osteopathic physicians, podiatrists, USA	28,369 (men)	42–77	10	Marital status, friends and relatives, church and group membership	HR=1.82† of fatal CHD incidence for low vs. high social network index

Table 18.2 (continued)

Author, published year study population, country	Sample size	Age at entry	Follow-up years	Social network measures	Relative risk
Rosengren et al (2004). Random sample of residents in Goteborg, Sweden	741 (men)	50	15	Relatives, friends and confidants	HR=0.45[+] of CHD incidence for highest vs. lowest quartile in social integration (P for trend=0.013)
Barefoot et al (2005). Random sample of residents in Copenhagen, Denmark	9,573 (men and women)	21–93	6	Marital status, and contact with children, relatives, neighbors and co-workers	HR=0.82[+] of CHD incidence for =3 types of contacts compared with <3 types
Mortality					
Orth-Gomer and Johnson (1987). Random sample of Swedish population.	17,433 (men and women)	29–74	6	Marital status, children and relatives, contacts with neighbors and co-workers	No association with cardiovascular mortality
Kaplan et al (1988). Residents of Kuopio and North Karelia, Finland.	13,301 (men and women)	39–59	5	Marital status, friends and relatives, group membership.	OR=1.54[+] of cardiovascular mortality for the first and second lowest vs. highest quintile of social connections index in men.
Olsen et al (1991). Random sample of elderly residents in Odense, Denmark	715 (men) 1,037 (women)	70–100	15–16	Contact with siblings, children, friends, grandchildren, and other relatives	No association with cardiovascular mortality No association with cardiovascular mortality
Welin et al (1992). Random sample of residents in Gothenburg, Sweden	989 (men)	50, 60	12	Social activities (visiting friends and relatives, participating social activities)	Cardiovascular mortality was related to a low level of social activities (β = -0.113[+] for cardiovascular deaths, by level of social activities)
Iwasaki et al (2002). Residents of Komochi Village and Isesaki City, Japan	11,565 (men and women)	40–65	7	Contact with relative and friends, participation in religious and other group activity	HR=1.63[+] of circulatory disease mortality for not participating in hobbies, club activities and community groups in men

Table 18.2 (continued)

Author, published year study population, country	Sample size	Age at entry	Follow-up years	Social network measures	Relative risk
Rutledge et al (2003). Elderly residents of Baltimore, Minneapolis, Portland, Monongahela Valley, USA	7,524 (women)	65+	6	Size and frequency of contact with family and friends, interdependent relationships	Higher social network scale predicted lower cardiovascular mortality rate in unmarried (HR=0.75[†] of cardiovascular mortality, by level of social network scale)
Berkman et al (2004). French employees of Electricity of France-Gas, France	12,347 (men)	40–50	10	Marital status, friends and family, voluntary group membership	No association with cardiovascular mortality
	4,352 (women)	35–50			Not conducted due to small number of cases
Survival					
Williams et al (1992). CAD patients diagnosed at Duke Medical Center, USA	1,368 (men and women)	52 (median)	<14.5	Marital status, contact with relatives and friends, confidant availability	HR=3.34[†] of cardiovascular death for non-married or without a confidant compared with married or a close confidant
Jenkinson et al (1993). MI patients participated in the Anglo-Scandinavian Study of Early Thrombolysis, UK	1,376 (men and women)	25–84	3	Group membership and visiting friends and relatives	HR=1.49[†] of mortality for socially isolated vs. not socially isolated
Irvine et al (1999). MI patients participated in the Canadian Amiodarone Myocardial Infarction Arrhythmia Trial, Canada	671 (men and women)	63.8 (means)	2	Contacts with family, friends and group membership, participation in social pleasurable activities	HR=1.04[†] of SCD for greater social network contacts and HR=0.98* for lower social participation
Horsten et al (2000). CHD patients participated in FemCorRisk study, Sweden	292 (women)	30–65	5	Relatives, friends and confidants	HR=2.3[†] of recurrent CHD for the lowest vs. highest quartile of social integration

Table 18.2 (continued)

Author, published year study population, country	Sample size	Age at entry	Follow-up years	Social network measures	Relative risk
Brummett et al (2001). CAD patients participated in Mediators of Social Support study, USA	430 (men and women)	63.6 (means)	3.9 (means)	Frequency of network visits, confidants, participation in religious activities	HR=2.43[†] of cardiac mortality and HR=2.11[†] of survival for =3 persons in their social support network
Rutledge et al (2004). CAD patients participated in the Women's Ischemia Syndrome Evaluation Study, USA	503 (women)	18+	2.3 (mean)	Marital status, family, children, friends, and coworkers, participation in volunteer or organizational activities	RR=2.4[†] of mortality for low vs. high quartile of social network index
Boden-Albala et al (2005). IS patients participated in the Northern Manhattan Stroke Study, USA	655 (men and women)	69 (means)	4.6 (mean)	Social isolation (knowing people well enough to visit their homes, socialization)	OR=1.4[†] of stroke, MI or death for social isolation
Rodríguez-Artalejo et al (2006). Heart failure patients admitted at emergency hospitals, Spain	371 (men and women)	65+	6.6 months (median)	Marital status, contact with family	No association with survival
Lett et al (2007). MI patients participated in the Enhancing Recovery in Coronary Heart Disease Trial, USA	1,296 (men and women)	61 (means)	2.1 (mean)	Frequency of contact with children, confidants, friends and acquaintances, participation in groups and religious meetings	No association with survival
Rutledge et al (2008). MI patients participated in the Women's Ischemia Syndrome Evaluation Study, USA	629 (women)	18+	5.9 (median)	Marital status, family, children, friends, and coworkers, participation in volunteer or organizational activities	HR=2.7[†] of stroke incidence for low vs. high social network index

CHD, coronary heart disease; MI, myocardial infarction; CAD, coronary artery disease; SCD, sudden cardiac death; IS, ischemic stroke as early stage prostate cancer or colorectal cancer. More detailed studies are called for that take account of tumor site, detailed tumor characteristics, as well as differences in treatment modality and background co-morbidity.

There are sparse data examining social networks and cancer survival, and once again the findings are hard to generalize because the studies included a heterogeneous mix of cancer types (Table 18.3). However, if we limit the focus to marital status (which is incorporated into almost every measure or index of social networks), there is evidence that married individuals have better survival following cancer diagnosis compared to the non-married. This has been reported across a range of tumor sites including breast cancer (Osborne et al, 2005; Waxler-Morrison et al, 1991), bladder cancer (Gore et al, 2005), colorectal cancer (Villingshøj et al, 2006), and melanoma (Reyes Ortiz et al, 2007).

3.4 Cognitive Decline

As Table 18.4 illustrates, a growing number of studies have found evidence of a protective effect of social networks on the maintenance of cognitive function and prevention of the onset of dementia (Crooks et al, 2008; Fratiglioni et al, 2000). The hypothesized mechanism is through the concept of social engagement described earlier, i.e., social ties challenge people to participate in interpersonal exchanges, to practice their skills of communication, and to mobilize the firing of gray matter synapses on a regular basis in such a way that promotes the maintenance of cognitive function with aging ("the use it or lose it" phenomenon) (Berkman, 2000). The beneficial influence of social networks on cognitive function may also provide insurance against future catastrophic events such as stroke (the "cognitive reserve" hypothesis). In the Families in Recovery from Stroke Trial (FIRST), both social networks and emotional social support independently predicted levels of cognitive functioning 6 months after a cerebrovascular accident

(Glymour et al, 2008). However, only emotional support predicted greater recovery (i.e., improvement) in post-stroke cognition, which is consistent with a main effects model for social networks versus a stress-buffering model for social support (see earlier discussion).

4 Future Directions

Many interesting questions remain to be addressed in social networks and health. We highlight three issues that deserve particular attention: (a) the role of culture, (b) gender differences, and (c) sociometric analysis.

Based on our summary tables, it is fair to characterize the state of the empirical literature on social networks and health as being heavily dominated by studies in Western populations. Whether social connectedness has similar effects on the health of other populations remains to be seen. Even within studies conducted in the United States, closer inspection of the data points to revealing heterogeneities. For example, in the three-community prospective study reported by Seeman and colleagues (1993), social networks were significant predictors of all-cause mortality in Iowa and New Haven (Connecticut), but not in East Boston (Massachusetts). The latter community originated as an island in Boston Harbor that was connected to the rest of the city only in the 19th century. The geographic isolation of East Boston and the history of settlement by Italian immigrants contributed to a high level of social cohesion in the community which may have diluted the influence of personal social ties on the health status of residents. Similarly, the only U.S. cohort study to date that did not find an association between social networks and CHD incidence was among Japanese-American males in Hawaii (Reed et al, 1983).

Culture may thus contribute to contextual heterogeneity in the effects of social networks on health in at least two ways: (a) by truncating the distribution (and the hence range of variability) of social connectedness among members of a

Table 18.3 Prospective studies of social network and cancer

Author, published year study population, country	Sample size	Age at entry	Follow-up years	Social network measures	Relative risk
Incidence					
Reynolds and Kaplan (1990). Residents of Alameda County, USA	6,848 (men and women)	30–69	17	Marital status, friends and relatives, church and group membership, social isolation	HR=1.1[†] of cancer incidence for few friends/relative contacts, HR=1.5[†] for socially isolated in women
Vogt et al (1992). Random sample of HMO members, USA.	2,603 (men and women)	18+	15	Scope, size and frequency of contact within and across family, friends, and community	HR=2.2[†] of cancer mortality for fewer social networks, HR=1.2[†] for few friend/relative contacts, HR=1.7[†] for socially isolated, HR=5.7[†] of smoking-related cancer mortality for fewer social networks in women. HR=3.4[†] of cancer survival for fewer social networks in men
					HR=0.69[†] of survival for high vs. low tertiles of network scope, HR=0.82* for network frequency and HR=0.79[†] for network size in cancer incidence cases
Mortality					
Welin et al (1992). Random sample of residents in Gothenburg, Sweden	989 (men)	50+	12	Social activities (visiting friends and relatives, participating group activities)	No association with cancer mortality
Kawachi et al (1996). Dentists, veterinarians, pharmacists, optometrists, osteopathic physicians, podiatrists, USA	32,624 (men)	42–77	4	Marital status, friends and relatives, church and group membership	No association with cancer mortality
Eng et al (2002). Dentists, veterinarians, pharmacists, optometrists, osteopathic physicians, podiatrists, USA	28,369 (men)	42–77	10	Marital status, friends and relatives, church and group membership	No association with cancer mortality

Table 18.3 (continued)

Author, published year study population, country	Sample size	Age at entry	Follow-up years	Social network measures	Relative risk
Iwasaki et al (2002). Residents of Komochi Village and Isesaki City, Japan	11,565 (men and women)	40–69	7	Contact with relative and friends, participation in religious and other group activity	HR=2.63[†] of cancer mortality for rarely/never met close relatives compared to often/sometimes in urban women
Berkman et al (2004). French employees of Electricity of France-Gas, France	12,347 (men)	40–50	10	Marital status, friends and family, voluntary group membership	RR=3.60* of cancer mortality for the least vs. most socially integrated men (P for trend=0.0089, by level of social integration)
	4,352 (women)	35–50			Not conducted due to small number of cases
Survival					
Waxler-Morrison et al (1991). Breast cancer patients referred to the A. Maxwell Evans Clinic in Vancouver, Canada	133 (women)	<55	4	Marital status, friends and relatives, church and group membership	Women with a large social network size had a longer survival after beast cancer. (Instantaneous relative death =1.59[†] for small vs. large social network size)
Kroenke et al (2006). Breast cancer patients diagnosed during the Nurses' Health Study follow-up periods (1992–2002), USA	2,835 (women)	46–71	6	Marital status, friends and relatives, church and group membership	HR=1.66[†] of mortality and HR=2.14[†] of breast cancer mortality for patients being socially isolated compared with those being socially integrated
Villingshøj et al (2006). Colorectal cancer patients identified in the Danish cancer registry, Denmark	770 (men and women)	18–80	<17	Contact frequency with relatives, friends and colleagues	HR=1.4[†] of mortality for patients having lost the partner before the operation, and HR=1.7[†] of mortality for those increased contact with children after operation
Marital status only and survival					
Gore et al (2005). Bladder carcinoma patients reported by the Surveillance, Epidemiology and End Results registries, USA	5,854 (men and women)	Not stated	3.3	Marital status	HR=1.26[†] of mortality for single compared with married

Table 18.3 (continued)

Author, published year study population, country	Sample size	Age at entry	Follow-up years	Social network measures	Relative risk
Osborne et al (2005). Breast cancer patients reported by the Surveillance, Epidemiology and End Results registries, USA	32,268 (women)	65+	3	Marital status	HR=1.25[†] of breast cancer mortality for non-married compared with married
Reyes Ortiz et al (2007). Melanoma patients reported by the Surveillance, Epidemiology and End Results registries, USA	14,630 (men and women)	65+	8	Marital status	OR=1.23[†] of melanoma mortality for widowed compared with married
Jatoi et al (2007). NSCLC patients diagnosed and treated at the Mayo Clinic in Rochester, USA	5,898 (men and women)	Not stated	≤9	Marital status	No association with survival
Saito-Nakaya et al (2008). NSCLC patients diagnosed at National Cancer Center Hospital East, Kashiwa, Japan	865 (men)	63.9 (means)	≤5	Marital status	HR=1.7[†] of mortality for widowed compared with married
	365 (women)				No association with survival

NSCLC, non-small cell lung cancer.

Table 18.4 Prospective studies of social network and cognitive decline

Author, published year study population, country	Sample size	Age at entry	Follow-up years	Social ntwork measures	Relative risk
Bickel and Cooper (1994). Random sample of elderly community residents & long-stay residential care residents, Mannheim, Germany	Community: 314 (men and women) Long-stay: 108 (men and women)	65+	Community: 7–8 Long-stay: 5–6	Frequency of contact within and outside the family circle	No association with dementia
Bassuk et al (1999). Multistage probability sample of non-institutionalized elderly residents in New Haven, USA	2,812 (men and women)	65+	12	Contact with friends and relatives, religious and other group membership, participation in social activities	The 3 years OR=2.24[†] of cognitive decline, the 6-years OR=1.91[†] and the 12-years OR=2.37[†] for no vs. five or six social tie
Fratiglioni et al (2000). Elderly resident of Kungsholmen district, Sweden	1,203 (men and women)	75+	3	Marital status, living arrangement, frequency of, and satisfaction with contact with children, relatives and friends	HR=1.6[†] of dementia for poor/limited vs. extensive or moderate social network
Seeman et al (2001). Elderly residents of Durham, East Boston, and New Haven, USA	1,189 (men and women)	70–79	7.4	Marital status, contact with close friends and relatives, church and group membership	No association with cognitive performance
Barnes et al (2007). Elderly residents of Baltimore, Minneapolis, Portland, and Monongahela Valley, USA	9,704 (women)	65+	15	Size and frequency of contact with relatives and friends, perceived general and confidant support	OR=1.20[†] of minor cognitive decline for poor Lubben Social Network Scale

Table 18.4 (continued)

Author, published year study population, country	Sample size	Age at entry	Follow-up years	Social ntwork measures	Relative risk
Crooks et al (2008). HMO elderly members participated in a longitudinal study of hormone replacement therapy, USA	2,249 (women)	78+	≤3	Size and frequency of contact with relatives and friends, perceived general and confidant support	HR=0.74[†] of dementia for high (12+) vs. low (<12) on Lubben Social Network Scale
Ertel et al (2008). Multistage probability sample of elderly population, USA	16,638 (men and women)	50+	6	Marital status, volunteer activities, contact with parents, children, and neighbors	High levels of social integration predicted a slower rate of memory decline (an average of 0.03[†] points/year faster decline for each decrease in number of domains of social integration)
Glymour et al (2008). Stroke patients admitted to Boston area hospitals and rehabilitation facilities, USA	272 (men and women)	45+	0.5	Contact with children, relatives and friends, participation in volunteer, community, paid work, religious and civic organizations	High levels of social integration predicted greater cognitive function after stroke (β=0.21[†] for 6 months Cognitive Summary Score, by level of social tie index)

community through higher or lower background levels of social cohesion; and (b) by moderating or altering the slope of the graded relationship between social ties and health. The notion that an individual's egocentric social ties are contingent on broader contextual characteristics – such as the extent of social cohesion within the community in which the individual resides – is one of the key insights of social capital theory (Kawachi and Berkman, 2000). Testing this idea formally would require some form of quantitative cross-cultural comparative analysis – e.g., assembling a multi-level pooled data set that uses consistent measures of social networks across different sites, and fits each context (e.g., community or country) as a random effect.

In addition to calling for a more nuanced appreciation of the role of culture, more studies are needed to understand gender differences in the relationship between social networks and health. These differences have been summarized by Deborah Belle (1987): women are more likely than men to maintain emotionally intimate relationships across the life-course; and they provide more frequent and effective social support to others within their networks. Adding these two observations results in the phenomenon that women are more susceptible to the "contagion of stress" (Belle, 1982) when alters within their networks experience an event. Indeed within marital dyads, researchers have remarked on the "social support gap" between husbands who tend to be net support recipients versus wives who tend to be net support providers. In turn, these observations have resulted in the conventional wisdom that men benefit more from marriage than do women (House et al, 1988). However, it may be time to re-examine the received wisdom. The balance of support provision/receipt within marital couples is likely to be *dynamic*, reflecting secular changes in norms and expectations about the household division of labor, as well as gendered patterns of labor force participation, fertility, and time use. Indeed, a recent meta-analysis of marital status and mortality based on 53 studies failed to detect a gender difference in the association with all-cause mortality (Manzoli et al, 2007). The pooled relative risk of mortality for mar-

ried versus unmarried men was 0.88 (95% CI: 0.84–0.93), and 0.90 (95% CI: 0.85–0.95) for women.[7] By contrast, an emerging pattern of evidence is beginning to suggest stark gender differences in the health benefit of marriage in the Asian population. For example, in a 10-year Japanese cohort study, being divorce/separated was associated with a 1.5- to 2.0-fold increase in risk of all-cause and cause-specific mortality among Japanese men, but there was no apparent adverse effect of widowhood/divorce on the health of Japanese women (Ikeda et al, 2007). As we have emphasized throughout, being socially connected is not uniformly beneficial to every group or for every health outcome. Social networks are not a panacea and their effects are likely to be historically and culturally contingent.

This brings us to the third and final observation, which is the need to move beyond studies that use the egocentric network perspective, towards a whole social network approach. As alluded to earlier, the assessment of whole social networks can be challenging not only because of the time and expense involved, but also on account of the need to define the boundaries of the network. Nevertheless, the potential power of the sociometric approach has been recently illustrated by two studies of the person-to-person ("epidemic") spread of obesity (Christakis and Fowler, 2007) as well as smoking behaviors (Christakis and Fowler, 2008). Both studies, based on analyses of the Framingham Offspring Study by Nicholas Christakis and colleagues, capitalized on serendipitous information about close personal contacts that happened to have been collected by the investigators for the purposes of longitudinal follow-up of cohort members. The first study found obesity was more likely to spread within a social network through close social ties – especially friends and siblings of the same sex. The second study found that

---

[7]No meta-analysis to our knowledge has examined gender differences in the effects of social networks on mortality. As indicated by our summary tables, the empirical data are heavily weighted toward males.

within social networks, groups of interconnected people tend to quit smoking together, and persons who remained smokers were observed to move to the outside of the network, so that over time the network became more polarized with respect to smokers and non-smokers.

5 Conclusion

Social networks are robustly associated with health outcomes (particularly, all-cause mortality and cardiovascular disease incidence and survival) in prospective epidemiologic studies. Growing evidence has pointed to the role of social networks in maintaining aspects of successful aging, such as cognitive functioning. The mechanisms of action that explain these diverse observations likely involve some combination of social influence, social engagement, access to social support, as well as material resources. There is a dose–response relationship between social networks and health outcomes: the more diverse the better, and some ties can substitute for others. We have also pointed to some gaps in the literature, including the need to understand the culturally and contextually contingent effects of social networks on health; gender differences in the effects of social networks; and the application of sociometric approaches to study both the positive and negative aspects of social integration.

References

Astrand, N. E., Hanson, B. S., and Isacsson, S. O. (1989). Job demands, job decision latitude, job support, and social network factors as predictors of mortality in a Swedish pulp and paper company. *Br J Ind Med*, 46, 334-340.

Barefoot, J. C., Grønbaek, M., Jensen, G., Schnohr, P., and Prescott, E. (2005). Social network diversity and risks of ischemic heart disease and total mortality: findings from the Copenhagen City Heart Study. *Am J Epidemiol*, 161, 960-967.

Barnes, D. E., Cauley, J. A., Lui, L. Y., Fink, H. A., McCulloch, C. et al (2007). Women who maintain optimal cognitive function into old age. *J Am Geriatr Soc*, 55, 259-264.

Bassuk, S. S., Glass, T. A., and Berkman, L. F. (1999). Social disengagement and incident cognitive decline in community-dwelling elderly persons. *Ann Intern Med*, 131, 165-173.

Berkman, L. F., and Syme, S. L. (1979). Social networks, host resistance, and mortality: a nine-year follow-up study of Alameda County residents. *Am J Epidemiol*, 109, 186-204.

Berkman, L. F. (2000). Which influences cognitive function: living alone or being alone? *Lancet*, 355, 1291-1292.

Berkman, L. F., and Glass, T. (2000). Social integration, social networks, social support, and health. In L. F. Berkman & I. Kawachi (Eds.), *Social Epidemiology* (pp. 137-173). New York: Oxford University Press.

Berkman, L. F., Blumenthal, J., Burg, M., Carney, R. M., Catellier, D. et al (2003). Effects of treating depression and low perceived social support on clinical events after myocardial infarction: the Enhancing Recovery in Coronary Heart Disease Patients (ENRICHD) Randomized Trial. *JAMA*, 289, 3106-3116.

Berkman, L. F., Melchior, M., Chastang, J. F., Niedhammer, I., Leclerc, A. et al (2004). Social integration and mortality: a prospective study of French employees of Electricity of France-Gas of France: the GAZEL Cohort. *Am J Epidemiol*, 159, 167-174.

Bearman, P. S., and Moody, J. (2004). Suicide and friendships among American adolescents. *Am J Public Health, 94*, 89-95.

Belle, D. (1982). *Lives in Stress: Women and Depression*. California: Sage.

Belle, D. (1987). Gender differences in the social moderators of stress. In R. C. Barnett, L. Biener, & G. K. Baruch (Eds.), *Gender and Stress* (pp. 257-277). New York: The Free Press.

Bickel, H., and Cooper, B. (1994). Incidence and relative risk of dementia in an urban elderly population: findings of a prospective field study. *Psychol Med*, 24, 179-192.

Blazer, D. G. (1982). Social support and mortality in an elderly community population. *Am J Epidemiol*, 115, 684-694.

Boden-Albala, B., Litwak, E., Elkind, M. S., Rundek, T., ad Sacco, R. L. (2005). Social isolation and outcomes post stroke. *Neurology*, 64, 1888-1892.

Brummett, B. H., Barefoot, J. C., Siegler, I. C., Clapp-Channing, N. E., Lytle, B. L. et al (2001). Characteristics of socially isolated patients with coronary artery disease who are at elevated risk for mortality. *Psychosom Med*, 63, 267-272.

Cerhan, J. R., and Wallace, R. B. (1997). Change in social ties and subsequent mortality in rural elders. *Epidemiology*, 8, 475-481.

Christakis, N. A., and Fowler, J. H. (2007). The spread of obesity in a large social network over 32 years. *N Engl J Med*, 357, 370-379.

Christakis, N. A., and Fowler, J. H. (2008). The collective dynamics of smoking in a large social network. *N Engl J Med*, 358, 2249-2258.

Cohen, S., and Wills, T. A. (1985). Stress, social support, and the buffering hypothesis. *Psychol Bull*, 98, 310-357.

Cohen, S., Doyle, W. J., Skoner, D. P., Rabin, B. S., and Gwaltney, J. M. Jr. (1997). Social ties and susceptibility to the common cold. *JAMA*, 277, 1940-1944.

Crooks, V. C., Lubben, J., Petitti, D. B., Little, D., and Chiu, V. (2008). Social network, cognitive function, and dementia incidence among elderly women. *Am J Public Health*, 98, 1221-1227.

Durkheim, E. (1951). *Suicide*: New York: Free Press. (originally published 1987.)

Eng, P. M., Rimm, E. B., Fitzmaurice, G., and Kawachi, I. (2002). Social ties and change in social ties in relation to subsequent total and cause-specific mortality and coronary heart disease incidence in men. *Am J Epidemiol*, 155, 700-709.

Eng, P. M., Kawachi, I., Fitzmaurice, G., and Rimm, E. B. (2005). Effects of marital transitions on changes in dietary and other health behaviours in US male health professionals. *J Epidemiol Community Health*, 59, 56-62.

Ertel, K. A., Glymour, M. M., and Berkman, L. F. (2008). Effects of social integration on preserving memory function in a nationally representative US elderly population. *Am J Public Health*, 98, 1215-1220.

Falk, A., Hanson, B. S., Isacsson, S. O., and Ostergren, P. O. (1992). Job strain and mortality in elderly men: social network, support, and influence as buffers. *Am J Public Health*, 82, 1136-1139.

Fratiglioni, L., Wang, H. X., Ericsson, K., Maytan, M., and Winblad, B. (2000). Influence of social network on occurrence of dementia: a community-based longitudinal study. *Lancet*, 355, 1315-1319.

Friedman, S. R., and Aral, S. (2001). Social networks, risk-potential networks, health, and disease. *J Urban Health*, 78, 411-418.

Fuhrer, R., Dufouil, C., Antonucci, T. C., Shipley, M. J., Helmer, C. et al (1999). Psychological disorder and mortality in French older adults: do social relations modify the association? *Am J Epidemiol*, 149, 116-126.

Giles, L. C., Glonek, G. F., Luszcz, M. A., and Andrews, G. R. (2005). Effect of social networks on 10 year survival in very old Australians: the Australian longitudinal study of aging. *J Epidemiol Community Health*, 59, 574-579.

Glass, T. A., Berkman, L. F., Hiltunen, E. F., Furie, K., Glymour, M. M. et al (2004). The families in recovery from Stroke Trial (FIRST): primary study results. *Psychosom Med*, 66, 889-897.

Glymour, M. M., Weuve, J., Fay, M. E., Glass, T., and Berkman, L. F. (2008). Social ties and cognitive recovery after stroke: does social integration promote cognitive resilience? *Neuroepidemiology*, 31, 10-20.

Gore, J. L., Kwan, L., Saigal, C. S., and Litwin, M. S. (2005). Marriage and mortality in bladder carcinoma. *Cancer*, 104, 1188-1194.

Granovetter, M. S. (1973). The strength of weak ties. *Am J Sociol*, 78, 1360-1380.

Hanson, B. S., Isacsson, S. O., Janzon, L., and Lindell, S. E. (1989). Social network and social support influence mortality in elderly men. The prospective population study of "Men born in 1914," Malmö, Sweden. *Am J Epidemiol*, 130, 100-111.

Ho, S. C. (1991). Health and social predictors of mortality in an elderly Chinese cohort. *Am J Epidemiol*, 133, 907-921.

Horsten, M., Mittleman, M. A., Wamala, S. P., Schenck-Gustafsson, K., and Orth-Gomér, K. (2000). Depressive symptoms and lack of social integration in relation to prognosis of CHD in middle-aged women. The Stockholm Female Coronary Risk Study. *Eur Heart J*, 21. 1072-1080.

House, J. S., Robbins, C., and Metzner, H. L. (1982). The association of social relationships and activities with mortality: prospective evidence from the Tecumseh Community Health Study. *Am J Epidemiol*, 116, 123-140.

House, J. S., Landis, K. R., and Umberson, D. (1988). Social relationships and health. *Science*, 241, 540-545.

Ikeda, A., Iso, H., Toyoshima, H., Fujino, Y., Mizoue, T. et al (2007). Marital status and mortality among Japanese men and women: the Japan Collaborative Cohort Study. *BMC Public Health*, 7, 73.

Irvine, J., Basinski, A., Baker, B., Jandciu, S., Paquette, M. et al (1999). Depression and risk of sudden cardiac death after acute myocardial infarction: testing for the confounding effects of fatigue. *Psychosom Med*, 61, 729-737.

Iwasaki, M., Otani, T., Sunaga, R., Miyazaki, H., Xiao, L. et al (2002). Social networks and mortality based on the Komo-Ise cohort study in Japan. *Int J Epidemiol*, 31, 1208-1218.

Jatoi, A., Novotny, P., Cassivi, S., Clark, M. M., Midthun, D. et al (2007). Does marital status impact survival and quality of life in patients with non-small cell lung cancer? Observations from the mayo clinic lung cancer cohort. *Oncologist*, 12, 1456-1463.

Jenkinson, C. M., Madeley, R. J., Mitchell, J. R., and Turner, I. D. (1993). The influence of psychosocial factors on survival after myocardial infarction. *Public Health*, 107, 305-317.

Kaplan, G. A., Salonen, J. T., Cohen, R. D., Brand, R. J., Syme, S. L. et al (1988). Social connections and mortality from all causes and from cardiovascular disease: prospective evidence from eastern Finland. *Am J Epidemiol*, 128, 370-380.

Kawachi, I., Colditz, G. A., Ascherio, A., Rimm, E. B., Giovannucci, E. et al (1996). A prospective study of social networks in relation to total mortality and cardiovascular disease in men in the USA. *J Epidemiol Community Health*, 50, 245-251.

Kawachi, I., and Berkman, L. F. (2000). Social cohesion, social capital, and health. In L. F. Berkman & I. Kawachi (Eds.), *Social Epidemiology* (pp 174-190). New York: Oxford University Press.

Kawachi, I., and Berkman, L. F. (2001). Social ties and mental health. *J Urban Health*, 78, 458-467.

Kiecolt-Glaser, J. K., and Newton, T. L. (2001). Marriage and health: his and hers. *Psychol Bull*, 127, 472-503.

Kroenke, C. H., Kubzansky, L. D., Schernhammer, E. S., Holmes, M. D., and Kawachi, I. (2006). Social networks, social support, and survival after breast cancer diagnosis. *J Clin Oncol*, 24, 1105-1111.

Lee, S., Cho, E., Grodstein, F., Kawachi, I., and Hu, F. B. et al (2005). Effects of marital transitions on changes in dietary and other health behaviours in US women. *Int J Epidemiol*, 34, 69-78.

Lett, H. S., Blumenthal, J. A., Babyak, M. A., Catellier, D. J., Carney, R. M. et al (2007). Social support and prognosis in patients at increased psychosocial risk recovering from myocardial infarction. *Health Psychol*, 26, 418-427.

Lillard, L. A., and Panis, C. W. A. (1996). Marital status and mortality: the role of health. *Demography*, 33, 313-327.

Loucks, E. B., Berkman, L. F., Gruenewald, T. L., and Seeman, T. E. (2006). Relation of social integration to inflammatory marker concentrations in men and women 70 to 79 years. *Am J Cardiol*, 97, 1010-1016.

Loucks, E. B., Sullivan, L. M., D'Agostino, R. B. Sr., Larson, M. G., Berkman, L. F. et al (2006). Social networks and inflammatory markers in the Framingham Heart Study. *J Biosoc Sci*, 38, 835–842.

Manzoli, L., Villari, P., Pirone, G. M., and Boccia, A. (2007). Marital status and mortality in the elderly: a systematic review and meta-analysis. *Soc Sci Med*, 64, 77–94

Olsen, R. B., Olsen, J., Gunner-Svensson, F., and Waldstrøm, B. (1991). Social networks and longevity. A 14 year follow-up study among elderly in Denmark. *Soc Sci Med*, 33, 1189–1195.

Orth-Gomér, K., and Johnson, J. V. (1987). Social network interaction and mortality. A six year follow-up study of a random sample of the Swedish population. *J Chronic Dis*, 40, 949–957.

Orth-Gomér, K., Rosengren, A., and Wilhelmsen, L. (1993). Lack of social support and incidence of coronary heart disease in middle-aged Swedish men. *Psychosom Med*, 55, 37–43.

Osborne, C., Ostir, G. V., Du, X., Peek, M. K., and Goodwin, J. S. (2005). The influence of marital status on the stage at diagnosis, treatment, and survival of older women with breast cancer. *Breast Cancer Res Treat*, 93, 41–47.

Penninx, B. W., van Tilburg, T., Kriegsman, D. M., Deeg, D. J., Boeke, A. J. et al (1997). Effects of social support and personal coping resources on mortality in older age: the Longitudinal Aging Study Amsterdam. *Am J Epidemiol*, 146, 510–519.

Reed, D., McGee, D., Yano, K., and Feinleib, M. (1983). Social networks and coronary heart disease among Japanese men in Hawaii. *Am J Epidemiol*, 117, 384–396.

Reyes Ortiz, C. A., Freeman, J. L., Kuo, Y. F., and Goodwin, J. S. (2007). The influence of marital status on stage at diagnosis and survival of older persons with melanoma. *J Gerontol A Biol Sci Med Sci*, 62, 892–898.

Reynolds, P., and Kaplan, G. A. (1990). Social connections and risk for cancer: prospective evidence from the Alameda County Study. *Behav Med*, 16, 101–110.

Rodríguez-Artalejo, F., Guallar-Castillón, P., Herrera, M. C., Otero, C. M., Chiva, M. O. et al (2006). Social network as a predictor of hospital readmission and mortality among older patients with heart failure. *J Card Fail*, 12, 621–627.

Rogers, R. G., Hummer, R. A., and Nam, C. B. (2000). *Living and Dying in the USA: Behavioral, Health, and Social Differentials of Adult Mortality.* San Diego: Academic Press.

Rosengren, A., Wilhelmsen, L., and Orth-Gomér, K. (2004). Coronary disease in relation to social support and social class in Swedish men. A 15 year follow-up in the study of men born in 1933. *Eur Heart J*, 25, 56–63.

Ross, C. E., Mirowsky, J., and Goldsteen, K. (1990). The impact of the family on health: the decade in review. *J Marr Fam*, 52, 1059–1078.

Rutledge, T., Matthews, K., Lui, L. Y., Stone, K. L., and Cauley, J. A. (2003). Social networks and marital status predict mortality in older women: prospective evidence from the Study of Osteoporotic Fractures (SOF). *Psychosom Med*, 65, 688–694.

Rutledge, T., Reis, S. E., Olson, M., Owens, J., Kelsey, S. F. et al (2004). Social networks are associated with lower mortality rates among women with suspected coronary disease: the National Heart, Lung, and Blood Institute-Sponsored Women's Ischemia Syndrome Evaluation study. *Psychosom Med*, 66, 882–888.

Rutledge, T., Linke, S. E., Olson, M. B., Francis, J., Johnson, B. D. et al (2008). Social networks and incident stroke among women with suspected myocardial ischemia. *Psychosom Med*, 70, 282–287.

Saito-Nakaya. K., Nakaya, N., Akechi, T., Inagaki, M., Asai, M. et al (2008). Marital status and non-small cell lung cancer survival: the Lung Cancer Database Project in Japan. *Psychooncology*, 17, 869–876.

Schoenbach, V. J., Kaplan, B. H., Fredman, L., and Kleinbaum, D. G. (1986). Social ties and mortality in Evans County, Georgia. *Am J Epidemiol*, 123, 577–591.

Seeman, T. E., Kaplan, G. A., Knudsen, L., Cohen, R., and Guralnik, J. (1987). Social network ties and mortality among the elderly in the Alameda County Study. *Am J Epidemiol*, 126, 714–723.

Seeman, T. E., Berkman, L. F., Kohout, F., Lacroix, A., Glynn, R. et al (1993). Intercommunity variations in the association between social ties and mortality in the elderly. A comparative analysis of three communities. *Ann Epidemiol*, 3, 325–335.

Seeman, T. E., Lusignolo, T. M., Albert, M., and Berkman, L. (2001). Social relationships, social support, and patterns of cognitive aging in healthy, high-functioning older adults: MacArthur studies of successful aging. *Health Psychol*, 20, 243–255.

Shye, D., Mullooly, J. P., Freeborn, D. K., and Pope, C. R. (1995). Gender differences in the relationship between social network support and mortality: a longitudinal study of an elderly cohort. *Soc Sci Med*, 41, 935–947.

Sugisawa, H., Liang, J., and Liu, X. (1994). Social networks, social support, and mortality among older people in Japan. *J Gerontol*, 49, S3–S13.

van der Gaag, M., and Webber, M. (2008). Measurement of individual social capital. In I. Kawachi, S. V. Subramanian, & D. Kim (Eds.), *Social Capital and Health* (pp. 29-49), New York: Springer.

Villingshøj, M., Ross, L., Thomsen, B. L., and Johansen, C. (2006). Does marital status and altered contact with the social network predict colorectal cancer survival? *Eur J Cancer*, 42, 3022–3027.

Vogt, T. M., Mullooly, J. P., Ernst, D., Pope, C. R., and Hollis, J. F. (1992). Social networks as predictors of ischemic heart disease, cancer, stroke and hypertension: incidence, survival and mortality. *J Clin Epidemiol*, 45, 659–666.

Waite, L. J. (1995). Does marriage matter? *Demography*, 32, 483-507.

Waxler-Morrison, N., Hislop, T. G., Mears, B., and Kan, L. (1991). Effects of social relationships on survival for women with breast cancer: a prospective study. *Soc Sci Med*, 33, 177–183.

Welin, L., Tibblin, G., Svärdsudd, K., Tibblin, B., Ander-Peciva, S. et al (1985). Prospective study of social influences on mortality. The study of men born in 1913 and 1923. *Lancet*, 1, 915–918.

Welin, L., Larsson, B., Svärdsudd, K., Tibblin, B., and Tibblin, G. (1992). Social network and activities in relation to mortality from cardiovascular diseases, cancer and other causes: a 12 year follow up of the study of men born in 1913 and 1923. *J Epidemiol Community Health*, 46, 127–132.

Williams, R. B., Barefoot, J. C., Califf, R. M., Haney, T. L., Saunders, W. B. et al (1992). Prognostic importance of social and economic resources among medically treated patients with angiographically documented coronary artery disease. *JAMA*, 267, 520–524.

Wilson, C. M., and Oswald, A. J. (2005). How does marriage affect physical and psychological health? A survey of the longitudinal evidence (June 2005). IZA Discussion Paper No. 1619. Available at SSRN http://ssrn.com.ezp-prod1.hul.harvard.edu/abstract=735205

Yasuda, N., Zimmerman, S. I., Hawkes, W., Fredman, L., Hebel, J. R. et al (1997). Relation of social network characteristics to 5-year mortality among young-old versus old-old white women in an urban community. *Am J Epidemiol*, 145, 516–523.

Chapter 19

Social Norms and Health Behavior

Allecia E. Reid, Robert B. Cialdini, and Leona S. Aiken

Psychologists, sociologists, and others interested in human behavior have long recognized the influence of the attitudes and behaviors of most others on one's own attitudes and behaviors (e.g., Durkheim, 1951; Sherif, 1936). Despite this history of research, the utility of normative information for influencing behavior has not gone unquestioned (e.g., Darley and Latané, 1970). More recently, researchers have raised concerns regarding the benefit of employing norms in the prediction of health behaviors (e.g., Godin and Kok, 1996). However, there appears to be consensus at present that norms are indeed a powerful "lever of social influence" (Goldstein and Cialdini, 2007).

1 Defining Norms

Social norms refer to common standards for behavior, set by and for members of a social group (Cialdini and Trost, 1998). Although the group must be, to some extent, definable, the degree to which individuals consider themselves to be members of the group and the group to be self-defining can vary. Certainly, norms are likely to exert the greatest influence on behaviors when they are representative of a group with which an individual strongly identifies (Terry and Hogg, 1996). However, the behaviors of others can also be influential in situations where the group identity itself is not particularly meaningful and individuals' self-concepts are not tied to membership in the group (Cialdini et al, 1990; Goldstein et al, 2008).

1.1 Differentiating Between Classes of Norms

Much of the early debate concerning the utility of norms focused on the lack of a commonly agreed upon definition of the construct. However, Cialdini et al's (1990) formulation classifying norms into two distinct categories, descriptive and injunctive, has set the standard for subsequent research. Additional characterizations of norms have been identified and studied (e.g., personal norms; Schwartz, 1977); however, the focus at present will be on descriptive and injunctive norms. Descriptive and injunctive norms distinguish, respectively, between perceptions of what *is* and what *ought* to be. While descriptive norms refer to perceptions of how others typically behave in a given situation, injunctive norms capture what is commonly approved or disapproved (Cialdini et al, 1990). For example, perceiving that the majority of individuals in one's immediate environment are smoking cigarettes, or that most of one's family, friends, coworkers, etc., are smokers, would be

A.E. Reid (✉)
Department of Psychology, Arizona State University, 950 S. McAllister Ave., P.O. Box 871104, Tempe, AZ 85287-1104, USA
e-mail: allecia.reid@asu.edu

A. Steptoe (ed.), *Handbook of Behavioral Medicine*, DOI 10.1007/978-0-387-09488-5_19,
© Springer Science+Business Media, LLC 2010

representative of a descriptive norm. However, considering the corresponding injunctive norm, one might perceive instead that most others disapprove of smoking, because of its negative health effects.

Each class of norms serves a distinct purpose. Descriptive norms provide a useful heuristic when accurate decision making is of importance and are likely to be particularly influential in novel situations or when the appropriate course of action is unclear (Cialdini and Trost, 1998). Injunctive norms aid in the formation and maintenance of social bonds and motivate behavior through the threat of social disapproval for inappropriate behavior or the promise of approval for conformity (Cialdini and Trost, 1998).

Questions have been raised as to the distinctiveness of descriptive and injunctive norms. Discriminant validity of the constructs has been supported by confirmatory factor analyses in the context of calcium consumption, exercise, and dieting, among others (Hagger and Chatzisarantis, 2005; Schmiege et al, 2007). Further, although what is typically done often reflects what is approved, descriptive and injunctive norms can also be opposing for a single behavior, as demonstrated in the smoking example given above. Many public service announcements depict unhealthy behaviors, such as smoking cigarettes and use of illicit drugs, as regrettably common (favorable descriptive norm), though widely disapproved (unfavorable injunctive norm; Cialdini, 2003). Reno et al (1993) devised situations in which the injunctive norm opposed littering but a heavily littered parking lot indicated a favorable descriptive norm. Although examining conflicting norms is useful for purposes of empirical inquiry and theoretical refinement, normative information is most powerful when the injunctive and descriptive norm correspond with, rather than contradict, one another (Cialdini, 2003). Indeed, Smith and Louis (2008) found that students held the most favorable attitudes toward signing a petition and reported the greatest willingness to do so when both the descriptive *and* the injunctive norm at their university supported the behavior.

2 Relationships of Norms to Health Behaviors

Descriptive and injunctive norms have both demonstrated relationships with a number of health behaviors. Much research has focused on demonstrating unique roles for both types of norms in predicting intentions and/or behavior (e.g., Rivis and Sheeran, 2003). Bolstering the argument for distinctiveness of the constructs, simultaneous roles for descriptive and injunctive norms have been observed across health-protective, health-risk, and screening behaviors.

Correlational research supports roles for descriptive and injunctive norms in the longitudinal prediction of both health-protective and health-risk behaviors. Etcheverry and Agnew (2008) documented relationships of both friends' use and approval of cigarettes with the number of cigarettes smoked over time. Similarly, in their meta-analysis, Sheeran et al (1999) observed relationships of both norms to condom use. However, descriptive norms exhibited a significantly larger relationship with the outcome than did injunctive norms. Research has also found only descriptive norms to be predictive of alcohol consumption and needle sharing among injection drug users (Carey et al, 2006; Davey-Rothwell et al, 2009). Additional research supports only a role for injunctive norms in the prediction of alcohol use (Larimer et al, 2004). Accordingly, it is unclear whether either category of norms consistently weighs more heavily than the other in decisions to perform health-protective or health-risk behaviors, though this question warrants future attention. Research does, however, support a greater role for descriptive norms in the prediction of intentions to engage in risky behaviors than in intentions to engage in protective behaviors (Rivis and Sheeran, 2003).

Both injunctive and descriptive norms are related to screening behaviors; however, research supports the superiority of injunctive norms in this realm. Smith-McLallen and Fishbein (2008) found that intentions to obtain a mammogram, colonoscopy, and screening test for prostate cancer were more strongly associated with injunctive norms than with descriptive norms. The recommendations of one's doctor likely weigh heavily when considering screening behaviors, though the desires and expectations of family and friends appear to play a role as well (Montaño et al, 1997).

As previously alluded to, questions remain regarding the utility of norms for predicting and ultimately changing health behaviors. This has, in part, resulted from the weak role of subjective norms, a form of an injunctive norm, in the Theories of Reasoned Action and Planned Behavior (Ajzen, 1991; Fishbein and Ajzen, 1975, see Chapter 2). In both theories, subjective norms, capturing perceptions of social pressure from important others to perform or not perform a behavior, are proposed as a determinant of intentions to engage in the behavior. However, the subjective norm–intention relationship has consistently been found to be the weakest of the proposed theoretical relationships (Ajzen, 1991; Godin and Kok, 1996). Stiff and Mongeau (2003) suggested that the weak role of subjective norms may result from a general focus on behaviors that are often performed in private. Such behaviors should be less responsive to injunctive norms as they lack the potential for social evaluation, the driving force behind conformity to injunctive norms. Further, accounting for either the type of behavior being examined or individual differences that may influence responsiveness to norms significantly alters the magnitude of the relationship between subjective norms and intentions (Trafimow and Finlay, 1996; Trafimow and Fishbein, 1994). Nonetheless, many have incorporated descriptive norms into the theories in response to the poor performance of subjective norms and the addition of descriptive norms significantly improves prediction of intentions (Rivis and Sheeran, 2003).

The literature discussed thus far has examined correlational relationships of descriptive and injunctive norms with a number of health behaviors. However, whether norms successfully bring about behavior change is ultimately of interest. Much research by Cialdini and colleagues (e.g., 1990, Reno et al, 1993) has demonstrated the utility of norms for motivating pro-

environmental behaviors. Such behaviors, often observed simultaneously with presentation of the normative manipulation (but see Schultz et al, 2007), may operate through different mechanisms than do health behaviors, which typically require prolonged effort and regulation. Accordingly, we will focus at present on social norms theory and its application to health behavior change.

3 Social Norms Theory

Perceptual biases can color both the encoding and the retrieval of information about the world around us, resulting in a widespread tendency to hold inaccurate perceptions of the behaviors and attitudes of most others. According to social norms theory, behavior is meaningfully influenced by these misperceptions (Perkins and Berkowitz, 1986). Accordingly, behavior change can be brought about by correcting misperceptions.

3.1 The Extent of Misperceptions

Social norms theory originated when Perkins and Berkowitz (1986) noted that undergraduate students were largely inaccurate in their perceptions of their peers' attitudes toward alcohol use. Students by and large reported that their own attitudes concerning heavy alcohol use were conservative, yet they believed that their classmates approved of and held liberal attitudes toward heavy alcohol use. Thus, although the actual injunctive norm favored controlled, moderate levels of drinking, it was perceived that most students were comfortable with heavy drinking. Such misperceptions have been repeatedly documented with respect to alcohol use. Perkins et al (2005) examined data from 76,145 students, representing 130 colleges nationwide, and found that, regardless of the magnitude of the actual drinking norms, students consistently overestimated the prevalence and approval of alcohol use on their campus. In a synthesis of the literature, Borsari and Carey (2003) found that undergraduates consistently reported that they drink less and are less approving of alcohol use than their peers. Erroneous perceptions of drinking norms are not localized to college students or collegiate settings. Young adults who do not attend college and middle and high school students hold similarly exaggerated views of the typical drinking behaviors of their peers (Linkenbach and Perkins, 2003a; Perkins and Craig, 2003b).

Although the social norms approach was developed in the context of alcohol use and, consequently, has focused extensively on this issue, discrepancies between perceived and actual norms have been documented across a number of health behaviors. Individuals generally overestimate the prevalence of risky behaviors and underestimate the prevalence of protective behaviors. This pattern of findings has been replicated for drug use, including the use of tobacco, marijuana, and other illicit drugs (Perkins and Craig, 2003b). With respect to sexual behavior, condom use is underestimated, while levels of sexual activity are overestimated (Scholly et al, 2005). Finally, having bearing for body image disturbance and self-esteem, most women believe that the average woman is thinner than she is (Sanderson et al, 2002), and women inaccurately believe that men find overly thin women attractive (Bergstrom et al, 2004).

3.2 Sources of Normative Misperceptions

Normative misperceptions have been attributed to four social psychological phenomena – the availability heuristic, the fundamental attribution error, the false consensus effect, and pluralistic ignorance. While the fundamental attribution error and the availability heuristic allow for consideration of others' behaviors as a source of misperception, the false consensus effect and pluralistic ignorance focus instead on personal attitudes and behaviors as sources of error. Errors in judgments of alcohol use and approval for

alcohol use are particularly useful for considering how these biases are likely to operate.

According to the fundamental attribution error, others' behaviors are typically inferred to reflect personal disposition, rather than situational forces (Ross, 1977), leading observers to view heavy alcohol use as indicative of the drinker's permissive attitude towards drinking. Simultaneously privately disapproving of heavy alcohol use, an individual's own dissent could serve as a basis for inferring the true attitudes of others. However, given pluralistic ignorance, the belief that one is alone in disagreeing with the perceived norms, individuals instead infer that their beliefs are highly discrepant from those of the majority (Miller and McFarland, 1987). As might be expected, individuals who engage in heavy alcohol use often believe that most others behave similarly, as the false consensus effect, the tendency to believe that others think and act as one does, biases perceptions of reality (Ross et al, 1977). Conversely, reliance on the availability heuristic can lead moderate drinkers and abstainers to misperceive rates of alcohol use as well. According to this heuristic, the ease with which an event is called to mind influences one's judgment of the probability of the occurrence of the event (Tversky and Kahneman, 1973). As most can easily recall instances of being in the presence of a highly intoxicated individual or watching movies or television shows depicting heavy alcohol use, such occurrences likely come to mind quite readily.

3.3 Consequences of Misperceptions for Behaviors

Misperceptions of the behaviors and beliefs of others function as a self-fulfilling prophecy. Although inaccurate, individuals conform to the perceived descriptive and injunctive norms in order to avoid feeling alienated from or rejected by their social group (Prentice and Miller, 1993). Through this process, erroneous perceptions of norms have real consequences for behaviors. Sher and colleagues (2001) examined college students' engagement in heavy drinking over 4 years of college. Perceptions of peer alcohol use and peer support for heavy drinking in years 1, 2, and 3 predicted heavy drinking in years 2, 3, and 4, respectively. Carey et al (2006) examined the influence of discrepancies between the perceived descriptive norm and personal drinking behavior on subsequent drinking behavior. Consistent with the social norms perspective, the degree to which individuals were discrepant from the descriptive norm positively predicted increases in drinking 30 days later.

Similar findings have been obtained in relation to other problematic behaviors. For example, perceptions of the prevalence of peer use of cigarettes and marijuana predict personal cigarette and marijuana use (Graham et al, 1991; Juvonen et al, 2007). The body image and disordered eating literatures have documented disturbing relationships of perceived norms for weight and body size with unhealthy behaviors among young women. Sanderson and colleagues (2002) found that women who had greater discrepancies between their own body mass index and the perceived average body mass index of their peers were at increased risk for both experiencing an extreme desire to be thin and engaging in behaviors that are symptomatic of bulimia, such as binging and purging. Similarly, Bergstrom et al (2004) documented greater unhealthy weight loss behaviors, including vomiting, fasting, and use of laxatives and diuretics, among women who overestimated men's endorsement of overly thin women as attractive.

3.4 Applications of Social Norms Theory to Behavior Change

As normative misperceptions are associated with a number of unhealthy behaviors, the social norms approach proposes that providing individuals with accurate information about the true norms in their environment should produce positive changes in behavior. Conducting research of this nature necessarily requires elicitation

research to determine the extent of misperceptions within a specific group and the true local norms (see Linkenbach, 2003 for an overview). Social norms based interventions have successfully reduced the prevalence of a number of problematic behaviors, and interventions have been conducted at the universal, selective, and indicated levels of prevention.

Universal interventions target an entire population or group, irrespective of the differing levels of risk that may exist within the group (Mrazek and Haggerty, 1994). Most social norms interventions have been conducted at this level, focusing often on alcohol use on college and high school campuses of varying sizes and geographic locations. State-wide interventions have also been conducted in areas where a single normative message was deemed to be widely applicable (Linkenbach and Perkins, 2003a). Messages correcting perceptions of peer cigarette and marijuana use have also significantly delayed initiation of cigarette and marijuana use among adolescents (Hansen and Graham, 1991; Linkenbach and Perkins, 2003a).

The social norms intervention conducted at Hobart and William Smith Colleges is perhaps the most comprehensive of the universal interventions conducted to date. Perkins and Craig (2003a) employed multiple channels for disseminating both descriptive and injunctive normative messages throughout a 4-year intervention period. Print media and screen savers on computers located in public, student used spaces delivered normative "factoids." Factoids included, "The majority of HWS seniors drink only 1–4 drinks or do not drink at all" and "91% of the entering class expressed the opinion that students should not drink to an intoxicating level that affects academic work or other responsibilities." In addition, an interactive website provided a forum for students to both respond to the factoids and watch videos of peers discussing drinking on campus. Finally, professors were trained to incorporate normative information into their lectures and class discussions, and an interdisciplinary alcohol safety course was offered. This multi-pronged approach appears to have been successful. After 1 year, perceptions of students' drinking behaviors and approval of drinking became more moderate, and the average number of drinks consumed at a bar or party declined significantly, from 5.1 to 4.4 drinks. Three and a half years into the program, results were more pronounced; the proportion of students consuming five or more drinks in a sitting declined by 32% and the number of student arrests for violations of liquor laws was reduced by nearly half.

While the arrests rates reported by Perkins and Craig (2003a) give some indication that social norms campaigns do affect actual behaviors, a common concern in this research is the reliance on self-report data. Indeed, repeated exposure to a message could potentially increase socially desirable responding, rather than produce true changes in behavior. However, intervention evaluations have also included objective behavioral measures. Foss et al (2003) recorded the blood alcohol content of students returning to their dormitories at night. Compared with pre-intervention rates 5 years prior, the proportion of students registering a blood alcohol content above 0.05 declined significantly, from 60 to 52%.

Selective social norms interventions, those targeting groups at an elevated risk for developing problematic behaviors (Mrazek and Haggerty, 1994), have also focused on a range of health behaviors. Targeting the thinness norms largely influenced and dictated by the media, Mutterperl and Sanderson (2002) provided college women with a brochure depicting accurate information about their peers' dieting and exercise behaviors. Particularly among women who did not compare themselves with celebrities, exposure to the brochure was associated with higher ideal weight and lower reports of disordered eating.

Selective interventions have also employed a small group format wherein misperceptions are addressed and corrected face to face. The "Small Group Norms-Challenging Model" often enlists respected peer leaders to provide information about both community-wide and group-specific norms in an interactive presentation (Far and Miller, 2003). Targeted groups have included fraternities, sororities, first year college students,

and athletes. Though some groups demonstrated significant reductions in alcohol consumption outcomes, others indicated more modest results. We will return to potential reasons for null findings in norms-based interventions.

Indicated interventions, those targeting individuals at high risk for engaging in risky behaviors (Mrazek and Haggerty, 1994), have proven effective as well. Marlatt and colleagues (1998) conducted brief individualized interventions addressing norms and personal alcohol use with freshmen who reported previous high risk drinking behaviors. At the 2-year follow-up, students who had received the brief intervention drank less frequently and consumed fewer drinks per sitting than a control group of high risk drinkers. Feedback regarding the magnitude of individual drinking relative to that of peers has also been delivered in computerized interventions, successfully reducing alcohol consumption (Neighbors et al, 2004). Similarly, personalized normative feedback mailed to at-risk students has effectively reduced engagement in heavy drinking episodes (Collins et al, 2002).

While most norm correction interventions have focused on adolescents and young adults, adults have been targeted as well. Peer alcohol use data has been employed with some success in reducing risk among middle aged individuals (Cunningham et al, 2001). In addition, a state-wide, norm-based media campaign demonstrated significant improvement in seatbelt use among adults (Linkenbach and Perkins, 2003b). Further, given Goldstein et al's (2008) success in motivating towel reuse among hotel patrons, presumably including young-, middle-, and later-aged adults, adults are similarly responsive to the norms in their environment.

3.5 Unsuccessful Social Norms Interventions: Problems and Solutions

As with any approach to behavior change, the social norms approach has not been without its null findings. Notably, Wechsler et al (2003) compared 37 colleges that had implemented social norms campaigns to reduce alcohol use with 61 colleges that had not. While significant decreases were not observed on any measure of alcohol consumption among schools with social norms campaigns, there appeared to be an increase in alcohol consumption on some outcomes. Similar increases were not observed among control campuses. Social norms interventions often fail for one of two reasons – either the intervention was unsuccessful in changing perceptions of the norm or misperceptions changed but did not result in decreases in risky behaviors.

Message recipients may not exhibit changes in misperceptions for several reasons. In some instances, individuals may question the authenticity of the normative information presented (e.g., Stewart et al, 2002). Accordingly, care must be taken to present information in a format that is believable. Conversely, message recipients may not respond favorably due to insufficient exposure to messages. Indeed, an 18-site randomized controlled trial indicated a dosage effect, such that campuses on which the greatest quantity of messages were presented over time exhibited the most pronounced decreases in alcohol use (DeJong et al, 2006). Thus, it is important to employ multiple channels for disseminating messages over a reasonable span of time (e.g., Perkins and Craig, 2003a).

Studies documenting increases in risky behaviors in response to altered misperceptions, pose a serious theoretical concern. In most cases, a majority of individuals do overestimate the prevalence of risky behaviors. There are, however, individuals whose estimates of the prevalence actually fall below the true norm (e.g., Perkins et al, 2005). Further, some who overestimate the norm may nonetheless exhibit behavior that falls below average. In either case, publicizing the true norm may produce a boomerang effect among individuals whose behavior falls below this threshold. Rather than remaining at a low level of behavior, such individuals may actually increase their behavior in response to learning the true descriptive norm.

Schultz and colleagues (2007) examined the boomerang effect in a sample of 290 households. Half of the households received a letter detailing both their own personal energy use and the average energy use, or descriptive norm, for their neighborhood. Energy meters were read prior to and 3 weeks following receipt of the normative feedback. Among these households, the boomerang effect was observed; households that initially fell below the norm significantly increased their energy use. The remaining households also received a letter detailing personal and average neighborhood energy use. However, an injunctive norm was added to the letter—a smiling emoticon if personal use fell below the neighborhood average or a frowning emoticon if personal use was above average. This coupling of the descriptive and injunctive norms eliminated the boomerang effect. Households that initially fell below the neighborhood average remained low in their energy use, while those that were above the average significantly decreased their energy use.

As suggested by Cialdini (2003), normative information is likely to be most effective in influencing behaviors when descriptive and injunctive norms correspond with one another. Perkins (2003) recommends inclusion of both descriptive and injunctive norms in attempts to change behavior. From the perspective of social norms theory, interventions should not overemphasize descriptive norms, but instead, would benefit from employing both injunctive and descriptive norms that jointly reinforce healthy behaviors.

4 Additional Applications of Norms to Behavior Change

Behaviors may exist for which normative perceptions are actually accurate or the magnitude of misperceptions less exaggerated. However, normative information can still be a useful tool for changing behavior under such circumstances. An interesting application of norms to behavior change has centered on labeling undesirable behaviors as normative among members of an out-group. Berger and Rand (2008) sought to decrease consumption of high-fat foods among undergraduates by providing information that such behavior is typical of an undesirable out-group (online gamers). This manipulation successfully increased selection of healthy foods among message recipients and was particularly effective among high self-monitors, individuals who are highly responsive to situational demands. Similar results have been obtained in motivating healthy behaviors among undergraduates by labeling heavy alcohol consumption and eating junk food as common among graduate students (Berger and Rand, 2008).

5 Media Influence on Health Behaviors

In our modern world, we are bombarded by mass communication and the communication matrix in which we are embedded has a profound impact on health behavior. From a psychological perspective, Bandura (2001) has provided a social cognitive theory formulation of the pathways through which communications systems operate. He includes a direct pathway to individuals and a socially mediated pathway through social networks. From a public health perspective, Abroms and Maibach (2008) characterized the dramatic change in media communication with the advent of the internet to blur the distinction between mass and interpersonal communication. They provide a broad agenda for mass communication and public health that argues for targeting social normative influences and social context for health behavior change. The dramatic change in communication pathways is accompanied by what has been described as a "shift" in the way patients acquire health information (Hesse et al, 2005).

Substantial concern has been expressed that for children and adolescents, at least, the media contribute to health problems including violence, sex, drugs, obesity, and eating disorders (Strasburger, 2009). Both correlational and experimental research support these claims. Perhaps the most mature area of research among these problems is on youth media exposure and violence. Conclusions include an increasing likelihood of aggressive behavior in younger

children (Browne and Hamilton-Giachristis, 2005) and an association with increased violence in youth that continues into adulthood (Anderson et al, 2003).

The media provide a significant source of standards of beauty, in the form of perceived body weight norms, collectively referred to as the "thin-ideal." Among women, research shows associations between media exposure and both body dissatisfaction and disordered eating (Grabe et al, 2008); these associations appear in preteen girls and continue into adulthood.

With regard to smoking, exposure to movie content in which people smoke, a media norm, is associated with the initiation of smoking in 10–14-year olds, an adjusted odds ratio of 2.6 for those in the highest versus lowest quartiles of such media exposure (Sargent et al, 2005). From the deterrent perspective, teens report that media messages about negative health consequences of smoking or that portray the tobacco industry as deceitful are a more powerful motivator to stop smoking or to not initiate smoking than are messages carrying social norms (Murphy-Hoefer et al, 2008). Most, however, underestimate the power of social norms in motivating their own behaviors (Nolan et al, 2008).

The media also serves as a source of information about sex and for modeling sexual behavior among teens (Brown et al, 2002), apparently encouraging early development of sexuality (Levin, 2009). For example, among 12–14-year olds, susceptibility to initiating intercourse and initiation of intercourse 2 years later were both associated with exposure to media and social norms for sexual behavior (L'Engle and Jackson, 2008). Media exposure to teen programming, of which over 80% has sexual content, is also associated with ongoing teen sexual activity (L'Engle et al, 2006).

Current literature on the international obesity epidemic, particularly among youth, targets the media as a significant force for poor diet and being overweight (Kumanyika and Brownson, 2007; Story et al, 2008). This literature illustrates the complexity of separating social normative influences as a single force of the media on behavior from other aspects of media. The media provide information on nutrition, diet, and food content, as well as normative messages about what attractive, happy, and successful people are eating. The same is so for media and sexual behavior, because adolescents acquire information on many aspects of sexual behavior, including contraception and sexually transmitted diseases, through mass media. Analysis of associations between media exposure and health-risk behaviors from the perspective of social normative influences requires parsing these aspects of media influence on health behavior.

Although the media contribute to undermining health, the media also provide support for a healthy lifestyle. Media depictions of aspirational peers engaged in healthy behavior can motivate behavior change. The influence of the media can be indirect, such as in Jackson and Aiken's (2006) intervention in which participants were shown that media norms had shifted towards favoring pale over tanned skin, which in turn, led to less positive attitudes to tanness and to greater sun protection. Alternatively, media influence can be direct, wherein aspirational peers are employed in active attempts to change behavior. For example, the "Got Milk" advertising campaign, launched in the United States in 1993 to encourage drinking of milk, often features extremely attractive female celebrities wearing a milk moustache, typically holding a glass of milk. Such media norms depicting aspirational peers engaged in health-protective behavior provide models for the adoption of healthier life styles.

6 Conclusion

Both correlational and experimental research has established a role for social norms in influencing health behaviors. Though unresolved issues remain in social norms research that require continued attention, descriptive and injunctive norms are indeed strong motivators of behavior that remain underutilized in health promotion. Although much of this chapter focused on normative misperceptions in the context of

social norms theory, we have addressed alternative applications of normative information that have successfully motivated behavior change as well. In sum, descriptive and injunctive norms have much to offer in both characterizing and changing health behaviors.

References

Abroms, L. C., and Maibach, E. W. (2008). The effectiveness of mass communication to change health behavior. *Annu Rev Public Health, 29*, 213–234.

Ajzen, I. (1991). The theory of planned behavior. *Organ Behav Hum Decis Process, 50*, 179–211.

Anderson, C. A., Berkowitz, L., Donnerstein, E., Huesmann, L. R., Johnson, J. D. et al (2003). The influence of media violence on youth. *Psychol Sci Public Interest, 4*, 81–110.

Bandura, A. (2001). Social cognitive theory of mass communication. *Media Psychol, 3*, 265–299.

Berger, J., and Rand, L. (2008). Shifting signals to help health: using identity signaling to reduce risky health behaviors. *J Consum Res, 35*, 509–518.

Bergstrom, R. L., Neighbors, C., and Lewis, M. A. (2004). Do men find "bony" women attractive? Consequences of misperceiving opposite sex perceptions of attractive body image. *Body Image, 1*, 183–191.

Borsari, B., and Carey, K. B. (2003). Descriptive and injunctive norms in college drinking: a meta-analytic integration. *J Stud Alcohol, 64*, 331–341.

Brown, J., Steele, J., and Walsh-Childers, K. (2002). *Sexual Teens, Sexual Media: Investigating Media's Influence on Adolescent Sexuality.* Mahwah, NJ: Lawrence Erlbaum.

Browne, K. D., and Himilton-Giachristis, C. (2005). The influence of violent media on children and adolescents: a public-health approach. *Lancet, 365*, 702–710.

Carey, K. B., Borsari, B., Carey, M. P., and Maisto, S. A. (2006). Patterns and importance of self-other differences in college drinking norms. *Psychol Addict Behav, 20*, 385–393.

Cialdini, R. B. (2003). Crafting normative messages to protect the environment. *Curr Dir Psychol Sci, 12*, 105–109.

Cialdini, R. B., and Trost, M. R. (1998). Social influence: social norms, conformity and compliance. In D. T. Gilbert, S. Fiske, & G. Lindzey (Eds.), *The Handbook of Social Psychology, 4th Ed* (pp. 151–192). New York: McGraw-Hill.

Cialdini, R. B., Reno, R. R., and Kallgren, C. A. (1990). A focus theory of normative conduct: recycling the concept of norms to reduce littering in public places. *J Pers Soc Psychol, 58*, 1015–1026.

Collins, S. E., Carey, K. B., and Sliwinski, M. J. (2002). Mailed personalized normative feedback as a brief intervention for at-risk college drinkers. *J Stud Alcohol, 63*, 559–567.

Cunningham, J. A., Wild, T. C., Bondy, S. J., and Lin, E. (2001). Impact of normative feedback on problem drinkers: a small-area population study. *J Stud Alcohol, 62*, 228–233.

Darley, J. M., and Latané, B. (1970). Norms and normative behavior: field studies of social interdependence. In J. Macaulay & L. Berkowitz (Eds.), *Altruism and Helping Behavior* (pp. 83–102). San Diego: Academic Press.

Davey-Rothwell, M. A., Latkin, C. A., and Tobin, K. E. (2009). Longitudinal analysis of the relationship between perceived norms and sharing injection paraphernalia. *AIDS Behaviour.* Advance online publication. doi: 10.1007/s10461-008-9520-z.

DeJong, W., Schneider, S. K., Towvim, L. G., Murphy, M. J., Doerr, E. E. et al (2006). A multisite randomized trial of social norms marketing campaigns to reduce college student drinking. *J Stud Alcohol, 67*, 868–879.

Durkheim, E. (1951). *Suicide: A Study in Sociology.* New York: Free Press.

Etcheverry, P. E., and Agnew, C. R. (2008). Romantic partner and friend influences on young adult cigarette smoking: comparing close others' smoking and injunctive norms over time. *Psychol Addict Behav, 22*, 313–325.

Far, J. M., and Miller, J. A. (2003). The small groups norms-challenging model: social norms interventions with targeted high-risk groups. In H. W. Perkins (Ed.), *The Social Norms Approach to Preventing School and College Age Substance Abuse: A Handbook for Educators, Counselors, and Clinicians* (pp. 111–132). San Francisco: Jossey-Bass.

Fishbein, M., and Ajzen, I. (1975). *Belief, Attitude, Intention, and Behavior: An Introduction to Theory and Research.* Reading, MA: Addison-Wesley.

Foss, R., Diekman, S., Goodwin, A., and Bartley, C. (2003). Enhancing a norms program to reduce high-risk drinking among first year students. http://www.hsrc.unc.edu/safety_info/alcohol/UNC SocialNormProject.pdf.

Godin, G., and Kok, G. (1996). The theory of planned behavior: a review of its applications to health related behaviors. *Am J Health Promot, 11*, 87–98.

Goldstein, N. J., and Cialdini, R. B. (2007). Using social norms as a lever of social influence. In A. Pratkanis (Ed.), *The Science of Social Influence: Advances and Future Progress* (pp. 167-192). Philadelphia: Psychology Press.

Goldstein, N. J., Cialdini, R. B., and Griskevicius, V. (2008). A room with a viewpoint: using social norms to motivate environmental conservation in hotels. *J Consum Res, 35*, 472–482.

Grabe, S., Ward, L. M., and Hyde, J. S. (2008). The role of the media in body image concerns among women:

a meta-analysis of experimental and correlational studies. *Psychol Bull, 134*, 460–476.

Graham, J., Marks, G., and Hansen, W. (1991). Social influence processes affecting adolescent substance use. *J Appl Soc Psychol, 16*, 291–298.

Hagger, M., and Chatzisarantis, N. (2005). First and higher-order models of attitudes, normative influence, and perceived behavioral control in the theory of planned behavior. *Br J Soc Psychol, 44*, 513–535.

Hansen, W. B., and Graham, W. J. (1991). Preventing alcohol, marijuana, and cigarette use among adolescents: peer pressure resistance training versus establishing conservative norms. *Prev Med, 20*, 414–430.

Hesse, B. W., Nelson, D. E., Kreps, G. L., Croyle, R. T., Arora, N. K. et al (2005). Trust and sources of health information: the impact of the internet and its implications for health care providers: findings from the first health information national trends survey. *Arch Intern Med, 165*, 2618–2624.

Jackson, K. M., and Aiken, L. S. (2006). Evaluation of a multicomponent appearance-based sun-protective intervention for young women: uncovering the mechanisms of program efficacy. *Health Psychol, 25*, 34–46.

Juvonen, J., Martino, S. C., Ellickson, P. L., and Longshore, D. (2007). "But others do it"! Do misperceptions of schoolmate alcohol and marijuana use predict subsequent drug use among young adolescents? *J Appl Soc Psychol, 37*, 740–758.

Kumanyika, S., and Brownson, R. (Eds.). (2007). *Handbook of Obesity Prevention: A Resource for Health Professionals.* New York: Springer.

Larimer, M. E., Turner, A. P., Mallett, K. A., and Geisner, I. M. (2004). Predicting drinking behavior and alcohol-related problems among fraternity and sorority members: examining the role of descriptive and injunctive norms. *Psychol Addict Behav, 18*, 203–212.

L'Engle, K. L., Brown, J. D., and Kenneary, K. (2006). The mass media are an important context for adolescents' sexual behavior. *J Adolesc Health, 38*, 186–192.

L'Engle, K. L., and Jackson, C. (2008). Socialization influences on early adolescents' cognitive susceptibility and transition to sexual intercourse. *J Res Adolesc, 18*, 353–378.

Levin, D. E. (2009). So sexy, so soon: the sexualization of childhood. In S. Olfman (Ed.), *The Sexualization of Childhood (Childhood in America)* (pp. 75–88). Westport, CT: Praeger.

Linkenbach, J. W. (2003). The Montana model: development and overview of a seven-step process for implementing macro-level social norms campaigns. In H. W. Perkins (Ed.), *The Social Norms Approach to Preventing School and College Age Substance Abuse: A Handbook for Educators, Counselors, and Clinicians* (pp. 182–206). San Francisco: Jossey-Bass.

Linkenbach, J. W., and Perkins, H. W. (2003a). Most of us are tobacco free: an eight-month social norms campaign reducing youth initiation of smoking in Montana. In H. W. Perkins (Ed.), *The Social Norms Approach to Preventing School and College Age Substance Abuse: A Handbook for Educators, Counselors, and Clinicians* (pp. 224–234). San Francisco: Jossey-Bass.

Linkenbach, J. W., and Perkins, H. W. (2003b, July). *Most of us wear seatbelts: the process and outcomes of a 3-year statewide adult seatbelt campaign in Montana.* Paper presented at the National Conference on the Social Norms Model, Boston, MA.

Marlatt, G. A., Baer, J. S., Kivlahan, D. R., Dimeff, L. A., Larimer, M. E. et al (1998). Screening and brief intervention for high-risk college student drinkers: results from a two-year follow-up assessment. *J Consult Clin Psychol, 66,* 604–615.

Miller, D. T., and McFarland, C. (1987). Pluralistic ignorance: when similarity is interpreted as dissimilarity. *J Pers Soc Psychol, 53,* 298–305.

Montaño, D. E., Thompson, B., Taylor, V. M., and Mahloch, J. (1997). Understanding mammography intention and utilization among women in an inner city public hospital clinic. *Prev Med, 26,* 817–824.

Mrazek, P. J., and Haggerty, R. J. (1994). *Reducing Risks for Mental Disorders: Frontiers for Preventive Intervention Research.* Washington, DC: National Academies Press.

Murphy-Hoefer, R., Hyland, A., and Higbee, C. (2008). Perceived effectiveness of tobacco countermarketing advertisements among young adults. *Am J Health Behav, 32,* 725–734.

Mutterperl, J. A., and Sanderson, C. A. (2002). Mind over matter: internalization of the thinness norm as a moderator of responsiveness to norm misperception information. *Health Psychol, 21,* 519–523.

Neighbors, C., Larimer, M. E., and Lewis, M. A. (2004). Targeting misperceptions of descriptive drinking norms: efficacy of a computer-delivered personalized normative feedback intervention. *J Consult Clin Psychol, 72,* 434–447.

Nolan, J. M., Schultz, P. W., Cialdini, R. B., Goldstein, N. J., and Griskevicius, V. (2008). Normative social influence is underdetected. *Pers Soc Psychol Bull, 34,* 913–923.

Perkins, H. W. (2003). The promise and challenge of future work using the social norms model. In H. W. Perkins (Ed.), *The Social Norms Approach to Preventing School and College Age Substance Abuse: A Handbook for Educators, Counselors, and Clinicians* (pp. 280–296). San Francisco: Jossey-Bass.

Perkins, H. W. and Berkowitz, A. D. (1986). Perceiving the community norms of alcohol use among students: some research implications for campus alcohol education programming. *Int J Addict, 21,* 961–976.

Perkins, H. W., and Craig, D. W. (2003a). The Hobart and William and Smith Colleges experiment: a synergistic social norms approach using print, electronic media, and curriculum infusion to reduce collegiate problem drinking. In H. W. Perkins (Ed.), *The Social Norms Approach to Preventing School and College Age Substance Abuse: A Handbook for Educators, Counselors, and Clinicians* (pp. 35–64). San Francisco: Jossey-Bass.

Perkins, H. W., and Craig, D. W. (2003b). The imaginary lives of peers: patterns of substance use and misperceptions of norms among secondary school students. In H. W. Perkins (Ed.), *The Social Norms Approach to Preventing School and College Age Substance Abuse: A Handbook for Educators, Counselors, and Clinicians* (pp. 209–223). San Francisco: Jossey-Bass.

Perkins, H. W., Haines, M. P., and Rice, R. (2005). Misperceiving the college drinking norm and related problems: a nationwide study of exposure to prevention information, perceived norms, and student alcohol misuse. *J Stud Alcohol, 66,* 470–478.

Prentice, D. A., and Miller, D. T. (1993). Pluralistic ignorance and alcohol use on campus: some consequences of misperceiving the social norm. *J Pers Soc Psychol, 64,* 243–256.

Reno, R. R., Cialdini, R. B., and Kallgren, C. A. (1993). The transsituational influence of social norms. *J Pers Soc Psychol, 64,* 104–112.

Rivis, A. and Sheeran, P. (2003). Descriptive norms as an additional predictor in the theory of planned behaviour: a meta-analysis. *Curr Psychol, 22,* 218–233.

Ross, L. (1977). The intuitive psychologist and his shortcomings: distortions in the attribution process. In L. Berkowitz (Ed.), *Advances in Experimental Social Psychology, vol. 10* (pp. 173–220). San Diego: Academic Press.

Ross, L., Greene, D., and House, P. (1977). The false consensus phenomenon: an attributional bias in self-perception and social perception processes. *J Exp Soc Psychol, 13,* 279–301.

Sanderson, C. A., Darley, J. M., and Messinger, C. S. (2002). "I'm not as thin as you think I am": the development and consequences of feeling discrepant from the thinness norm. *Pers Soc Psychol Bull, 28,* 172–183.

Sargent, J. D., Beach, M. L., Adachi-Mejia, A. M., Gibson, J. J., Titus-Ernstoff, L. T. et al (2005). Exposure to movie smoking: its relation to smoking initiation among US adolescents. *Pediatrics, 116,* 1183–1191.

Schmiege, S. J., Aiken, L. S., Sander, J. L., and Gerend, M. A. (2007). Osteoporosis prevention among young women: psychosocial models of calcium consumption and weight-bearing exercise. *Health Psychol, 26,* 577–587.

Scholly, K., Katz, A. R., Gascoigne, J., and Holck, P. S. (2005). Using social norms theory to explain perceptions and sexual health behaviors of undergraduate college students: an exploratory study. *J Am Coll Health, 53,* 159–166.

Schultz, P. W., Nolan, J. M., Cialdini, R. B., Goldstein, N. J., and Griskevicius, V. (2007). The constructive, destructive, and reconstructive power of social norms. *Psychol Sci, 18*, 429–434.

Schwartz, S. H. (1977). Normative influences on altruism. In L. Berkowitz (Ed.), *Advances in Experimental Social Psychology, vol. 10* (pp. 221–279). New York: Academic Press.

Sheeran, P., Abraham, C., and Orbell, S. (1999). Psychosocial correlates of heterosexual condom use: a meta-analysis. *Psychol Bull, 125*, 90–132.

Sher, K. J., Bartholow, B. D., and Nanda, S. (2001). Short- and long-term effects of fraternity and sorority membership on alcohol use: a social norms perspective. *Psychol Addict Behav, 15*, 42–51.

Sherif, M. (1936). *The Psychology of Social Norms*. New York: Harper Collins.

Smith, J. R., and Louis, W. R. (2008). Do as we say and as we do: the interplay of descriptive and injunctive group norms in the attitude-behaviour relationship. *Br J Soc Psychol, 47*, 647–666.

Smith-McLallen, A., and Fishbein, M. (2008). Predictors of intentions to perform six cancer-related behaviours: roles for injunctive and descriptive norms. *Psychol Health Med, 13*, 389–401.

Stewart, L. P., Lederman, L. C., Golubow, M., Cattafesta, J. L., Goodhart, F. W. et al (2002). Applying communication theories to prevent dangerous drinking among college students: the R U sure campaign. *Commun Stud, 53*, 381–399.

Stiff, J. B., and Mongeau, P. A. (2003). *Persuasive Communication, 2nd Ed.* New York: Guilford.

Story, M., Kaphingst, K. M., Robinson-O'Brien, R., and Glanz, K. (2008). Creating healthy food and eating environments: policy and environmental approaches. *Annu Rev Public Health, 29*, 253–272.

Strasburger, V. C. (2009). Media and children: what needs to happen now? *JAMA, 301*, 2265–2266.

Terry, D., and Hogg, M. (1996). Group norms and the attitude-behavior relationship: a role for group identification. *Pers Soc Psychol Bull, 22*, 776–793.

Trafimow, D., and Finlay, K. A. (1996). The importance of subjective norms for a minority of people: between-subjects and within-subjects analyses. *Pers Soc Psychol Bull, 22*, 820–828.

Trafimow, D., and Fishbein, M. (1994). The moderating effect of behavior type on the subjective norm-behavior relationship. *J Soc Psychol, 134*, 755–763.

Tversky, A., and Kahneman, D. (1973). Availability: a heuristic for judging frequency and probability. *Cogn Psychol, 5*, 207–232.

Wechsler, H., Nelson, T., Lee, J. E., Seiberg, M., Lewis, C. et al (2003). Perception and reality: a national evaluation of social norms marketing interventions to reduce college students' heavy alcohol use. *J Stud Alcohol, 64*, 484–494.

Chapter 20

Social Marketing: A Tale of Beer, Marriage, and Public Health

Gerard Hastings and Ray Lowry

Down at the King's Head

Bethany was getting irritated. She kept glancing at the door of the King's Head and furtively checking her watch. She explained, a little sharply, that her husband Steve was supposed to have joined her at 6 pm. It was now 6:25. A full half an hour later, I was standing near the door when Steve appeared. By this time it was nearly 7 pm and he looked hunted. He knew that he was in trouble and was preparing to face Bethany's wrath. But before he could cross the room to join her, the landlady, Helen, intervened. Despite his obvious hurry she insisted he came over to the bar first. She then said just one sentence to him: "Remember, Bethany has had her hair done".

Steve's face relaxed and his eyes smiled in gratitude: Helen had provided his get out of jail free card. He floated across to Bethany and swept aside her irritation with an unanswerable "darling, your hair looks lovely".

Helen is a consummate marketer. She had worked out what her customer needed and provided it just in time. As a publican one might assume that she sells beer; in reality, on this occasion, she was selling marital harmony - but rest assured the beer sales will follow. Her sensitivity and customer focus will result in deep loyalty from Steve (with Bethany also acquiring pleasant associations with the King's Head); as a result he won't just buy her beer tonight but for weeks and probably years to come.

G. Hastings (✉)
Institute for Social Marketing, University of Stirling, Stirling FK9 4LA, Scotland, UK
e-mail: gerard.hastings@stir.ac.uk

1 Introduction: It Is About People

It may seem a long stretch from Helen's success in running a local pub to a text book on public health, but she does have a crucial common agenda with those working in infant immunization, smoking cessation, and obesity prevention; she too is dealing in voluntary behavior change. She wants – needs – people to visit her pub, buy her beer, tell their friends and family what a good pub it is, visit her pub again, organize their wedding receptions with her... And she knows they have a choice; she cannot compel them to do these things, so she has to seduce them. This means she has to understand their needs absolutely and cater to them at every opportunity. She has to avoid the trap of taking refuge in the technicalities of her work, focusing purely on the science of good beer or minutiae of stock management. These things matter, but only in so far as they help her meet her customers' needs.

As with the King's Head, so with smoking cessation. Case Study A shows how a service in the North East of England succeeded in building links with pregnant smokers from very low-income communities and persuading them through their doors. The first step was qualitative research to dig down and understand the perspective of the women and how they felt about their smoking and the possibility of quitting. This revealed a remarkable degree of ambivalence in both arenas. They knew smoking to be harmful for them and their baby, but they also valued the indulgence, affirmation, and "me-time" it provided – rewards

A. Steptoe (ed.), *Handbook of Behavioral Medicine*, DOI 10.1007/978-0-387-09488-5_20,
© Springer Science+Business Media, LLC 2010

that were only enhanced by their constrained lives. Corresponding research with health professionals revealed that they fully understood this ambivalence among the low-income smokers and it made them reluctant to broach the idea of quitting and reticent in their approach when they did. The resulting initiative built on these insights and comparison with neighboring providers demonstrated their striking success – attendance at the local cessation service shot up.

Case Study A: Using Social Marketing to Increase Recruitment of Pregnant Smokers to Smoking Cessation Service

Problem Definition

The impacts of smoking in pregnancy are well documented. Funding in the United Kingdom city of Sunderland was used to appoint a local champion to coordinate services for pregnant women who wanted to give up smoking. In Sunderland between April 2001 and March 2002 only 19 women set a quit date and 8 successfully quit smoking at the 4-week stage through the mainstream service.

Stakeholder Analysis

Detailed work was done with stakeholders in the pregnancy-smoking condition: with the women themselves and their "significant others" (partners, parents, friends); health professionals (obstetric, medical, health promotion), as well as service providers, clinical managers, and support groups. At the time the intervention was being planned, background work was being done developing the social marketing foundations, including research with many stakeholders in this and other areas of health-related issues.

Aims and Objectives

The aim of the intervention was to increase the number of women in Sunderland who were accessing smoking cessation services and achieving formal quitting target.

The objectives were to

- Use social marketing to design a user-friendly service.
- To re-engineer the local service to meet customer needs.
- To implement the service and achieve targets.
- To record activity accurately and feedback to service providers.
- To adjust practice in relation to feedback.

Formulation of Strategy

Four Ps:

Product A customer-focused smoking cessation service
Price Ease of access for the target (including free of charge)
Place Concentrate on the target population's preferred locations
Promotion Enthuse and skill up health professionals in contact with the target audience
Consumer research Focus groups with target audience, in-depth interviews with professionals
Testing Materials and approach in groups
Specific channels Antenatal clinics

Paid and voluntary agents Clinicians and supporters of target women
Incentives Health and self-esteem related

Research

Although it has long been known that smoking during pregnancy is undesirable, and that many women still find it difficult to abstain, many health-care professionals are at loss to help. Therefore to start the social marketing process, wide-ranging market research was undertaken with the target population. The research adopted a qualitative focus group method. Subjects were recruited to take part in 1 of 12 focus groups on a door-to-door basis by trained and experienced market research interviewers according to a strict code of conduct. The research spans 10 years from 1992. The majority of focus groups took place at the beginning and the final two more recently. A total of 12 groups were segmented in relation to age, social class, smoking behavior/history, and cohabitation status.

Analysis of Barriers and Interventions to Overcome Them

Barriers	Interventions
Difficulty recruiting women	Proactive recruiting, dedicated worker, home visits
Poor existing information	Design and pretest new marketing/information material with target population
Health professionals lack of engagement	Role play to engage health professionals
No nagging/make them feel worse	Consumer-friendly cessation support (including dedicated worker)

Outcomes

Recruitment of pregnant (and non-pregnant) smokers to the new smoking cessation intervention increased ten-fold during intervention phase and the Sunderland stop smoking service is now one of the top performers in the UK: Sunderland pregnancy stop smoking service was highlighted in the Department of Health's "Best practice in smoking cessation services for pregnant smokers" (November 2005), and is one of top three beacon services in England, and is the *most cost effective* (quitters per member of staff, clarity of data collection and reporting procedures).

Recruitment of pregnant smokers also increased after actor/role play sessions with health-care professionals (especially midwives) (Fig. 20.1) and was higher than the neighboring services (in which different smoking cessation interventions targeted at pregnant women were being undertaken) in all the parameters measured.

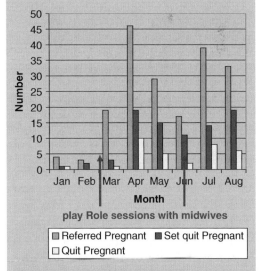

Fig. 20.1 Sunderland smoking cessation activity (pregnancy) by month (referral to service, quit date, and 4-week quit rates)

Market research identified a number of barriers that women face in relation to smoking cessation during pregnancy: unsatisfactory information, lack of enthusiasm/empathy from health-care professionals, short-term support, all showing as a reluctance to be recruited.

The difficulty of recruiting women to take part in smoking cessation meant the researchers had to concentrate effort where women might be recruitable (in this case, in the antenatal clinic at first booking). Support was designed to be consumer friendly by using information from focus groups, recruitment of skilled and empathic dedicated worker, and using feedback techniques. Apart from designing and pretesting posters and leaflets that would meet women's needs, a whole-time worker was specially recruited for providing long-term, home-based, user-friendly support. The major barrier to overcome was health-care professional enthusiasm/empathy and to do that the researchers used professional actor/role players.

By studying the transcripts of the focus groups, actor/role players were able to bring to groups of health-care workers the chance to interact with the target women as they had never before. Using active participation in group work, professional staff were able to get direct feedback on what it felt to be the target women, and what approaches might work more effectively. These sessions evaluated well with participants and proved to be very effective in the intervention.

They had done a Helen. They had focused on the women's needs and honed the offering to meet them, rather than becoming trapped in the technicalities of addiction or a myopic preoccupation with targets. As with Helen's stock keeping these matter, but they are only a means to the end of providing a people-centered service and thereby engaging them in a long-term process of not just moving away from tobacco, but toward health improvement.

What Helen does on a small scale and by instinct, larger companies do by training and systems. Major corporations have succeeded because they have adopted marketing ideas to make sure that customers are at the core of their activities. This has driven their growth by enabling them to remain public facing and at least appear approachable and responsive, despite their often immense size. Marketing is defined by the American Marketing Association (2007) as "the activity, set of institutions, and processes for creating, communicating, delivering, and exchanging offerings that have value for customers, clients, partners, and society at large." This takes matters beyond the individual customer, recognizing an important upstream agenda to which we will return, but at this point let us just note that it reinforces the point that marketing is about people and their voluntary behavior – as of course is public health.

The AMA definition also emphasizes the complexity of marketing. Helen's instincts work at the level of a small business, but something more systematic and thought-through is needed when the scale increases and the stakes multiply. The core goal of being people centered depends on the coordinated deployment of a package of principles and practices.

In this chapter we will examine what these are, and how, in the form of social marketing, such "knowledge, concepts, and techniques" can be used "to enhance social as well as economic ends" (Lazer and Kelley, 1973: p. *ix*) – and specifically to benefit public health. We have already established the most fundamental precept of marketing: consumer orientation and this idea underpins all that follows. To deliver this, eight subordinate principles are followed (see Fig. 20.2).

These emphasize that successful social marketing needs to start with clearly defined behavioral objectives and target groups: *what* do we want *who* to do? Achieving these will depend on a continuous stream of research intelligence and theoretical insight about the behavior, the target group and the progress being made with

Fig. 20.2 How social
marketing puts people first

> Good social marketing:
> 1. Sets clear behavioral objectives
> 2. Uses 'navigational' research
> 3. Builds on theory
> 4. Creates attractive motivational exchanges with the target group
> 5. Recognizes that one size does not always fit all
> 6. Thinks beyond communications
> 7. Thinks beyond the individual
> 8. Pays careful attention to the competition *Source: Hastings 2007*

both. This thinking also needs to recognize the importance of motivation and emotion in human decision making: the brand values of Marlboro can and frequently do trump the positivist reality of lung cancer, and social marketers need to recognize this.

Satisfying people's needs also requires a move beyond the assumption that we are all alike, opening the way for customized approaches to cohesive sub-groups or segments of the wider population. And these approaches have to involve more than communication – behavior change needs facilitation, encouragement, and opportunity as well as mere instruction.

It also depends on more than the individual; social marketing has to build on the well-established truth that human behavior is strongly influenced by social context and hence should target stakeholders and policy makers – and indeed competitors (whether in the form of attractive alternative behaviors or the World Health Organization's "hazard merchants") – as well as individual citizens.

Each of these principles will be discussed in turn. The chapter will then explain the need to pull these ideas into a coherent strategic plan. Helen wants Steve to become a regular, to keep his custom for as long as she is running the King's Head; similarly large companies like Tesco or Walmart seek our loyalty and they reward us continuously when we provide it – public health needs to be equally far sighted. Ultimately our interest is not in smoking, or other individual health behaviors, it is in lifestyles.

Finally the chapter returns to the core focus of marketing (and public health) and thinks again about the importance of people.

2 Eight Ways of Putting People First

2.1 Clear Behavioral Objectives

Social marketing has to begin with a definitive statement of behavioral objectives: exactly *what* we want *who* to do (or to stop doing). Without this clarity it is impossible to either decide about methods or monitor progress. Behavioral objectives are often incremental, building gradually to the final, and often longer term goal. For example, if we want to help people stop smoking, intermediate objectives might include attending quit services; setting quit dates; stopping smoking; or staying quit for a target time with proof (as with carbon monoxide monitors).

In each case objective needs to be both realistic and measurable. The first keeps our feet on the ground and recognizes that change is difficult and takes time. A commercial marketer does not expect to dominate the market overnight; Coca-Cola, for instance, would be delighted with a couple of percentage points improvement in its market share vis-à-vis Pepsi and their other rivals – and has been working at the task for a century. By the same token we should not expect to eliminate smoking in a few weeks or get everyone jogging with one intervention.

Measurability makes sure we can gauge progress. Case Study A shows how clearly laid out initial objectives made it possible to demonstrate the success of the intervention.

Good objectives have the additional benefit of clarifying communications between all those involved in the social marketing effort. Funders, agents, team members can all sign up to a transparent statement of intent – minimizing the risk of subsequent disagreements. A recent project that the Institute for Social Marketing was involved in illustrates the hazards of getting this wrong. In this case a major UK Government drugs prevention initiative suffered from mission creep: the funder thought they were conducting a trial; the research team was still sticking to the initially agreed pilot study agenda. Because this mismatch was not identified and dealt with by agreeing clear objectives, the status of the resulting research findings could not be agreed, to everyone's discomfort.

Thus research is not an ad hoc addition to social marketing activity, but an integral and continuous part of it. And this gestalt matters, it moves the emphasis beyond the intervention and the development of tools and focuses it on understanding people. It also ensures, like the Chinese taxi driver in Fig. 20.3, that social marketers focus on where their clients are coming from, rather than rushing to determine where they should be going. Case Study A shows how this organic approach to research helped enable the social marketing team to build up a real understanding of their customers.

2.2 Navigational Research

Research is the eyes and ears of social marketing. It is used much as an explorer uses a map and compass: to plot the direction of travel and continuously check on progress. In public health terms the first research task is to define the problem and identify intelligent solutions – taking us back to the "who needs to do what" of the objectives. Research can then contribute to the development of the solution through concept and pretesting. In particular, qualitative research makes it possible to flexibly explore options for different offerings. Next "process evaluation" can be used to ensure the initiative is implemented as intended and then outcome evaluation can measure success against the agreed objectives.

2.3 Building on Theory

Social marketing is founded on exchange theory (Bagozzi, 1974; Houston and Gassenheimer, 1987), which argues that given behavioral options people will ascribe values to the alternatives and select the one that offers greatest benefit – or enhancement – to themselves. This process may be prolonged and considered, as with a career decision, or truncated and virtually automatic as with the purchase of a chocolate bar. The values ascribed to the marketer's offering during an exchange may be tangible (e.g., monetary) or psychological (e.g., status), immediate (e.g., nicotine now) or deferred (e.g., better health later), but they will always be subjective.

Chi Li is taxi driver at Beijing airport, who beat all his colleagues in the stiff competition for fares. Like all taxi drivers, he would stand in the arrivals hall and approach tourists as they looked for a ride to town. Unlike his rivals, however, who asked the obvious "where are you going", he would ask: "where are you from?" When they replied, he would produce a letter of recommendation from a satisfied customer from their home town. He would secure their services for their whole stay by giving them a fixed price (no hidden extras) and asking for their own letter of recommendation if entirely satisfied. How could they refuse? His customer based approach was a winner: people trust their own background most, especially when in unfamiliar situations.

Chi Li's approach of asking "where are you from?" is also a good formula for finding the customer approach in social marketing.

Fig. 20.3 The Chinese taxi driver

The priorities of the consumer will differ from those of the manufacturer as will those of the health promoter and their target. Commercial marketers have therefore long accepted that if they are going to influence behavior (e.g., by encouraging purchase or brand loyalty) they must adopt a consumer perspective and be prepared to compromise. The same applies to social marketers.

The notion of compromise, of adjusting the offering to meet the target group's needs, can be a difficult one for public health which puts such emphasis on the evidence base and expert-driven solutions. A marketer might be able to change his chocolate bar in response to consumer concerns about obesity – by making it less calorific, for instance – but smoking cessation services are selling one non-negotiable product: quitting. Closer examination, however, suggests that what seems like a dichotomy is actually more nuanced. Drugs prevention has long been – and tobacco control increasingly is – moving away from an absolutist position and offering harm reduction options. And the reformulation of the chocolate manufacturer is still going to make its customers fat.

Exchange also implies mutual benefit – in other words that the social marketer gets something out of the deal. This again can be difficult for public health practitioners, who often prefer to think of their work in more altruistic terms (Rothschild, 1999). However, this ignores the obvious reality that, especially in an era of ubiquitous targets, social marketers do get something more than a warm fuzzy feeling from their clients. It also presumes a rather asymmetrical view of the world where the health worker has something of value to offer, but his or her client does not.

Exchange theory does not replace or supersede other behavioral theories, nor does social marketing limit itself to this one theoretical perspective. Rather it is eclectic and pragmatic, adopting those insights that offer most hope of success. For example, a social marketing intervention on low-income smoking (Stead et al, 2001) used social cognitive theory to explain the origins of smoking, stages of change theory to assess proximity to quitting and exchange theory to inform attempts to encourage quitting.

2.4 Creating Attractive Motivational Exchanges with the Target Group

Social marketers do not make any assumptions about what their clients want; they ask them – and then determine how this benefit can be made as attractive as possible. This takes in the notion of subjectivity and adds in the idea of emotion – that feelings matter. The power of branding in commercial marketing is increasingly being recognized in public health – and a few baby steps are being made toward emulating it (Farrelly et al, 2002; Hastings et al, 2008).

Thus we move from a place where public health solutions are evidence-based givens being sold to a passive populace to one where they are compromises negotiated with an active one. Furthermore, in these post-modern times, the process of negotiation and compromise is becoming increasingly overt. Consumers recognize those marketers who are most inclined to move toward them and respond more positively as a result. Social marketers ignore this increasingly sophisticated public at their peril.

2.5 Recognizing that One Size Does Not Always Fit All

People differ. We all have varying experiences, needs, and expectations. This has direct implications for social marketing: if customer needs are going to be properly met, then heterogeneous mass markets have to be broken down into more homogeneous segments and offerings honed accordingly. In Case Study B it is clear that the various stakeholder groups for water fluoridation see the issue differently and if fluoridation is going to proceed then these alternative needs have to be met.

Case Study B: Working to Extend Water Fluoridation

Water fluoridation is a safe, effective, and cost-effective way to prevent tooth decay and it is particularly valuable at reducing dental health inequalities due to social deprivation. Despite this, at present only about 10% of the population of the UK drink fluoridated water at the optimal one part per million, some where it occurs naturally, most through water treatment. Best current estimates are that for about 25% of the population water fluoridation would be cost-effective where water treatment plants serve large numbers of people with high caries rates. These would include areas of social deprivation which in practice means the major conurbations.

Existing fluoridation schemes in the UK were implemented in the 1960s when the bulk of the water supply industry was in public ownership, i.e., under the management of local government. Both private and state-owned water suppliers were persuaded, at the time, to fluoridate water for the public good under a nonprofit-making arrangement whereby the state met all the appropriate costs.

Social marketing was used to try to increase coverage of water fluoridation to the population by leading strategic development of new water fluoridation schemes, after 1987, undertaking 3 months successful consultation with the public, local authorities, and community health councils, negotiating with local water companies and achieving unprecedented progress using sophisticated social marketing techniques. A failure to progress at the time was investigated using social marketing principles, and "up-stream" remedies were identified; a subsequent change in primary legislation in the UK parliament has resolved many of the structural and procedural issues impeding further implementation of new water fluoridation schemes and social marketing principles and practice contributed to the success of this intervention.

With recent changes in the law, it has now become feasible to consider implementing new water fluoridation schemes, including in the North East of England. Subject to detailed implementation plans, such a program would extend the benefits to approximately 1.7 million more people in the North East through seven new schemes. This would result in more than 75% of people in the North East receiving fluoridated water once the schemes were implemented. So up-stream social marketing has produced a foundation for progress in implementing this health promotion intervention.

2.6 Thinking Beyond Communications

Some readers may be surprised to get this far into a chapter about social marketing with barely a mention having been made of communication campaigns. This is quite deliberate: marketing and advertising are not synonyms; marketing is a way of thinking about the challenge of influencing consumer behavior which may – or may not – use advertising as one of its tools. Similarly, social marketing is a way of thinking about social and health behavior change that may – or may not – make use of communications.

In both cases there are three other tools to consider: the product (this may be the behavior or a related service) that the target group will be offered; its price (what they have to give up to make the proffered changes) and the place (where they access the offering). Classically, commercial marketers meet their consumer's needs by offering a product that is highly valued, appropriately priced, made available in convenient and attractive outlets, and backed by relevant and engaging communications. This mix of variables (the so-called marketing mix) is manipulated to maximize satisfaction. Again the rubric can be applied to social and health behaviors. Case Study C demonstrates how the marketing mix was used to think through a strategy for encouraging doctors to prescribe sugar-free medicines.

Case Study C: Changing Consumption of Sugared Liquid Oral Medicines

Problem Definition

With the high rates of dental decay in the North East of England, there was a desire to promote the use of sugar-free medications. In 1994 a conventional communication approach to the problem was tried in the North West of England. It was aimed at all the groups who might have an influence on behavior: general medical practitioners, pharmacists, health visitors, dentists, and parents of young children. The evaluation of the campaign showed a marked attitude change in favor of sugar-free medication by the health professionals but no sustained change in prescribing behavior took place.

It was therefore decided to tackle the problem using a social marketing approach.

Objective

The objective of the initiative was to produce a significant reduction in the consumption by young children of sugar-containing, liquid, oral medication obtained by prescription, with the long-term aim of improving their dental health.

Development

Four potential target groups were identified: pharmaceutical manufacturers and distributors, pharmacists, parents, and general medical practitioners (GPs). However, limited resources meant that only one initiative was possible, so these groups had to be prioritized. Qualitative research was therefore conducted with each group (segment) to establish which showed greatest potential and guide the development of an appropriate offering for this group.

Research with pharmaceutical manufacturers and distributors revealed that the industry is demand led, and that attempts to impose sugar-free medicine through the supply chain would meet resistance and be prohibitively expensive. Pharmacists are also demand led. Their job is to fill the prescription as determined by the general practitioner. Furthermore, sugar-free alternatives are generally more expensive, so if the pharmacist changes the prescription they have to bear the difference in price.

Attention therefore focused on the two remaining targets: parents and GPs. Over-the-counter medicines were excluded because qualitative research indicated a resistance to change beyond the means of the initiative to influence. The attitude of parents to the sugar-free issue was related to social class: lower social class (IV and V) mothers expected their general medical practitioner to prescribe the sugar-free alternative without prompting if it was available and appropriate; higher social class (I and II) mothers were more engaged with the issue, although some were wary of artificial sweeteners.

This suggested that family doctors were the key: if they could be persuaded to prescribe sugar-free alternatives, pharmacists and most parents would co-operate. Furthermore, research showed that the doctors were open to persuasion and pretesting made it possible to develop an appropriate marketing mix:

Product: This was "the prescribing by general medical practitioners of sugar-free medicines." It was basically acceptable to the GP, especially if backed by appropriate evidence of effectiveness. However, they had many other priorities and concerns, with the resulting danger that it would get overlooked.

Price: It was therefore very important to keep the price low by making prescribing the sugar-free version of any medication as easy as possible. Information helped here (see promotion), but perhaps more important was the adjustment of prescribing software to favor sugar-free alternatives.

Place: Information and prescribing alternatives were needed at the point of prescription to provide convenient reminders and cues.

Promotion: This helped highlight the issue, by providing information on mothers' views and dental decay in the area, as well ease change by suggesting and cueing alternatives. A personal selling approach was adopted, using a specially trained health authority "representative" to promote sugar-free options on a one-to-one basis, backed up by targeted written materials. This mimicked the standard way that GP's learn about new medicines.

The Evaluation

Method

Test and control areas were chosen for the intervention matched for population size and socio-economic characteristics, GP, and pharmacist numbers. The initiative took place over 3 years: 1995 pre-intervention, 1996 the intervention year, 1997 post-intervention.

The campaign was evaluated in two ways: by questionnaires distributed before and after the campaign and by quantitative analysis of prescription and sales of target medicines before and after the campaign, in both the test and the control areas.

Agreement was obtained from the health authorities and their medical and pharmaceutical advisors for the circulation of pre- and post-campaign questionnaires to GPs and community pharmacists in both the test and the control areas. In addition, agreement was obtained for access to "prescribing analysis and cost" (PACT) data for GPs in both areas.

Results

The questionnaire analysis showed there was a non-statistically significant increase in the knowledge and awareness of both pharmacists and general medical practitioners in relation to the role of sugared medicines in dental caries and the desirability of using sugar-free substitutes in both the test and the control areas. So, for example, the percentage of GPs who thought sugar in medicines was important in relation to dental decay rose from 63 pre-campaign to 66 post-campaign.

Quantitative analysis of the PACT data showed there was an overall increase in the prescribing of sugar-free medicines in both test and control areas between 1995 and 1997 ($p<0.01$) and this increase was significantly greater in the test area ($p<0.0001$).

2.7 Thinking Beyond the Individual

No man or woman is an island. John Donne's observation is backed by numerous theories of behavior change – social cognitive theory, social norms, the theory of planned behavior to name but a few – as well as common sense (see Chapter 2). Furthermore, ignoring this not only undermines effectiveness, but also raises serious moral questions. If we simply go after individuals to change behaviors over which they have limited control we risk blaming them for their own predicament – so-called victim blaming. Given what is now known about the link between inequalities and ill health this is particularly unacceptable.

Social marketing, then, recognizes the collective determinants of human behavior and one of the first decisions to be made in any intervention, as we have already noted, is *whose* behavior has to change. Sometimes this will be individuals. For example, attempts to improve dental health might consider targeting parents to encourage tooth brushing and reduced sugar consumption. However, as Case Study B shows, water fluoridation is likely to be much more effective – and the individual's control over this is very limited; fluoridation of water supplies easily trumps the potential health promotion power of other, more individual-based, health promotion interventions.

2.8 Paying Careful Attention to the Competition

This final principle recognizes that people – whether parents or water providers – have a choice. They can – and often do – continue with their current behavior. It is therefore very important to look closely at this "competition" in order to understand what benefits it is perceived to bring and how our alternative behavior can be made more attractive. In Case Study C, for example, the doctors were not prescribing sugar-free alternatives because it was easier to go with the option automatically suggested by their software. As in so many other aspects of life, convenience matters. The solution was to get rid of the competition and change the software so that it favored sugar-free.

These current behavior patterns might be termed *passive competition*. There is, however, an important additional sense in which social marketers need to address the competition. As well as current behaviors, there are also organizations that are actively pushing in the opposite direction. One of the key reasons that so many people continue to smoke, eat, and drink unhealthily is that tobacco, fast food, and alcohol companies are using marketing to encourage them to do so. And we know that their efforts are successful (Anderson et al, 2009; Hastings et al, 2006; National Cancer Institute, 2008).

Social marketers have to look critically at this activity if they are going to do a thorough job of addressing the context, which as we have just noted, is so important. It also brings a major additional benefit: understanding the efforts of Philip Morris or Diageo, and consumer response to them, provides us with invaluable intelligence about how to engage and retain our customers. Indeed this is how social marketing came into existence in the first place. Over 50 years ago an American academic called Wiebe (1951/52) used an analysis of commercial marketing campaigns to conclude that "you can sell brotherhood like soap." The success of the tobacco, alcohol, and food industries also provides a rich – if salutary – seam of evidence that marketing works. This reminds us that if marketing can get us to buy a Ferrari it can also encourage us to drive it safely – and resist the temptation to steal one.

3 The Vital Role of Strategic Planning

Thus the eight principles outlined in Fig. 20.2 help social marketers to deliver on the idea of customer orientation: they ensure that people are at the heart of their efforts. However, social marketing must do more than institute these principles in isolation if it is to succeed; it has to bring them together in a long-term vision. Ultimately, as we have already noted, our interest is not just in nudging this or that behavior a few degrees in the right direction; we do not just want more people to visit cessation services, or a few GPs to prescribe sugar-free medicines – we want to help everyone to become smoke-free and all doctors to offer healthier medicines. More broadly our interest is improving the public health of whole societies; not just behavior change, but social change.

Strategic planning (see Fig. 20.4) helps ensure that we keep this bigger picture in view.

It takes the eight principles and sets them within a systematic process for guiding decision making. In this way the whole becomes more than the sum of the parts and social marketing moves beyond ad hoc interventions toward an ongoing means of learning more about the market place and the particular exchanges it incorporates. This fits with the earlier discussion of research being a conduit to understanding people not just a means of honing tools

or interventions: good carpenters know about chisels; great ones know about wood. Strategic planning can make the difference between the two.

This learning can take place within particular public health silos – this year's teen cycling proficiency initiative can be used to inform next year's. But it can also move between topics: research on teenager cycling will provide valuable insights into their priorities, concerns, and aspirations which can be equally relevant for smoking prevention or sexual health.

This longer term perspective also gels perfectly with recent thinking in commercial marketing which has increasingly put the emphasis on building relationships with customers; not just generating transactions. At its crudest level this leads on from the simple calculus that it is much cheaper to keep existing customers than continually win new ones. Dissatisfied customer also complain volubly – and, very harmfully, they are much more likely to do so to family and friends than to the marketer. Consumer marketing then – whether in the hands of Helen at the King's Head or a behemoth like Tesco – becomes fundamentally about keeping people happy, about service, satisfaction, and loyalty – about building trust (Morgan and Hunt, 1994; Hastings and Saren, 2003).

Moving upstream, this reasoning is even more compelling: stakeholders are fewer in number and more powerful. Like ordinary citizens they have needs that can be satisfied, and just as on the high street, transactions can be converted into relationships.

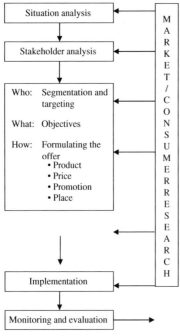

Adapted from Hastings and Elliott (1993)

Fig. 20.4 A social marketing plan Adapted from Hastings and Elliott (1993)

4 Final Thoughts

This chapter began with a discussion of a well-run pub – not a conventional focus for a public health text book, but a useful one because we wanted to demonstrate how insights used by commercial marketing to influence consumer behavior can be applied to social and health behavior. At the core of this thinking is the idea that the person you want to do business with – be it the individual citizen or the stakeholder – has to be the center of your attention. We then saw how eight key principles can help ensure this is the case and how these can be applied in practice through the three case studies.

Finally we examined the importance of long-term thinking and strategic planning that is so necessary if social marketers are to raise their eyes above ad hoc interventions and begin to address the possibility of wide-ranging social change. Given that even in developed countries poor people are now dying up to 20 years before their wealthier peers (Marmot, 2004), such ambition is surely needed.

References

American Marketing Association (2007). Definition of Marketing. http://www.marketingpower.com/AboutAMA/Pages/DefinitionofMarketing.aspx.

Anderson, P., de Bruijn, A., Angus, K., Gordon, R., and Hastings, G. (2009). Impact of alcohol advertising and media exposure on adolescent alcohol use: a systematic review of longitudinal studies. *Alcohol Alcohol, 44*, 229–243.

Bagozzi, R. P. (1974). Marketing as an organised behavioral system of exchange. *J Marketing, 38*, 77–81.

Farrelly, M. C., Healton, C. G., Davis, K. C., Messeri, P., Hersey, J. C. et al (2002). Getting to the truth: evaluating national tobacco countermarketing campaigns. *Am J Public Health, 92*, 901–907.

Hastings, G. (2007). *Social Marketing: Why Should the Devil Have All the Best Tunes?* Oxford: Butterworth-Heinemann.

Hastings, G. B., and Elliott, B. (1993). Social marketing practice in traffic safety. In OECD-Road Transport Research (Ed.), *Marketing of Traffic Safety* (pp. 35–53). Paris: Organisation for Economic Co-operation and Development (OECD).

Hastings, G., and Saren, M. (2003). The critical contribution of Social Marketing: theory and application. *Marketing Theory, 3*, 305–322.

Hastings, G., Freeman, J., Spackova, R., and Siquier, P. (2008). HELP: A European public health brand in the making. In D. W. Evans & G. Hastings (Eds.), *Public Health Branding: Applying Marketing for Social Change* (pp. 93–108). Oxford: Oxford University Press.

Hastings, G., McDermott, L., Angus, K., Stead, M., and Thomson, S. (2006). *The Extent, Nature and Effects of Food Promotion to Children: A Review of the Evidence. Technical Paper prepared for the World Health Organization*. Geneva: World Health Organization.

Houston, F. S., and Gassenheimer, J. B. (1987). Marketing and exchange. *J Marketing, 51*, 3–18.

Lazer, W., and Kelley, E. (1973). *Social Marketing: Perspectives and Viewpoints*. Homewood, IL: Richard D. Irwin.

Marmot, M. G. (2004). *Status Syndrome: How Your Social Standing Directly Affects Your Health and Life Expectancy*. London: Bloomsbury Publishing Plc.

Morgan, R. M., and Hunt, S. D. (1994). The commitment-trust theory of relationship marketing. *J Marketing, 58*, 20–38.

National Cancer Institute (2008). *The Role of the Media in Promoting and Reducing Tobacco Use*. Tobacco Control Monograph No. 19. Bethesda, MD: U.S. Department of Health and Human Services, National Institutes of Health, National Cancer Institute.

Rothschild, M. L. (1999). Carrots, sticks, and promises: a conceptual framework for the management of public health and social issue behaviors. *J Marketing, 63*, 24–37.

Stead, M., MacAskill, S., MacKintosh, A. M., and Eadie, D. R. (2001). Tackling smoking in low income communities through a social marketing framework. *Presentation at Academy of Marketing Science 10th Biennial World Marketing Congress – Global Issues at the Turn of the Millennium*, Cardiff, 28 June–1 July 2001.

Wiebe, G. D. (1951/52). Merchandising commodities and citizenship in television. *Public Opin Q, 15*, 679–691.

Part IV
Epidemiological and Population
Perspectives

Chapter 21

Assessment of Psychosocial Factors in Population Studies

Susan A. Everson-Rose and Cari J. Clark

1 Overview

It is widely recognized that psychosocial factors influence health and well-being. Broadly speaking, *psychosocial factors* refer to a variety of psychological characteristics, including emotional states and personality factors, social networks and support, as well as socioenvironmental characteristics. Thus, it can be argued that psychosocial factors reflect genetic predispositions, learned habits, and shared experiences. Historical and clinical anecdotes about the influences of psychosocial factors on health have existed for centuries. Empirical evidence validating these relations has accumulated rapidly over the past 50 years across many scientific disciplines including epidemiology, psychology, psychiatry, sociology, and physiology. Since the purpose of this chapter is to discuss issues related to and methods of assessing psychosocial factors in large, population-based studies, a special focus on epidemiology, particularly social epidemiology, is warranted. Research conducted within the context of social epidemiology – the branch of epidemiology that investigates the social distribution and determinants of health and illness (Berkman and Kawachi, 2000b) –

has generated much knowledge about the influence of various psychological and social factors on states of health and illness. Research from a social epidemiologic perspective has examined morbidity and mortality due to cardiovascular diseases, diabetes, and cancer, as well as outcomes such as disability and Alzheimer's disease. Findings from this discipline form the bulk of the literature examined in this chapter.

We begin by providing a historical perspective and then discuss the rationale for selecting particular psychosocial constructs for inclusion in population-based studies. Next, we discuss the most commonly used methods for assessing psychosocial factors, including the strengths and challenges associated with these assessment methods. We briefly describe some research diagnostic interview measures used in studies focused on mental health and then devote much of the chapter to a description of commonly used self-report measures of psychosocial factors. We conclude with a discussion of issues likely to be important for furthering the study of psychosocial factors within populations.

2 Historical Perspective on Psychosocial Factors in Population Health

Research on psychosocial factors and health outcomes largely has focused on affective states or emotions, personality characteristics, acute and chronic stress/stressors, and various aspects of

S.A. Everson-Rose (✉)
Department of Medicine, Program in Health Disparities Research, University of Minnesota Medical School, 717 Delaware Street SE, Suite 166, Minneapolis, MN 55414, USA
e-mail: saer@umn.edu

A. Steptoe (ed.), *Handbook of Behavioral Medicine*, DOI 10.1007/978-0-387-09488-5_21,
© Springer Science+Business Media, LLC 2010

social relationships.[1] The focus on these particular psychosocial factors derives mainly from three sources: (1) historical anecdotes and clinical observations that supported the idea that certain personality features and emotions were prominent in certain disease states – e.g., the classic psychosomatic hypothesis of a "hypertensive personality"; (2) specific disciplinary foci of the scientific traditions that have contributed to this literature; and (3) key scientific discoveries or advances that have contributed to the knowledge base.

Historical observations and anecdotal information have long contributed to the belief that strong emotional states and personality characteristics related to hostility, anger, aggressiveness, and a need to be hard driving contributed to heart disease and high blood pressure (Alexander, 1939; Dunbar, 1943). This knowledge provided an important impetus to the now-classic work on coronary-prone behavior conducted in the 1950s and 1960s by Rosenman and Friedman (Friedman and Rosenman, 1971; Rosenman et al, 1975) that identified the Type A behavior pattern as a risk factor for coronary heart disease (CHD). Based on this seminal work, Type A was the first psychosocial factor to be accepted by the medical community as an established risk factor for CHD (Cooper et al, 1981). Subsequently, the hostility component of Type A has been identified as a particularly "toxic" feature (Dembroski and Czajkowski,

1989) and has received much attention in the literature on psychosocial factors and health (see Chapter 13).

In the early half of the 20th century, the initial reports linking depression to subsequent CHD-related mortality in psychiatric patients appeared in the literature (Fuller, 1935; Malzberg, 1937). Later work confirmed the importance of depression in the prognosis of cardiac patients, showing that depression and elevated depressive symptoms in the absence of depressive disorder both contributed to greater morbidity and mortality in patients with CHD (Frasure-Smith et al, 1995a, b). Several psychiatric epidemiology studies designed to establish prevalence of mental disorders and psychopathology in the general population also found that a core dimension of non-specific psychological distress common to a wide range of mental disorders was related to excess mortality risk (Kessler et al, 2002; Pratt, 2009).

These developments occurred as the science of public health was expanding. Indeed, the recognized health impact of poor sanitation, harsh-working conditions, and poverty, widely documented and reported in the mid-to-late 1800s and early part of the 1900s, provided a strong impetus for the development of the science of public health and epidemiology in particular (Berkman and Kawachi, 2000a). One focus of much of the early work in epidemiology was understanding the spread of infectious diseases (e.g., cholera); this work was critical in drawing attention to the importance of social conditions on health and illness.

Sociology, with its focus on social interactions and relationships, also has made unique contributions to understanding the relation between social factors and health. Indeed, Durkheim's renowned work on suicide identified lack of social integration as a critical feature of persons who commit suicide (Durkheim, 1979). Subsequently, a number of epidemiologic studies documented increased mortality rates and greater morbidity related to infectious diseases, accidents as well as mental illness among persons who were unmarried or socially isolated (see House et al, 1988 for a review). In the mid-

---

[1] While the term 'psychosocial factors' describes many different psychological and social characteristics, we focus our discussion on the constructs that have been most commonly included in population-based studies: emotions, personality, stress, and qualitative and quantitative features of social connections. The importance of the broader social contexts in which people live their lives is well-recognized; however, other chapters within this volume address the critical socio-environmental characteristics of socioeconomic position and neighborhoods as well as significant ethnic and cultural issues and thus those constructs are not explicitly addressed in this chapter.

1970s, now-classic work by Cassel (1976) and Cobb (1976) reported on the protective effects of social relationships. These lines of work have contributed greatly to an ever expanding and remarkably rich literature on the health benefits of social support, social capital, and both qualitative and quantitative features of social relationships.

Finally, advances in physiology in the first half of the 20th century – most notably the pioneering work of Walter Cannon and Hans Selye – provided critical theoretical and empirical evidence for understanding how stressors lead to physiological perturbations and ultimately to disease states. Cannon identified the "fight-or-flight" response (Cannon, 1935), physiologic reactions to threat or challenge, and postulated that poor health could result from dysregulation of the system not only at physiological levels but also at higher levels related to psychological and sociocultural functioning. Selye, following the work of Cannon, was the first to observe that while a core stress response was adaptive, severe, prolonged stress responses would lead to tissue damage and disease (Selye, 1956). Together, the work of Cannon and Selye provided a critical model for investigating physiological mechanisms that link various psychological states and social factors with poor health.

Thus, converging evidence from these varied disciplines has laid the foundation for the scientific investigation of the relationship between psychosocial factors and health within population-based epidemiological studies.

3 Rationale for Assessment of Psychosocial Constructs

The rationale for selecting psychosocial factors for assessment within population-based studies, as well as which assessment methods to use, varies widely. While some studies have focused on a particular psychosocial factor, others have measured a broad array of constructs. Lengthier and/or more in-depth assessments of a single construct would be appropriate if the goal is to increase depth of understanding of that construct. In contrast, shorter, less burdensome assessments are appropriate if the goal is to increase breadth of constructs assessed.

One issue that has been strongly debated in the literature on psychosocial factors and health is whether assessments include measures of clinical diagnoses (e.g., major depressive disorder, panic disorder) or measures of symptom severity or both. Within the context of studying the health impact of negative emotions and personality, questions have been raised as to whether assessment of symptoms without assessment of clinical conditions is sufficient. An example is the assessment of depressive symptoms versus major depressive disorder (i.e., clinical depression). The initial studies examining whether depression was linked to increased morbidity and mortality were conducted within psychiatric populations, so an early emphasis in the literature was on clinically diagnosed depression. However, because it is uncommon to have time or resources to complete clinical interviews within the context of large, population-based studies, much of the epidemiologic research on the relation of depression and health outcomes has utilized checklist-type measures that assess symptoms of depression (see Table 21.1 for examples of such measures). While these measures of depressive symptoms cannot be used to diagnose major depressive disorder, they do provide a picture of the level, and in certain cases severity, of symptomatology experienced by participants. Detailed presentation of the findings of such studies is beyond the scope of this chapter but is discussed elsewhere in this volume (see Chapter 12). In brief, such studies largely have shown that higher levels of depressive symptoms are associated with increasing risk of cardiovascular morbidity and mortality and poorer health outcomes in general. This pattern of findings suggest that the impact of depression on health is not a threshold phenomenon – but rather, lies along a continuum with increasing risk conferred with increasing numbers and severity of symptoms. Similar patterns of association exist for anxiety (e.g., symptoms

Table 21.1 Scales measuring psychosocial constructs in population-based studies

Psychosocial construct	Scale	Notes	Source
Personality characteristics			
Type A	Jenkins Activity Scale	Research on Type A personality has shifted toward hostility as it is particularly health-damaging component	Jenkins et al (1979)
	Framingham Type A Scale		Haynes et al (1978)
	Bortner Rating Scale		Bortner (1969)
Hostility	Cook–Medley Hostility Scale: Total Scale and Cynicism Subscale	Subsets of this scale are typically used, notably (Barefoot et al, 1989; Everson et al, 1997; Greenglass and Julkunen, 1989)	Cook and Medley (1954)
Trait anger	State-Trait Anger Expression Inventory-2 (STAXI-2)	This scale can measure state anger with the State Anger Scale (S-Anger)	Spielberger (1999)
Trait anxiety	State-Trait Anxiety Inventory (STAI-Form Y)	This scale can measure state anxiety with the State Anxiety Scale (S-Anxiety)	Spielberger (1983)
Neuroticism Extraversion Openness to experience Agreeableness Conscientiousness	NEO Five-Factor Inventory (NEO-FFI)	Measures neuroticism, extraversion, openness to experience, agreeableness, and conscientiousness. Longer form available	Costa and McCrae (1992)
Type D	DS14	At present, measure more frequently used outside of the USA	Denollet (2005)
Optimism	Life Orientation Test (LOT)	Half of the items of this measure assess optimism and half assess pessimism. A revised version of this scale is available	Scheier and Carver (1985)
Emotional states			
Negative			
Depression	Beck Depression Inventory (BDI)	Many earlier studies use the original BDI, however, the BDI-II is becoming widely used	Beck et al (1961)

Table 21.1 (continued)

Psychosocial construct	Scale	Notes	Source
	Center for Epidemiologic Studies Depression Scale (CES-D)	The scale is widely used and has well-developed short forms	Radloff (1977)
	Patient Health Questionnaire-9 (PHQ-9)	Items track DSM-IV depressive disorder diagnosis criteria	Kroenke et al (2001)
	Hospital Anxiety and Depression Scale (HADS)	Measures depression and anxiety	Zigmond and Snaith (1983)
Distress	General Health Questionnaire-30 (GHQ-30)	Measures aspects of depression, anxiety, social impairment, and hypochondriasis. Shorter and longer forms available	Goldberg (1972)
	Hopkins Symptom Checklist-25 (HSCL-25)	Measures aspects of depression and anxiety. Shorter and longer forms available	Derogatis et al (1974); Winokur et al (1984)
	Mental Health Inventory-5 (MHI-5)	Items assess multiple domains (anxiety, depression, loss of behavioral or emotional control, and psychological well-being)	Berwick et al (1991)
	K-6 and K-10	Measures of non-specific psychological distress; designed specifically for large population-based studies and to be particularly sensitive to individuals at the highest end of the distribution	Kessler et al (2002)
Hopelessness	Kuopio Ischemic Heart Disease Risk Factor (KIHD) Study Hopelessness Scale	Brief efficient measure of hopelessness	Everson et al (1996)
	Beck Hopelessness Scale (BHS)	Performs better in populations where at least a moderate level of hopelessness is anticipated	Beck et al (1974)
Positive	Positive and Negative Affect Schedule (PANAS)	Short form available that has been validated on multi-cultural samples	Watson et al (1988)
Chronic stress and stressors			
Perceived stress	Perceived Stress Scale	Widely used global measure of stress	Cohen et al (1983)
Life events	Psychiatric Epidemiology Research Interview (PERI)	Measures of life events frequently rely on one or more of these scales for a subset of items that are relevant to the study population. Frequently though, the source scales for the life events measured are not explicitly mentioned	Dohrenwend et al (1978)
	Impact of Event Scale – Revised (IES-R)		Weiss (2004)

Table 21.1 (continued)

Psychosocial construct	Scale	Notes	Source
	Life Experiences Survey (LES)		Sarason et al (1978)
	Social Readjustment Rating Scale (SRRS)		Holmes and Rahe (1967)
Job strain	Job Content Questionnaire (JCQ)	Based on the Demand/Control Model. Measures psychological demands, decision latitude, social support, physical demands, and job insecurity	Karasek et al (1998)
	Effort-Reward Imbalance Questionnaire (ERI)	Based on the Effort-Reward Imbalance Model and measures effort, reward, and overcommitment	Siegrist et al (2004)
Perceived discrimination	Experiences of Discrimination (EOD)	Explicitly measures racial discrimination	Krieger et al (2005)
	Perceived Unfair Treatment and Everyday Discrimination	This scale is known by many names, although frequently as the Perceived Discrimination Scale. It was framed as a measure of unfair treatment without specific mention of race	Williams et al (1997)
Social relationships			
Social network	Social Network Index (SNI)	Frequently used as the conceptual basis of measurements of social integration/social networks	Berkman and Syme (1979)
Perceived support	Interpersonal Support Evaluation List (ISEL)	Measures perceived support conceptualized as tangible, belonging, self-esteem, and appraisal	Cohen and Hoberman (1983)
	MOS Social Support Survey	Measures emotional/informational, tangible, and affectionate social support and positive social interaction	Sherbourne and Stewart (1991)
	Social Support Questionnaire 6 (SSQ6)	Measures availability and satisfaction with social support. Longer version available	Sarason et al (1987)
Isolation/loneliness	R-UCLA Loneliness Scale (R-UCLA)	Standard measure of loneliness	Russell et al (1980)
	Three-Item Loneliness Scale	Based on the R-UCLA scale but shortened and formatted for use with telephone survey administration	Hughes et al (2004)

of tension and anxiety versus diagnoses of panic disorder or phobias). Together, this type of evidence indicates that symptoms related to negative emotional states, as well as clinical conditions, importantly influence health. Thus, within the context of population-based studies, there is convincing rationale to include assessments of psychosocial factors that focus on non-clinical levels and/or symptom counts. Such assessments are worthwhile and can provide crucial information to characterize and understand the health of populations, even if clinical assessments of psychiatric conditions are not feasible.

4 Methods of Assessing Psychosocial Factors

Within population-based studies, there are two primary methods of assessing psychosocial factors: (1) structured or semi-structured research diagnostic interviews and (2) self-administered or interviewer-administered questionnaires or surveys (i.e., "self-report"). Studies in which the primary focus is on mental health and psychosocial functioning (e.g., psychiatric epidemiology studies) tend to favor fully structured or semi-structured diagnostic interviews over self-report instruments to assess psychopathology symptoms and diagnoses. Three of the most commonly used diagnostic interviews include the Diagnostic Interview Schedule (House et al, 1988; Robins et al, 1981), the Composite International Diagnostic Interview (CIDI) (WHO, 1990), and the Structured Clinical Interview for DSM Disorders (SCID) (Spitzer et al, 1992). The DIS was developed nearly 30 years ago in conjunction with the National Institute of Mental Health in the U.S. to address the need for a comprehensive diagnostic interview for use in a large, multi-site epidemiologic study known as the Epidemiologic Catchment Area (ECA) study (Robins and Regier, 1991). The DIS is based solely on the criteria and descriptions for mental disorders put forth by the American Psychiatric Association

(APA) in their Diagnostic and Statistical Manual (DSM) (APA, 1987). Though specialized training is required, the DIS is a fully structured interview that is designed to be administered by lay interviewers, which was a unique feature at the time of its development. It has been used widely across a variety of studies throughout the world and adapted for use in cross-cultural studies (Bravo et al, 1991; Compton et al, 1991; Lee et al, 1990). The DIS also served as the basis for the CIDI, which was developed in response to concerns that the DSM system for diagnoses of mental disorders was not applicable internationally across disparate cultures. International diagnostic standards are based on the International Classification of Diseases (ICD) rather than the DSM, so the CIDI expanded the DIS by using ICD criteria, thereby allowing for cross-national comparisons of mental health.

The CIDI is a fully structured, non-clinical interview and is used worldwide in general population surveys. The most recent version of the CIDI (version 2.1) (Kessler and Ustun, 2004; WHO, 1997) is used in the World Mental Health Study, which is an initiative by the WHO to examine the prevalence and correlates of mental disorders, behavioral disorders, and substance-abuse disorders from all regions of the world (Kessler and Ustun, 2008). The CIDI has both computerized and paper and pencil versions, both of which have been modularized, giving investigators the option of choosing only the modules most relevant to their research goals. The SCID is a semi-structured psychiatric interview used to identify lifetime history of and current psychiatric disorders. Like the DIS, the SCID is based on APA criteria for mental disorders, as defined in the DSM; however, administration of the SCID is done only by highly trained clinical interviewers. The SCID has been widely used in clinical settings as well as research studies and has demonstrated reliability for diagnoses of psychiatric disorders in multiple race/ethnicity groups (Bromberger et al, 2009; Williams et al, 1992).

Each of these diagnostic interviews offers in-depth assessment of psychosocial functioning vis-a-vis mental health. However, each requires substantial specialized training to administer. The time, training, and costs involved to develop expertise in these interviews, as well as the extra participant burden such time-intensive interviews create, very often make it prohibitive to use such interviews in large, population-based studies, particularly those in which mental health is not a primary focus. The need for less time-consuming measures has prompted the development of self-report questionnaires based on diagnostic interviews. These types of questionnaires increasingly are being used as screening tools for common mental disorders in clinical research and in population-based studies. For example, the Primary Care Evaluation of Mental Disorders (PRIME-MD) (Spitzer et al, 1994) was developed as a clinician-administered interview for use in primary care to diagnose five common disorders based on criteria set forth in the APA's DSM. Subsequently, a self-administered version was developed as the Patient Health Questionnaire (PHQ) (Spitzer et al, 1999). Two short forms, the PHQ-9 (Kroenke et al, 2001) and PHQ-8 (Kroenke et al, 2009), specifically assess depressive symptoms based on DSM-IV criteria and are increasingly used in both clinical and research settings (Cannon et al, 2007; Strine et al, 2009).

Studies in which physical health outcomes are of primary interest tend to rely predominantly on self-report, by far the most commonly used method of assessing a wide range of psychosocial constructs. Table 21.1 lists 35 self-report questionnaires that assess psychosocial constructs that have been rigorously tested in terms of their relation to morbidity and mortality outcomes and have shown very consistent, if not unequivocal, associations with health outcomes (Bruce et al, 2009; Egan et al 2008; Everson-Rose and Lewis, 2005; Hemingway and Marmot, 1999) including personality characteristics, emotional states (negative and positive), chronic stress and stressors, and structural and functional features of social relationships. Our focus in this table is on objective measures of these constructs – that is, measures with standardized and specific items that are presented with fixed or limited response options (Segal and Coolidge, 2004). While not an exhaustive

listing, the self-report instruments described in Table 21.1 were selected for inclusion based on their relatively widespread use in previous population-based health studies. Promising measures that are likely to feature in future population-based studies also are presented.

A thorough evaluation of the strengths and weaknesses of various self-report instruments in order to recommend a particular set of measures or assessment approaches for future work is well beyond the scope of this chapter. The table is intended to be used as a resource for investigators seeking to understand the types of self-report questionnaires commonly used to assess personality, emotions, stress, and social relationships. We include measures for each specific construct, provide citations to each measure, and include a column labeled "Notes" that is meant to offer readers some general insight into the use of the measures. Below we provide further detail about many of the measures noted in the table. We emphasize that although the extant literature related to these measures is well developed, new measures and revised versions of older ones are continuously being developed; therefore, interested readers are encouraged to consult the literature for any new developments prior to choosing a scale for future research.

4.1 Personality Characteristics

Investigations of personality characteristics were at the forefront of research-linking psychosocial risk factors to physical health. Type A, as mentioned earlier, was the first recognized psychosocial risk factor for CHD. Common measures of Type A have been listed in the table; however, the field of inquiry has predominantly shifted its attention to hostility as the likely health damaging Type A component. Hostility can be measured with several different instruments; by far the most frequently used measure is the Cook–Medley Hostility Scale (Cook and Medley, 1954), which is derived from the Minnesota Multiphasic Personality Inventory

(Hathaway and McKinley, 1940). Shortened versions of this scale are most often employed, the most common of which are listed in Table 21.1. As with measurement of hostility, population-based measurement of most of the other personality characteristics listed in Table 21.1 are frequently accomplished with a dominant measure, namely the Spielberger scales for trait anger and anxiety (Spielberger, 1983, 1999), the NEO Five Factor Inventory (NEO-FFI) for the five empirically identified broad dimensions of personality (Costa and McCrae, 1992), and the Life Orientation Test (LOT) (Scheier and Carver, 1985) for the measurement of optimism. The measurement of Type D personality (the letter "D" refers to "distressed" and this is a trait characterized by both negative affectivity and social inhibition) is similarly accomplished with the DS14 (Denollet, 2005); however, this measure predominantly has been used in studies based in western Europe.

4.2 Emotional States

While personality characteristics lead the investigation of psychosocial factors and health, the measurement of negative emotional states, particularly depression, is among the most studied psychosocial risk factors for poor physical health. In population-based studies, depression is most frequently measured by the Center for Epidemiological Studies Depression Scale (CES-D) (Radloff, 1977) or the Beck Depression Inventory (BDI) (Beck et al, 1961) and more recently the BDI-II (Dozois and Covin, 2004). The Hospital Anxiety and Depression Scale (HADS) (Zigmond and Snaith, 1983) was designed for use in medical settings; its psychometric properties seem to apply to population-based studies as well (Bjelland et al, 2002), although it has been less frequently used in population-based studies compared to the CES-D or BDI. Because the PHQ-9 (Kroenke et al, 2001) and PHQ-8 (Kroenke et al, 2009) are both short and track DSM-IV depressive disorder diagnosis criteria, their use likely will increase in population-based studies.

Distress is a construct that entails components of depression and anxiety among other emotional and behavioral components. Hence, measures tapping into this construct frequently involve items representing two or more related constructs, such as anxiety and depression, and are sometimes used to measure those dimensions, particularly depression. Widely used measures include the GHQ-30 (Goldberg, 1972) and the Hopkins Symptom Checklist-25 (HSCL-25) (Derogatis et al, 1974; Winokur et al, 1984). The Mental Health Inventory-5 (MHI-5) (Berwick et al, 1991) is of note not only because of its brevity but also because it is contained in the very popular Short Form-36 measurement of health and well-being (Ware and Sherbourne, 1992). The K-6 and K-10 (Kessler et al, 2002) measures are promising as they have been included in large population-based surveys in the USA and Australia and have been incorporated into the World Mental Health Surveys, thereby providing a unique opportunity to standardize the scoring and to establish internationally valid calibration rules.

The measurement of hopelessness in population-based studies has frequently been via the Kuopio Ischemic Heart Disease Risk Factor (KIHD) Study hopelessness scale (Everson et al, 1996), which with only two items is a highly efficient measure of a psychosocial risk. The Beck Hopelessness Scale (BHS) (Beck et al, 1974) also is used outside the clinical setting. However, the scale demonstrates greater reliability among those with at least moderate levels of hopelessness (Dozois and Covin, 2004). Recent research suggests that hopelessness may be a particularly health damaging component of depression as was the case for hostility and Type A (Whipple et al, 2009). The measurement of positive emotional states and their relationship to health has gained prominence recently (see Chapter 14). In population-based studies, the Positive and Negative Affect Scale (PANAS) (Watson et al, 1988) is very frequently employed to measure positive well-being; it is also used to measure negative affect. The measurement of optimism, mentioned above, and its relationship to health contributes to this growing body of literature.

4.3 Chronic Stress and Stressors

In population-based studies, stress is frequently conceptualized in one or more ways. Very frequently these measurements reflect a more global measure of perceived stress, using the Perceived Stress Scale (Cohen et al, 1983), or measurements of life events. Life events measures are frequently based on one or more underlying measures, the source of which is sometimes cited. The most prominent of these underlying scales are listed in Table 21.1. The choice of life events is in large part determined by space available on the questionnaire as well as the relevance of the particular life event to the study population. Similarly, role-specific measures of chronic stress are also dependent in large part on the study population. Outside of measures of job strain, namely the Job Content Questionnaire (Karasek et al, 1998) and the Effort-Reward Imbalance Questionnaire (Siegrist et al, 2004), the choice of role-specific measures in population-based studies is considerably more variable. More recently, discrimination has received attention as a measure of psychosocial stress. Two of the most commonly used measures are listed in Table 21.1, one without specific reference to race, the Perceived Unfair Treatment and Everyday Discrimination Scale (Williams et al, 1997), and one anchored to racial discrimination, the Experiences of Discrimination Scale (Krieger et al, 2005). Scale development and refinement is underway to examine non-racial sources of discrimination as well as to better examine racial discrimination in a variety of racial/ethnic groups.

the distinction between measurements of social network structure and function predominates. Most measurements of social network structure in the last 30 years are conceptually based on the Social Network Index (Berkman and Syme, 1979), which incorporates measurements of marital status, contact with friends and relatives, and church and group membership. Functional support is conceptualized as several types such as emotional, informational, tangible, and belonging (Uchino, 2004). While the exact domains differ across instruments, many of them include more than one such as the Interpersonal Support Evaluation List (Cohen and Hoberman, 1983) and the MOS Social Support Survey (Sherbourne and Stewart, 1991). The Social Support Questionnaire-6 (Sarason et al, 1987) is a promising measure that taps into the perceived availability of and satisfaction with social support utilizing only six items. A related construct, isolation or loneliness, is also featured among measures of social relations. The most commonly used measure is the R-UCLA Loneliness Scale (Russell et al, 1980), although a shorter version of this measure has recently been developed specifically for surveys administered over the telephone (Hughes et al, 2004).

Together, these measures provide good examples of self-report instruments available for population-based studies. As has been demonstrated, well-developed instruments are available for a range of constructs, providing valid measurements within the time constraints typically involved in large population-based studies. However, their use should be considered within the larger frame of advantages and disadvantages to self-report psychosocial assessments.

4.4 Social Relationships

The measurement of social relationships or lack thereof continues to be a component of most population-based studies. While there is an entire literature on the characterization of various aspects of social relationships that are relevant to health (Laireiter and Baumann, 1992),

5 Advantages and Disadvantages of Self-Report Psychosocial Assessments

Both self-report formats and interview-based methods for assessing psychosocial factors have distinct advantages and disadvantages. The advantages and disadvantages of interview methods have been described above. Perhaps the greatest advantages of self-report formats are the ease of administration and relatively low costs, which make it possible to administer self-report questionnaires to large numbers of participants – clearly a strength when conducting a population-based study with a large sample. Self-report instruments allow the respondent privacy in terms of answering questions, which is a particular advantage when asking questions about what many consider sensitive or personal information. Questions are highly structured and have standardized response formats. Response options typically are on a true/false, visual analog, or Likert-type scale, making scoring of items relatively straightforward. In addition, many questionnaires have been translated into multiple languages and validated, allowing use of these measures in ethnically diverse samples and in cross-country comparisons.

However, these advantages need to be weighed against recognized disadvantages or challenges associated with self-report questionnaires and surveys. Concerns have been noted that self-report is subjective, based on a person's perceptions, rather than an objective indicator of a particular construct. However, psychosocial factors, by their very nature, are experiential and so reliance on self-report to denote these characteristics is valid. Self-report measures can be prone to error, which may be introduced in several ways. For example, questions may be misunderstood, may ask information that the respondent cannot accurately report or inquire about information that a respondent may be unwilling to accurately report (Fowler and Mangione, 1990). These issues can be magnified with self-report questionnaires precisely because there is not an interviewer present to clarify questions, to probe to see if the respondent understood the question as intended, or to gauge the respondent's ability or willingness to provide accurate responses. As a whole, the method of self-report has both strengths and weaknesses that must be considered in light of the research question involved. For research questions in which

self-report instruments are sufficient, the survey methodology literature should be consulted for insight into how to minimize the disadvantages of self-report.

6 Future Directions

Although the study of psychosocial factors in population-based studies of health has grown exponentially over the last several decades, there remain several important issues that need to be addressed. The five issues briefly described below may provide a useful framework for future research that seeks to better understand the impact of psychosocial factors on health and well-being of populations.

6.1 Multiple Psychological and Social Influences on Population Health

Many individual psychological characteristics and social factors have been associated with a broad range of health outcomes. Indeed, the approach of many epidemiologic studies has been to attempt to identify the *independent* contributions of such characteristics. However, it is widely recognized that psychosocial risk factors rarely occur in isolation (e.g., persons who experience depression often are socially isolated), and yet, to date, very few studies have attempted to examine whether health risks are exacerbated in the presence of multiple psychosocial risk factors or whether psychological characteristics and social factors interact in a synergistic fashion to elevate health risks. To further this field of study, it is necessary to expand the breadth of studies to address this issue of multiplicity of psychosocial risk. Several socio-ecological models (c.f., Glass and McAtee, 2006; Kaplan et al, 2000; Krieger, 2001) exist that can inform this type of work.

6.2 Factors Unique to Immigrant Groups and Minority Populations

Historically, much of the research on the role of psychosocial factors in health was limited to study cohorts that were predominantly white (e.g., Whitehall Civil Service study, KIHD Study) or had too few participants of color to reliably examine whether any differences in the relation of psychosocial factors to health outcomes existed between race/ethnicity groups. A growing number of published studies have included minority groups – notably, African Americans and, more recently, Hispanics; however, much remains to be learned about cultural, psychological, and social factors that may be unique and/or particularly relevant to the health experience of minority populations and immigrant groups. This is a significant issue, given that minorities tend to bear a disproportionate burden of disease in the USA and in most westernized countries. One example is the impact of unfair treatment and discrimination on health. There is growing evidence that these stressors have a significant impact on cardiovascular functioning in particular (Krieger and Sidney, 1996; Lewis et al, 2006, 2009), but there is a clear need for systematic study of the long-term health consequences of chronic stress exposure. In addition, more work is needed to understand how acculturation as well as the stress that may be experienced during that process (i.e., acculturative stress) impacts the trajectories of health among immigrant populations over time.

6.3 Cultural Framework of Assessment Tools

Further work is needed to ensure that the assessment tools used to study psychosocial factors in relation to health outcomes are culturally sensitive as well as specific. Increasingly, questionnaires have been translated and administered in multiple languages, which increases the utility of such measures across many race/ethnicity groups. However, such translations by themselves do not explicitly address the cultural relevance of various psychosocial constructs across multiple and varied cultures. For example, the manifestation of symptoms of depression or anxiety in different cultures will reflect culturally accepted modes of expression but this issue is rarely addressed in research studies. Expanding our understanding of the impact of psychosocial factors on the health of populations in an increasingly multi-cultural world will require greater attention to such issues.

6.4 Measurement and Modeling Issues

The collective evidence supporting the significant influence that psychosocial factors have on various aspects of health, using varied assessment approaches, is fairly compelling. A major criticism that has been raised regarding epidemiologic studies of psychosocial factors and health outcomes is the lack of a standardized assessment approach to psychosocial factors, which limits the ability to make quantitative comparisons across studies (Hemingway and Marmot, 1999). A standardized assessment approach would increase the comparability of data, thereby potentially allowing for more definitive conclusions regarding the relation of psychosocial factors to health across multiple populations. Nevertheless, we believe the rationale for choosing particular psychosocial constructs to assess in a given study, as well as which particular assessment tools to use, should ultimately be driven by the goals and resources of the study. An additional measurement issue that warrants future research attention relates to the fact that some of the psychosocial constructs noted here have less well developed and/or inconsistent approaches to assessment. Specifically, assessment of life events and social networks and support has been less rigorous, with investigators creating their own measures in many instances, and/or providing little documentation about the measures used. This lack of consistency and lack of pertinent information in many publications make it challenging to know what measures may be best in terms of assessing structural and functional aspects of social relationships and hampers our understanding of the ways in which significant social stressors influence health. Moreover, despite the existence of a rich literature on the assessment and health impact of chronic psychosocial stressors within the work setting (e.g., Levi et al, 2000), measures of non-work-related chronic daily stressors are rather poorly developed. Exceptions to this are the more recent scales assessing perceptions of unfair treatment and discrimination; however, much more work is needed to adequately address the measurement of chronic stress.

6.5 Pathways from Psychosocial Factors to Health and Illness

A final area that holds much opportunity for future investigations is to more comprehensively examine the pathways by which psychosocial factors influence health and illness. Psychosocial factors may operate through direct mechanisms, such as alterations in sympatho-adrenal-medullary functioning or brain neurotransmitters (e.g., serotonin, dopamine), or they may operate indirectly through behavioral pathways (e.g., poorer health habits related to diet, activity, and smoking). Few studies have comprehensively examined both behavioral and pathophysiological pathways and their interactions. Greater knowledge about such pathways will serve to inform interventions that can reduce psychosocial risk and promote health.

7 Summary

The study of psychosocial factors and health has expanded greatly in the past several decades, with important contributions and converging

lines of evidence coming from psychology, epidemiology, public health, sociology, and physiology. In this chapter, we have presented an overview of two primary assessment methods used to assess psychosocial factors, focusing on measures of emotional states, personality, chronic stress and stressors and both qualitative and quantitative features of social relationships. While population studies focused on mental health have strongly favored structured or semi-structured interviews to assess various aspects of psychosocial functioning, vis-a-vis mental health, those focused on physical health outcomes have predominantly relied on self-report questionnaires or surveys and it is this latter method to which we have devoted most of this chapter. Our intent is for readers to be able to use the information presented as a resource when designing new studies and considering which psychosocial constructs and associated assessment methods may be most relevant to their research goals and to the health outcomes of interest. Population-based measurement of psychosocial factors using epidemiological research techniques will continue to play a vital role in the investigation of the relationship between psychosocial factors and mental and physical health and well-being.

References

American Psychiatric Association. (1987). *Diagnostic and Statistical Manual of Mental Disorders, Third Edition-Revised (DSM-III-R)*. Washington, DC: American Psychiatric Association.

Alexander, R. (1939). Emotional factors in essential hypertension. *Psychosom Med, 1*, 173–179.

Barefoot, J. C., Dodge, K. A., Peterson, B. L., Dahlstrom, W. G., and Williams, R. B. Jr. (1989). The Cook-Medley hostility scale: item content and ability to predict survival. *Psychosom Med, 51*, 46–57.

Beck, A. T., Ward, C. H., Mendelson, M., Mock, J., and Erbaugh, J. (1961). An inventory for measuring depression. *Arch Gen Psychiatry, 4*, 561–571.

Beck, A. T., Weissman, A., Lester, D., and Trexler, L. (1974). The measurement of pessimism: the hopelessness scale. *J Consult Clin Psychol, 42*, 861–865.

Berkman, L. F., and Kawachi, I. (2000a). A historical framework for social epidemiology. In L. F. Berkman

& I. Kawachi (Eds.), *Social Epidemiology* (pp. 3–12). New York, NY: Oxford University Press.

Berkman, L. F., and Kawachi, I. (Eds.). (2000b). *Social Epidemiology*. New York, NY: Oxford University Press.

Berkman, L. F., and Syme, S. L. (1979). Social networks, host resistance, and mortality: a nine-year follow-up study of Alameda County residents. *Am J Epidemiol, 109*, 186–204.

Berwick, D. M., Murphy, J. M., Goldman, P. A., Ware, J. E. Jr., Barsky, A. J. et al (1991). Performance of a five-item mental health screening test. *Med Care, 29*, 169–176.

Bjelland, I., Dahl, A. A., Haug, T. T., and Neckelmann, D. (2002). The validity of the Hospital Anxiety and Depression Scale. An updated literature review. *J Psychosom Res, 52*, 69–77.

Bortner, R. W. (1969). A short rating scale as a potential measure of pattern A behavior. *J Chronic Dis, 22*, 87–91.

Bravo, M., Canino, G. J., Rubio-Stipec, M., and Woodbury-Farina, M. (1991). A cross-cultural adaptation of a psychiatric epidemiologic instrument: the diagnostic interview schedule's adaptation in Puerto Rico. *Cult Med Psychiatry, 15*, 1–18.

Bromberger, J. T., Kravitz, H. M., Matthews, K., Youk, A., Brown, C. et al (2009). Predictors of first lifetime episodes of major depression in midlife women. *Psychol Med, 39*, 55–64.

Bruce, M. A., Beech, B. M., Sims, M., Brown, T. N., Wyatt, S. B. et al (2009). Social environmental stressors, psychological factors, and kidney disease. *J Investig Med, 57*, 583–589.

Cannon, D. S., Tiffany, S. T., Coon, H., Scholand, M. B., McMahon, W. M. et al (2007). The PHQ-9 as a brief assessment of lifetime major depression. *Psychol Assess, 19*, 247–251.

Cannon, W. B. (1935). Stresses and strains of homeostasis (Mary Scott Newbold Lecture). *Am J Med Sci, 189*, 1–14.

Cassel, J. (1976). The contribution of the social environment to host resistance: the Fourth Wade Hampton Frost Lecture. *Am J Epidemiol, 104*, 107–123.

Cobb, S. (1976). Presidential Address-1976. Social support as a moderator of life stress. *Psychosom Med, 38*, 300–314.

Cohen, S., and Hoberman, H. M. (1983). Positive events and social supports as buffers of life change stress. *J Applied Soc Psychol, 13*, 99–125.

Cohen, S., Kamarck, T., and Mermelstein, R. (1983). A global measure of perceived stress. *J Health Soc Behav, 24*, 385–396.

Compton, W. M., 3rd, Helzer, J. E., Hwu, H. G., Yeh, E. K., McEvoy, L. et al (1991). New methods in cross-cultural psychiatry: psychiatric illness in Taiwan and the United States. *Am J Psychiatry, 148*, 1697–1704.

Cook, W., and Medley, D. (1954). Proposed hostility and pharasaic virtue scales for the MMPI. *J. Appl. Psychol, 38*, 414–418.

Cooper, T., Detre, T., and Weiss, S. M. (1981). Coronary-prone behavior and coronary heart disease: a critical review. The review panel on coronary-prone behavior and coronary heart disease. *Circulation, 63*, 1199–1215.

Costa, P. T., and McCrae, R. R. (1992). *Revised NEO Personality Inventory (NEO-PI-R) and NEO Five-Factor Inventory (NEO-FFI) Professional Manual*. Odessa, FL: Psychological Assessment Resources.

Dembroski, T. M., and Czajkowski, S. M. (1989). Historical and current developments in coronary-prone behavior. In A. W. Siegman & T. M. Dembroski (Eds.), *In Search of Coronary-Prone Behavior: Beyond Type A* (pp. 21–39). Hillsdale, NJ: Erlbaum.

Denollet, J. (2005). DS14: standard assessment of negative affectivity, social inhibition, and Type D personality. *Psychosom Med, 67*, 89–97.

Derogatis, L. R., Lipman, R. S., Rickels, K., Uhlenhuth, E. H., and Covi, L. (1974). The Hopkins Symptom Checklist (HSCL): a self-report symptom inventory. *Behav Sci, 19*, 1–15.

Dohrenwend, B. S., Krasnoff, L., Askenasy, A. R., and Dohrenwend, B. P. (1978). Exemplification of a method for scaling life events: the Peri Life Events Scale. *J Health Soc Behav, 19*, 205–229.

Dozois, D. J. A., and Covin, R. (2004). The Beck Depression Inventory-II (BDI-II), Beck Hopelessness Scale (BHS), and the Beck Scale for Suicide Ideation. In M. J. Hilsenroth & D. L. Segal (Eds.), *Comprehensive Handbook of Psychological Assessment, Vol. 2*, Personality Assessment (pp. 50–69). Hoboken, NJ: John Wiley and Sons, Inc.

Dunbar, F. (1943). *Psychosomatic Diagnosis*. New York, NY: Hoeber.

Durkheim, E. (1979). *Suicide: A Study in Sociology*. New York, NY: Free Press.

Egan, M., Tannahill, C., Petticrew, M., and Thomas, S. (2008). Psychosocial risk factors in home and community settings and their associations with population health and health inequalities: a systematic meta-review. *BMC Public Health, 8*, 239.

Everson-Rose, S. A., and Lewis, T. T. (2005). Psychosocial factors and cardiovascular diseases. *Annu Rev Public Health, 26*, 469–500.

Everson, S. A., Goldberg, D. E., Kaplan, G. A., Cohen, R. D., Pukkala, E. et al (1996). Hopelessness and risk of mortality and incidence of myocardial infarction and cancer. *Psychosom Med, 58*, 113–121.

Everson, S. A., Kauhanen, J., Kaplan, G. A., Goldberg, D. E., Julkunen, J. et al (1997). Hostility and increased risk of mortality and acute myocardial infarction: the mediating role of behavioral risk factors. *Am J Epidemiol, 146*, 142–152.

Fowler, F. J., and Mangione, T. W. (1990). Standardized survey interviewing: minimizing interview-related error. In *Applied Social Research Methods Series, Vol 18*. Newbury Park, CA: Sage Publications, Inc.

Frasure-Smith, N., Lesperance, F., and Talajic, M. (1995a). Depression and 18-month prognosis after myocardial infarction. *Circulation, 91*, 999–1005.

Frasure-Smith, N., Lesperance, F., and Talajic, M. (1995b). The impact of negative emotions on prognosis following myocardial infarction: is it more than depression? *Health Psychol, 14*, 388–398.

Friedman, M., and Rosenman, R. H. (1971). Type A Behavior Pattern: its association with coronary heart disease. *Ann Clin Res, 3*, 300–312.

Fuller, R. G. (1935). What happens to mental patients after discharge from the hospital?. *Psychiatr Q, 9*, 95–104.

Glass, T. A., and McAtee, M. J. (2006). Behavioral science at the crossroads in public health: extending horizons, envisioning the future. *Soc Sci Med, 62*, 1650–1671.

Goldberg, D. P. (1972). *The Detection of Psychiatric Illness by Questionnaire*. London: Oxford University Press.

Greenglass, E. R., and Julkunen, J. (1989). Construct validity and sex differences in Cook-Medley hostility. *Person Indiv Diff, 10*, 209–218.

Hathaway, S. R., and McKinley, J. C. (1940). A multiphasic personality schedule (Minnesota): I. Construction of the schedule. *J Psychol, 10*, 249–254.

Haynes, S. G., Levine, S., Scotch, N., Feinleib, M., and Kannel, W. B. (1978). The relationship of psychosocial factors to coronary heart disease in the Framingham study. I. Methods and risk factors. *Am J Epidemiol, 107*, 362–383.

Hemingway, H., and Marmot, M. (1999). Evidence based cardiology: psychosocial factors in the aetiology and prognosis of coronary heart disease. Systematic review of prospective cohort studies. *BMJ, 318*, 1460–1467.

Holmes, T. H., and Rahe, R. H. (1967). The Social Readjustment Rating Scale. *J Psychosom Res, 11*, 213–218.

House, J. S., Landis, K. R., and Umberson, D. (1988). Social relationships and health. *Science, 241*, 540–545.

Hughes, M. E., Waite, L. J., Hawksley, L. C., and Cacioppo, J. T. (2004). A Short Scale for Measuring Loneliness in Large Surveys: results from two population-based studies. *Res Aging, 26*, 655–672.

Jenkins, C. D., Zyzanski, S. J., and Rosenman, R. H. (1979). *Manual for the Jenkins' Activity Survey*. New York: Psychological Corporation.

Kaplan, G. A., Everson, S. A., and Lynch, J. W. (2000). The contribution of social and behavioral research to an understanding of the distribution of disease: a multilevel approach. In B. Smedley & S. L. Syme (Eds.), *Promoting Health: Intervention Strategies From Social And Behavioral Research* (pp. 37–80). Washington, DC: National Academy Press.

Karasek, R., Brisson, C., Kawakami, N., Houtman, I., Bongers, P. et al (1998). The Job Content Questionnaire (JCQ): an instrument for internationally comparative assessments of psychosocial job characteristics. *J Occup Health Psychol, 3*, 322–355.

Kessler, R. C., Andrews, G., Colpe, L. J., Hiripi, E., Mroczek, D. K. et al (2002). Short screening scales to monitor population prevalences and trends in nonspecific psychological distress. *Psychol Med, 32*, 959–976.

Kessler, R. C., and Ustun, T. B. (2004). The World Mental Health (WMH) Survey initiative version of the World Health Organization (WHO) Composite International Diagnostic Interview (CIDI). *Int J Methods Psychiatr Res, 13*, 93–121.

Kessler, R. C., and Ustun, T. B. (Eds.). (2008). *The WHO Mental Health Surveys: Global Perspectives on the Epidemiology of Mental Disorders*. New York, NY: Cambridge University Press and the World Health Organization.

Krieger, N. (2001). Theories for social epidemiology in the 21st century: an ecosocial perspective. *Int J Epidemiol, 30*, 668–677.

Krieger, N., and Sidney, S. (1996). Racial discrimination and blood pressure: the CARDIA Study of young black and white adults. *Am J Public Health, 86*, 1370–1378.

Krieger, N., Smith, K., Naishadham, D., Hartman, C., and Barbeau, E. M. (2005). Experiences of discrimination: validity and reliability of a self-report measure for population health research on racism and health. *Soc Sci Med, 61*, 1576–1596.

Kroenke, K., Spitzer, R. L., and Williams, J. B. (2001). The PHQ-9: validity of a brief depression severity measure. *J Gen Intern Med, 16*, 606–613.

Kroenke, K., Strine, T. W., Spitzer, R. L., Williams, J. B., Berry, J. T. et al (2009). The PHQ-8 as a measure of current depression in the general population. *J Affect Disord, 114*, 163–173.

Laireiter, A., and Baumann, U. (1992). Network structures and support-functions-theoretical and empirical analyses. In H. O. Veiel & U. Baumann (Eds.), *The Meaning and Measurement of Social Support* (pp. 33–55). New York, NY: Hemisphere Publishing Corporation.

Lee, C. K., Kwak, Y. S., Yamamoto, J., Rhee, H., Kim, Y. S. et al (1990). Psychiatric epidemiology in Korea. Part I: Gender and age differences in Seoul. *J Nerv Ment Dis, 178*, 242–246.

Levi, L., Bartley, M., Marmot, M., Karasek, R., Theorell, T. et al (2000). Stressors at the workplace: theoretical models. *Occup Med, 15*, 69–106.

Lewis, T. T., Barnes, L. L., Bienias, J. L., Lackland, D. T., Evans, D. A. et al (2009). Perceived discrimination and blood pressure in older African American and white adults. *J Gerontol A Biol Sci Med Sci, 64*, 1002–1008.

Lewis, T. T., Everson-Rose, S. A., Powell, L. H., Matthews, K. A., Brown, C. et al (2006). Chronic exposure to everyday discrimination and coronary artery calcification in African-American women: the SWAN Heart Study. *Psychosom Med, 68*, 362–368.

Malzberg, B. (1937). Mortality among patients with involutional melancholia. *Am J Psychiatry, 93*, 1231–1238.

Pratt, L. A. (2009). Serious psychological distress, as measured by the K6, and mortality. *Ann Epidemiol, 19*, 202–209.

Radloff, L. S. (1977). The CES-D scale: a self-report depression scale for research in the general population. *Applied Psychological Measurement*, 385–401.

Robins, L. N., Helzer, J. E., Croughan, J., and Ratcliff, K. S. (1981). National Institute of Mental Health Diagnostic Interview Schedule. Its history, characteristics, and validity. *Arch Gen Psychiatry, 38*, 381–389.

Robins, L. N., and Regier, D. A. (Eds.). (1991). *Psychiatric Disorders in America: The Epidemiologic Catchment Area Study*. New York, NY: Free Press.

Rosenman, R. H., Brand, R. J., Jenkins, D., Friedman, M., Straus, R. et al (1975). Coronary heart disease in Western Collaborative Group Study. Final follow-up experience of 8 1/2 years. *JAMA, 233*, 872–877.

Russell, D., Peplau, L. A., and Cutrona, C. E. (1980). The revised UCLA Loneliness Scale: concurrent and discriminant validity evidence. *J Pers Soc Psychol, 39*, 472–480.

Sarason, I. G., Johnson, J. H., and Siegel, J. M. (1978). Assessing the impact of life changes: development of the Life Experiences Survey. *J Consult Clin Psychol, 46*, 932–946.

Sarason, I. G., Sarason, B. R., Shearin, E. N., and Pierce, G. R. (1987). A brief measure of social support: practical and theoretical implications. *J Soc Person Relat, 4*, 497–510.

Scheier, M. F., and Carver, C. S. (1985). Optimism, coping, and health: assessment and implications of generalized outcome expectancies. *Health Psychol, 4*, 219–247.

Segal, D. L., and Coolidge, F. L. (2004). Objective assessment of personality and psychopathology: an overview. In M. J. Hilsenroth & D. L. Segal (Eds.), *Comprehensive Handbook of Psychological Assessment, Vol. 2*, Personality Assessment (pp. 3–13). Hoboken, NJ: John Wiley and Sons, Inc.

Selye, H. (1956). *The Stress of Life*. New York, NY: McGraw-Hill.

Sherbourne, C. D., and Stewart, A. L. (1991). The MOS social support survey. *Soc Sci Med, 32*, 705–714.

Siegrist, J., Starke, D., Chandola, T., Godin, I., Marmot, M. et al (2004). The measurement of effort-reward imbalance at work: European comparisons. *Soc Sci Med, 58*, 1483–1499.

Spielberger, C. D. (1983). *Manual for the State-Trait Anxiety Inventory: STAI (Form Y)*. Palo Alto, CA: Consulting Psychologists Press.

Spielberger, C. D. (1999). *Professional Manual for the State-Trait Anger Expression Inventory-2 (STAXI-2)*. Odessa, FL: Psychological Assessment Resources.

Spitzer, R. L., Kroenke, K., and Williams, J. B. (1999). Validation and utility of a self-report version of PRIME-MD: the PHQ primary care study. Primary Care Evaluation of Mental Disorders. Patient Health Questionnaire. *JAMA, 282*, 1737–1744.

Spitzer, R. L., Williams, J. B., Gibbon, M., and First, M. B. (1992). The Structured Clinical Interview for DSM-III-R (SCID). I: History, rationale, and description. *Arch Gen Psychiatry, 49*, 624–629.

Spitzer, R. L., Williams, J. B., Kroenke, K., Linzer, M., deGruy, F. V., 3rd, et al (1994). Utility of a new procedure for diagnosing mental disorders in primary care. The PRIME-MD 1000 study. *JAMA, 272*, 1749–1756.

Strine, T. W., Kroenke, K., Dhingra, S., Balluz, L. S., Gonzalez, O. et al (2009). The associations between depression, health-related quality of life, social support, life satisfaction, and disability in community-dwelling US adults. *J Nerv Ment Dis, 197*, 61–64.

Uchino, B. N. (2004). *Social Support and Physical Health: Understanding the Health Consequences of Relationships*. New Haven, CT: Yale University Press.

WHO (1990). *Composite International Diagnostic Interview (CIDI), Version 1.1* Geneva, Switzerland: World Health Organization.

WHO (1997). *Composite International Diagnostic Interview (CIDI), Version 2.1*. Geneva, Switzerland: World Health Organization.

Ware, J. E. Jr., and Sherbourne, C. D. (1992). The MOS 36-item short-form health survey (SF-36). I. Conceptual framework and item selection. *Med Care, 30*, 473–483.

Watson, D., Clark, L. A., and Tellegen, A. (1988). Development and validation of brief measures of positive and negative affect: the PANAS scales. *J Pers Soc Psychol, 54*, 106–1070.

Weiss, D. (2004). The Impact of Event Scale-Revised. Assessing psychological trauma and PTSD. In J. P. Wilson & T. M. Keane (Eds.), *Assessing Psychological Trauma and PTSD, 2nd Ed.* (pp. 168–190). London: The Guilford Press.

Whipple, M. O., Lewis, T. T., Sutton-Tyrrell, K., Matthews, K. A., Barinas-Mitchell, E. et al (2009). Hopelessness, depressive symptoms, and carotid atherosclerosis in women: the Study of Women's Health Across the Nation (SWAN) heart study. *Stroke, 40*, 3166–3172.

Williams, D. R., Yu, Y., Jackson, J. S., and Anderson, N. B. (1997). Racial differences and mental health: socio-economic status, stress and discrimination. *J Health Psychol, 2*, 335–351.

Williams, J. B., Gibbon, M., First, M. B., Spitzer, R. L., Davies, M. et al (1992). The Structured Clinical Interview for DSM-III-R (SCID). II. Multisite test-retest reliability. *Arch Gen Psychiatry, 49*, 630–636.

Winokur, A., Winokur, D. F., Rickels, K., and Cox, D. S. (1984). Symptoms of emotional distress in a family planning service: stability over a four-week period. *Br J Psychiatry, 144*, 395–399.

Zigmond, A. S., and Snaith, R. P. (1983). The hospital anxiety and depression scale. *Acta Psychiatr Scand, 67*, 361–370.

Chapter 22

Socio-economic Position and Health

Tarani Chandola and Michael G. Marmot

1 Introduction

Socio-economic position (SEP) and health are intimately linked and this association results in social inequalities in health. The systematic unequal distribution of power, prestige and resources among groups in society results in health inequalities. Although SEP is just one aspect of the distribution of power relations and resources in society, there is overwhelming evidence that people of lower socio-economic position have poorer health and higher death rates (Marmot, 2004). Such socio-economic inequalities in mortality rates are observed in almost every country and for most major causes of death. Furthermore, these socio-economic inequalities in health are observed at different stages of the life course, for all age groups, although the magnitude of these health inequalities varies between populations and across time.

Despite these universal observations, there are a number of debates on socio-economic status and health. This chapter will reflect on a number of such debates which include discussions on concepts and measures of SEP in relation to health and health inequalities, explanations for the association between SEP and health and potential policy responses. Much of the material and references for this chapter has been taken from the World Health Organization Commission on the Social Determinants of Health (CSDH, 2007, 2008; CSDH Measurement and Evidence Knowledge Network, 2007).

2 Social Stratification and Social Class

Social stratification is the ranking of individuals into social groups. However, measures of social stratification are usually not explicit about how and why unequal power relations are distributed in society. Most social stratification measures do not say anything about how the mechanisms generate social inequality. For example, people may be ranked by their educational qualifications but this ranking does not tell us anything about the social mechanism generating educational inequalities. One could hypothesize that intelligence or family background or the status of educational institutions could be the source of educational inequalities. However, the measure of qualifications in itself does not have any explicit theoretical framework that explains how these educational inequalities are generated. Measures of social class, on the other hand, have explicit theories underlying them, which are explicit about how power and resources get allocated to different social groups.

Social class can be defined by relations of ownership or control over productive resources (i.e. physical, financial, organizational) (Muntaner et al, 2003). Much of the literature

T. Chandola (✉)
Professor in Medical Sociology, CCSR, School of Social Sciences, Kantorovich Building, Humanities Bridgeford Street, University of Manchester, Manchester, M13 9PL, UK
e-mail: tarani.chandola@manchester.ac.uk

A. Steptoe (ed.), *Handbook of Behavioral Medicine*, DOI 10.1007/978-0-387-09488-5_22,
© Springer Science+Business Media, LLC 2010

on theoretical basis of socio-economic position starts with the Marxist position that socio-economic position is entirely determined by "social class". Social class is defined by an individual's relation to the "means of production" (in capitalist societies, factories and raw materials). The two main social classes are the capitalists who own and control the means of production and the labourers who sell their labour power. The capitalists are able to enjoy better health as a result of their control over material resources, while health equity (and other forms of equality) would only be able to arise as a result of changing an individual's relation to the "means of production".

Max Weber added other dimensions and more classes to Marx's view of social class. For Weber, society is stratified on the basis of class, status and party (or power). The Weberian concept of social class is similar to Marx in that it is about ownership and control of material resources. Status is the respect with which a person or status position is regarded by others and is influenced by their "access to life chances" based on social and cultural factors such as family background, lifestyle and social networks. Power is not just about membership of political parties or unions, but also about a person's ability to get their own way. "Thus, class, status and party are each aspects of the distribution of power within a community"(Hurst, 2007). Most modern day conceptualizations of social class reflect the three separate but linked dimensions of class, status and power.

Discussions of power and the underlying distribution of power in different dimensions of SEP are often neglected and not explicitly theorized in most of the literature linking SEP with health. Power, like SEP, is not an individual property, but a characteristic of groups. If power relations are not explicitly theorized in measures of SEP, then there is the danger of recommending improvement in SEP for individuals (through higher educational attainment, for example) as key for reducing social inequalities in health. However, taking power explicitly into consideration suggests that empowering disadvantaged individuals will not reduce inequalities in health.

The key to reducing inequalities in health lies in the empowerment of disadvantaged social groups (CSDH, 2007).

2.1 Measures of Socio-economic Position

The most commonly used indicators for socio-economic position in high-income countries are occupational class and status, level of education and income level (CSDH Measurement and Evidence Knowledge Network, 2007). Each indicator covers a different aspect of social stratification and some argue that it is therefore preferable to use all three instead of only one (Kunst and Mackenbach, 1995). Another conceptualization of SEP is in terms of an aggregate concept (Krieger et al, 1997) that includes both resource-based (material and social resources and assets) and prestige-based measures (individuals' rank or status in a social hierarchy). For example, occupational class position could reflect the status of being members of a particular profession, as well as access to financial and material resources. Disentangling the two concepts from a single measure may be problematic and so it may be preferable to use separate measures of SEP that differentiate between resource-based and prestige-based measures.

2.2 Education

Many epidemiological studies only measure education as a measure of SEP either in terms of years spent in education or in terms of highest qualifications obtained. There are a number of advantages to use education. The population coverage of education is more complete than other measures of SEP. It is usually simpler to collect data on education than occupation or income. Educational attainment is usually acquired by early adulthood and so reflects their SEP upon entry into adulthood. A person's highest achieved level of education is a good indicator of his or her acquired skills and intellectual and cultural resources; this in turn is likely to lead to better conditions in which people live and work and healthier lifestyles. Education thus combines dimensions of social status (through the prestige of having higher qualifications or attending prestigious educational institutions) as well as increases access to resources through enhancing ability to process information.

There are, however, several limitations to using education as a measure of SEP. Some argue that while education is a determinant of social class, by itself it is not a measure of social class but merely a proxy. This brings us back to the idea that education, like income, is a measure of social stratification, but it does not necessarily tell us about the mechanism that generates the stratification in the first place. One characteristic that measures of SEP share is social mobility – people can be upwardly or downwardly mobile over the life course. However, education is largely invariant over the adult life course and also it is hard to conceptualize of downward social mobility using education as a measure of SEP (at least intra-generationally). Furthermore, there are strong cohort and period effects in education, as older populations tended to live in times when fewer people had higher qualifications. Hence the meaning of not having any qualifications or having university qualifications may have changed over time.

2.3 Income, Wealth and Consumption

Income is a good indicator of a person's position in the labour market as well as their material standard of living. Higher levels of income enable greater access to and greater consumption of health-promoting resources and services. While income may be measured at the individual level, a more sensitive measure of the latter can be obtained by calculating the equivalent household disposable income which adjusts for the size of household after adding up the disposable incomes (total income after tax and social security deductions) of all household members. This requires data from multiple sources of income (formal employment, informal employment, savings, remittances, benefits, etc.). Such accurate measurements of income require detailed information from all income streams of all individuals in the same household which is not always possible in surveys. Furthermore, current income levels are not always an accurate measure of long-term standard of living as there may be considerable variation in income levels from 1 month to the next.

Data on income are often sensitive. People are not willing to disclose how much they earn. So there is usually a large proportion of non-response or missing data from surveys on income. Many studies use proxy measures of material living standards such as entitlements to social security benefits, possession of consumer goods and assets, wealth, car ownership and house ownership (or "consumption" measures) which are less prone to non-response bias. Wealth represents the total value of a person or household's assets. These can be a wide variety of assets and requires valuation of non-monetary assets such as land, housing, which are difficult to estimate and measure. Furthermore, there are marked variations in wealth between households with the same income. Racial differences in wealth in the USA are far wider than racial differences in income (Lynch and Kaplan, 2000). Some argue that consumption expenditure is a more accurate representation of long-term economic status than income (Friedman, 1957). This is because income is subjective to greater fluctuations, whereas individuals and households may base their consumption decisions on their planned and anticipated ("permanent") income rather than their current income levels.

2.4 Occupational Class

In the developed world, some authors argue that occupational class is the key measure of SEP

(Rose and Pevalin, 2002). Employment is central to understanding social structures and occupational conditions highlight divisions in society that are not captured by other nonoccupational indices of social inequality such as household income, housing tenure or education. A review of measurements of social circumstances concluded that a classification based on occupation was essential to understanding social inequality (Rose and Pevalin, 2002). There are compelling theoretical reasons, supported by a mass of empirical research, for believing that an individual's position within employment relations (that is, labour markets and production units as determined by skill, career prospects, authority and other aspects of both work and market situations and as proxied by an occupationally based social classification) is a key determinant of life chances, access to other types of social good and subjective quality of life.

Occupationally based classifications have been shown to be associated with a wide variety of social outcomes in diverse areas such as health, education, political behaviour, fertility and social mobility. No other measure of inequality has been developed which matches its scope. Some argue that occupation is the key variable in the accumulation of advantages and disadvantages over a person's life course. Occupation can be regarded as the means by which a persons' principal resource (education) is converted into an important reward (income). As occupation links these two sets of advantages, it is a greater measure of accumulated advantages than either one alone.

However, epidemiological studies have tended to shy away from using theoretically based occupational classifications for a number of reasons. One of them being the lack of comprehensive population coverage – vulnerable groups such as children, women and the elderly often have to be classified by proxy measures of social class in which case these social class measures no longer reflect differences between occupations in employment relations, but rather they reflect differences between households in membership of particular occupations.

Another problem associated with using occupational class relates to the changing meaning and life experiences of social classes over time. People in professional and manual occupations today are in very different social and occupational circumstances compared to 50 years ago. A related problem is the changing class sizes with a huge increase of people in professional and other non-manual occupations and a decline in numbers (especially among men) in unskilled manual occupations. It is possible that with greater numbers at the top, there has been a dilution of the elite social status. Similarly, with the more mobile members of the unskilled manual class moving up to more skilled occupations, it is possible that there has been a concentration of more disadvantaged people at the bottom than ever before. Furthermore, if equality is measured on the basis of differences between social groups, is greater equality achieved if the size of the privileged classes increases while the numbers in the poorer groups decline even though the death rates in the classes remain the same? Such questions necessitate analyses of the changes in the distribution of social classes over time in relative and absolute terms.

Occupational class schemes have tended to neglect women's occupations and have either lumped diverse women's occupations into one big non-manual unskilled group or classified them on the basis of their head of household's occupation. Both methods are unsatisfactory in terms of the dismissal of the specific nature of women's employment and associated factors that may generate inequalities in women's health. The changing, increasingly flexible labour market means that an increasing number of people (especially women) are employed part time or temporarily. While these people can be classified by both their own occupation and their head of household's occupation, either method by itself does not produce a satisfactory summary of their occupational and socio-economic position. People who have never been employed and living alone such as unemployed lone parents and those living on disability benefit cannot be classified by occupational class schemes. Yet these are often people who are most vulnerable to adverse health outcomes and should be included in any analysis of health inequalities.

2.5 Adjusting for Socio-economic Position

Taking account of confounding is one of the major concerns of epidemiology, in order to improve causal inference. SEP is linked to most health outcomes. So most epidemiological studies routinely "control" for SEP in analyses linking a particular exposure to health outcomes. However, on deeper investigation, the measure of SEP controlled for often turns out to be poorly measured, representing a single dimension of social stratification, and may be of little relevance to measuring social inequality in the population at that stage of the life course. For example, education is a measure that is commonly used to control for SEP. Many studies conceptualize this as a binary variable having no school qualifications vs having some school qualifications. This, however, is a crude binary classification and ignores more detailed social stratification processes and other aspects of SEP. Measures of qualifications attained upon leaving full-time education may not be strongly correlated with early life or later life SEP. And yet, many epidemiological studies confidently state that they adjust for SEP using a crude measure of qualification (or any other single measure of SEP). Given the number of different ways in which different measures of SEP can affect health, it is unlikely that adjusting for a crude measure of SEP can truly control for the effects of SEP in analyses.

A related problem that is also common in the epidemiological literature is that measures of SEP will be used at different levels without an understanding of how their meaning changes when measured at an individual, household or area level. Education and occupational class are typically measured at an individual level – they are measures of SEP that are characteristic of individuals describing a particular set of qualifications or a particular kind of occupation.

Income and wealth are typically measured at the household level, although they can also be described for individuals. Measures of area-level SEP, such as area deprivation indices, may be aggregates of individuals and households living in an area or they may be truly ecological characteristics such as pollution or graffiti which cannot be reduced down to the individual level. Most individual measures of SEP can be aggregated up to household or area levels, although the meaning of these SEP measures changes. So, for example, a person's occupational class may not correspond with their head of household's occupational class. Similarly, someone who does not earn an income may live in a very wealthy household. Just as different measures of SEP are not proxies of each other, different levels of SEP may not correlate well.

2.6 Relative or Absolute Differences

Just as there is no single "gold standard" measure of SEP, there is no single measure of the association between SEP and health. Kunst et al (2001) reviewed the different summary indices of the magnitude of health inequalities. They distinguish broadly between absolute measures of inequality which measure differences between social groups in the occurrence of health problems (e.g. Rate Difference and Slope Index of Inequality) and relative measures of inequality which express the absolute differences in terms of a proportion (e.g. Rate Ratio and Relative index of inequality). Absolute difference measures tend to be easier to calculate and interpret, but relative difference measures are often necessary to demonstrate the magnitude of inequalities.

Measures of absolute differences give us an estimate of the burden attributable to lower SEP. This is important for public health decisions and resource allocation – it is important to know whether a reduction in the exposure to low SEP would save 10 lives or 1000 lives. Measures of relative differences are more helpful in understanding the aetiology of disease. Explanations of the mechanisms underlying the association between low SEP and disease are often described in terms of relative differences between SEP groups.

Some argue against using relative difference measures such as rate ratios to measure and monitor inequalities, as relative inequalities tend to increase when overall mortality decreases (Scanlan, 2000). There are mathematical reasons underlying the observation that relative inequalities using the rate ratio tend to be larger at lower mortality levels (Houweling et al, 2007). This problem is avoided when using absolute measures of inequality like rate differences (Clarke et al, 2002). However, others argue the low relative ratios (small relative differences between social groups) at high levels of mortality are not a result of equitable policies, but a function of the necessity that in order to have high overall mortality rates, all social groups contribute to high mortality. Houweling et al (2007) provide examples of countries where declining relative inequalities are coupled with improving health (in terms of mortality rates for children aged under 5) and argue that both absolute and relative measures of inequality are meaningful for measuring socio-economic health inequalities.

It is widely accepted that socio-economic position plays a large role in influencing social processes and outcomes. The measurement of SEP is key to understanding social inequalities in health. A single measure cannot be assumed to capture all relevant aspects of SEP for health. Figure 22.1 shows the association between education and occupational grade with mortality from the Whitehall II study of civil servants. Within high-grade civil servants, there is an educational gradient in mortality. However, among low-grade civil servants, age of leaving full-time education does not affect the risk of mortality. Thus the effect of education on the risk of mortality differs by occupational class and neither measure of SEP can be taken to be proxies of each. All epidemiological studies need to take into account the different dimensions and levels of SEP in their analyses. Failure to do so will result in an underestimation of confounding

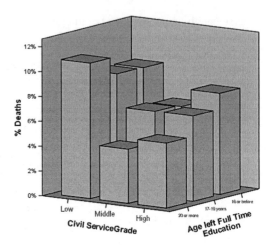

Fig. 22.1 Proportion of deaths by civil service employment grade and education, in the Whitehall II civil service cohort (1985–2007)

biases generated by the effect of different socio-economic factors on health.

3 Explanations for the Association Between Socio-economic Position and Health

It has been conventional to start explanations of the association between SEP and health with the four described in the Black Report (Black, 1980): measurement artefact, natural or social selection, materialist, and cultural behavioural differences. Years on, the debates on explaining health inequality are still shaped by these explanations. The first two types of explanation largely deny causal connections between the factors specifically related to social class (such as poverty, education) and subsequent levels of health. The last type of explanation (behavioural explanations) stresses the importance of individual behaviour (such as smoking, exercise) in producing health outcomes. The authors of the Black Report downplayed the role of these three types of explanations and expressed their preference for materialist explanations which see class differences in health as the result of economic and socio-structural factors. Since the

Black Report was published, there have been a number of developments and elaborations on explanations of health inequalities which include psychosocial, neo-material, life course and ecological explanations.

While the debates surrounding these issues have moved on to consider other possible factors, these explanations still are a useful basis for discussions on the reasons for the association between SEP and health. It is unlikely that a complex phenomenon like social inequality can be reduced to a single explanation and others have argued that there has been a tendency in the literature to use "hard" versions of the debate and exclude "softer" explanations that acknowledge the contribution of many factors that result in health inequalities. Such debates around the relative importance, these explanations also carry important implications for research and policy mechanisms on reducing health inequalities. The specification of the underlying mechanisms of inequality in health and their relative importance is a necessary step in the reduction of such inequality.

3.1 Health-Selection Explanations

In its simplest and strongest form, the health-selection explanation for the mortality differentials across social classes emphasizes the poor health (and disability) of individuals in early life as the primary causal factor which results in their increased risk of mortality as well as their non-participation in the workforce or their participation in low skill, low paying jobs. So low SEP does not cause ill health, rather ill health in earlier life causes low SEP. In many low income countries, the cost of health care for low SEP groups is very expensive relative to their incomes. Hence having poor health requiring expensive treatment is often a major cause of poverty in those countries.

However, others argue that such health or social selection explanations are "Social Darwinist" because the social class structure is seen as resulting from the redistribution of

individuals on the basis of their "health, i.e. physical strength, vigour, or agility" (Black Report (Black, 1980):156). In this struggle of the fittest, the healthiest individuals go to the top of the social class ladder and the least fit people drift down to the bottom rung of the SEP. Empirical studies have tended to show that health is not a major determinant of such social mobility and changes in socio-economic position (Blane, 1985). A number of studies have now shown that greater social mobility corresponds to reductions in health inequalities, rather than a widening of health inequalities as might be hypothesized from a social Darwinist perspective (Bartley and Plewis, 2007).

3.2 Cultural/Behavioural Explanations

Cultural/behavioural explanations view social gradients in health as the result of social class differences in individual behaviours such as the excessive consumption of harmful commodities (alcohol, tobacco, refined foods), lack of exercise and the under-utilization of preventive health care (vaccination, contraception). There is strong epidemiological evidence that links some of these behaviours to major causes of death such as coronary heart disease, lung cancer and chronic bronchitis as well as a social gradient in such behaviours (Wardle and Griffith, 2001). One of the implications of emphasizing cultural/behavioural explanations of social inequalities in health is that health behaviours are largely under individual control. Some have argued (Fuchs, 1986) that the systematic variations in health behaviours across social classes is a consequence of a lack of education or individual thoughtlessness. Explanation for health inequalities in welfare societies with compulsory education then takes an individual form. The policy implications for reducing inequalities in health would stress the need for comprehensive health education and the publicizing of health risks of certain behaviours (like warning smokers of the hazards of tobacco on cigarette packets).

A variant of the cultural/behaviours explanations is the hypothesis that intelligence is the root cause of social inequalities in health. This argument suggests that intelligence stratifies people into SEP groups as well as confers health benefits. Children with lower ability are not able to attain high SEP in adulthood and their lower ability also translates into greater health risk due to a lack of health literacy such as an inability to comprehend health education messages. Intelligence thus confounds the association between SEP and health. However, others contend that intelligence in itself is not the causal agent, but a product of poor SEP in childhood. Feinstein shows that family SEP is a strong determinant of changes in childhood ability. Children with high ability scores at 22 months who have a disadvantaged family background have lower than average ability by age 10. On the other hand, less able children at age 22 months from advantaged family backgrounds are able to attain higher than average ability by age 10.

The Black Report criticized the individual nature of cultural/behavioural explanations. Instead, the authors of the Report saw healthy and unhealthy behaviours as conditioned by the social and material context in which individuals live. In other words, health behaviours are intervening variables between the social/material structure and health outcomes. They point out that reducing social inequalities in health is not just a matter of changing individual lifestyles as these healthy lifestyles are influenced by social and material conditions. For example, healthy lifestyles are determined by personal tastes, behaviours, and preferences as well as access to good food and sports facilities.

3.3 Materialist Explanations

Materialist explanations of the social inequalities in health are concerned with the effects of the social structure on health. Social class differences in health are the result of "structurally determined differences in the spheres of production and consumption" (Blane, 1985). The Black Report favoured these kind of explanations and recommended policies to decrease the health gap between social classes which focused on material and social-structural factors.

Morris and colleagues estimated the "minimum cost of healthy living" for single young British men in 1999 to be £131.86 per week (Morris et al, 2000). This figure included the costs of healthy nutrition, recreational activities, housing, personal care, transport and psychosocial relationships like social networks and caring. This cost was greater than the minimum wage (in April 1999) for a standard week and far exceeded basic social security allowances. They repeated these calculations for older populations and found that the minimum income requirement for healthy living in England is 50% greater than the state pension (Morris et al, 2007). Clearly, material and financial constraints restrict the ability to live healthily.

Studies of occupational health show that many occupations have direct deleterious effects on health and these are clustered in lower SEP. Many workplace hazards include physical, chemical, ergonomic and psychosocial stressors and their effects on health have been detailed (CSDH Employment Conditions Knowledge Network, 2007). In many developing countries, much of the labour force are in the informal economy and outside the scope of whatever little protective legislation on health and safety in the workplace. This is particularly true of self-employed workers, the majority of whom are women.

3.4 Psychosocial Factors

Marmot (2004) has emphasized the role of psychosocial factors, and in particular the social conditions that generate feelings of powerlessness and lack of control, in influencing ill health. These psychosocial stressors largely accumulate in disadvantaged groups over a lifetime and are hypothesized to cause physiological and psychological damage.

One psychosocial approach highlights the role of social capital in generating health. Authors such as Robert Putnam, Richard Wilkinson and James Coleman emphasize the role of social networks and social trust and social relationships that influences health through supportive relationships or negative stressful relationships. Greater socio-economic inequality (and income inequality in particular) results in less social trust, less social reciprocity and lower levels of civic participation and this leads to a loss of social capital and social cohesion. Social capital can affect health through (a) negative psychological responses to perceptions of inequality and unfairness, such as stress and anxiety, (b) the formation of shared norms that promote healthy or unhealthy behaviours or supportive relationships (c), the formation of political mobilization, activist groups for resources that have a health impact.

Wilkinson (1996) proposed that health inequalities are associated more strongly with relative rather than absolute material standards. He hypothesizes the existence of psychosocial pathways such as stress as the mechanism that links people's feelings of being relatively deprived to higher mortality rates. The existence of social networks and support that can buffer the effects of stress is also hypothesized to play a role in linking feelings of relative deprivation to adverse health outcomes. Income inequality is used as an indicator of the degree to which society is unequal (Wilkinson and Pickett, 2006). More unequal societies generate greater psychosocial stressors, which result in poorer overall health and lower life expectancy. Others, however, disagree with this view (Lynch et al, 2004).

Another type of psychosocial explanation involves stressors from living and working conditions which are assumed to have direct biological effects on stress reactions. Repeated activation of the stress biology systems are assumed to have a deleterious effect on health, especially mental health and cardiovascular functioning

(Brunner, 2000). A number of observational studies have shown that stressors generated from poor working conditions affect coronary heart disease independently of cardiovascular risk factors (Eller et al, 2009). Moreover, these stressors are socially graded so that over a life course, those who have lower SEP have increased exposure to these stressors (Chandola and Marmot, in press).

3.5 Neo-material Explanations

The neo-material approach adopts a materialistic perspective and suggests that there is a danger in promoting social capital as a substitute for structural change when facing health inequity (Lynch et al, 2000). The neo-material perspective views the relationship between SEP and health as a consequence of how society is structured and organized and the extent to which governments invest in economic resources and human capital (Kavanagh et al, 2006). The Commission on Social Determinants of Health (CSDH, 2007) acknowledges the role of such explanations and identifies the socio-economic political context as crucial in understanding health inequalities. These are the social and political mechanisms that generate, configure and maintain social hierarchies, such as the labour market, the educational system and political institutions including the welfare state.

However, the debate between neo-material and psychosocial explanations for health inequalities is a false dichotomy as these explanations are closely bound up with each other. These explanations are not "either/or". Improvements in stressful social and environmental conditions would almost certainly require improvements in neo-material factors such as better (health) services and environmental conditions. Similarly, providing more equitable distribution of services such as health care may not lead to improved health among poorer groups if health-care providers treat the patients with disdain and disrespect. The Commission on Social Determinants of

Health's (CSDH, 2007) conceptual framework emphasizes the role of structural, material, psychosocial and behavioural factors in health equity and does not prioritize one over the other.

3.6 Life Course Factors

Studies on the effects of the life course on health have shown that health is a result of factors that occur throughout the life course (Kuh and Ben-Shlomo, 1997, see Chapter 34). Such factors may accumulate throughout a person's lifetime, such as the accumulation of poor living conditions in childhood and adulthood, or there may be critical periods in the life course during which some factors are particularly important, for example qualifications obtained when someone leaves compulsory full time education. A life course explanation thus incorporates many of the Black Report explanations. It takes into account health selection, by stressing the importance of (poor) health experiences and illnesses in earlier life (such as in childhood). It also stresses the importance of looking at the pathways linking adult health behaviours to earlier psychosocial and material living conditions.

Biologically it seems plausible that important aspects of early life health and development affect adult health. Hence taking action on adverse social factors that affect children's health and development is important in reducing adult social inequalities in health. Furthermore, a disadvantaged family background in childhood affects educational attainment and later life SEP. So although biological programming may determine a range of adult health parameters, the social and family circumstances of childhood are the beginnings of pathways which will be protective to health or increase vulnerability to ill health (Wadsworth, 1997).

3.7 Ecological Factors

The analyses of the effect of areas on health have had a long and distinguished history in epidemiology. Many ecological studies have shown that deprived areas have higher mortality rates and poorer health. However, the ecological fallacy (inferring individual level relationships from relationships observed at the aggregate level) has limited the interpretation that area deprivation is a cause of poor health over and above individual and family level SEP. However, methodological developments in statistics, computing and survey methods have improved the ability to analyse and infer ecological effects on the health of individuals.

There are three types of explanation for area differences in health: compositional, contextual and collective (MacIntyre et al, 2002). Compositional explanations focus on the characteristics of individuals concentrated in particular places and are typically concerned with individual level risk factors for health such as behaviours. Contextual explanations examine the local physical and social environment such as physical features of the environment (quality of air and water, latitude, climate), availability of healthy environments at home, work and play, and services provided to support people in their daily lives. Collective explanations emphasize the importance of shared norms, traditions, values and interests, such as the political, economic, ethnic and religious history of communities and the reputation of areas, how they are perceived, by residents, planners and investors.

4 Policy Implications

4.1 Health Gaps or Gradients

Although reducing health inequalities is a major public health goal in many countries, there is a dearth of evidence on effective policies to reduce health inequalities. Some policies urge action on health gaps, which focuses on poverty and absolute deprivation. In most countries, there is a social gradient in infant mortality, although in some countries, the association of SEP with infant mortality may not resemble a gradient so much as a gap between the very poorest and the rest of society. Victora et al (2003) for example highlight the "bottom inequity" pattern which is found where most children do have access to interventions, but there is a clear group which lags behind (e.g. Brazil and Nicaragua). Others argue that we need to look at the social gradient across all of society (CSDH, 2007). Targeting extreme groups for specific diseases may have the unintended consequence of disadvantaging other relatively deprived groups for other diseases and health problems. We need to be cautious before advocating a health inequalities policy targeted only at the very poorest even for these bottom inequity pattern countries. Dedicating policy resources to just the health gap may disadvantage other deprived groups in society and miss most of the health problem distributed across the rest of society.

Graham describes three different ways that health inequalities have been conventionally described in the literature (Graham, 2004). The health disadvantage/disparities approach describes differences between social groups, without any explicit reference to social injustice or a moral dimension. The health gaps approach focuses on the very poorest vs the rest of society. This approach may or may not assume that everyone who is not the poorest enjoys good health, but it is mostly concerned with levelling up the good health among the most disadvantaged in society. The social gradient in health approach describes health inequalities across the whole of the population, not just the most deprived. This means a focus not just on the second-most deprived group, but also on groups in the population who may not be considered deprived at all, but who are relatively doing worse off in terms of their health than those at the very top.

The Commission on the Social Determinants of Health (CSDH, 2007) argues "an approach which considers the whole of the gradient in health equity in a society should be the starting point for an analysis of the structure of health inequities in that society". If we only consider and target the most disadvantaged groups, this ignores the rest of society, and is not holistic. It is important to start the policy implications of

health inequalities by looking at all members of society, the social gradient in health,-only then can you see the systemic process of inequality. If we just focus on the very poorest, we may miss the structural drivers of inequality.

Policy goals tend to be targeted at the poorest and most deprived. In order to narrow such health gaps, the health of the poorest has to improve faster than the population average. This is seldom if ever achievable. What is more realistic and common is that the very poorest improve but not as fast the rest of society. Thus, if policies only address those at the bottom of the social hierarchy, inequities in health will still exist (CSDH, 2007), and it will also mean that the association of SEP with other non-targeted measures of health will continue and widen. The founding principle of the World Health Organization was that the enjoyment of the highest attainable standard of health is a fundamental human right and should be within reach of all "without distinction for race, religion, political belief, economic or social condition". This does not single out the very poorest or disadvantaged as being the most deserving- the standards of health enjoyed by the best-off should be attainable by all.

4.2 Social Mobility

An extension of the policy debate about whether to focus on health gaps or health gradients is the suggestion that increasing social mobility will lead to reducing health inequalities. This argument suggests that the focus on health gaps misses the important dimension of reducing inequalities, as social mobility can only be examined in the context of the whole of society, not just in terms of taking action on an extreme deprived group.

Bartley and Plewis (2007) show, using evidence from a number of empirical studies, that social class mobility leads to a reduction in health inequalities. This is because people who are not socially mobile at the highest SEP have the best levels of health, while people who are not mobile at the lowest SEP have the poorest health. If health selection was the main driver of health inequalities, upwards mobile people should display better health than the class they join and downwards movers worse health that the class they are joining, so that the overall social gradient would be wider than that of the socially static. However, it has been repeatedly shown that there is a tendency for those who are socially mobile to have levels of health somewhere between that of their social class at birth and in adulthood. For those who are upwardly mobile, the effect of such mobility is to reduce the average levels of health in the adult destination social class. For those who are downwardly mobile, the effect of social mobility is to improve average levels of health in the adult destination social class. The UK experienced a reduction in social mobility for cohorts born between 1958 and 1970 (Blanden and Machin, 2007). Such declining social mobility is suggested as an explanation for widening trend in health inequalities in the UK.

4.3 The Role of Health Services and Inter-sectoral Government Action

Lower SEP groups in general have poorer access to health services and poorer outcomes from health service utilization. At all stages of health service utilization (preventative care, diagnosis, treatment and follow up), lower SEP groups have poorer experiences. This contributes to their higher burden of disease and mortality rates. Where there is some debate is the role of health services in reducing health inequalities. Some argue that as the origins of social inequalities in health are in social processes, tacking health inequalities only through healthcare delivery would be like putting a band aid over a festering wound. Better health-care delivery for poorer SEP groups would not tackle the underlying causes of health inequalities. In some countries with nominally free access to health care, there are widening inequalities in health. Others argue that health systems have a crucial

role in reducing health inequalities by ensuring that ill health does not adversely impact on a person's SEP, through supporting the rehabilitation of sick workers back into employment, through providing better preventative and primary care services.

The Commission on the Social Determinants of Health (CSDH, 2008) explicitly recommended that action on health inequalities needs the active engagement of not just the health sector, but other governmental agencies that affect people's living, working and growing conditions such as in housing, finance, local government and education. Policies on reducing health inequalities cannot just be confined to the health sector – coordinated inter-sectoral approaches from different government departments are crucial in order to build health equity.

5 Conclusion

This chapter has shown that although SEP and health are linked, measures of SEP are not proxies of each other and have effects on health through different pathways. Studies that claim to control for the effect of SEP on health ignore biases that arise from inappropriate measures of SEP. The association of SEP with health results in social inequalities in health. Explanations for such health inequalities lie in the socioeconomic political context, as well as in the living, working and growing conditions that affect people's behaviour, material and psychosocial resources and neighbourhoods. Moreover such explanations operate over the life course (and inter-generationally) and this results in health-selection processes for some social groups and also increasing vulnerabilities or resilience for other groups. Policies to address such social inequalities in health need to address the whole of the social gradient, not just target the extreme poor and disadvantaged. Actions by the health sector alone will not reduce health inequalities – this needs coordinated action across different government agencies that affect people's living, working and growing conditions.

References

Bartley, M. and Plewis, I. (2007). Increasing social mobility: an effective policy to reduce health inequalities. *J Royal Stat Soc A*, 170, 469–481.

Black, D. (1980). *Inequalities in Health: Report of a Research Working Group*. London: DHSS.

Blanden, J., Machin, S. (2007). *Recent Changes in Intergenerational Mobility in Britain Centre for Economic Performance at LSE*. London: Sutton Trust, December 2007.

Blane, D. (1985). An assessment of the Black Report's "explanation of health inequalities". *Soc Health*, 7, 421–445.

Brunner, E. J. (2000). Toward a new social biology. In L. F. Berkman & I. Kawachi (Eds.), *Social Epidemiology* (pp. 306–331). New York: Oxford University Press.

Chandola, T. and Marmot, M. G. (in press). Socioeconomic Status and Stress. In A. Baum & R. Contrada (Eds.), *Handbook of Stress Science* Springer.

Clarke, P. M., Gerdtham, U. G., Johannesson, M., Bingefors, K., and Smith, L. (2002). On the measurement of relative and absolute income-related health inequality. *Soc Sci Med*, 55, 1923–1928.

CSDH (2007). *A Conceptual Framework for Action on the Social Determinants of Health*. Geneva: Commission on the Social Determinants of Health: WHO. http://www.who.int/entity/social_determinants/resources/csdh_framework_action_05_07.pdf

CSDH (2008). *Closing the Gap in a Generation: Health Equity Through Action on the Social Determinants of Health*. Final Report of the Commission on Social Determinants of Health. Commission on Social Determinants of Health: WHO. http://whqlibdoc.who.int/hq/2008/WHO_IER_CSDH_08.1_eng.pdf

CSDH Employment Conditions Knowledge Network (2007). *Final Report of the Economic Conditions Knowledge Network - Employment Conditions and Health Inequalities*. Commission on Social Determinants of Health: WHO. http://www.who.int/entity/social_determinants/resources/articles/emconet_who_report.pdf

CSDH Measurement and Evidence Knowledge Network (2007). *Final Report of the Measurement and Evidence Knowledge Network - The Social Determinants of Health: Developing an Evidence Base for Political Action*. Commission on the Social Determinants of Health: WHO. http://www.who.int/entity/social_determinants/resources/mekn_final_report_102007.pdf

Eller, N. H., Netterstrom, B., Gyntelberg, F., Kristensen, T. S., Nielsen, F., Steptoe, A. et al (2009). Work-related psychosocial factors and the development of ischemic heart disease: a systematic review. *Cardiol Rev*, 17, 83–97.

Friedman, M. (1957). *A Theory of the Consumption Function*. Princeton, NJ: Princeton University Press.

Fuchs, V. R. (1986). Time preference and health: and exploratory study. In V. R. Fuchs (Ed.), *Economic Aspects of Health*. Chicago: The University of Chicago Press.

Graham, H. (2004). Social determinants and their unequal distribution: clarifying policy understandings. *Milbank Q*, 82, 101–124.

Houweling, T. A., Kunst, A. E., Huisman, M., and Mackenbach, J. P. (2007). Using relative and absolute measures for monitoring health inequalities: experiences from cross-national analyses on maternal and child health. *Int J Equity Health*, 6, 15.

Hurst, C. E. (2007). *Social Inequality Forms, Causes, and Consequences, 6th Ed*. Boston, MA: Allyn and Bacon.

Kavanagh, A. M., Turrell, G., and Subramanian, S. V. (2006). Does area-based social capital matter for the health of Australians? A multilevel analysis of self-rated health in Tasmania. *Int J Epidemiol*, 35, 607–613.

Krieger, N., Williams, D. R., and Moss, N. E. (1997). Measuring social class in US public health research: concepts, methodologies and guidelines. *Ann Rev Public Health*, 18, 341–378.

Kuh, D. and Ben-Shlomo, Y. (1997). *A Life Course Approach to Chronic Disease Epidemiology*. Oxford: Oxford University Press.

Kunst, A. E., Bos, V., Mackenbach J.P., and EU Working Group on Socio-economic Inequalities in Health (2001). *Monitoring Socio-economic Inequalities in Health in the European Union: Guidelines and Illustrations. A Report for the Health Monitoring Program of the European Commission*. Rotterdam: Erasmus University. http://ec.europa.eu/health/ph_projects/1998/monitoring/fp_monitoring_1998_frep_06_a_en.pdf

Kunst, A. E. and Mackenbach, J. P. (1995). *Measuring Socio-economic Inequalities in Health*. Copenhagen: Regional Office for Europe. http://www.euro.who.int/document/PAE/Measrpd416.pdf

Lynch, J., Davey Smith, G., Harper, S., Hillemeier, M., Ross, N., Kaplan, G. A. et al (2004). Is income inequality a determinant of population health? Part 1. A systematic review. *Millbank Q*, 82, 5–99.

Lynch, J. and Kaplan, G. (2000). Socioeconomic position. In L. F. Berkman & I. Kawachi (Eds.), *Social Epidemiology* (pp. 13–35). New York: OUP.

Lynch, J. W., Davey-Smith, G., Kaplan, G. A., and House, J. S. (2000). Income inequality and mortality: importance to health of individual income, psychosocial environment, or material conditions. *Br Med J*, 320, 1200–1204.

MacIntyre, S., Ellaway, A., and Cummins, S. (2002). Place effects on health: how can we conceptualise, operationalise and measure them? *Soc Sci Med, 55*, 125–139.

Marmot, M. (2004). *The Status Syndrome*. New York: Henry Holt.

Morris, J. N., Donkin, A. J. M., Wonderling, D., Wilkinson, P., and Dowler, E. A. (2000). A minimum income for healthy living. *J Epidemiol Commun Health, 54*, 885–889.

Morris, J. N., Wilkinson, P., Dangour, A. D., Deeming, C., and Fletcher, A. (2007). Defining a minimum income for healthy living (MIHL): older age, England. *Int. J Epidemiol., 36*, 1300–1307.

Muntaner, C., Borrell, C., Benach, J., Pasarin, M. I., and Fernandez, E. (2003). The associations of social class and social stratification with patterns of general and mental health in a Spanish population. *Int J Epidemiol, 32*, 950–958.

Rose, D. and Pevalin, D. (2002). The National Statistics Socio-economic Classification: unifying official and sociological approaches to the conceptualisation and measurement of social class. *Sociétés Contemporaines, 45/46*, 75–106.

Scanlan, J. P. (2000). Race and mortality. *Society, 37*, 19–35.

Victora, C. G., Wagstaff, A., Schellenberg, J. A., Gwatkin, D., Claeson, M., and Habicht, J. P. (2003). Applying an equity lens to child health and mortality: more of the same is not enough. *Lancet, 362*, 233–241.

Wadsworth, M. E. (1997). Health inequalities in the life course perspective. *Soc Sci Med, 44*, 859–869.

Wardle, J. and Griffith, J. (2001). Socioeconomic status and weight control practices in British adults. *J Epidemiol Commun Health, 55*, 185–190.

Wilkinson, R. G. and Pickett, K. E. (2006). Income inequality and population health: a review and explanation of the evidence. *Soc Sci Med, 62*, 1768–1784.

Wilkinson, R. G. (1996). *Unhealthy Societies: The Afflictions of Inequality*. London: Routledge.

Chapter 23

Race, Ethnicity, and Health in a Global Context

Shawn D. Boykin and David R. Williams

1 Introduction

Race/ethnic disparities in health have been documented extensively in countries with diverse population groups. These disparities are profound and exhibit similar and consistent patterns across time and geography. Quite simply, the trend across many multi-racial and multi-ethnic societies is that socially advantaged white population groups generally report being in better health and display better health outcomes than socially disadvantaged non-whites.

It is of no surprise then that an important question in the social sciences, clinical practice, and public health globally is "how do 'race' and 'ethnicity' get under the skin differentially for health?" Historically, genetics was the dominant explanatory framework for race/ethnic differences in health (Krieger, 1987). Consistent evidence shows that low-frequency genetic mutations are typically more common in some race/ethnic populations and could underlie some differences in disease susceptibility and health outcomes (e.g., sickle-cell disease among some populations of African and Mediterranean descent). Strong evidence also exists, however, that socioeconomic factors serve as fundamental causes of race/ethnic disparities because they

shape the social and physical environments that individuals negotiate and also determine access to resources – all of which either promote health or pose risks to it (Nazroo and Williams, 2006; Williams and Collins, 1995). The recent melding of these approaches has led researchers to focus on the interactions of genes and environments to explain race/ethnic disparities in more socially and genetically complex disease states such as atherosclerosis, diabetes, and asthma. Despite the conceptual and methodological differences in these approaches, the unifying theoretical premise across them is that negative exposures to causal factors result in biologic taxation of the body with adverse health consequences. Moreover, repeated negative exposures of the same type or the accumulation of multiple types of negative exposures potentially accelerate declines in health status.

Exposures vary among individuals in type and frequency, although some trends are evident for particular race/ethnic groups. For example, certain genetic mutations are known to occur at higher frequency in some race/ethnic groups. They are relatively rare, however, providing minimal contribution to explanations of race/ethnic differences in morbidity and mortality (Cooper et al, 2003). In contrast, evidence shows that most non-white groups are more likely to be exposed to adverse conditions associated with socioeconomic factors that predispose individuals to poorer health outcomes (Bhopal, 2007; Boykin et al, 2010; Kozol, 1991; Massey, 2004; Nazroo, 1999; Smedley et al, 2003; Williams, 1997). Relative to white populations, such conditions for non-whites may include (1) lower

S.D. Boykin (✉)
Department of Epidemiology, Center for Integrative
Approaches to Health Disparities, University of
Michigan School of Public Health, 109 South
Observatory St, Ann Arbor, MI 48109, USA
e-mail: sdhb@umich.edu

A. Steptoe (ed.), *Handbook of Behavioral Medicine*, DOI 10.1007/978-0-387-09488-5_23,
© Springer Science+Business Media, LLC 2010

probability of employment in higher status occupations; (2) lower rates of high school completion and college degree attainment; and (3) higher rates of poverty, fewer assets owned, and lower per capita income. For some groups these conditions are compounded by the added effects of racism and discrimination. These effects can result in (1) blocked opportunities for education, income, and wealth attainment; (2) greater exposures to environmental hazards, stress, and fewer health-promoting resources; (3) limited access to medical care, inferior quality of care, and lower rates of treatment; and (4) the rapid depletion of health-promoting resources among non-white immigrants.

These effects are further exacerbated by the fact that compared to whites, non-whites report experiencing greater cumulative exposures to stress and other adverse conditions, including discrimination throughout the life course (Hatch and Dohrenwend, 2007; Williams and Mohammed, 2009; Williams et al, 2008). Across countries such as the USA, the UK, Australia, Brazil, and South Africa, these exposures often manifest in higher infant and adult mortality, greater risks for chronic and acute diseases, lower self-assessments of health, and higher levels of functional limitation for non-whites compared to white populations (Australian Bureau of Statistics, 2008; Bradshaw et al, 2004; World Health Organization, 2003; Matijasevich et al, 2008; Mensah et al, 2005; National Center for Health Statistics, 2009; Parliamentary Office of Science and Technology, 2007).

In this chapter we consider the definitions and uses of the concepts of race and ethnicity for classifying groups of people in several countries with diverse populations. We also provide examples of the ways in which health status varies by race/ethnicity. These examples are hardly meant to be exhaustive. Rather, our use of them is intended for illustrative purposes. Additionally, we discuss some of the potential mechanisms through which race and ethnicity may differentially affect health. Finally, we offer directions for future research.

2 Definitions and Uses of "Race" and "Ethnicity"

Racial assignment has served the purpose of categorizing individuals based upon various shared heritable characteristics presumed to reflect common ancestry. In common discourse the term "race" connotes groups of people with shared biological traits that are often reflected by phenotype as a marker of some underlying shared genetic attribute. A biologic conception of race, however, is a misnomer in both its historical and its modern applications. Strong evidence exists that differences in phenotype do not always directly reflect underlying genetic differences. Moreover, "genes underlying phenotypic differences used to assign race categories are atypical, and vary between races much more than genes in general…[and] do not reflect genome-wide differences between groups" (Feldman et al, 2003). Additionally, scientific comparisons of genetic diversity show that humans have much less genetic variability than other mammalian species (Kaessmann et al, 2001).

Furthermore, the use of race categories predates hypotheses regarding genetic differences between population groups (Smedley, 1999). Taken together, these factors negate any scientific motivation for categorizing persons by race based on biological criteria. Instead, they point to a social motivation. Over time, race has served largely as a relational category, denoting institutionalized socio-political relations between groups used to reify the superiority and inferiority of these groups relative to one another (American Sociological Association [ASA], 2003; Geronimus, 2000; Krieger, 2000; Williams, 1997).

Given this motivation for racial classification across diverse societies, intuitively it makes sense that non-biologic attributes have held central importance along with phenotypic characteristics for the purpose of categorizing population groups. For example, population classification in Brazil has been historically determined by skin color in combination with social position (Travassos and Williams, 2004). In South Africa, race categorization currently reflects descent and social standing (Bradshaw et al, 2004). In the USA, racial assignment in the early 19th century was determined not only by physical appearance, but also by blood fraction (percentage of non-white blood) and social affiliation (Sweet, 2005). Race in the USA now reflects personal identification with such historically created categories.

The term "ethnicity" is often interchanged with "race" in modern usage because it also presumes common ancestry. Ethnicity is a much broader concept than race; however, it includes recognition of common and defining characteristics of groups such as culture, language, religion, physical traits, and other factors. Thus, ethnic variation exists within all race groups. Given the lack of evidence supporting a biologic foundation for race, race categories essentially exist as socio-ethnic categories because the defining characteristics of ethnicity along with social position are what hold such categories together.

The term "ethnicity" is more commonly used in the UK and Canada than in the USA. In the UK, the terms "ethnic group" and "ethnic minority" largely refer to population groups that emigrated in the latter half of the 20th century from former British colonies and are used to differentiate these immigrants based upon ancestral origin from white British and Irish groups. Similarly in Canada, "ethnicity" is used to designate groups with common ancestral origins as opposed to citizenship, nationality, or language spoken (Statistics Canada, 2004). In Australia, the term "ancestry" is employed in similar fashion to designate ethnic or cultural origin (Australian Bureau of Statistics, 2006b).

Thus, the concepts and uses of the terms "race" and "ethnicity" garner significance in relational situations such as among population groups in multi-racial and multi-ethnic societies. Although one's individual race/ethnic identity is established based, in part, upon self-determined beliefs, practices, and behaviors, for some persons its creation may also invoke the internalization of stereotypical characteristics associated with externally assigned racial categories. Generally speaking, groups with political and economic power historically assigned race and

ethnicity. The tendency was to ascribe more positive aesthetic, social, behavioral, and intellectual attributes to their own groups and less desirable and more inferior ones to others. Although mostly unfounded, these attributes came to be accepted by many as inherent to the various race/ethnic groups to which they were historically ascribed as a result of longstanding societal institutions and policies and a way of life that justified the subjugation of groups deemed "inferior." Oppression, exploitation, discrimination, racism, inequality, and blocked access to societal rewards and resources were, and continue to serve as some of the predominant forms of race/ethnic subjugation in many diverse societies (Williams, 1997). These practices are most notably recorded in modern history as being used to justify the colonization, killing, enslavement, and creation of castes of native people in countries of the Americas, Africa, Asia, and Australia; validate the practices of African slave trading, slavery, and inhumane treatment of slaves in North and South America and the Caribbean; and substantiate systems of apartheid and racial segregation in South Africa and the USA.

Although race/ethnic classification predates population census taking in most countries, examples from censuses across localities uniformly provide evidence of the fluidity of the conceptions and uses of race and ethnicity, as well as how they have been socio-politically determined over time. The USA provides a good example of this given that race categories have never remained the same in any census. Four distinct political periods mark census data collection efforts in the USA from the first census in 1790 to the most recent census in 2000.

The first period extended from 1790 to 1840 and was shaped by slavery, representational apportionment in government, and racial ideology (Nobles, 2000). Enumerators assigned race according to official definitions in the census and by means of observation. They often relied upon characteristics such as skin color, hair texture, and facial contour to differentiate blacks from other groups (Linné, 1806; United States Census, 1854). Differentiation of blacks during this time was significant. The large number of southern black slaves served as a point of contention for congressional representation between northern and southern states and the first article of the US constitution stipulated that black slaves were to be counted as only three-fifths of a person.

The second period was marked by the advancement of racialized scientific theory emphasizing polygenism from 1850 to 1920. Political wielding led to the addition of "mulatto," "quadroon," and "octoroon" categories in the census for persons of mixed lineage to distinguish how much black blood one had (1/2, 1/4, 1/8, respectively) (Nobles, 2000). The prevailing thought of the time was that the census provided evidence of the existence of discreet races of people with varying moral and intellectual capacities that would be evident in graded fashion where higher levels would be associated with less black blood (Nobles, 2000). Race categories were also expanded during this period to include Chinese, Japanese, and (tax paying) Indians. Additionally, birthplace began to be documented to distinguish between foreign and native-born populations as the influx of immigrants began to increase.

Throughout the third period from 1930 to 1960, definitions for race categories in the US Census were changed to be consistent with statues in southern states, including "jim crow" laws. These laws mandated separation of the races and defined blacks as any person having a trace of black blood. Other mixed race persons were accorded the race of their non-white parent. No legal definition existed for "white," however, in the statues or in the census.

The fourth period, 1970 to the present, included changes to the number of race categories, the race categories included, and the assignment of race in the census. These changes occurred after landmark civil rights legislation when the U.S. Office of Management and Budget (OMB) implemented Statistical Directive number 15 (Office of Management and Budget [OMB], 1978). The OMB oversees all governmental statistical reporting and Directive 15 established the minimum race

categories to be collected by US government agencies including the census (OMB, 1978). It also added a Hispanic ethnic category which could be associated with any race. A revision in the 1990s allowed for the endorsement of as many racial categories as apply to an individual. The current racial categories that OMB requires the US Census to assess are white, African American/black, American Indian or Alaska Native, Asian (referring to descendents from the Far East, Southeast Asia, or the Indian subcontinent), Native Hawaiian or other Pacific Islander, and one ethnic category: Hispanic/Latino or not. Data from the most recent US Census (2000) indicated that 75.1% of the population racially identified as white alone, 12.3% as black or African American alone, 0.9% as American Indian or Alaskan Native alone, 3.6% as Asian alone, 0.1% as Native Hawaiian or other Pacific Islander alone, 5.5% some other race, and 2.4% as two or more races. Additionally, 12.5% of the total US population identified their ethnicity as Hispanic or Latino.

In South Africa, the first comprehensive census after the abolishment of apartheid was taken in 1996. Similarly to the USA, population groups are classified according to race. Race is self-reported in the South African census according to the following categories: black/African, colored, white, Asian/Indian, and other. These categories evolved from the 1950 Population Registration Act which mandated racial classification for the apartheid system. They reflect both descent and social standing (Bradshaw et al, 2004). According to the 2001 South African Census, 79% identified as black African, 8.9% as colored, 2.5% as Indian or Asian, and 9.6% as white (Statistics South Africa, 2001).

In contrast to the USA and South Africa, in the UK Census, a question pertaining to racial/ethnic identification was asked for the first time in 1991. This ethnicity question serves the purpose of identifying white population groups as well as non-whites including blacks, South Asians (descendents from the Indian subcontinent), and Chinese (Bhopal, 2007). Nativity data were collected in the UK Census to designate population groups – primarily British and Irish, for 150 years prior to the addition of the ethnicity question, but allowed for looking at many non-white first generation immigrants. Nativity data continue to be collected. Data from the 2001 UK Census indicated that 92.1% of the population identified as white, 1.2% as mixed ethnicity, 4.0% as all Asian or Asian British, 2.0% as all black or black British, 0.4% as Chinese, and 0.4% as other ethnic groups (National Statistics Online UK, 2001).

In Brazil, racial assignment in the census has always been based primarily upon skin color. Skin color is connected to race and ancestry to the extent that skin color reflects the admixture of the three original population groups in the country prior to the implementation of the census – Europeans, Indians, and Africans (Nobles, 2000). Current census categories include branca (white), parda (brown/mixed), preta (black), amarela (yellow), and indigenous groups (Instituto Brasilleiro de Geografia e Estatitsica, 2006a). These color categories came into existence as the result of acknowledgment by Brazilian political and intellectual elites of the widespread mixing of population groups and the need for fluid categories in the census to capture it (Nobles, 2000). According to the 2006 Brazilian Census 49.9% identified as branca (white), 6.3% as preta (black), 43.2% as parda (mixed), and 0.7% as amarela (yellow), or indigenous (Instituto Brasilleiro de Geografia e Estatitsica, 2006b).

Similarly in Canada, racial classification prior to the 1986 census was also based upon skin color and included white, black, red, and yellow categories (Statistics Canada, 2001). The Canadian Census now includes questions about ethnicity as it relates to a person's ancestry. In the 2006 Canadian Census more than 200 ethnic groups were reported. The largest "visible" minority groups as a percentage of the total Canadian population included 4.0% South Asian (descendents from the Indian subcontinent), 3.9% Chinese, and 2.5% black (Statistics Canada, 2006). Roughly 4.0% of the Canadian population reported belonging to more than one "visible" minority group (Statistics Canada, 2006).

Questions about ancestry have been asked in the Australian Census since 1986. Additionally in Australia, questions pertaining to markers of ethnicity, including language spoken in the home and parental birthplace, have been asked in the census since 2001 (Australian Bureau of Statistics, 2006b). According to the 2006 Australian Census, greater than 70% of the population reported ancestral origin other than Australian (Australian Bureau of Statistics, 2006c).

Racial and ethnic data are not unproblematic and major reliability and validity problems exist. Such problems include miscounting and misclassification of persons by race and ethnicity; differences in individual responses to race/ethnic questions depending upon time, indicator, and survey; variation in procedures to collect race/ethnic data within and between data collection agencies; and the absence of definitions of race and ethnicity for data collection (Hahn, 1992). The result is that the accuracy of race/ethnic statistical information may be compromised and inconsistent across time and place.

In addition to the issues of reliability and validity, the present use of race/ethnic categories to disaggregate scientific data has been questioned by some because of the social nature of the concept as opposed to being more biologically based and the possibility that continued use will reify stereotypes and encourage further race/ethnic fragmentation in societies (Bhopal, 2007; Fullilove, 1998). Speculation also exists as to the current significance of race categories in modern multi-racial and multi-ethnic societies given the greater numbers of later generation immigrants born in host countries and their acculturation, higher levels of interracial marriage and children born of more than one race, increased race/ethnic residential and workplace integration in some areas, the expansion of the global economy, and greater inter-country economic dependence compared to previous time periods (Parliamentary Office of Science and Technology, 2007). The historic and contemporary reality, however, is that of the perpetual reinforcement of power relations in historically racialized societies via race/ethnic assignment.

Accordingly, race remains a consequential *social* variable that is a key determinant of access to power, privilege, and societal resources (ASA 2003; Williams, 1997).

3 The Significance of Race and Ethnicity for Health

The health consequences of race/ethnic classification are born out in data from multiple countries with heterogeneous populations. As Krieger (2000) states,

> Throughout our life course we likewise embody these social realities – whether oppression or privilege, depending on our ascribed and internalized race/ethnic identity – and in doing so manifest what can be called 'biological expression of race relations.' (p. 212)

Data from the USA, UK, Canada, Australia, Brazil, and South Africa consistently show that most non-white groups in each of these countries experience more health problems, rate their health lower, and have lower overall life expectancies and higher all-cause mortality than whites.

For example, for the 15 leading causes of death in the USA, blacks have higher death rates than whites for nine causes including heart disease, stroke, flu/pneumonia, septicemia, homicide, cancer, diabetes, kidney diseases, and hypertension (National Center for Health Statistics, 2009). Moreover, the white–black gap in life expectancy in the USA has widened over the past 25 years due to slower improvements in black health status compared to the overall population (Mensah et al, 2005). American Indians also have markedly poorer health than whites for a number of outcomes including infant mortality, diabetes and injury related mortality, activity limitation, and self-assessed fair/poor health (National Center for Health Statistics, 2009). Although the health of US Hispanic and Asian immigrants, as reflected in overall mortality rates, tends to be comparable or better than that of whites, research suggests that their health

advantage declines with longer length of US residency, number of generations in the USA, and US nativity (Frisbie et al, 2001; Fujimoto et al, 2000; Koya and Egede, 2007; Lutsey et al, 2008; Sundquist and Winkleby, 1999). This pattern has been well documented for cardiovascular disease and related biomedical and behavioral risk factors, but exists for a broad range of outcomes.

Although US race/ethnic disparities in health are compelling, the data are not without problems. Studies show that 10–25% of Hispanics, American Indians, and Asian/Pacific Islanders are misclassified on death certificates, with the problem being greatest for American Indians (Williams, 2005). This numerator undercount leads to an underestimate of mortality and suggests that mortality rates for these groups are higher than the officially reported ones. Demographic analyses conducted by the U.S. Census Bureau have long indicated that the census fails to count over 10% of middle-aged black males. Denominator undercounts inflate reported rates. Some evidence from post-enumeration surveys of the US Census indicates that there may also be an undercount problem for American Indians and Hispanics (Williams, 2005).

In the UK, Pakistani, Bangladeshi, and black Caribbean people report the poorest health of all population groups and the absolute percentages of people reporting poor health increases dramatically with age for these ethnic groups compared to whites (Nazroo and Williams, 2006). Additionally, Bangladeshi and Pakistani men are 50% more likely to have a heart attack or angina and Caribbean men are 50% more likely to die of stroke despite lower levels of coronary artery disease than the general population (Parliamentary Office of Science and Technology, 2007). Results from the Health Survey of England indicate that hypertension and diabetes prevalence rates are also higher among Caribbeans than whites (Nazroo, Jackson, Karlsen, and Torres, 2007).

Similarly, studies from Brazil confirm significantly higher hypertension rates among blacks than whites. Interestingly, they also show striking color gradients in age-adjusted cerebrovascular disease mortality where rates increase with darker skin color (Lotufo et al, 2007; Sichieri et al, 2001). Data from the Pan-American Health Organization (PAHO) (2007a) indicate that indigenous and black Brazilian populations have a higher incidence of mortality from vaccine preventable diseases than whites. Additionally, the PAHO (2007a) data show that blacks have a greater risk of death than whites from endocrine diseases and complications of pregnancy/child birth and greater prevalence rates for hypertension and diabetes. Persons of mixed descent also have a higher risk of death from pregnancy/child birth than whites, but lower death rates associated with neoplasms, circulatory, respiratory, and digestive diseases. Data for the "mixed" racial group may be unreliable; however, due to the relatively high rate of race misclassification for this group (Pan-American Health Organization, 2007a).

In contrast, data from the Canadian National Population Health Survey indicate that black Canadians, Southeast Asians, and South Asians experience high levels of functional and self-rated health that are comparable to levels for white Canadians (Wu and Schimmele, 2005). Indigenous, Arabic, and mixed raced groups experience health outcomes that are poorer than the Canadian sample average (Wu and Schimmele, 2005). PAHO (2007b) data show that the indigenous population, known as the Canadian First Nation, has a disproportionately high prevalence of chronic disease. These conditions including hypertension, heart disease, tuberculosis, HIV infection, fetal alcohol syndrome, and diabetes which are five times higher than the Canadian national average. The data also indicate that death rates due to injury and poisoning for the First Nation group are four times higher than for the overall Canadian population. Additionally, babies born to First Nation mothers are more likely to be born preterm and infant mortality is twice the rate for other Canadian populations. Moreover, life expectancy among First Nation men and women is between 5 and 7 years shorter than the Canadian national average (PAHO, 2007b).

In South Africa, results from several studies provide evidence of health disparities among race groups resulting, in part, from the differential impact of the epidemiologic transition in the country. Results show that among older adults, Africans are at greatest risk of death from infectious diseases such as tuberculosis and diarrhea. Additionally, the prevalence rate for HIV among Africans over 2 years of age is 13.3% (Human Sciences Research Council, 2009). This is nearly seven times greater than the HIV infection rate for colored and Indian groups (1.9 and 1.6%, respectively) and nearly 22 times greater than the rate for whites (0.6%) (Human Sciences Research Council, 2009). Results from the South African Stress and Health Study also indicate that black groups report higher levels of self-rated ill health and higher levels of psychological distress than whites (Williams et al, 2008). Moreover, Africans and other non-whites are approximately two times more likely to die at younger ages of adulthood (45–59 years of age) than whites which may reflect differences in underlying causes of mortality associated with the epidemiologic transition.

In contrast, white adults are at greatest risk of death from chronic diseases such cardiovascular disease (CVD) and cancer, but have greater longevity, on average, than non-whites. Results from the South Africa Adult Demographic and Health Survey indicate that age-adjusted hypertension rates and stroke deaths are higher among whites, Asians, and coloreds compared to Africans (Bradshaw et al, 2004). Additionally, these groups are also significantly more likely to smoke heavily (Bradshaw et al, 2004).

Health disparities exist in Australia as well. For example, the infant mortality rate for aborigines persists at greater than two times the Australian national average (Australian Bureau of Statistics, 2007). Additionally, life expectancy is nearly 20 years shorter for aboriginal people than the general population. This largely reflects the higher prevalence rates of heart disease, stroke, diabetes, alcohol consumption, and smoking among members of this group (Australian Bureau of Statistics, 2008; 2007).

4 Race/Ethnic Heterogeneity in Health Status

Despite the relatively high degree to which race/ethnic categories capture health disparities between population groups, some of the monolithic categories developed for census taking across countries fail to reflect race/ethnic heterogeneity in cultural factors, migration status, and ancestry. These factors potentially give rise to important health differences within race/ethnic groups. For example, data from the US National Health Interview Survey show that among Latinos, Puerto Ricans more frequently report "poor" or "fair" self-rated health than Cubans and Mexican Americans (Hajat et al, 2000). Additionally, Puerto Ricans report greater levels of functional limitation, higher levels of restricted activity and bed disability days, and greater overall numbers of hospitalizations compared to other Latinos. Data from the same survey also indicate that among Asian Americans, Vietnamese and Korean persons are more likely to report lower health status than Chinese, Japanese, or Filipinos (Kuo, 1997). Chinese persons are also less likely to report experiencing activity limitations compared to other Asian groups. Heterogeneity also exists among persons of African descent in the USA. For example, data from the National Survey of American Life indicate that black Caribbean men are at higher risk of experiencing psychiatric disorders than African American men, while the reverse trend is evident for Caribbean and African American women (Williams et al, 2007a).

Ethnic heterogeneity in health status is also evident among some groups in the UK. Research suggests that South Asians (including people with ancestral origins from India, Sri Lanka, Bangladesh, Nepal, and Pakistan) have significantly higher risk of coronary heart disease than other ethnic groups in the UK, although the prevalence of cardiovascular disease risk factors varies significantly among South Asian sub-groups. For example, results from a study conducted in Newcastle indicate that Bangladeshi men compared to Indians and Pakistanis are more likely to smoke, have the highest triglyceride and fasting plasma glucose levels, the lowest concentration of high density lipoprotein (HDL) cholesterol, and the lowest median blood pressure levels (Bhopal et al, 1999). CVD risk factor prevalence varies further among Indians. For example, Punjabi Sikhs from North India have lower rates of smoking compared to Gujarati Hindu men from West India, largely because of religious prohibitions on smoking. Punjabis, however, have higher blood pressure and cholesterol levels (Forouhi and Sattar, 2006).

5 Mechanisms Through Which Race and Ethnicity May Affect Health

5.1 Socioeconomic status

Race/ethnic differences in health continue to be evident even after adjustment for socioeconomic status, although there is evidence that SES indicators are not equivalent across race (Williams and Collins, 1995). Compared to whites, US blacks have less income at every level of education and less wealth at every level of income. Additionally they possess less purchasing power for goods and services because of higher costs in the residential areas where they are disproportionately located. Generally speaking, the socioeconomic status of non-white race/ethnic groups in the USA, the UK, Canada, Australia, and South Africa is lower on average than whites, whether measured by educational attainment, income, wealth, or occupational grade. Although research suggests that persistent low SES is a strong predictor of morbidity and mortality, studies from the UK, Canada, and the USA show that race/ethnic disparities in health status exist even after adjustment for socioeconomic status (Nazroo, 1999; Williams, 1997; Wu and Schimmele, 2005).

Some evidence indicates that the association between socioeconomic status and health is modified by immigrant status. There appears to be inconsistent socioeconomic patterning of health status among non-white immigrants despite fairly consistent patterns among native-born groups. In the UK, for example, results from a study conducted by Marmot et al (1984) showed that mortality was inversely and strongly associated with occupational grade in native-born populations in England but was inconsistently associated with social class among immigrants from South Asia and the Caribbean. Additionally, results from the Multi-Ethnic Study of Atherosclerosis in the USA showed minimal and inconsistent education and income patterning of major CVD risk factors, including hypertension, diabetes, obesity, low density lipoprotein cholesterol, high density lipoprotein cholesterol, and smoking among a sample of majority foreign-born Hispanics and Asians (Boykin et al, 2010). It may be the case that immigrants carry the social patterning of diseases with them from their countries of origin to their host countries. Studies show that the social patterning of cardiovascular risk factors in some developing countries exhibits positive associations such that CVD risk increases with greater socioeconomic status (Steyn et al, 2005; Yu et al, 2002). These patterns appear to change over time to those of host countries for immigrants with greater length of stay and acculturation. Patterns evident in industrialized countries are generally inverse in direction such that lower SES groups experience greater CVD morbidity and mortality.

5.2 Discrimination, Racism, and Stress

Discrimination includes actions targeted to reinforce symbolic boundaries separating social groups from one another and can occur at both institutional and personal levels (Jackman, 1994). Institutional discrimination involves efforts on the part of societal institutions such as government, businesses, and neighborhood organizations to prevent certain groups from gaining access, employment, advancement, or participation within their jurisdiction. Such efforts can be informal, enforced by law, or both. Moreover, discriminatory acts are often racially charged or motivated by other factors such as gender or socioeconomic status.

Residential race/ethnic segregation is one example of institutional discrimination and serves as the predominant factor responsible for the creation of disparities in socioeconomic status between whites and non-whites, particularly in the USA and South Africa. To the extent that socioeconomic status predicts race/ethnic disparities in health in various societies, residential race/ethnic segregation may be considered a fundamental cause of these disparities because segregation determines individual, household, neighborhood, and community socioeconomic conditions (Williams and Collins, 2001). This includes the quality of education, employment opportunities, and neighborhoods. Furthermore, residential racial segregation often determines opportunities for amassing wealth via homeownership. Homes are important assets for many individuals and families in industrialized countries because their value usually appreciates over time. In racially segregated residential areas, however, housing values are often much lower and less likely to appreciate significantly compared to non-segregated areas. The influx of new residents seeking to buy homes in these areas is low and fewer opportunities exist to obtain loans to purchase homes while predatory lending in certain segregated areas is high relative to non-segregated places.

Examples of politically and institutionally enforced residential racial segregation include discriminatory governmental policies mandating physical separation of blacks and whites in some areas of the USA prior to the middle of the 20th century and in South Africa during the apartheid era. Although laws supporting residential racial segregation in both places have been overturned, high levels of black–white segregation remain stable since the peak of their enforcement. Currently, the index of dissimilarity, the percentage of blacks that would have to move to create evenness among white and black races in the area, is estimated to be 90% in South Africa and between 80 and 85% in large US cities such as Detroit (MI), Chicago (IL), New York (NY), Newark (NJ), and Milwaukee (WI) (Massey, 2004). These areas are overwhelmingly poor and surrounded by other impoverished areas with sub-standard housing. Additionally these areas have greater resident density per housing unit, fewer available municipal and medical services, low numbers of recreational facilities and fresh food markets, fewer economic opportunities, and higher crime rates. They are also more likely to be exposed to environmental hazards including pollutants, allergens, and landfills. Furthermore, racially segregated areas in the USA are significantly more likely to be targeted for marketing campaigns for alcohol, tobacco, and fast food.

Life in these areas can be extremely stressful, physically and psychologically, because of the lack of available resources and potential hazards, including violence, financial stress, high unemployment, and higher levels of chronic illness. Additionally, school facilities are often dilapidated and resources are inadequate. For example, post-apartheid government spending per white pupil in South Africa is four times the amount spent on black students who mostly live in segregated areas (Chisholm et al, 1998). Similarly in the USA, spending on students in large predominantly non-white school districts in cities such as New York can be as much as 50% lower than in mostly white-surrounding suburban areas (Kozol, 1991). Moreover, dropout rates for students in schools in extremely poor and racially segregated inner cities in the USA such as in Baltimore, Maryland, approach 65%. Similarly in South Africa, attrition approaches 60% among students who start school and leave prior to completing high school (Department of Education, 2003).

Consequently, blacks in the USA and in South Africa live in areas that have been designated as being "extremely segregated," are overwhelmingly represented at the lowest end of the socioeconomic spectrum, and display poorer health outcomes compared to other race/ethnic groups. Historically, many white immigrant groups as well as Latinos and Asians have lived in segregated residential conditions and ethnic enclaves, but no US immigrant group has lived under the high levels of segregation that currently characterize the black population (Williams and Collins, 2001). Moreover, the wealthiest blacks

in the USA are more likely to live in racially segregated areas than the poorest Latinos and Asians (Massey, 2004).

Residential segregation is also evident in the UK but it appears to be less extreme than in the USA. Ethnic minorities in the UK are more likely to live in areas where the total ethnic minority population exceeds 40% (Nazroo, 2004). Furthermore, 45% of the ethnic minority population in the UK resides in the city of London compared to only 10% of whites (Nazroo, 2004). Nearly half of all South Asian adults over the age of 60 years live in fairly large households with very low income. Many also live in areas with high-ethnic minority concentrations (Nazroo, 2004). Such conditions are potentially detrimental to health, particularly in advanced stages of life.

Personal experiences of racism and discrimination are also potentially deleterious to health although the numbers of experiences vary among members of race/ethnic groups across countries. Results from the South African Stress and Health Study indicated that Africans and coloreds were twice as likely as whites to report an experience of racial discrimination and Indians were three times more likely to report racial discrimination (Williams et al, 2008). Africans and Indians also reported twice the level of non-racial discrimination as whites although the overall level of reported discrimination in the study was less than 10%.

In contrast, a study conducted in the UK showed that greater than 10% of nonwhite individuals reported experiencing some form of racial harassment and 25% reported being fearful of harassment (Modood, 1997). Furthermore, 70% of indigenous persons in an Australian study reported at least one experience of race-based discrimination (Paradies and Cunningham, 2009). Three quarters of blacks recently polled by The Washington Post/ABC News (2009) in the USA and 68% of other nonwhites reported personal experiences of racial discrimination. Experiences most often cited by US blacks in the poll included being made to feel unwelcome in a store, being stopped by the police, being denied a job, and being denied housing because of their race. The reporting of discrimination experiences may depend upon individual and group perceptions of what is considered to be "discriminatory" in various domains as well as what is considered acceptable to report. Improvements in measuring and capturing experiences of race/ethnic discrimination across societies are needed to better understand the implications of these experiences for health among various population groups (Williams and Mohammed, 2009).

Discrimination can affect health in many ways. It can result in reduced access to necessary goods and services, lead to the internalization of negative stereotypes, increase stress, and trigger behavioral responses such as substance use, excessive eating, and failure to adhere to medical regimens that can have adverse consequences for health. For example, findings from a national study in South Africa suggested that perceived chronic discrimination was positively associated with psychological distress (Williams et al, 2008). In the USA, results from several studies showed that racial discrimination was associated with cardiovascular and physiological reactivity among blacks in laboratory settings, worse physical and mental health, higher risk of low birth weight and preterm birth, and engagement in negative health behaviors such as smoking, alcohol consumption, and illicit drug use (Paradies, 2006; Williams et al, 2003). Moreover, studies from the USA, South Africa, Australia, and New Zealand found that consideration of experiences of racial discrimination in statistical analyses provided additional incremental contribution in accounting for race/ethnic disparities in health beyond the effects of socioeconomic status (Williams and Mohammed, 2009).

5.3 Medical Care

Differences in health-care access, quality, and treatment rates for non-whites compared to whites have been documented extensively in the USA, the UK, Australia, and Canada. They are likely attributed to residential racial segregation and experiences of racism and discrimination within health-care systems. Racial and ethnic minorities in the USA are overrepresented among the almost 50 million Americans who lack health insurance and thus face major challenges in obtaining access to medical care. A report from the Institute of Medicine in the USA showed consistent race disparities in the quality and intensity of care for numerous health conditions that persisted after differences in clinical need, appropriateness of treatment, SES, and insurance are controlled (Smedley et al, 2003). Discrimination on the part of health-care providers, much of it probably below their conscious awareness, but based on negative stereotypes of their ethnic minority patients likely plays a role in these patterns (Smedley et al, 2003). Other research indicates that US physicians who provide care to non-white patients are less likely to be board certified (accredited by a medical governing body in their area of specialization) and are also more likely to report difficulties in arranging access for their patients to specialists, diagnostic testing services, and hospitals for non-emergency admissions (Bach et al, 2004). Furthermore, in racially segregated areas in the USA, physicians are less likely to accept Medicaid payment (low-income governmental health-care insurance) for services, pharmacies are less likely to be stocked with adequate medical supplies, and hospitals are more likely to close (Buchmueller et al, 2006; Greene et al, 2006; Morrison et al, 2000). The result is that race-based disparities in health-care access and quality are significantly associated with poorer health outcomes, including higher mortality, among non-whites in the US health-care system (Smedley et al, 2003). In contrast, US whites generally have greater access to health care, experience higher quality care, and have higher rates of treatment – all of which are presumed to provide additional benefit for maintaining health.

Race/ethnic differences in health-care access are also evident in other countries. Ethnic differences in access to health care in the UK vary within parts of the National Health Service (NHS). Although research suggests that blacks and other non-white groups receive primary care at a rate equivalent to the general UK population relative to need, access to tertiary care for disease-specific treatments is lower among non-whites (Parliamentary Office of Science and Technology, 2007). Non-whites also report greater levels of dissatisfaction with multiple aspects of health-care delivery in the NHS (Parliamentary Office of Science and Technology, 2007). Moreover, findings from Australian studies comparing treatment rates for cardiovascular disease among indigenous and non-indigenous patients suggest that indigenous patients admitted to public hospitals are nearly 50% less likely to receive diagnostic or therapeutic procedures (Cunningham, 2002). Additionally, indigenous patients are less likely to receive invasive coronary procedures after acute myocardial infarction than non-indigenous patients with similar presentation even after controlling for co-morbidities (Coory and Walsh, 2005; Cunningham, 2002). Other studies also show that indigenous Australians receive lower levels of care for cancer and renal transplantation (Cass et al, 2003; Hall et al, 2004).

Similarly, research suggests that indigenous Canadian populations are also significantly less likely to receive renal transplantation (Tonelli et al, 2004). They are also less likely to obtain adequate prenatal care even after holding potential confounders constant across groups (Heaman et al, 2005). Additionally, Canadian immigrants are less likely than native-born Canadians to receive preventive care, including cervical cancer screenings, although screening rates among immigrants with longer residency in Canada are nearly double for those recent immigrants (Lofters et al, 2007). Thus, culture and language may serve as major barriers to health-care access for Canadian immigrants and indigenous population groups (Lai and Chau, 2007).

5.4 Immigration and Resources for Health

Immigration involves the relocation of people from one country to another usually for the purposes of work or political asylum and immigrants can either be legally recognized in their new host country or not. Recent data suggest that net migration rates are positive and highest for highly industrialized countries and negative for less developed countries. Thus, the net flow of migrants tends to be from less developed areas of eastern Europe, central and north Africa, Asia, South America, Mexico, and the Caribbean to developed countries with advanced economies such as the USA, Canada, Russia, western European countries, Australia, and South Africa (Central Intelligence Agency, 2009). Implicit in this migratory trend are differences in patterns of disease prevalence, morbidity, and mortality between immigrants' countries of origin and their host countries due to differences in the rates at which the epidemiologic transition is occurring between these places. Morbidity and mortality in non-developed countries are most often attributed to infectious and maternal diseases associated with poverty, while death rates and morbidity associated with chronic diseases are greatest in industrialized countries.

First generation immigrants to developed countries bring with them personal health behaviors, cultural practices, beliefs, and other resources from their former country. The usual result is that mortality rates are often lower for newer immigrants once in their host country than for the host's general population, particularly if the host is a developed country. Mortality rates for communicable, maternal, and poverty-related diseases associated with immigrants' countries of origin rapidly decline to host levels due to decreased exposure in the host country. Additionally, a lag usually takes place after immigrants' arrival in the host country prior to any acculturation processes occurring. Thus, a time delay often exists before new immigrants begin to adopt the health behaviors of the host country, including the adoption of common health behaviors in industrialized countries that may lead to elevated risks for chronic diseases. Both immigration and length of residency in a host country may further contribute to race/ethnic heterogeneity in health outcomes between population groups and within them. Moreover, the effects of acculturation may widen race/ethnic disparities, particularly between white and non-white groups.

For example, recent data from the US Multi-Ethnic Study of Atherosclerosis show that carotid plaque prevalence and mean carotid intima media thickness, both markers of atherosclerosis, an antecedent to clinical cardiovascular disease, were greater among US-born than foreign-born study participants. Markers of atherosclerosis were also greater among persons in the study with greater numbers of familial generations that had lived in the USA (Lutsey et al, 2008). In Australia, data concerning chronic disease prevalence indicate that recent immigrants are less likely to report having arthritis, asthma, diabetes, heart disease, vascular diseases, and stroke or mental health problems compared with immigrants with longer length of residence in the country (Australian Bureau of Statistics, 2006a). Similarly, data from the Canadian Community Health Survey and Canadian Population Health Survey confirm that immigrants to Canada with fewer than 30 years of residence in the country are less likely to report having a chronic health condition than native-born persons and the health advantage is greatest among recent immigrants (Perez, 2002). More refined analyses also show that among men who immigrated to Canada in the past 20 years compared to native-born men, the odds of heart disease incidence are lower and not fully explained by differences in dietary patterns, smoking, physical activity, alcohol consumption, body mass index, or place of origin (Perez, 2002).

While health-promoting behaviors are most often cited as the greatest health resources immigrants bring with them, it is plausible that immigrants bring other resources as well. Resources vary significantly by group but may include higher levels of socioeconomic status, material resources such as money, social networks providing instrumental and emotional social support, and professional training for employment opportunities in the host country. Some studies show, however, that socioeconomic status combines with immigrant status in complex ways to affect health outcomes of some immigrant groups. For example, the Latino health paradox in the USA provides an example of this for several health outcomes including infant and overall mortality, cardiovascular diseases, cancer, and self-reported physical and mental health status. The paradox is that the health status of Latinos in the USA is more comparable to that of whites despite lower overall socioeconomic status in this group. However, second generation Latinos in the USA face major challenges with regard to socioeconomic mobility and the combination of low SES and acculturation leads to a marked decline in health status. In contrast, many Asian immigrants have higher income and education levels than US whites and declines in their health over time appear to be less steep than those of the Latino population (Williams, 2005).

The better health of immigrants, generally, and new immigrants in particular, is sometimes dismissed in the literature as the result of selection or bias. Some studies suggest that the "healthy migrant" effect results from self-selection or other selection of healthier persons for immigration prior to arrival in the host country. Others hypothesize that some less healthy and elderly immigrants in host countries may return to their countries of origin and their deaths are not counted in the mortality statistics of the host country resulting in biased counts and race/ethnic disparities that are artificially lessened. Exploratory data from the USA suggest that return migration rates are relatively high for certain Latino immigrant groups. However, tests of the healthy migrant and return migration hypotheses using data from the US National Longitudinal Mortality Study showed that neither hypothesis explained the lower overall mortality among Cuban and Puerto Rican immigrants in the USA compared to non-Latino immigrants and US-born whites (Albraido-Lanza et al, 1999). It has been hypothesized that the social and cultural capital that immigrants bring with them, including health-promoting behaviors and extended kin networks, may contribute to the health paradox because of their strong protective effects for immigrants' health in host countries. More research is needed to investigate how the health status that immigrants bring with them combines with their human capital resources at arrival, and their exposures, risks, and resources in their host society to create particular trajectories of health for immigrants and their children.

Evidence that the global epidemiologic transition is currently taking place at a highly accelerated rate in mostly non-white developing regions of the world such as East Asia/Pacific, Latin America/Caribbean, Middle East/North Africa, South Asia, and sub-Saharan Africa compared to the rates at which it occurred in developed countries suggests that morbidity and mortality patterns will inevitably change for population groups in developing regions. Moreover, it is also likely that the health advantage experienced by immigrants from these regions upon arriving in a host country will narrow. It is estimated that coronary heart disease will increase between 120 and 140% in developing countries through the year 2020 (Leeder et al, 2004). The rapid pace of the transition is the result of the quick and far-penetrating importation of the "western" lifestyle and its associated commodities (refined sugar drinks, cigarettes, and processed foods) coupled with a lack of preventative interventions. The unfortunate result in developing countries is earlier onset of disease, increased demands on health-care delivery systems, loss of worker productivity, and increased family poverty due to health-related job loss. These societal and economic burdens threaten the sustainability of developing countries (Gaziano, 2007). Thus, the impact of the current epidemiologic transition in developing countries may lead to greater numbers of people who want to immigrate to other places, but immigrants may possess fewer resources for health and have poorer health status that could be further exacerbated by acculturation processes after immigration. Moreover, the potential exists that the unintended by-product of the transition will be that race/ethnic disparities in industrialized host countries will increase.

6 Future Research Directions

In this chapter we reviewed conceptions and uses of race and ethnicity across several countries with diverse population groups. Additionally, we illustrated the global context of race/ethnic disparities in health and outlined some of the mechanisms through which disparities become manifest. Although these topics have been examined extensively in many countries, race/ethnic disparities continue to persist and are, for some outcomes, widening in many societies. Thus, more research is needed to further elucidate factors that contribute to race/ethnic disparities in health. Moreover, translational research is also needed to effectively convey existing findings for the development of public policies targeted to eliminate these disparities. We suggest five directions for future research globally to achieve these aims.

(1) *Investigating health-promoting factors.* While much of the existing research on race/ethnic disparities in health has taken the "glass half empty" approach, we suggest an expansion in focus to include a complimentary "glass half full" approach. In other words, future research should investigate factors contributing to better health among various race/ethnic groups. Ideally, this approach will lead to greater understanding of factors that preserve and/or promote health for specific populations. For example, blacks in the USA have lower lifetime prevalence of major depressive disorders compared to other race/ethnic groups (Williams et al, 2007). Future investigations of individual and environmental factors that are protective for black mental health are needed to advance the literature on this topic.

Attention must be paid to heterogeneity within race/ethnic groups by nativity, nationality, and gender. Additionally, a life course approach is warranted to investigate the incremental contributions of potentially positive health exposures across the lifespan. Such exposures might include increased social and material resources; wealth; residential integration; neighborhood resources; positive psychological attributes and resources; certain health behaviors (i.e., increased physical activity, low-fat diet); religiosity and belief systems. Improved understanding of how these factors contribute to health could potentially lead to expedient policy development in an effort to protect, create, or expand health-promoting structures within societies.

(2) *Developing better measures of the social context for health.* Improvements over existing research on race/ethnic disparities in health must include better measures of the social contexts individuals negotiate on a daily basis. These measures are necessary to assess the specific risks and resources that individuals may be exposed to and that may vary systematically by race and ethnicity. It may be the case that existing SES measures such as education, income, wealth, and occupational status do not fully capture important aspects of social status that may matter for health in certain population groups. For example, extensive familial and social networks in ethnic immigrant communities may serve as key resources for preservation of health-promoting cultural factors and for pooling economic resources. Thus, it may be the interactive effect of the absence of such networks in some communities simultaneously with low SES that leads to a greater negative impact on the health status of some ethnic immigrants. Incorporating measures of the social and environmental contexts and changes in them over time may allow for better understanding of the pathways through which traditional measures, such as education and income affect health over the life course. Similarly, there has been inadequate attention paid to the ways in which chemical and physical environmental exposures in residential and occupational environments of ethnic minorities combine with psychosocial risks and resources to affect health.

(3) *Examining cumulative exposures over the life course.* Future research must also examine the impact of cumulative exposures throughout the life course. These investigations should consider both positive and negative exposures that affect health. Additionally, study objectives should include determining stages of the life course where certain exposures may be most health promoting or eroding. For example, an important question to be investigated is to what extent do childhood socioeconomic circumstances (including those of immigrants) contribute to the onset of specific diseases, such as cardiovascular disease, associated biologic risk factors, and the clustering of risk factors at various stages of the life course. By way of extension, are low-SES children and adolescents of particular race/ethnic backgrounds more likely to develop risk factors for certain diseases earlier in life? Natural experiments, such as the relocation of people from low-income housing projects to higher SES areas or school choice programs where parents can send children to higher performing schools within districts, may prove extremely useful for investigating such questions. Results from these studies may provide compelling evidence regarding the types of effective interventions that could be implemented on a larger scale.

(4) *Elucidating biologic pathways through which social determinants affect health.* Translational and multidisciplinary research is essential for developing creative approaches for understanding how "upstream" causal factors that may be sociological or economic in nature contribute to more "downstream" biologic pathways that create or prevent specific disease states in various race/ethnic groups. For example, "allostatic load" refers to the process where chronic experiences of psychological stress lead to the deregulation of multiple physiologic systems that ultimately give rise to disease (McEwen, 1998; see Chapter 42). Future research is necessary to link such alterations in biological processes to specific disease states and to determine if certain race/ethnic groups are more susceptible to such alterations. Other biologic pathways also need to be uncovered. Additionally,

studies should investigate the importance of specific gene×environment interactions to the progression of disease processes and their contribution to alterations of natural aging processes for various race/ethnic groups.

(5) *Ensuring greater levels of accuracy in the collection and use of race/ethnic data.* Significant reliability and validity problems plague race/ethnic data and often result from miscounting and misclassifying persons due to the lack of unifying definitions for race/ethnic groups across place and time and variations in race/ethnic data collection procedures among data collection agencies. For example, the Asian race category in the US Census refers to descendents from the Far East, Southeast Asia, and the Indian subcontinent and has evolved over time from its original form, whereas ethnic categories in the UK Census distinguish between some Asian ethnic groups. This example illustrates that (a) the interpretation of study results and their meaningfulness, using the Asian US race category must carefully reflect the fact that multiple groups with different ancestral origins are combined in one category; and that (b) race/ethnic classifications across countries may not be comparable. A rethinking of current race/ethnic categories and the creation of new categories may be warranted in order to better reflect the changing demographic compositions of race/ethnic groups within localities. Additionally, greater emphasis needs to be placed on unifying definitions of race/ethnicity across place, while still reflecting the unique demographic compositions of countries in order to provide for greater data comparability and to better identify the social determinants of race/ethnic differences in health. Even with consistent race/ethnic definitions across locations, one must still take into consideration the ethnic heterogeneity within categories and the unique social, environmental, and immigration factors that shape the individual experiences of persons identifying with a particular race/ethnic group.

Race/ethnic disparities in health violate norms of equal opportunity and systematically restrict the quality of life and productive capacity of many individuals. They warrant immediate attention in research and policy domains. Although research designs need to be sophisticated, investigators must take a "common sense" approaches to frame research questions and to develop measures in racially and ethnically relevant contexts. Moreover, results must provide key messages for policy makers that can be easily translated into high-impact policies ensuring the promotion of health for all race/ethnic groups across diverse societies.

References

ABC News/Washington Post (2009). Poll: race relations. *http:/abcnews.com/pollingunit.*

Albraido-Lanza, A., Dohrenwend B., Daisy, S., Ng-Mak, M., and Blake Turner, J. (1999). The Latino mortality paradox: a test of the "salmon bias" and healthy migrant hypotheses. *Am J Public Health, 89,* 1543–1548.

Australian Bureau of Statistics. (2008). 4704.0 – The Health and Welfare of Australia's Aboriginal and Torres Strait Islander Peoples.

Australian Bureau of Statistics. (2007). 1301.0 – Year Book Australia 2007, Infant Mortality Over the Past 100 Years.

Australian Bureau of Statistics. (2006a). 4364.0 – National Health Survey: Summary of Results, 2004–2005.

Australian Bureau of Statistics. (2006b). 29140.0—2006 Census of Population and Housing Fact Sheets: Ancestry.

Australian Bureau of Statistics (2006c). 2068.0—2006 Census Tables: Ancestry (Full Class) by Sex.

Bach, P., Pham, H., Schrag, D., Tate, R., and Hargraves, L. (2004). Primary care physicians who treat blacks and whites. *NEMJ, 351,* 575–584.

Bhopal, R. (2007). *Ethnicity, Race and Health in Multicultural Societies.* New York: Oxford University Press.

Bhopal, R., Unwin, N., White, M., Yallop, J., Walker L. et al (1999). Heterogeneity of coronary heart disease risk factors in Indian, Pakistani, Bagladeshi, and European origin populations: cross sectional study. *BMJ, 319,* 215–220.

Boykin, S., Diez-Roux, A., Carnethon, M., Shrager, S., Ni, H. et al (2010). Education and income patterning of major CVD risk factors in U.S. White Black, Hispanic, and Chinese: The Multi-Ethnic Study of Atherosclerosis. Unpublished.

Bradshaw, D., Norman, R., Laubscher, R., Schneider, M., Mbananga, N. et al (2004). An exploratory investigation into racial disparities in the health of older South Africans. In N. Anderson, R. Bulatao, & B. Cohen (Eds.), *Critical Perspectives on Racial and Ethnic Differences in Health in Late Life* (pp. 703–736). Washington, DC: National Academies Press.

Buchmueller, T. C., Jacobson, M., and Wold, C. (2006). How far to the hospital? The effect of hospital closures on access to care. *J Health Econ, 2*, 740–761.

Cass, A., Cunningham, J., Snelling, P., Wang, Z., and Hoy, W. (2003). Renal transplantation for indigenous Australians: identifying the barriers to equitable access. *Ethn Health, 8*, 111–119.

Central Intelligence Agency (United States). (2009). The World Factbook, Country Comparisons-Net Migration Rates. http://www.cia.gov/library/publications/the-world-factbook/rankorder/2112rank.html.

Chisholm, L., Vally, S., and Motala, S. (1998). *Review of South African Education 1994–1997.* Johannesburg: Education Policy Unit, University of the Witwatersrand.

Coory, M., and Walsh, W. (2005). Rates of percutaneous coronary interventions and bypass surgery after acute myocardial infarction in indigenous patients. *Med J Aust, 182*, 507–512.

Cooper, R., Kaufman, J., and Ward, R. (2003). Race and genomics. *NEMJ, 348*, 1166–1170.

Cunningham, J. (2002). Diagnostic and therapeutic procedures among Australian hospital patients identified as indigenous. *Med J Aust, 176*, 58–62.

Department of Education (South Africa). (2003). *Education Statistics in South Africa At A Glance in 2001.* Pretoria, South Africa: South Africa Department of Education.

Feldman, M., Lewontin, R., and King, M. (2003). Race: a genetic melting pot. *Nature, 424*, 374.

Forouhi, N., and Sattar, N. (2006). CVD risk factors and ethnicity – a homogenous relationship? *Atheroscler Suppl, 7*(1), 11–19.

Frisbie, W., Cho, Y., and Hummer, R. (2001). Immigration and the Health of Asian and Pacific Islander Adults in the United States. *Am J Epidemiol, 153*, 372–380.

Fujimoto, W., Bergstrom, R., Boyko, E., Chen, K., Kahn, S., and Leonetti, D. (2000). Type 2 diabetes and the metabolic syndrome in Japanese Americans. *Diabetes Res Clin Pract, 50*, S73–S76.

Fullilove, M. (1998). Comment: abandoning 'race' as a variable in public health research – an idea whose time has come. *Am J Public Health 88*, 1297–1298.

Gaziano, T. (2007). Reducing the growing burden of cardiovascular disease in the developing world. *Health Aff, 26*, 13–24.

Geronimus A. (2000). To mitigate, resist or undo: addressing structural influences on the health of urban populations. *Am J Public Health, 90*, 867–872.

Greene J., Blustein J., and Weitzman B. (2006). Race, segregation, and physician's participation in Medicaid. *Milbank Q, 84*, 239–272.

Hahn, R. (1992). The state of federal health statistics on racial and ethnic groups. *JAMA, 267*, 268–71.

Hatch, S., and Dohrenwend, B. (2007). Distribution of traumatic and other stressful life events by race/ethnicity, gender, SES and age: a review of the research. *Am J Community Psychol, 30*, 313–332.

Heaman, M., Gupton, A., and Moffatt, M. (2005). Prevalence and predictors of inadequate prenatal care: a comparison of aboriginal and non-aboriginal women in Manitoba. *J Obstet Gynaecol Can, 27*, 237–46.

Hajat, A., Lucas J., and Kington R. (2000). *Health Outcomes Among Hispanic Subgroups: Data from the National Health Interview Survey, 1992–1995.* Advance Data from Vital and Health Statistics; no. 310. Hyattsville, MD: National Center for Health Statistics.

Hall, S., Bulsara, C., Bulsara, M., Leahy, T, Culbong, M. et al (2004). Treatment patterns for cancer in western Australia: does being indigenous make a difference? *Med J Aust, 181*, 191–194.

Human Sciences Research Council. (2009). Factsheet 2 : National HIV prevalence in South Africa - the graphics. http://www.hsrc.ac.za/Factsheet-40.phtml.

Instituto Brasileiro de Geografia e Estatitsica (IBGE). (2008a). *Pesquisa Nacional Por Amostra de Domicílios 2007.* Rio de Janeiro, RJ, Brazil: IBGE.

Instituto Brasileiro de Geografia e Estatitsica (IBGE). (2008b). *Síntese de Indicadores Sociais—Cor: Tabela 8.1 - População total e respectiva distribuição percentual, por cor ou raça, segundo as Grandes Regiões, Unidades da Federação e Regiões Metropolitanas – 2007.* ftp://ftp.ibge.gov.br/Indicadores_Sociais/Sintese_de_Indicadores_Sociais_2008/Tabelas/

Jackman, M. (1994). *The Velvet Glove: Paternalism and Conflict in Gender, Class, and Race Relations.* Los Angeles, CA: University of California Press.

Kaessmann H., Wiebe, V., Weiss, G., and Pääbo, S. (2001). Great ape DNA sequences reveal a reduced diversity and an expansion in humans. *Nat Genet, 27*, 155–156.

Kozol, J. (1991). *Savage Inequalities: Children in America's Schools.* New York: Crown Publishers.

Koya, D., and Egede, L. (2007). Association between length of residency and cardiovascular risk factors among an ethnically diverse group of United States immigrants. *J Gen Int Med 22*, 841–846.

Krieger, N. (2000). Refiguring "race": epidemiology, racialized biology, and biological expressions of race relations. *Int J Health Serv, 30*, 211–216.

Krieger, N. (1987). Shades of difference: theoretical underpinnings of the medical controversy on black/white differences in the United States, 1830–1870. *Int J Health Serv, 17,* 259–278.

Kuo, J. (1997). *Health Status of Asian Americans: United States, 1992–1994.* Advance Data from Vital and Health Statistics; no. 298. Hyattsville, MD: National Center for Health Statistics.

Lai, D., and Chai, S. (2007). Effects of service barriers on health status of older Chinese immigrants in Canada. *Social Work 52,* 261–269.

Leeder, S., Raymond S., and Greenberg, H. (2004). *A Race Against Time: The Challenge of Cardiovascular Disease in Developing Economies.* New York: Trustees of Columbia University.

Linné, C. (1806). *A General System of Nature Through the Three Grand Kingdoms of Animals, Vegetables, and Minerals Systematically Divided Into Their Several Classes, Orders, Genera, Species, and Varieties With Their Habitations, Manners, Economy, Structure, and Peculiarities.* London: Lackington, Allen, and Company.

Lofters, A., Glazier, R., Agha, M., Creatore, M., and Mioinedden, R. (2007). Inadequacy of cervical cancer screening among urban recent immigrants: a population based study of physician and laboratory claims in Toronto Canada. *Prev Med, 44,* 536–542.

Lutsey, P., Diez Roux, A., Jacobs, D., Burke, G., Harman, J. et al (2008). Associations of acculturation and socioeconomic status with subclinical cardiovascular disease in the Multi-Ethnic Study of Atherosclerosis. *Am J Public Health, 98,* 1963–1970.

Marmot, M. G., Adelstein, A. M., and Bulusu, L. (1984). Lessons from the study of immigrant mortality. *Lancet, 1,* 1455–1457.

Massey, D. (2004). Segregation and stratification: a biosocial perspective. *DuBois Rev: Soc Sci Res Race, 1,* 7–25.

Matijasevich, A., Victora, C., Barros, A., Santos, I., Marco, P. et al (2008). Widening ethnic disparities in infant mortality in southern Brazil: Comparison of 3 birth cohorts. *Am J Public Health, 98,* 692–698.

McEwen, B. (1998). Protective and damaging effects of stress mediators. *New England J Med 338,* 171–179.

Mensah, G., Mokdad, A., Ford, E., Greenlund, K., and Croft, J. (2005). State of disparities in cardiovascular health in the United States. *Circulation, 111,* 1233–1241.

Modood T. (1997). Employment. In T. Modood, R. Berthoud, J. Lakey, et al (Eds.), *Ethnic Minorities in Britain: Diversity and Disadvantage* (pp. 83–149). London: Policy Studies Institute.

Morrison, S., Wallenstein, S., Natale, D., Senzel, R., and Huang, L. (2000). "We Don't Carry That" – failure of pharmacies in predominantly nonwhite neighborhoods to stock opioid analgesics. *NEMJ, 342,* 1023–26.

National Center for Health Statistics. (2009). Health, United States, 2008 with Chartbook. Hyattsville, MD: United States Department of Health and Human Services.

National Statistics Online, U.K. (2001). Ethnicity and identity. http://www.statistics.gov.uk/cci/nugget.asp?id=455.

Nazroo, J. (2004). Ethnic disparities in aging health, what can we learn from the United Kingdom? In N. Anderson, R. Bulatao, and B. Cohen (Eds.), *Critical Perspectives on Racial and Ethnic Differences in Health in Late Life* (pp. 677–702). Washington, DC: The National Academies Press.

Nazroo, J. (1999). Demography of multicultural Britain. In J. Nazroo (Ed.), *Health and Social Research in Multiethnic Societies* (pp. 1–19). New York: Routledge.

Nazroo, J. and Williams, D. (2006). The social determination of ethnic/racial inequalities in health. In M. Marmot & R. Wilkinson (Eds.), *Social Determinants of Health* (pp. 238–266). New York: Oxford University Press.

Nazroo, J., Jackson, J., Karlsen, S., and Torres, M. (2007). The Black diaspora and health inequalities in the US and England: does where you go and how you get there make a difference? *Sociology of Health and Illness, 29,* 811–830.

Nobles, M. (2000). History counts: a comparative analysis of racial/color categorization in US and Brazilian Censuses. *Am J Public Health, 90,* 1738–1745.

Office of Management and Budget. (1978). U.S. Directive No. 15: Race and Ethnic Standards for Federal Statistics and Administrative Reporting. Washington, DC: Office of Federal Statistical Policy Standards, U.S. Department of Commerce.

Pan-American Health Organization. (2007a). Health in the Americas. Volume II- Countries- Brazil. http://www.paho.org/hia/archivosvol2/paisesing/Brazil%20English.pdf.

Pan-American Health Organization. (2007b). Health in the Americas. Volume II- Countries- Canada. http://www.paho.org/hia/archivosvol2/paisesing/Canada%20English.pdf.

Paradies, Y. (2006). A systematic review of empirical research on self-reported racism and health. *Int J Epidemiol, 35,* 888–901.

Paradies, Y. and Cunningham, J. (2009). Experiences of racism among urban Indigenous Australians: findings from the DRUID study. *Ethn Racial Stud, 32,* 548–573.

Parliamentary Office of Science and Technology (United Kingdom). (2007). Postnote No. 276. Ethnicity and Health.

Perez, C. (2002). Health status and health behavior among immigrants. *Health Rep, 13,* 89–100.

Sichieri, R., Oliveira, M., and Pereira, R. (2001). High prevalence of hypertension among black and mulatto women in a Brazilian survey. *Ethn Dis, 11,* 412–418.

Smedley, A. (1999). *Race in North America: Origin and Evolution of A Worldview, 2nd Ed.* Boulder, CO: Westview Press.

Smedley, B., Stith, A., and Nelson, A. (2003). *Unequal Treatment: Confronting Racial and Ethnic Disparities in Health Care.* Washington, DC: National Academies Press.

Statistics Canada. (2006). Canada's Ethnocultural Mosaic, 2006 Census National Picture.

Statistics Canada. (2004). 2001 Census Ethnic Origin User Guide. http://www12.statcan.ca/english/census01/Products/Referece/tech_rep/ethnic.cfm.

Statistics South Africa. (2001). Census 2001, Census in Brief. Report no. 03-02-03.

Steyn, K., Sliwa, K., Hawken, S., Commerford, P., Onen, C. et al (2005). Risk factors associated with myocardial infarction in Africa: the INTERHEART Africa Study. *Circulation, 112,* 3554–3561.

Sundquist, J., and Winkleby, M. A. (1999). Cardiovascular risk factors in Mexican American adults: a transcultural analysis of NHANES III: 1988–1994. *Am J Public Health, 89,* 723–730.

Sweet, F. (2005). *Legal History of the Color Line.* Palm Coast, FL: Backintyme Publishers.

Tonelli, M., Hemmelgarn, B., Manns, B., Pylypchuk, G., Bohm, C. et al (2004). Death and renal transplantation among aboriginal people undergoing dialysis. *CMAJ, 171,* 577–82.

Travassos, C., and Williams, D. R. (2004). The concept and measurement of race and their relationship to public health: a review focused on Brazil and the United States. *Saúde Pública, 20,* 660–678.

United States Census Bureau. (2000). Overview of Race and Hispanic Origin. Census 2000 Brief.

United States Census Bureau. (1854). Statistical View of the United States, Compendium of the Seventh Census.

Williams, D. R. (1997). Race and health: basic questions, emerging directions. *Ann Epidemiol. 7,* 322–333.

Williams, D. R. (2005). The health of U.S. racial and ethnic populations. *J Gerontol B, 60B,* 53–62.

Williams, D. R., and Mohammed, S. (2009). Discrimination and racial disparities in health: evidence and needed research. *J Behav Med, 32,* 20–47.

Williams, D. R., and Collins, C. A. (2001). Racial residential segregation: a fundamental cause of racial disparities in heath. *Public Health Rep, 116,* 404–415.

Williams, D. R., and Collins, C. A. (1995). U.S. socioeconomic and racial differences in health: patterns and explanations. *Annu Rev Sociol, 21,* 349–386.

Williams, D. R., Gonzalez, H., Williams, S., Mohammed, S., Moomal, H. et al (2008). Perceived discrimination, race and health in South Africa. *Soc Sci Med, 67,* 441–452.

Williams, D. R., Haile, R., Gonzalez, H., Neighbors, H., Baser, M. et al (2007a). The mental health of Black Caribbean Immigrants: results from the National Survey of American Life. *Am J Pub Health, 97,* 52–58.

Williams, D. R., Gonzalez, H. M., Neighbors, H., Nesse, R., Abelson, J. et al (2007b). Prevalence and distribution of major depressive disorder in African Americans, Caribbean Blacks, and Non-Hispanic Whites: results from the National Survey of American Life. *Arch Gen Psychiatry, 64,* 305–315.

Williams, D. R., Neighbors, H. W., and Jackson, J. S. (2003). Racial/ethnic discrimination and health: findings from community studies. *Am J Pub Health, 93,* 200–208.

World Health Organization. (2003). World health report– Statistical Annex: List of Member States by WHO Region and Mortality Stratum.

Wu, Z., and Schimmele, C. (2005). Racial/ethnic variation in functional and self-reported health. *Am J Public Health 95,* 710–716.

Yu, Z., Nissinen, A., Vartiainen, E., Hu, G., Tian, H. et al (2002). Socioeconomic status and serum lipids: a cross-sectional study in a Chinese urban population. *J Clin Epidemiol, 55,* 143–149.

Chapter 24

Neighborhood Factors in Health

Mahasin S. Mujahid and Ana V. Diez Roux

1 Introduction

Although the notion that "place matters" has ample historical roots in the public health and epidemiologic literature (Kawachi and Berkman, 2003a; Macintyre et al, 2002; Smith et al, 2001), there has been a resurgence of interest in the health effects of place in the last decades. This increased interest, as demonstrated by the explosion of the neighborhood health effects literature, is in part a function of three converging themes. First, researchers are beginning to recognize that variations in health cannot be solely explained by individual-level factors. In fact, human disease and illness arise from complex interactions of genetic, biological, social, and environmental factors operating at multiple levels of organization (Diez-Roux, 1998b; Schwartz et al, 1999). Moreover, the more proximal individual-level causes of disease are nested within organizational structures and contexts that are as important as individual-level characteristics for understanding disease etiology. The traditional practice of descriptive epidemiology, including the simple documentation of variations in health across places (i.e., countries, regions, states, and neighborhoods), is insufficient, and researchers have begun to explicitly investigate how and why place matters for health (Diez-Roux, 1998a; Schwartz et al, 1999).

The ability to investigate the multi-level determinants of disease has also been a function of advances in statistical methods. For example, multi-level modeling (Diez-Roux, 2000; Subramanian et al, 2003) provides a comprehensive approach to simultaneously studying neighborhoods or other contexts and individuals, allowing investigators to document effects of features of places (i.e., contextual factors) above and beyond the characteristics of the individuals that reside within them (i.e., compositional factors) (see Chapter 56). Other spatial analysis tools such as geographic information systems (Rushton, 2003), systems that can be used to capture, manage, and analyze spatially referenced data, also allow for more sophisticated examinations of the spatial patterning of health and its determinants.

A third factor contributing to recent interest in neighborhood health effects is the global and national commitment to understanding and eliminating social inequalities in health (CSDH, 2008; Davis, 1998). Public health researchers have drawn on literature in the social sciences (geography, sociology, urban planning) that provides both relevant theory and empirical documentation of how neighborhoods are socially patterned (Sampson, 2003). For example, theories on the concentration of poverty and patterns of residential segregation explain the spatial sorting and stratification of individuals across places. These theories highlight the notion that people of different socioeconomic and racial/ethnic backgrounds do not live in

M.S. Mujahid (✉)
Division of Epidemiology, University of California Berkeley, School of Public Health, 50 University Hall, #7360, Berkeley, CA 94720-7360, USA
e-mail: mmujahid@berkeley.edu

A. Steptoe (ed.), *Handbook of Behavioral Medicine*, DOI 10.1007/978-0-387-09488-5_24,
© Springer Science+Business Media, LLC 2010

the same areas (Jargowsky, 1997; Massey and Denton, 1993; Wilson, 1987). This differential sorting coupled with the differential distribution of health-enriching resources across these areas provides a lens for understanding how places contribute to health inequalities (Block et al, 2004; Moore and Diez Roux, 2006; Moore et al, 2008a).

Continued emphasis on the study of neighborhoods in relation to health may improve our understanding of disease processes and the manifestation of health inequalities. However, the study of neighborhood health effects also raises a number of theoretical and methodological challenges. A major challenge in the study of neighborhood health effects pertains to separating context from composition, or in other words determining whether differences in health outcomes across neighborhoods are due to the effects of neighborhood-level characteristics (sometimes referred to as contextual effects) or result simply from the fact that individuals with certain characteristics tend to live in certain types of neighborhoods (sometimes referred to as compositional effects). The ability to separate the two is crucial to drawing causal inferences regarding neighborhood effects (Duncan et al, 1998). Improved inferences regarding neighborhood effects will require addressing a series of challenges including: (1) defining and operationalizing neighborhood boundaries, (2) measuring neighborhood exposures, (3) improving study design and causal inference, and (4) accounting for time and life-course effects.

In this chapter, we briefly review selected past work on neighborhoods and health with a focus on behavioral outcomes. We then discuss challenges related to estimating these effects and provide examples of novel approaches to address these challenges. We illustrate our discussion drawing primarily on the literature on cardiovascular disease (CVD) risk factors and outcomes, which has been extensively studied in the neighborhood health effects literature (Chaix, 2009; Diez Roux, 2003). We highlight key issues and refer the reader to other sources for a more comprehensive review and discussion (Diez Roux,

2007; Kawachi and Berkman, 2003b; O'Campo, 2003; Oakes, 2004; Sampson et al, 2002).

2 Brief Summary of Past Work on Neighborhoods and Behavioral Outcomes

The neighborhood health effects literature is rapidly expanding. Early work was dominated by investigations of neighborhood socioeconomic environments in relation to a variety of health outcomes including: maternal and child health, chronic disease, health behaviors, mental health, and mortality (Kawachi and Berkman, 2003b; Leventhal and Brooks-Gunn, 2000; Pickett and Pearl, 2001; Truong and Ma, 2006). In general, this research suggests that living in socioeconomically disadvantaged neighborhoods is associated with worse health outcomes, independent of many individual-level factors. More recent work has examined specific features of neighborhood environments in relation to health. These features include measures of the neighborhood: (1) built/physical environment including land use patterns, density and access to destinations, street connectivity, access to healthy foods, and recreational resources and (2) social environment including safety/violence, social cohesion/social capital, collective efficacy, and signs of disorder. We briefly summarize this research in relation to a selection of behavioral and other related outcomes below.

2.1 Physical Activity

There have been several critical reviews of studies linking neighborhood physical and social environments to physical activity (Humpel et al, 2002; Kaczynski and Henderson, 2008; Saelens and Handy, 2008; see also Chapter 1). A review by Humpel and colleagues (2002) identified 19 studies between 1989 and 2001 examining the relationship between environmental attributes including perceived and objective measures of neighborhood physical environments in relation to physical activity behaviors. Physical activity behaviors were most consistently associated with the accessibility of facilities, opportunities for physical activity, and aesthetic quality. A later review in 2008 examined studies investigating the role of features of the built environments of neighborhoods in relation to physical activity function and intensity (Saelens and Handy, 2008). Fifty articles were indentified between 1998 and 2005 and the majority of these found significant positive relationships between the presence of resources for physical activity and residents physical activity levels. A final review in 2008 identified 29 new original articles and 13 in prior reviews published between 2002 and 2006 that investigated features of neighborhood built environments in relation to walking behavior (Kaczynski and Henderson, 2008). Results indicated that greater population density, more land use mix, and distance to non-residential destinations are linked to more walking for transportation. Additionally, better pedestrian infrastructure and aesthetic quality were also consistently associated with more walking for recreation.

Evidence regarding the relationship between features of the social environment of neighborhoods and physical activity is less consistent. For example, a recent review in 2008 identified 41 studies examining neighborhood safety/crime or other related measures (i.e., collective efficacy) and physical activity outcomes (Foster and Giles-Corti, 2008). Study results have been inconsistent, mostly likely because of measurement error due to the difficulties in assessing the social environment. However, more recent studies using more novel measurement techniques have documented associations (Bennett et al, 2007; McGinn et al, 2008; Sallis et al, 2007) between neighborhood safety and physical activity.

2.2 Diet

Studies examining the local food environment in relation to dietary habits have focused on the presence or absence of supermarkets as a proxy for healthy food availability. These studies have consistently documented associations between the presence of a supermarket and other retail stores and healthier dietary behaviors (i.e., high intake of fruits and vegetables, low calories from dietary fat, low total caloric intake) (Larson et al, 2009). Recent work has also documented associations between the presence of fast food restaurants and poor diet quality (Moore et al, 2009). An emerging body of work has begun to examine and document associations between the actual availability of healthy foods in retail stores and higher intake of healthy foods and greater home availability of healthy foods (Larson et al, 2009).

2.3 Body Mass Index and Obesity

Several reviews highlight the growing body of research examining features of the physical and social environments of neighborhoods in relation to body mass index (BMI) (Black and Macinko, 2008; Larson et al, 2009; Papas et al, 2007). For example, a review in 2007 identified 20 studies between 2002 and 2006 investigating associations between the built environments of neighborhoods in relation to BMI (Papas et al, 2007). The majority of these studies (17 out of 20) documented significant associations between an array of built environment measures and BMI. The most consistent associations were between greater walkability and access to recreational resources. There have also been recent studies linking the local retail environment to BMI/obesity. The results of this work suggested that poor access to supermarkets was associated with greater BMI (Larson et al, 2009).

A smaller body of work has examined features of the social environment of neighborhoods in relation to BMI with mixed results. While some studies have reported associations between poorer social environments (i.e., low collective efficacy/social cohesion, greater crime/violence, poorer aesthetic quality) and higher levels of BMI (Boehmer et al, 2007; Cohen et al, 2006;

Glass et al, 2006), several studies have also found no association or associations in the unexpected direction (Burdette et al, 2006; Mujahid et al, 2008a).

2.4 Summary

In general, studies investigating neighborhood physical environments in relation to behavioral outcomes suggest that residing in better environments (i.e., more access to healthy foods and resources for physical activity) is cross-sectionally associated with greater physical activity, healthier diets, and, to a lesser extent, lower BMI. The results are far less consistent regarding aspects of neighborhood social environments in relation to these outcomes. Many theoretical and methodological challenges exist to determine if these associations are causal. These challenges are discussed in the remainder of the chapter.

3 Theoretical and Methodological Considerations

3.1 Conceptualization and Measurement of Neighborhoods

The term "neighborhood" is widely used in public health research, and throughout this chapter, in part because it is a component of the popular contemporary lexicon. However, it is a concept that is difficult to precisely define and measure and many definitions exist across various disciplines. For example, in the sociological tradition, a neighborhood is an ecologic structure nested within a local community and includes a collection of people and institutions occupying a spatially defined area (Park, 1915; Suttles, 1972). This area is influenced by both internal and external forces such as historical, cultural, ecological, environmental, geographical, and political forces (Park, 1915; Suttles, 1972). Based on traditional definitions, neighborhoods are often

assumed to be nested and bounded structures that are discrete and non-overlapping (Chaskin, 1997). Additionally it is often assumed that neighborhoods need to be relatively homogeneous with respect to the exposures of interest (Pickett and Pearl, 2001). We will discuss alternative conceptualizations of neighborhoods that rely on a more "relational" as opposed to "spatial" understanding of neighborhoods (see Section 3.1.1).

In practice, neighborhoods are most often operationalized using administrative boundaries constructed by administrative agencies. In the US context, these boundaries are most consistently provided by the US Census Bureau and include counties, tracts, and block groups that vary in size between an average of 100,000 individuals per area (counties) to 1000 individuals per area (block groups) (U.S. Bureau of the Census, 1994). Zip codes, derived from the US Postal Service to facilitate efficient mail delivery, are also frequently used in the US context (U.S. Postal Service, 2003). There are a number of limitations to the use of administrative boundaries and a continuing debate over which of these areas is most appropriate and if they should be used at all (Krieger et al, 2002). Administrative boundaries are imperfect and considered mere proxies for the true geographical areas based on resident perceptions or historical and local knowledge. Additionally, different administrative boundaries vary dramatically in spatial scale. For example, census counties and zip codes are generally considered too large especially in trying to define homogeneous neighborhood exposures, a fundamental assumption of the statistical techniques used to create neighborhood variables and to relate them to health. Specifically, these methods require exposures that are more homogeneous than not in order to isolate neighborhood effects from the effects of compositional (individual-level) characteristics (Diez-Roux, 2000; Subramanian et al, 2003). In this regard, census tracts and block groups are preferred because they are smaller and were designed to be relatively homogeneous with respect to census-derived population and socioeconomic indicators. However, physical changes (i.e., changes in street patterns, highway construction, and other developments) as well as population growth and migration patterns cause the composition and boundaries of tracts and block groups to change over time. Moreover, because these areas are defined based on having an average number of individuals located within them, less densely populated areas are much larger in spatial scale as compared with more densely populated areas. For example, based on the 2000 US Census, tracts in more densely populated urban areas such as New York City, New York, are as small as 0.01 square miles. However, tracts in more rural and sparsely populated areas such as Santa Barbara, California, are as large as 1168 square miles (U.S. Bureau of the Census, 2000).

There are a number of benefits to using administratively defined neighborhood boundaries, which explains their wide use in the literature. Administrative data are readily available at no additional cost to researchers providing easy links to health outcomes data. In addition to pre-specified neighborhood boundaries, censuses also provide information on the sociodemographic characteristics of residents and these aggregate socioeconomic status (SES) measures are often used as proxies for neighborhood features in analyses. Measures based on administrative areas can also be obtained for very large geographic regions allowing for national analyses. Despite the fact that neighborhoods based on administrative definitions are likely to be very imperfect proxies for the spatial areas relevant to health, the fact that they have allowed detection of health-relevant associations suggests that features of these areas may be correlated with the true area-level constructs of interest.

Researchers have also attempted to characterize neighborhoods based on historical roots or resident perceptions. For example, mental maps have been developed as a technique of creating neighborhood boundaries based on residents' perceptions (Downs and Stea, 1973; Gould and White, 1974). This approach requires individuals to construct cognitive maps representing their relationship to space including the geographic boundaries that defined their daily lives based on physical (i.e., streets, highways, rivers, landmarks) and social elements (i.e., relationship and networks of friends and neighbors). These maps remain underused in the public health literature because it is hard to conduct them on a large scale and because there is a great deal of variability in resident perceptions. Studies have documented that perceptions of neighborhood boundaries vary significantly by individual characteristics such as age, gender, race/ethnicity, and social class (Anderson, 1990; Chaskin, 1997). Moreover, this approach is often dismissed as being overly subjective and impractical because of the difficulty in obtaining objective measures for these subjectively defined areas.

3.1.1 Spatial Scale

A more fundamental issue related to defining and operationalizing neighborhood boundaries is identifying the appropriate spatial scale. The different spatial scales represented in the literature are in part driven by data availability such that the most common option is the use of administrative sources with pre-specified boundaries at various spatial scales. However, the most relevant spatial scale for investigation depends on many other factors including: (1) the processes through which area features are hypothesized to affect specific health outcome, (2) the neighborhood exposures being measured, and (3) the most appropriate spatial scale for intervention or policy-relevant solutions. Different spatial scales may be more or less relevant for specific health processes under investigation. For example, the immediate area (i.e., smaller neighborhood boundaries) may be important for understanding how environmental exposures (i.e., toxins) relate to asthma. Alternatively, larger areas may be more appropriate for understanding how the presence of fast food restaurants shapes dietary behaviors. Misspecifying the spatial scale can result in bias consistent with exposure misclassification in epidemiologic research. Specifically, neighborhood exposures may be misclassified if the spatial scale most relevant to the process of interest is not used. This may result in spurious associations or lack of associations between neighborhood exposures and health outcomes. This problem is often referred to as the modifiable area unit problem (MAUP), the fact that the association detected between a geographic unit and an outcome is a function of the spatial scale used (Openshaw, 1984). Thus, using the wrong spatial scale or the wrong boundary within a correct spatial scale can produce biased results.

Because public health researchers are interested not only in studying problems but also in implementing solutions, decisions regarding the relevant spatial scale may be based on the potential for interventions or policy solutions. In some states (with more populated counties), local county governance determines how important resources such as courts, judicial systems, public transportation, welfare services, child and family services, hospitals, food and safety regulations, and environmental health services are distributed. As such, examining variations in health by counties may lead to results that are more amenable to local policy solutions. Similarly, considering definitions based on urban planning may also be useful. For example the city of New York consists of five boroughs and 59 community districts (New York City Department of City Planning, 2005). There are also hundreds of neighborhoods within these community districts with strong historical underpinning. However, goods and services are distributed at the community district level. Specifically, the department of city planning promotes strategic growth and development within each of the community districts providing an added incentive for investigating how features of these areas may relate to health.

Future research may benefit from a more careful consideration of the relevant spatial scale. However, there is limited theory available to inform our understanding on the appropriate spatial scale. For some research questions, multiple spatial scales may operate to affect the health processes under investigation. Additionally, although neighborhoods are most often studied in relation to health, there may

be features of larger geographic areas such as metropolitan areas, states, and regions that have important health implications. Thus, it is important to understand how neighborhoods are located within surrounding areas and how features of these non-residential or surrounding environments may also matter for health. To this end, a growing body of research has examined neighborhood processes in relation to multiple spatial scales and has considered both local neighborhoods and surrounding neighborhoods in relation to health (Auchincloss et al, 2007; Chaix et al, 2005; Morenoff, 2003; Robert and Ruel, 2006). For example, Auchincloss and colleagues (2007) investigated associations between neighborhood poverty and insulin resistance, considering both neighborhood poverty within the local neighborhood and the distance to a wealthy neighborhood. They found that although neighborhood poverty was positively associated with insulin resistance, the distance to a wealthy area was also positively associated with insulin resistance. These findings suggest that while living in a poor neighborhood is problematic, so is living in close proximity to other poor neighborhoods.

In a similar vein, researchers are also beginning to conceptualize and operationalize neighborhoods based on more relational considerations. For example, some researchers argue that contrary to popular belief, neighborhoods are actually unstructured and unbounded constellations of connections and interactions between people (Castree, 2004; Graham and Healey, 1999). This conceptualization highlights the fluid and dynamic nature of neighborhood environments and challenges assumptions regarding our ability to tease out contextual versus compositional effects. The reality is that neighborhoods shape people and people shape neighborhoods and these relationships change over time (Cummins et al, 2007).

As a final note, neighborhoods and other geographic areas represent only one of many important contexts that may have health-relevant properties. Other important contexts such as school and work environments have also been studied in relation to health. Future research may benefit from considering how individuals exist within multiple overlapping contexts which may matter for health (Muntaner et al, 2006; Szapocznik et al, 2006). Statistical methods such as cross-classified random effects models make this type of investigation possible (Subramanian et al, 2003).

3.2 Measuring Neighborhood Exposures

Another important challenge in the study of neighborhood heath effects is the measurement of neighborhood exposures. Two important questions illustrate the scope of this challenge: (1) What are the relevant features of neighborhoods important for health? (2) How does one obtain information on these features? With regard to the first question, most studies examining neighborhoods in relation to health investigate the socioeconomic characteristics of neighborhoods. These census-derived indicators are readily available and easily linked to health outcomes data and have been studied in relation to CVD risk factors and outcomes. Specifically studies have consistently documented associations between neighborhood

disadvantage or deprivation and increased CVD risk, morbidity, and mortality (Diez Roux et al, 2001; Sundquist et al, 2004). However, documenting associations between neighborhood socioeconomic indicators and health provides few clues as to the underlying important health-relevant features. It also does not shed light on the pathways by which neighborhoods impact a particular health outcome (Diez Roux, 2001). Establishing evidence of these pathways is important to drawing causal inferences and to identifying important interventions.

The specific features of neighborhoods that are most health relevant are likely to differ for each health outcome. For this reason, beginning with a clear conceptual framework is an important pre-requisite for delineating these features and the pathways by which they impact health. Figure 24.1 shows a conceptual framework of neighborhood environments in relation to CVD. The framework highlights features of the physical and social features of neighborhood environments and the hypothesized pathways by which they may impact CVD risk. For example, neighborhood availability and relative cost of health foods may impact diet quality which in turn may impact more proximate biological risk factors such as BMI and hypertension. Alternatively, neighborhood crime may have a direct impact on

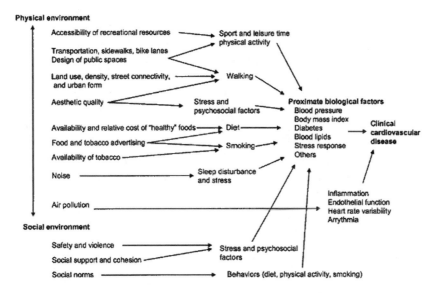

Fig. 24.1 Schematic representation of possible pathways linking residential environments to cardiovascular risk

CVD through stress processes. Such frameworks have been an important omission in the literature. An increased usage of conceptual frameworks may serve to address important critiques regarding the atheoretical and data-driven nature of some research in this area (Macintyre et al, 2002; O'Campo, 2003).

Consistent with the aforementioned conceptual framework, researchers have begun to measure potentially health-relevant features of neighborhoods. These include measures of physical environment such as access to health-enriching resources including the density and accessibility of opportunities for engaging in physical activity and purchasing affordable healthy foods (Mujahid et al, 2007). Measures of the built environment have also been measured such as land use patterns (mix of commercial and residential spaces), the presence and amount of green space, street connectivity, and housing density (Handy et al, 2002). Finally measures of the presence of ill-health promoting facilities (i.e., the presence and density of liquor stores and fast food restaurants) and features of the social environment such as collective efficacy, social cohesion, and informal social control have also been considered (Mujahid et al, 2007). These novel measures have been increasingly studied in relation to health in general and cardiovascular health in particular (Auchincloss et al, 2009; Augustin et al, 2008; Moore et al, 2009; Mujahid et al, 2008b).

A major challenge in measuring specific health-relevant features of neighborhood environments involves the second issue, obtaining data on these features. Administrative data sources can sometimes be used to obtain information on specific health-relevant features. For example, proprietary data sources can provide information on the presence of businesses and facilities in a given area. The linkages of these geo-referenced data sources to health study data are made possible through Geographical Information System (GIS) technology (Rushton, 2003). In addition to linking data sources, GIS can be used to create sophisticated measures of spatial accessibility including density measures such as kernel densities which allow for smoothing densities over space to create neighborhood specific measures for various spatial scales and various neighborhood definitions.

Neighborhood environments can also be assessed using data from individuals. There are three general approaches to this type of investigation. The first two approaches involve asking individuals to report on neighborhood characteristics via a self-administered survey. In the first approach, each health study participant provides an assessment of his or her neighborhood. These measures of neighborhoods can then be examined in relation to a particular health outcome. Information on neighborhood environments can also be obtained from an informant sample of individuals who reside in the same areas as the health study participants but who themselves are not participants (Mujahid et al, 2007). Through administration of a neighborhood survey, information can be obtained on various dimensions of neighborhood environments and can then be linked to study participants. While the first approach has the benefit of feasibility, it is limited by the potential for same-source bias, the process by which obtaining information on self-reported neighborhood features and self-reported outcomes may result in spurious associations if both types of reports are affected by underlying propensities of the individual. Moreover, the outcome may affect an individual's assessment of the neighborhood exposure. For example, individuals who are physically inactive may report few opportunities for physical activity provided by the neighborhood, irrespective of the actual availability. The use of an information sample can reduce this source of bias. An additional benefit of the second approach is that there can be a more detailed assessment of the neighborhood environment. The often broad scope of health studies usually limits the ability of an in-depth investigation of any given area. Moreover, the use of informants allows denser sampling and multiple responses can be aggregated across areas to obtain more reliable and valid estimates of neighborhood properties. (Mujahid et al, 2007).

A final approach to obtaining information on neighborhood environments is the use of systematic social observation by which a team of trained investigators assess the neighborhood environments based on a set of systematic criteria (Sampson and Raudenbush, 1999). While this approach may allow for more objective and systematic characterizations of neighborhood environments, it can be very time and labor intensive limiting its feasibility and use in the public health literature. Additionally, this approach may not provide an accurate assessment of the social environments of neighborhoods because it is very difficult as an outsider to observe features such as neighborhood social cohesion or crime.

Recent studies have begun to compare associations between specific features of neighborhood environments in relation to health using multiple methods of collecting neighborhood measures (Moore et al, 2008). For example, Moore and colleagues examined measures of neighborhood food environments in relation to diet quality. They found that the food environment as measured by a proprietary data source, perceptions of health study participants, and perceptions of an informant sample produced comparable results in terms of the direction and magnitude of associations with diet quality.

3.2.1 From Psychometrics to Ecometrics

As more researchers are developing neighborhood measures based on individual assessments (i.e., informant sample or systematic social observation), advanced methods have been developed to examine the measurement properties of these approaches. Because these measures are obtained via questionnaire, neighborhood measures are constructed by aggregating survey items within a particular construct to create a summary measure. Traditional psychometric assessments can only characterize the validity and reliability of measures based on two levels of data (i.e., scale items nested within individuals). For example, the internal consistency has been used to assess the extent to which responses to scale items are consistent

within individuals. However, ecometrics, developed as an extension of psychometrics, considers the additional nested structure of the data (i.e., scale items nested within individuals, nested within neighborhoods) (Raudenbush and Sampson, 1999). Thus, these methods can allow investigators to additionally assess the extent to which individuals within the same neighborhood agree on their assessment of neighborhood conditions (Raudenbush and Sampson, 1999). These approaches are increasingly being used in the literature (Mujahid et al, 2007).

3.3 Improving Study Design and Causal Inference

Another major challenge in neighborhood health research relates to the fact that the majority of studies are observational which limits the ability to draw causal inferences. One limitation of observational studies is their inability to randomly assign individuals to be exposed versus unexposed and thereby balance the distribution of measured and unmeasured confounding variables. This problem, common to all observational studies, is often referred to as the "selection problem" in the neighborhood health effects literature (Oakes, 2004). The selection issue represents the phenomenon by which individuals residing in different neighborhoods also differ in their individual-level characteristics that may also impact the health outcome. For example, it is well known that disease and illness are socially patterned such that individuals with less education and income have a worse health profile. Because these same individuals are also more likely to reside in disadvantaged neighborhoods, any association between neighborhood disadvantage and health can be attributed to individual-level socioeconomic position.

Regression methods allow investigators to adjust for confounding, however, problems arise when there is residual confounding due to the inability to collect information on all confounding variables or when those included are measured with error. Statistical models assume exchangeability of exposed and unexposed, individuals conditional on covariates in the model. This assumption may be violated when there is limited overlap between the confounders and the exposures of interest resulting in estimates based on extrapolations to sections of the distribution with very little data. For example, if there is very little overlap in the distribution of neighborhood poverty between individuals of low and high socioeconomic position (i.e., poor individuals live only in poor neighborhoods and wealthy individuals live only in wealthy neighborhoods), then estimates of the associations of neighborhood poverty with health outcomes after "statistically adjusting" for individual-level socioeconomic position will be based on extrapolations because there are few if any poor individuals in wealthy neighborhoods (and vice versa) on which to base these estimates. Other methods such as propensity score matching allow investigators to empirically test for non-overlapping distributions (Rubin, 1997; Wooldridge, 2002) and therefore better determine the assumptions implicit in the comparisons.

3.4 Causal Diagrams

Statistical analyses of observational data may benefit from systematic approaches to determine the variables that should and should not be adjusted for. Tools such as directed acyclic graphs (DAGs) which represent the causal relationships between exposures, outcomes, and other covariates can be very useful in this regard (Greenland et al, 1999). DAGs are useful in identifying the appropriate statistical specifications of controlling and stratifying variables in order to achieve causal estimates of a particular exposure in relation to an outcome. Often there is an over-control for variables that are on the causal pathway between an exposure and a disease especially when dealing with such distal factors such as neighborhood environments. In some situations, adjustment can introduce rather than control for confounding (Fleischer and Diez Roux, 2008). DAGS can be used to explore

different situations and help develop an analytic plan.

3.4.1 Randomization

There has been one attempt to study neighborhood effects in a randomized trial setting, the Moving to Opportunity Project (Goering and Feins, 2003). In this study, individuals in poor neighborhoods were randomized to either stay in that area or move to a non-poor area (based on a pre-specified set of criteria). The obvious advantage of this approach is that it randomizes individuals to living in different neighborhoods and therefore improves our ability to draw causal inferences. However, even in this randomized design, questions remain. For example, the extent to which persons randomized to move to a non-poor area actually experienced a significant improvement in neighborhood conditions has been questioned (Clark, 2008). A bigger issue is the fact that this was an experiment on the effect of moving and not the effect of improving neighborhood environments. Given the complexities of randomized experiments in this field, a number of researchers have called for better use of natural experiments and quasi-experimental designs to identify the health impact of changes in neighborhood conditions.

3.5 Accounting for Time and Life-Course Effects

Although a number of longitudinal studies of neighborhood health effects have been published (Auchincloss et al, 2009; Diez Roux, 2001; Sundquist et al, 2004), most studies in neighborhood health effects are cross-sectional and measure neighborhood exposures and health outcomes at a single point in time. In addition to the inability to avoid endogeneity (i.e., the possibility that health is causally related to residential location), these studies are unable to answer questions regarding the timescale over which neighborhood health effects operate or the time lags involved. Some concerns regarding endogeneity are addressed with the increasing number of cohort studies that have examined neighborhood environments in relation to changes in health behaviors or conditions over time or in relation to incident disease (Auchincloss et al, 2009; Diez Roux, 2001; Mujahid et al, 2005; Sundquist et al, 2004). However, these studies often do not provide any insight into the timescales most relevant for neighborhood health effects, especially for conditions that are chronic in nature and develop over long periods. Moreover, few studies have investigated neighborhood environment over the life course (Chichlowska et al, 2009; Pollitt et al, 2007, 2008). Future research may benefit from investigations of neighborhood environments early in the life course in addition to the cumulative effect of neighborhood environments in relation to health.

4 Conclusion

As research continues to grow in the area of neighborhood health effects, it is important to continue to address the theoretical and methodological challenges. In this chapter we have highlighted a few of these challenges and provided examples of the novel and creative methods that researchers are using to overcome them. As we seek to improve our understanding of how neighborhoods are causally related to health, continued efforts need to consider multidisciplinary approaches and solutions that bring together epidemiologists, sociologists, geographers, urban planners, and policy makers in an effort to understand how neighborhoods affect health and develop strategies to create healthy sustainable neighborhoods.

References

Anderson, E. (1990). *Streetwise: Race, Class, and Change in an Urban Community*. Chicago: University of Chicago Press.

Auchincloss, A. H., Diez Roux, A. V., Brown, D. G., O'Meara, E. S., and Raghunathan, T. E. (2007). Association of insulin resistance with distance to wealthy areas: the multi-ethnic study of atherosclerosis. *Am J Epidemiol, 165*, 389–397.

Auchincloss, A. H., Diez Roux, A. V., Mujahid, M. S., Shen, M., Bertoni, A. G. et al (2009). Neighborhood resources for physical activity and healthy foods and incidence of type 2 diabetes mellitus: the Multi-Ethnic study of Atherosclerosis. *Arch Intern Med, 169*, 1698–1704.

Augustin, T., Glass, T. A., James, B. D., and Schwartz, B. S. (2008). Neighborhood psychosocial hazards and cardiovascular disease: the Baltimore Memory Study. *Am J Public Health, 98*, 1664–1670.

Bennett, G. G., McNeill, L. H., Wolin, K. Y., Duncan, D. T., Puleo, E. et al (2007). Safe to walk? Neighborhood safety and physical activity among public housing residents. *PLoS Med, 4*, 1599–1606.

Black, J. L., and Macinko, J. (2008). Neighborhoods and obesity. *Nutr Rev, 66*, 2–20.

Block, J. P., Scribner, R. A., and DeSalvo, K. B. (2004). Fast food, race/ethnicity, and income: a geographic analysis. *Am J Prev Med, 27*, 211–217.

Boehmer, T. K., Hoehner, C. M., Deshpande, A. D., Brennan Ramirez, L. K., and Brownson, R. C. (2007). Perceived and observed neighborhood indicators of obesity among urban adults. *Int J Obes, 31*, 968–977.

Burdette, H. L., Wadden, T. A., and Whitaker, R. C. (2006). Neighborhood safety, collective efficacy, and obesity in women with young children. *Obesity, 14*, 518–525.

Castree, N. (2004). Differential geographies: place, indigenous rights and 'local' resources. *Political Geogr, 23*, 133–167.

Chaix, B. (2009). Geographic life environments and coronary heart disease: a literature review, theoretical contributions, methodological updates, and a research agenda. *Annu Rev Public Health, 30*, 81–105.

Chaix, B., Merlo, J., and Chauvin, P. (2005). Comparison of a spatial approach with the multilevel approach for investigating place effects on health: the example of healthcare utilisation in France. *J Epidemiol Community Health, 59*, 517–526.

Chaskin, R. J. (1997). Perspectives on neighborhood and community: a review of the literature. *Soc Serv Rev, 71*, 521–547.

Chichlowska, K. L., Rose, K. M., Diez-Roux, A. V., Golden, S. H., McNeill, A. M. et al (2009). Life course socioeconomic conditions and metabolic syndrome in adults: The Atherosclerosis Risk in Communities (ARIC) Study. *Ann Epidemiol, 19*, 875–883.

Clark, W. A. (2008). Reexamining the moving to opportunity study and its contribution to changing the distribution of poverty and ethnic concentration. *Demography, 45*, 515–535.

Cohen, D. A., Finch, B. K., Bower, A., and Sastry, N. (2006). Collective efficacy and obesity: the potential influence of social factors on health. *Soc Sci Med, 62*, 769–778.

CSDH. (2008). *Closing the Gap in a Generation: Health Equity Through Action on the Social Determinants of Health. Final Report of the Commission on Social Determinants of Health.* Geneva: World Health Organization.

Cummins, S., Curtis, S., Diez-Roux, A. V., and Macintyre, S. (2007). Understanding and representing 'place' in health research: a relational approach. *Soc Sci Med, 65*, 1825–1838.

Davis, R. M. (1998). "Healthy people 2010": national health objectives for the United States. *BMJ, 317*, 1513–1517.

Diez-Roux, A. V. (1998a). Bringing context back into epidemiology: variables and fallacies in multilevel analysis. *Am J Public Health, 88*, 216–222.

Diez-Roux, A. V. (1998b). On genes, individuals, society, and epidemiology. *Am J Epidemiol, 148*, 1027–1032.

Diez-Roux, A. V. (2000). Multilevel analysis in public health research. *Annu Rev Public Health, 21*, 171–192.

Diez Roux, A. V. (2001). Investigating neighborhood and area effects on health. *Am J Public Health, 91*, 1783–1789.

Diez Roux, A. V. (2003). Residential environments and cardiovascular risk. *J Urban Health, 80*, 569–589.

Diez Roux, A. V. (2007). Neighborhoods and health: where are we and were do we go from here? *Rev Epidemiol Sante Publique, 55*, 13–21.

Diez Roux, A. V., Merkin, S. S., Arnett, D., Chambless, L., Massing, M. et al (2001). Neighborhood of residence and incidence of coronary heart disease. *N Engl J Med, 345*, 99–106.

Downs, R. M., and Stea, D. (1973). Cognitive maps and spatial behavior: process and products. In R. M. Downs & D. Stea (Eds.), *Image and Environment*. Chicago: Aldine Publishing Company.

Duncan, C., Jones, K., and Moon, G. (1998). Context, composition and heterogeneity: using multilevel models in health research. *Soc Sci Med, 46*, 97–117.

Fleischer, N. L., and Diez Roux, A. V. (2008). Using directed acyclic graphs to guide analyses of neighborhood health effects: an introduction. *J Epidemiol Community Health, 62*, 842–846.

Foster, S., and Giles-Corti, B. (2008). The built environment, neighborhood crime and constrained physical activity: an exploration of inconsistent findings. *Prev Med, 47*, 241–251.

Glass, T. A., Rasmussen, M. D., and Schwartz, B. S. (2006). Neighborhoods and obesity in older adults: the Baltimore Memory Study. *Am J Prev Med, 31*, 455–463.

Goering, J. M., and Feins, J. D. (2003). *Choosing a Better Life?: Evaluating the Moving to Opportunity Social Experiment*. Washington, DC: Urban Institute Press.

Gould, P., and White, R. R. (1974). *Mental Maps*. New York: Penguin.

Graham, S., and Healey, P. (1999). Relational concepts of space and place: issues for planning theory and practice. *Euro Planning Studies, 7*, 623–646.

Greenland, S., Pearl, J., and Robins, J. M. (1999). Causal diagrams for epidemiologic research. *Epidemiology, 10*, 37–48.

Handy, S. L., Boarnet, M. G., Ewing, R., and Killingsworth, R. E. (2002). How the built environment affects physical activity: views from urban planning. *Am J Prev Med, 23*(2 Suppl), 64–73.

Humpel, N., Owen, N., and Leslie, E. (2002). Environmental factors associated with adults' participation in physical activity: a review. *Am J Prev Med, 22*, 188–199.

Jargowsky, P. A. (1997). *Poverty and Place: Ghettos, Barrios, and the American City*. New York: Russell Sage Foundation.

Kaczynski, A. T., and Henderson, K. A. (2008). Parks and recreation settings and active living: a review of associations with physical activity function and intensity. *J Phys Act Health, 5*, 619–632.

Kawachi, I., and Berkman, L. F. (2003a). Introduction. In I. Kawachi & L. F. Berkman (Eds.), *Neighborhoods and Health* (pp. 1–42). Oxford; New York: Oxford University Press.

Kawachi, I., and Berkman, L. F. (2003b). *Neighborhoods and Health*. Oxford; New York: Oxford University Press.

Krieger, N., Chen, J. T., Waterman, P. D., Soobader, M. J., Subramanian, S. V. et al (2002). Geocoding and monitoring of US socioeconomic inequalities in mortality and cancer incidence: does the choice of area-based measure and geographic level matter?: the Public Health Disparities Geocoding Project. *Am J Epidemiol, 156*, 471–82.

Larson, N. I., Story, M. T., and Nelson, M. C. (2009). Neighborhood environments: disparities in access to healthy foods in the U.S. *Am J Prev Med, 36*, 74–81.

Leventhal, T., and Brooks-Gunn, J. (2000). The neighborhoods they live in: the effects of neighborhood residence on child and adolescent outcomes. *Psychol Bull, 126*, 309–337.

Macintyre, S., Ellaway, A., and Cummins, S. (2002). Place effects on health: how can we conceptualise, operationalise and measure them? *Soc Sci Med, 55*, 125–139.

Massey, D. S., and Denton, N. A. (1993). *American Apartheid: Segregation and the Making of the Underclass*. Cambridge, MA: Harvard University Press.

McGinn, A. P., Evenson, K. R., Herring, A. H., Huston, S. L., and Rodriguez, D. A. (2008). The association of perceived and objectively measured crime with physical activity: a cross-sectional analysis. *J Phys Act Health, 5*, 117–131.

Moore, L. V., and Diez Roux, A. V. (2006). Associations of neighborhood characteristics with the location and type of food stores. *Am J Public Health, 96*, 325–331.

Moore, L. V., Diez Roux, A. V., Evenson, K. R., McGinn, A. P., and Brines, S. J. (2008a). Availability of recreational resources in minority and low socioeconomic status areas. *Am J Prev Med, 34*, 16–22.

Moore, L. V., Diez Roux, A. V., Nettleton, J. A., Jacobs, D. R., and Franco, M. (2009). Fast-food consumption, diet quality, and neighborhood exposure to fast food: the multi-ethnic study of atherosclerosis. *Am J Epidemiol, 170*, 29–36.

Moore, L. V., Diez Roux, A. V., Nettleton, J. A., and Jacobs, D. R. Jr. (2008b). Associations of the local food environment with diet quality--a comparison of assessments based on surveys and geographic information systems: the multi-ethnic study of atherosclerosis. *Am J Epidemiol, 167*, 917–924.

Morenoff, J. D. (2003). Neighborhood mechanisms and the spatial dynamics of birth weight. *Am J Soc, 108*, 976–1017.

Mujahid, M. S., Diez Roux, A. V., Borrell, L. N., and Nieto, F. J. (2005). Cross-sectional and longitudinal associations of BMI with socioeconomic characteristics. *Obes Res, 13*, 1412–1421.

Mujahid, M. S., Diez Roux, A. V., Morenoff, J. D., and Raghunathan, T. (2007). Assessing the measurement properties of neighborhood scales: from psychometrics to ecometrics. *Am J Epidemiol, 165*, 858–867.

Mujahid, M. S., Diez Roux, A. V., Morenoff, J. D., Raghunathan, T. E., Cooper, R. S. et al (2008b). Neighborhood characteristics and hypertension. *Epidemiology, 19*, 590–598.

Mujahid, M. S., Diez Roux, A. V., Shen, M., Gowda, D., Sanchez, B. et al (2008a). Relation between neighborhood environments and obesity in the Multi-Ethnic Study of Atherosclerosis. *Am J Epidemiol, 167*, 1349–1357.

Muntaner, C., Li, Y., Xue, X., Thompson, T., O'Campo, P., Chung, H. et al (2006). County level socioeconomic position, work organization and depression disorder: a repeated measures cross-classified multilevel analysis of low-income nursing home workers. *Health Place, 12*, 688–700.

New York City Department of City Planning. (2005). New York: a city of neighborhoods. http://www.nyc.gov/html/dcp/html/neighbor/neigh.shtml

O'Campo, P. (2003). Invited commentary: advancing theory and methods for multilevel models of residential neighborhoods and health. *Am J Epidemiol, 157*, 9–13.

Oakes, J. M. (2004). The (mis)estimation of neighborhood effects: causal inference for a practicable social epidemiology. *Soc Sci Med, 58*, 1929–1952.

Openshaw, W. (1984). *The Modifiable Area Unit Problem. Concepts and Techniques in Modern Geography No. 38. Geo Books.* Norwich, CT.

Papas, M. A., Alberg, A. J., Ewing, R., Helzlsouer, K. J., Gary, T. L. et al (2007). The built environment and obesity. *Epidemiol Rev, 29*, 129–143.

Park, R. E. (1915). The city: suggestions for the investigation of human behavior in the city environment. *Am J Soc, 20*, 577.

Pickett, K. E., and Pearl, M. (2001). Multilevel analyses of neighborhood socioeconomic context and health outcomes: a critical review. *J Epidemiol Community Health, 55*, 111–122.

Pollitt, R. A., Kaufman, J. S., Rose, K. M., Diez-Roux, A. V., Zeng, D. et al (2007). Early-life and adult socioeconomic status and inflammatory risk markers in adulthood. *Eur J Epidemiol, 22*, 55–66.

Pollitt, R. A., Kaufman, J. S., Rose, K. M., Diez-Roux, A. V., Zeng, D. et al (2008). Cumulative life course and adult socioeconomic status and markers of inflammation in adulthood. *J Epidemiol Community Health, 62*, 484–491.

Raudenbush, S. W., and Sampson, R. J. (1999). Ecometrics: towards a science of assessing ecological settings, with applications to the systematic social observation of neighborhoods. *Soc Methodol, 29*, 1–41.

Robert, S. A., and Ruel, E. (2006). Racial segregation and health disparities between black and white older adults. *J Gerontol B Psychol Sci Soc Sci, 61*(4), S203–211.

Rubin, D. B. (1997). Estimating causal effects from large data sets using propensity scores. *Ann Intern Med, 127*, 757–763.

Rushton, G. (2003). Public health, GIS, and spatial analytic tools. *Annu Rev Public Health, 24*, 43–56.

Saelens, B. E., and Handy, S. L. (2008). Built environment correlates of walking: a review. *Med Sci Sports Exerc, 40*(7 Suppl), S550–566.

Sallis, J. F., King, A. C., Sirard, J. R., and Albright, C. L. (2007). Perceived environmental predictors of physical activity over 6 months in adults: activity counseling trial. *Health Psychol, 26*, 701–709.

Sampson, R. J. (2003). Neighborhood-level context and health: lessons from Sociology. In I. Kawachi & L. F. Berkman (Eds.), *Neighborhoods and Health* (pp. 132–146). Oxford; New York: Oxford University Press.

Sampson, R. J., Morenoff, J. D., and Gannon-Rowley, T. (2002). Assessing "Neighborhood Effects": social processes and new directions in research. *Annu Rev Soc, 28*, 443–478.

Sampson, R. J., and Raudenbush, S. W. (1999). Systematic social observation of public spaces: a new look at disorder in urban neighborhoods. *Am J Soc, 105*, 603–651.

Schwartz, S., Susser, E., and Susser, M. (1999). A future for epidemiology? *Annu Rev Public Health, 20*, 15–33.

Smith, G. D., Dorling, D., and Shaw, M. (2001). *Poverty, Inequality and Health in Britain, 1800–2000: A Reader*. Bristol: Policy Press.

Subramanian, S. V., Jones, K., and Duncan, C. (2003). Multilevel methods for public health research. In I. Kawachi & L. F. Berkman (Eds.), *Neighborhoods and Health* (pp. 65–111). Oxford; New York: Oxford University Press.

Sundquist, K., Winkleby, M., Ahlen, H., and Johansson, S. E. (2004). Neighborhood socioeconomic environment and incidence of coronary heart disease: a follow-up study of 25,319 women and men in Sweden. *Am J Epidemiol, 159,* 655–662.

Suttles, G. D. (1972). *The social Construction of Communities.* Chicago: University of Chicago Press.

Szapocznik, J., Lombard, J., Martinez, F., Mason, C. A., Gorman-Smith, D. et al (2006). The impact of the built environment on children's school conduct grades: the role of diversity of use in a Hispanic neighborhood. *Am J Community Psychol, 38,* 299–310.

Truong, K. D., and Ma, S. (2006). A systematic review of relations between neighborhoods and mental health. *J Ment Health Policy Econ, 9,* 137–154.

U.S. Bureau of the Census. (1994). Geographic areas reference manual. http://www.census. gov/geo/www/garm.html

U.S. Bureau of the Census. (2000). American fact finder. http://factfinder.census.gov

U.S. Postal Service. (2003). *The United States Postal Service: An American History 1775–2002*: U.S. Postal Serviceo. Document Number

Wilson, W. J. (1987). *The Truly Disadvantaged: The Inner City, the Underclass, and Public Policy.* Chicago: University of Chicago Press.

Wooldridge, J. (2002). Inverse probability weighted M-estimators for sample selection, attrition, and stratification. *Portuguese Econ J, 1,* 117–139.

Chapter 25

Health Literacy: A Brief Introduction

Michael S. Wolf, Stacy Cooper Bailey, and Kirsten J. McCaffery

1 Introduction

Clear and effective communication is a fundamental component of quality healthcare. There is
an assumption that patients possess an adequate
set of skills to understand the health information provided to them and to take the appropriate actions in response. While individuals must
have the motivation to engage in various health
roles, they must also be able to access, understand, and eventually apply health information to
support actions. Comprehension of health information is therefore a highly important outcome
and arguably a necessary "precondition" for the
later adoption of sustainable health behaviors; it
is often described as such in prominent health
behavior theories (Ajzen, 1991; Janz et al, 2003).
However, possessing knowledge alone will not
necessarily directly link to recommended behaviors (Wolf et al, 2006a). Rather, intrinsic and
extrinsic motivational influences assume prominent roles in determining whether or not one
engages in a particular action. Regardless, the
value of health literacy as a public health concept
is undeniable, and it has been framed as a matter
of clear health communication, and also health
literacy addresses issues of healthcare equity,
safety, and quality (Institute of Medicine, 2004,
2009).

In this chapter, we review the meaning of
health literacy, its associations with health outcomes, and recommended approaches for intervention. A conceptual framework deconstructing
the health literacy skill set is specifically identified and guidance offered for incorporating this
relatively new construct into the design of robust
and complimentary strategies applicable to the
field of behavioral medicine.

2 Definition and Measurement

The definition of health literacy widely accepted
by the Institute of Medicine (IOM) and also
National Library of Medicine (NLM) in the
United States is the "degree to which individuals have the capacity to obtain, process, and
understand basic health information and services
needed to make appropriate health decisions"
(Institute of Medicine, 2004). It is a multi-
faceted concept, although reading ability has
been viewed as its most fundamental component. An individual's ability to read, comprehend, and take action based on health-related
material may be closely related to a more general ability to read comprehend and take action
based on other types of materials (Rudd, 2007).
However, the context of healthcare is likely to
be an especially challenging environment for
many due to its changing nature and complexity. What one must do to promote, protect, and

M.S. Wolf (✉)
Division of General Internal Medicine, Feinberg School
of Medicine, Northwestern University, 750 N. Lake
Shore Drive, 10th Floor, Chicago, IL 60611, USA
e-mail: mswolf@northwestern.edu

A. Steptoe (ed.), *Handbook of Behavioral Medicine*, DOI 10.1007/978-0-387-09488-5_25,   355
© Springer Science+Business Media, LLC 2010

manage health is likely to be more difficult and often less familiar than what may be required of an individual in other settings, with far more serious consequences associated with inadequate performance.

At the individual level, health literacy involves one's ability to apply existing functional literacy skills toward learning and communicating effectively in the context of healthcare (Baker, 2006). Functional literacy, however, includes far more than one's ability to read text in print materials. Rather, literacy and *health literacy* skills encompass a broad range of cognitive and social processes involved in the act of comprehending and responding to both oral and print communication. Individuals therefore need to have adequate listening and speaking skills, numeracy ability, reasoning and conceptual knowledge to engage in routine self-care and way-finding activities to navigate complex healthcare systems.

In its seminal 2004 health literacy report *A Prescription to End Confusion*, the IOM recognized that patients' health-related knowledge, skills, and subsequent behaviors are heavily influenced by (1) cultural background, (2) prior learning opportunities, and (3) health system demands (Institute of Medicine, 2004). Given the latter, it is difficult to truly isolate with precision the knowledge and skills one must possess to have "adequate" health literacy, as the complexity of the health system is a major determinant. To this end, the IOM report appropriately has framed limited health literacy not as a problem situated within the individual, rather as a challenge to healthcare providers and health systems to reach out and more effectively communicate with patients and families.

While the accepted definition is basically the same in the United Kingdom as in the United States, it should be noted that many studying the topic in continental Europe have expanded the concept of health literacy to not only include basic health competencies but also citizen competencies. This means individuals must share in the public health responsibility of promoting and protecting health in a society, suggesting that each individual must play the role of an empowered and informed consumer of healthcare services (Kickbusch et al, 2006; Nutbeam, 2008).

3 Epidemiology of Limited Health Literacy

Typically, estimates of limited health literacy have been based on national functional literacy assessments, which are prevalent among many countries (Rudd, 2007). In the United States, the National Assessment of Adult Literacy (NAAL) of 2003 reported that 14% of American adults possess skills in the lowest level of prose and document literacy ("below basic"), and 22% are at the lowest level for quantitative literacy (Kutner et al, 2005). These individuals can perform only the most simple and concrete tasks associated with each of these domains. However, those with only "basic" literacy proficiency have limited abilities and are likely to be hindered in routine daily activities. When considering individuals with basic and below basic skills combined, as many as 34 55% of adults in the United States have limited literacy skills. Estimates are significantly higher among the elderly; 60% of individuals over the age of 65 have limited levels of prose and document literacy.

These general estimates may not give the full picture for health literacy. As described earlier, reading fluency and the full range of literacy skills are likely to vary with an individual's familiarity with content (Rudd et al, 2004). Health materials and encounters may be more likely to use difficult and often-unclarified medical terms that are unfamiliar to many individuals (Castro et al, 2007). Therefore, estimates of limited health literacy based on general functional literacy surveys are likely to underestimate the problem. As a response to this concern, The NAAL (2003) included the first national health literacy assessment. The report showed the average health literacy scores of Americans to be lower than average general literacy scores of adults, as measured by the NAAL.

In fact, only 12% of adults were identified as having "proficient" health literacy skills, as most (53%) fell into an intermediate classification. The NAAL report concluded that a large numbers of American adults – especially the elderly, socioeconomically disadvantaged, and those belonging to racial/ethnic minority groups or living in rural areas – lack the health literacy skills to effectively access, understand, and use health materials to accomplish challenging health-related tasks.

3.1 Extent and Associations

While the relationship between health literacy and health outcomes is not entirely clear, there are plausible mechanisms by which literacy could directly affect health behaviors, compliance with medications, and other pathways to health (Baker, 1999; DeWalt et al, 2004; Institute of Medicine, 2004; Paasche-Orlow and Wolf, 2007). Empirical data collected over the past two decades also support these links. Limited health literacy has been associated with less health knowledge (Gazmararian et al, 2003), worse self-management skills (Schillinger et al, 2002), higher hospitalization rates (Baker et al, 1998, 2002), poorer health (Wolf et al, 2005), and greater mortality (Sudore et al, 2006; Wolf et al, 2006b). Literacy is more strongly associated with these outcomes than years of education (Baker et al, 2002; Elo and Preston, 1996; Kitigawa and Hauser, 1973; Wolf et al, 2005, 2006b; Yen and Moss, 1999).

3.1.1 Health Knowledge

Individuals with limited health literacy possess less health knowledge, access fewer preventive services, and have poorer self-management skills. Williams and colleagues (1998a) interviewed patients presenting to an urban hospital asthma clinic and/or emergency department and found those with low health literacy had poorer asthma knowledge. In a similar study, lower literate patients with hypertension and diabetes were also reported to have poorer knowledge of disease (Williams et al, 1998b). Other research studies have since confirmed this relationship in a multitude of contexts. Among individuals living with HIV/AIDS, those with limited literacy were less able to define CD4 lymphocyte count and viral load and to identify antiviral medications in their regimen even with the aid of pictures (Kalichman et al, 1999; Wolf et al, 2004). A great deal of attention has also highlighted the association between low health literacy and treatment misunderstanding, including medication names, indications, and instructions. Davis and colleagues (2006a) conducted a multisite study among adults and found those with limited literacy had higher rates of misunderstanding the directions for medications provided by either the physician or the pharmacist. The problem extended to text messages and icons used for medication warnings and precautions. Finally, in perhaps one of the most indicting studies linking literacy skills to medical understanding, Gazmararian et al (2003) interviewed patients with asthma, hypertension, diabetes, or congestive heart failure and found that low health literacy was an independent predictor of poor knowledge across all of the studied chronic conditions.

3.1.2 Health Behavior

Scott and colleagues (2002) found individuals with low health literacy to be less likely to have received an influenza or pneumococcal vaccination, mammogram, or Papanicolaou smear, if eligible. Dolan and colleagues (2004) found that low literacy was significantly associated with poor knowledge and negative attitudes toward use of colon cancer screening tests. Davis et al (1996a) had found earlier that knowledge, attitudes, and screening intention for mammography were strongly associated with literacy skills in a group of screening eligible women. Bennett and colleagues (1998) reported that racial disparities in advanced stage presentation of prostate cancer were partly explained by lower literacy levels among African-Americans, suggesting that low literacy may be associated with late or less frequent screening. These findings were confirmed using more recent data in the current era where a blood test to measure Prostate Specific Antigen (PSA) is widely used for determining the extent of disease at time of diagnosis (Wolf et al, 2006c).

In another study by Williams and colleagues (1998a), asthma patients' technique for using a metered dose inhaler (MDI) was evaluated. Those with low-health literacy skills were less able to demonstrate proper MDI technique compared to those with adequate literacy. Three additional studies found individuals with limited health literacy to report poorer medication adherence compared to those with adequate health literacy (Gazmararian et al, 2006; Kalichman et al, 1999; Wolf et al, 2006a). Schillinger et al (2002) found that among diabetic patients, those with low-health literacy skills were less able to achieve tight glycemic control and reported higher rates of retinopathy as the result of poor diabetes self-care.

3.1.3 Health Status

Individuals with limited health literacy experience poorer health outcomes. Baker et al (1998) examined the relationship between health literacy and self-reported health among patients presenting to the emergency department or ambulatory clinic at one of two urban public hospitals. Patients with low health literacy were more than twice as likely to self-report poor health on a single-item question, even after adjusting for age, gender, race, and markers of economic deprivation. Wolf and colleagues (2005) investigated the relationship between inadequate health literacy and self-reported functional health status among older adults. Those with low health literacy had a higher prevalence of diabetes and congestive heart failure, reported worse physical and mental health, greater difficulties with activities of daily living and limitations due to physical

health. Likewise, Mancuso and Rincon (2006) reported that among adult asthma patients, limited health literacy was associated with poorer physical health, worse quality of life, and a greater number of emergency department visits. Two studies by Baker and colleagues (1999, 2002) had previously reported that patients with inadequate health literacy had a greater risk of hospital admission compared to those with adequate literacy.

Most recently, research has identified low health literacy as a significant risk factor for greater mortality. Sudore and colleagues (2006) reported that low health literacy was associated with a 75% increased risk for all-cause mortality compared to those with adequate health literacy. Similarly, Baker, Wolf and colleagues (2007) found low health literacy to be significantly and independently associated with a 51% greater mortality risk; the association was found to be significant for cardiovascular causes but not for cancer.

3.2 Causal Pathways

This review of the evidence suggests health literacy to be one of the strongest known socioeconomic indicators of health outcomes. While the causal pathways linking limited health literacy to poorer health are not entirely clear, hypotheses are available (Fig. 25.1). For instance, regardless of whether lower literate individuals have more limited access to healthcare services, the quality of their experience may be compromised due to ineffective communication within the medical encounter. This is compounded by a lack of accessible health information resources to supplement what was or was not understood during the physician–patient encounter. For instance, it has been noted previously that physicians often do not communicate at a level that is understood by patients with lower literacy skills (Davis et al, 2000; Lindau et al, 2001; Weiss et al, 1998). Yet patients with limited literacy may also feel shame as a result of their poor reading ability, not understand terms

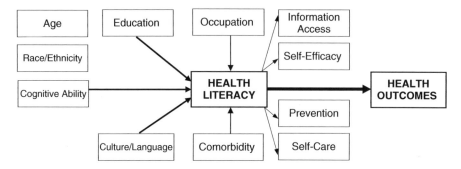

Fig. 25.1 Simplified conceptual model linking health literacy to health outcomes
Note: Only primary described pathways associated with health literacy are identified among a select list of variables

used by the physician, and consequently lack the self-efficacy to seek out clarification or acquire information elsewhere. The majority of patient education materials that are distributed in physicians' offices or other health-related settings have repeatedly been found to be too complex, written on too high a level or not organized from the patient's perspective (Davis et al, 1996a,b; Hearth-Holmes et al, 1998; Zion and Aiman, 1989). Over time, these factors contribute to worse health status, as a result of inadequate use of preventive services, negative health behaviors, and poorer self-management of acquired illness.

4 Health Literacy Interventions

Promoting health literacy means helping individuals better comprehend health information, make appropriate decisions, and ultimately take action. Over the past decade, few interventions have been formulated to address the problem of limited health literacy. The majority of interventions have focused on rewriting health materials at a simpler reading level or following other design techniques to improve patient reading comprehension (Davis et al, 1998; Gerber et al, 2005; Pignone et al, 2005; Rothman et al, 2004). While there is a need for additional research on how to appropriately respond to limited health literacy, certain health communication "best practices" have been recommended. These are relatively simple steps that will assist healthcare providers in identifying patients at

risk for limited health literacy and potentially poor health outcomes and will improve the quality and effectiveness of communication during clinical encounters and an individual's ability to retain that information for later use. Targets for intervention generally include health materials, oral communication skills of healthcare providers, and healthcare practices themselves. An overall, if not long-term goal should also be to better familiarize individuals and families to the healthcare system and their role within it.

4.1 Enhancing Print Materials

The value of print health materials is that they are tangible and can ideally reinforce verbal communication or information provided by other, less-tangible sources (i.e., video). However, many print materials utilized in healthcare settings today are written at a level that is too complex for the majority of patients to comprehend; such health materials should be simplified so that they are easier to understand among patients across all literacy levels. Printed materials such as postcards, fact sheets, brochures, and booklets should be created in a format that promotes patient understanding. There are numerous resources available that describe "best practices" for writing healthcare materials. Table 25.1 describes some key techniques identified by prominent practitioners in the field (Doak et al, 1996). Studies have shown that the majority of patients, even those without

Table 25.1 Techniques to simplify print materials

Technique	Explanation
Write in short sentences	Short sentences tend to be easier to read and understand for patients. Sentence length should be less than 15 words, and ideally less than 10 words. Sentences should be written in a conversational style
Print in large, Sans-Serif font	Text should be written in Sans-Serif font (i.e., Arial) with a minimum font size of 12 pt. Use of all capital letters should be avoided; only the first letter of words in text should be capitalized
Include sufficient white space	Large margins and adequate spacing between sentences and paragraphs will provide sufficient white space and prevent a document from appearing to be solid text. In general, text should be left justified for easy reading
Select simple words	Words that are commonly used in conversation are the best to include in health messages. Shorter words tend to be easier to understand and more familiar to patients
Provide information in bulleted lists	Bullets help to separate information from the rest of the text. Information provided in lists is often easier and faster for patients to read and comprehend
Highlight or underline key information	Bolding and highlighting phrases or words can draw attention to essential information for patients. It should be used sparingly to differentiate key sentences or phrases from the rest of the text
Design passages to be action and goal oriented	Written passages should be action and goal oriented and should provide readers with a clear explanation of the purpose of the written material. Passages should clearly define what actions should be taken by the reader and why these actions are necessary
Group and limit instructional content	Consider grouping information under common headings to promote understanding. Place key information in the beginning of a paragraph and be sure to limit the amount of instructional content that is given to what is essential for the patient to know and understand
Use active voice	Information written using active voice is easier to understand and more likely to motivate the patient to action
Avoid unnecessary jargon	Unnecessary jargon can be distracting to patients and often provides little information. Medical terminology should be used as infrequently as possible and, if used, should always be clearly defined and explained to the patient

limited health literacy, prefer to have print materials provided in clear and concise formats like those described above. Ensuring that print materials are simplified is a practice that should be universally adopted to promote the transfer to health information to all patients, regardless of literacy level.

4.1.1 Utilizing Visual Aids

Healthcare providers should also consider using visual aids within print material and during clinical encounters to help patients remember and process health information. One study demonstrated that subjects who listened to medical instructions accompanied by a pictograph remembered 85% of what they heard in contrast to 14% for patients who did not receive a visual

aid (Houts et al, 2001). Visual materials are useful to teach patients about health conditions that cannot be seen easily (for example, cholesterol in the blood vessels) and to demonstrate how to follow steps to complete a task. Visual materials should be tailored to reflect the culture, age, and background of the patient population and should be simple, recognizable, and clear. Photographs and visual materials depicting how to correctly engage in health activities can be very effective methods for delivering health information.

4.2 Improving Oral Communication Skills

It may not always be possible to identify patients with limited health literacy. A best practice for health communication is to adopt a universal precaution approach, always use plain language with all patients, and to try to avoid the use of medical jargon (Paasche-Orlow et al, 2006a). This is not always possible, so terms and concepts should be defined and clarified when they arise. Healthcare providers should also verify that information provided verbally has been effectively understood by the patient by incorporating interactive communication strategies, such as confirming the understanding using the "teach back" technique or through guided imagery approaches during clinical encounters with patients.

The "teach back" technique is a particularly useful and simple way to confirm patient understanding during the encounter (Schillinger et al, 2003). After describing a diagnosis and or recommending a course of treatment, the healthcare provider should ask the patient to reiterate what has been discussed by reviewing the core elements of the encounter thus far. The healthcare provider should be specific about what the patient should teach back, and should limit instruction to 1 or 2 main points. If a patient provides incorrect information, the healthcare provider should review the information again and give the patient another opportunity to demonstrate understanding. In this manner, the healthcare provider can gain assurance that the patient has adequately understood the health information presented (Fig. 25.2).

In contrast, guided imagery requires the patient to not only teach back information and instructions but also describe how a recommended behavior (i.e., medication use) will be specifically performed within the patient's own situation. This might include explicitly asking a patient when they will take a prescribed medicine, where they will store the medicine, and how they will remind themselves of the activity. A study by Park and colleagues found the use of guided imagery to significantly improve adherence (Park et al, 2007).

4.3 Simplifying Health Systems

More intensive care-management strategies have been found to be effective at reducing health literacy barriers among patients with certain chronic conditions, such as heart failure and diabetes, and at a fairly low cost (Pignone et al, 2005; Rothman et al, 2004). These include minimizing, whenever possible, the patient's role and responsibilities in managing health. For instance, healthcare practices can streamline tasks, more closely track and follow-up chronically ill patients, use "navigators" or other forms of care coordination to deliver preventive services or set action plans for disease management. These broad strategies have incorporated several of these approaches to address system complexity, unfortunately making it difficult to elucidate the true cause for any reduction in the effect of health literacy on outcomes. It is also unclear whether these comprehensive interventions involving system change can be sustained and/or translated to other settings. More research is needed to provide more conclusive evidence as to how to optimally modify clinical practices to overcome the problem of health literacy, in terms of health promotion, disease prevention, chronic disease management, and healthcare navigation.

4.4 Long-Term Strategies

To address problems with health literacy in the long term, efforts should be made to orient

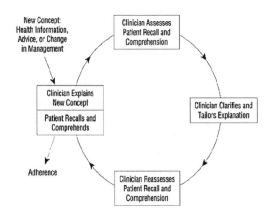

Fig. 25.2   The teach back technique

individuals to the healthcare system, such as medical terminology, and the tasks they must complete to manage their health. This could include training people early on (i.e., through schools) on how to more effectively communicate with healthcare providers or giving explicit guidance on what typical questions one should always ask (Davis et al, 2002, 2006b; Mika et al, 2007). These activities can increase an individual's self-efficacy to seek and obtain health information in a more productive manner and develop strategies to handle new healthcare experiences.

4.5 To Screen or Not to Screen

Currently, routine health literacy screening in clinical care is not recommended. Controversies remain on whether there is sufficient evidence to support clinical screening. Opposition to screening programs has primarily been based on the potential for inducing shame and stigma, coupled with a lack of viable responses (Sobel et al, 2008). However, many of the approaches described have been implemented and individual differences by literacy level still remained among the outcomes under study (Davis et al, 2009; Shaywitz and Shaywitz, 2005). Acceptable screening tools and methods that more comprehensively assess the health literacy skill set would still need to be created before this could be a possibility. This would also require a clear plan for incorporating this information into clinical decisions and establishing robust interventions.

For now, healthcare providers should seek to identify patients with limited health literacy through informal measures. There are several "clues" that may suggest a greater probability that a patient has limited health literacy. Patients with limited health literacy may be less likely to complete intake forms and histories and may be more likely to leave paperwork incomplete due to reading and writing difficulties. Additionally, patients with less than a high school graduate level of education, those who are older that age 65, are socioeconomically disadvantaged or

are members of a racial/ethnic minority have a greater risk of having low health literacy (Kutner et al, 2005). If limited health literacy is suspected in a particular patient, providers should be compelled to address the concern. Simple, direct questions can alleviate much of the shame and stigma a patient may feel with regards to such limitations. For instance, a healthcare provider may ask "How often do you have any trouble reading print forms?" or "How often do you have someone help you read health materials?" If the patient responds affirmatively, healthcare providers may need to spend additional time with the patient reviewing pertinent health information and verifying that the patient understands the information presented.

5 Conclusion

Limited health literacy is a serious barrier to communication in healthcare and may impact an individual's ability to manage health. Clinicians and other health professionals should seek to communicate with all patients in a clear and concise manner and to provide easy-to-understand print and visual materials to reinforce health messages. Utilizing the "teach back" technique and guided imagery during clinical encounters and incorporating adult education design standards into the creation of health materials will promote the effective transfer of information between healthcare providers and patients. As healthcare becomes increasingly complex with new technologies and cost restraints, problems will become even more apparent with greater burdens placed on patients when attempting to access health services (Parker et al, 2008). We must continue to strive to increase the health literacy of individuals and families and empower all to better understand their health roles and to take action on health information for the benefit of their own physical and mental well-being.

References

Ajzen, I. (1991). The theory of planned behavior. *Org Behav Hum Dec*, 50, 179–211.

Baker, D. W., Parker, R. M., Williams, M. V., Clark, W. S. (1998). Health literacy and the risk of hospital admission. *J Gen Intern Med, 13,* 791–798.

Baker, D. W. (1999) Reading between the lines: deciphering the connections between literacy and health. *J Gen Intern Med, 14,* 315–317.

Baker, D. W., Gazmararian, J. A., Williams, M. V., Scott, T., Parker, R. M. et al (2002). Functional health literacy and the risk of hospital admission among Medicare managed care enrollees. *Am J Public Health, 92,* 1278–1283.

Baker, D. W. (2006). The meaning and the measure of health literacy. *J Gen Intern Med, 21,* 878–883.

Baker, D. W., Wolf, M. S., Feinglass, J., Gazmararian, J. A., Thompson, J. A., et al (2007). Health literacy and mortality among elderly persons. *Arch Intern Med, 167,* 1503–1509.

Bennett, C. L., Ferreira, M. R., Davis, T. C., Kaplan, J., Weinberger, M. et al (1998). Relation between literacy, race, and stage of presentation among low-income patients with prostate cancer. *J Clin Oncol, 16,* 3101–3104.

Castro, C. M., Wilson, C., and Schillinger, D. (2007). Babel Babble: Physicians' use of unclarified medical jargon with patients who have type 2 diabetes and limited health literacy. *Am J Health Behav, 31,* S885–895.

Davis, T. C., Arnold, C., Berkel, H. J., Nandy, I., Jackson, R. H. et al (1996a). Knowledge and attitude on screening mammography among low-literate, low-income women. *Cancer, 78,* 1912–1920.

Davis, T. C., Bocchini, J. A. Jr., Fredrickson, D., Arnold, C., Mayeaux, E. J., et al (1996b). Parent comprehension of polio vaccine information pamphlets. *Pediatrics, 97*(6 Pt 1), 804–810.

Davis, T. C., Fredrickson, D. D., Arnold. C., Murphy. P. W., Herbst, M. et al (1998). A polio immunization pamphlet with increased appeal and simplified language does not improve comprehension to an acceptable level. *Pat Ed Couns, 35,* 25–33.

Davis, T. C., Williams, M. V., Branch, W, T., Jr., and Green, K. W. (2000) Explaining illness to patients with limited literacy. In D. A. Whaley & B. Bryan (Eds.). *Explaining Illness: Research, Theory, and Strategies* (pp. 123–146). Mahway, NJ: Lawrence Erlbaum Associates.

Davis, T. C., Fredrickson, D. D., Bocchini, C., Arnold, C., Green, K. W. et al (2002) Improving vaccine risk/benefit communication with an immunization education package: a pilot study. *Ambul Pediatr, 2,* 193–200.

Davis, T. C., Wolf, M. S., Bass, P. F., Tilson, H., Neuberger, M., et al (2006a). Literacy and misunderstanding of prescription drug labels. *Ann Intern Med, 145,* 887–894.

Davis, T. C., Wolf, M. S., Bass, P. F., Middlebrooks, M., Kennan, E., et al (2006b). Low literacy impairs comprehension of prescription drug warning labels. *J Gen Intern Med, 21,* 847–851.

Davis, T. C., Federman, A. D., Bass, P. F., Jackson, R. H., Middlebrooks, M. et al (2009). Improving patient understanding of prescription drug instructions. *J Gen Intern Med, 24,* 57–62.

Dewalt, D. A., Berkman, N. D., Sheridan, S., Lohr, K. N., Pignone, M. P. (2004). Literacy and health outcomes: a systematic review of the literature. *J Gen Intern Med, 19,* 1228–1239.

Doak, C. C., Doak, L. G., and Root, J. H. (1996). *Teaching Patients with Low Literacy Skills, 2nd Ed.* Philadelphia: Lippincott.

Dolan, N. C., Ferreira, M. R., Davis, T. C., Gorby, N., Rademakar, A. et al (2004). Colorectal cancer screening knowledge, attitudes, and beliefs among veterans: does literacy make a difference? *J Clin Oncol, 22,* 2617–2622.

Elo, I. T., and Preston, S. H. (1996). Educational differentials in mortality: United States, 1979–85. *Soc Sci Med, 42,* 47–57.

Gazmararian, J. A., Williams, M. V., Peel, J., and Baker, D. W. (2003). Health literacy and knowledge of chronic disease. *Patient Educ Couns, 51,* 267–275.

Gazmararian, J. A., Kripalani, S., Miller, M. J., Echt, K. V., Ren, J. et al (2006). Factors associated with medication refill adherence in cardiovascular-related diseases: a focus on health literacy. *J Gen Intern Med, 21,* 1215–1221.

Gerber, B. S., Brodsky, I. G., Lawless, K. A., Smolin, L. I., Arozullah, A. M. et al (2005). Implementation and evaluation of a low-literacy diabetes education computer multimedia application. *Diabetes Care, 28,* 1574–1580.

Hearth-Holmes, M., Murphy, P. W., Davis, T. C., Nandy, I., Elder, C. G., et al (1998). Literacy in patients with a chronic disease: systemic lupus erythematosus and the reading level of patient education materials. *J Rheumatol, 25,* 1649–1650.

Houts, P. S. Witmer, J. T., Egeth, H. E., Loscalzo, M. J., and Zabora, J. R. (2001). Using pictographs to enhance recall of spoken medical instructions. *Patient Educ Couns, 43,* 231–242

Institute of Medicine. (2004). *Health Literacy: A Prescription to End Confusion.* In L. Nielsen-Bohlman, A. Panzer, & D. A. Kindig (Eds.). Washington, DC: National Academies Press.

Institute of Medicine (2009). *Integrative Medicine and Patient Centered Care.* Washington, DC: National Academies Press.

Janz, N. K., Champion, V. L., and Strecher, V. J. (2003). The health belief model. In: K. Glanz, F. M. Lewis, & B. K. Rimer (Eds.), *Health Education Behavior.* San Francisco: Jossey-Bass.

Kalichman, S. C., Ramachandran, B., and Catz, S. (1999). Adherence to combination antiretroviral therapies in HIV patients of low health literacy. *J Gen Intern Med, 14,* 267–273.

Kickbusch, I., Wait, S., and Maag, D. (2006). Navigating health: the role of health literacy. Healthy Choices Forum, European Public Health Centre, London, UK.

Kitigawa, E., and Hauser, P. M. (1973). *Differential Mortality in the United States: A Study in Socioeconomic Epidemiology.* Cambridge, MA: Harvard University Press.

Kutner, M., Greenberg, E., and Baer, J. (2005). *A First Look at the Literacy of America's Adults in the 21st Century (NCES 2006–470).* U.S. Department of Education. Washington, DC: National Center for Education Statistics.

Kutner, M., Greenberg, E., Jin, Y., and Paulsen, C. (2006). *The Health Literacy of America's Adults: Results from the 2003 National Assessment of Adult Literacy (NCES 2006–483).* U.S. Department of Education. Washington, DC: National Center for Education Statistics.

Lindau, S., Tomori, C., McCarville, B. A., and Bennett, C. L. (2001). Improving rates of cervical cancer and pap smear follow-up for low-income women with limited health literacy. *Cancer Invest, 19,* 316–323.

Mancuso, C. A., and Rincon, M. (2006). Impact of health literacy on longitudinal asthma outcomes. J *Gen Intern Med, 21,* 813–817.

Mika, V. S., Wood, P. R., Weiss, B. D., and Treviño, L. (2007). Ask Me 3: improving communication in a Hispanic pediatric outpatient practice. *Am J Health Behav, 31,* S115–21.

Nutbeam, D. (2008). The evolving concept of health literacy. *Soc Sci Med, 67,* 2072–2078.

Paasche-Orlow, M. K., Schillinger, D., Greene, S. M., and Wagner, E. H. (2006). How health care systems can begin to address the challenge of limited literacy. *J Gen Intern Med, 21(8),* 884–887.

Paasche-Orlow, M. K., Cheng, D. M., Palepu, A., Meli, S., Faber, V. et al (2006). Health literacy, antiretroviral adherence, and HIV-RNA suppression: a longitudinal perspective. *J Gen Intern Med, 21,* 835–840.

Paasche-Orlow, M. K., and Wolf, M. S. (2007). The causal pathways linking health literacy to health outcomes. *Am J Health Behav, 31,* S19–26.

Park, D. C., Gutchess, A. H., Meade, M. L., and Stine-Morrow, E. A. (2007). Improving cognitive function in older adults: nontraditional approaches. *J Gerontol, 62B,* 45–52.

Parker, R. M., Wolf, M. S., and Kirsch, I. (2008). Preparing for an epidemic of limited health literacy: weathering the perfect storm. *J Gen Intern Med, 23,* 1273–1276.

Pignone, M., DeWalt, D. A., Sheridan, S., Berkman, N., and Lohr, K. N. (2005). Interventions to improve health outcomes for patients with low literacy: a systematic review. *J Gen Intern Med, 20,* 185–192.

Rothman, R. L., DeWalt, D. A., Malone, R., Bryant, B., Shintani, A. et al (2004). Influence of patient literacy on the effectiveness of a primary care-based diabetes disease management program. *JAMA, 292,* 1711–1716.

Rudd, R. E., Kirsch, I., and Yamamoto, K. (2004). *Literacy and Health in America.* Princeton, NJ: Educational Testing Service.

Rudd, R. E. (2007). Health literacy skills of U.S. adults. *Am J Health Behav, 31,* S8–18.

Schillinger, D., Grumbach, K., Piette, J., Wang, F., Osmond, D. et al (2002). Association of health literacy with diabetes outcomes. *JAMA, 288,* 475–482.

Schillinger, D., Piette, J., Grumbach, K., Wang, F., Wilson, C. et al (2003). Closing the loop: physician communication with diabetic patients who have low health literacy. *Arch intern Med, 163,* 83–90.

Scott, T. L., Gazmararian, J. A., Williams, M. V., and Baker, D. W. (2002). Health literacy and preventive health care use among Medicare enrollees in a managed care organization. *Med Care, 40,* 395–404.

Shaywitz, S. E., and Shaywitz, B. A. (2005). Dyslexia (specific reading disability). *Biol Psychiatry, 57,* 1301–1309.

Sobel, R., Waite, K., Paasche-Orlow, M. K., Federman, A. D., Rittner, S., et al (2009). Asthma 1-2-3: a low-literacy multimedia tool to educate African American adults about asthma. *J Community Health, 34,* 321–327.

Sudore, R. L., Yaffe, K., Satterfield, S., Harris, T. B., Mehta, K. M. et al (2006). Limited literacy and mortality in the elderly: the health, aging, and body composition study. *J Gen Intern Med, 21,* 806–812.

Weiss, B. D., Coyne, C., Michielutte, R., Davis, T. C., Meade, C. D. et al (1998). Communicating with patients who have limited literacy skills: consensus statement from the National Work Group on Literacy and Health. *J Family Practice, 46,* 168–176

Williams, M. V., Baker, D. W., Honig, E. G., Lee, T. M., and Nowlan, A. (1998a). Inadequate literacy is a barrier to asthma knowledge and self-care. *Chest, 114,* 1008–1015.

Williams, M. V., Baker, D. W., Parker, R. M., and Nurss, J. R. (1998b). Relationship of functional health literacy to patients' knowledge of their chronic disease. A study of patients with hypertension and diabetes. *Arch Intern Med, 158,* 166–172.

Wolf, M. S., Davis, T. C., Cross, J. T., Marin, E., Green, K. M. et al (2004). Health literacy and patient knowledge in a Southern US HIV clinic. *Int J STD AIDS, 15,* 1144–1150.

Wolf, M. S., Davis, T. C., Skripkauskas, S., Bennett, C. L., and Makoul, G. (2006a). Literacy, self-efficacy, and HIV medication adherence. *Pat Educ Couns, 65,* 253–260.

Wolf, M. S., Feinglass, J. M., Carrion, V., Gazmararian, J., and Baker, D. (2006b). Literacy and mortality among Medicare enrollees. *J Gen Intern Med, 21,* 81–92.

Wolf, M. S., Gazmararian, J. A., and Baker, D. W. (2005). Health literacy and functional health status among older adults. *Arch Intern Med, 165,* 1946–1952.

Wolf, M. S., Knight, S. J., Lyons, E. A., Durazo-Arvizu, R., Pickard, S. A. et al (2006c). Literacy, race, and PSA level among low-income men newly diagnosed with prostate cancer. *Urology, 68,* 89–93.

Yen, I. H., and Moss, N. (1999). Unbundling education: a critical discussion of what education confers and how it lowers risk for disease and death. *Ann N Y Acad Sci, 896,* 350–351.

Zion, A. B., and Aiman, J. (1989). Level of reading difficulty in the American College of Obstetricians and Gynecologists patient education pamphlets. *Obstet Gynecol, 74,* 955–960.

Chapter 26

Screening and Early Detection of Cancer: A Population Perspective

Laura A.V. Marlow, Jo Waller, and Jane Wardle

1 The Public Health Context of Screening

The 20th century saw a dramatic change in the landscape of public health, most notably in developed countries, with the decline of infectious diseases and the rise in the proportion of deaths attributable to non-communicable disease including cardiovascular disease, diabetes, and cancer. While methods of preventing communicable disease continue to progress, in many countries there has been a new emphasis on prevention of non-communicable disease. One of the cornerstones of this effort has been screening for early stage disease or disease precursors.

The aim of screening is to "discover those among the apparently well who are in fact suffering from disease" (Wilson and Junger, 1968). By identifying disease at an early stage, treatment to reduce morbidity and mortality is expected to be more successful. Screening has been applied to a wide range of conditions, including common cancers, sexually transmitted infections, hearing problems in newborn infants, and cardiovascular risk factors. It can be population-based and targeted at "average-risk" groups (e.g., cytological screening of all women within a certain age range for signs of pre-cancerous cervical lesions) or targeted at "high-risk" groups (e.g., genetic testing for Huntington's disease among relatives of those known to have the disease).

2 Screening and Cancer Control

This chapter focuses on the use of screening for cancer. Cancer is a leading cause of death worldwide, and in 2007 accounted for 7.9 million deaths (around 13% of all deaths), a figure that is predicted to rise to 12 million by 2030 (WHO, 2009). Screening represents a major part of the cancer control effort, particularly in developed countries. The Papanicolaou (Pap) test for the detection of pre-cancerous cervical lesions is the most widely used cancer screening test. It was developed in 1928 and is now available to women across the globe; albeit with different technologies and test frequencies. Some cervical cancer screening programs now also incorporate DNA testing for human papillomavirus (HPV), the viral precursor to cervical cancer. Mammography screening was developed in the 1950s for early diagnosis of breast cancer and involves taking a low-energy X-ray of the breast which is then examined for signs of calcification or soft tissue masses. More recently, colorectal cancer (CRC or bowel cancer) screening in the form of colonoscopy, sigmoidoscopy, or fecal occult blood (FOB) testing has been widely implemented. Screening for cervical, breast, and colorectal cancer is widely recommended for developed countries (e.g., by the US Preventive Services Task Force and the European Council). In addition, prostate-specific antigen (PSA) testing is used to detect prostate cancer in some

J. Wardle (✉)
Health Behaviour Research Centre, Department of Epidemiology & Public Health, University College London, Gower Street, London WC1E 6BT, UK
e-mail: j.wardle@ucl.ac.uk

A. Steptoe (ed.), *Handbook of Behavioral Medicine*, DOI 10.1007/978-0-387-09488-5_26,
© Springer Science+Business Media, LLC 2010

settings, although evidence for its efficacy is less clear. Throughout this chapter, examples from screening for these four common cancers will be used.

3 Characteristics of Good Screening Tools

Wilson and Junger (1968) outlined ten criteria for the appraisal of screening (see Table 26.1). A good screening test should be for a disease that is a common cause of morbidity and mortality and for which treatment is available, efficacious, safe, and cost-effective. At the most basic level, a screening test must be demonstrated to do more good than harm, and for national screening programs, it is important that the test is cost-effective in reducing morbidity and mortality at a population level. This will depend on a number of characteristics of the test. First, the reliability of the test (sensitivity and specificity) is crucially important. Sensitivity relates to the proportion of people who have the disease and have it detected in the screening test; a sensitive test will pick up the majority of cases of disease, giving few false negative results. In a test with high specificity, a positive result will almost always indicate the presence of disease. The sensitivity and specificity of a test, together with the prevalence of the disease within a given population, can be used to calculate the positive and negative predictive value of the test. The positive predictive value is the probability that the disease is present given a positive test result and the negative predictive value is the probability that the disease is absent given a negative test result. High sensitivity is a prerequisite of a good screening test but if specificity is low in a primary screening tool (e.g., FOB testing) this can be overcome by introducing further tests (e.g., colonoscopy) following a positive result.

It is also important to consider the possible side effects of screening. Clearly a test with common and harmful side effects would not be useful; for example, the risk of bowel perforation during colonoscopy must be considered when deciding whether it is suitable as a population-based screening tool. Consequences of screening follow-up must also be considered; one reason why cervical screening is often deemed inappropriate for women under 25 years is that many HPV-related abnormalities regress spontaneously at this age while treatment can compromise future pregnancies. Distress and anxiety should also be considered when the costs and benefits of a screening test are evaluated. Another potential harm, which is gathering more attention at present, is the risk of over-diagnosis, i.e., detecting disease that may never have resulted in significant morbidity or mortality. Topical examples of screening tests that have attracted concern regarding possible over-diagnosis include PSA testing to detect prostate cancer (Schroder et al, 2009) and mammography screening for breast cancer, especially in women under 50 years old (Gotzsche and Nielsen, 2009).

Table 26.1 Ten criteria for the appraisal of screening (Wilson and Junger, 1968)

1. The condition sought should be an important health problem
2. There should be an accepted treatment for patients with recognized disease
3. Facilities for diagnosis and treatment should be available
4. There should be a recognizable latent or early symptomatic stage
5. There should be a suitable test or examination
6. The test should be acceptable to the population
7. The natural history of the condition (including development from latent to declared disease) should be adequately understood
8. There should be an agreed policy on whom to treat as patients
9. The cost of case finding (including diagnosis and treatment of patients diagnosed) should be economically balanced in relation to possible expenditure on medical care as a whole
10. Case finding should be a continuing process and not a "once and for all" project

Finally, a successful screening program relies on good systems of quality assurance so that performance can be monitored at all levels of the process from sample taking to carrying out the laboratory tests. In organized screening programs (see below), quality assurance is often undertaken by the body responsible for screening, but where screening is opportunistic, monitoring is more difficult.

4 Provision of Cancer Screening Services

Most cancer screening across the world is opportunistic, but some countries have regionally or nationally organized programs, in which every stage of the screening process from the invitation to participate, to the follow-up of abnormal results is organized and monitored by a central body. Opportunistic screening is dependent on the individual requesting a screening test or the health-care provider offering it, whereas organized screening depends on databases with information on the target population from which invitations are produced automatically. Both systems have advantages and disadvantages, but in general, organized programs usually offer free or subsidized tests, are able to achieve greater coverage, and minimize social inequalities in access (although not necessarily in uptake), by making sure everyone in the population who is eligible is invited (Miles et al, 2004). However, they could be criticized for reducing the opportunity for patient–provider interaction to discuss the test and for lacking the flexibility to match screening recommendations to patient characteristics – organized programs will occasionally issue invitations for cervical screening to women who have no cervix, or FOB test kits to people who have just been treated for colorectal cancer; something that would be much less likely in an opportunistic screening context.

Information on the availability of screening services worldwide is collated by the International Cancer Screening Network (ICSN) which is sponsored by the National Cancer Institute (http://appliedresearch.cancer. gov/icsn/). Starting in 1988 with just 11 countries, the ICSN now reports on screening services that are available across 28 countries in Europe, Asia, Australasia, and the Americas. Even in countries without an organized program, most publicize recommendations on which cancers to screen for, the age of the population to be screened, and the optimal frequency of testing. For example, the US Centers for Disease Control and Prevention advocates screening as recommended by the US Preventive Services Task Force (http://www. ahrq.gov/clinic/uspstfix.htm), and the European Council provides screening guidelines for all the countries in the European Union (http:// ec.europa.eu/health/ph_determinants/genetics/ cancer_screening_en.pdf).

Cervical screening is currently offered to women in most developed countries. This is usually by Pap testing, but there has recently been a move to using liquid-based cytology in some countries. The USA and Canada offer cervical screening opportunistically, but organized programs are offered in Australia, the UK, and some other European countries. In a survey of 25 European screening centers (from 18 countries), organized screening was offered by 15 and opportunistic screening by 10 centers (Anttila et al, 2004). The age that cervical screening starts ranges from 18 to 30 years, and screening usually finishes between 60 and 69 years. Recommended screening intervals vary widely across countries (from 1 to 10 years) and in some countries depend on the age of the woman and whether she has had a previous abnormal result. Across Europe, the number of Pap tests a woman has in her life time therefore ranges from 7 to 50 (Anttila et al, 2004).

Organized breast screening with mammography is offered in Canada, Australia, New Zealand, Japan, Korea, and most of Europe, with opportunistic screening in the USA and Brazil. The age ranges for screening vary, but the lower limit is between 40 and 50 years, and the upper limit between 69 and 74 years. Recommended screening intervals also vary, ranging from 1 to 3 years (Shapiro et al, 1998; Klabunde and Ballard-Barbash, 2007). In the USA, the Preventive Services Task Force recently changed its mammography guidelines and now recommends against breast screening for women below the age of 50 and suggests biennial rather than annual screening (USPSTF, 2009).

Colorectal cancer screening most commonly uses FOB testing, but can include sigmoidoscopy or colonoscopy. Screening is offered to men and women from 45 to 60 years up until 64–80 years of age, with no upper age limit in some countries. The interval depends on the type of test: for FOB testing most screening is every 1–2 years, but flexible sigmoidoscopy or colonoscopy is only required once or every 5–10 years (Benson et al, 2008). Screening for colorectal cancer is available in the USA, Australia, the UK, and several countries in Europe and Asia. Only 12 countries currently offer national organized screening programs (Australia, Cyprus, Czech Republic, England, Finland, France, Israel, Japan, Korea, Poland, Portugal, Scotland, and Slovenia) but other countries have organized regional programs (Power et al, 2009).

Controversy surrounding the specificity of the PSA test means there are currently no organized prostate cancer screening programs. In combination with the Digital Rectal Exam, PSA testing is offered opportunistically to men over the age of 50 years in several countries including the USA, Canada, the UK, and Australia. In the USA, men are offered the test annually as part of a regular health check. The UK allows any man over the age of 50 who asks for a PSA test to have one, but only after discussion of the implications with the provider.

5 Optimizing Screening Uptake

Monitoring screening uptake rates is vital to ensure that tests are cost-effective and are reaching the majority of the eligible population. In countries with organized screening (e.g., the UK), objective uptake rates can be calculated, but in countries that do not have these systems in place, uptake is usually determined from population-based surveys of self-reported participation. These surveys offer the best available estimates, although self-selection bias in survey participation and biases in self-reported screening are likely to mean these figures are overestimates.

In most developed countries, uptake of cervical screening is good. The most recent figures in the UK show that 79% of women aged 25–64 years have been screened within the last 5 years (2008–2009 figures: NHSCSP, 2009), and in Australia the equivalent figure for women aged 20–69 years is 86% [2006–2007 figures: Australian Institute of Health and Welfare (AIHW), 2009b]. Across Europe, uptake of cervical screening at the recommended intervals ranges from 30 to 93% and is greater than 75% for six countries: Finland, Sweden, UK, Denmark, Iceland, and the Netherlands (Anttila et al, 2004). In the US National Health Interview Survey, 83% of American women aged 18 or older reported having had a Pap test in the preceding 3 years (2000 data: Solomon et al, 2007). Similarly in the Canadian National Population Health Survey, 79% of women aged 20–69 said they had had a Pap test within the previous 3 years (data from 1998–1999).

Mammography coverage is similar to cervical screening, with most studies suggesting high uptake. In population surveys in Canada, 72% of women aged 50–69 reported having had a mammogram in the past 2 years (Shields and Wilkins, 2009) and data from the 2006 Behavioral Risk Factor Surveillance System in the USA found 76% self-reported mammography in women over 40 years within the preceding 2 years (Ryerson et al, 2008). Similar levels are recorded in the UK screening program (74% for women aged 50–64 years having a mammogram within 3 years: 2007–2008 figures), with records in Australia showing slightly lower uptake: 57% of women aged 50–69 years have had a mammogram in the past 2 years (AIHW, 2009a).

The figures presented above suggest that the majority of eligible women participate in breast and cervical screening whether in organized or opportunistic contexts. Colorectal cancer screening has not achieved such high uptake rates, with figures ranging from 20 to 71% (Power et al, 2009). Self-reported uptake in the USA showed that in 2005 only 50% of adults over 50 years had had either an FOB test within the last year or endoscopy (colonoscopy or sigmoidoscopy) in the last 10 years (Shapiro et al, 2008). This is similar to uptake rates for FOB testing from the pilot centers for the UK national program (Steele et al, 2009; Weller et al, 2007).

Prostate cancer screening using PSA testing is only offered opportunistically. The most recent estimates from the US suggest that around half of 50–79 year olds have had a PSA test in the past 2 years (Ross et al, 2008; Weller et al, 2007). UK estimates based on a survey of general practitioners suggest that the rate of PSA testing in asymptomatic men is only 2% (Melia et al, 2004).

6 Predictors of Uptake

Despite relatively good coverage, at least for cervical and breast screening, a significant minority of the eligible population do not attend for screening, and there is a considerable body of work exploring demographic and psychosocial predictors of non-attendance. A systematic review published in 2000 identified research that had explored determinants of screening for breast (35 studies), cervical (12 studies), colorectal (12 studies), and prostate cancer (4 studies) and gives a detailed discussion of predictors of uptake (Jepson et al, 2000).

6.1 Demographic Factors

Examining demographic factors associated with uptake of screening has been important in trying to understand variation in cancer mortality and in tackling social disparities. Demographic factors including sex, age, marital status, socio-economic status (SES), and ethnicity have all been associated with uptake of cancer screening.

6.1.1 Sex

Most cancer screening programs target gender-specific cancers, but gender differences are of interest in colorectal cancer screening. Evidence for gender differences is mixed and seems to depend on the test that is used. An international review of participation in endoscopy concluded that men are more likely to be screened than women (Stock et al, 2010), although data from a small trial in England with female nurse endoscopists found the reverse effect (Brotherstone et al, 2007). In contrast, there is evidence that women are more likely to complete FOB tests than men (Seeff et al, 2004; Steele et al, 2009; Weller et al, 2007). Across all procedures, men in the USA are more likely to be screened than women, but the difference is small at around 3% (Seeff et al, 2004; Shapiro et al, 2008).

6.1.2 Age

Age appears to be associated with uptake of all types of cancer screening, but the pattern varies. Cervical screening is offered across the widest age range and uptake seems to follow an inverted U curve, with lowest uptake among the younger and older age groups. On average, compared to the group in the mid age range, uptakes in the youngest and oldest screening age groups are 10 and 5% lower, respectively (AIHW, 2009b; Health Canada, 2002; Hewitt et al, 2004; NHSCSP, 2009). In the UK, there have been recent concerns that coverage is falling among young women, with suggestions that this is a cohort effect (Lancuck et al, 2008).

Similarly, for breast screening, women aged 50–69 have higher uptake rates than those who are younger (40–50 years) or older (Meissner et al, 2007; Ryerson et al, 2008). A similar pattern is seen for PSA testing among men, with greater use among those aged 65–80 years than among younger (50–64 years) or older men (Ross et al, 2004, 2008).

Participation in colorectal cancer screening tends to be higher among those aged over 60 years compared to those aged 50–60 years. This appears to be the case for both men and women and across all types of test (Seeff et al, 2004; Meissner et al, 2006; Weller et al, 2007).

6.1.3 Marital Status

Being married is associated with higher uptake of cervical (Hewitt et al, 2004; Sutton and Rutherford, 2005), breast (Ryerson et al, 2008), and colorectal cancer screening (Seeff et al, 2004; van Jaarsveld et al, 2006), as well as with use of PSA testing (Ross et al, 2008). Across these studies, marriage was associated with a 7–22% increase in screening participation.

6.1.4 Socio-economic Status

There is evidence of variation in uptake by SES across breast, cervical, colorectal, and prostate cancer screening, with poorer coverage in more deprived populations. Disproportionate uptake of screening by affluent groups could widen existing inequalities in cancer mortality, so this is a cause for concern. In 1997, an international review of socio-economic inequalities in breast and cervical cancer screening concluded that women from deprived backgrounds were less likely to be screened (Segnan, 1997). The review focused on studies using education and income as markers of SES, and despite the passage of time, the main conclusions still stand. More recent studies in the USA continue to show that compared to those with a college education, women who did not graduate high school have a screening uptake around 10% lower for mammography (CDC, 2005) and 14–18% lower for cervical screening (Hewitt et al, 2004; Coughlin et al, 2006). US studies also show significant associations when income is used as a marker of SES. For example, data on mammography screening from the Behavioral Risk Factor Surveillance System (2000–2006) show a consistent uptake gradient across five income groups, ranging from around 60% in the lowest income group to 80% uptake in the highest group. In other countries, income shows a less consistent association with screening attendance and this may be partially explained by the use of free organized screening programs. Uptake of colorectal cancer screening using endoscopy or FOB testing also varies by education level, income, and area-level deprivation (Meissner et al, 2006; Seeff et al, 2004; Stock et al, 2010; von Wagner et al, 2009), as does use of PSA testing in the USA (Ross et al, 2008).

Although SES gradients may be explained partly by issues of cost and access, it should be remembered that socio-economic disparities exist even in the context of organized programs that are free at the point of delivery, pointing to more complex underlying causes. One UK study found that cognitive factors (beliefs and expectations about the screening test) explained much of the SES variation in interest in sigmoidoscopy screening (Wardle et al, 2004). A more recent analysis confirmed that cognitive factors are strongly associated with screening intentions, but once a positive intention has been formed, they show much less association and do not mediate the socio-economic gradient in participation (Power et al, 2008).

Other individual-level indicators of SES including car ownership, house ownership and occupational class have shown associations with screening uptake, but study findings are sometimes mixed, with some indicators showing associations and others not. This is a particular issue in multivariate analyses, because different SES indicators are likely to share a considerable amount of variance. In addition some studies have considered area-level SES, and a recent review of 19 studies concluded that there was no consistent pattern in the association between area SES and cancer screening (Pruitt et al, 2009). A better understanding of the mediators of the association between SES and cancer screening is an important prelude to developing interventions to reduce inequalities.

6.1.5 Ethnicity

In both the USA and the UK, being from a non-white ethnic background is associated with non-attendance at cancer screening. In the USA, women from white and black backgrounds have similar self-reported attendance for cervical screening, but women from Hispanic and other backgrounds have uptake levels around 10% lower (Hewitt et al, 2004). Mammography screening uptake follows the same pattern, although the differences are smaller (Ryerson et al, 2008). In the UK, women from non-white backgrounds are less likely to go for cervical screening, even when controlling for SES, although mammography attendance is not associated with ethnicity after controlling for other variables (Moser et al, 2009).

For colorectal cancer screening, attendance also appears to be lower among the non-white population in the USA, UK, Australia, and The Netherlands and this is the case when controlling for education and income (Power et al, 2009; von Wagner et al, 2009). Finally, participation in PSA testing among 50–79 year olds in the USA is highest among men from non-Hispanic white and African American backgrounds. Among 40–49 year olds, African Americans have the highest rate of PSA testing (23% compared to 13–15%), which may be due to a higher rate of physician recommendation reflecting the increased risk of prostate cancer in this ethnic group (Ross et al, 2008).

6.2 Psychosocial Predictors

In addition to examining demographic patterning of screening attendance, much work has been done to try to identify potentially modifiable psychosocial predictors of screening uptake, with a view to optimizing screening-related information and designing interventions to increase coverage.

6.2.1 Cognitive Factors

There is some evidence that awareness and knowledge of cancer and cancer screening are associated with participation in cervical, breast, and CRC screening (Power et al, 2009; Royse and Dignan, 2009; Schueler et al, 2008), although this has not always been observed (Weinberg et al, 2009). But it is widely acknowledged that simply knowing about a screening program is not enough to ensure uptake, even in countries where screening is free.

Men and women with higher levels of perceived risk of cancer seem to be more likely to participate in cancer screening (Katapodi et al, 2004; Shavers et al, 2009; Sutton et al, 2000), although a review of risk perception and cancer screening behaviors concluded that there was only sufficient evidence for this with mammography and not cervical or colorectal screening (Vernon, 1999). Belief that the screening test is "not necessary" is cited as a common reason for not taking part among non-attenders and this is sometimes explained in terms of absence of any symptoms that could be indicative of disease (Seeff et al, 2004; Shields and Wilkins, 2009). Belief in the efficacy of screening tests also appears to be important: women who believe that mammography is ineffective or inaccurate, or believe it is only needed in the presence of cancer symptoms, are less likely to participate in breast screening (Schueler et al, 2008).

6.2.2 Emotional Factors

Feeling some fear or concern about cancer has been shown to motivate screening behavior (Haque et al, 2009), although when levels of worry are high this can have the opposite effect (Sutton et al, 2000). Conversely, fear of pain, discomfort, or embarrassment as a result of the screening test itself appears to be a barrier to participation (Seeff et al, 2004; Shields and Wilkins, 2009).

6.3 Practical and Service-Level Factors

In countries where cancer screening tests are not free at the point of use, the cost of the test could be an important barrier. US studies have shown that those with health insurance are more likely to have screening for cervical (Coughlin et al, 2006), breast (Ryerson et al, 2008), prostate (Ross et al, 2008), and colorectal cancer (Seeff et al, 2004). Physician-related factors also appear to be important, with those who report having a "usual source of care" and those who have seen a doctor recently more likely to attend for cervical or CRC screening in countries where screening is opportunistic (Hewitt et al, 2004; Meissner et al, 2006). In a systematic review of breast cancer screening, the authors concluded that improving access to screening and recommendations from physicians would be the most effective way to increase mammography utilization (Schueler et al, 2008).

7 Intention Versus Action

One of the common reasons given by people who do not go for screening tests is that they "did not get round to it" (Seeff et al, 2004; Shields and Wilkins, 2009; Waller et al, 2009). Seeing a doctor who recommends cancer screening may act as a prompt to overcome this inertia, but this barrier is still cited by women in countries with organized screening programs (who receive a personal invitation) so "prompting" may be insufficient to encourage some women to be screened. In these situations the intention to be screened may be there, but translation of this intention into behavior never occurs. A review of research into the "intention-behavior gap" suggests this is the case for a significant proportion (around 40%) of individuals (Sheeran, 2002). A recent study in the context of CRC screening showed that while psychosocial predictors were strongly associated with intention to be screened, factors relating to life difficulties (e.g., SES, stress and social support) played a larger role in predicting actual attendance (Power et al, 2008). Researchers are now beginning to consider ways to bridge the intention–behavior gap, and one way is to encourage individuals to plan when and where the behavior will take place. Such

interventions have been shown to be successful for cervical screening attendance (Sheeran and Orbell, 2000).

8 Interventions to Promote Uptake

Research that identifies predictors of screening attendance is useful in informing the development of interventions aimed at increasing uptake. A review of intervention studies across various types of screening (for cancer and other illnesses) concluded that invitation appointments, letters, telephone calls and counseling, reduction of financial barriers, and physician reminders all showed some evidence of effectiveness, while most educational interventions failed to increase uptake (Jepson et al, 2000).

Cochrane systematic reviews of breast (16 studies: Bonfill et al, 2001) and cervical screening interventions (35 studies: Forbes et al, 2002) were carried out at around the same time. Invitation letters and phone calls increased uptake in both reviews. For cervical screening there was evidence that having letters sent from a physician (rather than an authority source) and offering a fixed versus open appointment were more effective. In terms of educational interventions, video and face-to-face interventions had some effect, with greater uptake in the intervention compared to control groups, but printed materials showed mixed findings.

A more recent series of reviews in the *American Journal of Preventive Medicine* evaluated interventions to increase client access to and demand for cancer screening services (Baron et al, 2008a, b), and provider recommendation and use of cancer screening tests (Sabatino et al, 2008). For client-based interventions there was strong evidence to support the use of reminders, small media interventions (video and printed materials), one-on-one interventions, and reducing structural barriers or out of pocket costs. For providers, offering feedback was an effective strategy (Task Force on Community Preventive Services, 2008).

9 Psychological Impact

When evaluating the efficacy of screening programs, their psychological impact must be taken into account and considered alongside potential health benefits. Psychological responses can be measured at different stages of the screening process: the introduction of a program, the receipt of an invitation to be screened, and the receipt of a normal or abnormal result. Psychological impact can be measured in terms of emotional well-being, but might also include potential changes in engagement in future health-related behaviors.

9.1 Overall Impact of Screening Programs

It seems intuitively possible that merely recommending screening for a particular cancer might raise awareness and thereby anxiety about the disease across the population, and critics have argued that for some screening programs, such negative effects outweigh the health benefits. This has rarely been examined empirically but one study found that people receiving information about CRC screening were actually less worried about CRC and considered themselves less at risk than a control group. The only adverse impact of the information was an increased tendency to report bowel symptoms (Wardle et al, 1999). However, receiving an invitation for an unfamiliar screening test has been found to cause anxiety and fear. One small study of cervical screening non-attenders found that merely receiving an invitation letter was interpreted by some women as meaning that they had cervical cancer, causing high levels of distress (Nathoo, 1988).

9.2 Impact of a Normal Screening Result

There is little evidence that taking part in screening and receiving a negative (normal) result have

any adverse impact on emotional well-being, and there is some evidence of a "relief" effect, with women receiving a normal mammography result showing lower levels of distress than unscreened women (Scaf-Klomp et al, 1997). In cervical screening, women who receive normal results have been found to feel more positive about their fertility, cancer risk, and health than women receiving abnormal results (Wardle et al, 1995).

A possible downside of a normal result is a "complacency effect," which may have an undesired impact on future screening attendance and other health-related behaviors. There is, for example, evidence from one study that people who take part in flexible sigmoidoscopy screening and have no polyps found may be less likely to give up smoking or to maintain a healthy weight than people who do have polyps found (Hoff et al, 2001) but this was not confirmed in another study in the UK (Miles et al, 2003).

9.3 Impact of Abnormal Results

There is little doubt that across types of cancer screening, receiving an abnormal result is a stressful experience (Brett et al, 2005; Parker et al, 2002; Rogstad, 2002). The exception to this is flexible sigmoidoscopy, where the discovery of polyps does not seem to be associated with increased anxiety, regardless of whether people are referred for further investigation or simply have the polyps removed (Wardle et al, 2003). This may be because of the provision of immediate clinical advice and reassurance, as well as a good explanation of what a "polyp" is. Following abnormal mammography, cytology or FOB test results, anxiety and distress tend to be highest while waiting for follow-up appointments, partly due to fear about cancer and future health, but also because of concerns about the follow-up procedures themselves. In countries like the USA with insurance-based health-care systems, concerns about insurance cover for follow-up procedures is likely to be an additional source of anxiety. However, most of the evidence suggests that if the abnormality is resolved, general anxiety quickly falls to normal levels in the majority of people, although cancer-specific concerns may be more enduring. This suggests either that measures of general anxiety are not sensitive enough to pick up concerns about cancer or that these concerns are not severe enough to have an impact on overall anxiety levels.

The introduction of HPV testing into cervical cancer screening brings with it the negative psychological consequences that are more often associated with testing for sexually transmitted infections, including feelings of stigma and shame as well as concerns about transmission, and questions about where the virus has come from, with the associated issues of trust and fidelity (McCaffery et al, 2006). In addition, poor understanding of the meaning of an HPV result can lead to heightened anxiety, at least in the short term (Maissi et al, 2004).

Abnormal screening results may also have desirable effects, including improvements in health behaviors and increased likelihood of attendance at future screening. However, although there is some evidence that a false positive mammography result increases the likelihood of future screening attendance in the USA, other findings are conflicting and may vary between countries (Brewer et al, 2007). As mentioned earlier, one study found that people who had polyps discovered at sigmoidoscopy screening were more likely to stop smoking and less likely to gain weight than people who were given the all-clear (Hoff et al, 2001).

9.4 Interventions to Reduce Negative Psychological Consequences of Screening

Much research has been devoted to exploring ways of minimizing anxiety associated with abnormal results and follow-up procedures. Studies have focused on information provision by leaflets, booklets, or DVDs. However, a recent Cochrane review of interventions to reduce anxiety at colposcopy concluded that such information provision is ineffective at reducing anxiety, although it does improve knowledge and reduce psychosexual dysfunction (Galaal et al, 2007). Similar findings have been reported in relation to colorectal cancer screening and more research is needed to optimize the information provided to people prior to screening. In addition to information provision, shorter waiting times, or see-and-treat clinics may help to reduce anxiety.

10 Issues for Future Research

Attending cancer screening can be an emotional experience because it involves facing up to the possibility of one of the most feared diseases, coping with an uncomfortable procedure, and tolerating a delay before the results are available. Research is needed not only to maximize participation rates but also to minimize adverse effects. It may also be possible to utilize the screening context to reinforce messages about prevention and early presentation. All these research areas will benefit from close collaboration between behavioral scientists and scientists with expertise in public health and epidemiology, as well as the oncology community. Below, we suggest a few areas that might benefit from this multidisciplinary focus.

10.1 Tackling Inequalities

Socioeconomic and ethnic inequalities in cancer screening uptake undermine health-care equity and are an important issue for behavioral research. There have been many local studies and initiatives that focus on specific "underserved" groups – often defined by ethnicity but sometimes by income status – directed either at exploring barriers to screening or at testing culturally sensitive interventions to promote uptake. While some of these initiatives produce very promising results, there can be problems of generalizability and sustainability. Research focused on one population sub-group also makes it hard to know whether barriers are genuinely specific or apply equally to other groups, albeit they might be less salient. A move toward identifying commonalities in the determinants of attendance that has currency across ethnic minority groups (e.g., language, cultural attitudes toward cancer), even if the level of each factor varies by ethnic group, could help to generate interventions that have wider application.

In the USA, the major emphasis in inequality research is on ethnicity or specific socio-economic groups whose economic/insurance status bars them from healthcare. In the UK, socio-economic status probably causes a higher attributable fraction of non-attendance than ethnicity because of the relatively small ethnic minority population (fewer than 8% of UK adults classify themselves as belonging to ethnic minority groups, although the proportions are higher at younger ages and lower in the elderly). Because all health care is free at the point of access in the UK, direct economic barriers do not play a role; nonetheless there are SES differences in screening uptake; and these are particularly striking in the newly introduced colorectal screening program (von Wagner et al, 2009). Importantly, the pattern is not one of exceptionally low attendance in the lowest SES groups, or exceptionally high attendance in the highest SES groups, but it is a gradient across SES levels. The greatest need is for research that explores the underlying determinants of the gradient and develops theoretically informed interventions to address them. There are almost no interventions that specifically aim to reduce inequalities. Designing methods of information and support which reduce the socio-economic gradient would be an interesting challenge as well as having the potential to make inroads on health inequalities.

10.2 Shift of Boundary Between Risk and Disease

Screening enthusiasts focus on the benefits in terms of cancer morbidity and mortality, and for a disease that is as much feared as cancer, this is a powerful motive for the public too. However expansion of screening programs may also increase people's sense of risk or to put it the other way, undermine the illusion of health. With some screening programs identifying precursor risks (e.g. HPV infection) in a much higher proportion of the population than would ever have been likely to develop cancer, then the barriers between health and disease are blurred further. This is striking in the metabolic field where huge proportions of the population are identified with hypertension, insulin resistance, or hyperlipidemia, potentially creating an almost population-wide perception of compromised health status. The growth in personalized genetic testing – which will increasingly offer quantitative risk feedback rather than just testing for the presence or absence of highly penetrant mutations, will also add to the blurring of boundaries between health, disease risk, and disease. Ultimately this might lead to a paradigm shift in understanding of the health–disease continuum, perhaps with positive consequences for health, but in the meantime, it is important to get a better understanding of how lay models of health and disease are changing and how screen-detected abnormalities fit into the picture.

10.3 Informed Decision-Making

In recent years there has been shift in attitudes toward screening, moving away from a paternalistic view that everyone should be encouraged to be screened to an informed decision-making approach, which aims to provide people with the appropriate information so that they can weigh up the costs and benefits of participating in screening and decide for themselves whether to have screening tests. This is particularly important for tests where the benefits are uncertain, for example, PSA testing for prostate cancer risk. In the UK, the national screening program has developed a "Prostate Cancer Risk Management" information pack to assist general practitioners in counseling men who are concerned about prostate cancer and to help them understand the 'pros' and 'cons' of PSA testing. The aim is to encourage men to make choices that are fully informed, rather than to persuade them to have (or not to have) the test. Informed decision-making may be particularly relevant where patients can make choices about which of a number of different tests to have, such as HPV test versus repeat cytology in follow-up of mild cytological abnormalities (McCaffery et al, 2008) or different options for CRC screening.

With any screening program, high coverage is essential to ensure greatest benefit to the population in terms of reductions in mortality and morbidity. With the move toward informed decision-making, this creates a tension between maximizing public health benefit and protecting the best interests of the individual. Informing people fully about the costs and benefits associated with taking part in screening might be expected to reduce levels of participation and thereby compromise the efficacy of the program as a whole. A recent paper accused the UK leaflet "Breast Screening: the Facts" of including only "one-sided propaganda" about mammography, at odds with notions of informed decision-making (Gotzsche et al, 2009) and argued for more balanced information, explaining the risk of over-diagnosis and psychological distress.

11 Conclusion

Screening for early stage disease (or disease precursors) makes a significant contribution to the reduction in morbidity and mortality from diseases such as cancer. The concept of screening the healthy population raises numerous issues including inequalities in uptake, informed consent, understanding of disease risk, and psychological consequences. These issues are likely to change as new screening tools are introduced and old screening technologies are updated, but there is no doubt that behavioral science makes an important contribution to the success

of screening and will continue to do so in the future.

References

Australian Institute of Health and Welfare (2009a). Breast Screen Australia monitoring report. www.aihw.gov.au/publications/can/can-44-10784/can-44-10784.pdf

Australian Institute of Health and Welfare (2009b). Cervical Screening in Australia 2006–2007. www.aihw.gov.au/publications/can/can-43-10676/can-43-10676.pdf

Anttila, A., Ronco, G., Clifford, G., Bray, F., Hakama, M. et al (2004). Cervical cancer screening programmes and policies in 18 European countries. Br J Cancer, 91, 935–941.

Baron, R. C., Rimer, B. K., Breslow, R. A., Coates, R. J., Kerner, J. et al (2008a). Client-directed interventions to increase community demand for breast, cervical, and colorectal cancer screening a systematic review. Am J Prev Med, 35, S34–S55.

Baron, R. C., Rimer, B. K., Coates, R. J., Kerner, J., Kalra, G. P. et al (2008b). Client-directed interventions to increase community access to breast, cervical, and colorectal cancer screening a systematic review. Am J Prev Med, 35, S56–S66.

Benson, V. S., Patnick, J., Davies, A. K., Nadel, M. R., Smith, R. et al (2008). Colorectal cancer screening: a comparison of 35 initiatives in 17 countries. Int J Cancer, 122, 1357–1367.

Bonfill, X., Marzo, M., Pladevall, M., Marti, J., and Emparanza, J. I. (2001). Strategies for increasing women participation in community breast cancer screening. Cochrane Database Syst Rev, CD002943.

Brett, J., Bankhead, C., Henderson, B., Watson, E., and Austoker, J. (2005). The psychological impact of mammographic screening. A systematic review. Psychooncology, 14, 917–938.

Brewer, N. T., Salz, T., and Lillie, S. E. (2007). Systematic review: the long-term effects of false-positive mammograms. Ann Intern Med, 146, 502–510.

Brotherstone, H., Vance, M., Edwards, R., Miles, A., Robb, K. A. et al (2007). Uptake of population-based flexible sigmoidoscopy screening for colorectal cancer: a nurse-led feasibility study. J Med Screen, 14, 76–80.

CDC (2005). Breast cancer screening and socioeconomic status – 35 metropolitan areas, 2000 and 2002. Morb Mortal Wkly Rep, 54, 981–985.

Coughlin, S. S., King, J., Richards, T. B., and Ekwueme, D. U. (2006). Cervical cancer screening among women in metropolitan areas of the United States by individual-level and area-based measures of socioeconomic status, 2000 to 2002. Cancer Epidemiol Biomarkers Prev, 15, 2154–2159.

Forbes, C., Jepson, R., and Martin-Hirsch, P. (2002). Interventions targeted at women to encourage the uptake of cervical screening. *Cochrane Database Syst Rev*, CD002834.

Galaal, K. A., Deane, K., Sangal, S., and Lopes, A. D. (2007). Interventions for reducing anxiety in women undergoing colposcopy. *Cochrane Database Syst Rev*, CD006013.

Gotzsche, P. C., Hartling, O. J., Nielsen, M., Brodersen, J., and Jorgensen, K. J. (2009). Breast screening: the facts--or maybe not. *Br Med J, 338*, b86.

Gotzsche, P. C., and Nielsen, M. (2009). Screening for breast cancer with mammography. *Cochrane Database Syst Rev*, CD001877.

Haque, R., Van Den Eeden, S. K., Jacobsen, S. J., Caan, B., Avila, C. C. et al (2009). Correlates of prostate-specific antigen testing in a large multiethnic cohort. *Am J Manag Care, 15*, 793–799.

Health Canada (2002). Cervical cancer screening in Canada 1998 surveillance report. www.phac-aspc.gc.ca/publicat/ccsic-dccuac/pdf/cervical-e3.pdf

Hewitt, M., Devesa, S. S., and Breen, N. (2004). Cervical cancer screening among U.S. women: analyses of the 2000 National Health Interview Survey. *Prev Med, 39*, 270–278.

Hoff, G., Thiis-Evensen, E., Grotmol, T., Sauar, J., Vatn, M. H. et al (2001). Do undesirable effects of screening affect all-cause mortality in flexible sigmoidoscopy programmes? Experience from the Telemark Polyp Study 1983–1996. *Eur J Cancer Prev, 10*, 131–137.

Jepson, R., Clegg, A., Forbes, C., Lewis, R., Sowden, A. et al (2000). The determinants of screening uptake and interventions for increasing uptake: a systematic review. *Health Technol Assess, 4*, 1–133.

Katapodi, M. C., Lee, K. A., Facione, N. C., and Dodd, M. J. (2004). Predictors of perceived breast cancer risk and the relation between perceived risk and breast cancer screening: a meta-analytic review. *Prev Med, 38*, 388–402.

Klabunde, C. N., and Ballard-Barbash, R. (2007). Evaluating population-based screening mammography programs internationally. *Semin Breast Dis, 10*, 102–107.

Lancuck, L., Patnick, J., and Vessey, M. (2008). A cohort effect in cervical screening coverage? *J Med Screen, 15*, 27–29.

Maissi, E., Marteau, T. M., Hankins, M., Moss, S., Legood, R. et al (2004). Psychological impact of human papillomavirus testing in women with borderline or mildly dyskaryotic cervical smear test results: cross sectional questionnaire study. *Br Med J, 328*, 1293.

McCaffery, K., Waller, J., Nazroo, J., and Wardle, J. (2006). Social and psychological impact of HPV testing in cervical screening: a qualitative study. *Sex Transm Infect, 82*, 169–174.

McCaffery, K. J., Irwig, L., Chan, S. F., Macaskill, P., Barratt, A. et al (2008). HPV testing versus repeat Pap testing for the management of a minor abnormal Pap smear: evaluation of a decision aid to support informed choice. *Patient Educ Couns, 73*, 473–481.

Meissner, H. I., Breen, N., Klabunde, C. N., and Vernon, S. W. (2006). Patterns of colorectal cancer screening uptake among men and women in the United States. *Cancer Epidemiol Biomarkers Prev, 15*, 389–394.

Meissner, H. I., Breen, N., Taubman, M. L., Vernon, S. W., and Graubard, B. I. (2007). Which women aren't getting mammograms and why? (United States). *Cancer Causes Control, 18*, 61–70.

Melia, J., Moss, S., and Johns, L. (2004). Rates of prostate-specific antigen testing in general practice in England and Wales in asymptomatic and symptomatic patients: a cross-sectional study. *BJU Int, 94*, 51–56.

Miles, A., Cockburn, J., Smith, R. A., and Wardle, J. (2004). A perspective from countries using organized screening programs. *Cancer, 101*, 1201–1213.

Miles, A., Wardle, J., McCaffery, K., Williamson, S., and Atkin, W. (2003). The effects of colorectal cancer screening on health attitudes and practices. *Cancer Epidemiol Biomarkers Prev, 12*, 651–655.

Moser, K., Patnick, J., and Beral, V. (2009). Inequalities in reported use of breast and cervical screening in Great Britain: analysis of cross sectional survey data. *Br Med J, 338*, b2025.

Nathoo, V. (1988). Investigation of non-responders at a cervical cancer screening clinic in Manchester. *Br Med J (Clin Res Ed), 296*, 1041–1042.

NHS Cervical Screening Programme (2009). *Cervical Screening Programme, England, 2008–2009*. London: The Health and Social Care Information Centre.

Parker, M. A., Robinson, M. H., Scholefield, J. H., and Hardcastle, J. D. (2002). Psychiatric morbidity and screening for colorectal cancer. *J Med Screen, 9*, 7–10.

Power, E., Miles, A., von Wagner, C., Robb, K., and Wardle, J. (2009). Uptake of colorectal cancer screening: system, provider and individual factors and strategies to improve participation. *Future Oncol, 5*, 1371–1388.

Power, E., van Jaarsveld, C. H., McCaffery, K., Miles, A., Atkin, W. et al (2008). Understanding intentions and action in colorectal cancer screening. *Ann Behav Med, 35*, 285–294.

Pruitt, S. L., Shim, M. J., Mullen, P. D., Vernon, S. W., and Amick, B. C. (2009). Association of area socioeconomic status and breast, cervical, and colorectal cancer screening: a systematic review. *Cancer Epidemiol Biomarkers Prev, 18*, 2579–2599.

Rogstad, K. E. (2002). The psychological impact of abnormal cytology and colposcopy. *BJOG, 109*, 364–368.

Ross, L. E., Berkowitz, Z., and Ekwueme, D. U. (2008). Use of the prostate-specific antigen test among U.S. men: findings from the 2005 National Health Interview Survey. *Cancer Epidemiol Biomarkers Prev, 17*, 636–644.

Ross, L. E., Coates, R. J., Breen, N., Uhler, R. J., Potosky, A. L. et al (2004). Prostate-specific antigen test use reported in the 2000 National Health Interview Survey. *Prev Med, 38*, 732–744.

Royse, D., and Dignan, M. (2009). Appalachian knowledge of cancer and screening intentions. *J Cancer Educ, 24*, 357–362.

Ryerson, A. B., Miller, J. W., Eheman, C. R., Leadbetter, S., and White, M. C. (2008). Recent trends in U.S. mammography use from 2000–2006: a population-based analysis. *Prev Med, 47*, 477–482.

Sabatino, S. A., Habarta, N., Baron, R. C., Coates, R. J., Rimer, B. K. et al (2008). Interventions to increase recommendation and delivery of screening for breast, cervical, and colorectal cancers by healthcare providers systematic reviews of provider assessment and feedback and provider incentives. *Am J Prev Med, 35*, S67–S74.

Scaf-Klomp, W., Sanderman, R., van de Wiel, H. B., Otter, R., and van den Heuvel, W. J. (1997). Distressed or relieved? Psychological side effects of breast cancer screening in The Netherlands. *J Epidemiol Community Health, 51*, 705–710.

Schroder, F. H., Hugosson, J., Roobol, M. J., Tammela, T. L., Ciatto, S. et al (2009). Screening and prostate-cancer mortality in a randomized European study. *N Engl J Med, 360*, 1320–1328.

Schueler, K. M., Chu, P. W., and Smith-Bindman, R. (2008). Factors associated with mammography utilization: a systematic quantitative review of the literature. *J Womens Health (Larchmt), 17*, 1477–1498.

Seeff, L. C., Nadel, M. R., Klabunde, C. N., Thompson, T., Shapiro, J. A. et al (2004). Patterns and predictors of colorectal cancer test use in the adult U.S. population. *Cancer, 100*, 2093–2103.

Segnan, N. (1997). Socioeconomic status and cancer screening. *IARC Sci Publ*, 369–376.

Shapiro, J. A., Seeff, L. C., Thompson, T. D., Nadel, M. R., Klabunde, C. N. et al (2008). Colorectal cancer test use from the 2005 National Health Interview Survey. *Cancer Epidemiol Biomarkers Prev, 17*, 1623–1630.

Shapiro, S., Coleman, E. A., Broeders, M., Codd, M., de Koning, K. H. et al (1998). Breast cancer screening programmes in 22 countries: current policies, administration and guidelines. International Breast Cancer Screening Network (IBSN) and the European Network of Pilot Projects for Breast Cancer Screening. *Int J Epidemiol, 27*, 735–742.

Shavers, V. L., Underwood, W., and Moser, R. P. (2009). Race/ethnicity, risk perception, and receipt of prostate-specific antigen testing. *J Natl Med Assoc, 101*, 698–704.

Sheeran, P. (2002). Intention-behaviour relations: a conceptual and empirical review. In M. Hewstone & W. Stroebe (Eds.), *European Review of Social Psychology* (pp. 1–36). Chichester, UK: John Wiley & Sons.

Sheeran, P., and Orbell, S. (2000). Using implementation intentions to increase attendance for cervical cancer screening. *Health Psychol, 19*, 283–289.

Shields, M., and Wilkins, K. (2009). An update on mammography use in Canada. *Health Reports, 20*, 7–19.

Solomon, D., Breen, N., and McNeel, T. (2007). Cervical cancer screening rates in the United States and the potential impact of implementation of screening guidelines. *CA Cancer J Clin, 57*, 105–111.

Steele, R. J., McClements, P. L., Libby, G., Black, R., Morton, C. et al (2009). Results from the first three rounds of the Scottish demonstration pilot of FOBT screening for colorectal cancer. *Gut, 58*, 530–535.

Stock, C., Haug, U., and Brenner, H. (2010). Population-based prevalence estimates of history of colonoscopy or sigmoidoscopy: review and analysis of recent trends. *Gastrointest Endosc, 71*, 366–381.

Sutton, S., and Rutherford, C. (2005). Sociodemographic and attitudinal correlates of cervical screening uptake in a national sample of women in Britain. *Soc Sci Med, 61*, 2460–2465.

Sutton, S., Wardle, J., Taylor, T., McCaffery, K., Williamson, S. et al (2000). Predictors of attendance in the United Kingdom flexible sigmoidoscopy screening trial. *J Med Screen, 7*, 99–104.

Task Force on Community Preventive Services (2008). Recommendations for client- and provider-directed interventions to increase breast, cervical, and colorectal cancer screening. *Am J Prev Med, 35*, S21–S25.

U.S. Preventive services task force. (2009). Screening for breast cancer: U.S. Preventive services task force recommendation statement. *Ann Intern Med, 151*, 716–236, W-236.

van Jaarsveld, C. H., Miles, A., Edwards, R., and Wardle, J. (2006). Marriage and cancer prevention: does marital status and inviting both spouses together influence colorectal cancer screening participation? *J Med Screen, 13*, 172–176.

Vernon, S. W. (1999). Risk perception and risk communication for cancer screening behaviors: a review. *J Natl Cancer Inst Monogr, 25*, 101–119.

von Wagner, C., Good, A., Wright, D., Rachet, B., Obichere, A. et al (2009). Inequalities in colorectal cancer screening participation in the first round of the national screening programme in England. *Br J Cancer, 101*, S60–S63.

Waller, J., Bartoszek, M., Marlow, L., and Wardle, J. (2009). Barriers to cervical cancer screening attendance in England: a population-based survey. *J Med Screen, 16*, 199–204.

Wardle, J., Pernet, A., and Stephens, D. (1995). Psychological consequences of positive results in cervical cancer screening. *Psychol Health, 10*, 185–194.

Wardle, J., McCaffery, K., Nadel, M., and Atkin, W. (2004). Socioeconomic differences in cancer screening participation: comparing cognitive and psychosocial explanations. *Soc Sci and Med, 59*, 249–261.

Wardle, J., Taylor, T., Sutton, S., and Atkin, W. (1999). Does publicity about cancer screening raise fear of cancer? Randomised trial of the psychological effect of information about cancer screening. *Br Med J, 319,* 1037–1038.

Wardle, J., Williamson, S., Sutton, S., Biran, A., McCaffery, K. et al (2003). Psychological impact of colorectal cancer screening. *Health Psychol, 22,* 54–59.

Weinberg, D. S., Miller, S., Rodoletz, M., Egleston, B., Fleisher, L. et al (2009). Colorectal cancer knowledge is not associated with screening compliance or intention. *J Cancer Educ, 24,* 225–232.

Weller, D., Coleman, D., Robertson, R., Butler, P., Melia, J. et al (2007). The UK colorectal cancer screening pilot: results of the second round of screening in England. *Br J Cancer, 97,* 1601–1605.

WHO (2009). Cancer. Fact sheet number 297. www. who.int/mediacentre/factsheets/fs297/en /print.html

Wilson, J. M. G., and Junger, G. (1968). *Principles and Practice of Screening for Disease.* Geneva: World Health Organization.

Chapter 27

The Impact of Behavioral Interventions in Public Health

Noreen M. Clark, Melissa A. Valerio, and Christy R. Houle

1 Introduction

The acceptance of the importance of social and behaviorally focused interventions is relatively new in public health, emerging in earnest little more than two decades ago. Several occurrences likely contributed to the recognition that behavior is the key element in improving the health status of individuals and populations. One is the worldwide increase in chronic disease and the cost of treating it. This has generated greater interest in prevention and greater understanding that the most powerful available means to avoid and manage disease are behavioral. Another factor also connected with the rise of chronic illness has been the dawning awareness among health care providers that control of long-term disease is in the hands of the individuals who experience the illness. As health systems, originally founded to rescue patients from threats posed by acute conditions, shifted more emphatically to address the clinical needs of those living with illness for extended periods of time, so too did recognition that what the person does away from the health care provider is the telling feature in disease control, that is, secondary prevention.

N.M. Clark (✉)
Center for Managing Chronic Disease, University of Michigan, 1415 Washington Heights, Ann Arbor, MI 48109, USA
e-mail: nmclark@umich.edu

2 The Public Health Case for Behavioral Interventions

A public health milestone in the United States supporting the idea that prevention and behavior are almost synonymous was the documentation in 1993 by McGinnis and Foege that behavior is the actual and dominant cause of premature death of Americans (see Table 27.1) (McGinnis and Foege, 1993). In other words, behavioral factors underlie the diseases and injuries that lead to death. Their analysis illustrated (see Fig. 27.1) that lifestyle (chosen or imposed) and environment (social and physical) account for more than 70% of early death while availability of health services and genetic predisposition account for the balance, that is, significantly less. Even with advancements in DNA and the gene-related knowledge base, researchers continue to emphasize that in almost every case, it is the gene–environment–behavior interaction that produces the positive or negative outcome.

Along with increasing acceptance of the role of social factors and behavior in public health have come many theories and methods attempting to account for the complexity of disease and the range of influences shaping well-being. As early as 1986, Wulff and colleagues seriously questioned the biomedical mechanical model of disease that for so long has dominated the scientific paradigm guiding research on human health in the United States. Critics of studies designed to accept or reject hypotheses about single factors have become more and more emphatic about the serious limitations of this approach as unable

A. Steptoe (ed.), *Handbook of Behavioral Medicine*, DOI 10.1007/978-0-387-09488-5_27,
© Springer Science+Business Media, LLC 2010

Table 27.1 Actual causes of death in the United States, 1990 (McGinnis and Foege, 1993)

Ten leading causes of death		Actual causes of death	
Heart disease	720,058	Tobacco	400,000
Cancer	505,322	Diet/inact. patterns	300,000
Cerebrovascular disease	144,088	Alcohol	100,000
Unintentional injuries	91,983	Certain infections	90,000
Chronic lung disease	86,679	Toxic agents	60,000
Pneumonia/influenza	79,513	Firearms	35,000
Diabetes	47,664	Sexual behavior	30,000
Suicide	30,906	Motor vehicles	25,000
Chronic liver disease	25,815	Drug use	20,000
HIV infection	25,188		
Total	1,757,188	Total	1,060,000

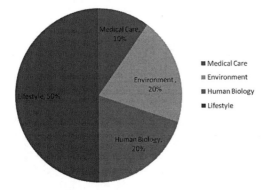

Fig. 27.1 Factors that could avoid premature mortality (McGinnis and Foege, 1993)

to accommodate multi-causal mechanisms (see, for example, Riley, 1993). New concepts in biological research including variation in response (House, 1981) and interaction of causal factors (Ory et al, 1992) have no doubt helped to broaden the perspective of scientists in general about the nature of antecedents influential in health and disease.

3 Creating the Evidence Base

Greater recognition about the population-wide social and behavioral causes of disease and health has been accompanied by a dramatic increase in related academic research. A quick look at research references for the key words "behavioral interventions and public health

impact" generates over 250,000 articles written in the past decade alone. These studies have varied dramatically and have ranged from disease-specific interventions, for example, effective behavioral interventions for children and adolescents with type 1 diabetes (Nansel et al, 2009) to methodological questions, for example, "Internal and external validity of cluster randomized trials" (Eldridge et al, 2008). With a few exceptions (e.g., smoking behavior, compliance with medical regimens, certain types of health care use), we have not seen concerted lines of inquiry regarding behavioral antecedents of health and health care. Rather, there have been a plethora of studies regarding various health problems, behaviors, and contexts for behavior.

The ultimate goal of public health is to achieve widespread and significant impact. One or two studies in an area do not always inspire confidence that a result was in fact valid and is reproducible. Accumulation of results of studies of sufficient scale and rigor is generally considered necessary to suggest adoption of a practice. In recent years, several major efforts in public health have attempted to address this need and to build such an evidence base for interventions.

The Cochrane Collaboration is an international, independent organization dedicated to making widely available, through systematic reviews, information about health-related interventions, primarily, but not exclusively, offered in the clinical setting. The Cochrane reviews are carried out using rigorous protocols to ensure the quality of studies included in analyses and health providers in more than 35 countries avail themselves of Cochrane-produced evidence. As noted, the appeal of these reviews, in the main, has been to clinicians seeking to improve their diagnosis and treatment of disease. Study of behavioral factors has been less evident. Only 2, of the 10 most accessed Cochrane reviews in 2007, concerned social or behavioral factors in disease management or prevention.

An analogous U.S. effort, but one focused specifically on providing evidence for preventive interventions, was the U.S. Centers for Disease Control (CDC) Guide to Clinical Preventive Services available until the late 1990s. It provided data examining 169 different types of disease-specific and clinically focused interventions for their effectiveness including screening,

counseling, and immunization. Dissemination of this type of information since 1998 has been through the Morbidity and Mortality Weekly Report also produced by the U.S. CDC. This channel for obtaining evidence for clinical practice is widely available and referenced in the public health literature.

A related effort much more focused on social and behavioral interventions and non-clinical settings is the Community Guide to Preventive Services. This unit of the U.S. CDC is devoted to creating the evidence base and has generated an impressive range of systematic reviews since its inception in 1996. These reviews touch on the behaviors shown in the McGinnis and Foege 1993 study to precipitate early death and significant morbidity among Americans. Table 27.2

Table 27.2 Summary of selected evidence conclusions of the Community Guide to Preventive Services (2000–2007) (CDC, 2008)

Health problem	Finding
Firearms	Insufficient[a] evidence to determine the effectiveness of any firearms laws on violent outcomes
Early childhood home visits to prevent violence	Strong evidence of effectiveness that early childhood home visitation prevents child abuse and neglect. Insufficient[a] evidence to determine effectiveness of visitation in preventing violence by children, parents, or intimate partners
Universal school-based programs to reduce violent behavior	Strong evidence that such programs decrease rates of violence and aggressive behavior among school-aged children
Effectiveness of HIV partner counseling and provider referral	Insufficient[a] evidence to determine if these changed behavior or reduced transmission. Sufficient evidence that they increased identification of high prevalence target population for HIV testing
Multicomponent school-based nutrition programs	Insufficient[a] evidence to determine effectiveness on children's dietary patterns
Skin cancer prevention	Sufficient evidence for "covering up." Insufficient[a] evidence to determine effectiveness of other population based interventions
Smoking bans	Strong evidence for bans of limits on tobacco smoking in workplaces and public areas in reducing consumption and exposures
Community education for Environmental Tobacco Smoke reduction	Insufficient[a] evidence to determine reduction of exposures
Mass media education to reduce tobacco use	Strong evidence for reducing use by adolescents
Diabetes self-management	Strong evidence for such interventions in community settings for adults and at home for children. Insufficient[a] evidence for interventions in other settings
Obesity in school children	Sufficient evidence for multicomponent interventions in weight loss reduction for adults in work sites. Insufficient[a] evidence to determine effectiveness for children in school settings
Increasing use of child safety seats	Strong evidence for laws requiring use of safety seats and seat belts, distribution of seats, and seat use education programs

[a]Insufficient evidence is not evidence of ineffectiveness

provides a summary of selected evidence conclusions of the Community Guide related to social and behavioral interventions after examination of those thought to have potential for public health impact. The Guide is quick to point out that insufficient evidence is not evidence of ineffectiveness. However, its compilation of studies point to interventions for which confidence for impact is significant.

4 What Has Deterred Wider Impact?

There have been significant improvements in the health of people worldwide in the past decades. At the same time, morbidity and premature mortality due to new conditions and failure to control old ones are at high levels, especially in ethnic and racial subpopulations, and the burden of cost and suffering is staggering. Much of this burden is a result of not applying what is known about disease prevention and control and not focusing on the social and behavioral aspects of well-being.

4.1 Translation of Evidence to Practice

Many argue that the impact of research on the public's health has been hampered less by what we do not know and more by failing to more broadly apply what we do know. Examples of the gap between what is known and population-wide behaviors are plentiful in public health (e.g., tobacco use, patterns of physical activity, and spread of infections) (Ginexi and Hilton, 2006; Glasgow et al, 2004). A major barrier in the translation of evidence to practice is the failure to link the work of academic researchers to the needs of practitioners and the ultimate beneficiaries: individuals and families. The translation process is fraught with problems such as how and when evidence becomes sufficient to recommend a change in practice, how valid findings can be effectively communicated beyond the

academy, and how quickly to gain wide acceptance of a new, more beneficial practice.

There is increasing public health focus on the identification of efficacious approaches for behavioral change and greater acceptance that complex problems require interdisciplinary interventions and therapies. Many health and medical experts posit that solutions drawing on the perspectives of different fields are more likely to be successfully translated into practice (Ginexi and Hilton, 2006; Glasgow et al, 2004). This line of reasoning is persuasive but has not been empirically tested. A further barrier to translation appears to be the general lack of information about the practicality and cost–benefits of a proposed change. Given that public health resources are limited, both efficacy and effectiveness of a change must be equal to or outweigh its cost. Similarly, an efficient means to introduce and maintain a new practice must be evident.

A number of observers (for example, Glasgow et al, 2004) have opined that most practice change requires modification of systems and policies to be truly integrated and maintained in the work of practitioners and behavior of people in general. Moving public health interventions proven through research into effective practice can take years to evolve. Society-wide changes often have been dependent on new or expanded policy (e.g., regarding smoking cessation: smoke-free public areas, tobacco sales taxes) (CDC, 2008; Warner, 2006). Some evidence also suggests that translation of findings into practice especially in low-income communities may be more successful when the individual and groups that experience the greatest burden of a health problem are involved in finding the solution for it (Israel et al, 2005).

Several factors, therefore, must be addressed in the translation of research to practice. One is a focus at the outset, in the initial design of research, on the issue of translation. Another is identification of means to communicate effectively to practitioners and other consumers in a timely manner regarding findings. Yet another is consideration of structural and organizational factors needed to encourage a new practice and addressing system and policy changes and resources needed to achieve translation. Finally, the process of moving from research to practice, itself, requires study and identification of the most powerful means to disseminate information and gain support for evidence. As in most important endeavors, without sufficient investment of time, energy, and money, effective translation of evidence into practice will certainly be slow and is likely to be unsuccessful.

4.2 Failure to be Holistic

Another reason for the lack of public health impact is the failure of practitioners, researchers, and policy makers to take a comprehensive or holistic view of problems. Public health interventions have often emphasized modifying the behavior of individuals, rather than the social and physical environments in which they function. However, a range of health risks have been shown to be related to structural aspects of the communities in which people live, over and above the personal characteristics of the individuals living there (Diez-Roux et al, 1999). That being said, large bodies of work in epidemiology as well as social science, fairly recently, have taken a more comprehensive view, positing both upstream and downstream determinants of population health (Kaplan, 2004). Figure 27.2 illustrates this perspective and the breadth of

the social and behavioral factors it encompasses. Such work has suggested that the best route to improving well-being and eliminating disparities in health status is enhancing social and economic conditions so that people are able to engage in healthy lifestyles, that is, behave in healthful ways.

4.3 Limited Use of Behavioral Models

The public health picture is more complicated when models for large-scale change are behavioral ones, that is, where behavior is the central feature in producing outcomes. Such models examine the behavior to health outcome trajectory and the dynamic nature of change. However, their very complexity can inhibit their use. For the sake of this discussion, we will present two models developed by the authors for circumventing or resolving health problems: one regarding individual behavior and one concerning community-wide behavior. These are by no means the only or necessarily the best models to be considered as explanation of behavior change conducive to improving public health. They are offered as illustrative and because of the authors' familiarity with them.

The model of self-regulation of chronic disease (Clark et al, 2001) (see Fig. 27.3) posits that individuals learn new behavior through a combination of observation, judgment, trial

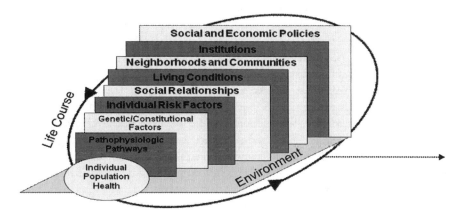

Fig. 27.2 Multilevel framework for reducing inequalities in health (Kaplan, 2004)

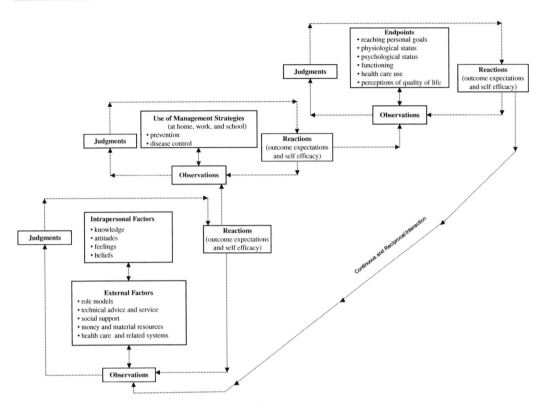

Fig. 27.3 The continuous and reciprocal nature of self-regulation processes in disease prevention and management (Clark et al, 2001)

behavior, and reaction (specifically outcome expectation – the behavior produced the desired result; and self-efficacy – the confidence to repeat the behavior). This self-regulation is the process through which behavior changes. The model has been used in large-scale asthma (Clark et al, 2005 et al, 2007) and heart disease (Clark et al, 2000, 2009a et al; Janz et al, 2004) management trials among other conditions. It is predicated on the idea that public health impact is achieved when large numbers of individuals are behaving in ways most conducive to health and disease control and are enabled to do so by the public health and wider societal systems. Although the process of self-regulation is individual and personal, the influences on it are external and often public. The model indicates that modifications of external influences (by the individual or by the public health system) are required to enhance a person's ability to self-regulate.

In the applications of such behavioral models, largely due to methodological constraints (see following section on new, promising evaluation methods), changes in individual and family behavior and social factors often have been observed. However the effect of changes in structural factors influencing behavior has been more difficult to assess.

When the behavior in question is community-wide actions and practices, the story is much the same. Figure 27.4 presents the Allies Against Asthma (Allies) model of community change (Clark et al, 2006) initiated through community-wide collaboration. When the goal is enhanced public health, collective efforts usually focus on enabling community structures and systems to facilitate behavior conducive to health. The Allies model indicates that tasks that a collective of stakeholders undertake are analogous to self-regulation (e.g., observation, planning, continuous monitoring). To achieve population-wide

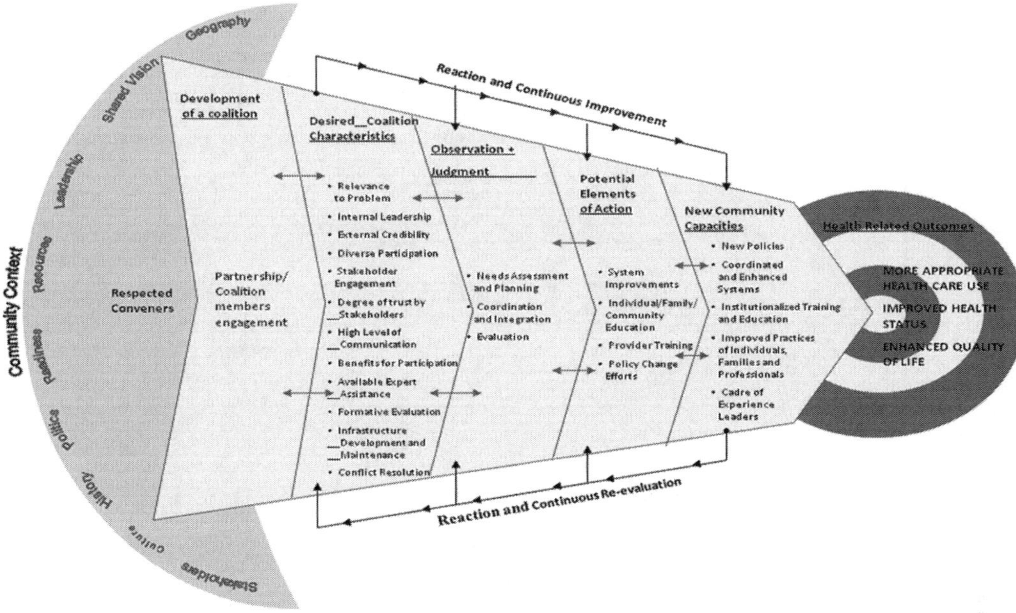

Fig. 27.4   Allies against asthma model (Clark et al, 2006)

change through collective action, collaborators must not only use skills similar to self-regulation but also develop and maintain their capacity to work together. Therefore, on top of their system and policy change efforts is layered the effort to keep community allies working effectively together. System and policy changes associated with the Allies model have been observed, as have health-related outcomes, for example, symptom reduction (Clark et al, 2009b). However, again largely because of methodological constraints, the links between collective efforts, system change, behavior change, and public health outcomes have been difficult to document.

5 Public Health as Social Movement

Given the varied and diverse influences inherent in large-scale behavioral change, it is possible to argue that the farthest reaching and most significant impact on the public's health in the United States has resulted from efforts that are essentially social movements. These movements have come closest to embodying the precepts of change discussed above. Bringing about widespread change takes time and requires multiple strategies, many, if not most, of which are behavioral in nature (Green and Kreuter, 2004). The most compelling example of public health as a social movement is the movement for tobacco control: the gradual reduction in cigarette smoking among Americans that over time led to dramatic decreases in heart disease and cancer, two of the country's most pernicious public health problems.

Figure 27.5 illustrates the critical events that have been associated with reductions in adult per capita cigarette smoking in America over the last 100 years. The increase in tobacco consumption and the attendant increases in heart disease and cancer began their rise at the turn of the last century. By the 1960s, cigarette consumption reached its highest level and strong evidence of the relationship between this habit and disease appeared in the public health literature (Freund and Ward, 1960; Hammond, 1960; Larson et al, 1960; Law et al, 1997; Miller, 1960; Ware, 1960). In 1964, the first U.S. surgeon general's report on the topic provided

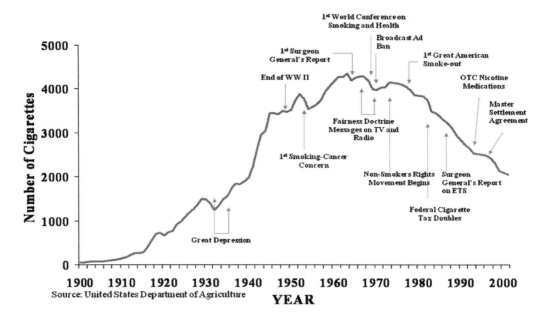

Fig. 27.5 Adult per capita cigarette consumption and major smoking and health events – U.S., 1900–2001 (Warner, 2006)

compelling information and underscored the relationship between smoking behavior and poor health, which then began in earnest the effort to change the national perspective on smoking, as well as personal practice. Contributing factors to the downward shift in behaviors have been documented by a number of observers (Mendez and Warner, 2004; Soliman et al, 2004). These included the first world conference on smoking and health held in 1967 that attempted to identify effective strategies for changing behavior and posited the expected effects of modifying the social environment to prohibit smoking. Dramatic changes in communication strategies ensued beginning with the fairness doctrine that required broadcasters to provide one anti-smoking public service announcement on American television for every three cigarette advertisements, and ending with a total ban on broadcast advertising. Smoker's rights collective action became national and visible and comprised local efforts to change policy, ensuring wide availability of "quit" options, encouragement of health professionals to counsel patients about smoking, and mobilization of the major health organizations for the first

"Great American Smoke-out" to change behavior. Community through national action was followed by the first serious efforts to raise tax on cigarettes and, eventually, legal action and the master settlement agreement between the government and cigarette producing companies. The U.S. surgeon general's report on environmental tobacco smoke reinforced local efforts to ban smoking in public places and many private sector organizations followed suit. It is interesting to note that only one clinical and pharmacological intervention, the availability of over-the-counter nicotine medications, is credited with contributing in a relatively small way (and fairly late in the game) to the decrease in smoking that transpired over time.

It was a range of intervention strategies in both the public and private sectors that produced this massive change in behavior (Andrews et al, 2007; Barth et al, 2008; Cofta-Woerpel et al, 2007; McDonald, 2004 et al; et alStack and Zillich, 2007; Valery et al, 2008). Much of the effort focused on modifying policy and systems to bring about the needed change. It took almost 40 years to reap significant public health benefits.

The most important lesson from the tobacco control experience may be that we need to take a longer term perspective on change than is usually evident in research and evaluation. We may need to conceive of strategies that can fit into or trigger a social movement hastening impact on the public's health. We need to undertake more focused lines of inquiry and with stronger research methods and tools and to place more emphasis on building the evidence base for promising interventions that accumulate to produce the outcomes we seek.

6 The Need for Robust Tools and Methods

An aim of public health efforts is to reach the largest number of people with the maximum level of benefit. Empirical studies that try to understand how to have such impact are few in number and are often methodologically questioned.

Several large-scale intervention trials occurring over the past three decades are conceptually close to social movements. These have related to cardiovascular disease risk (e.g., the North Karelia Project, the Stanford Five-City Project) (Fortmann and Varady, 2000), smoking behavior (e.g., COMMIT study, Project ASSIST) (Stillman et al, 1999), and cancer risk (5-A-Day Program) (Campbell et al, 1999). Such projects have targeted whole communities, used multiple strategies to modify individual behaviors and concurrently change the social environment in which behaviors are shaped (Elder et al, 1993; Goodman et al, 1996; Merzel and D'Afflitti, 2003). However, available evaluations of multistrategy, community-wide, large-scale interventions have shown limited effect on population health risks (Merzel and D'Afflitti, 2003). As noted, person–environment response and accommodation to health-related experiences is difficult to measure and analyze. Indeed, outside of bona fide ineffectiveness or poor implementation of strategies, it is believed that the modest effects of such trials may be attributable to inadequate

evaluation methods (Craig et al, 2008; Hawe et al, 2004a; Merzel and D'Afflitti, 2003).

Although experimental design and its quasi-experimental approximations are considered the most robust means to establish a causal link between public health interventions and observed effects (Zaza et al, 2000), these are often difficult to use or inappropriate in community-based research. A particular hurdle for studies at the community or population level is that often there are insufficient numbers of subjects for statistical power to detect anything other than large intervention effects. Further, amassing data to discern financial, legal, or ethical effects associated with an approach can be prohibitively expensive or practically infeasible (Lipsey and Cordray, 2000). Beyond design and power questions, appropriate and valid measures and evaluative tools are not always available. However, new means hold promise.

6.1 Social Network Analysis

Social network analysis, or the study of social structures, is becoming increasingly popular as researchers better appreciate the linkages between social relationships and health status and/or health behavior. Network analysis is quantitative and assesses the composition, patterning, and function of social relationships (e.g., size, density or reciprocity, resources drawn upon by the network) among people, groups, or organizations (see Hawe et al, 2004; Heaney and Israel, 1997). In population health, network analysis is believed by some to be an important means to understand how individual actions and interactions affect health outcomes at the community or population level (Cattell, 2001; Hawe et al, 2004).

6.2 Hierarchical Linear Modeling

Advances in statistical procedures, including hierarchical linear modeling (HLM), have provided a fuller understanding of the relationships between intervention activities and changes in health (see Chapter 56). HLM analysis can account for variation that exists at the individual level (e.g., age, race/ethnicity, treatment group) while examining effects at the population level (Weinfurt, 2000). To date, however, few studies have sufficient data from process and outcome evaluation activities to examine whether lack of effect was explained by the failure of strategy, implementation, or theory (Lipsey and Cordray, 2000).

6.3 Geographical Information Systems

Geographical Information Systems (GIS) are computer-based tools that can enhance understanding of the spatial and temporal relationships that affect health risks and outcome by digitally linking data and geography, often in the form of a map. Given that patterns among data are often easier to observe when presented in map format, GIS is thought to facilitate hypothesis formation about causal relationships and promote evidence-based decision-making among a wider range of stakeholders (Boulos, 2005). Applications of GIS in the public health arena are wide-ranging and are being used to identify patterns of disease, strengthen emergency preparedness, assess the impact of health initiatives, and track health and social service resources (CDC, 2009; WHO, 2009).

6.4 Health Impact Assessment (HIA)

HIA is defined as a blend of procedures, methods, and tools to provide decision-makers with information about the potential effects of a policy, program, or project on population health and the distribution of such effects between population sub-groups (Dannenberg et al, 2006; European Center for Health Policy, 1999).

Interest in HIA methods has grown out of recognition that the advancement of many public health objectives requires effective communication and action among stakeholders within and outside of traditional public health arenas (e.g., urban planners, city governmental officials, health department officials). HIA processes to assess cross-sector interests, actions, and collaborations can be prospective, concurrent, or retrospective and incorporate qualitative and quantitative evidence. They can include the use of tools ranging from simple checklists to complex collaborative tracking (Parry and Kemm, 2005; Taylor et al, 2003). Examples of policies, programs, and projects examined using an HIA approach include those related to residential redevelopment, walk-to-school programs, land-use planning, wage policies, and home energy subsidies (Dannenberg et al, 2006; WHO, 2009). Evidence accumulated in Europe, Canada, and elsewhere that health impact assessments can be a useful tool to improve public health fueled recent interest in the development and use of HIAs in the United States (Dannenberg et al, 2006).

6.5 Social Movement Assessment

Given parallels between large-scale interventions and social movements, methodological approaches or tools used by social movement researchers and activists may prove particularly useful in public health arenas. One such tool, for example, is the Movement Action Plan (MAP), a framework designed to help stakeholders understand and evaluate social movements by describing stages through which they progress (Moyer, 2001). The MAP framework comprises eight stages: (1) Critical Social Problem Exists; (2) Proven Failure of Official Institutions; (3) Ripening Conditions; (4) Take Off; (5) Perception of Failure; (6) Majority Public Opinion; (7) Success; and (8) Continuation. For each stage, the MAP outlines related advocacy and implementation roles and goals.

7 Conclusion

The role of behavior, often overlooked, has become more prominent in both public health-related research and practice. As health problems have become increasingly complex, more holistic efforts to understand them have become necessary and more evident. Recognition of the influence of the social and physical environment on behavior has also increased, particularly, as disparities in health outcomes have become a national concern. More robust and reliable tools to assess behavior–environment–outcome relationships will be needed to determine the full value of sociobehavioral approaches for improving the public's health.

Acknowledgements The authors wish to thank Minal R. Patel for her assistance with preparation of this chapter.

References

Andrews, J. O., Bentley, G., Crawford, S., Pretlow, L., and Tingen, M. S. (2007). Using community-based participatory research to develop a culturally sensitive smoking cessation intervention with public housing neighborhoods. *Ethn Dis, 17*, 331–337.

Barth, J., Critchley, J., and Bengel, J. (2008). Psychosocial interventions for smoking cessation in patients with coronary heart disease. *Cochrane Database Syst Rev, 23*, CD006886.

Boulos, M. N. (2005). Research protocol: EB-GIS4HEALTH UK - foundation evidence base and ontology-based framework of modular, reusable models for UK/NHS health and healthcare GIS applications. *Int J Health Geogr, 4*, 2.

Campbell, M. K., Reynolds, K. D., Havas, S., Curry, S., Bishop, D. et al (1999). Stages of change for increasing fruit and vegetable consumption among adults and young adults participating in the national 5-a-day for better health community studies. *Health Educ Behav, 26*, 513–534.

Cattell, V. (2001). Poor people, poor places, and poor health: the mediating role of social networks and social capital. *Soc Sci Med, 52*, 1501–1516.

Centers for Disease Control and Prevention (CDC). Community guide to preventive services. Accessed on November 26, 2008 at http://www.thecommunityguide.org/.

Centers for Disease Control and Prevention (CDC). GIS and public health. Accessed on January 30, 2009 at http://www.cdc.gov/nchs/gis.htm.

Clark, N. M., Janz, N. K., Dodge, J. A., Schork, M. A., Fingerlin, T. E. et al (2000). Changes in functional health status of older women with heart disease: evaluation of a program based on self-regulation. *J Gerontol B Psychol Sci Soc Sci, 55*, S117–S126.

Clark, N. M., Gong, M., and Kaciroti, N. (2001). A model of self-regulation for control of chronic disease. *Health Educ Behav., 28*, 769–782.

Clark, N. M., Gong, M., Kaciroti, N., Yu, J., Wu, G. et al (2005). A trial of asthma self-management in Beijing schools. *Chronic Illn, 1*, 31–38.

Clark, N. M., Doctor, L. J., Friedman, A. R., Lachance, L. L., Houle, C. R. et al (2006). Community coalitions to control chronic disease: allies against asthma as a model and case study. *Health Promot Pract, 7* (2 Suppl), 14S–22S.

Clark, N. M., Gong, Z. M., Wang, S. J., Lin, X., Bria, W. F. et al (2007). A randomized trial of a self-regulation intervention for women with asthma. *Chest, 132*, 88–97.

Clark, N. M., Janz, N. K., Dodge, J. A., Lin, X., Trabert, B. L. et al (2009a). Heart disease management by women: does intervention format matter? *Health Educ Behav. 36*, 394–409.

Clark, N. M, Doctor, L. J., Gilmore, L., Kelly, C., Krieger, J. et al (2009b). Policy and system change and community coalitions: outcomes from allies against asthma. Unpublished manuscript, University of Michigan.

Cofta-Woerpel, L., Wright, K. L., and Wetter, D. W. (2007). Smoking cessation 3: multicomponent interventions. *Behav Med, 32*, 135–149.

Craig, P., Dieppe, P., Macintyre, S., Michie, S., Nazareth, I., Petticrew, M. et al (2008). Developing and evaluating complex interventions: the new medical research council guidance. *BMJ, 337*, a1655.

Dannenberg, A. L., Bhatia, R., Cole, B. L., Dora, C., Fielding, J. E. et al (2006). Growing the field of health impact assessment in the United States: an agenda for research and practice. *Am J Public Health, 96*, 262–270.

Diez-Roux, A. V., Nieto, F. J., Caulfield, L., Tyroler, H. A., Watson, R. L. et al (1999). Neighbourhood differences in diet: the atherosclerosis risk in communities (ARIC) study. *J Epidemiol Community Health, 53*, 55–63.

Elder, J. P., Wildey, M., de Moor, C., Sallis, J. F., Jr, Eckhardt, L. et al (1993). The long-term prevention of tobacco use among junior high school students: classroom and telephone interventions. *Am J Public Health, 83*, 1239–1244.

Eldridge, S., Ashby, D., Bennett, C., Wakelin, M., and Feder, G. (2008) Internal and external validity of cluster randomized trials: systematic review of recent trials. *BMJ, 336*, 876–880.

European Centre for Health Policy, World Health Organization Regional Office for Europe (1999). Health Impact Assessment: Main Concepts and Suggested Approach. Gothenburg Consensus

Paper. Available at http://www.who.dk/document/PAE/Gothenburgpaper.pdf. Accessed November 19, 2008.

Fortmann, S. P., and Varady, A. N. (2000). Effects of a community-wide health education program on cardiovascular disease morbidity and mortality: The Stanford five-city project. *Am J Epidemiol, 152,* 316–323.

Freund, J., and Ward, C. (1960). The acute effect of cigarette smoking on the digital circulation in health and disease. *Ann N Y Acad Sci, 90,* 85–101.

Ginexi, E. M., and Hilton, T. F. (2006). What's next for translation research? *Eval Health Prof, 29,* 334–347.

Glasgow, R. E., Klesges, L. M., Dzewaltowski, D. A., Bull, S. S., and Estabrooks, P. (2004). The future of health behavior change research: what is needed to improve translation of research into health promotion practice? *Ann Behav Med, 27,* 3–12.

Goodman, R. M., Wandersman, A., Chinman, M., Imm, P., and Morrissey, E. (1996). An ecological assessment of community-based interventions for prevention and health promotion: approaches to measuring community coalitions. *Am J Community Psychol, 24,* 33–61.

Green, L. W., and Kreuter, M. W. (2004). *Health Promotion Planning: An Educational and Environmental Approach, 4th Ed.* New York: McGraw-Hill.

Hammond, E. C. (1960). Smoking in relation to heart disease. *Am J Public Health Nations Health, 50,* 20–26.

Hawe, P., Shiell, A., Riley, T., and Gold, L. (2004a). Methods for exploring implementation variation and local context within a cluster randomized community intervention trial. *J Epidemiol Community Health, 58,* 788–793.

Hawe, P., Webster, C., and Shiell, A. (2004b). A glossary of terms for navigating the field of social network analysis. *J Epidemiol Community Health, 58,* 971–975.

Heaney, C. A., and Israel, B. A. (1997) Social networks and social support. *Health Behavior & Health Education.* San Francisco: Jossey-Bass Publishers.

House, J. S. (1981). *Work Stress and Social Support.* Reading, MA: Addison-Wesley.

Israel, B. A., Eng, E., Schulz, A. J., and Parker, E. A. (2005). *Methods in Community-Based Participatory Research for Health* (pp. 404–405). Jossey Bass.

Janz, N. K., Dodge, J. A., Janevic, M. R., Lin, X., Donaldson, A. E. et al (2004). Understanding and reducing stress and psychological distress in older women with heart disease. *J Women Aging, 16,* 19–38.

Kaplan, G. A. (2004). What's wrong with social epidemiology, and how can we make it better? *Epidemiol Rev, 26,* 124–135.

Larson, P. S., Haag, H. B., and Silvette, H. (1960). Changing concepts of the role of tobacco in the management of disease. *Am J Med Sci, 240,* 613–635.

Law, M. R., Morris, J. K., and Wald, N. J. (1997). Environmental tobacco smoke exposure and ischaemic heart disease: an evaluation of the evidence. *BMJ, 315,* 973–980.

Lipsey, M. W., and Cordray, D. S. (2000). Evaluation methods for social intervention. *Annu Rev Psychol, 51,* 345–375.

McDonald, P. W. (2004). A low-cost, practical method for increasing smokers' interest in smoking cessation programs. *Can J Public Health, 95,* 50–53

McGinnis, J. M., and Foege, W. H. (1993). Actual causes of death in the United States. *JAMA, 270,* 2207–2212.

Mendez, D., and Warner, K. E. (2004). Adult cigarette smoking prevalence: declining as expected (not as desired). *Am J Public Health, 94,* 251–252.

Merzel, C., and D'Afflitti, J. (2003). Reconsidering community-based health promotion: promise, performance, and potential. *Am J Public Health, 93,* 557–574.

Miller, W. F. (1960). The role of tobacco smoking in disease of the respiratory tract. *Tuberculol Thorac Dis, 19,* 8–13.

Moyer, B. (2001). *Doing Democracy: The MAP Model for Organizing Social Movements.* Tennessee: New Society.

Nansel, T. R., Anderson, B. J., Laffel, L. M., Simons-Morton, B. G., Weissberg-Benchell, J. et al (2009). A multisite trial of a clinic-integrated intervention for promoting family management of pediatric type 1 diabetes: feasibility and design. *Pediatr Diabetes, 10,* 30–40.

Ory, M. G., Abeles, R. P., and Lipman, P. D. (1992). *Introduction*: *Aging, Health and Behavior.* Newbury Park, CA: Sage.

Parry, J. M., Kemm, J. R., and Evaluation of Health Impact Assessment Workshop. (2005). Criteria for use in the evaluation of health impact assessments. *Public Health, 119,* 1122–1129.

Riley, M. W. (1993). A theoretical basis for research on health. In K. Dean (Ed.), *Population Health Research: Linking Theory and Methods* (pp. 37–53). London, England: Sage.

Soliman, S., Pollack, H. A., and Warner, K. E. (2004). Decrease in the prevalence of environmental tobacco smoke exposure in the home during the 1990s in families with children. *Am J Public Health, 94,* 314–320.

Stack, N. M., and Zillich, A. J. (2007). Implementation of inpatient and outpatient tobacco-cessation programs. *Am J Health Syst Pharm, 64,* 2074–2079.

Stillman, F., Hartman, A., Graubard, B., Gilpin, E., Chavis, D. et al (1999). The American Stop Smoking Intervention Study. Conceptual framework and evaluation design. *Eval Rev, 23,* 259–280.

Taylor, L., Gowman, N., and Quigley, R. (2003). Evaluating health impact assessment. London, England: Health Development Agency. Available at http://www.iaia.org/Non_Members/Pubs_Ref_Material/Evaluating%20HIA%20pdf. Accessed November 19, 2008.

Valery, L., Anke, O., Inge, K. K., and Johannes, B. (2008). Effectiveness of smoking cessation interventions among adults: a systematic review of reviews. *Eur J Cancer Prev, 17*, 535–544.

Ware, G. W. (1960). "Tobaccosis" or the pathologic effects of tobacco on the human body. *Med Ann Dist Columbia, 29*, 333–340.

Warner, K. E. (2006). Tobacco policy research: insights and contributions to public health policy. In K. E. Warner (Ed.), *Tobacco Control Policy* (pp. 3–86). San Francisco: Jossey-Bass.

Weinfurt, K. P. (2000). Repeated measures analyses: ANOVA, MANOVA, and HLM. In L. G. Grimm & P. R. Yarnold (Eds.), *Reading and Understanding More Multivariate Statistics*. American Psychological Association.

World Health Organization (WHO) (2009). GIS and public health mapping. Accessed on January 30, 2009. At http://www.who.int/health_mapping/gisandphm/en/index.html.

Wulff, H. R. (1986). Rational diagnosis and treatment. *J Med Philos, 11*, 123–134.

Zaza, S., Wright-De Aguero, L. K., Briss, P. A., Truman, B. I., Hopkins, D. P. et al (2000). Data collection instrument and procedure for systematic reviews in the guide to community preventive services. Task Force on Community Preventive Services. *Am J Prev Med, 18*(1 Suppl), 44–74.

Part V
Genetic Process in Behavioral Medicine

Chapter 28

Quantitative Genetics in Behavioral Medicine

Eco de Geus

1 Introduction

A striking characteristic of almost all of the traits of interest in behavioral medicine is that they show large individual differences, which often follow an approximate normal distribution. For behavioral traits this distribution is thought to derive from a number of nature/nurture variance components, schematically depicted in Fig. 28.1. Starting with the *genes* block, this scheme posits that individual differences in the development of physiological systems, including the central nervous system governing behavioral disposition, depend in part on the variation in the genetic code stored in the deoxyribonucleic acid (DNA) molecules of all cells. In parallel, individual differences depend on the specific experiential history of each person that involves exposure to a multilayered *environment* that includes the intrauterine environment (fetal programming), diet, climate, parental rearing styles (harsh discipline, parental monitoring), peer affiliation, illness and accidents, lifestyle factors, stressful life events (e.g., abuse, neglect, poverty, parental discord, residential instability, sibling or parental psychopathology) and many other factors.

Genetic and environmental factors may exert independent main effects on variation in behavioral traits, but they can also interact to create various forms of *gene–environment interaction*. From the first cell division onward, regulation of gene expression at the right time and in the right cells is strongly dependent on the appropriate cues. Environmental stressors, either physical (e.g., infection) or mental (e.g., trauma), can directly influence gene expression through glucocorticoids, nutrient molecules, oxygen radicals, or cytokines which are known to exert powerful genomic effects. Hence, behavioral outcomes can reflect an interaction of genetic variation with environmental stressors.

Through the long entwined action of genetic variation, environmental effects, and their interactions, each individual will develop a unique set of behavioral dispositions that predict the behavior of the individual across a number of situations. These dispositions are summarized as intelligence, empathy, extraversion, creativity, neuroticism, hostility, etc. Ongoing behavior will be determined by the interaction of these dispositions and the subjects' current environment, most prominently the social environment. Since the variation in disposition is partly genetically driven, this creates a second-order gene–environment interaction.

Importantly, the past and current environments themselves are not independent of behavior as indicated by the *gene–environment correlation* loops in Fig. 28.1. Three different forms of gene–environment correlation have been described (Plomin et al, 2000). Active correlation occurs when individuals with a certain genetic makeup actively select certain environments over others. For instance, children that are of above average intelligence because of a

E. de Geus (✉)
Department of Biological Psychology, VU University,
Van der Boechorststraat 1, 1081 BT, Amsterdam,
The Netherlands
e-mail: jcn.de.geus@psy.vu.nl

A. Steptoe (ed.), *Handbook of Behavioral Medicine*, DOI 10.1007/978-0-387-09488-5_28,
© Springer Science+Business Media, LLC 2010

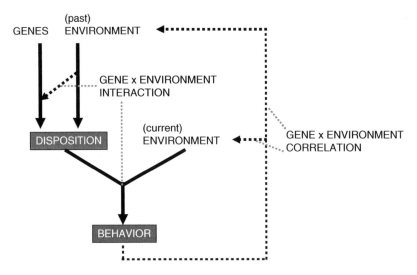

Fig. 28.1 Genetic and environmental factors that cause individual differences in behavioral traits

small genetic advantage in brain development will do well at school, will more actively seek out new knowledge, and be selected for higher and longer education. This increases their exposure to materials that will further enhance brain development.

Reactive correlation refers to the reaction of others to the (partly genetically driven) behavior of an individual that may give rise to individual-specific social environments that are correlated with their genotype. For instance, children that are mildly obese because of small genetic disadvantages in energy metabolism and/or behavioral responses to the current overabundance in food may develop poor exercise abilities compared to more lean children. Some emphatic teachers or coaches may be able to compensate the poor performance during sports activities, but peers will be relentless and the child/adolescent may start to dislike and actively avoid exercise activities. Non-exercising may then get correlated to the genetic disadvantage in body build with both contributing to a further development of obesity. Reactive gene–environment correlation remains at work in adults too. Higher innate levels of aggression and hostility will lead to more marital conflicts and conflicts with colleagues at work than seen in more agreeable colleagues and may lead the individual to end up with

a smaller social network to buffer adverse life events.

Cultural transmission finally gives rise to passive gene–environment correlation when parents provide genes as well as environments to their offspring. The classic example is again from the field of intelligence, where the double advantage hypothesis states that children from highly educated parents receive genes that favor their cognitive development as well as intellectually more enriched environments (Jencks et al, 1972).

The scheme in Fig. 28.1 is not limited to behavioral traits but also applies well to physiological traits. Blood pressure, for instance, evolves as a function of genetic endowment and environmental influences during development, including the intrauterine environment (fetal programming), family diet, and stress exposure. There are many possible sources of gene–environment interaction in blood pressure regulation where some genetic variants influence blood pressure most strongly when dietary sodium levels are high or when chronic psychosocial stress is present (Ge et al, 2009). In addition, dispositional factors like hostility and lifestyle choices like smoking or exercise behavior can influence blood pressure levels (Pickering, 2001), and any of the gene–environment interactions and correlations that affect these behavioral traits can also become determinants of blood pressure.

We can formalize the scheme in Fig. 28.1 by first defining the value of a trait for individual i as the population mean plus a genetic effect, an environmental effect, and an interaction term:

$$\text{Phenotype } (P_i) = \mu + G_i + E_i + G_i \times E_i. \tag{28.1}$$

In Eq. (28.1), we use the term *phenotype* rather than trait, in keeping with the terminology in genetics. Following standard rules of variance computation, the phenotypic variance (V_P) in a group of individuals consists of genetic and environmental variance and variance due to the interaction term. In addition, if the genotype and the environment are not independent (gene–environment correlation), the non-zero covariance terms should be added:

$$\begin{aligned}\text{Variance } (P) &= \text{variance } (\mu + G + E + G \times E) \\ &= \text{variance } (G) + \text{var}(E) \\ &\quad + \text{var}(G \times E) + 2 \times \text{Cov}(G, E). \end{aligned} \tag{28.2}$$

Below we first focus on the genetic variance term.

2 Genetic Variance

Biobehavioral scientists typically observe the effects of genetic variance at the far downstream stage, for instance, as variation in blood pressure levels or personality. It is important to keep in mind that such variation starts upstream with variation in the quantity and quality of proteins. This protein variation then translates into variation in the organization of physiological systems, like the endothelial function of blood vessels or connectivity within limbic nervous system structures, and finally into variation in the observed biobehavioral traits. Protein function variation can arise from genotypic variation in the coding parts (exons) of a gene, yielding functionally less, or more, efficient isoforms. Most of this

variation is at the level of single base substitutions or single nucleotide polymorphisms (SNPs). For SNPs causing disease, the severity of the clinical manifestations often depends on the location of the SNP in the coding triplets (codons). SNPs in the first or second base of a codon have usually more consequences than mutations in the third base. More dramatic variations are the insertion of a stop codon (abolishing translation), frame shift mutations (disturbing the complete polypeptide sequence following the codon change), insertions or deletions of one or more bases, or repeat expansions that do not just create normal variability in efficiency but lead to absence of proteins (e.g., phenylketonuria, or PKU) or dysfunctional proteins and even toxic proteins (e.g., Huntington disease).[1]

2.1 Monogenetic Trait Variation

Although important, variation in the isoform of proteins may actually make up only a very small part of functional allelic variation. Much variation in physiology and behavior arises from a difference in expression of the gene. That is, much allelic variation may lead to more or less of a protein, rather than a different form of the protein. To illustrate the *quantitative* effects of allelic variation we use a modification of the example in the classical textbook on quantitative genetics by Falconer (Falconer and Mackay, 1996) and hypothesize a bi-allelic gene for systolic blood pressure (SBP) that has a decreaser allele "b" which causes lower blood pressure and an increaser allele "B" which causes higher blood pressure (see Fig. 28.2). For now, let us assume that the mean effect of all other factors translates into a SBP of 129 mm Hg and that none of these factors leads to variation between

---

[1] What was left out here is large-scale genetic variation, including loss or gain of chromosomes or breakage and rejoining of chromatids. This variation is rare but often leads to profound developmental problems.

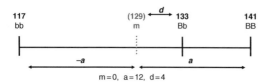

m = 0, a = 12, d = 4

Fig. 28.2 A hypothetical "SBP gene" with a bi-allelic polymorphism that influences systolic blood pressure level

individuals. We observe three types of individuals, one with a SBP of 117 mm Hg and genotype "bb," one with a SBP of 133 mm Hg and genotypes "Bb," and one with a SBP of 141 mm Hg and genotype "BB." The allelic effects are typically defined with respect to the difference between the homozygotes (bb, BB). They can be formalized as "+a" and "−a," which is the difference between each of the two homozygotes and the homozygote midpoint (m), and d, which is the dominance deviation of the heterozygote from the homozygote midpoint. If the alleles were perfectly additive, the heterozygote (Bb) should have been equal to the homozygote midpoint (129 mm Hg). However, the increaser allele B of this SBP gene appears to "dominate" the decreaser allele d. The SBP gene is said to display dominance ($d \neq 0$).

Now suppose we would do the following breeding experiment (please note that this is a *thought* experiment!). We select pairs of heterozygous parents for the SBP locus (both have genotype Bb). Such parents will yield an offspring with genotypes BB, Bb, and bb and the expected frequencies and genotypic effects as in Table 28.1.

The contribution of this locus to the mean SBP in the offspring (mean genetic effect μ_g) is the sum of the genotypic effects multiplied by their appropriate population frequencies, or

$$\mu_g = \Sigma f_i \times x_i. \qquad (28.3)$$

In the SBP gene example ($a=12$, $d=4$) the μ_g in the offspring is $\frac{1}{4} \times 12 + \frac{1}{2} \times 4 + -\frac{1}{4} \times 12 = 2$ mm Hg. The mean population SBP will be $129 + 2 = 131$ mm Hg. The genetic variance (V_G) around this mean is computed according to standard variance rules as the sum over all genotypes of the squared differences between the genetic effect of the genotype and the mean genetic effect weighted by the frequency of each genotype, or

$$V_G = \Sigma(f_i \times (x_i - \mu_g)^2). \qquad (28.4)$$

In the example, the V_G for SBP in the offspring is $\frac{1}{4} \times (12 - 2)^2 + \frac{1}{2} \times (+4 - 2)^2 + \frac{1}{4} \times (-12 - 2)^2 = 76$ mm Hg^2.

Selective breeding and inbreeding are daily practice in animal and plant genetics, but of course completely unthinkable in human research, which must always be observational. In a human sample all possible matings (e.g., BB×BB, BB×Bb, BB×bb) can occur and the three genotype frequencies in the offspring will not be $\frac{1}{4}$, $\frac{1}{2}$, and $\frac{1}{4}$ but something else. Common notation for the frequency of a bi-allelic gene in a population is p for the frequency of one allele and q for the frequency of the second allele, with p, q probabilities varying between 0 and 1, and summing to 1 ($p = 1 - q$). The genotype frequencies for BB, Bb, and bb are then p^2, $2pq$, and q^2. The mean genetic effect and genetic variance can still be derived exactly as before, but now p and q are additional unknowns that need to be estimated from a sample of the population (see Table 28.2).

Under the assumption of random mating, lack of selection according to genotype and absence of mutation or migration, the frequencies of the genotypes in the population are perfectly predicted by the frequencies of the alleles, which is referred to as Hardy–Weinberg equilibrium (HWE). As an example consider the SBP gene

Table 28.1 Expected frequency and genotypic effects of a heterozygous mating Bb × Bb

Genotype (i)	BB	Bb	Bb
Frequency (f_i)	$\frac{1}{4}$	$\frac{1}{2}$	$\frac{1}{4}$
Genotypic effects (x_i)	a	d	−a
Frequency × genotypic effect ($f_i \times x_i$)	$\frac{1}{4}$ a	$\frac{1}{2}$ d	$-\frac{1}{4}$ a

Table 28.2 Expected frequency and genotypic effects for a gene with frequency p for the B allele and frequency q for the b allele

Genotype (i)	BB	Bb	bb
Frequency (f_i)	p^2	$2pq$	q^2
Genotypic effects (x_i)	a	d	$-$a
$f_i \times x_i$	p^2a	$2pq$d	$-q^2$a

where we let the least frequent, or minor, allele B take up 40% of all alleles in the population ($p=0.4$). The expected frequencies for the three genotypes BB, Bb, bb are then p^2 (0.16), $2pq$ (0.48), and q^2 (0.36), respectively. We now genotype the 500 subjects in our sample and observe them to have genotypes BB, Bb, bb at frequencies 75, 235, 190, respectively (expected frequencies are 0.16×500, 0.48×500, and 0.36×500, or 80, 240, and 180). A χ^2 test for HWE simply compares the expected genotype frequencies to the observed genotype frequencies with a significant χ^2 value indicating that HWE does not hold. In the example the $\chi^2 = 0.97$ with a p-value of 0.61, which means that the HWE assumption is not violated.

Under the HWE assumption, the mean genetic effect (μ_g) of Eq. (28.3) can now be more generally computed as

$$\begin{aligned} \mu_g &= p^2a + 2pqd - q^2a \\ &= (1-q)^2a + 2pqd - q^2a \qquad (28.5) \\ &= a(p-q) + 2pqd. \end{aligned}$$

The genetic variance around this genetic mean will have two terms, reflecting additive genetic effects and dominance effects respectively or

$$\begin{aligned} V_G &= p^2 \times (2q(a-dp))^2 + 2pq \times (a(q-p) \\ &\quad + d(1-2pq))^2 + q^2 \times (-2p(a+dq))^2 \\ &= 2pq(a + (q-p)d)^2 + 4(pqd)^2. \end{aligned}$$
$$(28.6)$$

where $2pq(a + (q-p)d)^2$ is the additive genetic variance (V_A) and $4(pqd)^2$ the dominance variance (V_D). The contribution of the additive genetic term to the total trait variance is often referred to as the *narrow sense* heritability, whereas the total contribution of additive plus dominance effects is the *broad sense* heritability.

2.2 Polygenetic Trait Variation

This monogenetic example applies well to diseases like Huntington and PKU but is obviously wrong for blood pressure that is, in reality, influenced by a great many genes (Newton-Cheh et al, 2009). However, the core principles for a single gene can be readily expanded to a polygenetic example (Mather and Jinks, 1971). Again, we use a thought experiment to illustrate this. Assume we cross double heterozygote parents for two additive SBP loci, in our SBP *gene B* and a second SBP *gene C*. The two heterozygous parents (both BbCc genotype), can segregate four different allele combinations to their offspring, listed in bold in Fig. 28.3. The combinatorial result of this mating yields 16 possible genotype combinations in the offspring. As extensively described by Punnett as early as 1905 (Punnett, 1905), a total of nine unique genotypes are actually observed (the general rule is 3^n, where n is the number of genes) because some genotypes have the same genotypic value (e.g., bBcC = BbcC = bBCc = bBCc). If the effect of both decreaser alleles ("b" and "c") is to add 0 to the mean blood pressure and the effect of both increaser alleles ("B" and "C") is to add +2 to the mean blood pressure, these two loci will increase the SBP in the various genotypes as depicted in the middle part of Fig. 28.3 (genotypic effects). We now encounter up to five different levels of the trait in the offspring (the general rule is $2n +1$, where n is the number of genes). A histogram of these genotypic effects is shown in the lower part of Fig. 28.3. For example, there are four genotypes that produce an increase in SBP of +2 mm Hg (bbcC, bBcc, bbCc, Bbcc) because they all have exactly one increaser (+2) allele.

This Punnett square illustrates two core principles in genetics: (1) Allelic variation is discrete

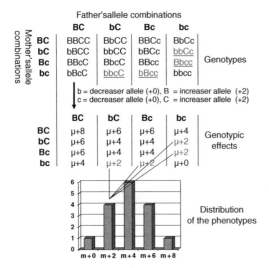

Fig. 28.3 Genotypes, genotypic effects, and distribution of phenotypes in a double heterozygous mating for two hypothetical SBP genes

Note that we still make the (unreasonable) assumptions that the parents are heterozygote for all loci, that increasing alleles of all three genes have the same effect size, that all alleles contribute additively such that there is no interaction within (dominance) or between loci (epistasis). If we, more realistically, move to a polygenic trait of 1500 genes or more with random allelic effect sizes and varying frequencies, also allowing for dominance and epistatic non-additivity while adding numerous environmental effects on the trait, empirical observation still overwhelmingly suggests that the summed effects of all determinants converge to a normal distribution for many biological and behavioral traits.

for all genes but when summed across multiple genes allelic effects lead to a (semi)continuous trait, (2) Segregation of parental allelic variation leads to resemblance within a family but at the same time allows children in the same family to differ substantially (one child may have m+0, whereas another may have m+8). Importantly, the Punnett square keeps working its magic at 3-genic, 4-genic, or 100-genic traits. As is already evident from the simple example in Fig. 28.3, adding more and more genes acts to create an increasingly normal-shaped distribution for the trait. This was the stroke of genius of Sir Ronald Fisher who invoked the central limit theorem to bring discontinuous Mendelian principles of heredity in line with the continuous trait variation observed for almost all traits (Fisher, 1918).

3 Heritability Estimation

Heritability, often abbreviated as h^2, is the relative contribution of all additive and dominant genetic effects to the total variation in a trait. To determine heritability we have to resort to family studies. The essence of all family studies is that they relate the degree of allelic resemblance to the degree of trait resemblance. To illustrate this we again make use of the imaginary SBP gene in Fig. 28.2. Table 28.3 shows the covariance in SBP between all nine possible combinations of the three genotypes found in the population.

To derive the covariance between the SBP values of two randomly drawn individuals with known genotypes we simply take the cross-product of the genotypic values for their two genotypes. For instance, the trait covariance of two BB homozygotes would be $(a - m) \times$

Table 28.3 Cross-products of genotypic values of two individuals for a gene with alleles b and B. Genotypic values are expressed in deviation from the heterozygote as depicted in Fig. 28.3. Note that the mean genetic effect "m" equals $a(p - q) + 2pqd$ (Eq. 28.5)

Individual 1 Individual 2	Genotype: **BB** genotypic value: $(a–m)$	Genotype: **Bb** genotypic value: $(d–m)$	Genotype: **bb** genotypic value: $(-a–m)$
BB$(a - m)$	$(a - m)^2$	$(d - m)(a - m)$	$(-a - m)(a - m)$
Bb$(d - m)$	$(a - m)(d - m)$	$(d - m)^2$	$(-a - m)(d - m)$
bb$(-a - m)$	$(a - m)(-a - m)$	$(d - m)(-a - m)$	$(-a - m)^2$

Table 28.4 Expected frequencies of the possible genotype combinations of two random drawn individuals from the population under Hardy–Weinberg equilibrium

Individual 1 Individual 2	Genotype: **BB** Frequency: p^2	Genotype: **Bb** Frequency: $2pq$	Genotype: **bb** Frequency: q^2
BBp^2 **Bb**$2pq$ **bb**q^2	BBBB p^4 BBBb $2p^3q$ BBbb p^2q^2	BbBB $2p^3q$ BbBb $4p^2q^2$ Bbbb $2pq^3$	bbBB q^2p^2 bbBb $2pq^3$ bbbb q^4

Table 28.5 Expected frequency of the possible genotype combinations in parent–offspring pairs for a single locus and, for each combination, the product of the frequency and the cross-products of genotypic values

Parent–offspring	BB	Bb	bb	Frequency × cross-products of genotypic values		
BB	p^3	p^2q	0	$p^3 \times (a-m)^2$	$p^2q \times (d-m)(a-m)$	0
Bb	p^2q	pq	pq^2	$p^2q \times (a-m)(d-m)$	$pq \times (d-m)^2$	$pq^2 \times (-a-m)(d-m)$
bb	0	pq^2	q^3	0	$pq^2 \times (d-m)(-a-m)$	$q^3 \times (-a-m)^2$

$(a-m)$ or $(a-m)^2$. The expected covariance between the trait values of two random genotypes is the weighted average of all nine cross-products, where each cross-product is weighted by the frequency of that genotype combination. Under HWE, the expected frequencies for the three genotypes are p^2, $2pq$, and q^2 and the frequencies of the genotype combinations are shown in Table 28.4.

Combining Tables 28.3 and 28.4 we predict the covariance in SBP between two randomly drawn individuals caused by our SBP gene as

Covariance (SBP$_{\text{individual 1}}$, SBP$_{\text{individual 2}}$) =

$$p^4(a-m)^2 + 2p^3q(d-m)(a-m)$$
$$+ q^2p^2(-a-m)(a-m)$$
$$+ 2p^3q(a-m)(d-m) + 4p^2q^2(d-m)^2$$
$$+ 2pq^3(-a-m)(d-m) + p^2q^2(a-m)$$
$$+ 2pq^3(d-m)(-a-m) + q^4(-a-m)^2.$$
$$(28.7)$$

When we solve this somewhat intimidating equation we find that the expectation for trait resemblance between two randomly drawn individuals turns out be exactly zero! In fact, this should not come as a surprise: when genes are the only source of variation in SBP, genetically unrelated individuals are not expected to show any resemblance in SBP.

Things change when the covariance is computed between individuals who *do* have a genetic relationship. Relatives will more often

have identical alleles than unrelated individuals.[2] Table 28.5 illustrates this for the expected covariance in parent–offspring pairs. The expected frequencies for the genotype combinations in the pairs are shown on the left. Derivation of the expected frequencies is non-trivial (Mather et al, 1971), but note that two of the cells are always zero since a homozygous BB parent cannot yield offspring without allele B and a homozygous bb parent cannot yield offspring without allele b.

The expected covariance between SBP in the parents and the offspring is the sum of the frequency×cross-products in the nine possible genotype combinations in the right-hand side of Table 28.5 or

Covariance (SBP$_{\text{parent}}$, SBP$_{\text{offspring}}$)
$$= p^3(a-m)^2 + 2p^2q(a-m)(d-m)$$
$$+pq(d-m)^2 + 2pq^2(-a-m)(d-m)$$
$$+q^3(-a-m)^2 = pq(a+(q-p)\text{d})^2.$$
$$(28.8)$$

---

[2] Alleles that are identical in family members fall into two groups. Alleles are identical by descent (IBD) in offspring when the same allele is received from a common ancestor in the grandparental generation. Alleles are identical by state (IBS) when the offspring shares alleles that are physically identical but not necessary came from the same grandparent. An AA homozygous father will give an "A" to all offspring but sometimes the "A" may be the grandpaternal "A" and at other times it may be the grandmaternal "A".

Table 28.6 Expected frequency of the possible genotype combinations in sibling pairs for a single locus

Sibling 1 Sibling 2	BB	Bb	bb
BB	$p^4 + p^3q + 1/4p^2q^2$	$p^3q + 1/2p^2q^2$	$1/4p^2q^2$
Bb	$p^3q + 1/2p^2q^2$	$p^3q + 3p^2q^2 + pq^3$	$1/2p^2q^2 + pq^3$
bb	$1/4p^2q^2$	$1/2p^2q^2 + pq^3$	$1/2p^2q^2 + pq^3 + q^4$

This example illustrates that the expected covariance between family members in traits that are partly under genetic control is non-zero. When we tie the expected covariance between parents and offspring back to Eq. (28.6), we see that it exactly equals half the additive genetic variance ($= \frac{1}{2} V_A$). Note that no dominance variance is passed from parent to offspring. Since only one allele is passed on per gene, parents and offspring cannot be identical by descent for both alleles. In contrast, the covariance between full siblings, i.e., brother, sister, or brother sister pairs, can contain both additive and dominance effects. Table 28.6 displays the expected frequencies for the genotype combinations of two full siblings.

The covariance again obtains as the sum of the frequency×cross-products in the nine possible genotype combinations or

$$
\begin{aligned}
&\text{Covariance (SBP}_{\text{sibling 1}}, \text{SBP}_{\text{sibling 2}}) \\
&= (p^4 + qp^3 + 1/4p^2q^2)(a-m)^2 \\
&\quad + (p^3q + 1/2p^2q^2)(a-m)(d-m) \\
&\quad + 1/4p^2q^2(d-m)^2 \\
&\quad + (p^3q + 1/2p^2q^2)(a-m)(d-m) \\
&\quad + (p^3q + 3p^2q^2 + pq^3)(d-m)^2 \\
&\quad + (1/2p^2q^2 + pq^3)(-a-m)(d-m) \\
&\quad + (1/4p^2q^2)(a-m) \\
&\quad + (1/2p^2q^2 + pq^3)(d-m)(-a-m) \\
&\quad + (1/2p^2q^2 + pq^3 + q^4)(-a-m)^2 \\
&= pq(a + (q-p)d)^2 + (pqd)^2.
\end{aligned}
$$

(28.9)

When we tie the expected covariance between full siblings back to Eq. (28.6), we see that it exactly equals half the additive genetic plus one quart of the dominance variance ($= 1/2 V_A + 1/4 V_D$). More generally, the genetic covariance varies systematically with the degree of genetic relatedness and a general formula for the genetic covariance between a trait measured in two relatives is

$$\text{Covariance } (P_1, P_2) = \mathbf{u} \times V_A \times \mathbf{r} \times V_D.$$
(28.10)

where P_1 is a trait measured in relative 1, P_2 the same trait measured in relative 2, $\mathbf{u}$ the coefficient of relationship representing the correlation between the relatives that would be found if all of the contributing loci acted additive, and $\mathbf{r}$ the coefficient of fraternity – the probability for all of the contributing loci that the relatives share both alleles identical by descent. For parent–offspring pairs, $u = \frac{1}{2}$ and $r = 0$, for full siblings $u = \frac{1}{2}$ and $r = \frac{1}{4}$, for uncles (aunts) with the nephews (nieces) $u = \frac{1}{4}$ and $r = 0$, for grandparent and grandchild $u = \frac{1}{4}$ and $r = 0$, and for single first cousins $u = 1/8$ and $r = 0$. When the covariance between family members in a trait is measured across many different family relationships (e.g., different values for $\mathbf{u}$ and $\mathbf{r}$) this yields a set of equations that can be algebraically solved to estimate V_A and V_D.

3.1 Twin Design

Studying family resemblance remains a powerful tool in genetics, but as already noted by Sir Francis Galton (Galton, 1869), a major shortcoming of this type of family studies is that the degree of genetic relatedness can be confounded with the degree of shared family environment. Full siblings, for instance, do not only share more genes than nieces and nephews but they are also typically raised in the same household. The shared family environment includes potentially important factors like parental SES, neighborhood, school, sports club, family diet, and parental attitudes and rearing style. The solution to separating the genetic and shared environmental effects on the trait resemblance of family members has been found in what Galton called "a unique experiment of nature": monozygotic and dizygotic twin pregnancies.

Monozygotic (MZ) twinning occurs when, for reasons that are still incompletely understood, a fertilized egg divides before it nestles in the uterus. MZ twins are usually said to inherit identical genetic material. This is not entirely correct. Genetic imprinting patterns can be found to differ in MZ twins as is illustrated, for instance, in an MZ twin pair discordant for Beckwith–Wiedemann syndrome due to differential imprinting (Martin, Boomsma, and Machin, 1997). A number of other occurrences can make the genetic identity of MZ twins less than 100%. Since these occurrences are all rare, the assumption that MZs have 100% genetic identity is quite defendable, particularly since deviation from perfect identity will lead to an *under*estimation of genetic effects (i.e., the assumption is a conservative one).

If more than one egg is released from the ovaries during a menstrual cycle and each egg is fertilized by a separate sperm, the result would be non-identical twins also known as dizygotic (DZ) or fraternal twins. DZ twinning rates have risen in the last decades in most countries because of artificial reproduction techniques and the higher age at which mothers get their first child which may be paired to higher levels of follicle stimulating hormone. Genetically, DZ twins do not differ from singleton brother–brother, sister–sister, or brother–sister pairs, that is, they share on average 50% of their genetic material. Opposite-sex (OS) twins are always DZ twins.

When twins are reared together they share part of their environment and this sharing of the family environment is the same for MZ and DZ twins. The important difference between MZ and DZ twins is that the former share (close to) all of their genotypes, whereas the latter share on average only half of the genotypes segregating in that family. This distinction is the basis of the classical twin study. In a twin study four possible components and their

interactions and correlations are thought to contribute to the total variance in a trait: unique environmental factors ("E"), shared environmental factors ("C"), additive genetic factors ("A"), and dominant genetic factors ("D"). Shared environmental factors ("C") and additive ("A") and dominant ("D") genetic factors can cause twin resemblance, whereas the extent to which twins do not resemble each other is ascribed to the unique (or non-shared) environmental factors. These include all unique experiences like differential jobs or lifestyle, accidents or other life events, and in childhood, differential treatment by the parents and non-shared peers.

For simplicity, we first will consider the case where there is no interaction between the A, C, E, and D components. The phenotypic value for a trait in individual i is now re-defined from Eq. (28.1) as

$$\text{Phenotype } (P_i) = \mu + A_i + D_i + Ci + E_i. \tag{28.11}$$

where A_i and D_i stand for the effects of the additive and dominant genetic factors and Ci and E_i for the effects of shared and unique environmental factors (with Ei also including the residual variance due to measurement error). Additionally assuming for the moment that the variance components are uncorrelated, the expectations for the total trait variance then become

$$\text{Variance } (P) = V_A + V_D + V_C + V_E. \tag{28.12}$$

The coefficients of relationship (**u**) and fraternity (**r**) are 1 and 1 in MZ twins and 0.5 and 0.25 in DZ twins, respectively. The shared environment is correlated as unity in both types of twins. Hence, Eq. (28.1) can now be used to derive the MZ and DZ twin covariances as

$$\text{Covariance } (P_1, P_2)_{MZ} = V_A + V_D + V_C. \tag{28.13}$$

$$\text{Covariance } (P_1, P_2)_{DZ} = 1/2 \, V_A + 1/4 \, V_D + V_C. \tag{28.14}$$

This leaves us with four unknowns in three equations and it is obvious that we cannot estimate $V_A + V_D + V_C + V_E$ at the same time. A practical solution is to set either V_C or V_D to zero. This is not to say that both V_C and V_D cannot contribute to the variance in a trait, rather that they cannot be estimated simultaneously with data from MZ and DZ twins alone. The practical approach in twin studies is to first inspect the MZ and DZ correlations to see whether dominance or shared environmental effects are actually likely to play a role. The presence of dominance can be recognized because it yields DZ correlations that are much lower than half the MZ correlation. In contrast, the presence of shared environmental effects yields DZ correlations that are much higher than half the MZ correlations.

A few rules of thumb can be used to estimate the contribution of additive genetic, shared, and unique environmental influences to the total variance by comparing the MZ and DZ twin correlations, when no evidence for dominance is found. Heritability or V_A/V_P can be estimated as twice the difference between the MZ and DZ correlations ($V_A/V_P = 2(r\text{MZ} - r\text{DZ})$). Unique environmentability or V_E/V_P is obtained by subtracting the MZ correlation from unit correlation ($V_E V_P = 1 - r\text{MZ}$). Shared environmentability or V_C/V_P is estimated subtracting the MZ correlation from twice the DZ correlation ($V_C V_P = 2r\text{DZ} - r\text{MZ}$). For example, the MZ correlation for exercise behavior of 14-year-old adolescents is 0.8 and DZ correlation is 0.6 (Stubbe et al, 2005) suggesting an influence of the shared family environment on adolescent exercise behavior. From these twin correlations, the estimates for the contribution of V_A, V_C, and V_E to the total phenotypic variance in exercise behavior would be 40, 40 and 20% respectively.

3.2 Structural Equation Models

Rather than relying on the rules of thumb above, twin researchers prefer to use structural equation modeling (SEM). In SEM, the relationships between several latent unobserved variables

(e.g., genetic and environmental factors) and observed variables are summarized by a series of structural equations. Additional equations can specify the correlation between the latent genetic and environmental factors if these are known. It is possible to derive the variance–covariance matrix implied by the total set of equations (*the model*) through the use of covariance algebra (Bollen and Long, 1993). When the complexity and number of the equations increases, the structural equation model can be formulated more easily by application of path tracing rules on the complete representation of all relationships between observed and unobserved variables in a so-called path diagram.

In a path diagram, observed variables are represented by square boxes, whereas independent variables are represented by circles. Causal effects are represented by unidirectional arrows, whereas correlations are represented by double-headed arrows. An example is depicted in Fig. 28.4 where SBP has been measured at rest in two twins and an additional non-twin sibling. Inspection of the twin correlations had suggested that dominance does not play a role and that all the genetic variance in SBP is additive genetic variance. Hence only the latent factors A, C, and E are used in the diagram and the latent D factor was omitted. Using our knowledge about the twin covariances in Eqs. (28.13) and (28.14) we

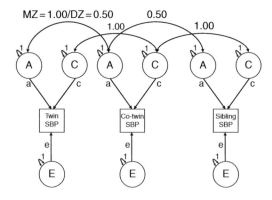

Fig. 28.4 Path diagram depicting correlated latent additive genetic (**a**) and shared environmental (**c**) factors that can cause sibling resemblance in SBP, as well as unique environmental (**e**) factors that are uncorrelated in the siblings

set the correlation of the latent genetic factors for MZ twins to 1 and for DZ twins to 0.5. The correlation of shared environmental factors is set to 1 for both types of twins and their siblings. The latent unique environmental factors are (per definition) uncorrelated. Unobserved latent variables have no scale: their variance is arbitrarily set to 1 (the double arrows that start and end in the latent factors). Path coefficients a, c, and e represent the factor loadings of SBP on the latent factors.

To derive the expected covariance between two observed variables we identify all pathways that start at one variable and end at the other, such that (1) a pathway begins by tracing backward, against the direction of one or more single or double-headed arrows; (2) a pathway changes direction at a double-headed arrow and moves thereafter only in the direction of single-headed arrows; (3) no pathway goes through more than one double headed arrow; (4) no pathway is counted twice. To obtain the covariance between two variables, we multiply the path coefficients along all distinct pathways connecting the two variables and sum these products. For instance, the derivation of the SBP covariance of two DZ twins begins by tracing backward from the SBP in twin 1 through the arrow labeled *a* to the latent genetic factor of twin 1. Through the double-headed arrow labeled *0.5* we reach the latent genetic factor of twin 2 and change direction to end up in the SBP of twin 2 through the forward *a* arrow. Multiplication yields $a \times 0.5 \times a$ or $1/2a^2$. When we repeat this for the only other pathway linking the two twins (through C) we find that the expected covariance for DZ twins is $1/2a^2 + c^2$. The covariance between a twin and a non-twin sibling is also $a \times 1 \times a + c \times 1 \times c$ or $a^2 + c^2$. The expected variance, which is the covariance between the variable and itself, derives as $a \times 1 \times a + c \times 1 \times c + e \times 1$ or $a^2 + c^2 + e^2$ for all twins and siblings alike.[3]

Using maximum likelihood estimation we can now iteratively test the fit of the expected covariances/ variance to the actual observed covariances/variance in a sample of hundreds of twins and siblings over a range of possible values for the path coefficients. From the best fitting model we take the estimates for the path coefficients (e.g., a, c, and e) and determine the relative contribution of the latent factors to the total variance in resting SBP. Heritability of SBP, for instance, obtains as the ratio of $a^2/(a^2 + e^2 + c^2)$ which is often expressed as a percentage. An additional round of iterations that varies the estimates for the path coefficients around the optimal level can be used to establish the confidence intervals around these estimates.

The huge advantage of SEM becomes apparent if we want to test various alternative descriptions of the observed data. Each model comes with a statistic of how likely the data are under the specified model and parameter estimates for the causes of familial resemblance, which can be expressed as a χ^2 or a log likelihood ratio. For instance in Fig. 28.4, we could hypothesize that the shared environment has no effect on SBP and simplify the ACE model to an AE model by dropping the latent C factor. The fit statistic of this AE model may indicate that the new model fits almost as good as the former but since it needs 1 degree of freedom (*df*) less to describe the data it is a more parsimonious model. The difference in fit statistics of various alternative models has a χ^2 distribution. Testing the loss of fit against the differences in *df*s of various models can determine which of the models is the most parsimonious description of the data. Because all model fitting are based on a set of regression equations, the effects of covariates like age or SES can be easily removed from the trait mean, before estimating the parameters a^2, c^2, and e^2.

Often the parameter estimates and the fit statistics of various models are displayed in tables like Table 28.7, which displays model fitting results for ambulatory measured SBP in the evening in adult Dutch twins and one or more of their non-twin siblings (Hottenga et al,

---

[3] The reasonable assumption that the trait variances in MZ twins, DZ twins, and non-twin siblings are the same is often explicitly tested before the actual ACE or ADE models are fitted.

Table 28.7 Proportion of variance in SBP explained by additive genetic factors and shared and unique environmental factors with goodness-of-fit parameters. Best model in bold face font

Model	Sex	a^2	c^2	e^2	$-2ll$	df	$\Delta\chi^2$	Δdf	p-value
ACE full	Males	0.39 (0.00;0.64)	0.05 (0.00;0.40)	o.56 (0.36;0.81)	7117	971			
	Females	0.51 (.17;.67)	0.00 (0.00;0.19)	0.49 (0.33;0.70)					
ACE nosex	M+F	0.48 (0.19;0.60)		0.52 (0.40;0.68)	7123	974	6	3	0.894
AE nosex	**M+F**	**0.48 (0.34;0.60)**		**0.52 (0.40;0.66)**	**7123**	**975**	**6**	**4**	**0.962**

2005). The first two rows show the full ACE model that estimates a^2, c^2, and e^2 separately for males and females on the raw data,[4] yielding a log likelihood value at 971 df. The third and fourth rows show the estimates and fits of two nested models. For instance, in the third row (ACE nosex), leaving out sex differences in the parameter estimates does not result in a model that fits significantly worse than the full ACE model.

There is a mild loss of fit ($\Delta\chi^2 = 7123 - 7117 = 6$) but the simpler model needs three parameters less to describe the data (it *gains* 3 df). This is indicated by the p-value for the test of a worsening of the fit, which remains well above the $p = 0.05$ threshold. The model in the fourth row has dropped the shared environmental factor leaving only additive genetic and unique environmental factors as causes of variation in evening SBP. This model again does not fit worse than a full ACE model and can be considered the most parsimonious model (which is indicated by the bold face font).

It is important to stress that the parameter estimates derived from twin studies are to be understood as applying to *a population*, not an individual. Heritability estimates do *not* give information on the contribution of genes to a trait in a single individual – a common misconception in the popular press. When we estimate the heritability of SBP to be 50% this does not mean that 70 mm Hg of the observed blood pressure of 140 mm Hg in a particular individual is determined by genes and 70 mm Hg by something else. It means that genetic variation explains 50% of the individual differences in blood pressure in this sample. Just like estimates for the mean SBP or the standard deviation of SBP, heritability and its environmental pendants (*shared environmentability* and *unique environmentability*) are descriptive statistics for the sampled population and should be regarded as such. They may or may not generalize to other samples, although empirically, a surprising stability of heritability estimates is found across cultures and age groups for many traits. Heritability estimates for resting SBP in the Netherlands, for instance, change only very little from adolescence to late adulthood (Hottenga et al, 2005, 2006) and are remarkable comparable to those in Australia (52%), Denmark (66%), Finland (53%), Sweden (54%), and the UK (53%) (Evans et al, 2003).

A second note of caution is that the twin method assumes that twins in the same household are exposed to shared environmental factors to the same extent whether they are MZ or DZ (*equal environment assumption*). If this is not the case, and MZ twin pairs are exposed to more similar environments than DZ pairs, then any excess similarity between MZ pairs compared with DZ pairs may be the result of shared environmental rather than genetic factors. The equal environment assumption has been a main target for skeptics of the twin method. All of its empirical tests, however, have shown that the assumption holds very well even for behavioral traits (e.g., intelligence and personality) that should be most sensitive to its effects (Bouchard, 1994; Derks et al, 2006; Kendler et al, 1993, 1994).

---

[4] It is also possible to fit the model directly to the variance and covariance matrices rather than the raw data but this has a number of disadvantages, including listwise deletion of families where one member has missing data.

4 Twin Studies on Cardiovascular Traits Often Used in Behavioral Medicine

Cardiovascular research in twin samples has suggested a clear-cut genetic contribution to hypertension (Kupper et al, 2005b; McCaffery et al, 2008), diabetes (Poulsen et al, 1999), stroke (Bak et al, 2002), and coronary heart disease (Zdravkovic et al, 2002). A landmark paper was published by twin researchers of the Karolinska Institute in Sweden (Marenberg et al, 1994). They searched the National Death Registry for death certificates on ~21,000 twins born in Sweden between 1886 and 1925, where both twins within a pair still lived within the country in 1961. The risk to have died from coronary heart disease when one's co-twin died before the age of 55 years was 8.1 among male monozygotic (MZ) twins as compared to 3.8 among male dizygotic (DZ) twins. Re-analysis using a correlated c-frailty model, which translates discrete yes/no traits into a continuously distributed latent liability, yielded a heritability to die from coronary heart disease of 57% in males and 38% in females (Zdravkovic et al, 2004).

The genetic contribution to cardiovascular disease end points most likely results from the joint effects of risk genes on the large number of biological and behavioral risk factors that impact on the atherosclerotic process. Table 28.8 summarizes the heritability estimates for many of these risk factors based on the study of twins and their family members registered in the Netherlands Twin Registry (NTR). The NTR was established in 1987 as a resource for prospective studies in behavior genetics and genetic epidemiology (www.tweelingenregister.org). The adult branch of register now includes over 23,000 participants that can be MZ or DZ twins, parents, siblings, children, or spouses of twins. They have been longitudinally assessed for a large number of behavioral and medical traits using biennial surveys and multiple visits to the laboratory or the university hospital. It is clear from Table 28.8 that *all* cardiovascular risk factors assessed were

significantly heritable and often more than half of the variance in the traits was explained by genetic factors.

Again, I stress that the heritability estimates in Table 28.8 are based on a single population in a single country. Many twin studies in different countries and ethnicities, however, have confirmed the importance of genetic factors not just in the established risk factors like smoking (Li et al, 2003), physical inactivity (Stubbe et al, 2006; Beunen and Thomis, 1999), blood pressure (Evans et al, 2003), cholesterol (Beekman et al, 2002; Iliadou et al, 2005), and BMI (Schousboe et al, 2003; Silventoinen et al, 2003) but also for insulin resistance (Poulsen et al, 2001), inflammation (Su et al, 2008; Worns et al, 2006), hemostasis (Peetz et al, 2004), cardiac autonomic control (Wang et al, 2009), personality (Wray et al, 2007), and depression (Sullivan et al, 2000), with very comparable heritability estimates to those in the Dutch population.

5 Multivariate Structural Equation Models

Structural equation models of twin family data can very easily be extended from the univariate to the multivariate case, which allows a whole new set of hypotheses to be tested because the observed information now includes all cross-twin cross-trait correlations. In addition to estimating the heritability of multiple traits, we can test the extent to which the heritability of these traits is caused by common genetic factors that influence all of the traits, and the extent to which heritability is caused by genetic factors that are specific to each trait. To illustrate this, Fig. 28.5 presents a bivariate extension of the ACE model of two different phenotypes: SBP measured at rest and SBP during mental stress. There are now two genetic factors, common genetic factor A influences SBP in both conditions, whereas specific genetic factor As influences only SBP under stress. Path coefficient a_{11} quantifies the effect of genetic factor A on SBP at rest, a_{21} quantifies the effect of A on SBP during stress. Coefficient a_{22}

Table 28.8 Heritability estimates for cardiovascular disease risk factors in the Netherlands

	Heritability[a]	Reference
Smoking		
– Initiation	44%	Vink et al (2005)
– Quantity smoked	51%	Vink et al (2004)
– Nnicotine dependence	75%	Vink et al (2005)
Physical inactivity		
– Exercise less than 60 min weekly	50–68%	Stubbe et al (2006)
Blood pressure		
– Systolic blood pressure	48–60%	Kupper et al (2005b); Hottenga et al (2005); de Geus et al (2007)
– Diastolic blood pressure	34–67%	Hottenga et al (2005); Kupper et al (2005b); de Geus et al (2007)
Lipids		
– LDL cholesterol	77–83%	Beekman et al (2002)
– HDL cholesterol	61–80%	Beekman et al (2002)
Obesity		
–Body Mass Index	64–81%	Schousboe et al (2003)
–Waist-to-Hip ratio	70%	*Unpublished*
Insulin resistance and beta cell function		
–Fasting glucose	38–66%	Simonis-Bik et al (2008)
–Insulin sensitivity (hyperinsulinemic euglycemic clamp)	60%	*Unpublished*
–Insulin response during hyperglycemic clamp	52%	*Unpublished*
First phase	77%	
Second phase		
Inflammation		
–Cytokine response to LPS	55–68%	Posthuma et al (2005)
–Fibrinogen	39%	de Lange et al (2006)
Coagulation and Fibrinolysis		
–Tissue plasminogen activator	67%	de Lange et al (2006)
–Von Willibrand factor	72%	de Lange et al (2006)
Cardiac autonomic control		
–Heart rate	37–68%	Kupper et al (2005a); Snieder et al (1997)
–Sympathetic control (pre-ejection period)	40–70%	Kupper et al (2006); de Geus et al (2007)
–Parasympathetic control (respiratory sinus arrhythmia)	28–55%	Kupper et al (2005a); Snieder et al (1997)
Personality		
–Type A behavior	45%	Rebollo and Boomsma (2006)
–Type D personality	52%	Kupper et al (2007)
Psychopathology		
–Major depression	36%	Middeldorp et al (2005)
–Anxiety disorders	36–51%	Distel et al (2008); Middeldorp et al (2005)

[a] Heritability estimates are ranged for some traits (e.g., 50–68%) because they were assessed in multiple studies in non-overlapping samples, e.g., young adults versus middle-aged, or by different assessment strategies, e.g., ambulatory recording versus laboratory-based measurements

quantifies the additional effect of genetic factor As on SBP during stress. In a similar way, path coefficients e_{11}, c_{11}, e_{21}, c_{21}, e_{22}, and c_{22} quantify the effects of common and specific factors E and C on SBP at rest and during stress. The heritability of SBP at rest is the variance due to the genetic factor A divided by the total variance in SBP at rest and obtains as the ratio of $a_{11}^2/(a_{11}^2 + c_{11}^2 + e_{11}^2)$. The heritability of SBP during stress is the variance due to the genetic factors A and As divided by the total variance

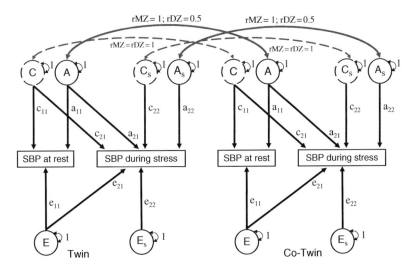

Fig. 28.5 A bivariate ACE model for SBP

in SBP under stress and obtains as the ratio of $(a_{21}^2 + a_{22}^2)/(a_{21}^2 + a_{22}^2 + c_{21}^2 + c_{22}^2 + e_{21}^2 + e_{22}^2)$.

We used the model depicted in Fig. 28.5 to test the hypothesis that stress increases the variance in SBP due to amplification of existing genetic variance and the emergence of new genetic variance (de Geus et al, 2007). Amplified genes are genes that have an effect on individual differences in a cardiovascular trait at rest, but these effects become stronger under stress. Emerging genes are genes that are expressed only during stress. To test for amplification (or *de*amplification) of genetic factors we compared the fit of a model in which a_{21} is freely estimated to the fit of a model in which a_{21} is constrained to be the same as a_{11}. If a_{11} and a_{21} are the same there is no evidence of amplification, but if a_{21} is significantly larger than a_{11} the effects of the genes acting on SBP at rest are amplified during stress. To test for emergence, we compared a model in which the path loading a_{22} is freely estimated to a model in which a_{22} was constrained to be zero.

Results first of all showed that the total variance in SBP increased from 59.5 mm Hg^2 at rest to 94 mm Hg^2 during stress. In both conditions DZ correlations were about half of the MZ correlations and model fitting confirmed that C did not influence SBP at rest or during stress and that an AE model fitted best. Under the AE model, the a_{21} coefficient was significantly larger than the a_{11} coefficient (ratio $a_{21}/a_{11} = 1.23$) providing evidence for the amplification of the genetic factors active at rest during times of stress. The a_{22} coefficient was significantly different from zero ($a_{22} = 4.0$) providing evidence for the emergence of stress-specific genetic variation in SBP in a cohort of adolescent twins. Total heritability of SBP was 59% at rest but increased to 72% during stress. The ratio of genetic variance at rest and under stress was $35.1/67.8 = 1.9$, whereas the ratio of unique environmental variance at rest and under stress was $24.4/26.4 = 1.1$. Hence the increase in heritability reflected a true increase in genetic variance, not simply a reduction in environmental variance (e.g., because stress is a more standardized condition).

5.1 Genetic and Environmental Correlation

Alternatively, the bivariate twin model in Fig. 28.5 can be used to decompose a phenotypic correlation between two traits into its three possible sources: overlapping genetic, overlapping shared environmental, or overlapping unique environmental factors. The word "overlapping" can be defined more precisely as the correlation between the latent genetic (Rg), shared environmental (Rc), or unique environmental (Re) factors influencing SBP at rest (A, C, E) and SBP under stress (As, Cs, Es). More generally Rg between two traits is derived as the genetic covariance between the traits divided by the square root of the product of their genetic variances:

$$Rg = (a_{11} \times a_{21})/\sqrt{(a_{11}^2)} \times \sqrt{(a_{21}^2 + a_{22}^2)} \tag{28.15}$$

If the genetic correlation is close to 1, the two genetic factors (A and As) overlap completely. In this case a_{22} will be zero and there are no genes that emerge specifically for the second trait. If the genetic correlation is significantly less than 1, there may be overlap in the genetic factors (A and As) that influence both traits but the overlap is imperfect and a_{22} will be non-zero (this was the case in our SBP example above). If the genetic correlation is close to 0, there is no overlap in the genetic factors that influence both traits and the heritability of the second trait is determined completely by a_{22}.

Analogously, the environmental correlations Rg and Rc between two traits are derived as the environmental covariance divided by the square root of the product of the environmental variances of the two traits:

$$R_c = (c_{11} \times c_{21})/\sqrt{(c_{11}^2)} \times \sqrt{(c_{21}^2 + c_{22}^2)}. \tag{28.16}$$

$$R_e = (e_{11} \times e_{21})/\sqrt{(e_{11}^2)} \times \sqrt{(e_{21}^2 + e_{22}^2)}. \tag{28.17}$$

The actual observed or phenotypic (Rp) correlation between two traits is a function of Rg, Rc, Re and the square roots of the standardized genetic (a^2), shared environmental (c^2), and unique environmental (e^2) variances of these two traits. In a general notation for traits x and y, the phenotypic correlation is

$$Rxy = \sqrt{a_x^2} \times Rg \times \sqrt{a_y^2} + \sqrt{c_x^2} \times Rc \times \sqrt{c_y^2} + \sqrt{e_x^2} \times Re\sqrt{} \times e_y^2. \tag{28.18}$$

In the adolescent sample used above, the observed phenotypic correlation between SBP at rest and during stress in our study was $Rp = 0.81$. Only additive genetic and unique environmental factors contributed to the variance in SBP at rest ($a_{rest}^2 = 0.59$ $e_{rest}^2 = 0.41$) and under stress ($a_{stress}^2 = 0.72$ $e_{stress}^2 = 0.28$) with $Rg = 0.874$, $Rc = 0$, and $Re = 0.707$. Hence, Eq. (28.18) correctly estimates the phenotypic correlation: $\sqrt{0.59} \times 0.874 \times \sqrt{0.72} + \sqrt{0} \times 0 \times \sqrt{0} + \sqrt{0.41} \times 0.707 \times \sqrt{0.28} = 0.81$. The extent to which the phenotypic correlation is explained by the correlation at the genetic level ($\sqrt{a_{rest}^2} \times Rg \times \sqrt{a_{stress}^2}$) is often reported as a percentage and represents the "heritability of the covariance." For the phenotypic correlation between SBP at rest and SBP under stress, the percentage explained by correlation at the genetic level is ($\sqrt{0.59} \times 0.874 \times \sqrt{0.72})/0.81 = 70\%$.

The bivariate model in Fig. 28.5 can be further expanded to a multivariate design when more than two measurements are available, e.g., during ambulatory blood pressure recording (Kupper et al, 2005b). More importantly, these multivariate models can also be used to compute genetic and environmental correlations between *different* traits, rather than the repeated measures of the same trait. A typical example is given in the left-hand side of Fig. 28.6, where three components of the metabolic syndrome, body mass index (BMI), SBP, and oral glucose tolerance test-derived insulin sensitivity (INS) have been assessed in Danish MZ and DZ twins. The study set out to detect the source of the clustering of a group of symptoms related to insulin resistance (obesity, glucose intolerance, hypertension, dyslipidemia) (Benyamin et al, 2007).[5] This cluster may be a better predictor of diabetes and cardiovascular disease than each of these risk factors separately.

---

[5] The original study computed genetic and environmental correlations between nine phenotypes, of which three were selected for the example figure used here.

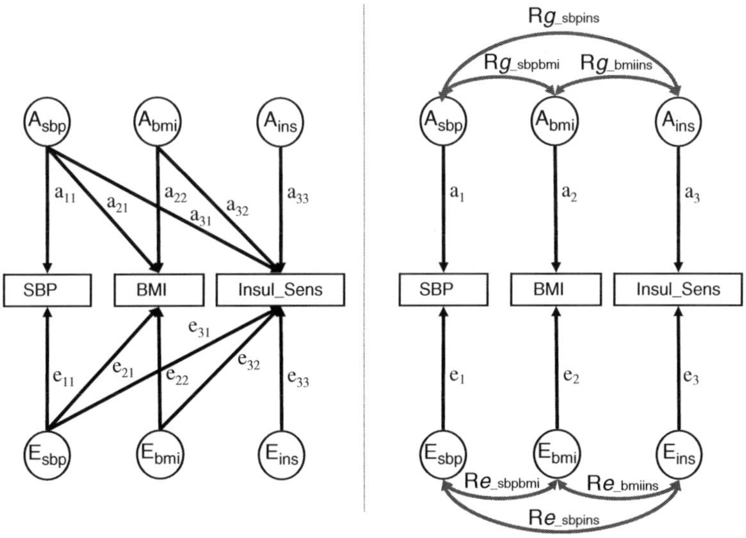

Fig. 28.6 A multivariate AE model for SBP, body mass index (BMI), and insulin sensitivity (Insul_Sens)

When multivariate models are depicted in a path diagram, the amount of arrows (and path loadings) can be become overwhelming so Fig. 28.6 differs from Fig. 28.5 in that only the part of *one* twin is depicted (the other twin and non-twin sibling is still used in the analyses with their latent factors correlated as before; they are just no longer drawn). The multivariate model drawn on the left is a so-called Cholesky decomposition, where *n* traits load on exactly *n* latent A, C, E factors with all traits loading on the first factor, *n–1* loading on the second factor, and so on. The right-hand side of Fig. 28.6 describes exactly the same model but it uses a different notation. In a correlated factors model the pathways from the latent factor of a trait to the observed value of the other traits are now replaced by correlations between the latent factors. The Cholesky model is the preferred model when there is a clear theoretical causal or temporal ordering of the traits (as in repeated measurements), but when the ordering of the traits is arbitrary a correlated factors model may be more appropriate.

Using the model on the right in Fig. 28.6 as the null model we can test the relative fit of various nested models. For instance, we can test a model that freely estimates Rg but fixes Rc and Re to zero. This would test the hypothesis

that the associations between SBP and BMI and between SBP and insulin sensitivity derive entirely from a common set of genetic factors. Empirical data showed this hypothesis to be false (Benyamin et al, 2007). The phenotypic correlations between SBP and INS ($r = -0.31$) as well as between SBP and BMI ($r = 0.26$) were due to not only genetic ($Rg = -0.23$ and 0.26) but also unique environmental ($Re = -0.26$ and 0.27) factors. Furthermore, the genetic correlations were rather modest which argues against the idea that all variables in the metabolic syndrome have a common (genetic) etiology.

6 Gene–Environment Interaction

Let us now return to Eq. (28.11), where the terms that capture the interactive effects between the genetic and environmental factors ($A \times E$, $A \times C$) were "conveniently" set to zero. The classical twin design needs to assume these terms to be zero simply because it is not possible to estimate the contribution of these effects to the total phenotypic variance with a twin study unless the environmental factors are measured or experimentally controlled. If the assumption on the absence of gene–environment interaction is wrong, the estimates for a^2, c^2, and e^2 may be biased. True A×C effects that are not modeled will inflate heritability estimates as well as the effects of the shared environment, whereas true A×E effects that are not modeled will act to inflate the estimates of the unique environmental contribution (Purcell, 2002). Perhaps counter-intuitively, the latter means that twin studies will underestimate the importance of genetic variance, if the relevant environmental factor is a person-specific factor, like the amount of life stress or level of job strain.

Fortunately, if the relevant environmental factors have been measured they can be readily incorporated in the twin design. Their interaction with genetic effects can be formally tested and the relative contribution of gene–environment interaction effects to the total trait variance estimated. There are a number of ways to do this. First, the classic twin analyses can be stratified for the measured environmental factor, such that the analyses are performed in subgroups of MZ and DZ twins that are concordant for the degree of environmental exposure (Heath et al, 1998). Significantly different heritability estimates in these subgroups signal gene–environment interaction. An example for blood pressure is provided by McCaffery and colleagues (2008) who investigated A×E gene–environment interaction in hypertension by examining the extent to which educational attainment modifies the heritability of hypertension in Vietnam-era twins. Thousands of MZ and DZ male twins provided data on their education and self-report physician diagnosis of hypertension or medication usage. From these, the MZ and DZ pairs were selected to be concordant for low or high educational attainment such that either both of them had received more than 14 years of education or both of them had received less than 14 years of education. Heritability of hypertension was 63% in the higher educated twins versus 46% in the lower educated twins. In view of the higher incidence of hypertension in lower educational attainment groups, individual differences in genetic vulnerability to hypertension seem to be swamped by the environmental risk factors in subjects with lower education levels. In contrast, in subjects

with high educational attainment only those at high genetic risk will develop hypertension.

A second way to test gene–environment interaction is to add the observed environmental factor as a moderator variable to the path loadings of the genetic factor on the observed variable. This extension of the twin model does not need to be restricted to the interaction of genetic with shared or unique environmental factors and can also be used to test for interaction within the two types of environment, i.e., C×E or E×E interactions (Purcell, 2002). Figure 28.7 depicts two ways of doing this. The left-hand side is a modified version of the models used by studies that aimed to detect possible moderating effects of regular physical activity on the genetic risk for obesity (McCaffery et al, 2009; Mustelin et al, 2009). A classical ACE decomposition is used, but now the effects of the latent factors are allowed to be modified by the measured environmental variable. Physical activity was allowed to act as an environmental modulator of the genetic effects on BMI ($\beta1$) as well as of the unique and shared environmental effects ($\beta2$, $\beta3$). Significance of, for instance, the gene–physical activity interaction can be tested by comparing this full model to a model with $\beta1$ set to zero.

The moderator variable in this model can be dichotomous, for instance, by contrasting non-exercisers (activity $= 0$) versus vigorous exercisers (activity $= 1$) based on the endorsement of one or more of five common vigorous intensity aerobic exercises (McCaffery et al, 2009).[6] The moderator can also be continuous for instance when a physical activity index is calculated from the product of self-reported exercise intensity, duration, and frequency as was done in thousands of Finnish twin pairs (Mustelin et al, 2009). Of note, both approaches showed that physical activity significantly modified the heritability of BMI, with a high level of physical activity decreasing the

---

[6] In the latter case the model resembles the approach above in that it computes the heritability separately in non-exercisers (a^2/V_P) versus and vigorous exercisers ($(a^2 + \beta_1*\text{activity})/V_P$).

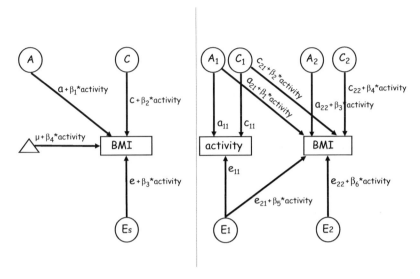

Fig. 28.7 Twin models testing the interaction of A, C, and E with physical activity on BMI, while accounting for potential correlation between A, C, or E and physical activity

additive genetic component in BMI (Mustelin et al, 2009; McCaffery et al, 2009). This suggests that genetic variation significantly influences variation in adiposity in sedentary subjects, but that in physically active individuals the effects of this genetic variation is diminished. The often-replicated effect of the *FTO* gene on BMI appears to be one of the genes modified by physical activity, as the association between *FTO* and BMI was blunted in people with high physical activity assessed either by self-report (Andreasen et al, 2008) or 7-day accelerometry (Rampersaud et al, 2008).

7 Gene–Environment Correlation

A new element in the left-hand side of Fig. 28.7 is the triangle with an effect of the moderator (physical activity) on the mean of the observed levels of BMI. This indicates that the effect of physical activity was regressed from the BMI level and that the ACE decomposition was performed on the residual BMI. In this way twin researchers try to deal with the possibility that the genes that influence BMI may also influence physical activity. This ties in directly with the second omission in Eq. (28.11) where we not

only assumed the absence of gene–environment interaction but also left out the terms that capture possible gene–environment (A–E, A–C) correlations. As indicated in the introduction, such gene–environment correlation is quite likely to occur, particularly in behavioral traits.

In both active and reactive gene–environment correlation the non-random aspects of the environment are a consequence of the genetic effects on the behavior of the individual and should be considered to reflect an *extended phenotype* (Dawkins, 1982). In this case the heritability of the phenotype meaningfully incorporates the effects of gene–environment correlation. For instance, the genes that cause individual differences in the drive to be physically active may also influence BMI because low levels of physical activity may *cause* high levels of BMI. In this case estimating heritability of the residual BMI, i.e., after regressing out (partly genetic) individual differences in physical activity may not be correct. In contrast, when parents transmit the genes for high BMI to their offspring together with low encouragement to engage in physical activity, it makes more sense to take this passive gene–environment correlation into account before attempting a genetic decomposition of the variance in BMI, because such gene–environment correlation may bias estimation of heritability and mask gene–environment interaction (Purcell, 2002).

To detect the gene–environment in the presence of potential gene–environment correlation, twin researchers first compute the genetic correlation between the moderating environmental variable and the trait of interest. If such a correlation is low or absent, the gene–environment correlation may be set to zero without dire effects on the estimates for the remaining final variance components. Both studies on BMI and physical activity, for instance, did not find a significant genetic correlation between BMI and physical activity in males. In females, however, a low but significant Rg of -0.22 was found. Such gene–environment correlation can be taken into account by regressing the effects of the moderator on the mean as is done in the left-hand side of Fig. 28.7. This removes genetic and environmental effects common to both physical activity and BMI. Similar reasoning applies to the potential E × activity and C × activity interactions.

A second approach is to perform combined test of gene–environment interaction and gene–environment correlation. This is shown in the right-hand side of Fig. 28.7, where the genetic factors that influence BMI are split up in those that are common to BMI and physical activity (A_1) and those that are not in common to these traits (A_2). Here A_1 is a hypothetical set of pleiotropic genes that lower BMI and increase the drive to exercise regularly. A_2 are genes specific to BMI. Importantly physical activity is now allowed to moderate the effects of the genetic and environmental factors it has in common with BMI (a_{21}, c_{21}, e_{21}) and/or the effects of the genetic or environmental factors that are specific to BMI (a_{22}, c_{22}, e_{22}). The test for gene–environment interaction is simply the test of a model with $\beta 1$ and $\beta 2$ freely estimated versus models that constrain these parameters to be zero.[7]

By far the best opportunity to test gene–environment interaction arises when the environment can be experimentally controlled (Falconer, 1952). The same trait is then measured repeatedly in MZ and DZ twins under different environmental conditions. This rules out gene–environment correlation since all subjects are exposed to all relevant environments. When the genetic correlation between the trait in different environments is found to be less than unity this constitutes robust evidence for gene–environment interaction. Figure 28.5 already presented an example of this approach where SBP was measured at rest and under stress. The genetic correlation was non-unity (0.87), signaling gene-by-stress interaction. Indeed the emergence of new genetic variance in a stressful environment versus a resting environment is exactly what geneticists mean by gene–environment interaction, namely that the effects of the individual's genotype on the phenotype are conditional on the environment.

8 Ongoing Evolution of Structural Equation Models for Twin Family Data

This chapter focused on quantitative traits, but virtually all models discussed can also be applied to measures that are categorical or dichotomous (e.g., diseased yes/no) by assuming some continuous underlying liability distribution of which the categories are a reflection (threshold models (Neale and Cardon, 1992)). In addition to estimating heritability, genetic and environmental correlations, and gene–environment interaction, twin studies can be used to detect differences in gene expression between the sexes, sibling rivalry or cooperation effects (Eaves, 1976),

---

[7] It should be noted that this solution seems to work well for A–E correlations but may not always work for A–C correlations that arise from cultural transmission where parents provide genes as well as a shared family environment to both twins (Purcell and Koenen, 2005). Also, nonlinear correlation of the environmental moderator and the trait of interest may sometimes be mistaken for gene–environment interaction (Rathouz et al 2008).

and rater bias, e.g., when father, mother, and teacher rate the behavior of a child (Bartels et al, 2003). Also, in longitudinal twin data, changes in genetic architecture over time can be modeled using Markov chains (simplex models) or growth curves (Neale and McArdle, 2000). There are various software packages available to fit different (nested) models to observed twin family data and to estimate all relevant parameters under these models. Often used packages include LISREL (Joreskog and Sorbom, 1999), Mplus (Muthén and Muthén, 2007), and Mx (Neale et al, 2006). For Mx, a large library of annotated jobs (http://www.psy.vu.nl/mxbib/) has been created that can deal with all models discussed in this chapter and many more.

The evolution of twin studies is still very much ongoing because the twin method makes a number of assumptions that, in contrast to the equal environment assumption, have been shown to be invalid for various traits (see Table 28.9). Twin researchers have expanded the twin design to involve a larger amount of family members than just the twins and their siblings to allow an explicit test of some of the assumptions in Table 28.9. (Eaves, 2009). The newer "cascade" models add the parents, spouses, and the offspring of DZ and MZ twins to obtain estimates of the genetic and environmental (interaction) effects that take potential violations of these assumptions into account as explained in detail elsewhere (Keller et al, 2009; Medland and Keller, 2009). Clearly, to maintain sufficient statistical power to test all assumptions at once, sufficient numbers of twins and of

these extra relatives are required. Hence, the need for a number of large-scaled well-organized Twin Family Registries worldwide remains high.

9 Conclusion

This chapter aimed to provide students in behavioral medicine with an introduction to the quantitative biometrical principles underlying the genetic variation in biological and behavioral traits. For a full treaty of quantitative genetics the interested readers are referred to the classic textbooks (Crow and Kimura, 1970; Falconer et al, 1996; Lynch and Walsh, 1997; Mather et al, 1971). This chapter further aimed to introduce the principles of twin studies since virtually all introductions of papers describing actual genetic and gene–environmental interactive effects on biobehavioral traits start by citing evidence for (multivariate) heritability on these traits from twin studies. Although a lot of ground was covered much was left untouched and the interested reader is referred to more detailed treaties of twin studies (Neale et al, 1992).

At this point it is good to stress that twin studies serve to tells us whether, how many and how strongly genetic factors contribute to the variation in biobehavioral traits and to their covariance. However, twin studies do not identify any actual genetic variants at the level of DNA. This requires molecular genetic approaches, which will be addressed in the next chapters.

Table 28.9 Examples of strong assumptions made in the classical twin design, which are amended by extended twin family designs that add the parents, spouses, or children of twins

Assumption	Violation
Random mating	There is "assortative" mating on the basis of (1) phenotypic resemblance between spouses or (2) similarity of social backgrounds (social homogamy)
No cultural transmission from parents to offspring	The behavior of the parents acts as a shared environment for the children and influences the offspring-phenotype directly. There may be additional sex differences in vertical transmission where father's behaviors have a different influence on sons and daughters than the behaviors of the mothers
Results from twins generalize to the non-twin population	There is a twin-specific shared environment that is not shared with singleton siblings. For instance twins may be at a disadvantage to singleton births because of fetal disadvantages specific to a twin pregnancy

References

Andreasen, C. H., Stender-Petersen, K. L., Mogensen, M. S., Torekov, S. S., Wegner, L. et al (2008). Low physical activity accentuates the effect of the FTO rs9939609 polymorphism on body fat accumulation. *Diabetes, 57*, 95–101.

Bak, S., Gaist, D., Sindrup, S. H., Skytthe, A., and Christensen, K. (2002). Genetic liability in stroke: a long-term follow-up study of Danish twins. *Stroke, 33*, 769–774.

Bartels, M., Hudziak, J. J., Boomsma, D. I., Rietveld, M. J., van Beijsterveldt, T. C. et al (2003). A study of parent ratings of internalizing and externalizing problem behavior in 12-year-old twins. *J Am Acad Child Adolesc Psychiatry, 42*, 1351–1359.

Beekman, M., Heijmans, B. T., Martin, N. G., Pedersen, N. L., Whitfield, J. B. et al (2002). Heritabilities of apolipoprotein and lipid levels in three countries. *Twin Res Hum Genet, 5*, 87–97.

Benyamin, B., Sorensen, T. I., Schousboe, K., Fenger, M., Visscher, P. M., and Kyvik, K. O. (2007). Are there common genetic and environmental factors behind the endophenotypes associated with the metabolic syndrome? *Diabetologia, 50*, 1880–1888.

Beunen, G., and Thomis, M. (1999). Genetic determinants of sports participation and daily physical activity. *Int J Obesity, 23*, S55–S63.

Bollen, K. A., and Long, J. S. (1993). *Testing Structural Equation Models*. Newbury Park, CA: Sage.

Bouchard, T. J. (1994). Genes, environment, and personality. *Science, 264*, 1700–1701.

Crow, J. F., and Kimura, M. (1970). *An Introduction to Population Genetics Theory*. New York, NY: Harper and Row.

Dawkins, R. (1982). *The Extended Phenotype: The Gene as the Unit of Selection*. Oxford: Oxford University Press.

de Geus, E. J. C., Kupper, N., Boomsma, D. I., and Snieder, H. (2007). Bivariate genetic modeling of cardiovascular stress reactivity: does stress uncover genetic variance? *Psychosom Med, 69*, 356–364.

de Lange, M., de Geus, E. J., Kluft, C., Meijer, P., van Doornen, L. J. et al (2006). Genetic influences on fibrinogen, tissue plasminogen activator-antigen and von Willebrand factor in males and females. *Thromb Haemost, 95*, 414–419.

Derks, E. M., Dolan, C. V., and Boomsma, D. I. (2006). A test of the equal environment assumption (EEA) in multivariate twin studies. *Twin Res Hum Genet, 9*, 403–411.

Distel, M. A., Vink, J. M., Willemsen, G., Middeldorp, C. M., Merckelbach, H. L. et al (2008). Heritability of self-reported phobic fear. *Behav Genet, 38*, 24–33.

Eaves, L. (1976). A model for sibling effects in man. *Heredity, 36*, 205–214.

Eaves, L. (2009). Putting the 'human' back in genetics: modeling the extended kinships of twins. *Twin Res Hum Genet, 12*, 1–7.

Evans, A., van Baal, G. C., McCarron, P., DeLange, M., Soerensen, T. I. et al (2003). The genetics of coronary heart disease: the contribution of twin studies. *Twin Res Hum Genet, 6*, 432–441.

Falconer, D. S. (1952). The problem of environment and selection. *Am Nat, 86*, 293–298.

Falconer, D. S., and Mackay, T. F. C. (1996). *Introduction to Quantitative Genetics, 4th Ed.* Essex: Pearson Education Limited.

Fisher, R. A. (1918). The correlation between relatives on the supposition of Mendelian inheritance. *Trans Roy Soc Edinburgh, 52*, 399–433.

Galton, F. R. S. (1869). *Heriditary Genius*. London: MacMillan and Co.

Ge, D., Su, S., Zhu, H., Dong, Y., Wang, X. et al (2009). Stress-induced sodium excretion: a new intermediate phenotype to study the early genetic etiology of hypertension? *Hypertension, 53*, 262–269.

Heath, A. C., Eaves, L. J., and Martin, N. G. (1998). Interaction of marital status and genetic risk for symptoms of depression. *Twin Res Human Genet, 1*, 119–122.

Hottenga, J. J., Boomsma, D. I., Kupper, N., Posthuma, D., Snieder, H. et al (2005). Heritability and stability of resting blood pressure. *Twin Res Hum Genet, 8*, 499–508.

Hottenga, J. J., Whitfield, J. B., de Geus, E. J., Boomsma, D. I., and Martin, N. G. (2006). Heritability and stability of resting blood pressure in Australian twins. *Twin Res Human Genet, 9*, 205–209.

Iliadou, A., Snieder, H., Wang, X., Treiber, F. A., and Davis, C. L. (2005). Heritabilities of lipids in young European American and African American twins. *Twin Res Human Genet, 8*, 492–498.

Jencks, C., Smith, M., Acland, H., Bane, M., Cohen, D. et al (1972). *Inequality: a Reassessment of the Effect of Family and Schooling in America*. New York: Basic Books.

Joreskog, K., and Sorbom, D. (1999). *LISREL 8: Structural Equation Modeling with the SIMPLIS Command Language*. Lincolnwood: Scientific Software International.

Keller, M. C., Medland, S. E., Duncan, L. E., Hatemi, P. K., Neale, M. C. et al (2009). Modeling extended twin family data I: description of the Cascade model. *Twin Res Hum Genet, 12*, 8–18.

Kendler, K. S., Neale, M. C., Kessler, R. C., Heath, A. C., and Eaves, L. J. (1993). A test of the equal-environment assumption in twin studies of psychiatric-illness. *Behav Genet, 23*, 21–27.

Kendler, K. S., Neale, M. C., Kessler, R. C., Heath, A. C., and Eaves, L. J. (1994). Parental treatment and the equal environment assumption in twin studies of psychiatric-illness. *Psychol Med, 24*, 579–590.

Kupper, N., Denollet, J., de Geus, E. J., Boomsma, D. I., and Willemsen, G. (2007). Heritability of type-D personality. *Psychosom Med, 69*, 675–681.

Kupper, N., Willemsen, G., Boomsma, D. I., and de Geus, E. J. (2006). Heritability of indices for cardiac contractility in ambulatory recordings. *J Cardiovasc Electrophysiol, 17*, 877–883.

Kupper, N., Willemsen, G., Posthuma, D., de Boer, D., Boomsma, D. I. et al (2005a). A genetic analysis of ambulatory cardiorespiratory coupling. *Psychophysiol, 42*, 202–212.

Kupper, N., Willemsen, G., Riese, H., Posthuma, D., Boomsma, D. I. et al (2005b). Heritability of day-time ambulatory blood pressure in an extended twin design. *Hypertension, 45*, 80–85.

Li, M. D., Cheng, R., Ma, J. Z., and Swan, G. E. (2003). A meta-analysis of estimated genetic and environmental effects on smoking behavior in male and female adult twins. *Addiction, 98*, 23–31.

Lynch, M., and Walsh, B. (1997). *Genetics and Analysis of Quantitative Traits*. Sunderland, MA: Sinauer Associates.

Marenberg, M. E., Risch, N., Berkman, L. F., Floderus, B., and de Faire, U. (1994). Genetic susceptibility to death from coronary heart disease in a study of twins. *New Engl J Med, 330*, 1041–1046.

Martin, N., Boomsma, D., and Machin, G. (1997). A twin-pronged attack on complex traits. *Nat Genet, 17*, 387–392.

Mather, K., and Jinks, J. L. (1971). *Biometrical Genetics*. London: Chapman and Hall.

McCaffery, J. M., Papandonatos, G. D., Bond, D. S., Lyons, M. J., and Wing, R. R. (2009). Gene X environment interaction of vigorous exercise and body mass index among male Vietnam-era twins. *Am J Clin Nutr, 89*, 1011–1018.

McCaffery, J. M., Papandonatos, G. D., Lyons, M. J., and Niaura, R. (2008). Educational attainment and the heritability of self-reported hypertension among male Vietnam-era twins. *Psychosom Med, 70*, 781–786.

Medland, S. E., and Keller, M. C. (2009). Modeling extended twin family data II: power associated with different family structures. *Twin Res Hum Genet, 12*, 19–25.

Middeldorp, C. M., Birley, A. J., Cath, D. C., Gillespie, N. A., Willemsen, G. et al (2005). Familial clustering of major depression and anxiety disorders in Australian and Dutch twins and siblings. *Twin Res Hum Genet, 8*, 609–615.

Mustelin, L., Silventoinen, K., Pietilainen, K., Rissanen, A., and Kaprio, J. (2009). Physical activity reduces the influence of genetic effects on BMI and waist circumference: a study in young adult twins. *Int J Obes (Lond), 33*, 29–36.

Muthén, L. K., and Muthén, B. O. (2007). *Mplus: Statistical Analysis with Latent Variables*. Los Angeles, CA: Muthen and Muthen.

Neale, M. C., Boker, S. M., Xie, G., and Maes, H. H. (2006). *Mx: Statistical Modeling, 7th Ed.* Richmond, VI: Department of Psychiatry, Virginia Commonwealth University.

Neale, M. C., and Cardon, L. R. (1992). *Methodology for Genetic Studies of Twins and Families*. Dordrecht: Kluwer Academic Publishers.

Neale, M. C., and McArdle, J. J. (2000). Structured latent growth curves for twin data. *Twin Res Human Genet, 3*, 165–177.

Newton-Cheh, C., Larson, M. G., Vasan, R. S., Levy, D., Bloch, K. D. et al (2009). Association of common variants in NPPA and NPPB with circulating natriuretic peptides and blood pressure. *Nat Genet, 41*, 348–353.

Peetz, D., Victor, A., Adams, P., Erbes, H., Hafner, G. et al (2004). Genetic and environmental influences on the fibrinolytic system: a twin study. *Thromb Haemost, 92*, 344–351.

Pickering, T. G. (2001). Mental stress as a causal factor in the development of hypertension and cardiovascular disease. *Curr Hypertens Rep, 3*, 249–254.

Plomin, R., DeFries, J. C., McClearn, G. E., and McGuffin, P. (2000). *Behavioral Genetics, 4th Ed.* New York: Worth.

Posthuma, D., Meulenbelt, I., de Craen, A. J., de Geus, E. J., Slagboom, P. E. et al (2005). Human cytokine response to ex vivo amyloid-beta stimulation is mediated by genetic factors. *Twin Res Hum Genet, 8*, 132–137.

Poulsen, P., Kyvik, K. O., Vaag, A., and Beck-Nielsen, H. (1999). Heritability of type II (non-insulin-dependent) diabetes mellitus and abnormal glucose tolerance--a population-based twin study. *Diabetologia, 42*, 139–145.

Poulsen, P., Vaag, A., Kyvik, K., and Beck-Nielsen, H. (2001). Genetic versus environmental aetiology of the metabolic syndrome among male and female twins. *Diabetologia, 44*, 537–543.

Punnett, R. C. (1905). *Mendelism*. Cambridge: Bowes and Bowes.

Purcell, S. (2002). Variance components models for gene-environment interaction in twin analysis. *Twin Res Human Genet, 5*, 554–571.

Purcell, S., and Koenen, K. C. (2005). Environmental mediation and the twin design. *Behav Genet, 35*, 491–498.

Rampersaud, E., Mitchell, B. D., Pollin, T. I., Fu, M., Shen, H. et al (2008). Physical activity and the association of common FTO gene variants with body mass index and obesity. *Arch Intern Med, 168*, 1791–1797.

Rathouz, P. J., Van Hulle, C. A., Rodgers, J. L., Waldman, I. D., and Lahey, B. B. (2008). Specification, testing, and interpretation of gene-by-measured-environment interaction models in the presence of gene-environment correlation. *Behav Genet, 38*, 301–315.

Rebollo, I., and Boomsma, D. I. (2006). Genetic and environmental influences on type a behavior pattern: evidence from twins and their parents in the Netherlands Twin Register. *Psychosom Med, 68*, 437–442.

Schousboe, K., Willemsen, G., Kyvik, K. O., Mortensen, J., Boomsma, D. I., Cornes, B. K. et al (2003). Sex differences in heritability of BMI: a comparative study of results from twin studies in eight countries. *Twin Res Hum Genet, 6*, 409–421.

Silventoinen, K., Sammalisto, S., Perola, M., Boomsma, D. I., Cornes, B. K. et al (2003). Heritability of adult body height: a comparative study of twin cohorts in eight countries. *Twin Res Hum Genet, 6*, 399–408.

Simonis-Bik, A. M. C., Eekhoff, E. M. W., Diamant, M., Boomsma, D. I., Heine, R. J. et al (2008). The heritability of HbA1c and fasting blood glucose in different measurement settings. *Twin Res Hum Genet, 11*, 597–602.

Snieder, H., Boomsma, D. I., van Doornen, L. J., and de Geus, E. J. (1997). Heritability of respiratory sinus arrhythmia: dependency on task and respiration rate. *Psychophysiol, 34*, 317–328.

Stubbe, J. H., Boomsma, D. I., and de Geus, E. J. C. (2005). Sports participation during adolescence: A shift from environmental to genetic factors. *Med Sci Sports Exerc, 37*, 563–570.

Stubbe, J. H., Boomsma, D. I., Vink, J. M., Cornes, B. K., Martin, N. G. et al (2006). Genetic influences on exercise participation: a comparative study in adult twin samples from seven countries. *PLoS ONE, 1*, e22.

Su, S., Snieder, H., Miller, A. H., Ritchie, J., Bremner, J. D. et al (2008). Genetic and environmental influences on systemic markers of inflammation in middle-aged male twins. *Atherosclerosis, 200*, 213–220.

Sullivan, P. F., Neale, M. C., and Kendler, K. S. (2000). Genetic epidemiology of major depression: Review and meta-analysis. *Am J Psychiat, 157*, 1552–1562.

Vink, J. M., Beem, A. L., Posthuma, D., Neale, M. C., Willemsen, G. et al (2004). Linkage analysis of smoking initiation and quantity in Dutch sibling pairs. *Pharmacogenomics J, 4*, 274–282.

Vink, J. M., Willemsen, G., and Boomsma, D. I. (2005). Heritability of smoking initiation and nicotine dependence. *Behav Genet, 35*, 397–406.

Wang, X., Ding, X., Su, S., Li, Z., Riese, H. et al (2009). Genetic influences on heart rate variability at rest and during stress. *Psychophysiol, 46*, 458–65.

Worns, M. A., Victor, A., Galle, P. R., and Hohler, T. (2006). Genetic and environmental contributions to plasma C-reactive protein and interleukin-6 levels--a study in twins. *Genes Immun, 7*, 600–605.

Wray, N. R., Birley, A. J., Sullivan, P. F., Visscher, P. M., and Martin, N. G. (2007). Genetic and phenotypic stability of measures of neuroticism over 22 years. *Twin Res Hum Genet, 10*, 695–702.

Zdravkovic, S., Wienke, A., Pedersen, N. L., Marenberg, M. E., Yashin, A. I. et al (2002). Heritability of death from coronary heart disease: a 36-year follow-up of 20 966 Swedish twins. *J Intern Med, 252*, 247–254.

Zdravkovic, S., Wienke, A., Pedersen, N. L., Marenberg, M. E., Yashin, A. I. et al (2004). Genetic influences on CHD-death and the impact of known risk factors: Comparison of two frailty models. *Behav Genet, 34*, 585–592.

Chapter 29

Candidate Gene and Genome-Wide Association Studies in Behavioral Medicine

Ilja M. Nolte, Jeanne M. McCaffery, and Harold Snieder

1 Introduction

Mapping of disease genes relies on the idea that patients more often carry a disease-predisposing DNA variant than healthy individuals do. Until 20 years ago genetic research mainly concentrated on rare so-called *Mendelian* diseases. Such diseases are characterized by aggregation of the phenotype of interest within families and are typically caused by a single gene with large effect. *Linkage* methods were developed to study the co-segregation of these Mendelian diseases with genetic variants or *markers* within pedigrees, which proved to be very successful, including, for example, the identification of genetic variation contributing to rare, familial forms of obesity such as variants within *MC4R* (Vaisse et al, 1998; Yeo et al, 1998) (see Chapter 33).

In the 1990s the focus shifted toward common diseases to which linkage analysis was applied as well. The success rate of identification of genes for complex traits and diseases through *positional cloning* (i.e., fine-mapping of linkage peaks) was disappointingly low, with the notable exception of the discovery of the diabetes risk *locus, TCF7L2* (Grant et al, 2006). The reasons for the limited success are that (i) many

genes play a role; (ii) these genes interact with each other and with various environmental factors; (iii) the gene variants that cause the disease, i.e., the *risk alleles*, are commonly observed in the general population; (iv) each individual risk allele confers low risk of the disease or trait. As such, affected individuals within a family might not carry a particular risk allele while unaffected individuals do. Hence the inheritance of the disease or trait does not fit a simple Mendelian pattern. As a consequence gene finding efforts for complex traits increasingly rely on *association* approaches, because linkage analysis has minimal power as shown by Risch and Merikangas (Risch and Merikangas, 1996). In contrast to linkage analysis, association studies compare unrelated individuals from the general population and test whether a particular allele and a trait co-occur more often than expected.

The conduct of association studies has been greatly facilitated by two large projects that were completed in the last decade. Early this century the Human Genome Project and Celera Genomics in parallel completed the human genome sequence of the four chemical building blocks (or *bases*) of the DNA (A, T, C, and G). These always occur in pairs (A with T; C with G) and are hence called *base pairs* (bp). In the process they identified and mapped the approximately 25,000 genes of the human genome (International Human Genome Sequencing Consortium 2004). Subsequently, the HapMap consortium (Frazer et al, 2007; International HapMap Consortium, 2005; The International HapMap Project, 2003) characterized millions of common DNA sequence variations of a single

H. Snieder (✉)
Unit of Genetic Epidemiology & Bioinformatics,
Department of Epidemiology, University Medical Center
Groningen, University of Groningen, Hanzeplein 1,
PO Box 30.001, 9700 RB Groningen, The Netherlands
e-mail: h.snieder@epi.umcg.nl

A. Steptoe (ed.), *Handbook of Behavioral Medicine*, DOI 10.1007/978-0-387-09488-5_29,
© Springer Science+Business Media, LLC 2010

base, called *single nucleotide polymorphisms (SNPs)*, across the genome in various human populations. Other major variation discovery efforts have a candidate gene focus (Crawford et al, 2005; Packer et al, 2006). These publicly available resources constitute the first steps toward a future where all variants of human genes will be known.

The increased availability of SNPs generated in projects such as the HapMap has already spawned two important developments in association studies. Rather than focusing on one or two functional SNPs candidate gene studies increasingly consider all common variants within the gene jointly (i.e., gene-wide) (Neale and Sham, 2004). The second development is that of the genome-wide association (GWA) study (Hirschhorn and Daly, 2005; Kruglyak, 2008; Pearson and Manolio, 2008; Wang et al, 2005). Rapid improvements in genotyping technology and reductions in cost have now made it feasible to conduct these studies, using sets of hundreds of thousands anonymous SNP markers distributed across the entire genome. This hypothesis-free GWA approach has led to an explosion in the number of newly identified genes for complex traits and diseases (Frayling, 2007; Manolio et al, 2008; The Wellcome Trust Case-Control Consortium, 2007) since its first successful application in 2005, which uncovered a functional SNP underlying age-related macular degeneration (Klein et al, 2005). By October 14, 2009, 417 studies on 482 diseases or traits (successful and unsuccessful) were recorded in the Catalog of Published Genome-Wide Association Studies of the National Human Genome Research Institute (www.genome.gov/gwastudies) (Hindorff et al, 2009a, b).

These recent developments in genetic association studies have also impacted the field of behavioral medicine, with the recent identification of new loci for obesity (Frayling et al, 2007; Loos et al, 2008; Thorleifsson et al, 2009; Willer et al, 2009), diabetes (Frayling, 2007; Saxena et al, 2007; Zeggini et al, 2008), blood pressure (Levy et al, 2009; Newton-Cheh et al, 2009), and cigarette smoking (Thorgeirsson and Stefansson, 2008) to name a few. Therefore, the aim of

the current chapter is to provide an overview of concepts and approaches used in candidate gene and GWA studies illustrated with examples of traits and genes relevant to behavioral medicine.

2 A (Very) Short Introduction to Molecular Genetics

The DNA between any two persons is almost exactly the same (99.9%). The 0.1% difference in the sequence of DNA among individuals is the source of all genetic variation and is responsible not only for, for example, eye color or blood group but also for susceptibility to disease. Variation in a single gene is responsible for Mendelian disorders such as cystic fibrosis and sickle cell disease (Ingram, 1956; Riordan et al, 1989). Variation in multiple genes, environmental factors, and gene–gene, and gene environment interactions is thought to account for complex traits, including most of those of interest in behavioral medicine (Burton et al, 2005; McCaffery et al, 2007).

The DNA is organized in 22 autosomal chromosomal pairs and one pair of sex chromosomes. Together they constitute the *genome*. Large-scale genetic variation includes loss or gain of chromosomes, or breakage and rejoining of different chromosomes. This variation is abnormal and often leads to profound developmental problems. On an intermediate scale, deleted or duplicated genomic regions of >1000 bp, which may contain (parts of) genes, are called *copy number variants* (CNVs) (Iafrate et al, 2004; Redon et al, 2006; Sebat et al, 2004) (see also Section 4.8). Smaller scale genetic variation is at the level of a single or small number of base pairs and contributes to most of the normal variation in the population. This variation can be classified into three groups: insertion/deletion polymorphisms, variable number of tandem repeats (VNTR), and SNPs. A deletion occurs when one or more nucleotides are eliminated from a sequence, whereas an insertion occurs when one or more nucleotides are duplicated and inserted into the sequence. VNTRs (which include very short repeats or *microsatellites*) are repetitions of short identical segments of DNA with the number of repeated segments varying between individuals. A SNP is defined as a single base substitution and is the most abundant form of DNA variation in the human genome, which harbors approximately 10 million common SNPs with a minor allele frequency (MAF) >5% (Frazer et al, 2007; International HapMap Consortium, 2005; Kruglyak, 2008).

For each chromosomal pair one chromosome is inherited from the father and one from the mother. If for a particular genetic marker a person inherited the same allele from both parents that person's *genotype* for that marker is *homozygous* and if he or she inherited different alleles it is *heterozygous*. Under a simple Mendelian inheritance model, and assuming random mating, lack of selection according to genotype, and absence of mutation or migration, the frequencies of the genotypes in the population are perfectly predicted by the frequencies of the two alleles, which is referred to as Hardy–Weinberg equilibrium (HWE) (Hardy, 1908; Weinberg, 1908). As an example consider a genetic marker with two alleles, denoted "short" (S) with frequency p and "long" (L) with frequency $q = 1-p$. Let the least frequent or *minor* allele S take up 40% of all alleles in the population ($p = 0.40$). There are three potential genotypes SS, SL, and LL with expected frequencies p^2 (0.16), $2 \cdot pq$ (0.48), and q^2 (0.36), respectively. A chi-square test with 1 degree of freedom for HWE compares these expected genotype frequencies to the observed genotype frequencies with a significant chi-square p-value indicating that HWE does not hold. This test is often used for quality control purposes and deviation of HWE may indicate genotyping error (Gomes et al, 1999; Hosking et al, 2004). Many of the association analyses discussed below require HWE to hold.

3 Candidate Gene Association Studies

For heritable traits and diseases genetic variants must exist that influence that trait or disease,

but which variants in which of the $\sim$25,000 genes does that concern? Candidate gene association studies test whether a particular allele in a candidate gene and a trait co-occur above chance level, given the frequency of the allele and the distribution of the trait in the population (Cordell and Clayton, 2005; McCaffery et al, 2007). These studies are hypothesis-based, which means that selection of genes as plausible candidates is required *a priori*. The selection may be based on the biological role of the gene in a causative pathway (physiological candidate) or a location close to a peak from a linkage or genetic mapping study (positional candidate). Ideally, the candidate gene fits both criteria. It should be noted that for most complex traits, our knowledge of underlying causative pathways is likely incomplete. Limiting the search for contributing genetic variation to known candidate genes will likely prevent the identification of potentially novel pathways that contribute to complex traits.

Two types of candidate gene association study designs can be distinguished (Fig. 29.1). In a *direct* association study, one or more putatively functional variants are typed and associated with the outcome of interest. It is presumed that the variants selected for genotyping are causative for the trait of interest. Genetic variants are prioritized by apparent functional significance or location within coding or promoter regions. Variability in coding regions can impact amino acid sequence and possibly protein structure (e.g., splice variants). Promoter variants located upstream of the gene may be associated with transcriptional efficiency and ultimately the amount of protein synthesized. One example of a putatively functional variant is the 44 bp insertion/deletion polymorphism (5HTTLPR) in the promoter region of the serotonin transporter gene (*SLC6A4*). In vitro studies suggest that the polymorphism affects transcriptional efficiency, resulting in altered transporter expression and serotonin uptake (Heils et al, 1995, 1996; Lesch et al, 1996). More recent work also suggests that a SNP within the inserted or long allele alters the functional significance of the marker, resulting in a version of the long allele that is functionally similar to the short allele and yielding the "tri-allelic" version of the marker (Wendland et al, 2006).

SNPs within a gene are often strongly associated (i.e., in *linkage disequilibrium* [LD]) with each other due to co-inheritance as a result of lack or absence of recombination events between the SNPs (Gabriel et al, 2002). A series of alleles at correlated SNPs on the same chromosome is called a *haploid genotype* or in short *haplotype*. Throughout the genome haplotype or LD blocks exist with SNPs from the same block being strongly and from different blocks being weakly correlated. If a haplotype block consists of k SNPs, 2^k possible haplotypes could exist. However, due to LD the number of observed haplotypes is often much lower implying that many SNPs can be predicted from a limited number of representative SNPs (*haplotype tagging SNPs* or *tagSNPs*) (Johnson et al, 2001). In an *indirect* association analysis only the tagSNPs have to be genotyped, hence reducing the genotyping costs, but these SNPs remain representative of and can be extrapolated to all common SNPs within a gene (Figs. 29.1 and 29.2). Such an approach affords gene-based replication and offers a promising solution to the lack of replicability that continues to plague association studies of complex diseases and traits (Neale and Sham, 2004).

TagSNPs are selected in such a way that all non-genotyped SNPs are strongly correlated with one or more of them (Fig. 29.2). The selection is ideally performed in a subset of the sample under study, but more often samples of the same ethnicity from freely available web

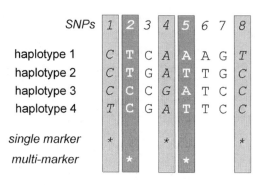

Fig. 29.2 Principle of tagSNPs selection. For eight SNPs four different haplotypes exist. In the single-marker tagging approach shown by the *light gray boxes* it would suffice to genotype SNPs 1, 4, and 8. SNP 1 discriminates haplotype 4 from the others, SNP 4 does the same for haplotype 3, and SNP 8 for haplotype 1. It is redundant to genotype SNP 6 as this SNP is highly correlated with SNP 8. In addition, SNP 3 is tagged by SNPs 4 and 8. However, in this case it is possible to tag all four haplotypes by only two SNPs. The more aggressive multi-marker approach shown by the *dark gray boxes* identifies SNPs 2 and 5 as tagSNPs discriminating all four haplotypes from each other through the combination of alleles. Combinations T-A, T-T, C-A, and C-T discriminate haplotypes 1 through 4, respectively

resources such as the HapMap are used. There are different approaches to identify tagSNPs (e.g., reviewed by Stram, 2005). Figure 29.2 shows the difference between single- and multi-marker tagging approaches. In a single marker approach each tagSNP discriminates one haplotype from the others. The more aggressive multi-marker approach allows haplotypes to be tagged by multiple SNPs and results in a further drop in number of SNPs needed for genotyping to cover all SNPs within the region of interest. In Fig. 29.2 the multi-marker approach used combinations of two SNPs, but more advanced methods use (many) more. They also allow for less than perfect correlation, usually a threshold for r^2 of 0.8 is regarded as a sufficiently strong correlation. The tagSNPs or their haplotype combinations inferred by estimation algorithms (Stephens and Donnelly, 2003) are then examined for association with the trait of interest in the total sample and the effects of unassayed SNPs would then be detected through LD with tagSNPs (Carlson

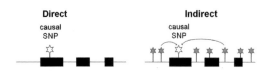

Fig. 29.1 Direct versus indirect association analysis. In direct association analysis the causal variant is genotyped and tested itself. In indirect association analysis multiple tagSNPs within a genic region are genotyped and tested in the hope that one or more of them are strongly correlated with the untyped causal variant

et al, 2004; Neale and Sham, 2004). Therefore, this procedure ensures reasonably good coverage of common variation throughout the gene. Even VNTRs and insertion/deletion polymorphisms can often be tagged. For example, a recent study by Wray and colleagues identified a two-SNP haplotype proxy for 5HTTLPR (Wray et al, 2009). The International HapMap project (http://www.hapmap.org) has characterized >3 million SNP markers on a genome-wide scale in multiple ethnic groups, greatly facilitating the use of tagSNPs in association studies (Frazer et al, 2007).

The statistical approach to candidate gene association studies depends on the research design of which cohort and case–control studies are the most common. For these designs we also discuss gene × gene and gene × environment interaction and provide some power and sample size considerations.

3.1 Cohort Studies: Continuous/Quantitative Traits

For individual diallelic polymorphisms such as SNPs, genotype is the unit of analysis and serves as the independent variable. Covariates and additional predictors of the dependent variable may also be incorporated. Within a regression framework, the most general model for genetic effects at a single locus includes a term for linear effects of a given allele and an additional parameter for the deviation from this linear effect, i.e., a *dominance* term (Cordell and Clayton, 2005). The general regression framework for a diallelic locus is given by

$$Y = \alpha + \beta_a A + \beta_d D + \beta_c C + e$$

where Y is a quantitative trait, α is the baseline mean of Y, A and D are dummy variables reflecting coding for linear (additive) and nonlinear (dominance) effects of the underlying genotype at a single locus, C represents other covariates such as age or sex, and e is

a residual error term assumed to be normally distributed.

For the linear term, genotypes (e.g., GG, GC, and CC) are assumed to function in an additive manner and the corresponding regression variable A is coded as 0, 1, and 2 reflecting dose of the C allele. The associated beta estimate is the additive effect of the C allele. This linear model alone predicts that the mean of the heterozygotes (GC) will be located at the midpoint between the means of the two types of homozygotes (GG, CC); however, in practice, this may not be the case. Deviation of the mean of the heterozygotes from the midpoint between the means of the homozygotes suggests that one allele is dominant over the other. To quantify this effect, an additional regression term is necessary. Specifically, the regression variable D for the dominance effect is coded 0, 1, and 0 with the associated beta estimate reflecting deviation of the heterozygotes from the midpoint of the two homozygous groups. One degree of freedom (df) is required to test each of the linear and nonlinear terms. In addition to the additive model ($D = 0$), other specific disease models with only 1 df are the (completely) dominant model (i.e., the effect is the same for GC and CC: $D = A$) and the recessive model (i.e., only CC is at increased risk: $D = -A$). In practice, when no hypothesis exists on the nature of the trait model, the 2 df model is often tested first and subsequently, the most appropriate and more powerful 1 df model is applied. Simply testing all 1 df models is inefficient because of the multiple testing penalty (see Section 4.4).

In genetic association studies of quantitative traits, assuming a simple additive model (i.e., no dominance effect), effect size of a locus is a function of mean trait differences between homozygotes (e.g., the CC versus GG genotype) and allele frequency (Blangero, 2004). It is usually described by the coefficient of determination R^2, in a regression analysis that is the percentage of variance explained by the genetic variant. An R^2 value >5% for a single gene is considered a large effect in genetic epidemiology, for complex diseases R^2 <2% are expected for each contributing gene.

3.2 Case–Control Studies: Disease Traits

Case–control genetic association studies are typically comprised of a group of cases with a disease of interest and well-matched controls. Ideally, the cases and controls should represent "identical" subsamples from a single population differing only on the trait of interest (Sullivan et al, 2001). Statistical analyses compare allele frequencies or genotypes across cases and controls. In samples well-matched for ethnicity, but possibly also for age, sex, or other predictors, differences in genotypes across cases and controls may be tested using chi-square tests. Alternatively, the risk of having the disorder may be modeled using logistic regression. The log odds of expressing the disease trait is modeled as a function of the additive effects of the dose of one of the alleles and a dominance term representing deviance from this additive pattern similar to the model for quantitative traits discussed in Section 3.1:

$$\ln (Y/(1 - Y)) = \alpha + \beta_a A + \beta_d D + \beta_c C + e$$

where Y is the binary expression of a phenotype, α is the baseline log odds of Y, and A, D, C, and e are the same as before. The term e^{β_a} reflects the change in odds of expression of the phenotype based on a unit increase in allele dose and is called the *odds ratio* (OR). The GG genotype becomes the reference group (0 alleles) and the effect of genotype is quantified by the additive beta estimate determining if there is a significant change in odds of the disease for each additional C allele and the dominance beta estimate reflecting the deviation of heterozygotes from the midpoint of the log odds for the two homozygous groups. Alternatively, genotypes are modeled by two dummy variables coded as 0, 1, 0 and 0, 0, 1 for GG, GC, CC, respectively, estimating separately the ORs for hetero- and homozygotes. Again, one of the more powerful 1 df models (dominant, recessive, or additive) can be tested based on the ORs observed in the 2 df model.

3.3 Gene × Gene and Gene × Environment Interaction

Nearly all traits in behavioral medicine are considered "complex," meaning that the causal pathways are likely to involve multiple genes of small effect, environmental factors, and gene × gene and gene × environment interaction (Burton et al, 2005; McCaffery et al, 2007). Interaction between two loci is termed *epistasis*. However, a distinction between epistasis referring to a statistical interaction and that referring to a physical interaction of gene products is warranted, as the presence of statistical interaction does not necessarily imply an underlying biological interaction (Cordell, 2002). Similarly, statistical gene × environment interactions should be interpreted with caution as the mathematical model may again have no obvious biological interpretation (Clayton and McKeigue, 2001). Finally, if the genotype is correlated to the environmental risk factor (e.g., genetic susceptibility to aggression and parental maltreatment), the interpretation of the statistical interaction is not straightforward (Turkheimer et al, 2005).

Modeling statistical gene × gene or gene × environment interaction may be accomplished by incorporating all interaction terms between two genetic predictors or between one genetic and one environmental predictor, respectively, into linear or logistic regression as described above (Cordell, 2002; Moffitt et al, 2005). Statistical epistasis implies that at least one of the gene × gene interaction coefficients differs significantly from zero.

3.4 Power and Sample Size Considerations

As mentioned in the previous paragraph, behavioral medicine traits are likely to be influenced by multiple genes and interactions. Therefore, effect sizes of individual genes are expected to be small. Consequently, required sample sizes to detect genetic main effects or gene × environment interactions with sufficient statistical power are expected to be relatively large. Excellent online resources specific to power and sample size calculations for genetic association studies exist (e.g., Quanto (Gauderman and Morrison, 2006) available at http://hydra.usc.edu/gxe or the Genetic Power Calculator (Purcell et al, 2003) at http://statgen.iop.kcl.ac.uk/gpc/).

As examples, we present sample size calculations for genetic main effects and gene × environment interactions for a continuous trait using Quanto (Gauderman and Morrison, 2006). In all models, statistical power is set at 0.80 and we assume additive genetic effects only. Effect sizes are quantified in terms of f, defined as the ratio of the standard deviation between genotype groups to the common standard deviation within genotype groups. Sample sizes for small ($f = 0.10$), medium ($f = 0.25$), and large effect sizes ($f = 0.40$) were calculated (Cohen, 1988). "Gene 1" is modeled after the 5HTTLPR upstream from the serotonin transporter gene (Caspi et al, 2003; Lesch et al, 1996; Risch et al, 2009) with an allele frequency of 0.40 for the risk allele. The outcome is depressive symptoms measured continuously (although binary traits can easily be accommodated) and the environmental risk is modeled after "severe adverse life events" with a prevalence of 30% (Caspi et al, 2003). Sample size requirements for gene main effects (Model A) and gene × environment interactions (Model B) by effect size are presented in Table 29.1.

As can be seen from the table, sample size required varies dramatically with effect size, desired significance level α, and the complexity of the model, as would be expected. A sample size of 500 affords sufficient power to detect a medium effect size for gene main effect models but may pose difficulty in detecting gene × environment interactions of even large effect size. To detect gene × environment interaction of a medium effect, a sample size of about 1500 is required. The required sample size will be even larger if the allele is relatively rare (e.g., 5–10%) or – as shown in Table 29.1 – a large number of markers is typed such as in GWA studies for which the statistical significance criterion is adjusted to 5.0×10^{-8} to take multiple comparisons into account (see Section 4.4). Differing modes of inheritance (additive, dominant, recessive) will also impact effect size and have resulting effects on power and sample size. On the other hand, careful selection and adjustment for environmental covariates may increase the trait heritability and improve power to detect main effects of the gene for a given sample size (Sabatti et al, 2009).

Table 29.1 Sample size calculations for a gene main effect and gene × environmental interaction with 80% power stratified by effect size and α level for additive genetic effects

Effect	Model A "Gene" only[a]			Model B "Gene × environment" interaction[b]		
size (f)[c]	$\alpha = 0.05$	$\alpha = 0.001$	$\alpha = 5.0 \times 10^{-8}$	$\alpha = 0.05$	$\alpha = 0.001$	$\alpha = 5.0 \times 10^{-8}$
0.10	1631	3549	8230	7667	16678	38681
0.25	258	561	1300	1200	2611	6055
0.40	98	214	496	453	986	2288

[a] Model A – main effect of one gene (risk allele frequency of 0.40)

[b] Model B – interaction effect of one genetic variant with a risk allele frequency of 0.40 and one environmental exposure with a prevalence of 30%, assuming main effect contributions of $f = 0.10$ for the variant and the environmental factor

[c] Effect size in f from Cohen (Cohen, 1988). In this example, f indicates the ratio of the standard deviation between genotype groups to the common standard deviation within genotype groups. Effect size of $f = 0.10$ corresponds to a small effect size, $f = 0.25$ corresponds to a medium effect size, and $f = 0.40$ corresponds to a large effect size (Cohen, 1988)

3.5 Non-significance, Non-replication, and Inconsistency

A negative finding does not necessarily mean that the candidate gene is not associated with the outcome. In this respect sample size plays an important role. Many prior studies used small samples and had little power to find true associations. Furthermore, note that even if a study is adequately sized (i.e., power = 80%), there is still 20% chance of not finding the association even if it truly exists. Negative results could also be due to inadequate coverage of a gene, for example, in studies of single variants. In addition, non-significant results may be attributable to a true lack of etiological relationship (Sullivan et al, 2001). Given the importance of non-replications in the literature, calls have been made for convenient formats to publish negative results (Colhoun et al, 2003; Moffitt et al, 2005; Sullivan et al, 2001).

Another issue in candidate gene studies is non-replication. Many initial significant associations could not be replicated by other studies or gave inconsistent results (Ioannidis, 2003; Ioannidis et al, 2001; Wacholder et al, 2004). A major reason is again that either the initial or the replication studies lacked sufficient statistical power (at least 80%). Low power could result in a false-positive finding in the first study or in false-negative ones in the replication studies. The latter in particular could be due to the "winner's curse" (Goring et al, 2001). This means that the initial study typically overestimates the effect size, which leads to non-replication in follow-up studies of similar sample size. Incomplete coverage of the gene could also lead to incorrect conclusions. The genetic marker showing significant association in the initial study may not be the causal variant, but only in strong LD with it. Follow-up studies in populations lacking this LD structure may be unable to confirm the association with the same marker locus and the initial finding will be falsely regarded as a replication failure. Non-replication could also arise from true heterogeneity, meaning that a gene variant might be associated in one population but not in another.

In conclusion, even if a candidate gene study is negative or if initial positive results are not replicated in follow-up studies it is very difficult to completely rule out the gene as a candidate.

4 Genome-Wide Association (GWA) Studies

In the last 5 years it has become feasible to perform large-scale GWA studies as a result of the development of high-throughput genome-wide genotyping arrays or chips (Affymetrix Inc., Santa Clara, CA, USA; Illumina Inc., San Diego, CA, USA) and the consequent reductions in cost per genotype. These chips contain hundreds of thousands of SNPs. The entire human genome has an approximate length of 3.3×10^9 base pairs, of which ~1 in 1000 is polymorphic. A well-selected sample of 300,000 tagSNPs already provides reasonable coverage of the European Caucasian genome (Illumina HumanHap 300 chip: correlation r^2 >0.8 with 77% of all HapMap Phase I SNPs) (The International HapMap Project, 2003; Manolio et al, 2008).

GWA studies allow interrogation of the entire genome (and thus every gene) at levels of resolution that were previously unattainable and aim to identify common genetic variations underlying disease. This GWA approach relies on the "common disease, common variant" hypothesis, which states that common disease susceptibility is the result of the joint action of multiple common variants (Pritchard and Cox, 2002). The alternative to this hypothesis is the "common disease, rare variant" or disease heterogeneity hypothesis, which claims that many low-frequent variants are the cause of common diseases with different variants present in different individuals (Smith and Lusis, 2002). The truth for complex diseases is likely to be somewhere in the middle.

4.1 Quality Control

An important aspect of GWA studies is that a huge amount of data is generated in a highly automated way. This requires strict quality control (QC) of the data before analyzing it for association with the disease or trait of interest. It is impossible to inspect each individual data point for its quality in a GWA study, therefore strict procedures have to be followed. Useful software packages facilitating the GWA QC are PLINK (Purcell et al 2007) or GenABEL (Aulchenko et al, 2007). In the next paragraphs we discuss the QC steps required to ensure reliable genotype data and association results.

- *Step 1: Inspection of genotype calling and signal intensity plots.* Genotypes are being called based on signal intensities of the two alleles of a SNP. The difficulty in calling genotypes is that the intensities may vary between chips because of DNA concentration or differences in probe affinities. Furthermore, all individuals should be analyzed together; otherwise bias may be introduced due to batch effects (Clayton et al, 2005). In particular when cases and controls are called separately, spurious associations as a result of differences in genotype calling may occur. Usually, only the plots from those SNPs that survive the other QC steps and that show some evidence of association in the statistical analysis are assessed through visual inspection.
- *Step 2: Reproducibility.* To assess the genotyping error rate a small number of individuals are usually re-genotyped. It is also possible to include HapMap individuals in your data set. The reproducibility of genotypes should be >99.5%.
- *Step 3: Missingness per individual.* A low percentage of successfully called genotypes (usually <95%) for an individual indicates low DNA quality and potentially dubious genotype calls. Individuals failing this criterion should be removed.

- *Step 4: Accidental mix-ups.* GWA data are well-suited to study relationships between individuals. The concordance rate between two individuals defined as the percentage of SNPs with identical genotypes can be used to identify accidental mix-ups in samples. A concordance rate of 1 indicates either sample duplication or monozygotic twins. If observed unexpectedly, either one or both individuals should be removed.
- *Step 5: Ethnicity.* Differential ethnic distribution between cases and controls, also known as population stratification, can lead to substantial inflation of the test statistic (Knowler et al, 1988). It is therefore essential to investigate the population structure of the sample for which several programs are available (e.g., STRUCTURE (Pritchard et al, 2000) or PLINK (Purcell et al, 2007)). Small numbers of individuals different from the non-dominant ethnic group should be removed. Otherwise stratified analyses may be performed. Association results should again be checked for evidence of population stratification (see Section 4.5).
- *Step 6: Heterozygosity per individual.* Based on their allele frequencies it can be determined how many autosomal SNPs are expected to be heterozygous. A typical approach is to estimate the mean and standard deviation (SD) of the heterozygosity across all individuals. If the heterozygosity of a single individual is $>3 \cdot SD$ below the mean it might indicate a uniparental disomy (i.e., when a person receives two copies of (a part of) a chromosome from one parent and none from the other); if it is $>3 \cdot SD$ above the mean it could point to DNA contamination. Deviating heterozygosity could also be evidence for low chip quality. Individuals with deviating heterozygosity should be excluded.

Once the sample is cleared of individuals failing one or more of the above criteria, SNPs can be subjected to quality checks in the remaining individuals.

- *Step 7: Missingness per SNP.* SNPs are of questionable quality when the genotype call rate (i.e., the percentage of individuals assigned a genotype) is low (<95%). It should be noted that SNPs can exhibit low genotype call rates as a result of a CNV (see Section 4.8). Signal intensity plots can be examined to determine if that is the case and if so, SNPs can be rescored as CNVs and analyzed accordingly (Franke et al, 2008).
- *Step 8: Minor allele frequency.* SNPs that are present on the genome-wide chip may not be polymorphic in all populations. In addition, SNPs that have low MAFs (<1% or <5%, depending on the sample size) are difficult to measure reliably and have low power to detect association with the trait of interest. Such SNPs need to be excluded.
- *Step 9: Violation of HWE.* Departure from HWE in controls or in a cohort may indicate genotyping errors (Gomes et al, 1999; Hosking et al, 2004). HWE testing must only be applied to controls, since cases might show deviation from HWE for SNPs associated to the disease. SNPs showing departure from HWE should be removed for classical diallelic association analysis. However, there is no consensus on the significance threshold to be used. It should be noted that SNPs can also show deviation from HWE as a result of a CNV (see also step 7).
- *Step 10: Comparison of control groups.* If the sample consists of multiple control groups, like in the Wellcome Trust Case Control Consortium (The Wellcome Trust Case-Control Consortium, 2007), genotype frequencies should be comparable between the groups. If these frequencies are different for a SNP, this SNP should be removed from the data set.

4.2 Imputation of SNPs

In order to be able to compare and combine GWA results generated from different genotyping platforms, imputation of non-genotyped SNPs, i.e., prediction of unknown genotypes based on LD with genotyped SNPs, is widely used. The HapMap Phase II database on 120 Caucasian, 120 African, or 180 Asian haplotypes consisting of ∼2,500,000 SNPs can be used as a reference set. The principle of imputation is the inverse of the selection of tagSNPs. If a SNP is not genotyped but it is strongly correlated in the reference set with one or a combination of genotyped SNPs, the genotypes of this SNP can be predicted with great accuracy. Imputation algorithms like those incorporated in MACH (Li and Abecasis, 2006), IMPUTE (Marchini et al, 2007), or BEAGLE (Browning and Browning, 2009) not only use information on haplotypes in the reference database but also account for the possibility of a recombination.

4.3 Association Analysis

Association with genotyped SNPs can be tested using linear or logistic regression as discussed in Sections 3.1 and 3.2 using PLINK (Purcell et al, 2007) or GenABEL (Aulchenko et al, 2007). The analysis of imputed SNPs is more complicated than for genotyped SNPs since the uncertainty of genotypes has to be taken into account. Such analysis can be performed using SNPTEST (Marchini et al, 2007), MACH2DAT (binary trait)/MACH2QTL (continuous trait) (Li and Abecasis, 2006), ProbABEL (Aulchenko et al, 2007), or BEAGLE (Browning and Browning, 2009). These programs also provide a quality score for each of the imputed SNPs and standard criteria for exclusion of SNPs based on low imputation quality are information score <0.5 (SNPTEST) and r^2 <0.3 (MACH2DAT/MACH2QTL and BEAGLE). Similar to genotyped SNPs, imputed SNPs with a low MAF or deviation from HWE should be discarded. Usually only the additive model is tested to reduce the number of tests and because this model has reasonable power to also detect dominant or recessive effects.

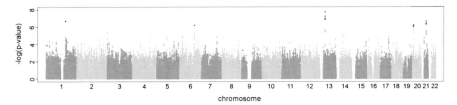

Fig. 29.3 Manhattan plot for QT interval based on GWAS meta-analysis of TwinsUK, BRIGHT, and DCCT/EDIC cohorts. SNPs are ordered along the chromosomes on the *x*-axis. The –log10 (*P*) results are plotted for 2,399,142 SNPs of the meta-analysis of TwinsUK, BRIGHT, and DCCT/EDIC cohorts for 3558 individuals. The *red dots* indicate SNPs with $p < 10^{-6}$. (From Nolte et al, 2009)

WGAViewer is a useful software package for visualizing GWA results (Ge et al, 2008) (Fig. 29.3 (Nolte et al, 2009)). It also facilitates zooming in on regions, making a selection of top hits (i.e., most significant SNPs), annotating SNPs or genomic regions in order to check for location of the SNPs with respect to genes that are located nearby, and looking for association with gene expression data, to name but a few of the options. Nice informative plots of associated regions incorporating information not only on significance but also on LD structure and gene positions can be created with the R script developed by De Bakker and colleagues (Saxena et al, 2007) or the web-based module SNAP (Fig. 29.4) (Johnson et al, 2008).

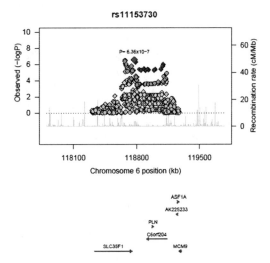

Fig. 29.4 Regional association plot for the SLC35F1/c6orf204/PLN locus on chromosome 6. Shown is the region extending to 500 kb either side of the most associated SNP rs11153730. The SNPs are illustrated on $-\log10(P)$ scale as a function of chromosomal position (NCBI build36.3). The sentinel SNP is illustrated in *blue*. Surrounding SNPs are colored according to their r^2 with rs11153730 (*red* indicates an $r^2 > 0.8$, *orange* an r^2 of 0.5–0.8, *yellow* an r^2 of 0.2–0.5, and *gray* an r^2 of less than 0.2). (From Nolte et al, 2009)

4.4 Multiple Testing

Next comes the crucial question regarding which *p*-values can be considered significant in a GWA study. In contrast to hypothesis-driven candidate gene association studies, GWA studies are hypothesis-free. This means that every SNP is tested without any assumption regarding genetic association with disease and hence, a huge multiple testing correction needs to be applied. For example, with 500,000 SNPs tested for association the standard significance level of 0.05 would already yield 25,000 false-positive results, assuming independence between all SNPs. Furthermore, in addition to the large number of SNPs a multiple testing correction should also be applied if multiple phenotypes or multiple genetic models are tested. However, as there is correlation between SNPs, between phenotypes, and between models, it is difficult to assess the true number of independent tests. Correction techniques for multiple comparisons based on the original Bonferroni criterion are in general too conservative (Manly et al, 2004). New procedures based on the false discovery rate effectively control the proportion of false discoveries without sacrificing the power to discover (Benjamini et al, 2001).

Recently, 5×10^{-8} has emerged as the consensus threshold for declaration of genome-wide significance (International HapMap Consortium, 2005). This threshold maintains a 5% genome-wide type I error rate based on estimations of the number of independent tests for common sequence variation (1 million tests), at least in Caucasians (Dudbridge and Gusnanto, 2008; Pe'er et al, 2008). Stricter thresholds are needed for populations with lower LD. For example, the genome-wide testing burden in Africans was estimated to be 2 million independent tests, which translates into a genome-wide significance threshold of 2.5×10^{-8} (Pe'er et al, 2008).

The downside of setting a stringent threshold for the type 1 error in order to avoid false-positive findings is that the probability of missing a true positive association (type II error or false-negative finding) becomes large, especially in small samples. Therefore a SNP is only considered a true positive result when it is replicated in other samples. In practice, a more lenient significance threshold (e.g., 10^{-6}) is often used for those SNPs taken forward for replication. Alternatively, the top 100 or 1000 SNPs are selected for follow-up and can be genotyped cost-effectively using custom-made chips.

4.5 Population Stratification

As mentioned in Section 4.1 cohort-based and case–control analysis of unrelated individuals may give rise to spurious genetic associations due to differences in both allele frequencies and the prevalence of the disease of interest among subgroups of different ancestry within the larger population, often reflecting racial or ethnic background (i.e., population stratification). It has been argued that there have been relatively few documented instances of bias due to population stratification reported in the literature and that population-based studies are relatively robust to this type of bias (Cardon and Palmer, 2003).

However, more recent empirical tests do find evidence of stratification effects, particularly among populations that recently originated from two or more distinct parental populations (genetic admixture), including African-Americans and Hispanic-Americans (Freedman et al, 2004).

If cases and controls are not matched for race, two methods are available to control for stratification using markers throughout the genome. In structure assessment, genetic markers, either anonymous markers or markers that differ substantially among ethnic groups, are used to predict membership to homogeneous subgroups within a stratified population (Hoggart et al, 2003; Price et al, 2006; Pritchard et al, 2000). Once identified, association analysis may be conducted within these subgroups to ensure a similar genetic background of cases and controls. A second method, genomic control, uses anonymous genetic markers to estimate the degree of inflation of the chi-square statistic due to population stratification and yields a correction factor lambda (λ) to account for the inflated significance (Devlin and Roeder, 1999).

In a GWA study both methods are applied. The first method, which identifies population substructures, is used as a QC step (see Section 4.1), while the second method is applied after the association analysis. A quantile–quantile (Q–Q) plot of test statistics or $-\log(p$-values) of non-associated SNPs visualizes the degree of inflation (Fig. 29.5). Deviation from the line of identity would indicate the presence of population stratification.

4.6 Interaction and Haplotype Analysis

In addition to single SNP tests, interaction of SNPs in different genes or haplotypes of SNPs within a gene can be analyzed. Analysis of interaction is to be performed in the same way as for candidate gene studies (see Section 3.3). However, since the number of SNPs in a GWA study usually is >100,000, the number of two-way interactions is >5 billion. Testing all

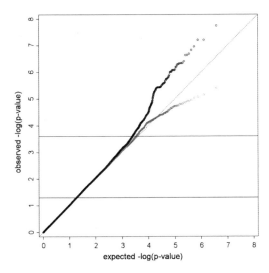

Fig. 29.5 Quantile–quantile plots of association results for QT interval of the meta-analysis from TwinsUK, BRIGHT, and DCCT/EDIC cohorts based on 2,399,142 SNPs in 3558 individuals from the combined cohorts. The $-\log10(P)$ of association test for QT interval is shown for all SNPs (*black diamonds*) and for all SNPs except those located within 1 Mb of the most significant SNPs of the five associated regions (*dark gray*). Genomic Control λ was 1.016. The lower *horizontal line* denotes the 95% percentile of the results of all SNPs, values lower than this threshold were used for calculating the λ. The *upper line* indicates the point from where *p*-values of the complete data set deviate from the expected line. (From Nolte et al, 2009)

these interactions would demand a huge multiple testing correction. Hence the set of gene × gene interactions to be tested should be selected wisely, for instance, looking only at genes in the same pathway or at SNPs that were at least suggestively associated ($p < 10^{-5}$) in the single SNP analysis.

Haplotype analysis of SNPs in LD with each other can also be used to further scan the genome for significant loci. Haplotype approaches rely on the hypothesis that chromosomal segments surrounding the disease mutation are still shared among cases and that disease mutation carrying haplotypes have a more recent common ancestor than other haplotypes (Nolte et al, 2007; Te Meerman et al, 1995). Exploiting the evolutionary history of haplotypes provides extra information on presence and location of a disease mutation in a genomic region and hence

haplotype analyses can be more powerful than single SNP analyses (Allen and Satten, 2007; Nolte et al, 2007).

To date most published GWA studies have focused on single SNP analyses and did not perform in-depth analyses like interaction or haplotype analyses implying that a potentially relevant source of information in GWA data is still unexplored.

4.7 Meta-analysis

GWA studies have identified large numbers of novel loci for complex traits and diseases, but these loci explain only a small fraction of the total genetic variation. For example, *NOS1AP* explains only 0.8–1.5% of the variance in QT interval (Arking et al, 2006; Nolte et al, 2009) whereas the total heritability is estimated to be around 50% (Dalageorgou et al, 2008). Typically, effect sizes of the newly identified common variants are modest requiring large sample sizes for detection. Thousand case–control pairs are needed to detect associations with 80% power of SNPs with a MAF of 35% and a OR of 1.51 or R^2 of 3.9% in a GWA, but this number increases rapidly to >10,000 for small effects (OR<1.14/R^2<0.39%) or low risk allele frequencies (<2.0%) (Gauderman and Morrison, 2006). Research groups involved in GWA studies quickly realized that collaborations in large consortia were a prerequisite for continued gene discovery through meta-analyses (Loos et al, 2008; Newton-Cheh et al, 2009; Nolte et al, 2009; Psychiatric GWAS Consortium Steering Committee, 2009; Saxena et al, 2007). These meta-analyses combine large numbers of cohorts to reliably show modest effects of susceptibility alleles (see Chapter 58). Although meta-analyses are useful for providing a composite effect measure for the genetic association, they may not properly capture the heterogeneity of designs, phenotype definitions, and variation in environmental exposures across studies (Arnett et al, 2007). Hence, a negative finding of a meta-analysis with significant results in some of the individual studies may indicate true heterogeneity between studies (see also Section 3.5).

4.8 Copy Number Variants (CNVs)

As already mentioned, identified risk variants underlying complex traits or diseases explain only a modest fraction of the heritable phenotypic variation. Increasing sample sizes by combining multiple GWA studies in meta-analyses will probably uncover more disease genes. However, the effects of such variants are expected to be even smaller than those found to date and the combined effects of these common SNPs will still only be able to explain a small part of the heritable variation in complex phenotypes (Lango et al, 2008). Discovering potential sources of this "missing" heritability constitutes a major challenge (Maher, 2008). CNVs may constitute one such source.

A few years ago two research groups first described the abundant presence of CNVs in the human genome (Iafrate et al, 2004; Sebat et al, 2004). Genomic regions of hundreds of thousands of bases are found to be either duplicated or deleted in multiple individuals. They affect as much as one-tenth of the human genome and encompass more nucleotide content per genome than SNPs (Redon et al, 2006). Many of these CNVs overlap with genes suggesting that CNVs might affect disease risk. Further evidence for this hypothesis comes from the correlation of CNVs with gene expression levels (Stranger et al, 2007) and associations of specific CNVs with clinical phenotypes (e.g., Aitman et al, 2006; Gonzalez et al, 2005). GWA studies facilitate the exploration of this hypothesis as genotyping arrays used to perform GWA studies increasingly include large numbers of CNVs.

4.9 Genetical Genomics

GWA studies are not limited to outcomes like diseases or traits, but they can also be applied to, for example, transcriptomic data. One of the first

GWA studies on global gene expression including ~400,000 SNPs and ~55,000 transcripts representing ~20,000 genes was published a few years ago (Dixon et al, 2007). Combinations of genome-wide with transcriptomic or proteomic data or the metabolic response to drugs will provide further insight into the role of genes in complex diseases.

5 Beyond Genome-Wide Association Studies

5.1 Rare Variants

GWA studies are often not capable of detecting risk variants with MAF <5% since this is commonly used as a QC exclusion criterion. Furthermore, these rare SNPs are never in strong LD ($r^2 > 0.8$) with more common variants, which limits detection of their signals through LD. Nevertheless, evidence is accumulating that these rare variants may be another important source of the "missing" heritability of common complex traits. For example, a recent study by Ji and colleagues (Ji et al, 2008) clearly showed that rare variants in renal salt handling genes known to be involved in Mendelian syndromes of salt wasting and hypotension can also produce clinically significant blood pressure reduction in the general population. Detection of such rare variants underlying common complex traits might be achieved using medical sequencing approaches in selections of individuals from large population-based cohorts such as the prospective LifeLines study, which will eventually encompass 165,000 individuals from the Northern Netherlands (Stolk et al, 2008). Furthermore, linkage analysis in large pedigrees may remain an efficient approach to map the location of such rare variants (Botstein and Risch, 2003).

5.2 Identification of Causal Variants

Confirmed signals emerging from GWA scans may not be causal themselves. Associated SNPs are often located in introns of genes or in intergenic regions that to date have no known function. Thus, they may simply be markers in LD with the causal variants. Replication samples from other ethnic groups with different LD structures may facilitate fine mapping of causal variants (McCarthy et al, 2008). In addition, bioinformatic tools may sometimes give a shortcut to functional (e.g., gene expression) information (Ge et al, 2008). In other cases sequencing of associated regions may be needed (McCarthy et al, 2008).

5.3 Clinical Relevance and Disease Prediction

As described by McCarthy and colleagues (McCarthy et al, 2008) clinical translation of recent GWA successes in the identification of susceptibility variants for complex diseases can take two routes. In the first, detection of novel loci – even with small effect sizes – may reveal new insights into disease pathogenesis leading to identification of new therapeutic targets. Such treatments may well be effective in individuals without the specific genetic variant that led to its discovery. Perhaps the best example is the development of HMG-CoA reductase inhibitors (statins) that effectively lower cholesterol levels in nearly everyone, except in individuals with homozygous absence of LDL-receptors who were instrumental in identifying this key metabolic pathway (Manolio et al, 2008).

The second translational route is through the use of genetic knowledge to develop more personalized approaches to disease prediction, prevention, and management. The major limitation here for most complex diseases is that the variants so far identified provide limited information on disease risk above and beyond conventional risk factors. For example, a recent study concluded that the combined impact of 18 risk variants for type 2 diabetes does not provide strong predictive value at the population level in addition to age, sex, and body mass index

(Lango et al, 2008). Before genetic profiling can be widely applied in clinical practice, the accuracy of risk prediction needs to be improved through identification of additional susceptibility variants and demonstration of their predictive value in prospective studies (Arnett et al, 2007; McCarthy et al, 2008).

6 Conclusions

In this chapter we aimed to provide a comprehensive overview of contemporary methodological approaches to identification of genes for complex traits and diseases. Nowadays association analysis, particularly through GWA scans, is the preferred tool. Within a few years it will be feasible to obtain complete human sequence data at relatively low cost (i.e., <$1000), which may render large-scale SNP genotyping – although developed only recently – a technique of the past. Future GWA studies will face major computational challenges in meaningfully relating complete sequence data to disease susceptibility traits, but offer the prospect of revealing parts of the missing heritability.

References

Aitman, T. J., Dong, R., Vyse, T. J., Norsworthy, P. J., Johnson, M. D. et al (2006). Copy number polymorphism in Fcgr3 predisposes to glomerulonephritis in rats and humans. Nature, 439, 851–855.
Allen, A. S., and Satten, G. A. (2007). Statistical models for haplotype sharing in case-parent trio data. Hum Hered, 64, 35–44.
Arking, D. E., Pfeufer, A., Post, W., Kao, W. H., Newton-Cheh, C. et al (2006). A common genetic variant in the NOS1 regulator NOS1AP modulates cardiac repolarization. Nat Genet, 38, 644–651.
Arnett, D. K., Baird, A. E., Barkley, R. A., Basson, C. T., Boerwinkle, E. et al (2007). Relevance of genetics and genomics for prevention and treatment of cardiovascular disease: a scientific statement from the American Heart Association Council on Epidemiology and Prevention, the Stroke Council, and the Functional Genomics and Translational Biology Interdisciplinary Working Group. Circulation, 115, 2878–2901.

Aulchenko, Y. S., Ripke, S., Isaacs, A., and van Duijn, C. M. (2007). GenABEL: an R library for genome-wide association analysis. *Bioinformatics, 23*, 1294–1296.

Benjamini, Y., Drai, D., Elmer, G., Kafkafi, N., and Golani, I. (2001). Controlling the false discovery rate in behavior genetics research. *Behav Brain Res, 125*, 279–284.

Blangero, J. (2004). Localization and identification of human quantitative trait loci: king harvest has surely come. *Curr Opin Genet Dev, 14*, 233–240.

Botstein, D., and Risch, N. (2003). Discovering genotypes underlying human phenotypes: past successes for mendelian disease, future approaches for complex disease. *Nat Genet, 33*(Suppl), 228–237.

Browning, B. L., and Browning, S. R. (2009). A unified approach to genotype imputation and haplotype-phase inference for large data sets of trios and unrelated individuals. *Am J Hum Genet, 84*, 210–223.

Burton, P. R., Tobin, M. D., and Hopper, J. L. (2005). Key concepts in genetic epidemiology. *Lancet, 366*, 941–951.

Cardon, L. R., and Palmer, L. J. (2003). Population stratification and spurious allelic association. *Lancet, 361*, 598–604.

Carlson, C. S., Eberle, M. A., Kruglyak, L., and Nickerson, D. A. (2004). Mapping complex disease loci in whole-genome association studies. *Nature, 429*, 446–452.

Caspi, A., Sugden, K., Moffitt, T. E., Taylor, A., Craig, I. W. et al (2003). Influence of life stress on depression: moderation by a polymorphism in the 5-HTT gene. *Science, 301*, 386–389.

Clayton, D., and McKeigue, P. M. (2001). Epidemiological methods for studying genes and environmental factors in complex diseases. *Lancet, 358*, 1356–1360.

Clayton, D. G., Walker, N. M., Smyth, D. J., Pask, R., Cooper, J. D. et al (2005). Population structure, differential bias and genomic control in a large-scale, case-control association study. *Nat Genet, 37*, 1243–1246.

Cohen, J. (1988). *Statistical Power Analysis for the Behavioral Sciences*. Hillsdale, NJ: Lawrence Erlbaum Associates.

Colhoun, H. M., McKeigue, P. M., and Davey Smith, G. (2003). Problems of reporting genetic associations with complex outcomes. *Lancet, 361*, 865–872.

Cordell, H. J. (2002). Epistasis: what it means, what it doesn't mean, and statistical methods to detect it in humans. *Hum Mol Genet, 11*, 2463–2468.

Cordell, H. J., and Clayton, D. G. (2005). Genetic association studies. *Lancet, 366*, 1121–1131.

Crawford, D. C., Akey, D. T., and Nickerson, D. A. (2005). The patterns of natural variation in human genes. *Annu Rev Genomics Hum Genet, 6*, 287–312.

Dalageorgou, C., Ge, D., Jamshidi, Y., Nolte, I. M., Riese, H. et al (2008). Heritability of QT interval: how much is explained by genes for resting heart rate? *J Cardiovasc Electrophysiol, 19*, 386–391.

Devlin, B., and Roeder, K. (1999). Genomic control for association studies. *Biometrics, 55*, 997–1004.

Dixon, A. L., Liang, L., Moffatt, M. F., Chen, W., Heath, S. et al (2007). A genome-wide association study of global gene expression. *Nat Genet, 39*, 1202–1207.

Dudbridge, F., and Gusnanto, A. (2008). Estimation of significance thresholds for genomewide association scans. *Genet Epidemiol, 32*, 227–234.

International Human Genome Sequencing Consortium. (2004). Finishing the euchromatic sequence of the human genome. *Nature, 431*, 931–945.

Franke, L., de Kovel, C. G., Aulchenko, Y. S., Trynka, G., Zhernakova, A. et al (2008). Detection, imputation, and association analysis of small deletions and null alleles on oligonucleotide arrays. *Am J Hum Genet, 82*, 1316–1333.

Frayling, T. M. (2007). Genome-wide association studies provide new insights into type 2 diabetes aetiology. *Nat Rev Genet, 8*, 657–662.

Frayling, T. M., Timpson, N. J., Weedon, M. N., Zeggini, E., Freathy, R. M. et al (2007). A common variant in the FTO gene is associated with body mass index and predisposes to childhood and adult obesity. *Science, 316*, 889–894.

Frazer, K. A., Ballinger, D. G., Cox, D. R., Hinds, D. A., Stuve, L. L. et al (2007). A second generation human haplotype map of over 3.1 million SNPs. *Nature, 449*, 851–861.

Freedman, M. L., Reich, D., Penney, K. L., McDonald, G. J., Mignault, A. A. et al (2004). Assessing the impact of population stratification on genetic association studies. *Nat Genet, 36*, 388–393.

Gabriel, S. B., Schaffner, S. F., Nguyen, H., Moore, J. M., Roy, J. et al (2002). The structure of haplotype blocks in the human genome. *Science, 296*, 2225–2229.

Gauderman, J., and Morrison, J. (2006). Quanto Version 1.1: A computer program for power and sample size calculations for genetic epidemiology studies, http://hydna.usc.edu/gxe

Ge, D., Zhang, K., Need, A. C., Martin, O., Fellay, J. et al (2008). WGAViewer: software for genomic annotation of whole genome association studies. *Genome Res, 18*, 640–643.

Gomes, I., Collins, A., Lonjou, C., Thomas, N. S., Wilkinson, J. et al (1999). Hardy-Weinberg quality control. *Ann Hum Genet, 63*, 535–538.

Gonzalez, E., Kulkarni, H., Bolivar, H., Mangano, A., Sanchez, R. et al (2005). The influence of CCL3L1 gene-containing segmental duplications on HIV-1/AIDS susceptibility. *Science, 307*, 1434–1440.

Goring, H. H., Terwilliger, J. D., and Blangero, J. (2001). Large upward bias in estimation of locus-specific effects from genomewide scans. *Am J Hum Genet, 69*, 1357–1369.

Grant, S. F., Thorleifsson, G., Reynisdottir, I., Benediktsson, R., Manolescu, A. et al (2006). Variant of transcription factor 7-like 2 (TCF7L2) gene confers risk of type 2 diabetes. *Nat Genet, 38*, 320–323.

Hardy, G. H. (1908). Mendelian proportions in a mixed population. *Science, 28*, 49–50.

Heils, A., Teufel, A., Petri, S., Seemann, M., Bengel, D. et al (1995). Functional promoter and polyadenylation site mapping of the human serotonin (5-HT) transporter gene. *J Neural Transm Gen Sect, 102*, 247–254.

Heils, A., Teufel, A., Petri, S., Stober, G., Riederer, P. et al (1996). Allelic variation of human serotonin transporter gene expression. *J Neurochem, 66*, 2621–2624.

Hindorff, L. A., Junkins, H. A., Mehta, J. P., and Manolio, T. A. (2009a). A catalog of published genome-wide association studies. Available at www.genome.gov/gwastudies

Hindorff, L. A., Sethupathy, P., Junkins, H. A., Ramos, E. M., Mehta, J. P. et al (2009b). Potential etiologic and functional implications of genome-wide association loci for human diseases and traits. *Proc Natl Acad Sci U S A, 106*, 9362–9367.

Hirschhorn, J. N., and Daly, M. J. (2005). Genome-wide association studies for common diseases and complex traits. *Nat Rev Genet, 6*, 95–108.

Hoggart, C. J., Parra, E. J., Shriver, M. D., Bonilla, C., Kittles, R. A. et al (2003). Control of confounding of genetic associations in stratified populations. *Am J Hum Genet, 72*, 1492–1504.

Hosking, L., Lumsden, S., Lewis, K., Yeo, A., McCarthy, L. et al (2004). Detection of genotyping errors by Hardy-Weinberg equilibrium testing. *Eur J Hum Genet, 12*, 395–399.

Iafrate, A. J., Feuk, L., Rivera, M. N., Listewnik, M. L., Donahoe, P. K. et al (2004). Detection of large-scale variation in the human genome. *Nat Genet, 36*, 949–951.

Ingram, V. M. (1956). A specific chemical difference between the globins of normal human and sickle–cell anaemia haemoglobin. *Nature, 178*, 792–794.

International HapMap Consortium. (2005). A haplotype map of the human genome. *Nature, 437*, 1299–1320.

The International HapMap Project. (2003). *Nature, 426*, 789–796.

Ioannidis, J. P., Ntzani, E. E., Trikalinos, T. A., and Contopoulos-Ioannidis, D. G. (2001). Replication validity of genetic association studies. *Nat Genet, 29*, 306–309.

Ioannidis, J. P. (2003). Genetic associations: false or true? *Trends Mol Med, 9*, 135–138.

Ji, W., Foo, J. N., O'Roak, B. J., Zhao, H., Larson, M. G. et al (2008). Rare independent mutations in renal salt handling genes contribute to blood pressure variation. *Nat Genet, 40*, 592–599.

Johnson, A. D., Handsaker, R. E., Pulit, S. L., Nizzari, M. M., O'Donnell, C. J. et al (2008). SNAP: a web-based tool for identification and annotation of proxy SNPs using HapMap. *Bioinformatics, 24*, 2938–2939.

Johnson, G. C., Esposito, L., Barratt, B. J., Smith, A. N., Heward, J. et al (2001). Haplotype tagging for the identification of common disease genes. *Nat Genet, 29*, 233–237.

Klein, R. J., Zeiss, C., Chew, E. Y., Tsai, J. Y., Sackler, R. S. et al (2005). Complement factor H polymorphism in age-related macular degeneration. *Science, 308*, 385–389.

Knowler, W. C., Williams, R. C., Pettitt, D. J., and Steinberg, A. G. (1988). Gm3;5,13,14 and type 2 diabetes mellitus: an association in American Indians with genetic admixture. *Am J Hum Genet, 43*, 520–526.

Kruglyak, L. (2008). The road to genome-wide association studies. *Nat Rev Genet, 9*, 314–318.

Lango, H., Palmer, C. N., Morris, A. D., Zeggini, E., Hattersley, A. T. et al (2008). Assessing the combined impact of 18 common genetic variants of modest effect sizes on type 2 diabetes risk. *Diabetes, 57*, 3129–3135.

Lesch, K. P., Bengel, D., Heils, A., Sabol, S. Z., Greenberg, B. D. et al (1996). Association of anxiety-related traits with a polymorphism in the serotonin transporter gene regulatory region. *Science, 274*, 1527–1531.

Levy, D., Ehret, G. B., Rice, K., Verwoert, G. C., Launer, L. J. et al (2009). Genome-wide association study of blood pressure and hypertension. *Nat Genet, 41*, 677–687.

Li, Y., and Abecasis, G. (2006). Mach 1.0: Rapid haplotype reconstruction and missing genotype inference. *Am J Hum Genet, S79*, 2290.

Loos, R. J., Lindgren, C. M., Li, S., Wheeler, E., Zhao, J. H. et al (2008). Common variants near MC4R are associated with fat mass, weight and risk of obesity. *Nat Genet, 40*, 768–775.

Maher, B. (2008). Personal genomes: the case of the missing heritability. *Nature, 456*, 18–21.

Manly, K. F., Nettleton, D., and Hwang, J. T. (2004). Genomics, prior probability, and statistical tests of multiple hypotheses. *Genome Res, 14*, 997–1001.

Manolio, T. A., Brooks, L. D., and Collins, F. S. (2008). A HapMap harvest of insights into the genetics of common disease. *J Clin Invest, 118*, 1590–1605.

Marchini, J., Howie, B., Myers, S., McVean, G., and Donnelly, P. (2007). A new multipoint method for genome-wide association studies by imputation of genotypes. *Nat Genet, 39*, 906–913.

McCaffery, J. M., Snieder, H., Dong, Y., and de Geus, E. (2007). Genetics in psychosomatic medicine: research designs and statistical approaches. *Psychosom Med, 69*, 206–216.

McCarthy, M. I., Abecasis, G. R., Cardon, L. R., Goldstein, D. B., Little, J. et al (2008). Genome-wide association studies for complex traits: consensus, uncertainty and challenges. *Nat Rev Genet, 9*, 356–369.

Moffitt, T. E., Caspi, A., and Rutter, M. (2005). Strategy for investigating interactions between measured genes and measured environments. *Arch Gen Psychiatry, 62*, 473–481.

Neale, B. M., and Sham, P. C. (2004). The future of association studies: gene-based analysis and replication. *Am J Hum Genet, 75*, 353–362.

Newton-Cheh, C., Johnson, T., Gateva, V., Tobin, M. D., Bochud, M. et al (2009). Genome-wide association study identifies eight loci associated with blood pressure. *Nat Genet, 41*, 666–676.

Nolte, I. M., de Vries, A. R., Spijker, G. T., Jansen, R. C., Brinza, D. et al (2007). Association testing by haplotype sharing methods applicable to whole genome analysis. *BMC Proc, 1*, S129.

Nolte, I. M., Wallace, C., Newhouse, S. J., Waggott, D., Fu, J. et al (2009). Common genetic variation near the phospholamban gene is associated with cardiac repolarisation: meta-analysis of three genome-wide association studies. *PLoS One, 4*, e6138.

Packer, B. R., Yeager, M., Burdett, L., Welch, R., Beerman, M. et al (2006). SNP500Cancer: a public resource for sequence validation, assay development, and frequency analysis for genetic variation in candidate genes. *Nucleic Acids Res, 34*, D617-621.

Pe'er, I., Yelensky, R., Altshuler, D., and Daly, M. J. (2008). Estimation of the multiple testing burden for genomewide association studies of nearly all common variants. *Genet Epidemiol, 32*, 381–385.

Pearson, T. A., and Manolio, T. A. (2008). How to interpret a genome-wide association study. *JAMA, 299*, 1335–1344. Erratum in: JAMA, 299, 2150.

Price, A. L., Patterson, N. J., Plenge, R. M., Weinblatt, M. E., Shadick, N. A. et al (2006). Principal components analysis corrects for stratification in genome-wide association studies. *Nat Genet, 38*, 904–909.

Pritchard, J. K., Stephens, M., and Donnelly, P. (2000). Inference of population structure using multilocus genotype data. *Genetics, 155*, 945–959.

Pritchard, J. K., and Cox, N. J. (2002). The allelic architecture of human disease genes: common disease-common variant.or not? *Hum Mol Genet, 11*, 2417–2423.

Psychiatric GWAS Consortium Steering Committee. (2009). A framework for interpreting genome-wide association studies of psychiatric disorders. *Mol Psychiatry, 14*, 10–17.

Purcell, S., Cherny, S. S., and Sham, P. C. (2003). Genetic power calculator: design of linkage and association genetic mapping studies of complex traits. *Bioinformatics, 19*, 149–150.

Purcell, S., Neale, B., Todd-Brown, K., Thomas, L., Ferreira, M. A. et al (2007). PLINK: a tool set for whole-genome association and population-based linkage analyses. *Am J Hum Genet, 81*, 559–575.

Redon, R., Ishikawa, S., Fitch, K. R., Feuk, L., Perry, G. H. et al (2006). Global variation in copy number in the human genome. *Nature, 444*, 444–454.

Riordan, J. R., Rommens, J. M., Kerem, B., Alon, N., Rozmahel, R. et al (1989). Identification of the cystic fibrosis gene: cloning and characterization of complementary DNA. *Science, 245*, 1066–1073.

Risch, N., and Merikangas, K. (1996). The future of genetic studies of complex human diseases. *Science, 273*, 1516–1517.

Risch, N., Herrell, R., Lehner, T., Liang, K. Y., Eaves, L. et al (2009). Interaction between the serotonin transporter gene (5-HTTLPR), stressful life events, and risk of depression: a meta-analysis. *JAMA, 301*, 2462–2471.

Sabatti, C., Service, S. K., Hartikainen, A. L., Pouta, A., Ripatti, S. et al (2009). Genome-wide association analysis of metabolic traits in a birth cohort from a founder population. *Nat Genet, 41*, 35–46.

Saxena, R., Voight, B. F., Lyssenko, V., Burtt, N. P., de Bakker, P. I. et al (2007). Genome-wide association analysis identifies loci for type 2 diabetes and triglyceride levels. *Science, 316*, 1331–1336.

Sebat, J., Lakshmi, B., Troge, J., Alexander, J., Young, J. et al (2004). Large-scale copy number polymorphism in the human genome. *Science, 305*, 525–528.

Smith, D. J., and Lusis, A. J. (2002). The allelic structure of common disease. *Hum Mol Genet, 11*, 2455–2461.

Stephens, M., and Donnelly, P. (2003). A comparison of bayesian methods for haplotype reconstruction from population genotype data. *Am J Hum Genet, 73*, 1162–1169.

Stolk, R. P., Rosmalen, J. G., Postma, D. S., de Boer, R. A., Navis, G. et al (2008). Universal risk factors for multifactorial diseases: LifeLines: a three-generation population-based study. *Eur J Epidemiol, 23*, 67–74.

Stram, D. O. (2005). Software for tag single nucleotide polymorphism selection. *Hum Genomics, 2*, 144–151.

Stranger, B. E., Forrest, M. S., Dunning, M., Ingle, C. E., Beazley, C. et al (2007). Relative impact of nucleotide and copy number variation on gene expression phenotypes. *Science, 315*, 848–853.

Sullivan, P. F., Eaves, L. J., Kendler, K. S., and Neale, M. C. (2001). Genetic case-control association studies in neuropsychiatry. *Arch Gen Psychiatry, 58*, 1015–1024.

Te Meerman, G. J., Van der Meulen, M. A., and Sandkuijl, L. A. (1995). Perspectives of identity by descent (IBD) mapping in founder populations. *Clin Exp Allergy, 25*(Suppl) 2, 97–102.

Thorgeirsson, T. E., and Stefansson, K. (2008). Genetics of smoking behavior and its consequences: the role of nicotinic acetylcholine receptors. *Biol Psychiatry, 64*, 919–921.

Thorleifsson, G., Walters, G. B., Gudbjartsson, D. F., Steinthorsdottir, V., Sulem, P. et al (2009). Genome-wide association yields new sequence variants at seven loci that associate with measures of obesity. *Nat Genet, 41*, 18–24.

Turkheimer, E., D'Onofrio, B. M., Maes, H. H., and Eaves, L. J. (2005). Analysis and interpretation of twin studies including measures of the shared environment. *Child Dev, 76*, 1217–1233.

Vaisse, C., Clement, K., Guy-Grand, B., and Froguel, P. (1998). A frameshift mutation in human MC4R is associated with a dominant form of obesity. *Nat Genet, 20*, 113–114.

Wacholder, S., Chanock, S., Garcia-Closas, M., El Ghormli, L., and Rothman, N. (2004). Assessing the probability that a positive report is false: an approach for molecular epidemiology studies. *J Natl Cancer Inst, 96*, 434–442.

Wang, W. Y., Barratt, B. J., Clayton, D. G., and Todd, J. A. (2005). Genome-wide association studies: theoretical and practical concerns. *Nat Rev Genet, 6*, 109–118.

Weinberg, W. (1908). Über den Nachweis der Vererbung beim Menschen. *Jahreshefte des Vereins für vaterländische Naturkunde in Württemberg, 64*, 368–382.

The Wellcome Trust Case-Control Consortium. (2007). Genome-wide association study of 14,000 cases of seven common diseases and 3,000 shared controls. *Nature, 447*, 661–678.

Wendland, J. R., Martin, B. J., Kruse, M. R., Lesch, K. P., and Murphy, D. L. (2006). Simultaneous genotyping of four functional loci of human SLC6A4, with a reappraisal of 5-HTTLPR and rs25531. *Mol Psychiatry, 11*, 224–226.

Willer, C. J., Speliotes, E. K., Loos, R. J., Li, S., Lindgren, C. M. et al (2009). Six new loci associated with body mass index highlight a neuronal influence on body weight regulation. *Nat Genet, 41*, 25–34.

Wray, N. R., James, M. R., Gordon, S. D., Dumenil, T., Ryan, L. et al (2009). Accurate, large-scale genotyping of 5HTTLPR and flanking single nucleotide polymorphisms in an association study of depression, anxiety, and personality measures. *Biol Psychiatry, 66*, 468–476.

Yeo, G. S., Farooqi, I. S., Aminian, S., Halsall, D. J., Stanhope, R. G. et al (1998). A frameshift mutation in MC4R associated with dominantly inherited human obesity. *Nat Genet, 20*, 111–112.

Zeggini, E., Scott, L. J., Saxena, R., Voight, B. F., Marchini, J. L. et al (2008). Meta-analysis of genome-wide association data and large-scale replication identifies additional susceptibility loci for type 2 diabetes. *Nat Genet, 40*, 638–645.

Chapter 30

Functional Genomic Approaches in Behavioral Medicine Research

Gregory E. Miller and Steve W. Cole

Since the completion of the Human Genome Project in 2003, interest in genetics has grown rapidly in the behavioral medicine community. Most of the research to date has focused on structural genomics and pursued questions such as To what extent are variations in specific genomic sequences, i.e., polymorphisms, responsible for individual differences in biobehavioral characteristics (Collado-Hidalgo et al, 2008; McCaffery et al, 2006; Wust et al, 2004)? Do these sequence variants accentuate the impact that major life stress has on risk for mental and physical illness (Binder et al, 2008; Capitanio et al, 2008; Caspi et al, 2003)? By contrast, relatively little attention had been paid to functional genomic processes in the behavioral medicine community. We know almost nothing about how thoughts, feelings, and stressors influence patterns of gene expression, despite the fact that most regulation of biological systems occurs at the level of transcription. Thus, functional genomic approaches have much to offer our field as it seeks to understand mechanisms linking the social world to biology and health outcomes. Gene expression studies also are fairly easily to undertake, are cost-effective, and yield high-quality data. In this chapter we provide a brief primer on functional genomics and then use our own research to illustrate how assessing those

processes can yield unique insights into mind–body mechanisms.

1 Genomics Primer

This section provides a simplified overview of functional genomics. It focuses on the basics of protein synthesis – how genes are "switched on" to produce messenger RNA (mRNA), which later serves as template for the assembly of proteins – and the methods that biologists use to measure these processes. Readers seeking more detailed accounts of these issues should consult other sources. For those seeking an accessible, nontechnical overview of genomics, we highly recommend the book *Molecular Biology Made Simple and Fun* (Clark and Russell, 2005). Textbooks such as *Human Molecular Genetics* (Strachan and Read, 2004) and *Molecular Biology of the Cell* (Alberts et al, 2002) are excellent resources for more advanced readers and so is a recent review by Johannes and colleagues (2008) on the significance of epigenetic processes.

1.1 Basics of Protein Synthesis

Francis Crick introduced the "central dogma" of molecular biology in 1958 to describe the flow of biological information within cells (for an elaborated version of this model, see Crick, 1970). He argued that DNA contains the blueprint for

G.E. Miller (✉)
Department of Psychology, University of British Columbia, 2136 West Mall, Vancouver BC, Canada V6T 1Z4
e-mail: gemiller@psych.ubc.ca

A. Steptoe (ed.), *Handbook of Behavioral Medicine*, DOI 10.1007/978-0-387-09488-5_30,
© Springer Science+Business Media, LLC 2010

assembling the protein molecules that carry out most cellular functions. These proteins are synthesized in two stages. First, the nucleotide sequence from a short string of DNA, called a gene, is transcribed into a complementary strand of mRNA. Next, the nucleotide sequence from the strand of mRNA is decoded, or translated, into a string of amino acids that are joined to form a protein.

Research over the past 50 years has shown that, in most cases, protein synthesis proceeds along the lines that Crick hypothesized. However, there are cases in which the flow of biological information diverges from the sequence outlined in the central dogma. For example, in retroviruses, RNA is the basic genomic material that encodes hereditary information. When these viruses enter a host cell, their RNA is reverse-transcribed into DNA. The DNA then integrates into the host genome and directs assembly of viral proteins. The virus that causes AIDS, human immunodeficiency virus, operates in this fashion. It has also been shown that some viral RNA molecules replicate themselves without any DNA involved in the process. And in recent years, scientists have recognized that RNA plays a much more versatile role in regulating cellular dynamics than the central dogma envisioned. While much of the RNA that gets transcribed is eventually translated into protein, RNA can serve other functions as well, including blocking the activity of other RNA molecules through a process called interference.

Finally, the central dogma's notion that protein synthesis entails a highly faithful transmission of biological information has been called into question. Crick argued that each gene codes for one specific mRNA molecule that has a non-fungible nucleotide sequence. And in turn, each mRNA molecule was thought to code for one specific protein with a non-fungible amino acid sequence. However, in recent decades it has become evident that this one gene/one protein hypothesis is inaccurate. After they have been transcribed, most mRNA molecules undergo an editing process, in which some segments are spliced out. This editing process enables a gene to give rise to more than one type of mRNA

molecule and, in turn, more than one type of protein. As a result human cells, which contain roughly 30,000 genes, can synthesize upward of 100,000 different proteins.

When a gene's DNA sequence has been transcribed into an mRNA molecule, biologists say that a "transcript" has been formed or that the gene has been "expressed." The actual process of transcription begins when a complex of molecules binds to a segment of DNA that is located upstream of the gene itself (its promoter). This complex is typically comprised of RNA polymerase and a transcription factor. RNA polymerase is an enzyme that unwinds the DNA double helix around the gene and then stitches together strings of nucleotides to form an mRNA strand. A transcription factor is a protein that shepherds RNA polymerase to a specific DNA segment so that it can initiate assembly of mRNA. (Or in some cases, blocks its access to a DNA segment in an effort to suppress activity of a gene.) After an mRNA molecule has been assembled, segments of it are edited through a splicing process, and the final transcript is transported to an organelle in the cell known as the ribosome. It is here that the nucleotide sequence of the mRNA molecule is translated into an amino acid sequence that is later joined and folded to form a protein.

1.2 Determinants of Gene Expression

How often protein synthesis takes place depends on a number of factors. Some genes are expressed in a steady-state fashion, or constitutively, because there is constant demand for the proteins they encode. Others are expressed according to a circadian schedule or induced on as-needed basis in response to stimuli, such as heat, light, hormones, or a signaling molecule from the host cell. In most cases these stimuli operate by activating transcription factors, which serve as the molecular switches on the genome, controlling which genes get expressed, at which rate, and in which tissue. Of special importance for readers of this chapter is the fact that many stimuli can activate transcription factors, including "signals" like hormones and cytokines which are themselves responsive to events in the social environment. For example, when epinephrine released from the adrenal medulla encounters a white blood cell, it can bind to a β2-adrenergic receptor on the cell surface, initiating a signaling cascade that eventually results in activation of the transcription factor cyclic AMP response element binding (CREB) protein. The activated CREB protein can then bind to specific segments of DNA (called cAMP response elements) located in promoters of some genes. Depending on the structure of the promoter and what other molecules are present, CREB could then serve to enhance or suppress transcription of that gene. Thus, CREB and other transcription factors can function as conduits through which the social world modulates activity of the genome. (Other hormones can influence gene expression in the same basic fashion. For example, cortisol can bind to glucocorticoid receptors located inside cells, and this newly formed complex can then attach to promoter segments specific for it.) Besides external triggers like hormones, there are also a number of more local regulatory factors that modulate gene expression. Their influences are important to consider because they could augment or curtail the effects that socially driven hormonal signals have on genome activity.

Variations in the nucleotide sequence of a gene's promoter can also influence its rate of expression. For example, there is a polymorphism in the promoter of the serotonin transporter gene, which influences how efficiently its DNA nucleotide sequence is transcribed into mRNA (and ultimately translated into protein). This differential transcription efficiency is thought to explain why people who carry a "short" allele are more prone to depression following major life stress than those who do not (Caspi et al, 2003). As this example illustrates, structural (DNA) and functional (RNA) genomics are closely intertwined, and in many cases the former only matters to the extent that it affects the latter. In other words, the biological significance of most of the polymorphisms

we study, particularly those located in promoter regions, is that they influence how efficiently a gene can be transcribed. When this is true, researchers may gain the most insight by assessing gene expression directly, rather than using genotype as a proxy for it. Of course, this approach is more plausible in some research contexts than others. For example, it is fairly easy for a researcher interested in genomic activity in the immune system to gain access to patients' white blood cells so as to assess mRNA production. This would be much more challenging for a researcher whose focus is on genes that regulate neurotransmitter metabolism in the central nervous system.

Genes are also subject to epigenetic alterations, defined as stable changes in expression, which arise without modifications to the DNA sequence (Jaenisch and Bird, 2003). This can occur in two main ways: methylation of the DNA itself or remodeling of the chromatin structure in which DNA is packaged. In DNA methylation, enzymes cause methyl groups to bind to cytosine residues in a gene's promoter. These methyl groups prevent transcription factors from interacting with DNA to modulate gene expression. In chromatin remodeling, various chemicals are attached to (or removed from) the histone proteins that package DNA within the cell's nucleus. These proteins cause the DNA near the gene to become more or less tightly coiled, which makes it more or less difficult for RNA polymerase and transcription factors to access its promoter (Whitelaw and Garrick, 2006).

In the last few years there has been mounting interest in epigenetics in the biomedical community (Feinberg, 2008). Much of this interest grows out of discoveries suggesting that epigenetic processes serve as pathways through which various chemical, biological, and social exposures can bring about long-term changes in the activity of genes and thereby contribute to the pathogenesis of disease. For example, studies in animal models have shown that some in utero or early-life exposures, like cigarette smoking, vitamin B12, and folic acid, result in epigenetic alterations to genes that regulate metabolism and other key biological processes. Over the long

term, these alterations can give rise to important phenotypic differences between organisms,
including vulnerability to medical conditions
like obesity, diabetes, and cancer (Jirtle and
Skinner, 2007; Richards, 2006).

Of particular interest to the behavioral
medicine community is a program of research
by Meaney and Szyf demonstrating that social
exposures in early life can have long-lasting
epigenetic and phenotypic influences (Meaney
and Szyf, 2005). This work shows that neonatal rodents who receive high levels of nurturing
from their mothers in the first week of life
exhibit diminished cortisol responses to stressful experience when they reach adulthood (Liu
et al, 1997). This hormonal resilience to stressors arises from nurturing-induced epigenetic
modifications, such as demethylation of DNA
and acetylation of histone proteins, that facilitate
expression of the gene that codes for the glucocorticoid receptor in hippocampal tissue (Weaver
et al, 2004). Greater expression of this receptor
enables tighter regulation of the hormonal system that controls release of cortisol. In summary,
this work shows that early social experiences
can get biologically embedded in the genome
through epigenetics and by doing so give rise
to important biobehavioral characteristics that
persist across the lifespan.

1.3 Measuring Gene Expression

Biologists use a variety of techniques to measure
gene expression, including quantitative reverse
transcriptase polymerase chain reaction (qPCR),
in situ hybridization, and an electrophoretic
method called Southern blotting. Of these methods, qPCR is the one likely to be of most use
to researchers in behavioral medicine, because
it is sensitive and reproducible, requires limited
technical expertise, can be done in large quantities, and is relatively inexpensive in terms of
reagents and manpower (approximately $15 per
sample). Another major advantage is that companies like Applied Biosystems have developed
extensive libraries of validated qPCR assays

(see http://www.appliedbiosystems.com). From
them, one can purchase kits that measure mRNA
from nearly any human gene of interest. Each
kit runs on the same platform under the same
conditions, so once a lab has mastered the
basic qPCR technique, it is simple to expand
the pool of outcomes a project is going to
assess.

qPCR is an extremely helpful technique in
cases where a study's primary outcome is the
expression of one (or a handful) of candidate genes for which there is a clear a priori
hypothesis. However, in the past 5 years newer
approaches have become available that allow
projects to measure the activity of tens of thousands of genes simultaneously. When they are
used in conjunction with advanced bioinformatic
strategies, these *microarrays* can provide deep
insights into cellular dynamics, which would
be difficult to achieve with a qPCR approach
that focuses on candidate genes. These deeper
insights are possible because microarrays can (a)
quantify the activity of networks of genes that
are biologically interrelated and (b) reveal new
genetic loci that are central to the phenomenon
of interest, but which the investigator may not
have considered previously. The downsides of
microarray technology are its high costs (which
are several hundred dollars per sample), its limited availability (the infrastructure may exist in
only a handful of core labs at a major university),
and the technical skills necessary to acquire and
analyze the data (a microarray operator and a
bioinformatics specialist).

2 Functional Genomics in Action

Having provided an overview of functional
genomic processes, we now turn to their application in behavioral medicine research. To do
so, we describe a project where genomic methods provided us with the leverage to address an
important mechanistic question, which did not
lend itself easily to approaches that are more
conventional in behavioral medicine.

2.1 Background

The goal of this work was to identify the mechanisms through which chronic psychological stressors – such as caring for a demented family member, having a severely troubled marriage, or working in a hostile environment – contribute to the development and progression of various medical illnesses (Cohen et al, 2007; Krantz and McCeney, 2002; Schneiderman et al, 2005). Historically, there has been much speculation that these effects are mediated by activation of the hypothalamic-pituitary-adrenocortical (HPA) axis, which releases the hormone cortisol into circulation following exposure to many life stressors (Dickerson and Kemeny, 2004; McEwen, 1998; Miller et al, 2007). Cortisol has wide-ranging effects on a variety of biological processes in the nervous, metabolic, skeletal, and immune systems. Because one of its most well-documented effects is to inhibit various leukocyte functions, e.g., cell proliferation and cytokine production (Webster et al, 2002), a prevailing assumption has been that it contributes to stress-evoked disease through immuno-suppressive mechanisms (Cohen, 1996). However, with increasing recognition that inflammation is a key pathogenic mechanism in many infectious, autoimmune, and cardiac diseases, the adequacy of this explanation has been called into question (Miller et al, 2002; Raison and Miller, 2003). This is because when taken to its logical end, this hypothesis suggests a paradoxical and inaccurate conclusion: that in boosting cortisol output and slowing immune activity, chronic stressors should ameliorate the symptoms of many diseases.

To resolve this paradox, we have proposed an alternative hypothesis focusing on cellular resistance to cortisol-mediated signaling (Miller et al, 2002). It specifies that chronic stressors elicit sustained elevations in cortisol which, over time, prompt immune cells to undergo a compensatory downregulation of glucocorticoid receptor (GR) activity. This adaptively limits cortisol's ability to further dampen immune responses. However, in cells like monocytes that are tightly regulated by cortisol, this dynamic also diminishes the potency of an important hormonal constraint, which acts to tonically inhibit the activity of signaling molecules that initiate and maintain inflammation. The long-term result of this process is mild, low-grade inflammation, fostered by monocytes that have acquired resistance to cortisol.

Support has emerged for the basic tenets of this hypothesis in studies of both humans and animals (Avitsur et al, 2001; Miller and Chen, 2006; Miller et al, 2002, 2009; Rohleder et al, 2001; Stark et al, 2001). Most of this work has made use of an ex vivo assay system, where leukocytes are stimulated with a bacterial product (endotoxin) in the presence of varying levels of cortisol, which is expected to suppress their ability to synthesize inflammatory cytokines. In most studies, cortisol does have this suppressive influence on cytokine production, but it is significantly attenuated in people and animals who are in the midst of a chronic stressor. While these findings are consistent with the cortisol resistance hypothesis we have articulated, we have found it difficult to draw definitive conclusions from them because they rely on ex vivo methods and used high doses of endotoxin and cortisol to stimulate white blood cells. To thoroughly evaluate the cortisol-resistance hypothesis, we needed a model system that captured the dynamics of the interactions of cortisol with leukocytes in vivo.

This dilemma led us to consider a functional genomics approach. One such approach uses microarray technology to monitor the activity of ~22,000 genes in a tissue of interest (e.g., immune cells collected from peripheral blood). This analysis identifies a subset of genes that are differentially expressed by two groups of patients, e.g., those who have and have not been exposed to some chronic stressor. Bioinformatics technology is then used to discern what these genes have in common. This can be done by grouping the differentially expressed genes into functional categories that correspond to their biological activities (e.g., metabolism, inflammation, motility). It can also be done by scanning the promoter regions of the differentially expressed genes to determine the prevalence of response elements (binding sites) for transcription factors (Cole et al, 2005). With these data in hand, one can make reverse inferences about how active certain signaling pathways have been in vivo. For example, if the genes that tend to be over-expressed in one set of patients show a disproportionate prevalence of transcription factor-binding motifs (TFBMs) for CREB, one can infer that their tissue has been exposed to greater adrenergic signaling. Hence, these methods enable researchers to quantify how "loudly" certain signals are being "heard" by the genome and what effect this is having on the ability of genes to get switched on to initiate protein synthesis. This approach was particularly appealing in our situation because the molecule that binds cortisol in leukocytes – the GR – is itself a transcription factor that upon activation can migrate into a cell's nucleus and switch genes on and off. Furthermore, because immunologists have extensively characterized the actions of glucocorticoids in leukocytes (Schoneveld and Cidlowski, 2007), we could easily form hypotheses about which pro-inflammatory transcription factors might be affected if cells had developed resistance to cortisol-mediated signaling. Of special importance in this regard was nuclear factor-kappa B (NF-κB), a transcription factor that is key to initiating and maintaining most inflammatory responses.

2.2 Differential Gene Expression

Recognizing the inferential leverage this functional genomic approach would provide, we conducted microarray assays on peripheral blood monocytes collected from two groups of subjects – those who were caring for a family member with brain cancer and controls who were similar demographically but free of major life stress (Miller et al, 2008). The first wave of our analyses indicated that a total of 614 genes were differentially expressed by the groups (defined as ≥1.5-fold difference in mRNA, corresponding to a false discovery rate of 5%), 127 (21%) of these transcripts were over-expressed in caregivers, and 488 (79%) were under-expressed, reflecting a net repressive effect of chronic stress on transcription in monocytes ($p < 0.0001$ by binomial test). The heatplot in Fig. 30.1 displays these findings visually. Red intensity indicates the magnitude of a gene's relative over-expression in caregivers versus controls and green intensity denotes the magnitude of under-expression.

Next, we used bioinformatics technology to discern what these differentially expressed genes had in common. We started by identifying common functional characteristics with the Gene Ontology Database (http://www.geneontology.org) and a software program called GOstat (http://gostat.wehi.edu.au) that finds statistically over-represented categories within it. These

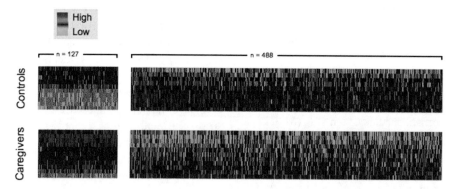

Fig. 30.1 Differential gene expression in chronically stressed individuals. Microarray analysis of gene expression in peripheral blood monocytes identified 614 transcripts showing >50% difference in mean expression levels across groups (*green* = under-expression in chronic stress, *red* = over-expression). Reprinted from Biological Psychiatry, vol. 64, G.E. Miller et al., pp. 266–272, 2008, with permission from Elsevier

analyses revealed that the Gene Ontology categories over-represented among genes upregulated in caregivers included wound healing (e.g., *THBS1, EREG;* GO:0042060), chemotaxis (e.g., *VEGF, IL8;* GO:0050918), and angiogenesis (e.g., *VEGF,* EREG; GO:0001525). Functional characteristics of the caregivers' downregulated genes included involvement in catabolism (e.g., *PSMB5, PRDX3;* GO:009056), lytic activity (e.g., *ASAHL, LIPA;* GO:0000323), and immune defense (e.g., *TLR1, HLA-DQA1,* GO:006952). These patterns suggest that chronic stress generally activates genes that not only support pro-inflammatory activities but may also inhibit some genes involved in microbial defense operations and monocyte pathogen catabolism.

We then used the TELiS bioinformatics procedure to evaluate our primary hypotheses about chronic stress and resistance to glucocorticoid signaling. TELiS (http://www.telis.ucla.edu) quantified the prevalence of 192 transcription factor-binding motifs in the promoters of differentially expressed genes (Cole et al, 2005). As noted above, these data enable the researcher to make reverse inferences about how active certain signaling pathways have been in vivo. The analyses indicated that among caregivers versus controls, there was a relative downregulation of glucocorticoid-responsive genes. Specifically, glucocorticoid receptor TFBMs occurred at 23.3% lower prevalence in the promoters of genes over-expressed by caregivers versus those over-expressed by controls (2.13 ± 0.21 versus 2.77 ± 0.11 sites/promoter for caregivers and controls; $p = 0.007$). These findings are consistent with our hypotheses in suggesting a stress-linked diminution of glucocorticoid-mediated transcription (see Fig. 30.2a).

Further TELiS analyses revealed a parallel upregulation of NF-κB-responsive transcription among caregivers. There was a 1.54-fold greater prevalence of NF-κB TFBMs in promoters of genes over-expressed by caregivers relative to those over-expressed by controls (1.66 ± 0.19 versus 1.08 ± 0.06 sites/promoter for caregivers and controls; $p = 0.005$; Fig. 30.2b). These findings are consistent with our hypothesis in suggesting that by blunting GR-mediated

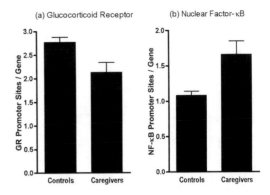

Fig. 30.2 Transcriptional activity of GR and NF-κB signaling pathways. In TELiS bioinformatics analysis of response element prevalence in promoters of differentially expressed genes, (**a**) GR response elements are under-represented in genes upregulated in stressed caregivers, whereas (**b**) transcripts bearing response elements for NF-κB are over-represented. Reprinted from Biological Psychiatry, vol. 64, G.E. Miller et al., pp. 266–272, 2008, with permission from Elsevier

signaling, chronic stress facilitates activation of the pro-inflammatory transcription factor NF-κB. In fact, with the coupling of increased NF-κB activity (1.54-fold difference) and decreased GR activity (0.77-fold difference), there is a net 2.01-fold skew toward inflammation in the structure of promoter TFBMs across genes over-expressed in caregivers versus controls.

2.3 Inflammatory Consequences

To determine whether these transcriptional disparities were manifested in systemic immune activation, we used ELISA methods to assess serum levels of three widely used protein biomarkers of inflammation: C-reactive protein, interleukin-1 receptor antagonist, and interleukin-6. As Fig. 30.3a illustrates, caregivers had about twice as much of the inflammatory biomarker C-reactive protein in circulation as controls (3.14 ± 0.65 versus 1.62 ± 0.54 mg/L; $t = 2.09$, $p = 0.05$). They also had more than twice as much serum interleukin-1 receptor antagonist (433.21 ± 61.87 versus 203.56 ± 29.19 pg/ml; $t = 3.25$, $p = 0.005$; Fig. 30.3b), a molecule released by monocytes

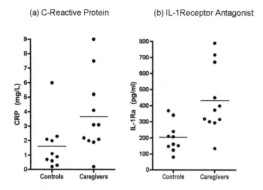

Fig. 30.3 Expression of inflammatory biomarkers in circulation. Caregivers display significantly higher concentrations of the inflammatory biomarkers (**a**) C-reactive protein and (**b**) interleukin-1 receptor antagonist than controls. Reprinted from Biological Psychiatry, vol. 64, G.E. Miller et al., pp. 266–272, 2008, with permission from Elsevier

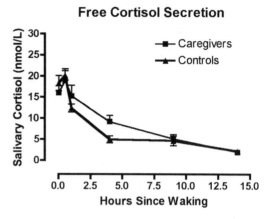

Fig. 30.4 Diurnal cortisol cycles in caregivers and controls. Caregivers showed higher cortisol than controls 4 h after waking ($t = 4.19$, $p = 0.029$), but did not differ significantly at other times of day or on global indices such as diurnal rhythm of secretion and total output over the day (p's >0.59). Reprinted from Biological Psychiatry, vol. 64, G.E. Miller et al., pp. 266–272, 2008, with permission from Elsevier

to neutralize the pro-inflammatory activities of interleukin-1. There were no caregiving-related differences in serum interleukin-6 ($1.18 + 0.20$ versus $0.96 + 0.14$ pg/ml in caregivers versus controls; $t = 0.88$, $p = 0.39$). However, much of the interleukin-6 found in circulation derives from adipose tissue, so any stress-related effects on monocytes are likely to have been obscured.

2.4 Underlying Mechanisms

To identify mechanisms linking chronic stress and differential transcription, we compared the diurnal output cortisol of caregivers and controls. Subjects collected saliva six times daily for a 3-day period, according to a schedule that captures the hormone's diurnal rhythm. Figure 30.4 illustrates that caregivers and controls displayed similar patterns of cortisol secretion over the day. Although caregivers showed higher cortisol than controls 4 h after waking ($t = 4.19$, $p = 0.029$), there were no significant differences at other times of day, and the groups were similar on global indices such as the diurnal rhythm of secretion and total output over the day (p's > 0.59). We also considered whether differences were attributable to reduced expression of the GR among caregivers; i.e., that glucocorticoid-mediated transcription arose because this group

simply had less bioavailable GR to bind cortisol. However, the groups showed similar quantities of monocyte GR mRNA both on the microarray (9.80 ± 0.12 versus 10.05 ± 0.18 log$_2$ relative gene expression units, $p = 0.29$) and in more sensitive RT-PCR analyses (4.88 ± 0.92 versus 4.65 ± 0.66 log$_2$ GAPDH-normalized relative expression units, $p = 0.12$). Together, these findings suggest that although caregivers are secreting normal volumes of cortisol and have sufficient GR available to transduce hormone signals, this message is not registered equivalently at the level of monocyte gene transcription.

2.5 Implications

The results of this project illustrate how a functional genomic approach can be used to address a difficult mechanistic question in behavioral medicine. They show that chronically stressed individuals had diminished expression of genes bearing response elements for GR, and at the same time heightened expression of transcripts with response elements for pro-inflammatory transcription factors like NF-κB. In other words, these data showed that caregivers' monocytes were registering fewer cortisol signals than were controls'. As a result, genes that cortisol usually switches on were not being expressed as strongly in monocytes from caregivers as those from controls and genes that cortisol usually silences were more active in caregivers than controls. This in vivo readout suggests an intriguing scenario for how chronic stressors influence disease: by interfering with cortisol's ability to deliver signals to white blood cells, stressors may facilitate the kinds of pro-inflammatory gene expression cascades that contribute to coronary disease, autoimmune disorders, and infectious diseases

The project also shows how functional genomic approaches can help researchers uncover patterns that may have been missed by focusing on traditional biological mechanisms. For example, in the above study we collected daily saliva samples from participants, but chronic stress was not associated with differential cortisol levels. Similarly, we measured the expression of GR in white blood cells, but this too was unrelated to chronic stress. If we had constrained our analysis to include only hormonal outputs or receptor expression, we would have mistakenly concluded that cortisol and the tissues it regulates are unaffected by caregiving. But as the gene expression profile revealed, this was not the case. Instead, we were able to discover that the monocytes of chronically stressed individuals are not "hearing" cortisol signals from the body as loudly as they should, even though this hormone is being secreted in sufficient quantities and there are a sufficient number of receptors available to bind it. As a consequence of that alteration, pro-inflammatory genes were over-expressed, leading to a change in circulating indicators of inflammation.

2.6 Applicability

One criticism sometimes leveled at microarrays is based on the assumption that they inherently involve non-hypothesis-driven exploratory analyses. However, the application we describe above shows how microarrays can be used to test a priori mechanistic hypotheses (i.e., that stress-induced alterations in inflammation are mediated by desensitization of the GR-mediated gene transcription control pathway). Of course, microarray technology can also be used for "unbiased discovery" studies to reveal patterns in the data that an investigator may not have previously considered. We believe that hypothesis-free discovery-based approaches can be quite useful, especially in areas where there is little pre-existing biological theory to guide research, and only a fraction of the potential mechanisms have been seriously explored. Theory-driven research is of course preferable in cases where strong theories exist. In that sense, microarrays are much like any other tools (e.g., an inferential statistical test or a blood pressure reading) – their epistemological strength derives from the research context in which they are used (e.g., in experimental studies or hypothesis-driven observational analyses) and is not a property of the methodology per se.

3 Conclusions

Though interest in genetics is growing rapidly in behavioral medicine, most of the work in this area to date has focused on structural genomic questions. In this chapter we have argued that functional genomic approaches have much to offer our field, particularly as it seeks to understand mechanisms that link the social world to biology and health outcomes. In the coming decade, these approaches are likely to become more widespread in behavioral medicine research as they help the field acquire deeper insights into the nature of mind–body relationships and ways in which they can be used to improve health and ameliorate disease.

References

Alberts, B., Johnson, A., Lewis, J., Raff, M., Roberts, K., and Walter, P. (2002). *Molecular biology of the cell.* London: Garland Science.

Avitsur, R., Stark, J. L., and Sheridan, J. F. (2001). Social stress induces glucocorticoid resistance in animals. *Hormones Behav, 39*, 247–257.

Binder, E. B., Bradley, R. G., Liu, W., Epstein, M. P., Deveau, T. C. et al (2008). Association of FKBP5 polymorphisms and childhood abuse with risk of posttraumatic stress disorder symptoms in adults. *JAMA, 299*, 1291–1305.

Capitanio, J. P., Abel, K., Mendoza, S. P., Blozis, S. A., McChesney, M. B. et al (2008). Personality and serotonin transporter genotype interact with social context to affect immunity and viral set-point in simian immunodeficiency virus disease. *Brain Behav Immun, 22*, 676–689.

Caspi, A., Sugden, K., Moffitt, T. E., Taylor, A., Craig, I. W. et al (2003). Influence of life stress on depression: moderation by a polymorphism in the 5-HTT gene. *Science, 301*, 386–389.

Clark, D. P., and Russell, L. D. (2005). *Molecular Biology Made Simple and Fun, 3rd Ed.* Saint Louis, MO: Cache River Press.

Cohen, S., Janicki-Deverts, D. L., and Miller, G. E. (2007). Psychological stress and disease. *JAMA, 298*, 1685–1687.

Cohen, S. (1996). Psychological stress, immunity, and upper respiratory infections. *Curr Direct Psychol Sci, 5*, 86–90.

Cole, S. W., Yan, W., Galic, Z., Arevalo, J., and Zack, J. A. (2005). Expression-based monitoring of transcription factor activity: the TELiS database. *Bioinformatics, 21*, 803–810.

Collado-Hidalgo, A., Bower, J. E., Ganz, P. A., Irwin, M. R., and Cole, S. W. (2008). Cytokine gene polymorphisms and fatigue in breast cancer survivors: early findings. *Brain Behav Immun*. Epub ahead of print.

Crick, F. (1970). Central dogma of molecular biology. *Nature, 227*, 561–563.

Dickerson, S. S., and Kemeny, M. E. (2004). Acute stressors and cortisol responses: a theoretical integration and synthesis of laboratory research. *Psychol Bull, 130*, 355–391.

Feinberg, A. P. (2008). Epigenetics at the epicenter of modern medicine. *JAMA, 299*, 1345–1350.

Jaenisch, R., and Bird, A. (2003). Epigenetic regulation of gene expression: how the genome integrates intrinsic and environmental signals. *Nat Genet, 33*, 245–254.

Jirtle, R. L., and Skinner, M. K. (2007). Environmental epigenomics and disease susceptibility. *Nat Rev Genet, 8*, 253–262.

Johannes, F., Colot, V., and Jansen, R. C. (2008). Epigenome dynamics: a quantitative genetics perspective. *Nat Rev Genet, 9*, 883–90.

Krantz, D. S., and McCeney, M. K. (2002). Effects of psychological and social factors on organic disease: a critical assessment of research on coronary heart disease. *Ann Rev Psychol, 53*, 341–369.

Liu, D., Diorio, J., Tannenbaum, B., Caldji, C., Francis, D. et al (1997). Maternal care, hippocampal glucocorticoid receptors, and hypothalamic-pituitary-adrenal responses to stress. *Science, 277*, 1659–1662.

McCaffery, J. M., Frasure-Smith, N., Dube, M. P., Theroux, P., Rouleau, G. A. et al (2006). Common genetic vulnerability to depressive symptoms and coronary artery disease: a review and development of candidate genes related to inflammation and serotonin. *Psychosom Med, 68*, 187–200.

McEwen, B. S. (1998). Protective and damaging effects of stress mediators. *N Engl J Med, 338*, 171–179.

Meaney, M. J., and Szyf, M. (2005). Environmental programming of stress responses through DNA methylation: life at the interface between a dynamic environment and a fixed genome. *Dialogue Clin Neurosci, 7*, 103–123.

Miller, G. E., Chen, E., Sze, J., Marin, T., Arevalo, J. M. G. et al (2008). A genomic fingerprint of chronic stress in humans: blunted glucocorticoid and increased NF-κB signaling. *Biol Psychiatry, 64*, 266–272.

Miller, G. E., Gaudin, A., Zysk, E., and Chen, E. (2009). Parental support and cytokine activity in childhood asthma: the role of glucocorticoid sensitivity. *J Aller Clin Immunol, 123*, 824–830.

Miller, G. E., and Chen, E. (2006). Life stress and diminished expression of genes encoding glucocorticoid receptor and beta2-adrenergic receptor in children with asthma. *Proc Natl Acad Sci U S A, 103*, 5496–5501.

Miller, G. E., Chen, E., and Zhou, E. (2007). If it goes up, must it come down? Chronic stress and the hypothalamic-pituitary-adrenocortical axis in humans. *Psychol Bull, 133*, 25–45.

Miller, G. E., Cohen, S., and Ritchey, A. K. (2002). Chronic psychological stress and the regulation of pro-inflammatory cytokines: a glucocorticoid resistance model. *Health Psychol, 21*, 531–541.

Raison, C. L., and Miller, A. H. (2003). When not enough is too much: the role of insufficient glucocorticoid signaling in the pathophysiology of stress-related disorders. *Am J Psychiatry, 160*, 1554–1565.

Richards, E. J. (2006). Inherited epigenetic variation - revisiting soft inheritance. *Nat Rev Genet, 8*, 395–401.

Rohleder, N., Schommer, N. C., Hellhammer, D. H., Engel, R., and Kirschbaum, C. (2001). Sex differences in the glucocorticoid sensitivity of proinflammatory cytokine production after psychosocial stress. *Psychosom Med, 63*, 966–972.

Schneiderman, N., Ironson, G., and Siegel, S. D. (2005). Stress and health: psychological, behavioral, and biological determinants. *Ann Rev Psychol, 1*, 607–628.

Schoneveld, O. J. L. M., and Cidlowski, J. A. (2007). Glucocorticoids and immunity: mechanisms and regulation. In R. Ader (Ed.), *Psychoneuroimmunology, 4th Ed* (pp. 45–61). Boston: Elsevier.

Stark, J. L., Avitsur, R., Padgett, D. A., Campbell, K. A., Beck, F. M. et al (2001). Social stress induces glucocorticoid resistance in macrophages. *Am J Physiol 280*, 1799–1805.

Strachan, T., and Read, A. P. (2004). *Human Molecular Genetics*. London: Garland Science.

Weaver, I. C. G., Cervoni, N., Champagne, F. A., D'Alessio, A. C., Sharma, S. et al (2004). Epigenetic programming by maternal behavior. *Nat Neurosci, 7*, 847–854.

Webster, J. I., Tonelli, L., and Sternberg, E. M. (2002). Neuroendocrine regulation of immunity. *Annu Rev Immun, 20*, 125–163.

Whitelaw, E., and Garrick, D. (2006). Epigenetic mechanisms. In P. Gluckman, & M. Hanson (Eds.), *Developmental Origins of Health and Disease* (pp. 62–74). New York, NY: Cambridge University Press.

Wust, S., Van, Rossum, E. F., Federenko, I. S., Koper, J. W., Kumsta, R. et al (2004). Common polymorphisms in the glucocorticoid receptor gene are associated with adrenocortical responses to psychosocial stress. *J Clin Endocrinol Metab, 89*, 565–573.

Chapter 31

Genetics of Stress: Gene–Stress Correlation and Interaction

Stephen B. Manuck and Jeanne M. McCaffery

1 Introduction

Psychological stress figures prominently in behavioral medicine research and, with the advent of new molecular technologies, has attracted interest as a key environmental component in gene–environment interactions affecting health. Here, we review two recent developments in behavioral genetics that are informative with respect to the role of stress in genetically influenced disease risk and behavior. The first addresses an unanticipated, but now well-established, observation that many environmental exposures have a heritable etiology. Thus, genetic factors influence many experiences of individuals, including the occurrence of traumatic or other stressful life events, self-appraisals of recent life circumstances, and environments of early rearing, as well as the availability of social resources for ameliorating reactions to stress. The second development involves an emerging literature describing interactions between measured features of the environment and specific genetic variation. While long serving as a conceptual model of genetically modulated vulnerability to disease (the diathesis-stress model) and, perhaps also, as a rhetorical truce between proponents of exclusively environmental and partly genetic perspectives

on development, gene–environment interaction is now routinely tested empirically. These efforts stem from widely cited findings of a few seminal studies published in the early 2000s (Caspi et al, 2002, 2003). As in the study of simple gene–behavior associations (genetic "main effects"), attempts to replicate these and similar reports of gene–environment interaction have met with mixed success, which may be due, at least in part, to methodological differences among studies. In this chapter, we review both evidence of gene–environment correlation and several recent literatures exploring gene–environment interactions, with an emphasis on environmental factors defined by adversity or stress.

1.1 Conceptualization and Measurement of Stress

Conceptualizations of stress vary, but most investigators would cite among its defining attributes environmental demands that challenge or surpass an organism's ability to adapt, along with ensuing behavioral and physiological responses that heighten risk for disease (Cohen et al, 1995, 2007; Lazarus and Folkman, 1984). Implicit in this definition is a distinction between antecedent events or circumstances (stressors) and consequent behavioral and biological reactions (stress responses). Hence, one longstanding tradition of stress research attempts to inventory naturally occurring stressors and to link their occurrence to clinical sequelae or

S.B. Manuck (✉)
Behavioral Physiology Laboratory, Department of Psychology, University of Pittsburgh, 506 OEH, 4015 O'Hara Street, Pittsburgh, PA 15260, USA
e-mail: manuck@imap.pitt.edu

A. Steptoe (ed.), *Handbook of Behavioral Medicine*, DOI 10.1007/978-0-387-09488-5_31,
© Springer Science+Business Media, LLC 2010

preclinical disease processes. In a second, experimental tradition, exposures to laboratory stressors are manipulated in order to evaluate their effects on aspects of behavior or physiology that might be implicated in psychiatric or physical illness.

Psychological models of stress also commonly postulate cognitive processes that intervene between stressor and stress response to determine the latter's likelihood, kind, chronicity, and magnitude. These processes involve evaluations of the threat or demands posed by a stressor (primary appraisal) and of the individual's ability and resources to cope with the stressor (secondary appraisal) (Lazarus and Folkman, 1984). Primary appraisals reflect both objective features of the stressor (e.g., potential for harm, intensity) and psychological attributes of the individual, such as expectations derived from prior experiences in the same or similar circumstances or traits of personality or temperament (e.g., threat sensitivity). In turn, secondary appraisals focus on means of removing or otherwise altering a stressor or of mitigating its emotional impact (Cohen et al, 1995). Efforts to cope are abetted, too, by external resources, such as social supports and networks of social engagement that may buffer an individual against the threat implied by a stressor. The stress response is therefore the outcome of encountering a situation that one both perceives as harmful or demanding and feels unable to counter or avoid. Appraisals are also recursive, because actions taken to deal with a stressor may prove effective or exposure to a stressor may be time limited. In both circumstances, reevaluating a previously stressful situation may return a benign appraisal that then terminates the stress response. In contrast, threat-affirming appraisals may occasionally persist long after removal of the stressor, as in posttraumatic stress reactions. And finally, physiological responses akin to those induced by stress can conceivably occur even when an environmental threat has been handled satisfactorily as a result (or correlate) of actions taken in coping with the stressor (Cohen et al, 1993; Manuck et al, 1978).

Stress is generally thought to affect health either through behavioral changes that increase disease risk (e.g., smoking, curtailed sleep, physical inactivity) or in conjunction with negative emotional states (e.g., depression) and their physiological concomitants. Among the latter, the most frequently studied stress responses are those of the body's principal neuroendocrine axes, particularly the sympathetic-adrenomedullary (SAM) and hypothalamic-pituitary-adrenal (HPA) systems. These, in turn, promote systemic biological changes conducive to disease, such as altered metabolic, immune, respiratory, and cardiovascular functioning. It is the impact of these processes on disease-specific pathophysiologies, along with changes in health behaviors, that is held to account for much of the association between stress and predicted clinical outcomes.

In practice, most stress research encompasses only selected components of this overall model. In epidemiologic investigations, for instance, stressful life events are commonly assessed using checklists of common life stressors or, to circumvent limitations of this method, life stress interviews that probe for details of reported events and their surrounding context (Cohen et al, 1995; Monroe and Kelley, 1995; Turner and Wheaton, 1995). Other approaches de-emphasize discrete events and, instead, focus on respondents' appraisals of their recent life circumstances along such dimensions as predictability, controllability, and overload (e.g., the Perceived Stress Scale) (Cohen et al, 1983; Monroe and Kelley, 1995) or, alternatively, concentrate on a particular category of stressful experience, such as trauma, marital discord, or work stress, and in developmental studies, physical or sexual abuse, family constellation (e.g., father absence, parental death or divorce), and psychosocial attributes of the family environment (e.g., conflict, emotional neglect) (Ellis, 2004; Lyons et al, 1993; Plomin, 1994; Spotts et al, 2004; Theorell and Karasek, 1996). Finally, laboratory studies of stress typically evaluate the physiological, affective, or behavioral responses of individuals exposed to punctate stressors, usually of standardized format and brief duration (see Chapter 41).

2 Gene–Environment Correlation

Perhaps because we often tend to reify the dualism of heredity and environment, as in nature versus nurture, our first impulse is to see environments as acting *on* people, somewhat as a hammer acts on a nail. Yet, scant reflection recalls that people commonly have a hand in their own experiences. If personal characteristics, such as dispositional attributes, lead individuals to create or select certain environmental experiences, and if these characteristics are genetically influenced, environmental "exposures" may also be genetically influenced. This circumstance is referred to as gene–environment correlation and, when involving the selection of environmental experiences based on heritable predispositions, as *active* gene–environment correlation (Plomin et al, 2008). For instance, a heritable propensity for impulsive risk taking might engender preferences for activities that increase the likelihood of experiencing such adverse events as financial loss (from gambling) or traumatic injury (reckless driving). A second pathway, termed *reactive* (or evocative) gene–environment correlation, occurs when individuals' heritable characteristics (e.g., an antagonistic temperament) create adverse environments (e.g., interpersonal problems) by leading others to respond in ways they do not respond to persons lacking these characteristics. And finally, a third form of gene–environment correlation is of particular interest in developmental contexts because it is specific to relationships among genetically related individuals. Consider, for example, that exposure to punitive parenting might predict later behavioral problems in children, not as a direct consequence of the parenting practice, but via shared genetic variation that is expressed in the parent as a proclivity to discipline harshly and in the child as a predisposition to oppositional or other problematic behavior. This is referred to as *passive*

gene–environment correlation. Thus, there are several means by which heritable qualities of individuals might shape the environments they experience.

3 Gene–Stress Correlation

Is there evidence of gene–environment correlation for environments definable as stressors, and if so, how pervasively do genetic factors influence exposure to stressors? These questions have been investigated extensively in twin and adoption studies of the past 2 decades, and much of this literature was evaluated recently in a systematic review by Kendler and Baker (2007). The short answer is that gene–environment correlation is now well documented and that genetic variation typically accounts for a small to moderate proportion of individual differences in environmental exposures, including stressful life events, traumatic experiences, interpersonal relationships, parenting and family environments, and stress-related appraisals. We briefly summarize these associations in the following sections. It should be noted that while genetic analyses reported in this literature can detect heritable influences on measures of stressor exposure or appraisal, generally they cannot discriminate among the various pathways to gene–environment correlation described above.

3.1 Stressful Life Events

Numerous twin investigations have examined the heritability of stressful life events using checklists or other inventories of diverse life stressors. Among studies that included a score reflecting the sum of all recently experienced events, Kendler and Baker (2007) report a mean heritability of 28% for total life events, when weighted for variation in sample sizes. A distinction is also commonly made between events that could be dependent, in part, on actions of the individual experiencing them (e.g., financial problems; marital discord, separation, or divorce; legal difficulties) and those that are truly adventitious (e.g., illness or death of a relative; natural disasters). When dependent (or controllable) events are examined separately, genetic influences account for an estimated 31% of the variation in their occurrence, whereas "independent" (or uncontrollable) events are much less heritable, with a weighted average heritability of 17%. Some life event scales include items that are clearly positive (e.g., marriage, improved financial circumstances), often based on a model of stress that emphasizes the amount of readjustment required to adapt to recent events, rather than the undesirability or threat implied by those events (Turner and Wheaton, 1995). The three studies that administered such scales nonetheless permit a distinction between positive and negative life events, and interestingly, when analyzed separately the aggregate heritability of positive events (34%) is nearly the same as that of negative events (39%) (Plomin et al, 1990; Thapar and McGuffin, 1996; Wierzbicki, 1989). This is seen also in relation to the specific domain of marriage, where having a spouse and having ever been married exhibit heritable variation (57 and 70%, respectively) (Johnson et al, 2004; Middeldorp et al, 2005), as does experiencing divorce (weighted average heritability, 35%) (Kendler and Baker, 2007; McGue and Lykken, 1992; Middeldorp et al, 2005). Finally, Kendler and Baker (2007) suggest that the true heritability of life events may be underestimated in this literature owing to reliance on event scales that commonly index exposures occurring within a single year. When events were reported over two 1-year intervals, for instance, the heritability of stable (as opposed to occasion specific) differences in the propensity to experience stressful life events (65%) was very much larger than customary estimates (Foley et al, 1996)

Because it is implausible that people possess genetic predispositions to have particular experiences, it must be asked how genetic factors might conceivably affect exposure to stressful life events. There is abundant evidence that heritable personality traits predict the likelihood of experiencing recent life events, as seen in studies employing event inventories that are the same or similar to those showing life events subject to genetic influence (Billig et al, 1996; Headey and Wearing, 1989; Kendler et al, 2003b; Magnus et al, 1993; Poulton and Andrews, 1992; Saudino et al, 1997). In multivariate models, moreover, Saudino and colleagues (1997) reported that genetic variance common to Neuroticism, Extraversion, and Openness to Experience accounted for all heritable influences on life events reported by women in the Swedish Adoption/Twin Study of Aging. These findings held for all life event categories exhibiting genetic covariance in unadjusted models – namely, dependent (controllable), negative (undesirable), and positive (desirable) life events. Similarly, Billig and colleagues (1996) found the phenotypic correlation of dependent life events with individual differences in Constraint largely mediated by overlapping genetic variation among late adolescent males. Although these associations could possibly reflect disposition-related reporting biases rather than actual event occurrences, personality traits have been shown to predict life events even in analyses restricted to events considered "objective" and verifiable (e.g., divorce, job loss) (Headey and Wearing, 1989; Magnus et al, 1993; Saudino et al, 1997). Using data from the Virginia Twin Registry, Kendler (2003a) also found many stressful life events (e.g., marital, financial, work-related, legal, and interpersonal difficulties) to be predicted by Neuroticism, whether self-reported or reported by an informant (co-twin). And among monozygotic (MZ) twin pairs, one twin's stressful life events could be predicted almost as well by their co-twin's self-reported Neuroticism as by their own, and when extended to the full sample, this cross-twin correlation was significantly greater for MZ than same-sex dizygotic (DZ) twin pairs. These results indicate that Neuroticism predicts life events beyond any personal reporting biases associated with this trait and, like preceding studies, suggest that genetic factors substantially mediate a dispositional influence on stressful life events.

3.2 Traumatic Experiences

Identifying the origins of individual differences in risk of encountering traumatic (or life-threatening) events is of particular importance since traumatic experiences are a predicate for posttraumatic stress reactions and their associated disorder. Analyses based on the Vietnam Era Twin Registry show, for instance, that twin-pair concordance for requesting service in Vietnam was greater for MZ than DZ twins enlisted in the US military during the Vietnam War, with genetic factors accounting for over a third of the variance in such volunteering (Lyons et al, 1993). And among those assigned to service in Southeast Asia, extent of self-reported combat experience had an estimated heritability of 47%. The latter finding was corroborated independently by the analysis of combat decorations received for service in the war, which showed 54% heritable variation. Lyons and colleagues (1993) note that requesting a Vietnam assignment is not a fortuitous event, but a personal act, yet much of the genetic variance associated with volunteering for service in Vietnam was shared with genetic variance in extent of combat exposure (57%). This suggests that whatever genetically influenced attributes prompted individuals to volunteer for Vietnam service also predisposed them to become more extensively involved in combat. Among these attributes may be prior conduct problems and substance abuse, which subsequent research found to predict combat exposure in this population (Koenen et al, 2002).

A second twin study examined the heritability of non-combat trauma in a sample comprised predominantly of women (Stein et al, 2002). Exposure to "assaultive" trauma (e.g., physical or sexual assault, robbery) was influenced by both genetic and environmental factors, whereas non-assaultive traumas (e.g., motor vehicle accidents, sudden death of a family member, natural disasters) showed no genetic influence. Among twin pairs in which both members had had a traumatic event, moreover, genetic factors accounted for 38% of the variance in total posttraumatic stress disorder (PTSD) symptoms (with individual symptom categories showing slightly lower heritabilities: reexperiencing [36%], avoidance [28%], numbing [36%], and hyperarousal [29%]). Although it is reasonable to think that etiologic factors affecting the likelihood of traumatic exposures might differ from those influencing PTSD symptomatology after the occurrence of a traumatic event, additive genetic effects on the experience of assaultive trauma correlated highly with genetic variance in PTSD symptoms (all r's > 0.70). These results suggest that liability to both trauma and PTSD symptomatology involves overlapping genetic influences. Finally, other research on this sample has shown personality variables, particularly adult and juvenile antisocial traits, to account for a significant proportion of the genetic variance in assaultive trauma (Jang et al, 2003). Like the literature on stressful life events, then, heritable personality characteristics and associated psychopathologies affect the likelihood of trauma exposure.

3.3 Parenting and Family Environments

Developmental studies have focused less on discrete events of childhood than on parenting behaviors and qualities of the family environment, some dimensions of which may reflect adversities of early rearing (Plomin, 1994). Parental warmth (and by its absence, affectless, chilly, or remote parental attention) has been studied extensively and shown to have substantial genetic variance. In their review, Kendler and Baker (2007) report weighted mean heritabilities of 37 and 34% for child-reported maternal and paternal warmth, respectively, and 35% for parents' descriptions of their own behaviors. Genetic influences appear to be substantially weaker for other parenting dimensions, such as negativity, control, and protectiveness, and again, whether reported by child (heritabilities of 15–26%) or parent (19–23%) (Kendler and Baker, 2007).

Along with absence of the father, family environments prone to discord and lacking in close interpersonal relationships have been of interest, in part, due to their association with girls' early pubertal development, which in turn increases the likelihood of a number of adolescent health outcomes, including problems of mood and conduct, early sexual activity, and teen pregnancy (Ellis, 2004). In twin studies, measures of family conflict and family cohesion show modest to moderate genetic influence, with weighted mean heritabilities in the Kendler and Baker (2007) review of 30 and 24%, respectively (Plomin et al, 1988, 1989; Jacobson and Rowe, 1999; Jang et al, 2001). In one other twin study, Krueger et al (2003) reported on the heritability of a retrospective measure of "perceived cohesion versus conflict in the family environment" derived from multiple environmental scales. The 16% of variance in this measure that could be attributed to heritable variation, moreover, was fully explained by genetic covariance with two personality factors, Negative Emotionality and Constraint. This finding suggests that people who, for genetic reasons, readily experience negative emotions and exhibit limited inhibitory control of their affect and behavior either tend to recollect their early family environments in ways colored by their personality (i.e., biased recall) or accurately recollect a family environment in which conflict was promoted and cohesion eroded via relatives' reactions to dispositional characteristics of the respondent, as expressed within the family. Unfortunately, the typical twin design is not well suited to detecting particular forms of gene–environment correlation, but adoption studies do provide examples of reactive gene–environment correlation. In one such study, for instance, antisocial and substance abuse disorders among biological parents predicted both adolescent antisocial behaviors in their adopted-away offspring and harsher discipline and less nurturant parenting in the adolescents' adoptive parents. Importantly, structural modeling indicated that the adoptees' conduct problems mediated the relationship between psychopathologies of the biological parent and parenting behaviors

of the adoptive parents (Ge et al, 1996; see also, O'Connor et al, 1998).

3.4 Perceived Stress and Social Support

As noted previously, most models of stress distinguish between stressors and their subjective evaluation (appraisals), even if this distinction is blurred in the wording of questions used to assess environmental exposures in specific instruments. Appraisals define the meaning of stressors to individuals, as in their perceptions of the threat or demands posed by a life event or circumstance, as well as individuals' sense of their capacity and resources to cope with a stressor effectively. Appraisal-based measures of stress tap these perceptions, either globally or within particular domains of activity. Compared with life event scales and early family environments, though, less is known about the heritability of stress appraisals. In a twin study of "organizational climate," genetic influences accounted for 22% of the variance in a composite measure of respondents' perceptions of their work environment as supportive (versus unsupportive) and 27% of the variance in reported "annoyance" associated with identified physical stressors in the work place (Hershberger et al, 1994). In contrast, respondents' perceptions of job-related time pressures showed no heritability in this study. Among more general measures of stress appraisals, the perceived stress scale (PSS) is perhaps the most widely used index of stressful experience referenced to the recent past (month) and the trier inventory for the assessment of chronic stress (TICS) is a prominent multidimensional measure of perceived stress referenced to the past year that has been shown to predict dysregulation of the HPA system (e.g., heightened cortisol response to awakening) (Cohen and Wills, 1985; Pruessner et al, 2003; Schlotz et al, 2004; Wust et al, 2000). Administering both measures to a young adult sample of MZ and DZ twins, Federenko and colleagues (2006) reported a heritability of 30% for the PSS and, among TICS scales, 23% for chronic worries and 45% for stress attributed to a "lack of social recognition." However, estimated heritabilities were consistently low for the remaining TICS scales – work overload (6%), social stress (5%), work discontent (16%), and intrusive memories (13%). Thus, there is significant genetic influence on the extent to which people generally perceive their recent life circumstances as stressful (PSS), but quite variable genetic variance among differentiated components of perceived chronic stressors (TICS scales).

Social support, perceived or tangible, represents an important resource for dealing with stressful life experiences, and so also, for appraising one's ability to cope (secondary appraisal) (Lazarus and Folkman, 1984). Framing social support as a resource encourages its interpretation as an environmental asset that promotes adaptation or ameliorates the impact of a stressor. Sources of support are not acquired fortuitously, though. They are embedded in interpersonal relationships that require effort to establish and maintain (e.g., the parents' admonition, "to have a friend, be a friend"), which may, in turn, depend on the heritable attributes of individuals. For instance, 59% of the variance in levels of social support indexed by one common support measure, the Interpersonal Support Evaluation List, was accounted for by genetic factors in a study of young adult MZ and DZ twins (Raynor et al, 2002). In the same investigation, participants having the least support reported a more hostile disposition and more depressive symptomatology than those scoring higher in social support, and shared genetic influence explained the major portion of these phenotypic associations (61–72%). Several analyses based on data of the Virginia Twin Registry show significant, if smaller, genetic effects on several support dimensions, with weighted mean heritabilities of 17% for support available from friends and 31% each for relative support, having a confidant with whom one can disclose private feelings, and social integration (defined by the density of friends, frequency of friend contacts, and involvements in clubs and recreational, religious, or other community organizations) (Agrawal et al, 2002; Kendler, 1997; Kendler and Baker, 2007; Kessler et al, 1992). As with stressful life events, moreover, the estimated heritability of stable variation in the these support indices, derived from measurements taken on two occasions 5-years apart, was much stronger than estimates based on single measurements (43–75%) (Kendler, 1997). It is also noteworthy that these genetic effects were greatest for social integration (75%) and the availability of confidants (66%), two dimensions of support that presumably are among the most objectively assessed. Finally, recent data on adolescent twins show heritable variation even in the fine structure of social networks, such as network transitivity (e.g., the likelihood that friends in a respondent's network are friends of each other) and centrality (where one is positioned between the center and periphery of a social network), for which genetic factors accounted for 47 and 29% of interindividual variability, respectively (Fowler et al, 2009).

3.5 Summary of Gene–Stress Correlation

In sum, biometric family studies document heritable variation in the likelihood of experiencing environmental stressors and do so across nearly all categories of stressors examined in this research. These associations include self-reported stressful life events (especially those that may be construed as controllable to some extent by the individual), exposure to traumatic (life-threatening) events, adverse parenting environments (particularly family conflict and absence of parental warmth), personal appraisals of recent life stress and some dimensions of perceived chronic stress, as well as resources for coping with stressors, such as confidants and engagement in social networks. The genetic variance in these environmental measures is relatively consistent across the several domains, but typically not large. The modest to moderate effect sizes describing genetic influences on exposure to stressors and resources for coping may reflect, in part, arbitrary reporting intervals that imperfectly capture stable individual differences in event occurrences and social support (Kendler and Baker, 2007). When these variables were assessed on even two occasions, estimated heritabilities were shown to be appreciably higher (~65%), suggesting that prevailing methodologies may significantly underestimate genetic effects (Foley et al, 1996; Kendler, 1997). Finally, heritable variation in the likelihood of experiencing various stressors does not appear to be an artifact of reporting biases and, where tested, genetic factors have been shown to mediate influences of personality on environmental exposures (e.g., Billig et al, 1996; Ge et al, 1996; Kendler et al, 2003a; Krueger et al, 2003; Raynor et al, 2002; Saudino et al, 1997).

4 Gene–Environment Interaction

Genotype-dependent interactions affecting health and behavior are emerging as a prominent focus of research in behavioral and psychiatric genetics, genetic epidemiology, and the new field of pharmacogenetics. This reflects an increasing recognition that the effects of genetic variation (polymorphisms) on measured phenotypes can differ greatly by context and circumstances, be they genetic (gene–gene interaction, or epistasis) or environmental (gene–environment interaction). Gene–environment interaction in this sense refers neither to the ecumenical platitude that development entails both nature *and* nurture nor to the genetic control of biochemical processes such as cell–cell communication or intracellular signaling cascades involving interdependent transduction molecules. Rather, it refers to a *statistical* interaction between genetic and environmental variables in which genetic factors affect measured phenotypes differently as a function of different environmental exposures, or alternatively, environments affect

phenotypes differently against different genetic backgrounds (Talmud, 2004).

4.1 Examples of Gene–Environment Interaction

Many examples of gene–environment interactions involving health-related behaviors may be cited. For instance, high density lipoprotein cholesterol (HDL) concentrations have been shown to vary by interaction of dietary fat intake and genetic variation in hepatic lipase, a key enzyme in HDL metabolism (Ordovas et al, 2002; Tai et al, 2003). In addition, the degree of cholesterol lowering achieved by consumption of a polyunsaturated, compared to saturated, fat diet may be predicted by polymorphic variation in genes encoding the cholesterol ester transfer protein (*CETP*) and lipoprotein lipase (*LPL*) (Wallace et al, 2000). An asparagine/aspartic acid substitution in *LPL* has also been shown to magnify effects of cigarette smoking on risk of incident ischemic heart disease (Talmud et al, 2000). Likewise, the ϵ4 allele of the apolipoprotein E gene (*APOE*) increases smoking-related risk for coronary disease events in prospective investigations (Humphries et al, 2001, 2003). A third health behavior, physical inactivity, has been found to moderate an association of the Pro12Ala polymorphism of paroxysome proliferator-activated receptor γ (PPAR-γ) on type 2 diabetes (Nelson et al, 2007). In African Americans (but not whites), each T allele of the 825 C>T polymorphism of the gene coding for the G-protein β3 subunit (*SNB3*) was found associated with a 20% lower prevalence of obesity among physically active individuals and a 23% increased prevalence of obesity in the physically inactive (Grove et al, 2007). Notably, on completion of a physical training program, African Americans homozygous for the T allele also achieved a greater reduction in body fat, compared to those of other 825 C>T genotypes (Rankinen et al, 2002).

It is noteworthy that genetic effects in some of these studies were magnified several fold when examined among individuals having certain health behaviors (Humphries et al, 2001, 2003; Talmud et al, 2000). In others, genetic effects were *only* seen when the study sample was stratified by relevant health behaviors (Nelson et al, 2007) or gene polymorphisms predicted opposite effects at high and low levels of a behavioral moderator (Grove et al, 2007; Ordovas et al, 2002; Tai et al, 2003). These context-dependent relationships, in turn, may help to explain the worrisome fragility of genetic "main effects" that characterizes candidate gene association studies generally (Munafo and Flint, 2004), since such effects may conceivably come and go when study cohorts are sampled from different locations along a gradient of environmental variation.

In view of the extensive gene–environment correlations described in the preceding section, though, it might be asked whether the environments party to these interactions – diet, smoking, physical activity – represent truly environmental moderators. It might be asked, but generally is not. Few reports of putative gene–environment interaction even acknowledge that their environmental variables may have some genetic origin. On this point, there is some evidence (albeit mixed) that caloric intake, dietary preference for fat, and fat consumption are heritable (e.g., Keskitalo et al, 2008; see McCaffery et al, 2001, for a summary review). Genetic factors are known to account for about half of interindividual variability in smoking initiation and for an even larger proportion of the variability in smoking rate, persistence of smoking, and nicotine dependence (Schnoll et al, 2007). And with respect to physical activity, participation in elective exercise exhibited a median heritability of 62% (48–71% across seven countries) in a multinational study of 37,000+ twin pairs (Stubbe et al, 2006). At the least, such findings render the interpretation of literatures on gene–environment interaction confusing, since one scientist's environmental variable often proves to be another's target of genetic influence. Because the potential contamination of gene–environment interaction by unappreciated gene–environment correlation extends also to studies

of gene–stress interactions, we will return to this issue in the final section of the chapter.

5 Gene–Stress Interaction

Gene–environment interaction can be detected by both quantitative genetic analyses and molecular studies of specific genetic variation (gene polymorphisms). Among the former, for instance, the heritability of body mass (body mass index) has been found lower among men who engage in vigorous exercise than in the less physically active (McCaffery et al, 2009), and the heritability of hypertension appears to rise with higher levels of educational attainment (McCaffery et al, 2008). Molecular studies of gene–stress interaction are more common than quantitative genetic studies, though, and these generally fall into two categories: (1) those that examine how naturally occurring stressors moderate genetic influences on aspects of disease risk and, in psychiatric genetics, liability to psychopathologies of mood or conduct; and (2) studies examining the genetic modulation of physiological responses to acute psychological stressors, as manipulated experimentally. The latter investigations add to a longstanding focus of research in behavioral medicine on psychophysiological reactivity as a possible risk factor for disease (Krantz and Manuck, 1984; Manuck, 1994; Marsland et al, 2002). Candidate genetic variation in these studies commonly targets genes encoding components of neurotransmitter systems acting in the brain or peripherally (e.g., enzymes effecting synthesis, release and reuptake, receptor activation, or metabolism), as well as intracellular signaling molecules, hormonal influences on gene expression (e.g., steroid receptors), and other elements of systemic physiology (e.g., inflammatory cytokines and other immune parameters). In the following sections, we discuss selected literatures involving genetic interactions with life events or other natural stressors and experimental studies of genetically modulated physiological responses to laboratory stressors.

5.1 Gene–Stress Interaction: Life Events and Other Natural Stressors

A dominant model of occupational stress posits the combination of high job demands and limited control over job-related decision making (low decision latitude) as pernicious attributes of the work environment, and job strain defined in this manner has been associated with both elevated blood pressure and heart disease (e.g., Kivimaki et al, 2006; Landsbergis et al, 2003; Ohlin et al, 2007). Because the sympathetic nervous system is a key determinant of cardiac and vascular function, obvious candidate genes for studies of gene–environment interactions affecting blood pressure are those of the several adrenergic receptors. In a large, middle-aged sample of employed individuals, for instance, homozygosity for the deletion allele of a common insertion/deletion polymorphism in the α_{2B}-adrenoreceptor (*ADRA2B*) was found associated with higher systolic and diastolic blood pressure in men, relative to those of other *ADRA2B* genotypes, but only when accompanied by job strain (Ohlin et al, 2007). In addition, the decision latitude component of job strain alone correlated inversely with systolic blood pressure in men. In another study of the same sample, job strain interacted only marginally with genotypes of an argenine/glycine substitution in the β_1-adrenoreceptor gene (*ADRB1*), although systolic blood pressure covaried inversely with extent of job demands among men carrying the glycine-encoding allele of this polymorphism (Ohlin et al, 2008). Another model of occupational stress construes the work environment as a balance of implied obligations whereby the employee's work effort is compensated by salary, recognition, security, and opportunities for advancement (Siegrist et al, 2004). Job stress is defined in this context as a relative imbalance between effort and reward. In the one study following this model, presence of hypertension was predicted by an interaction of job stress and another argenine/glycine substitution, in the β_2-adrenoreceptor gene (*ADRB2*:

β_2-*AR-16*) (Yu et al, 2008). Hypertension was about 3.5 times more prevalent among individuals with any glycine-encoding allele than in those homozygous for the alternate argenine allele, but only in conjunction with high job stress (effort/reward imbalance) and, again, only in men. All three of these studies suggest that attributes of the work environment moderate effects of adrenoreceptor gene variation on blood pressure and do so in men alone, although variability in their operational definitions of job stress (job strain, effort-reward imbalance) and in the components of genotype-dependent job strain associated with blood pressure (latitude, job demands) leaves these gene–environment interactions preliminary.

Activation or dysregulation of the HPA system is the most frequently invoked mechanism to explain effects of psychological stress on disease, both physical and psychiatric (see Chapter 43). This is undoubtedly due to actions of the glucocorticoid hormone, cortisol, on diverse physiological functions and tissues of the body, including metabolism and activities of the cardiovascular, immune, and central nervous systems. Some HPA phenotypes are also heritable. For instance, genetic variance appears to account for half or more of interindividual variability in basal cortisol levels aggregated across multiple measurements in the morning (Bartels et al, 2003; Meikle et al, 1988) and similar, if somewhat lesser, heritabilities are seen in the cortisol response to morning awakening (Kupper et al, 2005; Wust et al, 2000). With respect to molecular variation, a series of investigations has focused on the corticotropin-releasing hormone type 1 receptor (*CRHR1*) gene. In the first of these, individual single nucleotide polymorphisms (SNPs) and a TAT haplotype at markers rs7209436, rs110402, and rs242924 were found associated with lower levels of depressive symptomatology, when compared to other *CRHR1* genotypes, among African American women who were abused in childhood (Bradley et al, 2008). The apparently protective effects of this *CRHR1* variation against early adversity/abuse were replicated in relation to lifetime history of major depressive disorder in an independent sample of predominantly Caucasian women (Bradley et al, 2008) and in relation to both past year and recurrent depression in a midlife sample of British women (Polanczyk et al, 2009). A similar interaction was not observed among participants of the Dunedin (New Zealand) Multidisciplinary Health and Development Study (Polanczyk et al, 2009). However, one other investigation has shown the "protective" alleles at rs110402 and rs242924 to mitigate the heightened cortisol responses to a dexamethasone/corticotropin-releasing hormone (dex/CRH) challenge otherwise seen among adults maltreated as children (Tyrka et al, 2009).

Another series of studies has examined polymorphic variation in *FKBP5*, which encodes a co-chaperone of heat stress protein-90, FK506 binding protein-5, that helps regulate binding affinity of the glucocorticoid receptor (GR). In a depressed patient sample, TT genotype at rs1360780 was found to be associated with a more rapid response to antidepressant treatment and greater recurrence of depressive episodes, higher levels of *FKBP5* expression in lymphocytes, and a blunted adrenocorticotropin hormone (ACTH) response to dex/CRH challenge, relative to those carrying one or more copies of the alternate C allele (Binder et al, 2004). This polymorphism and another *FKBP5* SNP, rs3800373, also predicted peritraumatic dissociation, a risk factor for PTSD, among medically injured children (Koenen et al, 2005), and these and two other SNPs analogously predicted adult PTSD symptomatology in interaction with childhood abuse (but not adult trauma exposure) among predominantly low-income, African American men and women (Binder et al, 2008). Interestingly, in the latter investigation, *CRHR1* SNPs previously reported to interact with childhood abuse in the prediction of depressive symptoms in the same study sample (Bradley et al, 2008) did not similarly predict PTSD symptoms here, suggesting some specificity of association.

Other recent studies have investigated PTSD risk in relation to varying exposure to hurricanes occurring in Florida in 2004. In one, the C allele of a SNP in the "regulator of G-protein signaling 2" (*RGS2*) gene, rs4606, predicted post-hurricane PTSD symptomatology, but only among individuals with high hurricane exposure (viz., a combination of hurricane force winds or flooding, material losses, and extended displacement) and low levels of social support (Amstadter et al, 2009). And in the same study, lifetime PTSD symptoms were likewise predicted by the interaction of *RGS2* variation with lifetime exposure to traumatic (life-threatening) events. Two prior investigations of the same study cohort genotyped common regulatory variation in the serotonin transporter gene-linked polymorphic region (5-HTTLPR), one variant of which (typically termed the short [S] allele) reduces transcriptional efficiency of the serotonin transporter gene compared to the alternate, long (L) allele. In one study, the low expression allele increased risk of post-hurricane PTSD in interaction with area-level socioeconomic indicators (crime and unemployment rates) (Koenen et al, 2009), and in the second, the same genetic variation predicted both PTSD and major depression in persons with high hurricane exposure and low social support, relative to all other combinations of genotype, exposure and support (Kilpatrick et al, 2007). To the extent that a high exposure to hurricanes, as defined by these investigators, is an impactful life event, it is perhaps surprising that the *RGS2* and 5-HTTLPR polymorphisms did not interact with exposure alone, but only in three-way interaction with social support or community characteristics. This may indicate that the presence of social support or socioeconomic advantage ameliorates genotype-dependent risk of PTSD and depression associated with hurricane exposure.

5.1.1 Gene–Stress Interaction and the Challenge of Replication

At present, studies of gene–stress interactions have produced only small literatures, often just one or two investigations addressed to a particular gene, environmental moderator, and phenotype or to phenotypes studied in multiple studies, but with respect to different genes (e.g.,

PTSD). Two exceptions are literatures generated by two early gene–environment studies (Caspi et al, 2002, 2003), in which a sufficient number of investigations testing the same hypothesis are available to evaluate the replicability of gene–stress interactions. In the first of these, the initial study found self-rated aggressiveness, conduct disorder, symptoms of adult antisocial personality disorder, and commission of a violent crime potentiated by childhood maltreatment among males with low-transcription variants of a functional promoter polymorphism of monoamine oxidase-A (*MAOA*), relative to men having an alternate, high-activity *MAOA* allele (Caspi et al, 2002). Two meta-analyses, the latter of which included the initial study and seven attempted replications, have now been reported (Kim-Cohen et al, 2006; Taylor and Kim-Cohen, 2007). In the second meta-analysis, the authors derived the correlation of adversity with antisocial outcomes for each *MAOA* genotype and expressed the *MAOA* × Adversity interaction as the difference in correlation between genotypes. The pooled estimate of effect size (correlation) across studies was 0.30 for the low-activity *MAOA* genotype and 0.13 for the high-activity genotype. The test of the interaction yielded a modest, but significant, effect size (for the difference in correlation) of 0.17 (95% CI: 0.09, 0.24; $p < 0.001$). This outcome was only minimally affected by the removal of either the original investigation or the two studies having effect sizes larger than the sentinel report, or by serial deletion of each study individually. This suggests the presence of a robust gene–stress interaction. More recent studies have tended also to confirm the interaction of *MAOA* variation and childhood maltreatment on later externalizing and antisocial behaviors (Ducci et al, 2008; Enoch et al, 2010), although this relationship may be less stable in women (Prom-Wormley et al, 2009) and less apparent at very severe levels of early adversity (Weder et al, 2009).

The second sizable literature on gene–stress interactions derives from a widely publicized study in which childhood maltreatment and recent stressful life events predicted depression in proportion to the number of S, relative to L, alleles of 5-HTTLPR that individuals possessed (Caspi et al, 2003). Over 30 investigations of widely varying design, methodology, and study population have been reported since, and this literature has been the subject of numerous commentaries, narrative reviews, and meta-analyses. With respect to the latter, two meta-analyses reported in 2009 covered largely (but not entirely) overlapping studies and both failed to confirm an interactive effect of 5-HTTLPR variation and life events on depression (Munafo et al, 2009; Risch et al, 2009). These results cast a long shadow over this most frequently cited instance of gene–stress interaction and may seem especially disconcerting given strong rationale for the hypothesis. For instance: (1) serotonergic dysregulation has long been implicated in depression and mood regulation (Thase, 2009); (2) the serotonin transporter is a primary target of pharmacotherapy for depression (Gitlin, 2009); (3) the S allele of orthologous 5-HTTLPR variation in the rhesus macaque lowers brain serotonin turnover in monkeys, but only among animals reared without maternal contact (Bennett et al, 2002); and (4) in vivo brain serotonergic responsivity (assessed by neuropharmacologic challenge) is attenuated in euthymic individuals with a history of depression (Bhagwagar et al, 2002; Flory et al, 1998) and among carriers of the 5-HTTLPR S allele (Reist et al, 2001; Whale et al, 2000). One environmental parameter, socioeconomic status, has also been shown to modulate the influence of 5-HTTLPR variation on central serotonergic responsivity (Manuck et al, 2004).

Stressful life events likewise warrant consideration as an environmental "pathogen" due to abundant evidence that they predict depression onset, particularly first episodes (Kendler et al, 2000; Uher and McGuffin, 2008) and, in twin research, have been found to do so in interaction with genetic liability (Kendler et al, 1995). A 30-year literature indicates that life events most germane to depression are those that occur abruptly and within 3–6 months preceding onset, that are impactful and directly affect the respondent, and that commonly involve situations of significant threat, loss, or humiliation (Brown and Harris, 1978; Brown, et al, 1995; Kendler et al, 2003; Monroe et al, 2009). Yet almost none of the studies of 5-HTTLPR-stress interactions for depression appear to have been informed by these observations. In reviewing the methodologies of 13 5-HTTLPR-life stress studies, for instance, Monroe and Reid (2008) found that only one study could appropriately distinguish acute stressors from chronic conditions, only three could appropriately distinguish major from minor events, only five restricted event assessments to the last 6 months (others extending measurements even to 5 years or lifetime exposure), only three assessed participant-focused events, and only one study satisfied all four of these conditions. They also report that instruments for assessing life events were diverse in format and content across studies, that nearly all lacked provenance in the life stress/depression literature, that procedures for determining total exposure to life events were different in every study, and that in only four studies could it be assumed that life events even preceded the onset of depression. Regarding this last consideration, a significant main effect of life events on depression, as reported in the two cited meta-analyses, could reflect, in part, reverse causation (events consequent on depression) or, where events and outcomes were assessed at the same time, biased event recall (Monroe and Reid, 2008).

Also addressing the heterogeneity of study methods, Uher and McGuffin (2010) recently stratified, by format of life event assessment, 34 studies that purposed to test interactive effects of 5-HTTLPR variation and environmental adversity on depression. By their analysis, the hypothesized interaction was demonstrated in 11 of 15 studies employing event measurements that were either "objective" (i.e., ascertained independently of participants' reports) or derived from contextually sensitive life stress interviews, while the four remaining studies reported at least partial replications (e.g., findings delimited by gender or event kind). On the other hand, all non-replications emerged in investigations using life event checklists or other self-report instruments, yielding a distribution of six replications, four partial replications, and ten non-replications. The authors note as well that the two previously cited meta-analyses (Munafo et al, 2009; Risch et al, 2009) included only a minority of all studies and, by sampling disproportionately from those relying on participants' self-reported life stress, may have confounded study outcomes with variability and quality of investigational methods (Uher and McGuffin, 2010).

As noted previously, the sentinel study in this literature (Caspi et al, 2003) reported that both childhood maltreatment and life events predicted depression in interaction with 5-HTTLPR variation. The interval of event reporting in this study was 5 years, suggesting that events per se were not a proximal cause of depression. In another recent commentary, Brown and Harris (2008) note that childhood maltreatment is itself a potent risk factor for depression and that in the study of Caspi and colleagues (2003) the genotype-dependent relationship between childhood adversity and depression appears to have been stronger than that for life events. Presenting evidence that early maltreatment also predicts the frequency of events experienced over a 4–5-year period in adulthood, Brown and Harris argue that life events occurring outside the canonical range for life event/depression associations may be a marker of early childhood adversities that, in interaction with allelic variation at 5-HTTLPR, affect neurodevelopmental processes. In turn, these neurodevelopmental changes may promote behaviors that increase the likelihood of experiencing stressful life events over the lifecourse and also heighten risk of depression in adulthood. In contrast, recent life events may predict depressive episodes independently or interact only minimally with 5-HTTLPR genotype. Such speculation is also consistent with a paucity of evidence showing allelic differences at 5-HTTLPR to affect serotonin transporter availability, binding, and mRNA expression in the adult brain (e.g., Mann et al, 2000; Parsey et al, 2006; Shioe et al, 2003; Sibille and Lewis, 2006; van Dyck et al, 2004).

5.2 Gene–Stress Interaction: Acute Stressors

Individual differences in the magnitude of cardiovascular reactions to laboratory stressors have attracted interest as a potential risk factor for cardiovascular disease and have been shown to predict extent and progression of preclinical atherosclerosis (e.g., Gianaros et al, 2002; Jennings et al, 2004; Krantz and Manuck, 1984). A number of investigators have also examined genetic effects on physiological responses to acute stressors in both twin studies and candidate gene association studies. In a recent meta-analysis of twin studies of heart rate and blood pressure responses to common experimental stressors (e.g., mental arithmetic or other cognitive challenges, video games, stressful interviews, or the Stroop color-word interference test), the pooled heritability estimate for change in heart rate was 43%, with no effects of gender or genetic dominance. For change in diastolic blood pressure, both additive genetic and dominance effects were observed, yielding a total heritability of 29%. Significant heritability was also observed for change in systolic blood pressure, although this was greater in females (38%) than males (26%) (Wu et al, in press).

Variation in genes within a number of pathways may moderate cardiovascular reactions to psychological stressors, with genes encoding components of the sympathetic nervous system, the renin–angiotensin–aldosterone system (RAAS), endothelial function, and serotonergic neurotransmission serving as potential examples (Snieder et al, 2002). At present, however, research on individual genes within these pathways is both sparse and mixed. In one study, for example, two SNPs that appear to affect adrenoreceptor function, the G allele of a C>G SNP at base pair (bp) 1165 of *ADRB1* and the G allele of an A>G substitution at bp 46 in *ADRB2*, were associated with higher resting systolic and diastolic blood pressure respectively, relative to the alternate alleles of these polymorphisms (McCaffery et al, 2002). In the same study, the variant at bp 1165 in *ADRB1*

also predicted elevated diastolic blood pressure responses to acute laboratory stressors (mental arithmetic, Stroop task). In contrast, higher resting systolic and diastolic blood pressure and heightened diastolic reactions to mental and physical stressors were associated with the A allele at bp 46 in *ADRB2* in a second study (Li et al, 2001). Among other preliminary studies, stress-elicited pressor responses have been found related to genetic variation in tyrosine hydroxylase, the dopamine type 1 receptor, the G-protein α subunit, and multilocus analyses of RAAS system polymorphisms (Ge et al, 2007; Lu et al, 2006; Rao et al, 2008).

Individual differences in cardiovascular reactions to psychological stressors have also been examined in relation to 5-HTTLPR variation. In a first study, individuals homozygous for the 5-HTTLPR S allele showed attenuated heart rate and blood pressure responses to an anger challenge (Williams et al, 2001), and a similar finding was later reported by the same group in a larger study sample (Williams et al, 2008). However, 5-HTTLPR genotype showed a main effect in the opposite direction in a study of young adult twins, and this association was qualified by gender (McCaffery et al, 2003). Whereas males showed no genotype-dependent variability in cardiovascular reactivity, females homozygous for the 5-HTTLPR S allele exhibited greater cardiac acceleration to cognitive stressors than females carrying any L allele. This association was also observed in genetically independent samples and corroborated by sib-pair linkage analysis. The paucity of studies overall and early inconsistencies among the few tests involving the same gene polymorphisms obviously precludes even interim interpretation, although the appreciable heritability of reactivity phenotypes demonstrated across multiple biometric studies should encourage further exploration of genetic variation moderating cardiovascular reactions to acute stressors.

Few investigations have examined the heritability of HPA responses to psychological stressors, although findings of gene association studies in this area are somewhat more consistent than those for cardiovascular responses. In children, genetic influences accounted for 55–60% of the variance in salivary cortisol measured at baseline and following performance of a challenging video game and for 44% of baseline-to-task cortisol reactivity (Steptoe et al, 2009). Also, similar heritability was observed for salivary and total cortisol, ACTH, and heart rate responses to the trier social stress test (TSST), a composite stress protocol involving mental arithmetic and public speaking before an audience, in an earlier study of adolescent/young adult twins (Federenko et al, 2004). Not surprisingly, one target of molecular studies has been the GR gene (NR3C1). Genotyping four putatively functional NR3C1 polymorphisms, labeled N363S, ER22/23EK, 9β, and an intronic marker of unknown function, Bcl1, Wust and colleagues (2004) found TSST-elicited salivary cortisol responses in males to be greatest among carriers of the 363S allele and blunted in participants homozygous for the Bcl1 GG allele. In a subsequent study, the Bcl1 GG genotype again predicted diminished HPA (ACTH) responses to the TSST in males, but heightened responses in females (Kumsta et al, 2007). Along with the GR, the mineralocorticoid receptor (MR) acts centrally in the coordination of HPA stress responses and enhanced salivary and plasma cortisol, as well as heart rate, reactions to TSST exposure have been found among carriers of the MR180V allele of the MRI180V polymorphism (DeRijk et al, 2006). Finally, the same variants of FKBP5 cited previously as predictors of recurrent depression, antidepressant response and, in interaction with childhood adversities, peritraumatic dissociation, and adult PTSD symptomatology (Binder et al, 2004, 2008; Koenen et al, 2005) retarded cortisol recovery following administration of the TSST (Ising et al, 2008). In the same study, effects of the GR and MR polymorphisms examined in earlier studies did not replicate, which the authors suggest may stem from the limited statistical power of this rather small investigation.

Finally, two studies have examined monoamine-regulating polymorphisms as predictors of HPA responses to laboratory stressors. In the first, rises in plasma ACTH among healthy volunteers administered a modified TSST (Groningen Acute Stress Test) were greater in those who were both homozygous for the met (methionine) allele of a val158met amino acid substitution in the catechol-O-methyl transferase (COMT) gene and of low activity MAOA genotype, when compared to individuals with any COMT val (valine) allele or those of high-activity MAOA genotype (Jabbi et al, 2007). In this study as well, stressor-induced plasma ACTH and cortisol responses were more pronounced among participants homozygous for the 5-HTTLPR S allele, compared to carriers of the L allele, although the cortisol effect was observed only in females. In a second investigation that also examined 5-HTTLPR variation, increases in salivary cortisol evoked by combined mental arithmetic and stressful interview were likewise greater in children homozygous for the S allele, relative to children with any L allele (Gotlib et al, 2008).

Genetic variation has also been shown to moderate behavioral responses to laboratory stimuli. When deprived by a study confederate of money earned in an experimental task, for instance, individuals of low-activity MAOA genotype were more likely to punish the confederate than were their high-activity MAOA counterparts (McDermott et al, 2009). This effect was seen when participants suffered an 80% earnings loss, but not at a more modest 20% loss, suggesting that MAOA variation is not related directly to an aggressive motivation, but to the disinhibited expression of such motivation when elicited by provocation.

As noted previously, a central component of most stress models is the primary appraisal of potential stressors along dimensions of threat or demand. A heightened sensitivity to threat-related cues might be expected therefore to enhance threat appraisals and potentiate stress responses. In this regard, genotypes containing the 5-HTTLPR S allele have been found to predict attentional biases toward words of negative emotional content (anxiety) in psychiatric inpatients (Beevers et al, 2007), pictures of phobic stimuli (spiders) in college students (Osinsky et al, 2008), and facial expressions of anger in adolescent volunteers (Perez-Edgar et al, 2010). In the corticolimbic circuitry of emotion processing, the amygdala plays a key role in detecting stimuli of psychological significance, including cues to environmental threats, and is readily engaged by emotional words and pictures or by facial displays of negative affect (see Chapter 52). Studies employing neuroimaging techniques have shown the 5-HTTLPR S allele to increase amygdala reactivity to such stimuli, compared to the L allele, and this association has been confirmed on meta-analysis of over a dozen investigations (Munafo et al, 2008). Moreover, polymorphic variations in several other relevant genes have been found to modulate threat-related amygdala reactivity as well, including those encoding the serotonin 1A receptor (Fakra et al, 2009); *MAOA* (Meyer-Lindenberg et al, 2006), neuronally active tryptophan hydroxylase (Brown et al, 2005; Canli et al, 2005); fatty acid amide hydrolase, a component of endocannabinoid signaling (Hariri et al, 2009), neuropeptide Y (Zhou et al, 2008); and the androgen receptor (Manuck et al, 2010).

6 Conclusions

We have addressed two topics in this chapter, gene–stress correlation and gene–stress interaction. This first of these – genetic influences on exposure to stressful environments – is now strongly supported, whereas research on the second topic – the moderation of genetic associations by stress-related environmental variation – has only recently emerged as an important focus of research in behavioral and health genetics. Thus, gene–stress correlation has been demonstrated for virtually all environmental dimensions investigated, from early family environments to stressful life events and traumatic experiences, and, with respect to protective factors, networks of social engagement and support. Genetic influence on these variables is not trivial and, when environmental measures are assessed more than once, can account for a half or more of individual differences in

exposures. Since heritable characteristics help determine the experiences people have, either as a result of their own actions or via reactions they elicit from others, it follows that studies that show measures of psychological stress to predict behavioral or health-related outcomes cannot be interpreted automatically as evidence of environmental impacts.

As noted, gene–stress interactions, and particularly those involving specific gene polymorphisms, are only beginning to be reported. Most literatures in this area contain only a few studies, often of diverse methodology or focusing on different genes in a common biological pathway. Nonetheless, several interesting and plausible gene–stress interactions have been reported, as in studies of adrenoreceptor variation, work stress, and blood pressure; HPA system polymorphisms, trauma, and PTSD; *MAOA* promoter variation, childhood maltreatment, and aggressive disposition; and genotype-dependent physiological responses to acute psychological stressors. The single most frequently investigated gene in studies of gene–stress interactions is that coding for the serotonin transporter and, within this gene, the 5-HTTLPR promoter polymorphism. 5-HTTLPR genotypes have been examined in relation to cardiovascular and HPA responses to laboratory stressors, attentional biases and neural sensitivity to threat, and a spectrum of psychopathologies (most notably, PTSD and depression). Interestingly, these 5-HTTLPR-dependent relationships may be detected more reliably with neuroimaging and experimental probes of emotional processing than in studies of distal behavioral phenotypes, such as depression. It is likely that investigations that examine genetic associations and gene–stress interactions for the purpose of predicting clinical outcomes require appreciably larger sample sizes than those in which the study phenotype lies closer to the gene's biological actions. In specific reference to the interaction of 5-HTTLPR variation and life events on depression, however, replication difficulties may be attributable as much to methodological deficiencies and dissimilarities among studies, and possibly, insufficiently refined hypothesis, as to inadequate statistical power (Brown and Harris, 2008; Monroe and Reid, 2008; Uher and McGuffin, 2008).

In concluding, we want to briefly address two additional considerations germane to gene–environment interactions, and so by implication, gene–stress interactions. The first concerns criteria for identification and selection of candidate genes, and the second, criteria for selecting candidate environmental moderators. It is argued, often by geneticists, that only genes already known to predict dependent variables of interest (that is, genes exhibiting strong main effects on study outcomes) should be interrogated for possible interaction with pertinent environmental exposures (Risch et al, 2009). In their thoughtful commentaries on strategies for studying gene–environment interactions, Moffitt and colleagues (2005, 2006) argue just the opposite, that exploiting environmental variation can aid in gene discovery since gene associations may be amplified in risk-enriched environments, and they point to many instances of gene–environment interaction in which genetic main effects were negligible. On the environmental side, in contrast, it is sometimes posited that only environmental factors already known to predict outcomes of interest should be entertained as potential moderators of genetic associations (Moffitt et al, 2005, 2006). Again in reference to studies of 5-HTTLPR variation, life events, and depression, for instance, the failure to assess life events in a manner informed by accumulated understanding of the environmental antecedents of depression may account for many inconsistencies seen in this literature (Monroe and Reid, 2008). On the other hand, the logic that suggests that testing for gene–environment interaction can unmask unrecognized genetic effects may be invoked equally to argue that testing for gene–environment interactions has the potential to unmask novel environmental effects. Moreover, predicating gene–environment analyses on variables having known main effects, either genetic or environmental, tends to presume an ordinal form of interaction in which outcomes differ only at the conjunction of a susceptibility allele and environmental risk factor (e.g., diathesis-stress models) (Manuck, in press).

Another possibility, however, is that genetic variation modulates susceptibility to environmental influences in general, so that some genotypes confer greater plasticity than others in the face of differing environments. Terming such genotype-dependent plasticity "differential susceptibility," Belsky and colleagues (2009) cite numerous studies in which people carrying putative "risk" alleles of several gene polymorphisms were more likely to experience negative outcomes in adverse environments and, conversely, less likely to experience the same outcomes in salutary environments, relative to individuals with other genotypes. Importantly, disordinal gene–environment interactions of this form will tend to be associated with smaller or absent main effects of both genetic and environmental predictors.

These arguments notwithstanding, proponents of a "strong" environmental predicate for gene–environment interaction maintain that candidate environmental variables should not only have mechanistic (e.g., biological) plausibility, but also exert a causal influence on the study outcome (Moffitt et al, 2005, 2006). The latter condition, although ignored by most investigators, tacitly acknowledges that putative environmental factors may be genetically influenced – that is, gene–environment correlation. As a result, an apparent gene–environment interaction might actually reflect, in part, an interaction of measured genotypes with unrecognized genetic variance in the "environmental" predictor. Obviously, this is not an interpretive problem when the environmental variable is manipulated experimentally, as in studies of acute stress responses or using other paradigms in which an experimental probe is evaluated in comparison to a control stimulus (e.g., functional neuroimaging) or to individuals not exposed to the experimental condition (e.g., placebo-controlled clinical trials). But as reported earlier, gene–environment correlation is well documented for many common environmental measures and, with respect to psychological stressors, pervasive. Quantitative genetic studies can potentially distinguish environmental effects that are causal from those associated with correlated genetic variation, and indeed, there is some evidence that stressful life events have both causal and non-causal effects on behavioral outcomes (e.g., depression) (Kendler et al, 1999). However, analogous claims cannot be made for most molecular genetic studies, which commonly examine population samples of unrelated individuals and are therefore ill-designed to identify causal environmental effects (Uher and McGuffin, 2008). Moreover, showing that candidate genes are unrelated to an environmental moderator in a given study, which some investigators have reported (e.g., Foley et al, 2004), is unpersuasive as a control for genetic confounding because it considers only a single source of potentially correlated genetic variation.

In the end, though, one might ask how important it is anyway to demonstrate "pure" gene–environment interaction if, to some extent, heritable influences contribute to interindividual variability in most all categories of experience, including exposure to psychological stressors. From a practical standpoint, for instance, genetic variance in behaviors or exposures detrimental to health does not preclude environmental interventions to ameliorate health risks by modifications of either behavior or environment. Similarly, recognizing that adversities of early rearing may have a heritable component is no more an argument against interventions to prevent the maltreatment of children than is the observation that individuals of high-activity *MAOA* genotype are resilient in the face of abuse. Finally, in view of the extent of demonstrated gene–stress correlations, it seems reasonable to assume that most dimensions of measured experience will have both environmental and genetic determinants and that most researchers addressing gene–environment interactions will not be able to fully account for the etiology of their environmental moderators. In this sense, it may be prudent to acknowledge the interpretative limitations of gene–environment (or gene–stress) interactions by referring instead, and more modestly, to interactions between genes and environmental *exposures*, where exposures denote experiences in the environment that may stem from a variety of undetermined causes.

Acknowledgments Preparation of this manuscript was supported, in part, by National Institutes of Health Grants PO1 HL040962 and RO1 HL065137 (SBM), and UO1 DK056993, RO1 AG018384, and RO1 HL072819 (JMM).

References

Agrawal, A., Jacobson, K. C., Prescott, C. A., and Kendler, K. S. (2002). A twin study of sex differences in social support. *Psychol Med, 32*, 1155–1164.

Amstadter, A. B., Koenen, K. C., Ruggiero, K. J., Acierno, R., Galea, S. et al (2009). Variant in *RGS2* moderates posttraumatic stress symptoms following potentially traumatic event exposure. *J Anxiety Disord, 23*, 369–373.

Bartels, M., de Geus, E. J. C., Kirschbaum, C., Sluyter, F., and Boomsma, D. (2003). Heritability of daytime cortisol levels in children. *Behav Genet, 33*, 421–433.

Beevers, C. G., Gibb, B. E., McGeary, J. E., and Miller, I. A. (2007). Serotonin transporter genetic variation and biased attention for emotional word stimuli among psychiatric inpatients. *J Abnorm Psychol, 116*, 208–212.

Belsky, J., Jonassaint, C., Pluess, M., Stanton, M., Brummett, B. et al (2009). Vulnerability genes or plasticity genes? *Mol Psychiatry, 14*, 746–754.

Bennett, A. J., Lesch, K. P., Heils, A., Long, J. C., Lorenz, J. G. et al (2002). Early experience and serotonin transporter gene variation interact to influence primate CNS function. *Mol Psychiatry, 7*, 118–122.

Bhagwagar, Z., Whale, R., and Cowen, P. J. (2002). State and trait abnormalities in serotonin function in major depression. *Br J Psychiatry, 180*, 24–28.

Billig, J. P. Hershberger, S. L., Iacono, W. G., and McGue, M. (1996). Life events and personality in late adolescence: genetic and environmental relations. *Beh Genet, 26*, 542–554.

Binder, E. B., Bradley, R. G., Liu, W., Epstein, M. P., Deveau, T. C. et al (2008). Association of FKBP5 polymorphisms and childhood abuse with risk of posttraumatic stress disorder symptoms in adults. *JAMA, 299*, 1291–1305.

Binder, E. B., Salyankina, D., Lichner, P., Wochnik, G. M., Ising, M., et al (2004). Polymorphisms in FDBP5 are associated with increased recurrence of depressive episodes and rapid response to antidepressant treatment. *Nat Genet, 36*, 1319–1325.

Bradley, R. G., Binder, E. B., Epstein, M. P., Tang, Y., Nair, H. P. et al (2008). Influence of child abuse on adult depression: moderation by the corticotrophin-releasing hormone gene. *Arch Gen Psychiatry, 65*, 190–200.

Brown, G. W., and Harris, T. (1978). *Social Origins of Depression*. New York: Free Press.

Brown, G. W., and Harris, T. O. (2008). Depression and the serotonin transporter 5-HTTLPR polymorphism: a review and a hypothesis concerning gene–environment interaction. *J Affect Disord, 111*, 1–12.

Brown, G. W., Harris, T. O., and Hepworth, C. (1995). Loss, humiliation and entrapment among women developing depression: a patient and non-patient comparison. *Psychol Med, 25*, 7–22.

Brown, S. M., Peet, E., Manuck, S. B., Williamson, D. E., Dahl, R. E. et al (2005). A regulatory variant of the human tryptophan hydroxylase-2 gene biases amygdala reactivity. *Mol Psychiatry, 10*, 884–888.

Canli, T., Congdon, E., Gutknecht, L., Constable, R. T., and Lesch, K. P. (2005). Amygdala responsiveness is modulated by tryptophan hydroxylase-2 gene variation. *J Neural Transm, 112*, 1479–1485.

Caspi, A., McClay, J., Moffitt, T. E., Mill, J., Martin, J. et al (2002). Role of genotype in the cycle of violence in maltreated children. *Science, 297*, 851–854.

Caspi, A., Sugden, K., Moffitt, T. E., Taylor, A., Craig, I. W. et al (2003). Influence of life stress on depression: moderation by a polymorphism in the 5-HTTLPR gene. *Science, 301*, 386–389.

Cohen, S., Janicki-Deverts, D., and Miller, G. E. (2007). Psychological stress and disease. *JAMA, 298*, 1685–1687.

Cohen, S., Kamarck, T., and Mermelstein, R. (1983). A global measure of perceived stress. *J Health Soc Behav, 24*, 385–396.

Cohen, S., Kessler, R. C., and Gordon, L. U. (1995). Strategies for measuring stress in studies of psychiatric and physical disorders. In S. Cohen, R.C. Kessler, & L. U. Gordon (Eds.), *Measuring Stress* (pp. 3–28). New York: Oxford University Press.

Cohen, S., Tyrrell, D. A. J., and Smith, A. P. (1993). Negative life events, perceived stress, negative affect, and susceptibility to the common cold. *J Pers Soc Psychol, 64*, 131–140.

Cohen, S., and Wills, T. A. (1985). Stress, social support and the buffering hypothesis. *Psychol Bull, 98*, 310–357.

DeRijk, R. H., Wust, S., Meijer, O. C., Zennaro, M.-C., Federenko, I. S. et al (2006). A common polymorphism in the mineralocorticoid receptor modulates stress responsiveness. *J Clin Endocrinol Metab, 91*, 5083–5089.

Ducci, F., Enoch, M.-A., Hodgkinson, C., Zu, K., Catena, M., Robin, R. W. et al (2008). Interaction between a functional *MAOA* locus and childhood sexual abuse predicts alcoholism and antisocial personality disorder in adult women. *Mol Psychiatry, 13*, 334–347.

Ellis, B. J. (2004). Timing of pubertal maturation I girls: an integrated life history approach. *Psychol Bull, 130*, 920–958.

Enoch, M.-A., Steer, C. D., Newman, T. K., Gibson, N., and Goldman, D. (2010). Early life stress, *MAOA*, and gene–environment interactions predict behavioral disinhibition in children. *Genes Brain Behav, 13*, 1122–1130.

Fakra, E., Hyde, L. W., Gorka, A., Fischer, P. M., Munoz, K. E. et al (2009). Effects of HTR1A C(-1019)G on amygdala reactivity and trait anxiety. *Arch Gen Psychiatry, 66*, 33–40.

Federenko, I. S., Nagamine, M., Hellhammer, D. H., Wadhwa, P. D., and Wust, S. (2004). The heritability of hypothalamus pituitary adrenal axis responses to psychosocial stress is context dependent. *J Clin Endocrinol Metab, 89*, 6244–6250.

Federenko, I. S., Schlotz, W., Kirschbaum, C., Bartels, M., Hellhammer, D. H. et al (2006). The heritability of perceived stress. *Psychol Med, 36*, 375–385.

Flory, J. D., Mann, J. J., Manuck, S. B., and Muldoon, M. F. (1998). Recovery from major depression is not associated with normalization of serotonergic function. *Biol Psychiatry, 43*, 320–326.

Foley, D. L., Eaves, L. J., Wormley, B., Silberg, J. L., Maes, H. H. et al (2004). Childhood adversity, monamine oxidase A genotype, and risk for conduct disorder. *Arch Gen Psychiatry, 61*, 738–744.

Foley, D. L., Neale, M. C., and Kendler, K. S. (1996). A longitudinal study of stressful life events assessed at interview with an epidemiological sample of adult twins: the basis of individual variation in event exposure. *Psychol Med, 26*, 1239–1252.

Fowler, J. H., Dawes, C. T., and Christakis, N. A. (2009). Model of genetic variation in human social networks. *Proc Natl Acad Sci USA, 106*, 1720–1724.

Ge, D., Zhu, H., Huang, Y., Treiber, F. A., Harshfield, G. A. et al (2007). Multilocus analyses of renin-angiotensin-aldosterone system gene variants on blood pressure at rest and during behavioral stress in young normotensive subjects. *Hypertension, 49*, 107–112.

Ge, X., Conger, R. D., Cadoret, R. J., Neiderhiser, J. M., Yates, W. et al (1996). The developmental interface between nature and nurture: a mutual influence model of child antisocial behavior and parent behaviors. *Dev Psychol, 32*, 574–589.

Gianaros, P. J., Bleil, M. E., Muldoon, M. F., Jennings, J. R., Sutton-Tyrrell, K. et al (2002). Is cardiovascular reactivity associated with atherosclerosis among hypertensives. *Hypertension, 40*, 742–747.

Gitlin, M. J. (2009). Pharmacotherapy and other somatic treatments for depression. In I. H. Gotlib & C. L. Hammen (Eds.), *Handbook of Depression, 2nd Ed* (pp. 554–585). New York: Guildford.

Gotlib, I. H., Joormann, J., Minor, K. L., and Hallmayer, J. (2008). HPA axis reactivity: a mechanism underlying the associations among 5-HTTLPR, stress, and depression. *Biol Psychiatry, 63*, 847–851.

Grove, M. L., Morrison, A., Folsom, A. R., Boerwinkle, E., Hoelscher, D. M. et al (2007). Gene–environment interaction and the GNB3 gene in the Atherosclerosis Risk in Communities Studies. *Int J Obes, 31*, 919–926.

Hariri, A. R., Gorka, A., Hyde, L. W., Kimak, M., Halder, I. et al (2009). Divergent effects of genetic variation in endocannabinoid signaling on human threat- and reward-related brain function. *Biol Psychiatry, 66,* 9–16.

Headey, B., and Wearing, A. (1989). Personality, life events, and subjective well-being: toward a dynamic equilibrium model. *J Pers Soc Psychol, 57,* 731–739.

Hershberger, S. L., Lichtenstein, P., and Knox, S. S. (1994). Genetic and environmental influences on perceptions of organizational climate. *J Appl Psychol, 79,* 24–33.

Humphries, S. E., Hawe, E., Dhamrait, S., Miller, G. J., and Talmud, P.J. (2003). In search of genetic precision. *Lancet, 361,* 1908–1909.

Humphries, S. E., Talmud, P. J., Hawe, E., Bolla, M., Day, I. N. M. et al (2001). Apolipoprotein E4 and coronary heart disease in middle-aged men who smoke: a prospective study. *Lancet, 358,* 115–119.

Ising, M., Depping, A.-M., Sliebertz, A., Lucae, S., Unschuld, P. G. et al (2008). Polymorphisms in the FDBP5 gene region modulate recovery from psychosocial stress in health controls. *Eur J Neurosci, 28,* 389–398.

Jabbi, M., Korf, J., Kema, I. P., Hartman, C., and van der Pompe, G. et al (2007). Convergent genetic modulation of the endocrine stress response involves polymorphic variations of 5-HTT, COMT and MAOA. *Mol Psychiatry, 12,* 483–490.

Jacobson, K. C., and Rowe, D. C. (1999). Genetic and environmental influences on the relationships between family connectedness, school connectedness, and adolescent depressed mood: sex differences. *Dev Psychol, 35,* 926–939.

Jang, K. L., Stein, M. B., Taylor, S., Asmundson, G. J., and Livesley, W. J. (2003). Exposure to traumatic events and experiences: aetiological relationships with personality function. *Psychiatry Res, 120,* 61–69.

Jang, K. L., Vernon, P. A., Livesley, W. J., Stein, M. B., and Wolf, H. (2001). Intra- and extra-familial influences on alcohol and drug misuse: a twin study of gene–environment correlation. *Addiction, 96,* 1307–1318.

Jennings, J. R., Kamarck, T. W., Everson-Rose, S. A., Kaplan, G. A., Manuck, S. B. et al (2004). Exaggerated blood pressure responses during mental stress are prospectively related to enhanced carotid atherosclerosis in middle-aged Finnish men. *Circulation, 110,* 2198–2203.

Johnson, W., McGue, M., Krueger, R. F., and Bouchard, T. J. (2004). Marriage and personality: a genetic analysis. *J Pers Soc Psychol, 86,* 285–294.

Kendler, K. S. (1997). Social support: a genetic-epidemiologic analysis. *Am J Psychiatry, 154,* 1398–1404.

Kendler, K. S., and Baker, J. H. (2007). Genetic influences on measures of the environment: a systematic review. *Psychol Med, 37,* 615–626.

Kendler, K. S., Gardner, C. O., and Prescott, C. A. (2003a). Personality and the experience of environmental adversity. *Psychol Med, 22,* 1193–1202.

Kendler, K. S., Hettema, J. M., Butera, F., Gardner, C. O., and Prescott, C. A. (2003b). Life event dimensions of loss, humiliation, entrapment, and danger in the prediction of onsets of major depression and generalized anxiety. *Arch Gen Psychiatry, 60,* 789–796.

Kendler, K. S., Karkowski, L. M., and Prescott, C. A. (1999). Causal relationship between stressful life events and the onset of major depression. *Am J Psychiatry, 156,* 837–841.

Kendler, K. S., Kessler, R. C., Walters, E. E., MacLean, C., Neale, M. C. et al (1995). Stressful life events, genetic liability, and onset of an episode of major depression in women. *Am J Psychiatry, 152,* 833–842.

Kendler, K. S., Thornton, L. M., and Gardner, C. O. (2000). Stressful life events and previous episodes in the etiology of major depression in women: an evaluation of the 'kindling" hypothesis. *Am J Psychiatry, 63,* 1113–1120.

Keskitalo, K., Tuorila, H., Spector, T. D., Cherkas, L. F., Knaapila, A. et al (2008). The three-factor eating questionnaire, body mass index, and responses to sweet and salty fatty foods: a twin study of genetic and environmental associations. *Am J Clin Nutr, 88,* 263–271.

Kessler, R. C., Kendler, K. S., Heath, A., Neale, M. C., and Eaves, L. J. (1992). Social support, depressed mood, and adjustment to stress: a genetic epidemiologic investigation. *J Pers Soc Psychol, 62,* 257–272.

Kilpatrick, D. G., Koenen, K. C., Ruggiero, K. J., Acierno, R., Galea, S. et al (2007). The serotonin transporter genotype and social support and moderation of posttraumatic stress disorder and depression in hurricane-exposed adults. *Am J Psychiatry, 164,* 1693–1699.

Kim-Cohen, J., Caspi, A., Taylor, A., Williams, B., Newcombe, R. et al (2006). MAOA, maltreatment, and gene–environment interaction predicting children's mental health: new evidence and a meta-analysis. *Mol Psychiatry, 11,* 903–913.

Kivimaki, M., Virtanen, M., Elovainio, M., Kouvonen, A., Vaanaanen, A. et al (2006). Work stress in the etiology of coronary heart disease – a meta-analysis. *Scand J Work Environ Health, 32,* 431–442.

Koenen, K. C., Aiello, A. E., Bakshis, E., Amstadter, A. B., Ruggiero, K. J. et al (2009). Modification of the association between serotonin transporter genotype and risk of posttraumatic stress disorder in adults by county-level social environment. *Am J Epidemiol, 169,* 704–711.

Koenen, K. C., Harley, R., Lyons, M. J., Wolfe, J., Simpson, J. C. et al (2002). A twin registry study of familial and individual risk factors for trauma exposure and posttraumatic stress disorder. *J Nerv Ment Dis, 190,* 209–218.

Koenen, K. C., Szxe, G., Purcell, S., Smoller, J. W., Bartholomew, D. et al (2005). Polymorphisms in FKBP5 are associated with peritraumatic dissociation in medically injured children. *Mol Psychiatry, 10,* 1058–1059.

Krantz, D. S., and Manuck, S. B. (1984). Acute psychophysiologic reactivity and risk of cardiovascular disease: a review and methodologic critique. *Psychol Bull, 96*, 435–463.

Krueger, R. F., Markon, K. E., and Bouchard, T. J. (2003). The extended genotype: the heritability of personality accounts for the heritability of recalled family environments in twins reared apart. *J Pers, 71*, 809–833.

Kumsta, R., Entringer, S., Koper, J. W., van Rossum, E. F. C., Hellhammer, D. H. et al (2007). Sex specific associations between common glucocorticoid receptor gene variants and hypothalamus-pituitary-adrenal axis responses to psychosocial stress. *Biol Psychiatry, 62*, 683–689.

Kupper, N., de Geus, E. J. C., van den Berg, M., Kirschbaum, C., Boomsma, E. I. et al (2005). Familial influences on basal salivary cortisol in an adult population. *Psychoneuroendocrinology, 30*, 857–868.

Landsbergis, P. A., Schnall, P. L., Pickering, T. G., Warren, K., and Schwartz, J. E. (2003). Life-course exposure to job strain and ambulatory blood pressure in men. *Am J Epidemiol, 157*, 998–1006.

Lazarus, R. W., and Folkman, S. (1984). *Stress, Appraisal and Coping*. New York: Springer.

Li, G. H., Faulhaber, H. D., Rosenthal, M., Schuster, H., Jordan, J. et al (2001). Beta-2 adrenergic receptor gene variations and blood pressure under stress in normal twins. *Psychophysiology, 38*, 485–489.

Lu, Y., Zhu, H., Wang, X., Snieder, H., Huang, Y. et al (2006). Effects of dopamine receptor type 1 and Gs Protein α subunit gene polymorphisms on blood pressure at rest and in response to stress. *Am J Hypertens, 19*, 832–836.

Lyons, M. J., Goldberg, J., Eisen, S. A., True, W., Tsuang, M. T. et al (1993). Do genes influence exposure to trauma? A twin study of combat. *Am J Med Genet, 48*, 22–27.

Magnus, K., Diener, E., Fujita, F., and Pavot, W. (1993). Extraversion and neuroticism as predictors of objective life events: a longitudinal analysis. *J Pers Soc Psychol, 65*, 1046–1053.

Mann, J. J., Huang, Y.-Y., Underwood, M. D., Kassir, S. A., Oppenheim, S. et al (2000). A serotonin transporter gene promoter polymorphism (5-HTTLPR) and prefrontal cortical binding I major depression and suicide. *Arch Gen Psychiatry, 57*, 729–738.

Manuck, S. B. (1994). Cardiovascular reactivity in cardiovascular disease. *Int J Behav Med, 1*, 4–31.

Manuck, S. B. (in press). The reaction norm in gene x environment interaction. *Mol Psychiatry*.

Manuck, S. B., Flory, J. D., Ferrell, R. E., and Muldoon, M. F. (2004). Socio-economic status covaries with central nervous system serotonergic responsivity as a function of allelic variation in the serotonin transporter gene-linked polymorphic region. *Psychoneuroendocrinology, 29*, 651–668.

Manuck, S. B., Harvey, A. H., Lechleiter, S. L., and Neal, S. K. (1978). Effects of coping on blood pressure responses to threat of aversive stimulation. *Psychophysiology, 15*, 544–549.

Manuck, S. B., Marsland, A. L., Flory, J. D., Gorka, A., Ferrell, R. E. et al (2010). Salivary testosterone and a trinucleotide (CAG) length polymorphism in the androgen receptor gene predict amygdala reactivity in men. *Psychoneuroendocrinology, 35*, 94–104.

Marsland, A. L., Bachen, E. A., Cohen, S., Rabin, B., Manuck, S. B. (2002). Stress, immune reactivity and susceptibility to infectious disease. *Physiol Behav, 77*, 711–716.

McCaffery, J. M., Bleil, M., Pogue-Geile, M. F., Ferrell, R. E., and Manuck, S. B. (2003). The association between a serotonin transporter gene variant and cardiovascular reactivity in young adult male and female twins. *Psychosom Med, 65*, 721–728.

McCaffery, J. M., Papandonatos, G. D., Bond, D. S., Lyons, M. J., and Wing, R. R. (2009). Gene X environment interaction of vigorous exercise and body mass index among male Vietnam-era twins. *Am J Clin Nutr, 89*, 1011–1018.

McCaffery, J. M., Papandonatos, G. D., Lyons, M. J., and Niaura, R. (2008). Educational attainment and the heritability of self-reported hypertension among male Vietnam-era twins. *Psychosom Med, 70*, 781–786.

McCaffery, J. M., Pogue-Geile, M. F., Ferrell, R. E., Petro, N., and Manuck, S. B (2002). Variability within alpha- and beta-adrenoreceptor genes as a predictor of cardiovascular function at rest and in response to mental challenge. *J Hypertens, 20*, 1105–1114.

McCaffery, J. M., Pogue-Geile, M. F., Muldoon, M. F., Debski, T. T., Wing, R. R. et al (2001). The nature of the association between diet and serum lipids in the community: a twin study. *Health Psychol, 20*, 341–350.

McDermott, R., Tingley, D., Cowden, J., Frazzetto, G., and Johnson, D. D. P. (2009). Monoamine oxidase A gene (MAOA) predicts behavioral aggression following provocation. *Proc Natl Acad Sci USA, 106*, 2118–2123.

McGue, M., and Lykken, D. (1992). Genetic influence on risk of divorce. *Psycho Sci, 3*, 368–373.

Meikle, A. W., Stringham, J. D., Woodward, M. G., and Bishop, D. T. (1988). Heritability of variation in plasma cortisol levels. *Metabolism, 37*, 514–517.

Meyer-Lindenberg, A., Buckholtz, S. W., Kolachana, B. R., Hariri, A. R., Pezawas, L. et al (2006). Neural mechanisms of genetic risk for impulsivity and violence in humans. *Proc Natl Acad Sci USA, 103*, 6269–6274.

Middeldorp, C. M., Cath, D. C., Vink, J. M., and Boomsma, D. I. (2005). Twin and genetic effects on life events. *Twin Res Hum Genet, 8*, 224–231.

Moffitt, T. E., Caspi, A., and Rutter, M. (2005). Strategy for investigating interactions between measured genes and measured environments. *Arch Gen Psychiatry, 62*, 473–481.

Moffitt, T. E., Caspi, A., and Rutter, M. (2006). Measured gene–environment interactions in psychopathology. *Perspectives on Psychological Science, 1*, 5–27.

Monroe, S. M., and Kelley, J. M. (1995). Measurement of stress appraisal. In S. Cohen, R. C. Kessler, & L. U. Gordon (Eds.), *Measuring Stress* (pp. 122–147). New York: Oxford University Press.

Monroe, S. M., and Reid, M. W. (2008). Gene–environment interactions in depression research: genetic polymorphisms and life-stress polyprocedures. *Psychol Sci, 19*, 947–956.

Monroe, S. M., Slavich, G. M., and Georgiades, K. (2009). The social environment and life stress in depression. In I. H. Gotlib & C. L. Hammen (Eds.), *Handbook of Depression, 2nd Ed* (pp. 340–360). New York: Guildford.

Munafo, M. R., Brown, S. M., and Hariri, A. R. (2008). Serotonin transporter (5-HTTLPR) genotype and amygdala activation: a meta-analysis. *Biol Psychiatry, 63*, 852–857.

Munafo, M. R., Durrant, C., Lewis, G., and Flint, J. (2009). Gene X environment interactions at the serotonin transporter locus. *Biol Psychiatry, 65*, 211–219.

Munafo, M. R., and Flint, J. (2004). Meta-analysis of genetic association studies. *Trends Genet, 20*, 439–444.

Nelson, T. L., Fingerlin, T. E., Moss, L. K., Barmada, M. M., Ferrell, R. E. et al (2007). Association of the peroxisome proliferator-activated receptor γ gene with type 2 diabetes mellitus varies by physical activity among non-Hispanic whites from Colorado. *Metabolism, 56*, 388–393.

O'Connor, T. G., Deater-Deckard, K., Fulker, D., Rutter, M., and Plomin, R. (1998). Genotype–environment correlations in late childhood and early adolescence: antisocial behavioral problems and coercive parenting. *Dev Psychol, 34*, 970–981.

Ohlin, B., Berglund, G., Nilsson, P., and Melander, O. (2007). Job strain, decision latitude and alpha2B-adrenergic receptor polymorphisms significantly interact and associate with higher blood pressures in men. *J Hypertens, 25*, 1613–1619.

Ohlin, B., Berglund, G., Nilson, P. M., and Melander, O. (2008). Job strain, job demands and adrenergic beta1-receptor-polymorphism: a possible interaction affecting blood pressure in men, *J Hypertens, 26*, 1583–1589.

Ohlin, B., Berglund, G., Rosvall, M., and Nilsson, P. M. (2007). Job strain in men, but not in women, predicts a significant rise in blood pressure after 6.5 years follow-up. *J Hypertens, 25*, 525–531.

Ordovas, J. M., Corella, D., Demissie, S., Cuupples, A., Couture, P. et al (2002). Dietary fat intake determines the effect of a common polymorphism in the hepatic lipase gene promoter on high-density lipoprotein metabolism. *Circulation, 106*, 2315–2321.

Osinsky, R., Reuter, M., Kupper, Y., Schmitz, A., Kozyra, E. et al (2008). Variation in the serotonin transporter gene modulates selective attention to threat. *Emotion, 8*, 584–588.

Parsey, R. V., Hastings, R. S., Oquendo, M. A., Hu, X., Goldman, D. et al (2006). Effect of a triallelic functional polymorphism of the serotonin-transporter-linked promoter region on expression of serotonin transporter in the human brain. *Am J Psychiatry, 163*, 48–51.

Perez-Edgar, K., Bar-Haim, Y., McDermott, J., Gerodetsky, E., Hodgkiinson, C. A. et al (2010). Variations in the serotonin-transporter gene are associated with attention bias patterns to positive and negative emotion faces. *Biol Psychol, 83*, 269–271.

Polanczyk, G., Caspi, A., Williams, B., Price, T. S., Danese, A. et al (2009). Protective effects of *CRHR1* gene variants on the development of adult depression following childhood maltreatment: replication and extension. *Arch Gen Psychiatry, 66*, 978–985.

Poulton, R. G., and Andrews, G. (1992). Personality as a cause of adverse life events. *Acta Psychiatr Scand, 85*, 35–38.

Plomin, R. (1994). *Genetics and Experience.* Thousand Oaks, CA: Sage.

Plomin, R., DeFries, J. C., McClearn, G. E., and McGuffin, P. (2008). *Behavioral Genetics, 5th Ed.* New York: Worth.

Plomin, R., Lichtenstein, P., Pedersen, N. L., McClearn, G. E. and Nesselroade, J. R. (1990). Genetic influence on life events during the last half of the life span. *Psychol Aging, 5*, 25–30.

Plomin, R., McClearn, G. E., Pedersen, N., Nesselroade, J. R., and Bergeman, C. S. (1988). Genetic influence on childhood family environment perceived retrospectively from the last half of the life span. *Dev Psychol, 24*, 738–745.

Plomin, R., McClearn, G. E., Pedersen, N., Nesselroade, J. R., and Bergeman , C. S. (1989). Genetic influence on adult's ratings of their current family environment. *J Marriage Fam, 51*, 791–803.

Prom-Wormley, E. C., Eaves, L. J., Foley, D. L., Gardner, C. O., Archer, K. J. et al (2009). Monoamine oxidase A and childhood adversity as risk factors for conduct disorder in females. *Psychol Med, 39*, 579–590.

Pruessner, M., Hellhammer, D. H., Pruessner, J. C., and Lupien, S. J. (2003). Self-reported depressive symptoms and stress levels in health young men: associations with the cortisol response to awakening. *Psychosom Med, 65*, 92–99.

Rankinen, T., Rice, T., Leon, A. S., Skinner, J. S., Wilmore, J. H. et al (2002). G protein β3 polymorphism and hemodynamic and body composition phenotypes in the HERITAGE family study. *Physiol Genom 8*, 151–157.

Rao, F., Zhang, L., Wessel, J., Zhang, K., Wen, G. et al (2008). Adrenergic polymorphism and the human stress response. *Ann NY Acad Sci, 1148*, 282–296.

Raynor, D. A., Pogue-Geile, M. F., Kamarck, T. W., McCaffery, J. M., and Manuck, S. B. (2002). Covariation of psychosocial characteristics associated with cardiovascular disease: genetic and environmental influences. *Psychosom Med, 64*, 191–203.

Reist, C., Mazzanti, C., Vu, R., Tran, D., and Goldman, D. (2001). Serotonin transporter promoter polymorphism is associated with attenuated prolactive response to fenfluramine. *Am J Med Genet, 105*, 363–368.

Risch, N., Herrell, R., Lehner, T., Liang, K. Y., Eaves, L. et al (2009). Interaction between the serotonin transporter gene (5-HTTLPR), stressful life events, and risk of depression: a meta-analysis. *JAMA, 301*, 2462–2471.

Saudino, K. J., Pedersen, N. L., Lichtenstein, P., McClearn, G. E., and Plomin, R. (1997). Can personality explain genetic influences on life events? *J Pers Soc Psychol, 72*, 196–206.

Schlotz, W., Hellhammer, D. H., Schulz, P., and Stone, A. A. (2004). Perceived work overload and chronic worrying predict weekend-weekday differences in cortisol awakening response. *Psychosom Med, 66*, 207–214.

Schnoll, R. A., Johnson, T. A., and Lerman, C. (2007). Genetics of smoking behavior. Curr *Psychiatry Rep, 9*, 349–357.

Shioe, K., Ichimiya, T., Suhara, T., Takano, A., Sudo, Y. et al (2003). No association between genotype of the promoter region of serotonin transporter gene and serotonin transporter binding in human brain measured by PET. *Synapse, 48*, 184–188.

Sibille, E., and Lewis, D. A. (2006). SERT-ainly involved in depression, but when? *Am J Psychiatry, 163*, 1–3.

Siegrist, J., Starke, D., Chandola, T., godin, I., Marmot, M. et al (2004). The measurement of effort-reward imbalance at work: European comparisons. *Soc Sci Med, 58*, 1483–1499.

Snieder, H., Harshfield, G. A., Barbeau, P., Pollock, D. M., Pollock, J. S., et al (2002). Dissecting the genetic architecture of the cardiovascular and renal stress response. *Biol Psychol, 61*, 73–95.

Spotts, E. L., Neiderhiser, J. M., Towers, S. H., Hansson, K., Lichtenstein, P. et al (2004). Genetic and environmental influences on marital relationships. *J Fam Psychol, 18*, 107–118.

Stein, M. B., Jang, K. L., Taylor, S., Vernon, P. A., and Livesley, W. J. (2002). Genetic and environmental influences. *Am J Psychiatry, 159*, 1675–1681.

Steptoe, A., van Jaarsveld, C. H. M., Semmler, C., Plomin, R., and Wardle, J. (2009). Heritability of daytime cortisol levels and cortisol reactivity in children. *Psychoneuroendocrinology, 34*, 273–280.

Stubbe, J. H., Boomsma, D. I., Vink, J. M., Cornes, B. K., Martin, H. G. et al (2006). Genetic influences on exercise participation in 37,051 twin pairs from seven countries. *PLos One 1*, e22.

Tai, E. S., Corella, D., Deurenberg-Yap, Cutter, J., Chew, S. K. et al (2003). Dietary fat interacts with the -514C>T polymorphism in the hepatic lipase gene promoter on plasma lipid profiles in a multiethnic Asian population: The 1998 Singapore National Health Survey. *J Nutr, 133*, 3399–3409.

Talmud, P. J. (2004). How to identify gene–environment interactions in a multifactorial disease: CHD as an example. *Proc Nutr Soc, 63*, 5–10.

Talmud, P. J., Bujac, S. R., Hall, S., Miller, G. J., and Humphries, S. E. (2000). Substitution of asparagines for aspartic acid at residue 9 (D9N) of lipoprotein lipase markedly augments risk of ischaemic heart disease in male smokers. *Atherosclerosis, 149*, 75–81.

Taylor, A., and Kim-Cohen, J. (2007). Meta-analysis of gene–environment interactions in developmental psychopathology. *Dev Psychopathol, 19*, 1029–1037.

Thapar, A., and McGuffin, P. (1996). Genetic influences on life events in childhood. *Psychol Med, 26*, 1675–1681.

Thase, M. E. (2009). Neurobiological aspects of depression. In I. H. Gotlib & C. L. Hammen (Eds.), *Handbook of Depression, 2nd Ed.* (pp. 187–217). New York: Guildford.

Theorell, T., and Karasek, R. A. (1996). Current issues relating to psychosocial job strain and cardiovascular disease research. *J Occup Health Psychol, 1*, 9–26.

Turner, R. J., and Wheaton, B. (1995). Checklist measurement of stressful life events. In S. Cohen, R. C. Kessler, & L. U. Gordon (Eds.), *Measuring Stress* (pp. 29–58). New York: Oxford University Press.

Tyrka, A. R., Price, L. H., Gelernter, J., Schepker, C., Anderson, G. M. et al (2009). Interaction of childhood maltreatment with the corticotrophin-releasing hormone receptor gene: effects on hypothalamic-pituitary-adrenal axis reactivity. *Biol Psychiatry, 66*, 681–685.

Uher, R., and McGuffin, P. (2008). The moderation by the serotonin transporter gene of environmental adversity in the aetiology of mental illness: review and methodological analysis. *Mol Psychiatry, 13*, 131–146.

Uher, R., and McGuffin, P. (2010). The moderation by the serotonin transporter gene of environmental adversity in the etiology of depression: 2009 update. *Mol Psychiatry, 15*, 18–22.

Van Dyck, C. H., Malison, R. T., Staley, J. K., Jacobsen, L. K., Seibyl, J. P. et al (2004). Central serotonin transporter availability measures with $[^{123}I]\beta$-CIT SPECT in relation to serotonin transporter genotype. *Am J Psychiatry, 161*, 525–531.

Wallace, A. J., Mann, J. I., Sutherland, W. H. F., Williams, S., Chisholm, A. et al (2000). Variants in the cholesterol ester transfer protein and lipoprotein lipase genes are predictors of plasma cholesterol response to dietary change. *Atherosclerosis, 152*, 327–336.

Weder, N., Yang, B. Z., Douglas-Palumberi, H., Massey, J., Krystal, J. H. et al (2009). MAOA genotype, maltreatment, and aggressive behavior: the changing impact of genotype at varying levels of trauma. *Biol Psychiatry, 65*, 417–424.

Whale, R., Quested, D. J., Laver, D., Harrison, P. J., and Cowen, P. J. (2000). Serotonin transporter (5-HTT) promoter genotype may influence the prolactin response to clomipramine. *Psychopharmacology, 150*, 120–122.

Wierzbicki, M. (1989). Twins' responses to pleasant, unpleasant, and life events. *J Genet Psychol, 150*, 135–145.

Williams, R. B., Marchuk, D. A., Gadde, K. M., Barefoot, J. C., Grichnik, K. et al (2001). Central nervous system serotonin function and cardiovascular responses to stress. *Psychosom Med, 63*, 300–305.

Williams, R. B., Marchuk, D. A., Siegler, I. C., Barefoot, J. C., Helms, M. J. et al (2008). Childhood socioeconomic status and serotonin transporter gene polymorphism enhance cardiovascular reactivity to mental stress. *Psychosom Med, 70*, 32–39.

Wu, T., Snieder, H., and de Geus, E. (in press). Genetic influences on cardiovascular stress reactivity. *Neurosci Biobeh Rev*

Wust, S., Federenko, I., Hellhammer, D.H., and Kirschbaum, C. (2000). Genetic factors, perceived chronic stress, and the free cortisol response to awakening. *Psychoneuroendocrinology, 25*, 707–720.

Wust, S., van Rossum, E. F. C., Federenko, I. S., Koper, J. W., Kumsta, R. et al (2004). Common polymorphisms in the glucocorticoid receptor gene are associated with adrenocortical responses to psychosocial stress. *J Clin Endocrinol Metab, 89*, 565–573.

Yu, S. F., Zhou, W. H., Jiang, K. Y., Gu, G. Z., and Wang, S. (2008). Job stress, gene polymorphism of beta2-AR, and prevalence of hypertension. *Biomed Environ Sci, 21*, 239–246.

Zhou, Z., Zhu, G., Hariri, A. R., Enoch, M.-A., Scott, D. et al (2008). Genetic variation in human *NPY* expression affects stress response and emotion. *Nature, 452*, 997–1002.

Chapter 32

Nicotine Dependence and Pharmacogenetics

Riju Ray, Robert Schnoll, and Caryn Lerman

1 Introduction

1.1 The Magnitude of the Problem

Nicotine dependence is among the most significant worldwide public health problems with approximately 1 billion current smokers worldwide (WHO, 2008). In the United States, the decline in smoking rates witnessed over the past several decades has stalled and, currently, 20.8% of American adults are current smokers (CDC, 2004, 2006); even worse, the rates of tobacco use in developing nations are rising rapidly (WHO, 2008). It is predicted that tobacco-related mortality will affect as many as 500 million people across the world (Levine and Kendler, 2004; WHO, 2008). Cigarette smoking causes 80–90% of all lung cancer deaths and increases the risk of other cancers, as well as cardiovascular disease, lung disease, and infectious diseases (CDC, 2004). The economic burden of tobacco-related morbidity and mortality worldwide is estimated to be several hundred billion dollars every year (Guindon, 2006). The current available treatment options for nicotine dependence are nicotine replacement therapy (NRT; transdermal patch, spray, inhaler, gum, or lozenge), bupropion (Zyban®, GlaxoSmithKline) and varenicline (Chantix®,

C. Lerman (✉)
Department of Psychiatry, Tobacco Use Research Center, University of Pennsylvania, 3535 Market Street, Suite 4100, Philadelphia, PA 19104, USA
e-mail: clerman@mail.med.upenn.edu

Pfizer). However, the long-term quit rates associated with these treatment options is only about 20%, with the majority of smokers relapsing to smoking within 1 year (Schnoll and Lerman, 2006).

1.2 The Neurobiology of Nicotine Dependence

Animal research has demonstrated that nicotine exerts its reinforcing effects via the ventrostriatal pathway by increasing dopamine (DA) release in the nucleus accumbens and the prefrontal cortex (PFC), in a similar way as other drugs of abuse (Nestler, 2005). Nicotine binds to the neuronal $\alpha4\beta2$ nicotinic acetylcholine receptors (nAChRs) located on the dopaminergic cell bodies in the ventral tegmental area (VTA) (Mifsud et al, 1989). Stimulation of these nAChRs by nicotine produces a shift from tonic firing of dopaminergic neurons to burst firing, resulting in increases in DA levels in the nucleus accumbens (Grenhoff et al, 1986; Mansvelder et al, 2003; Nisell et al, 1994). The meso-limbic dopaminergic pathway is under the influence of other neurochemical modulators such as GABA-ergic interneurons (Kalivas, 1993) and GABA-ergic innervations from the nucleus accumbens (Walaas and Fonnum, 1980), both of which provide inhibitory control over DA neurons. In addition, glutamergic projections from the prefrontal cortex (PFC) (Sesack and Pickel, 1992) and cholinergic inputs from the tegmental pedunculopontine nucleus (TPP)

A. Steptoe (ed.), *Handbook of Behavioral Medicine*, DOI 10.1007/978-0-387-09488-5_32,
© Springer Science+Business Media, LLC 2010

(Chen et al, 2006) have stimulatory effects on DA firing in the VTA. The GABA-ergic neurons are predominantly α4β2 nAChR subtype (Klink et al, 2001) causing them to desensitize quickly, whereas the presynaptic nAChRs on the glutamergic terminals are mainly α7 nAChR subtype (Jones and Wonnacott, 2004), which are slower to desensitize (Mansvelder et al, 2002). Thus, with continuous nicotine exposure, the inhibitory GABA-ergic control is reduced while the positive glutamergic control increases, contributing to long-term plasticity of behavior. The α5 subunit can also combine with the α4 and β2 nAChR subunits, and the inclusion of the α5 subunit may increase conductance of the α4β2 receptors and cause a higher rate of desensitization (Ramirez-Latorre et al, 1996). Lastly, there is evidence of involvement of the endogenous opioid pathway in nicotine dependence as nicotine administration causes release of endogenous opioid peptides (e.g.,: β-endorphin) that binds to mu-opioid receptors (MOR), which are located on the GABA interneurons in the VTA (Davenport et al, 1990). This stimulation of the mu-opioid receptors also produces disinhibition of the GABA-ergic interneurons thereby increasing DA release in the nucleus accumbens (Bergevin et al, 2002).

2 Heritability of Nicotine Dependence

2.1 Smoking Initiation and Dependence

Several twin studies have demonstrated that there are strong genetic factors that contribute to smoking behavior (Hopfer et al, 2003; Li, 2003). Meta-analyses of twin studies suggest that 50–60% of the variability in smoking initiation is attributable to genetic factors (Li et al, 2003; Sullivan and Kendler, 1999; Vink et al, 2005). There is evidence to suggest that the heritability estimate for smoking initiation might be greater for males (Hamilton et al, 2006),

though the opposite has also been observed (Li et al, 2003). Adoption studies (that control for confounding factors) have demonstrated that adoptees raised in separate environments had a greater likelihood of being a current smoker if their biological siblings were smokers (OR = 3.2) or ex-smokers (OR = 2.6) (Osler et al, 2001). In addition, genetic factors account for 60–70% of the variability in smoking rate and level of nicotine dependence (Haberstick et al, 2007; True et al, 1999; Vink et al, 2005), with greater heritability among men (Hopfer et al, 2003). Osler and colleagues also demonstrated that an adoptee was twice as likely to be a heavy smoker if their biological sibling was also a heavy smoker (Osler et al, 2001).

2.2 Smoking Cessation and Persistence

Results from recent twin studies and a meta-analysis indicate that heritability estimates associated with smoking persistence range from 60 to 70% (Hamilton et al, 2006; Hardie et al, 2006; Sullivan and Kendler, 1999). Genetic factors also contribute significantly toward determining the results of cessation attempts and self-reported level of withdrawal symptoms (Xian et al, 2003), as well as the duration of cessation (Hardie et al, 2006). Adoptee smokers who had quit smoking had a three times greater odds that their biological siblings were ex-smokers as well (Osler et al, 2001).

3 Genetic Studies of Smoking Among Adolescents

3.1 Pharmacokinetic Candidate Genes

The primary enzyme responsible for breakdown of nicotine is cytochrome P450 2A6 (CYP2A6), which has several well-characterized variants that decrease enzymatic activity either partially or completely (http://www.imm.ki.se/ CYPalleles/cyp2a6.html). Studies have compared individuals with variants associated with slower nicotine metabolism (one or two copies of the null alleles (*CYP2A6*2* or *CYP2A6*4*), or with two copies of the reduced activity alleles (*CYP2A6*9* or *CYP2A6*12*)), intermediate nicotine metabolism (carriers of a single *CYP2A6*9* or *CYP2A6*12* allele), and normal nicotine metabolism (those with *CYP2A6*1* alleles) (Benowitz et al, 2006).

A few longitudinal studies of smoking adoption have examined associations with *CYP2A6* alleles. In a cross-sectional study, adolescents carrying the slow or reduced activity alleles of *CYP2A6* had an increased odds of being smokers at 18 years of age; however, no association was observed at 13–15 years (Huang et al, 2005). A second prospective study following 7th grade students in Montreal for 54 months demonstrated that the carriers of null alleles for *CYP2A6* genotype (*2 or *4) had significantly greater likelihood of progressing to tobacco dependence (Karp et al, 2006; O'Loughlin et al, 2004). However, findings differed in a recent study of smoking adoption among adolescents followed from 9th to 12th grade (Audrain-McGovern et al, 2007). Specifically, adolescents with *CYP2A6* genotypes associated with normal metabolism exhibited faster and steeper acceleration in nicotine dependence compared with slower metabolizers. Adolescents who were normal metabolizers also smoked more cigarettes at grade 12 compared to the slow metabolizers. The results reported by Audrain and colleagues (Audrain-McGovern et al, 2007) differ in direction of association from the prior studies (Huang et al, 2005; O'Loughlin et al, 2004). While the reason for the divergence in findings is not entirely clear, there were differences across studies in the age of samples (early to mid-adolescence vs. mid- to late adolescence), how nicotine dependence was measured (ICD-10 vs. mFTQ), analytic approaches (survival analysis vs. latent growth modeling), and the conceptualization of nicotine dependence (binary vs. continuous). For example, the earlier studies utilized a dichotomous measure of nicotine

dependence and Cox Proportional Hazards models (Karp et al, 2006; O'Loughlin et al, 2004), while the latter study (Audrain-McGovern et al, 2007) used latent growth modeling and a continuous measure. The Huang et al study used a cross-sectional study design and measured associations that also included never smokers; plus the adolescents in the age groups (18 years and 13–15 years) were different. The genotype groups between the studies also differed as slow metabolizers in the Audrain-McGovern study were adolescents with either one or two copies of the null variants or two copies of the decreased activity variants; the prior study only included individuals with one or two copies of the null variants in the slowest metabolizers group. Further, Audrain-McGovern and colleagues (2007) combined individuals with reduced activity (intermediate metabolizers, i.e., one copy of either *CYP2A6*9* or *CYP2A6*12*) or null activity (slowest metabolizers, i.e., one or two copies of inactive variants (*CYP2A6*2* and *CYP2A6*4*) or two copies of *CYP2A6*9* and/or *CYP2A6*12*) alleles into one group while the previous study (Karp et al, 2006; O'Loughlin et al, 2004) examined slow metabolizers based on the presence of null activity alleles (one or two copies of inactive variants *CYP2A6*2* and *CYP2A6*4*). Additional research will be required to fully understand the role of the *CYP2A6* gene in smoking adoption.

3.2 Pharmacodynamic Candidate Genes

3.2.1 Nicotinic Pathway Genes

The genes encoding the nAChR α5-α3-β4 subunits (*CHRNA5, CHRNA3, CHRNB4*) are located in a locus on chromosome 15q24 (Duga et al, 2001). Polymorphisms from the conserved region on this gene cluster and their haplotypes have been associated with an earlier age of tobacco initiation in a sample of young adults (ages 17–21) (Schlaepfer et al, 2008). An independent set or markers from the *CHRNA5-CHRNA3-CHRNB4* locus and their haplotypes have been associated with the severity of nicotine dependence if daily smoking was initiated by or before 16 years of age (Weiss et al, 2008). This genetic association was lost among the smokers who started daily smoking after 16 years of age pointing toward a link between haplotypes on this locus and early nicotine exposure. Ehringer et al (2007) observed that a SNP located upstream of the *CHRNB2* gene was associated with initial subjective response to tobacco, however, failed to observe any association of the *CHRNA4* gene and nicotine dependence among young adults.

3.2.2 Dopaminergic Pathway Genes

The neurotransmitter, dopamine, is considered to be centrally involved in nicotine addiction. Thus, several studies have examined the associations of smoking with members of the dopaminergic pathway among adolescents. The *ANKK1* gene, located upstream of the dopamine receptor 2 gene (*DRD2*), has a common variant referred to as Taq1A (rs1800497). This variant has been associated with nicotine dependence (Laucht et al, 2008), as well as smoking progression in adolescents, with each minor (A1, or T) allele doubling the odds of smoking progression (Audrain-McGovern et al, 2004). Another intronic SNP in *DRD2* has been associated with smoking progression among adolescents (Laucht et al, 2008). The dopamine receptor 4 (*DRD4*) has a 7-repeat functional polymorphism that decreases dopamine binding and blunts the intracellular response. Adolescents with the 7-repeat allele had a greater odds of lifetime smoking and initiated tobacco smoking at an earlier age (Laucht et al, 2008); however, a previous study observed these effects only among male smokers (Laucht et al, 2005). The dopamine transporter (*SLC6A3*), which transports extra-cellular dopamine out of the synapse, has a 40 bp functional repeat polymorphism, and the 9-repeat allele lowers transporter expression and protein levels. Young adults with the 9-repeat allele have a greater likelihood of being a non-smoker and

there is evidence of greater transmission of the 9-repeat allele among never and non-smokers (Timberlake et al, 2006). Conversely, adolescents who are homozygous for the 10-repeat allele smoke daily at an earlier age and express lower levels of interest in quitting (Laucht et al, 2008). The presence of both the *ANKK1* */T (Taq1A) allele and the *SLC6A3* 10-repeat allele is related to greater risk of smoking among adolescents who did not participate in team sports (Audrain-McGovern et al, 2006). Tyrosine hydroxylase (*TH*) is the rate-limiting step for DA synthesis and also has a functional repeat polymorphism that affects meso-limbic transmission. The 4-repeat allele (K4) at *TH* is protective against the development of nicotine dependence (Anney et al, 2004), as adolescents with K-4 allele have a threefold lower odds of developing nicotine dependence (Olsson et al, 2004).

3.2.3 Serotonergic Pathway Genes

The promoter region of the serotonin transporter has a repeat polymorphism (*5-HTTLPR*), and the short (S) form decreases the rate of transcription compared with the long (L) form. High-school students who were homozygous for the S-form were more likely to be smokers, have had an earlier onset of smoking behavior, and to be heavier smokers (Gerra et al, 2005). Skowronek et al (2006) observed an interaction between the *5-HTTLPR* and the *DRD4* 7-repeat polymorphism with smoking among adolescent girls (Skowronek et al, 2006); girls who did not possess the 7-repeat allele and were homozygous for the L allele at *5-HTTLPR* had the highest smoking activity (Skowronek et al, 2006).

4 Genetic Studies of Smoking Among Adults

4.1 Linkage Studies

Linkage studies help to identify susceptibility loci for nicotine dependence using polymorphic markers that are distributed across the entire genome. There have been several linkage studies from various populations that have been published in the literature. Here, we focus only on findings that have been successfully replicated. Linkage findings have been replicated on regions on chromosomes 9 (91.9–136.5 cM), 10 (62–158 cM), 11 (2–76.1 cM), and 17 (31.9–65 cM) (Li, 2008). The regions on these chromosomes have been associated with nicotine dependence in both Caucasian and African American populations in four or more independent studies (Li, 2008). These regions contain biologically relevant genes such as GABA-B receptor subunit 2 (*GABBR2*), neurotrophic tyrosine kinase receptor 2 (*NTRK2*), and Src homology domain-containing transforming protein C3 (*SHC3*), B-arrestin 1 (*ARRB1*), GABA-A receptor-associated protein (*GABARAP*), and Beta-arrestin 2 (*ARRB2*). Other chromosomes that have suggestive areas of linkage include chromosomes 1, 5, 10, 11, 12, 16, 20, and 22, but these findings have not been fully replicated possibly due to differences across studies in terms of sample size and ethnicity, density of markers, definition and assessment of the nicotine dependence phenotype, and statistical approaches used.

4.2 Pharmacokinetic Candidate Genes

Case–control association studies have documented significant associations between *CYP2A6* genotype and smoking status (Munafo et al, 2004). Individuals who were slow nicotine metabolizers were less likely to be smokers (Malaiyandi et al, 2005; Pianezza et al, 1998; Schoedel et al, 2004) and reported smoking fewer cigarettes per day (Kubota et al, 2006; Malaiyandi et al, 2006; Schoedel et al, 2004). Faster nicotine metabolizers had greater levels of nicotine dependence (Kubota et al, 2006; Malaiyandi et al, 2006), smoked their first cigarette of the day earlier in the day, and experienced greater nicotine withdrawal symptoms after a quit attempt (Kubota et al,

2006). In contrast, slow nicotine metabolizers had smoked for fewer years (Schoedel et al, 2004), were more likely to quit smoking (Gu et al, 2000), and were less likely to experience nicotine withdrawal symptoms after a quit attempt (Kubota et al, 2006). The lower rate of cigarette consumption among slow metabolizers is associated with lower plasma cotinine and lower expired breath carbon monoxide (CO) levels (Rao et al, 2000). These lower CO levels among slow metabolizers could be due to smoking fewer cigarettes per day or a decreased puff volume (Strasser et al, 2007). Methoxsalen, an inhibitor for CYP2A6 activity, has been shown to decrease smoking rate and desire to smoke (Sellers et al, 2000; Sellers et al, 2003). There is no evidence linking *CYP2B6* (which plays a minor role in nicotine metabolism) to nicotine dependence or self-reported smoking rate among treatment seeking smokers (Lee et al, 2007b).

4.3 Pharmacodynamic Candidate Genes

4.3.1 Nicotinic Pathway Genes

Several recent studies have identified and replicated associations between markers in the *CHRNA5-A3-B4* gene cluster and nicotine dependence. A large genome wide and candidate gene association study simultaneously identified a non-synonymous SNP (rs16969968) located on *CHRNA5* associated with nicotine dependence (Bierut et al, 2007; Saccone et al, 2007). In vitro and binding studies have demonstrated that this polymorphism causes a decrease in transcription level of the *CHRNA5* gene (Wang et al, 2008a) and dampens response of the receptor to a nicotine agonist (Bierut et al, 2008). Subsequent studies have identified other markers on this *CHRNA5-A3-B4* gene cluster associated with nicotine dependence (Berrettini et al, 2008; Bierut et al, 2008; Chen et al, 2009; Saccone et al, 2009; Sherva et al, 2008; Spitz et al, 2008; Thorgeirsson et al, 2008), cigarettes per day (Caporaso et al, 2009), and susceptibility to heavy smoking (Stevens et al, 2008). A separate study reported no association between the *CHRNA5-A3-B4* cluster and ability to quit smoking, suggesting that smoking cessation and nicotine dependence have different genetic influences (Breitling et al, 2008). Other neuronal nicotinic receptor genes that have been associated with nicotine dependence are *CHRNB3* (Bierut et al, 2007; Saccone et al, 2007), *CHRNA4* (Hutchison et al, 2007; Li et al, 2005), *CHRNB1* (Lou et al, 2006; Saccone et al, 2009), and *CHRNA6* (Hoft et al, 2009). Polymorphisms on the *CHRNB3* gene also have been associated with number of quit attempts (Hoft et al, 2009).

4.3.2 Dopaminergic Pathway Genes

Associations between dopaminergic genes and nicotine dependence have been evaluated in several studies. The *ANKK1* gene has been associated with nicotine dependence (Gelernter et al, 2006). However, associations of the common Taq1A (T) allele, described above, with smoking behavior have not been consistent (Bierut et al, 2000; Comings et al, 1996; Johnstone et al, 2004a; Radwan et al, 2007); association of this polymorphism with smoking behavior was also not confirmed in a meta-analysis (Munafo et al, 2009b). Another functional variant (rs2734849) located in the c-terminal of *ANKK1* has been associated with nicotine dependence in an African-American population (Huang et al, 2009). Dopamine receptor 3 (*DRD3*) has a functional non-synonymous polymorphism that has been associated with nicotine dependence (Huang et al, 2008b) and time to first cigarette and heaviness of smoking index (Vandenbergh et al, 2007) among Caucasians. Individual SNPs and a 3-SNP haplotype on the dopamine receptor 1 (*DRD1*) have also been associated with measures of nicotine dependence in an African-American population (Huang et al, 2008a). Results linking the *SLC6A3* repeat polymorphism with smoking have been mixed (Lerman et al, 1999; Vandenbergh et al, 2002).

The catechol *o*-methyl transferase enzyme (*COMT*) is responsible for the breakdown of DA in the brain and a common Val/Met polymorphism affects enzymatic activity. The Val (high activity) allele has been associated with nicotine dependence (Redden et al, 2005) and smoking persistence amongst Caucasian women (Colilla et al, 2005). In addition, several studies have confirmed the relationship of the *COMT* Val allele with risk of smoking relapse (Johnstone et al, 2007; Munafo et al, 2008). Other studies, however, have failed to observe any associations with the Val/Met polymorphism and smoking status (David et al, 2002; McKinney et al, 2000).

Dopamine decarboxylase (*DDC*) is involved in the synthesis of DA; several SNPs and their haplotypes on *DDC* have been associated with nicotine dependence in both Caucasians and African-American populations (Ma et al, 2005; Yu et al, 2006; Zhang et al, 2006a). Individuals with the *DRD4* 7-repeat allele had a greater risk for smoking (only among African-Americans) (Shields et al, 1998) and greater craving symptoms and attention to smoking cues (Hutchison et al, 2002). Depressed smokers homozygous with the *DRD4* S allele were more likely to smoke for self-medication purposes (stimulation and negative affect reduction) (Lerman et al, 1998). Other dopaminergic genes that have been associated with smoking are the *MAO-A* (monoamine oxidase A), VNTR (Wiesbeck et al, 2006), and *TPH1* and *TPH2* (tryptophan hydroxylase 1 and 2) (Reuter et al, 2007).

4.3.3 Serotonergic Pathway Genes

The L allele (greater transcription) at the *5-HTTLPR* was more common among current smokers vs. never smokers (Ishikawa et al, 1999; Kremer et al, 2005); however, subsequent studies have failed to observe any association between the *5-HTTLPR* polymorphism and smoking behavior (Rasmussen et al, 2008; Trummer et al, 2006). Two studies also observed that the interaction between the S allele at the *5-HTTLPR* locus and neuroticism was positively correlated with smoking behavior (Hu et al, 2000; Lerman et al, 2000).

4.3.4 Endogenous Opioid Pathway Genes

The endogenous opioid system underlies the development and persistence of nicotine dependence. The reduced activity allele (G) at the functional A118G polymorphism on the mu-opioid receptor gene (*OPRM1*) has been associated with level of nicotine dependence (Schinka et al, 2002). Another study observed that a 3-SNP haplotype (lacking the A118G polymorphism) on *OPRM1* was associated with risk for smoking initiation but only marginally associated with level of nicotine dependence (Zhang et al, 2006b). In a human laboratory study, the *OPRM1* A118G was associated with nicotine reward and self-administration via smoking (Ray et al, 2006). Haplotypes on two genes, β-arrestin 1 (*ARRB1*) and β-arrestin 2 (*ARRB2*), that interact and regulate the trafficking of the mu-opioid receptors, have been associated with nicotine dependence among Caucasians (Sun et al, 2008).

4.3.5 GABA-ergic Pathway

The GABA-ergic system plays an important role in controlling the DA levels in the meso-limbic system, suggesting that genes in this pathway may influence smoking phenotypes. Several SNPs located on GABA type A receptor subunit 4 (*GABRA4*) and subunit 2 (*GABRA2*) have been associated with nicotine dependence at a single-marker and haplotype level (Agrawal et al, 2008, 2009). The GABA-A receptor-associated protein (*GABARAP*) has been linked to measures of nicotine dependence in a Caucasian sample (Lou et al, 2007). Significant associations between SNPs on the GABA type B receptor subunit 2 (GABA-B2) and smoking have been observed in Caucasian and African-American populations (Beuten et al, 2005a).

4.3.6 Miscellaneous Genes

Genome wide association studies (GWAS) examining markers across the entire human genome have nominated several genes that are involved in cell adhesion, intra-cellular signaling, transcription regulators, and molecules that regulate DNA, RNA, and proteins (Bierut et al, 2007; Uhl et al, 2008). Src homology 2 domain-containing transforming protein C3 (*SHC3*) lies within the region containing a linkage peak on chromosome 9. SNP and haplotype analyses of markers on *SHC3* are associated with nicotine dependence in both Caucasians and African-Americans and account for 40–59% of the signal from the linkage peak on chromosome 9 (Li et al, 2007). Neurexin-1 (*NRXN-1*), which plays a key role in synaptogenesis and synaptic maintenance, has been associated with nicotine dependence from a GWAS (Bierut et al, 2007) and a candidate gene (Nussbaum et al, 2008) study. A functional (Val66Met) polymorphism on the brain-derived neurotrophic factor (*BDNF*) gene predisposes individuals to initiate and maintain smoking (Lang et al, 2007), and a haplotype that lacks the functional SNP has a gender-specific association with nicotine dependence among Caucasians (Beuten et al, 2005b). Other genes that have been associated with nicotine dependence include the cannabinoid receptor 1 (*CNR-1*) (Chen et al, 2008b), neurotrophic tyrosine kinase receptor 2 (*NTRK2*) (Beuten et al, 2007b), protein phosphatase 1 regulatory subunit 1B (*PPP1R1B*) (Beuten et al, 2007a), Rho GTPAase (*RHOA*) (Chen et al, 2007), and amyloid precursor protein-binding protein family B member 1 (*APBB1*) (Chen et al, 2008a).

5 Pharmacogenetic Studies of Nicotine Replacement Therapy

5.1 Pharmacokinetic Candidate Genes

Studies have examined the role of variability in nicotine metabolism on treatment outcome after NRT. Treatment seeking smokers who were slow metabolizers (carriers of one null allele or two reduced activity alleles of the *CYP2A6* gene) had significantly greater levels of plasma nicotine from the nicotine patch than normal metabolizers, despite equivalent rates of patch usage between both groups (Malaiyandi et al, 2006). In addition, fast metabolizers used the nicotine nasal spray more to obtain equal levels of plasma nicotine, compared to slow metabolizers (Malaiyandi et al, 2006). In a separate trial, the rate of nicotine metabolism estimated using the phenotypic marker of CYP2A6 activity (3-hydroxycotinine/cotinine or nicotine metabolite ratio; NMR) predicted quitting success using the nicotine patch (Lerman et al, 2006b). Among individuals who used the nicotine patch, there was a 30% drop in the odds of remaining abstinent with each increasing quartile of the metabolite ratio (measured in quartiles) (Lerman et al, 2006b). There was no association of the nicotine metabolite ratio with smoking cessation in the nasal spray arm of this study, which may be explained by the greater variability in nasal spray use (Lerman et al, 2006b). Further, the CYP2A6 genotype data from this trial (Malaiyandi et al, 2006) indicated that the normal metabolizers had significantly greater usage of the nasal spray than the slow metabolizers, suggesting that this variability in use is related to metabolism rate. The association of nicotine metabolism rate and smoking cessation was replicated in an open-label nicotine patch study with participants in the first quartile for nicotine metabolite ratio (slow metabolizers) more likely to be abstinent vs. those in the other three quartiles (Schnoll et al, 2009). The nicotine metabolite ratio also predicted abstinence at 6-month follow-up, indicating that nicotine metabolism rate may influence quitting success independent of treatment (Lerman et al, 2006b). There was no effect of CYP2B6 genotype on quit rates after NRT (Lee et al, 2007b).

5.2 Pharmacodynamic Candidate Genes

5.2.1 Nicotinic Pathway Genes

A functional polymorphism on the CHRNA4 gene (rs2236196) has been associated with response to NRT (Hutchison et al, 2007).

Compared to participants with a TC genotype at this SNP locus, participants in other genotype groups were more likely to be abstinent on the nicotine nasal spray, but not the nicotine patch (Hutchison et al, 2007).

5.2.2 Dopaminergic Pathway Genes

The ANKK1 T allele was associated with greater response to the nicotine patch among women (Yudkin et al, 2004), as well as individuals who had the A/* genotype for dopamine beta-hydroxylase (DBH) (Johnstone et al, 2004b). However, these findings were not confirmed in a larger cohort study (Munafo et al, 2009a). Two functional polymorphisms on DRD2 (-141 Ins/DelC & C957T) were tested for association with response to NRT. At the end of treatment participants homozygous for the DelC allele had a more favorable response to NRT (Lerman et al, 2006a); and, there was evidence for an interaction between this polymorphism and a dopamine receptor interacting gene (FREQ) for predicting abstinence after NRT (Dahl et al, 2006). For the C957T polymorphism, participants possessing the C/* allele were more likely to be abstinent after NRT regardless of treatment form (patch vs. spray) (Lerman et al, 2006a). The Met/Met (low activity) COMT genotype group was associated with greater likelihood of abstinence with nicotine patch (Johnstone et al, 2007; Munafo et al, 2008) and a threefold increase in quitting success in women regardless of NRT form (patch vs. spray) (Colilla et al, 2005). The DRD4 7-repeat allele has been associated with lower abstinence rates on the nicotine patch (David et al, 2008), while no effect on abstinence was observed for the –521 promoter polymorphism located on DRD4 (Munafo et al, 2006b). Smokers carrying the 9-repeat allele for the SLC6A3 VNTR were more likely to be abstinent than individuals that possessed the 10/10 genotype (O'Gara et al, 2007; Stapleton et al, 2007).

5.2.3 Serotonergic Pathway Genes

The 5-HTTLPR VNTR repeat polymorphism has not demonstrated any pharmacogenetic associations with NRT in two published studies (David et al, 2007b; Munafo et al, 2006a).

5.2.4 Endogenous Opioid Pathway Genes

The *OPRM1* gene has been associated with NRT treatment outcome in two studies. The first study observed that the G allele at the A118G locus was associated with better quit rates on the nicotine patch, quicker recoveries from a cigarette lapse, significant decline in negative mood symptoms during the first two weeks of abstinence, and lower weight gain compared to A/A genotype individuals (Lerman et al, 2004). The second study observed an opposite finding in that participants with the A/A genotype had higher quit rates on nicotine patch, compared with placebo, with no difference in quit rates on either nicotine patch or placebo for the */G allele participants (Munafo et al, 2007). However, when these results were examined by gender, female participants with the */G allele were more likely to quit on nicotine patch compared to placebo patch (Munafo et al, 2007). Further, the discrepancy between the two studies could be due to the fact that the latter study (Munafo et al, 2007) was able to only collect genetic information retrospectively on 50% of the original population that participated in the clinical trial whereas Lerman and colleagues collected genotype data prospectively on all participants in their study; partial ascertainment in a genetic study can contribute bias. Additional reasons for the opposing findings could be the differing ancestries of the two populations tested; however, the similar minor allele frequencies across the populations argue against this. The two studies also differ in terms of study design as all the study population studied by Lerman and colleagues received NRT (patch vs. spray) while the population studied by Munafo and colleagues compared active NRT (i.e., nicotine patch) to placebo treatment. Lastly, the differing findings between one or both studies could be reflective of a type 1 error. Mu-opioid receptor interacting proteins *ARRB2* and protein kinase-c inhibiting proteins (*HINT1*) did not show any evidence for interaction with *OPRM1* genotype and quitting success on NRT (Ray et al, 2007a).

6 Pharmacogenetic Studies of Bupropion

6.1 Pharmacokinetic Candidate Genes

The NMR phenotypic marker of CYP2A6 activity was recently examined in a placebo-controlled bupropion study (Patterson et al, 2008). The results indicated that there was a dose–response effect of nicotine metabolism in the placebo arm in terms of quit rates at the end of treatment. Specifically, the quit rates across the NMR quartiles for those in the placebo group, from slowest to fastest metabolizer, were 32, 25, 20, and 10%. In contrast, bupropion increased the quit rate for the fastest metabolizers (4th quartile) to 34% at the end of treatment. Thus, there was a significant interaction effect between NMR status and treatment group, indicating a significant benefit from bupropion for the fast metabolizers and no incremental benefit for the slow metabolizers.

The CYP2B6 enzyme is the primary enzyme involved in the metabolism of bupropion to its metabolites and the *CYP2B6*5 (C1459T) variant has been associated with reduced bupropion metabolism. In a placebo-controlled clinical trial of bupropion, smokers with one or two *CYP2B6*5 T alleles who received placebo reported higher levels of abstinence-induced cravings and were less likely to be abstinent at the end of treatment (Lerman et al, 2002). Bupropion helped to overcome this increased relapse risk among female carriers of the T allele at the end of treatment, with quit rates for bupropion for female T allele carriers of 54%, compared to 15% for female T allele carriers on placebo (Lerman et al, 2002). The T allele at *CYP2B6*5 also moderated the effect of the *ANKK1* polymorphism on abstinence in a placebo-controlled bupropion trial (David et al, 2007a). The *CYP2B6*6 (G516T and A785G) polymorphism has also been found to be associated with response to bupropion, although this effect is driven by a poorer placebo response in the *6 group (Lee et al, 2007a).

6.2 Pharmacodynamic Candidate Genes

6.2.1 Nicotinic Pathway Genes

A Bayesian analysis nominated SNPs located in the *CHRNA5, CHRNA2*, and *CHAT* (choline acetyltransferase) genes as potential pharmacogenetic associations with bupropion response (Heitjan et al, 2007). A system-based genetic approach also identified a SNP located on 3′ untranslated region of *CHRNB2* as a potential pharmacogenetic correlate of smoking cessation with bupropion among smokers that possessed the wild-type allele (Conti et al, 2008).

6.2.2 Dopaminergic Pathway Candidate Genes

In contrast to the findings with NRT, a pharmacogenetic analysis of response to bupropion indicated that participants with the *ANKK1* C/C genotype had a greater reduction in cravings and higher quit rates with bupropion treatment (David et al, 2007a; David et al, 2007c). Individuals with the */T allele did not report reductions in their withdrawal symptoms with bupropion (David et al, 2003) and had a greater likelihood of withdrawing from treatment due to side effects, although these effects were only found among female participants (Swan et al, 2005). Participants with the *ANKK1* */T allele receiving bupropion were more likely to be non-abstinent at the end of the treatment if they were lacking the *SLC6A3* 9-repeat allele (Swan et al, 2007). In a separate placebo-controlled bupropion trial, individuals with the C/C genotype at *ANKK1* and 9-repeat allele for *SLC6A3* VNTR were more likely to be abstinent regardless

of treatment assignment (Lerman et al, 2003). Smokers that were homozygous for the InsC allele at the *DRD2* -141 locus had a more favorable response to bupropion treatment, compared to smokers with the DelC allele (Lerman et al, 2006a). Though the *COMT* Val/Met was not associated with bupropion treatment response, a haplotype comprising two *COMT* SNPs was associated with higher quit rates with bupropion, compared to placebo (Berrettini et al, 2007).

6.3 Summary of Pharmacogenetic Findings

Consistent associations with smoking cessation have been observed for genotypic and phenotypic measures of variation in nicotine metabolism (Lerman et al, 2006b; Malaiyandi et al, 2006; Patterson et al, 2008; Schnoll et al, 2009). Findings for association of the *COMT* val158met polymorphism with response to nicotine patch therapy are also largely consistent, suggesting that smokers who carry the val allele have a greater risk for relapse (Colilla et al, 2005; Johnstone et al, 2007; Munafo et al, 2008). Findings for association of *OPRM1* with smoking cessation warrant further attention.

Although associations of the *CHRNA5-A3-B4* gene cluster with nicotine dependence have been replicated in several studies (Bierut et al, 2008; Saccone et al, 2007; Thorgeirsson et al, 2008), evidence for association with smoking cessation is not consistent across studies (Baker et al, 2009; Breitling et al, 2008; Conti et al, 2008).

7 Genetic Studies of Nicotine Dependence Endophenotypes

7.1 Genetic Associations with Nicotine Reward

The relative reinforcing value of nicotine can be evaluated using the cigarette choice paradigm. In this procedure, participants are given the opportunity to choose between smoking a regular nicotine cigarette vs. a denicotinized cigarette, but they are blinded as to which cigarette contains nicotine. Female participants with the low-activity (G or Asn40) allele at the *OPRM1* gene showed reduced reinforcement from cigarettes in this paradigm since they chose equally between the nicotine and the denicotinized cigarette (Ray et al, 2006). Individuals with the G allele were also less likely to distinguish between either cigarette based on self-report measures of satisfaction and strength (Ray et al, 2006). In a separate trial, haplotypes on the cyclic AMP binding protein 1 (*CREB1*) interacted with *OPRM1* genotype to effect nicotine reward; specifically, while the *CREB1* genotype had little effect on nicotine reinforcement between naltrexone and placebo for those with the *OPRM1* G allele, there was a reduction in the reinforcing value of smoking (i.e., fewer puffs from the nicotine cigarette) for those homozygous for the OPRM1 A allele and possessing *CREB1* rs2551640 A/A genotypes (Ray et al, 2007b).

7.2 Genetic Associations with Nicotine Sensitivity

Nicotine sensitivity was tested by administering nicotine nasal spray to non-smokers and recording self-reported mood changes. Individuals with the *DRD4* 7-repeat allele reported higher levels of aversive reactions to nicotine exposure as well as reduced nicotine choice (Perkins et al, 2008a). Men with the TT genotype at *DRD2* C957T had greater subjective effects after nasal spray administration (Perkins et al, 2008a). In a separate study, the non-synonymous SNP located on *CHRNA5*, which has been linked with nicotine dependence, was associated with self-reported pleasurable rush or 'buzz' during the first cigarette of the day (Sherva et al, 2008). Two polymorphisms on *CHRNB3* also have been associated with subjective responses to initial tobacco use among adolescents (Zeiger et al,

2008). A functional SNP on *CHRNA4* has been associated with nicotine sensitivity with smokers possessing the TC genotype, compared to the CC genotype, reporting increased physiological and cognitive effects after smoking a single high-nicotine (1.1 mg) cigarette (Hutchison et al, 2007).

7.3 Genetic Associations with Mood-Related Measures

There has been limited research investigating the effects of genetic variants on smoking-related changes in mood states. A recent study published by Perkins and colleagues (2008b) observed that cigarette liking was greater during negative vs. positive mood induction among participants that had the *ANKK1* */T allele and the *OPRM1* AA genotype. Latency to first puff was significantly shorter after negative vs. positive mood induction among smokers with the SLC6A3 9-repeat allele and the *ANKK1* */T allele (Perkins et al, 2008b). Individuals with *SLC6A3* 9-repeat allele and the *DRD2* C957T CC genotype also took a greater number of puffs during negative vs. positive mood induction (Perkins et al, 2008b).

7.4 Genetic Associations with Smoking Phenotypes in Neuroimaging Studies

A recent PET study examined associations of dopaminergic gene variants with smoking-induced DA release using the radio-tracer [^{11}C]raclopride and observed that smokers carrying variants associated with reduced dopaminergic tone (i.e., *SLC6A3* 9-repeat allele, *DRD4* S allele, or the *COMT* Val/Val genotypes) had greater smoking-induced decreases in raclopride binding in the striatum, indicative of greater DA release in this region (Brody et al, 2006). A perfusion-MRI study after overnight abstinence found that genetic variants associated with reduced dopaminergic tone (*DRD2*-141

DelC variant and *COMT* Val/Val genotype) and increased endogenous opioid binding (*OPRM1* AA genotype) had greater regional abstinence-induced rCBF increases that may increase risk for relapse (Wang et al, 2008b). Jacobsen and colleagues (2006) investigated the association between the *DRD2* C957T polymorphism and brain activation during a working memory task called the N-back task following pretreatment with either nicotine or placebo patch. The N-back task requires responses based on certain rules if the current stimulus is identical to the stimuli that have appeared previously. For example in the 1-back condition the participant is required to respond if the stimulus on the screen is identical to the one that appeared right before the current one. The task is progressively more difficult as the participant has to keep in their working memory stimuli that have appeared 2 (2-back) or 3 (3-back) times before the current one, increasing their working memory load (Loughead et al, 2009). Carriers of the 957T allele had greater activation during the most challenging condition of the task in the left anterior insula, left cerebellum, right and middle occipital gyri, right fusiform, and the right middle temporal gyrus while they were on the nicotine patch. Conversely, individuals with the *DRD2* 957 C/C genotype showed decreased activation in these areas on the nicotine patch. This difference by genotype could be due to imbalances in levels of dopamine among participants with the */T allele after nicotine patch administration (Jacobsen et al, 2006). A subsequent study examined the effects of *COMT* genotype on abstinence-induced cognitive deficits using a visual N-back task (Loughead et al, 2009). During abstinence the Val/Val homozygotes had lower activation in the bilateral dorsolateral prefrontal cortices and medial prefrontal cortex while they performed the toughest condition of the task, compared to the other genotype groups. The Val/Val homozygotes also had slower reaction times during this condition of the N-back task (Loughead et al, 2009). Abstinence-induced cognitive deficits in the Val/Val group may contribute to the greater relapse risk observed in this group (Colilla et al, 2005). McClernon

and colleagues (2007) observed an association between the *DRD4* VNTR and smoking cue-reactivity; individuals with the longer-repeat alleles had greater BOLD (blood oxygen-level dependent) activation to the smoking cues in the right superior frontal gyrus and the right insula (McClernon et al, 2007).

8 Conclusions and Future Directions

This review highlights the important role of genetics as one factor in determining the acquisition of smoking, the transition to nicotine dependence, and response to standard smoking cessation pharmacotherapies. The genetic studies examining associations with pharmacokinetic and pharmacodynamic targets of nicotine add support to the basic understanding of the neurobiology of nicotine dependence.

8.1 Nicotine Dependence

In studies of adolescent smoking, associations of the *ANKK1* Taq1A and *SLC6A3* repeat polymorphism and smoking acquisition are suggestive. However, there is also evidence that environmental factors moderate this effect. Evidence for association of *CYP2A6* with smoking progression in adolescents is not completely consistent and requires further research to clarify.

In studies of adult smokers, there is strong evidence linking the *CYP2A6* gene with nicotine dependence, with fast metabolizers being at greater risk for developing dependence. There is also substantial evidence linking the *CHRNA5-A3-B4* gene cluster to nicotine dependence in several different populations. The dopaminergic system is thought to play a key role in the experience of nicotine reward, and this is supported by some genetic evidence for associations of nicotine dependence with the *ANKK1* gene. Associations of the *DRD4*, *COMT*, and *OPRM1* genes with nicotine dependence remain suggestive and additional studies are needed to confirm these results. Inconsistent results across these studies could be due to variability across studies in terms of sex, race, and additional undiscovered genetic variants.

8.2 Smoking Cessation

The phenotypic marker for CYP2A6 activity, the nicotine metabolite ratio, is differentially associated with treatment response to both NRT and bupropion. These findings suggest that slower metabolizers derive greater nicotine from a standard dose of nicotine patch and have greater success with this treatment, compared to faster metabolizers. Alternatively, bupropion is an effective medication with efficacy for this risk group. Thus, one mechanism is likely to focus on the reduced dose of treatment achieved from nicotine replacement products in the slow vs. fast metabolizers, while bupropion targets a different neurobiological mechanism (dopaminergic system). The CYP2B6 enzyme is responsible for bupropion metabolism, and polymorphisms that are known to decrease CYP2B6 activity have been associated with a more favorable treatment response with bupropion across studies.

The *COMT* val158met polymorphism has been related to success with nicotine replacement therapy in independent studies. Nicotine increases dopamine release and genetic differences in brain dopamine levels are one plausible mechanism for this genetic association. The val allele is the high-activity allele associated with increased enzyme and decreased brain dopamine levels (Chen et al, 2004), as well as with dopamine release following smoking. Associations of other genes, such as *OPRM1*, with smoking cessation and treatment response are suggestive and warrant further attention.

8.3 Future Directions

Moving forward, pharmacogenetic studies that prospectively randomize participants based on

genotype should be conducted in order to replicate the 'retrospective' findings obtained thus far in the context of treatment trials. Studies that investigate whether randomizing participants to different treatments based on nicotine metabolite ratio (as a pretreatment screening) increases smoking cessation rates would be a vital step toward extending the field from controlled clinical trials to clinical practice. Further, since varenicline is the most efficacious medication available, pharmacogenetic studies are needed to identify sub-groups of smokers who would benefit most from this treatment. Pharmacogenetic studies that focus on treatment efficacy should also focus on other longitudinal outcome measures such as lapses, relapses, and changes in smoking rate over time. Since treatment compliance is a significant issue in the context of treating nicotine dependence, pharmacogenetic studies of nicotine dependence trials should focus on medication side effects or discontinuation of therapy to help tailor medication choice or dose in an attempt to improve long-term quit success. Lastly, additional genetic studies are needed to examine more biologically promixal markers (i.e., endophenotypes) to help increase our understanding of nicotine dependence and identify novel candidates that can be potential targets for medication development (Lerman et al, 2007). Conducting these studies may eventually help researchers, clinicians, and policy makers to capitalize on the understanding of the genetics of nicotine dependence to develop more effective approaches to treating smokers and reducing the global public health impact of nicotine addiction.

References

Agrawal, A., Pergadia, M. L., Balasubramanian, S., Saccone, S. F., Hinrichs, A. L. et al (2009), Further evidence for an association between the gamma-aminobutyric acid receptor A, subunit 4 genes on chromosome 4 and Fagerstrom Test for Nicotine Dependence. *Addiction, 104*, 471–477.

Agrawal, A., Pergadia, M. L., Saccone, S. F., Hinrichs, A. L., Lessov-Schlaggar, C. N. et al (2008). Gamma-aminobutyric acid receptor genes and nicotine dependence: evidence for association from a case-control study. *Addiction, 103*, 1027–1038.

Anney, R. J., Olsson, C. A., Lotfi-Miri, M., Patton, G. C., and Williamson, R. (2004). Nicotine dependence in a prospective population-based study of adolescents: the protective role of a functional tyrosine hydroxylase polymorphism. *Pharmacogenetics, 14*, 73–81.

Audrain-McGovern, J., Koudsi, N., Rodriguez, D., Wileyto, E. P., Shields, P. G. et al (2007). The role of CYP2A6 in the emergence of nicotine dependence in adolescents. *Pediatrics, 119*, e264–e274.

Audrain-McGovern, J., Lerman, C., Wileyto, E. P., Rodriguez, D., and Shields, P. G. (2004). Interacting effects of genetic predisposition and depression on adolescent smoking progression. *Am J Psychiatry, 161*, 1224–1230.

Audrain-McGovern, J. Rodriguez, D., Wileyto, E. P., Schmitz, K. H., and Shields, P. G. (2006). Effect of team sport participation on genetic predisposition to adolescent smoking progression. *Arch Gen Psychiatry, 63*, 433–441.

Baker, T. B., Weiss, R. B., Bolt, D., von Niederhausern, A., Fiore, M. C. et al (2009). Human neuronal acetylcholine receptor A5-A3-B4 haplotypes are associated with multiple nicotine dependence phenotypes. *Nicotine Tob Res*

Benowitz, N. L., Swan, G. E., Jacob, P. 3rd, Lessov-Schlaggar, C. N., and Tyndale, R. F. (2006). CYP2A6 genotype and the metabolism and disposition kinetics of nicotine. *Clin Pharmacol Ther, 80*, 457–467.

Bergevin, A., Girardot, D., Bourque, M. J., and Trudeau, L. E. (2002). Presynaptic mu-opioid receptors regulate a late step of the secretory process in rat ventral tegmental area GABAergic neurons. *Neuropharmacology, 42*, 1065–1078.

Berrettini, W., Wileyto, E. P., Epstein, L., Restine, S., Hawk, L. et al (2007). Catechol-O-methyltransferase (COMT) gene variants predict response to bupropion therapy for tobacco dependence. *Biol Psychiatry, 61*, 111–118.

Berrettini, W., Yuan, X., Tozzi, F., Song, K., Francks, C. et al (2008). Alpha-5/alpha-3 nicotinic receptor subunit alleles increase risk for heavy smoking. *Mol Psychiatry, 13*, 368–373.

Beuten, J., Ma, J. Z., Lou, X. Y., Payne, T. J., and Li, M. D. (2007a). Association analysis of the protein phosphatase 1 regulatory subunit 1B (PPP1R1B) gene with nicotine dependence in European- and African-American smokers. *Am J Med Genet B Neuropsychiatr Genet, 144B*, 285–290.

Beuten, J., Ma, J. Z., Payne, T. J., Dupont, R. T., Crews, K. M. et al (2005a). Single- and multilocus allelic variants within the GABA(B) receptor subunit 2 (GABAB2) gene are significantly associated with nicotine dependence. *Am J Hum Genet, 76*, 859–864.

Beuten, J., Ma, J. Z., Payne, T. J., Dupont, R. T., Lou, X. Y. et al (2007b). Association of specific haplotypes of neurotrophic tyrosine kinase receptor 2 gene

(NTRK2) with vulnerability to nicotine dependence in African-Americans and European-Americans. *Biol Psychiatry, 61*, 48–55.

Beuten, J., Ma, J. Z., Payne, T. J., Dupont, R. T., Quezada, P. et al (2005b). Significant association of BDNF haplotypes in European-American male smokers but not in European-American female or African-American smokers. *Am J Med Genet B Neuropsychiatr Genet, 139B*, 73–80.

Bierut, L. J., Madden, P. A., Breslau, N., Johnson, E. O., Hatsukami, D. et al (2007). Novel genes identified in a high-density genome wide association study for nicotine dependence. *Hum Mol Genet, 16*, 24–35.

Bierut, L. J., Rice, J. P., Edenberg, H. J., Goate, A., Foroud, T. et al (2000). Family-based study of the association of the dopamine D2 receptor gene (DRD2) with habitual smoking. *Am J Med Genet, 90*, 299–302.

Bierut, L. J., Stitzel, J. A., Wang, J. C., Hinrichs, A. L., Grucza, R. A. et al (2008). Variants in nicotinic receptors and risk for nicotine dependence. *Am J Psychiatry, 165*, 1163–1171.

Breitling, L. P., Dahmen, N., Mittelstrass, K., Illig, T., Rujescu, D. et al (2008). Smoking cessation and variations in nicotinic acetylcholine receptor subunits alpha-5, alpha-3, and beta-4 Genes. *Biol Psychiatry, 65*, 691–695.

Brody, A. L., Mandelkern, M. A., Olmstead, R. E., Scheibal, D., Hahn, E. et al (2006). Gene variants of brain dopamine pathways and smoking-induced dopamine release in the ventral caudate/nucleus accumbens. *Arch Gen Psychiatry, 63*, 808–816.

Caporaso, N., Gu, F., Chatterjee, N., Sheng-Chih, J., Yu, K. et al (2009). Genome-wide and candidate gene association study of cigarette smoking behaviors. *PLoS ONE, 4*, e4653.

CDC. (2004). *The Health Consequences of Smoking: A Report of the Surgeon General. 2004*. Atlanta: Department of Health and Human Services, Centers for Disease Control and Prevention, National Center for Chronic Disease Prevention and Health Promotion, Office on Smoking and Health.

CDC. (2006). Tobacco use among adults—United States, 2005 [Electronic Version], *Vol. 55*, 1145–1148 from http://www.cdc.gov/mmwr/preview/mmwrhtml/mm5542a1.htm.

Chen, G. B., Payne, T. J., Lou, X. Y., Ma, J. Z., Zhu, J. et al (2008a). Association of amyloid precursor protein-binding protein, family B, member 1 with nicotine dependence in African and European American smokers. *Hum Genet, 124*, 393–398.

Chen, J., Lipska, B. K., Halim, N., Ma, Q. D., Matsumoto, M. et al (2004). Functional analysis of genetic variation in catechol-O-methyltransferase (COMT): effects on mRNA, protein, and enzyme activity in postmortem human brain. *Am J Hum Genet, 75*, 807–821.

Chen, J., Nakamura, M., Kawamura, T., Takahashi, T, and Nakahara, D. (2006). Roles of pedunculopontine tegmental cholinergic receptors in brain stimulation reward in the rat. *Psychopharmacology (Berl), 184,* 514–522.

Chen, X., Che, Y., Zhang, L. Putman. A. H., Damaj, I. et al (2007). RhoA, encoding a Rho GTPase, is associated with smoking initiation. *Genes Brain Behav, 6,* 689–697.

Chen, X., Chen, J., Williamson, V. S., An, S. S., Hettema, J. M. et al (2009). Variants in nicotinic acetylcholine receptors alpha5 and alpha3 increase risks to nicotine dependence. *Am J Med Genet B Neuropsychiatr Genet.*

Chen, X., Williamson, V. S., An, S. S., Hettema, J. M., Aggen, S. H. et al (2008b). Cannabinoid receptor 1 gene association with nicotine dependence. *Arch Gen Psychiatry, 65,* 816–824.

Colilla, S., Lerman, C., Shields, P. G., Jepson, C., Rukstalis, M. et al (2005). Association of catechol-O-methyltransferase with smoking cessation in two independent studies of women. *Pharmacogenet Genomics, 15,* 393–398.

Comings, D. E., Ferry, L., Bradshaw-Robinson, S., Burchette, R., Chiu, C. et al (1996). The dopamine D2 receptor (DRD2) gene: a genetic risk factor in smoking. *Pharmacogenetics, 6,* 73–79.

Conti, D. V., Lee, W., Li, D., Liu, J., Van Den Berg, D. et al (2008). Nicotinic acetylcholine receptor beta2 subunit gene implicated in a systems-based candidate gene study of smoking cessation. *Hum Mol Genet, 17,* 2834–2848.

Dahl, J. P., Jepson, C., Levenson, R., Wileyto, E. P., Patterson, F. et al (2006). Interaction between variation in the D2 dopamine receptor (DRD2) and the neuronal calcium sensor-1 (FREQ) genes in predicting response to nicotine replacement therapy for tobacco dependence. *Pharmacogenomics J, 6,* 194–199.

Davenport, K. E., Houdi, A. A., and Van Loon, G. R. (1990). Nicotine protects against mu-opioid receptor antagonism by beta-funaltrexamine: evidence for nicotine-induced release of endogenous opioids in brain. *Neurosci Lett, 113,* 40–46.

David, S. P., Brown, R. A., Papandonatos, G. D., Kahler, C. W., Lloyd-Richardson, E. E. et al (2007a). Pharmacogenetic clinical trial of sustained-release bupropion for smoking cessation. *Nicotine Tob Res, 9,* 821–833.

David, S. P., Johnstone, E., Griffiths, S. E., Murphy, M., Yudkin, P. et al (2002). No association between functional catechol O-methyl transferase 1947A>G polymorphism and smoking initiation, persistent smoking or smoking cessation. *Pharmacogenetics, 12,* 265–268.

David, S. P., Munafo, M. R., Murphy, M. F., Proctor, M., Walton, R. T. et al (2008). Genetic variation in the dopamine D4 receptor (DRD4) gene and smoking cessation: follow-up of a randomised clinical trial of transdermal nicotine patch. *Pharmacogenomics J, 8,* 122–128.

David, S. P., Munafo, M. R., Murphy, M. F., Walton, R. T., and Johnstone, E. C. (2007b). The serotonin transporter 5-HTTLPR polymorphism and treatment response to nicotine patch: follow-up of a randomized controlled trial. *Nicotine Tob Res, 9,* 225–231.

David, S. P., Niaura, R., Papandonatos, G. D., Shadel, W. G., Burkholder, G. J. et al (2003). Does the DRD2-Taq1 A polymorphism influence treatment response to bupropion hydrochloride for reduction of the nicotine withdrawal syndrome? *Nicotine Tob Res, 5,* 935–942.

David, S. P., Strong, D. R., Munafo, M. R., Brown, R. A., Lloyd-Richardson, E. E. et al (2007c). Bupropion efficacy for smoking cessation is influenced by the DRD2 Taq1A polymorphism: analysis of pooled data from two clinical trials. *Nicotine Tob Res, 9,* 1251–1257.

Duga, S., Solda, G., Asselta, R., Bonati, M. T., Dalpra, L. et al (2001). Characterization of the genomic structure of the human neuronal nicotinic acetylcholine receptor CHRNA5/A3/B4 gene cluster and identification of novel intragenic polymorphisms. *J Hum Genet, 46,* 640–648.

Ehringer, M. A., Clegg, H. V., Collins, A. C., Corley, R. P., Crowley, T., et al (2007). Association of the neuronal nicotinic receptor beta2 subunit gene (CHRNB2) with subjective responses to alcohol and nicotine. *Am J Med Genet B Neuropsychiatr Genet, 144B,* 596–604.

Gelernter, J., Yu, Y., Weiss, R., Brady, K., Panhuysen, C. et al (2006). Haplotype spanning TTC12 and ANKK1, flanked by the DRD2 and NCAM1 loci, is strongly associated to nicotine dependence in two distinct American populations. *Hum Mol Genet, 15,* 3498–3507.

Gerra, G., Garofano, L., Zaimovic, A., Moi, G., Branchi, B. et al (2005). Association of the serotonin transporter promoter polymorphism with smoking behavior among adolescents. *Am J Med Genet B Neuropsychiatr Genet, 135B,* 73–78.

Grenhoff, J., Aston-Jones, G., and Svensson, T. H. (1986). Nicotinic effects on the firing pattern of midbrain dopamine neurons. *Acta Physiol Scand, 128,* 351–358.

Gu, D. F., Hinks, L. J., Morton, N. E., and Day, I. N. (2000). The use of long PCR to confirm three common alleles at the CYP2A6 locus and the relationship between genotype and smoking habit. *Ann Hum Genet, 64,* 383–390.

Guindon, G. E. (2006). *The Cost Attributable to Tobacco Use: A Critical Review of the Literature.* Geneva: World Health Organization.

Haberstick, B. C., Timberlake, D., Ehringer, M. A., Lessem, J. M., Hopfer, C. J. et al (2007). Genes, time to first cigarette and nicotine dependence in a general population sample of young adults. *Addiction, 102,* 655–665.

Hamilton, A. S., Lessov-Schlaggar, C. N., Cockburn, M. G., Unger, J. B., Cozen, W. et al (2006). Gender differences in determinants of smoking initiation and persistence in California twins. *Cancer Epidemiol Biomarkers Prev, 15*, 1189–1197.

Hardie, T. L., Moss, H. B., and Lynch, K. G. (2006). Genetic correlations between smoking initiation and smoking behaviors in a twin sample. *Addict Behav, 31*, 2030–2037.

Heitjan, D. F., Guo, M., Ray, R., Wileyto, E. P., Epstein, L. H. et al (2007). Identification of pharmacogenetic markers in smoking cessation therapy. *Am J Med Genet B Neuropsychiatr Genet, 147B*, 712–719.

Hoft, N. R., Corley, R. P., McQueen, M. B., Schlaepfer, I. R., Huizinga, D. et al (2009). Genetic association of the CHRNA6 and CHRNB3 genes with tobacco dependence in a nationally representative sample. *Neuropsychopharmacology, 34*, 698–706.

Hopfer, C. J., Crowley, T. J., and Hewitt, J. K. (2003). Review of twin and adoption studies of adolescent substance use. *J Am Acad Child Adolesc Psychiatry, 42*, 710–719.

Hu, S., Brody, C. L., Fisher, C., Gunzerath, L., Nelson, M. L. et al (2000). Interaction between the serotonin transporter gene and neuroticism in cigarette smoking behavior. *Mol Psychiatry, 5*, 181–188.

Huang, S., Cook, D. G., Hinks, L. J., Chen, X. H., Ye, S. et al (2005). CYP2A6, MAOA, DBH, DRD4, and 5HT2A genotypes, smoking behaviour and cotinine levels in 1518 UK adolescents. *Pharmacogenet Genomics, 15*, 839–850.

Huang, W., Ma, J. Z., Payne, T. J., Beuten, J., Dupont, R. T. et al (2008a). Significant association of DRD1 with nicotine dependence. *Hum Genet, 123*, 133–140.

Huang, W., Payne, T. J., Ma, J. Z., Beuten, J., Dupont, R. T. et al (2009). Significant association of ANKK1 and detection of a functional polymorphism with nicotine dependence in an African-American sample. *Neuropsychopharmacology, 34*, 319–330.

Huang, W., Payne, T. J., Ma, J. Z., and Li, M. D. (2008b). A functional polymorphism, rs6280, in DRD3 is significantly associated with nicotine dependence in European-American smokers. *Am J Med Genet B Neuropsychiatr Genet, 147B*, 1109–1115.

Hutchison, K. E., Allen, D. L., Filbey, F. M., Jepson, C., Lerman, C. et al (2007). CHRNA4 and tobacco dependence: from gene regulation to treatment outcome. *Arch Gen Psychiatry, 64*, 1078–1086.

Hutchison, K. E., LaChance, H., Niaura, R., Bryan, A., and Smolen, A. (2002). The DRD4 VNTR polymorphism influences reactivity to smoking cues. *J Abnorm Psychol, 111*, 134–143.

Ishikawa, H., Ohtsuki, T., Ishiguro, H., Yamakawa-Kobayashi, K., Endo, K. et al (1999). Association between serotonin transporter gene polymorphism and smoking among Japanese males. *Cancer Epidemiol Biomarkers Prev, 8*, 831–833.

Jacobsen, L. K., Pugh, K. R., Mencl, W. E., and Gelernter, J. (2006). C957T polymorphism of the dopamine D2 receptor gene modulates the effect of nicotine

on working memory performance and cortical processing efficiency. *Psychopharmacology (Berl), 188*, 530–540.

Johnstone, E. C., Elliot, K. M., David, S. P., Murphy, M. F., Walton, R. T. et al (2007). Association of COMT Val108/158Met genotype with smoking cessation in a nicotine replacement therapy randomized trial. *Cancer Epidemiol Biomarkers Prev, 16*, 1065–1069.

Johnstone, E. C., Yudkin, P., Griffiths, S. E., Fuller, A., Murphy, M. et al (2004a). The dopamine D2 receptor C32806T polymorphism (DRD2 Taq1A RFLP) exhibits no association with smoking behaviour in a healthy UK population. *Addict Biol, 9*, 221–226.

Johnstone, E. C., Yudkin, P. L., Hey, K., Roberts, S. J., Welch, S. J. et al (2004b). Genetic variation in dopaminergic pathways and short-term effectiveness of the nicotine patch. *Pharmacogenetics, 14*, 83–90.

Jones, I. W., and Wonnacott, S. (2004). Precise localization of alpha7 nicotinic acetylcholine receptors on glutamatergic axon terminals in the rat ventral tegmental area. *J Neurosci, 24*, 11244–11252.

Kalivas, P. W. (1993). Neurotransmitter regulation of dopamine neurons in the ventral tegmental area. *Brain Res Brain Res Rev, 18*, 75–113.

Karp, I., O'Loughlin, J., Hanley, J., Tyndale, R. F., and Paradis, G. (2006). Risk factors for tobacco dependence in adolescent smokers. *Tob Control, 15*, 199–204.

Klink, R., de Kerchove d'Exaerde, A., Zoli, M., and Changeux, J. P. (2001). Molecular and physiological diversity of nicotinic acetylcholine receptors in the midbrain dopaminergic nuclei. *J Neurosci, 21*, 1452–1463.

Kremer, I., Bachner-Melman, R., Reshef, A., Broude, L., Nemanov, L. et al (2005). Association of the serotonin transporter gene with smoking behavior. *Am J Psychiatry, 162*, 924–930.

Kubota, T., Nakajima-Taniguchi, C., Fukuda, T., Funamoto, M., Maeda, M. et al (2006). CYP2A6 polymorphisms are associated with nicotine dependence and influence withdrawal symptoms in smoking cessation. *Pharmacogenomics J, 6*, 115–119.

Lang, U. E., Sander, T., Lohoff, F. W., Hellweg, R., Bajbouj, M. et al (2007). Association of the met66 allele of brain-derived neurotrophic factor (BDNF) with smoking. *Psychopharmacology (Berl), 190*, 433–439.

Laucht, M., Becker, K., El-Faddagh, M., Hohm, E., and Schmidt, M. H. (2005). Association of the DRD4 exon III polymorphism with smoking in fifteen-year-olds: a mediating role for novelty seeking? *J Am Acad Child Adolesc Psychiatry, 44*, 477–484.

Laucht, M., Becker, K., Frank, J., Schmidt, M. H., Esser, G. et al (2008). Genetic variation in dopamine pathways differentially associated with smoking progression in adolescence. *J Am Acad Child Adolesc Psychiatry, 47*, 673–681.

Lee, A. M., Jepson, C., Hoffmann, E., Epstein, L., Hawk, L. W. et al (2007a). CYP2B6 genotype alters abstinence rates in a bupropion smoking cessation trial. *Biol Psychiatry, 62*, 635–641.

Lee, A. M., Jepson, C., Shields, P. G., Benowitz, N., Lerman, C. et al (2007b). CYP2B6 genotype does not alter nicotine metabolism, plasma levels, or abstinence with nicotine replacement therapy. *Cancer Epidemiol Biomarkers Prev, 16*, 1312–1314.

Lerman, C., Caporaso, N., Main, D., Audrain, J., Boyd, N. R. et al (1998). Depression and self-medication with nicotine: the modifying influence of the dopamine D4 receptor gene. *Health Psychol, 17*, 56–62.

Lerman, C., Caporaso, N. E., Audrain, J., Main, D., Bowman, E. D. et al (1999). Evidence suggesting the role of specific genetic factors in cigarette smoking. *Health Psychol, 18*, 14–20.

Lerman, C., Caporaso, N. E., Audrain, J., Main, D., Boyd, N. R. et al (2000). Interacting effects of the serotonin transporter gene and neuroticism in smoking practices and nicotine dependence. *Mol Psychiatry, 5*, 189–192.

Lerman, C., Jepson, C., Wileyto, E. P., Epstein, L. H., Rukstalis, M. et al (2006a). Role of functional genetic variation in the dopamine D2 receptor (DRD2) in response to bupropion and nicotine replacement therapy for tobacco dependence: results of two randomized clinical trials. *Neuropsychopharmacology, 31*, 231–242.

Lerman, C., LeSage, M. G., Perkins, K. A., O'Malley, S. S., Siegel, S. J. et al (2007). Translational research in medication development for nicotine dependence. *Nat Rev Drug Discov, 6*, 746–762.

Lerman, C., Shields, P. G., Wileyto, E. P., Audrain, J., Hawk, L. H., Jr. et al (2003). Effects of dopamine transporter and receptor polymorphisms on smoking cessation in a bupropion clinical trial. *Health Psychol, 22*, 541–548.

Lerman, C., Shields, P. G., Wileyto, E. P., Audrain, J., Pinto, A. et al (2002). Pharmacogenetic investigation of smoking cessation treatment. *Pharmacogenetics, 12*, 627–634.

Lerman, C., Tyndale, R., Patterson, F., Wileyto, E. P., Shields, P. G. et al (2006b). Nicotine metabolite ratio predicts efficacy of transdermal nicotine for smoking cessation. *Clin Pharmacol Ther, 79*, 600–608.

Lerman, C., Wileyto, E. P., Patterson, F., Rukstalis, M., Audrain-McGovern, J. et al (2004). The functional mu opioid receptor (OPRM1) Asn40Asp variant predicts short-term response to nicotine replacement therapy in a clinical trial. *Pharmacogenomics J, 4*, 184–192.

Levine, R., and Kendler, M. (2004). *Millions Saved: Proven Success in Global Health.* Washington, DC: Center for Global Development.

Li, M. D. (2003). The genetics of smoking related behavior: a brief review. *Am J Med Sci, 326*, 168–173.

Li, M. D. (2008). Identifying susceptibility loci for nicotine dependence: 2008 update based on recent genome-wide linkage analyses. *Hum Genet, 123*, 119–131.

Li, M. D., Beuten, J., Ma, J. Z., Payne, T. J., Lou, X. Y. et al (2005). Ethnic- and gender-specific association of the nicotinic acetylcholine receptor alpha4 subunit gene (CHRNA4) with nicotine dependence. *Hum Mol Genet, 14*, 1211–1219.

Li, M. D., Cheng, R., Ma, J. Z., and Swan GE. (2003). A meta-analysis of estimated genetic and environmental effects on smoking behavior in male and female adult twins. *Addiction, 98*, 23–31.

Li, M. D., Sun, D., Lou, X. Y., Beuten, J., Payne, T. J. et al (2007). Linkage and association studies in African- and Caucasian-American populations demonstrate that SHC3 is a novel susceptibility locus for nicotine dependence. *Mol Psychiatry, 12*, 462–473.

Lou, X. Y., Ma, J. Z., Payne, T. J., Beuten, J., Crew, K. M. et al (2006). Gene-based analysis suggests association of the nicotinic acetylcholine receptor beta1 subunit (CHRNB1) and M1 muscarinic acetylcholine receptor (CHRM1) with vulnerability for nicotine dependence. *Hum Genet, 120*, 381–389.

Lou, X. Y., Ma, J. Z., Sun, D., Payne, T. J., and Li, M. D. (2007). Fine mapping of a linkage region on chromosome 17p13 reveals that GABARAP and DLG4 are associated with vulnerability to nicotine dependence in European-Americans. *Hum Mol Genet, 16*, 142–153.

Loughead, J., Wileyto, E. P., Valdez, J. N., Sanborn, P., Tang, K. et al (2009). Effect of abstinence challenge on brain function and cognition in smokers differs by COMT genotype. *Mol Psychiatry, 14*, 820–826.

Ma, J. Z., Beuten, J., Payne, T. J., Dupont, R. T., Elston, R. C. et al (2005). Haplotype analysis indicates an association between the DOPA decarboxylase (DDC) gene and nicotine dependence. *Hum Mol Genet, 14*, 1691–1698.

Malaiyandi, V., Lerman, C., Benowitz, N. L., Jepson, C. Patterson, F. et al (2006). Impact of CYP2A6 genotype on pretreatment smoking behaviour and nicotine levels from and usage of nicotine replacement therapy. *Mol Psychiatry, 11*, 400–409.

Malaiyandi, V., Sellers, E. M., and Tyndale, R. F. (2005). Implications of CYP2A6 genetic variation for smoking behaviors and nicotine dependence. *Clin Pharmacol Ther, 77*, 145–158.

Mansvelder, H. D., De Rover, M., McGehee, D. S., and Brussaard, A. B. (2003). Cholinergic modulation of dopaminergic reward areas: upstream and downstream targets of nicotine addiction. *Eur J Pharmacol, 480*, 117–123.

Mansvelder, H. D., Keath, J. R., and McGehee, D. S. (2002). Synaptic mechanisms underlie nicotine-induced excitability of brain reward areas. *Neuron, 33*, 905–919.

McClernon, F. J., Hutchison, K. E., Rose, J. E., and Kozink, R. V. (2007). DRD4 VNTR polymorphism is associated with transient fMRI-BOLD responses to smoking cues. *Psychopharmacology (Berl), 194*, 433–441.

McKinney, E. F., Walton, R. T., Yudkin, P., Fuller, A., Haldar, N. A. et al (2000). Association between polymorphisms in dopamine metabolic enzymes and tobacco consumption in smokers. *Pharmacogenetics, 10*, 483–491.

Mifsud, J. C., Hernandez, L., and Hoebel, B. G. (1989). Nicotine infused into the nucleus accumbens increases synaptic dopamine as measured by in vivo microdialysis. *Brain Res, 478*, 365–367.

Munafo, M., Clark, T., Johnstone, E., Murphy, M., and Walton, R. (2004). The genetic basis for smoking behavior: a systematic review and meta-analysis. *Nicotine Tob Res, 6*, 583–597.

Munafo, M. R., Elliot, K. M., Murphy, M. F., Walton, R. T., and Johnstone, E. C. (2007). Association of the mu-opioid receptor gene with smoking cessation. *Pharmacogenomics J, 7*, 353–361.

Munafo, M. R., Johnstone, E. C., Guo, B., Murphy, M. F., and Aveyard, P. (2008). Association of COMT Val108/158Met genotype with smoking cessation. *Pharmacogenet Genomics, 18*, 121–128.

Munafo, M. R., Johnstone, E. C., Murphy, M. F., and Aveyard, P. (2009a). Lack of association of DRD2 rs1800497 (Taq1A) polymorphism with smoking cessation in a nicotine replacement therapy randomized trial. *Nicotine Tob Res.*

Munafo, M. R., Johnstone, E. C., Wileyto, E. P., Shields, P. G., Elliot, K. M. et al (2006a). Lack of association of 5-HTTLPR genotype with smoking cessation in a nicotine replacement therapy randomized trial. *Cancer Epidemiol Biomarkers Prev, 15*, 398–400.

Munafo, M. R., Murphy, M. F., and Johnstone, E. C. (2006b). Smoking cessation, weight gain, and DRD4 -521 genotype. *Am J Med Genet B Neuropsychiatr Genet, 141B*, 398–402.

Munafo, M. R., Timpson, N. J., David, S. P., Ebrahim, S., and Lawlor, D. A. (2009b). Association of the DRD2 gene Taq1A polymorphism and smoking behavior: a meta-analysis and new data. *Nicotine Tob Res, 11*, 64–76.

Nestler, E. J. (2005). Is there a common molecular pathway for addiction? *Nat Neurosci, 8*, 1445–1449.

Nisell, M., Nomikos, G. G., and Svensson, T. H. (1994). Systemic nicotine-induced dopamine release in the rat nucleus accumbens is regulated by nicotinic receptors in the ventral tegmental area. *Synapse, 16*, 36–44.

Nussbaum, J., Xu, Q., Payne, T. J., Ma, J. Z., Huang, W. et al (2008). Significant association of the neurexin-1 gene (NRXN1) with nicotine dependence in European- and African-American smokers. *Hum Mol Genet, 17*, 1569–1577.

O'Gara, C., Stapleton, J., Sutherland, G., Guindalini, C., Neale, B. et al (2007). Dopamine transporter polymorphisms are associated with short-term response to smoking cessation treatment. *Pharmacogenet Genomics, 17*, 61–67.

O'Loughlin, J., Paradis, G., Kim, W., DiFranza, J., Meshefedjian, G. et al (2004). Genetically decreased CYP2A6 and the risk of tobacco dependence: a prospective study of novice smokers. *Tob Control, 13*, 422–428.

Olsson, C., Anney, R., Forrest, S., Patton, G., Coffey, C. et al (2004). Association between dependent smoking and a polymorphism in the tyrosine hydroxylase gene in a prospective population-based study of adolescent health. *Behav Genet, 34*, 85–91.

Osler, M., Holst, C., Prescott, E., and Sorensen, T. I. (2001). Influence of genes and family environment on adult smoking behavior assessed in an adoption study. *Genet Epidemiol, 21*, 193–200.

Patterson, F., Schnoll, R., Wileyto, E., Pinto, A., Epstein, L. et al (2008). Toward personalized therapy for smoking cessation: a randomized placebo-controlled trial of bupropion. *Clin Pharmacol Ther, 84*, 320–325.

Perkins, K. A., Lerman, C., Coddington, S., Jetton, C., Karelitz, J. L. et al (2008a). Gene and gene by sex associations with initial sensitivity to nicotine in nonsmokers. *Behav Pharmacol, 19*, 630–640.

Perkins, K. A., Lerman, C., Grottenthaler, A., Ciccocioppo, M. M., Milanak, M. et al (2008b). Dopamine and opioid gene variants are associated with increased smoking reward and reinforcement owing to negative mood. *Behav Pharmacol, 19*, 641–649.

Pianezza, M. L., Sellers, E. M., and Tyndale, R. F. (1998). Nicotine metabolism defect reduces smoking. *Nature, 393*, 750.

Radwan, G. N., El-Setouhy, M., Mohamed, M. K., Hamid, M. A., Azem, S. A. et al (2007). DRD2/ANKK1 TaqI polymorphism and smoking behavior of Egyptian male cigarette smokers. *Nicotine Tob Res, 9*, 1325–1329.

Ramirez-Latorre, J., Yu, C. R., Qu, X., Perin, F., Karlin, A. et al (1996). Functional contributions of alpha5 subunit to neuronal acetylcholine receptor channels. *Nature, 380*, 347–351.

Rao, Y., Hoffmann, E., Zia, M., Bodin, L., Zeman, M. et al (2000). Duplications and defects in the CYP2A6 gene: identification, genotyping, and in vivo effects on smoking. *Mol Pharmacol, 58*, 747–755.

Rasmussen, H., Bagger, Y., Tanko, L. B., Christiansen, C., and Werge, T. (2008). Lack of association of the serotonin transporter gene promoter region polymorphism, 5-HTTLPR, including rs25531 with cigarette smoking and alcohol consumption. *Am J Med Genet B Neuropsychiatr Genet.*

Ray, R., Jepson, C., Patterson, F., Strasser, A., Rukstalis, M. et al (2006). Association of OPRM1 A118G variant with the relative reinforcing value of nicotine. *Psychopharmacology (Berl), 188*, 355–363.

Ray, R., Jepson, C., Wileyto, E. P., Dahl, J. P., Patterson, F. et al (2007a). Genetic variation in mu-opioid-receptor-interacting proteins and smoking cessation in a nicotine replacement therapy trial. *Nicotine Tob Res, 9*, 1237–1241.

Ray, R., Jepson, C., Wileyto, P., Patterson, F., Strasser, A. A. et al (2007b). CREB1 haplotypes and the relative reinforcing value of nicotine. *Mol Psychiatry, 12*, 615–617.

Redden, D. T., Shields, P. G., Epstein, L., Wileyto, E. P., Zakharkin, S. O. et al (2005). Catechol-O-methyl-transferase functional polymorphism and nicotine dependence: an evaluation of nonreplicated results. *Cancer Epidemiol Biomarkers Prev, 14*, 1384–1389.

Reuter, M., Hennig, J., Amelang, M., Montag, C., Korkut, T. et al (2007). The role of the TPH1 and TPH2 genes for nicotine dependence: a genetic association study in two different age cohorts. *Neuropsychobiology, 56*, 47–54.

Saccone, N. L., Saccone, S. F., Hinrichs, A. L., Stitzel, J. A., Duan, W. et al (2009). Multiple distinct risk loci for nicotine dependence identified by dense coverage of the complete family of nicotinic receptor subunit (CHRN) genes. *Am J Med Genet B Neuropsychiatry Genet, 150B*, 453–466.

Saccone, S. F., Hinrichs, A. L., Saccone, N. L., Chase, G. A., Konvicka, K. et al (2007). Cholinergic nicotinic receptor genes implicated in a nicotine dependence association study targeting 348 candidate genes with 3713 SNPs. *Hum Mol Genet, 16*, 36–49.

Schinka, J. A., Town, T., Abdullah, L., Crawford, F. C., Ordorica, P. I. et al (2002). A functional polymorphism within the mu-opioid receptor gene and risk for abuse of alcohol and other substances. *Mol Psychiatry, 7*, 224–228.

Schlaepfer, I. R., Hoft, N. R., Collins, A. C., Corley, R. P., Hewitt, J. K. et al (2008). The CHRNA5/A3/B4 gene cluster variability as an important determinant of early alcohol and tobacco initiation in young adults. *Biol Psychiatry, 63*, 1039–1046.

Schnoll, R. A., and Lerman, C. (2006). Current and emerging pharmacotherapies for treating tobacco dependence. *Expert Opin Emerg Drugs, 11*, 429–444.

Schnoll, R. A., Patterson, F., Wileyto, E. P., Tyndale, R. F., Benowitz, N. et al (2009). Nicotine metabolic rate predicts successful smoking cessation with transdermal nicotine: a validation study. *Pharmacol Biochem Behav, 92*, 6–11.

Schoedel, K. A., Hoffmann, E. B., Rao, Y., Sellers, E. M., and Tyndale, R. F. (2004). Ethnic variation in CYP2A6 and association of genetically slow nicotine metabolism and smoking in adult Caucasians. *Pharmacogenetics, 14*, 615–626.

Sellers, E. M., Kaplan, H. L., and Tyndale, R. F. (2000). Inhibition of cytochrome P450 2A6 increases nicotine's oral bioavailability and decreases smoking. *Clin Pharmacol Ther, 68*, 35–43.

Sellers, E. M., Tyndale, R. F., and Fernandes, L. C. (2003). Decreasing smoking behaviour and risk through CYP2A6 inhibition. *Drug Discov Today, 8*, 487–493.

Sesack, S. R., and Pickel, V. M. (1992). Prefrontal cortical efferents in the rat synapse on unlabeled neuronal targets of catecholamine terminals in the nucleus accumbens septi and on dopamine neurons in the ventral tegmental area. *J Comp Neurol, 320*, 145–160.

Sherva, R., Wilhelmsen, K., Pomerleau, C. S., Chasse, S. A., Rice, J. P. et al (2008). Association of a single nucleotide polymorphism in neuronal acetylcholine receptor subunit alpha 5 (CHRNA5) with smoking status and with 'pleasurable buzz' during early experimentation with smoking. *Addiction, 103*, 1544–1552

Shields, P. G., Lerman, C., Audrain, J., Bowman, E. D., Main, D. et al (1998). Dopamine D4 receptors and the risk of cigarette smoking in African-Americans and Caucasians. *Cancer Epidemiol Biomarkers Prev, 7*, 453–458.

Skowronek, M. H., Laucht, M., Hohm, E., Becker, K., and Schmidt, M. H. (2006). Interaction between the dopamine D4 receptor and the serotonin transporter promoter polymorphisms in alcohol and tobacco use among 15-year-olds. *Neurogenetics, 7*, 239–246.

Spitz, M. R., Amos, C. I., Dong, Q., Lin, J., and Wu, X. (2008). The CHRNA5-A3 region on chromosome 15q24-25.1 is a risk factor both for nicotine dependence and for lung cancer. *J Natl Cancer Inst, 100*, 1552–1556.

Stapleton, J. A., Sutherland, G., and O'Gara, C. (2007). Association between dopamine transporter genotypes and smoking cessation: a meta-analysis. *Addict Biol, 12*, 221–226.

Stevens, V. L., Bierut, L. J., Talbot, J. T., Wang, J. C., Sun, J. et al (2008). Nicotinic receptor gene variants influence susceptibility to heavy smoking. *Cancer Epidemiol Biomarkers Prev, 17*, 3517–3525.

Strasser, A. A., Malaiyandi, V., Hoffmann, E., Tyndale, R. F., and Lerman, C. (2007). An association of CYP2A6 genotype and smoking topography. *Nicotine Tob Res, 9*, 511–518.

Sullivan, P. F., and Kendler, K. S. (1999). The genetic epidemiology of smoking. *Nicotine Tob Res, 1*(Suppl 2), S51–S57; discussion S69-S70.

Sun, D., Ma, J. Z., Payne, T. J., and Li MD. (2008). Beta-arrestins 1 and 2 are associated with nicotine dependence in European American smokers. *Mol Psychiatry, 13*, 398–406.

Swan, G. E., Jack, L. M., Valdes, A. M., Ring, H. Z., Ton, C. C. et al (2007). Joint effect of dopaminergic genes on likelihood of smoking following treatment with bupropion SR. *Health Psychol, 26*, 361–368.

Swan, G. E., Valdes, A. M., Ring, H. Z., Khroyan, T. V., Jack, L. M. et al (2005). Dopamine receptor DRD2 genotype and smoking cessation outcome following treatment with bupropion SR. *Pharmacogenomics J, 5*, 21–29.

Thorgeirsson, T. E., Geller, F., Sulem, P., Rafnar, T., Wiste, A. et al (2008). A variant associated with nicotine dependence, lung cancer and peripheral arterial disease. *Nature, 452,* 638–642.

Timberlake, D. S., Haberstick, B. C., Lessem, J. M., Smolen, A., Ehringer, M. et al (2006). An association between the DAT1 polymorphism and smoking behavior in young adults from the National Longitudinal Study of Adolescent Health. *Health Psychol, 25,* 190–197.

True, W. R., Xian, H., Scherrer, J. F., Madden, P. A., Bucholz, K. K. et al (1999). Common genetic vulnerability for nicotine and alcohol dependence in men. *Arch Gen Psychiatry, 56,* 655–661.

Trummer, O., Koppel, H., Wascher, T. C., Grunbacher, G., Gutjahr, M. et al (2006). The serotonin transporter gene polymorphism is not associated with smoking behavior. *Pharmacogenomics J, 6,* 397–400.

Uhl, G. R., Liu, Q. R., Drgon, T., Johnson, C., Walther, D. et al (2008). Molecular genetics of successful smoking cessation: convergent genome-wide association study results. *Arch Gen Psychiatry, 65,* 683–693.

Vandenbergh, D. J., Bennett, C. J., Grant, M. D., Strasser, A. A., O'Connor, R. et al (2002). Smoking status and the human dopamine transporter variable number of tandem repeats (VNTR) polymorphism: failure to replicate and finding that never-smokers may be different. *Nicotine Tob Res, 4,* 333–340.

Vandenbergh, D. J., O'Connor, R. J., Grant, M. D., Jefferson, A. L., Vogler, G. P. et al (2007). Dopamine receptor genes (DRD2, DRD3 and DRD4) and gene-gene interactions associated with smoking-related behaviors. *Addict Biol, 12,* 106–116.

Vink, J. M., Willemsen, G., and Boomsma, D. I. (2005). Heritability of smoking initiation and nicotine dependence. *Behav Genet, 35,* 397–406.

Walaas, I., and Fonnum, F. (1980). Biochemical evidence for gamma-aminobutyrate containing fibres from the nucleus accumbens to the substantia nigra and ventral tegmental area in the rat. *Neuroscience, 5,* 63–72.

Wang, J. C., Grucza, R., Cruchaga, C., Hinrichs, A. L., Bertelsen, S. et al (2008a). Genetic variation in the CHRNA5 gene affects mRNA levels and is associated with risk for alcohol dependence. *Mol Psychiatry, 14,* 501–510.

Wang, Z., Ray, R., Faith, M., Tang, K., Wileyto, E. P. et al (2008b). Nicotine abstinence-induced cerebral blood flow changes by genotype. *Neurosci Lett, 438,* 275–280.

Weiss, R. B., Baker, T. B., Cannon, D. S., von Niederhausern, A., Dunn, D. M. et al (2008). A candidate gene approach identifies the CHRNA5-A3-B4 region as a risk factor for age-dependent nicotine addiction. *PLoS Genet, 4,* e1000125.

WHO. (2008). *WHO Report on the Global Tobacco Epidemic, 2008: The MPOWER package.* Geneva: World Health Organization.

Wiesbeck, G. A., Wodarz, N., Weijers, H. G., Dursteler-MacFarland, K. M., Wurst, F. M. et al (2006). A functional polymorphism in the promoter region of the monoamine oxidase A gene is associated with the cigarette smoking quantity in alcohol-dependent heavy smokers. *Neuropsychobiology, 53,* 181–185.

Xian, H., Scherrer, J. F., Madden, P. A., Lyons, M. J., Tsuang, M. et al (2003). The heritability of failed smoking cessation and nicotine withdrawal in twins who smoked and attempted to quit. *Nicotine Tob Res, 5,* 245–254.

Yu, Y., Panhuysen, C., Kranzler, H. R., Hesselbrock, V., Rounsaville, B. et al (2006). Intronic variants in the dopa decarboxylase (DDC) gene are associated with smoking behavior in European-Americans and African-Americans. *Hum Mol Genet, 15,* 2192–2199.

Yudkin, P., Munafo, M., Hey, K., Roberts, S., Welch, S. et al (2004). Effectiveness of nicotine patches in relation to genotype in women versus men: randomised controlled trial. *BMJ, 328,* 989–990.

Zeiger, J. S., Haberstick, B. C., Schlaepfer, I., Collins, A. C., Corley, R. P. et al (2008). The neuronal nicotinic receptor subunit genes (CHRNA6 and CHRNB3) are associated with subjective responses to tobacco. *Hum Mol Genet, 17,* 724–734.

Zhang, H., Ye, Y., Wang, X., Gelernter, J., Ma, J. Z. et al (2006a). DOPA decarboxylase gene is associated with nicotine dependence. *Pharmacogenomics, 7,* 1159–1166.

Zhang, L., Kendler, K. S., and Chen, X. (2006b). The mu-opioid receptor gene and smoking initiation and nicotine dependence. *Behav Brain Funct, 2,* 28.

Chapter 33

Genetics of Obesity and Diabetes

Karani S. Vimaleswaran and Ruth J.F. Loos

Abbreviations

ADAMTS9	ADAM metallopeptidase with thrombospondin type I motif 9
ADIPOQ	Adiponectin, C1Q and collagen domain containing
ADRB2	β-adrenergic receptor 2
ADRB3	β-adrenergic receptor 3
BAT2	HLA-B-associated transcript 2
BCDIN3D	BCDIN3 domain containing
BDNF	Brain-derived neurotrophic factor
CAMK1D	Calcium/calmodulin-dependent protein kinase 1D
CDKAL1	CDK5 regulatory subunit associated protein 1-like 1
CDKN2A	Cyclin-dependent kinase inhibitor 2A
CNR1	Endocannabinoid receptor 1
CTNNBL1	Catenin (cadherin-associated protein), β-like 1
DGI	Diabetes genetics initiative
DGKG	Diacylglycerol kinase
DIAGRAM	Diabetes genetics replication and meta-analysis
ENPP1	Ectonucleotide pyrophosphatase/phosphodiesterase 1
ETV5	Ets variant gene 5
FAIM2	Fas apoptotic inhibitory molecule 2
FTO	Fat mass and obesity associated
FUSION	Finland-United States Investigation of NIDDM Genetics
GIANT	Genomic investigation of anthropometric traits
GNB3	Guanine nucleotide binding protein (G protein), beta polypeptide 3
GNPDA2	Glucosamine-6-phosphate deaminase 2
HHEX	Hematopoietically expressed homeobox
HTR2C	5-Hydroxytryptamine (serotonin) receptor 2C
IDE	Insulin-degrading enzyme
IL6	Interleukin 6
JAZF1	Juxtaposed with another zinc finger gene 1
KCTD15	Potassium channel tetramerisation domain containing 15
KIF11	Kinesin family member 11
LEP	Leptin
LEPR	Leptin receptor
LGR5	Leucine-rich repeat-containing G-protein coupled
MC4R	Melanocortin 4 receptor
MTCH2	Mitochondrial carrier homolog 2
MTNR1B	Melatonin receptor 1B
NEGR1	Neuronal growth regulator 1
NOTCH2	Notch homologue 2, Drosophila
NPC1	Niemann-Pick disease, type C1
NR3C1	Nuclear receptor subfamily 3, group C, member 1
PFKP	Phosphofructokinase
PPARG	Peroxisome proliferator-activated receptor gamma
PTER	Phosphotriesterase related

K.S. Vimaleswaran (✉)
Medical Research Council (MRC) Epidemiology Unit,
Institute of Metabolic Science, Addenbrooke's
Hospital – Box 285, Hills Road, Cambridge,
CB2 0QQ, UK
e-mail: vimaleswaran.karani-santhanakrishnan@mrc-epid.cam.ac.uk

A. Steptoe (ed.), *Handbook of Behavioral Medicine*, DOI 10.1007/978-0-387-09488-5_33,
© Springer Science+Business Media, LLC 2010

QTL	Quantitative trait loci
ROC	Receiver operating characteristics
SEC16B	SEC16 homolog B
SH2B1	SH2B adaptor protein 1
SLC30A8	Solute carrier family 30 (zinc transporter), member 8
SNP	Single nucleotide polymorphism
THADA	Thyroid adenoma associated
TMEM18	Transmembrane protein 18
TCF7L2	Transcription factor 7-like 2
TSPAN8	Tetraspanin 8
UCP	Uncoupling protein
WFS1	Wolfram syndrome 1
WTCCC	Wellcome trust case control consortium

1 Introduction

The continuing rise in obesity and diabetes prevalence is becoming an increasingly important clinical and public health challenge throughout the world (see Chapter 46). Obesity has reached epidemic proportions and is the major cause of the vast increase in the prevalence of type 2 diabetes. By current estimates, nearly 70% of adults in the USA and more than 60% in the UK are overweight; half of these are obese (International Association for the Study of Obesity). Changes in diet and physical activity habit are likely the main drives of the rise in obesity and diabetes prevalence during the last three decades (Hill et al, 2003). However, the contribution of hereditary influences cannot be ignored, especially at a time when we are beginning to develop an understanding of the molecular pathways involved in the control of energy homeostasis and of how variation in genes encoding proteins in these pathways can influence common obesity and type 2 diabetes.

The genetic contribution to obesity and diabetes has been established through family, twin and adoption studies (Maes et al, 1997; Stunkard et al, 1986; Permutt et al, 2005). Results from twin studies have suggested that genetic factors explain 40–80% of the variance in body mass

index (BMI) and in risk of obesity (Allison et al, 1996; Herskind et al, 1996), while family studies have typically reported lower heritabilities of 20–50% (Luke et al, 2001; Rice et al, 1999). Data from adoption studies confirm the importance of a genetic contribution (20–60%) to obesity as evidenced by stronger correlations in BMI between adoptees and biological parents than between adoptive parents and adoptees (Stunkard et al 1986). The considerable range in heritability estimates is likely not only due to the differences in study design but also due to sample size, characteristics of the population (such as age) and the environment they live in, such as their dietary and physical activity habits (Maes et al, 1997).

There is also ample evidence that diabetes has a substantial genetic component. The concordance of type 2 diabetes in monozygotic twins ranges between 50 and 70% compared to 20–37% in dizygotic twins (Kaprio et al, 1992; Newman et al, 1987; Poulsen et al 1999). Further evidence comes from studies that compare the risk in offspring with a family history of type 2 diabetes with offspring without such a family history. While the lifetime risk of developing type 2 diabetes is 7% in the general population, this risk is four- to sixfold (30–40%) higher in offspring of whom one parent had type 2 diabetes and almost 10-fold (70%) if both parents had diabetes (Köbberling and Tillil, 1982).

Despite serious efforts over the past two decades to identify genetic variants that contribute to the predisposition to obesity and type 2 diabetes using traditional genetic epidemiological approaches, such as candidate gene approach and linkage studies, progress until recently has been slow and success limited. The availability of genome-wide association studies through the advancements of the International HapMap Project, the Human Genome Project and the progress in high-throughput genotyping has accelerated the potential to uncover genetic variants influencing common traits and diseases (Manolio et al, 2008).

In this chapter, we review the main findings of candidate gene studies, genome-wide linkage and genome-wide association studies for common obesity and type 2 diabetes. We, then, discuss how lifestyle factors such as diet and physical activity can influence the genetic susceptibility to obesity and diabetes. Finally, we discuss the impact of validated obesity and diabetes loci on public health and conclude by speculating about the discoveries that the future might bring.

2 Obesity

2.1 Candidate Gene Studies

The number of candidate gene studies (Box 33.1) for common obesity has grown steadily over the past 15 years. The latest update of Human Obesity Gene Map, which covers the literature available at the end of October 2005, reports 127 candidate genes associated with obesity-related traits (Rankinen et al, 2006). Among those, findings for 12 genes (*ADIPOQ, ADRB2, ADRB3, GNB3, HTR2C, NR3C1, LEP, LEPR, PPARG, UCP1, UCP2* and *UCP3*) were replicated in 10 or more studies. Despite this number of replications, many other studies have shown no or even opposite association, and thus the overall conclusion for most of these genes remains inconclusive (Rankinen et al, 2006).

Box 33.1 – Candidate Gene Approach

- The candidate gene approach, which has been used since the early 1990s, is a hypothesis-driven approach that relies on current understanding of the biology and pathophysiology of the disease. Genes that are thought to be involved in the pathogenesis of the disease based on animal models, cellular systems or extreme/monogenic cases are considered candidates.

- The candidacy of a gene is based on the following sources:

  (i) Linkage and positional cloning studies using extreme cases (e.g. morbidly obese/severe insulin resistance) and their families have provided evidence that several genes are implicated in monogenic forms of a disease.

  (ii) Animal models using gene knockout and transgenic approaches have identified the functional aspects of genes in relation to disease.

  (iii) Cellular model systems are used to identify biological networks and provide insight into molecular and regulatory aspects of genes responsible for phenotypes of interest, such as obesity and diabetes.

- Genetic variations in these candidate genes are then studied for association with the disease (obesity/diabetes) in the general population.

- For detecting the expected small effects of genetic variants involved in common traits and diseases, candidate gene studies need to be large scale (such as meta-analysis) and well powered.

The major problem that has plagued the candidate gene approach is that many studies are small and thus often underpowered (see Chapter 29). Obesity is a heterogeneous condition and it is expected that many common genetic variants contribute to BMI and obesity, each conferring only modest risk. Thus, large sample sizes are required to identify such variants. This can be achieved by combining the previously published studies or by doing large-scale studies.

Large-scale analyses were instrumental in more firmly establishing the role of genetic variation in the *MC4R* (melanocortin 4 receptor), *ADRB3* (beta 3 adrenergic receptor), *PCSK1* (prohormone convertase 1/3), *BDNF* (Brain-derived neurotrophic factor) and *CNR1* (endocannabinoid receptor 1) genes in common obesity.

MC4R encodes a seven-transmembrane, G protein-linked receptor that is widely expressed in the central nervous system and plays a key role in the regulation of food intake and energy homeostasis (Huszar et al, 1997). Mutations in *MC4R* are the most common monogenic cause of obesity, with approximately 5% of severely obese children carrying pathogenic mutations in the *MC4R* gene (Farooqi et al, 2003). Its role in common forms of obesity remained unexplained until recently. The two most frequently studied and most common non-synonymous *MC4R* variants are the V103I and I251L, which have been shown to have potential functional implications (Xiang et al, 2006). Both variants have been studied frequently for association with BMI and obesity. So far, only one sizeable population-based study (7937 individuals) on the V103I variant has reported a significantly reduced risk of obesity in 103I allele carriers [odds ratio (OR): 0.69, 95% confidence interval (CI) 0.50–0.96; $p = 0.03$] (Heid et al, 2005), whereas other smaller studies found no evidence of such association. However, a meta-analysis including 29,563 individuals from 25 populations (Young et al, 2007) confirmed the protective effect of the 103I allele (OR: 0.82, 95% CI 0.70–0.96; $p = 0.015$) on obesity risk, which was further established with the latest meta-analyses (Stutzmann et al, 2007), including a total of 39,879 individuals (OR: 0.80, 95% CI: 0.70–0.92; $p = 0.002$). In addition, strong evidence for a protective effect of the I251L *MC4R* variant on BMI and risk for adult and childhood obesity was obtained in eight out of nine populations examined (Stutzmann et al, 2007). The meta-analysis of all case–control studies found a nearly 50% reduced risk for obesity among carriers of the 251L-allele (OR: 0.52, 95% CI 0.38–0.71; $p = 3.6 \times 10^{-5}$).

The Arg64Trp *ADRB3* variant is one of the first genetic variants for which association with obesity was reported (Clement et al, 1995; Widen et al, 1995; Walston et al, 1995). *ADRB3* is an obvious candidate gene given its involvement in the regulation of lipolysis and thermogenesis. A meta-analysis of 97 studies ($n = 44,833$) examining the association between *ADRB3* Trp64Arg variant and BMI showed significant association in East Asians between the Arg64Trp variant and BMI, with Arg64 allele carriers having a 0.31 kg/m^2 ($p = 0.001$) higher BMI compared to non-carriers, but not in populations of white European origin (0.08 kg/m^2, $p = 0.36$) (Kurokawa et al, 2008). In vitro experiments in rodent and human cell lines showed that stimulation of cell lines with the Arg64 variant had a reduced ability to stimulate adenyl cyclase activity compared with cell lines stimulated with the Trp variant (Pietri-Rouxel et al, 1997). Also, lipolysis in human adipocytes was lower in cells with the Arg64 variant compared with cells with the Trp variant (Umekawa et al, 1999).

The *PCSK1* gene is another candidate for obesity as it encodes the prohormone convertase 1/3 enzyme that converts prohormones into functional hormones involved in energy metabolism regulation. Rare mutations in the *PCSK1* gene have been found to cause monogenic obesity (Jackson et al, 1997). In a comprehensive large-scale study, the role of common variants in the *PCSK1* gene was studied in relation to the risk of obesity (Benzinou et al, 2008b). Two non-synonymous variants, N221D (located in the catalytic domain of prohormone convertase 1/3) and the Q665E-S690T pair, were consistently associated with obesity in adults and children. Each additional minor allele (frequency: 4-7%) of the N221D variant increased the risk of obesity 1.34-fold, while each additional minor allele (frequency: 25-30%) of the Q665E-S690T pair increased the risk 1.22-fold. Functional characterization of these variants showed a significant impairment of the N221D mutant PC1/3 protein catalytic activity, but no significant functional role for the Q665E-S690T amino acid substitutions (Benzinou et al, 2008).

Rodent studies have shown that *BDNF* is involved in eating behaviour, body weight regulation and hyperactivity (Rios et al, 2001). Rare mutation in *BDNF* likely causes severe obesity and hyperphagia (Gray et al, 2006). A large-scale study, including 10,109 women, found that individuals homozygous for Met allele (frequency: 4.5%) of the Val66Met variant have a significantly lower BMI (-0.76 kg/m^2) than Val66 allele carriers (Shugart et al, 2009). Genome-wide association studies have further confirmed the association of *BDNF* variant with BMI (Thorleifsson et al, 2009).

Because of the physiological role in the regulation of energy metabolism and food intake, *CNR1* has been considered as a biological candidate for human obesity. A study on 5750 individuals showed that *CNR1* variations increase the risk of obesity and modulate BMI in European children (odds ratio (OR): 1.52. $p = 3 \times 10^{-5}$) and adults (OR: 1.85, $p = 1.1 \times 10^{-6}$) (Benzinou et al, 2008).

Large-scale studies have also been well powered to prove that an association is truly negative. In this regard, the role of *ENPP1* (ectoenzyme nucleotide pyrophosphate phosphodiesterase) in the development of obesity was shown to be likely limited. Four studies each with more than 5000 participants and with a combined sample size of 27,781 individuals found no association between the Lys121Gln variant and the obesity-related traits (Meyre et al, 2007; Grarup et al, 2006; Lyon et al, 2006; Weedon et al, 2006). Also, the association between the -174G→C *IL6* (interleukin-6) variant and the obesity was challenged by a large meta-analysis (Qi et al, 2007) combining data from 26,944 individuals from 25 populations, which showed no association between the -174G→C *IL6* variant and obesity risk. In a large meta-analysis (Jalba et al, 2008), the Glu27Gln and the Arg16Gly polymorphisms of the beta 2-adrenergic receptor (*ADRB2*) gene were examined for their association with obesity in 10,404 and 4328 individuals, respectively. The presence of the Glu27 allele in the *ADRB2* gene was found to be a significant risk factor for obesity in Asians, Pacific Islanders and American Indians, but not in Europeans. However, the Arg16 allele was not associated with obesity. Although it might be premature to fully discount the involvement of *ENPP1, IL6* and *ADRB2* in obesity development, it would take more large-scale studies and meta-analyses to reverse current observations. For other genes tested in large-scale studies or in meta-analyses and for most of the candidate genes reported in the Human Obesity Gene Map (Rankinen et al, 2006), further studies will be required to prove or refute their role in obesity susceptibility.

In summary, by means of large-scale studies and meta-analyses, at least five variants in four candidate genes have been found to be robustly associated with obesity-related traits (Loos, 2009). The candidate gene approach will continue to contribute to our understanding of obesity susceptibility, as it is useful for determining the association of a genetic variant with obesity and for identifying genes of modest effect.

2.2 Genome-Wide Studies

2.2.1 Genome-Wide Linkage Studies

Although genome-wide linkage studies (Box 33.2) have proven to be successful for monogenic disorders with large genetic effects (Dean, 2003), its success in common diseases and continuous traits such as obesity and BMI has been limited (Saunders et al, 2007). Results of the first genome-wide linkage scan on body fat percentage were published in 1997 (Norman et al, 1997) and, similar to the candidate gene approach, the number of studies and QTLs (Quantitative trait loci) has grown exponentially over the past 10 years. The latest Human Obesity Gene map (Rankinen et al, 2006) reported more than 250 genetic regions, distributed across all chromosomes (except the Y chromosome), from more than 60 genome-wide linkage scans of which 15 loci have been replicated in at least three studies. Thus far, however, none of these loci could be narrowed down sufficiently to pinpoint the genes or variants that underlie the linkage to the obesity-related traits. This is likely due to lack of power and resolution to identify genetic variants of small effects that we expect for common obesity. A meta-analysis of 37 genome-wide linkage studies containing data on over 31,000 individuals from more than 10,000 families showed only a nominal evidence for linkage at chromosomes 13q13.2-q33.1, 12q23-q24.3, 11q13.3-22.3 and 16q12.2, of which the latter harbours the *FTO* (fat mass and obesity-associated) locus (Saunders et al, 2007).

Box 33.2 – The Genome-Wide Approaches

Genome-wide approaches are hypothesis generating and aim to identify new, unanticipated genetic variants associated with traits or diseases through screening of the whole genome.

Genome-Wide Linkage Approach

- The genome-wide linkage approach, used since the mid-1990s, tests whether certain chromosomal regions across the genome co-segregate with a trait or disease of interest from one generation to the next.
- The approach requires populations of related individuals, such as siblings, nuclear families or extended pedigrees, hence, limiting the likelihood of achieving large sample sizes.
- Genome-wide linkage can only identify broad chromosomal regions that harbour hundreds of genes and it is often impossible to pinpoint which variant is causing the linkage with the disease.

Genome-Wide Association Approach

- The genome-wide association approach, which was first published in 2005, also examines the entire genome with no prior assumptions and aims to identify previously unsuspected genetic loci associated with a disease or trait of interest.
- It does not rely on familial relatedness and can therefore achieve larger sample sizes than typical family-based linkage studies.
- This approach screens the whole genome at higher resolution levels than genome-wide linkage studies and, thus, is able to narrow down the associated locus more accurately.
- Two major advances have set the stage for genome-wide association studies. First are the recent advancements in the International HapMap Project (International HapMap Consortium et al, 2007) and the completion of the human genome project and second is the substantial progress in high-throughput genotyping, which has made it possible to genotype more than 1 million genetic variants in a single analysis. Together, these breakthroughs have enabled production of single nucleotide polymorphism (SNP) chips that can capture more than 80% of the common genetic variation reported in the HapMap (Magi et al, 2007).
- *Study design*: Genome-wide association studies typically comprise two stages; a discovery stage, followed by at least one replication stage. The discovery stage involves high-density genotyping of hundreds of thousands of genetic variants across the genome. Each variant is tested for association with a trait or disease

of interest. Studies with large sample sizes at this stage tend to be more successful, in particular for common traits such as obesity and diabetes as, they are better powered to identify associations of small effect size. Associations that meet the genome-wide significance threshold ($p < 5.0\times10^{-8}$) are taken forward for replication to validate the initial observation. Only variants of loci for which the association observed at the discovery stage is confirmed at the replication stage are considered "true hits".

Genome-wide linkage has now largely been replaced by genome-wide association as the hypothesis-generating approach, at least for common diseases and traits. This is because not only the latter has become more affordable to the general scientific community but it also has much greater resolution and does not require recruitment of related individuals, which is often a tedious task that limits sample size and thus power.

2.2.2 Genome-Wide Association Studies

Genome-wide association is the latest gene-finding tool in genetic epidemiology (Box 33.2) and has already resulted in an unprecedented chain of discoveries in the genomics of complex diseases. Since the introduction of the genome-wide association approach, three waves of discoveries based on large-scale high-density genome-wide association studies for obesity-related traits have been performed. The first wave, in 2007, comprised two high-density genome-wide association studies that each confirmed *FTO* as the first gene, incontrovertibly associated with common obesity and related traits. Interestingly, the first study (Frayling et al, 2007) identified *FTO* through a genome-wide association study for type 2 diabetes in which a cluster of common variants in the

first intron of the *FTO* gene showed a highly significant association with type 2 diabetes mediated through BMI. Subsequently, the association with BMI and obesity was unequivocally replicated in 13 cohorts comprising more than 38,000 individuals. The second study (Scuteri et al, 2007) was the first large-scale high-density genome-wide association study of BMI, conducted in more than 4000 Sardinians. In the initial analyses, variants in the *FTO* and *PFKP* (platelet-type phosphofructokinase) genes showed the strongest association, but only those in *FTO* were significantly replicated in European Americans and Hispanic Americans. Each risk allele increased BMI by 0.10–0.13 standard deviations (equivalent to about 0.40–0.66 kg/m^2) and the risks for overweight and obesity by 1.18-fold and 1.32-fold, respectively. Taken together, homozygotes for the risk allele weighed about 3 kg more and had a 1.67-fold increased risk for obesity compared with those who did not inherit a risk allele (Frayling et al, 2007; Scuteri et al, 2007). The frequency of the *FTO* risk alleles is high in populations of European decent; 63% carry at least one risk allele and 16% are homozygous. Although the population attributable risk for obesity ($\sim$20%) and overweight ($\sim$13%) was rather high, the *FTO* variants explained only 1% of the variation in BMI (Frayling et al, 2007).

In the second wave of discoveries, collaborative efforts were initiated to combine individual genome-wide association studies, thereby increasing sample size and power to identify more common variants with small effects. The GIANT (Genomic Investigation of Anthropometric Traits) consortium is an international collaborative initiative that brings together research groups specifically focussing on anthropometric traits from across Europe and the USA. In their first meta-analysis, data of 7 genome-wide association scans for BMI including 16,876 individuals were combined (Loos et al, 2008). Despite a quadrupling increase in sample size compared to the first wave of genome-wide association studies, only *FTO* and one new locus – out of 10 loci that were taken forward for replication – were unequivocally confirmed. The newly identified locus mapped at 188 kb downstream of *MC4R* (near-*MC4R*). The same locus was also identified by a genome-wide association study in 2684 Indian Asians and confirmed in 11,955 individuals of Indian Asian and European ancestry (Chambers et al, 2008). While the effect size is the same in both ethnic groups, the frequency of the risk allele in Asian Indians (36%) is higher than in white Europeans (27%). This explains in part why this locus could be identified with a relatively small sample of Asian Indians in the discovery stage.

For the third wave of discoveries, the GIANT consortium increased the sample size to 32,387 adults of European ancestry from 15 cohorts (Willer et al, 2009). Of the 35 loci that were taken forward for follow-up in an independent series of 59,082 individuals, eight loci were firmly replicated. These include the previously established *FTO* and near-*MC4R* loci and six new loci, i.e. near *NEGR1*, near *TMEM18*, in *SH2B1*, near *KCTD15*, near *GNPDA2* and in *MTCH2*. In parallel with the analyses of the GIANT consortium, deCODE genetics performed a meta-analysis of four genome-wide association studies for BMI, including 30,232 Europeans and 1,160 African Americans (Thorleifsson et al, 2009). A total of 43 single nucleotide polymorphisms (SNPs) in 19 chromosomal regions were taken forward for replication genotyping in 5,586 Danish individuals and for confirmation in discovery stage data of the GIANT consortium. Besides the *FTO* and near-*MC4R* loci, eight additional loci reached genome-wide significance. Of these, four loci (near *NEGR1*, near *TMEM18*, in *SH2B1*, near *KCTD15)* had also been identified by the GIANT consortium, whereas four loci were novel, i.e. in *SEC16B*, between *ETV5* and *DGKG*, in *BDNF* and between *BCDIN3D* and *FAIM2*. Variation in the *BAT2* gene was consistently associated with weight, but not BMI, suggesting that this locus might contribute to overall size rather than adiposity. While the studies by the GIANT consortium and deCODE genetics focused on BMI as the main outcome, a third genome-wide association study examined association with the risk of early-onset and morbid adult

obesity in 1380 cases and 1416 controls (Meyre et al, 2009). A total of 38 highly significant markers were taken forward for genotyping in 14,186 adults and children to test for replication with BMI and obesity risk. In addition to *FTO* and near-*MC4R*, three new markers were identified; in *NPC1*, near *MAF* and near *PTER* (Table 33.1).

The discovery of these novel loci has already started to provide valuable insights into pathophysiological mechanisms and pathways that underlie obesity development, in particular for the first discovered *FTO* gene. Two studies (Gerken et al, 2007; Sanchez-Pulido and Andrade-Navarro, 2007) pointed out that *FTO* is a member of the non-heme dioxygenase superfamily, encodes a 2-oxoglutarate-dependent nucleic acid demethylase and localizes to the nucleus. Studies in rodents indicated that *Fto* mRNA is most abundant in the brain, particularly in the hypothalamic nuclei governing energy balance (Gerken et al, 2007). Another study (Fischer et al, 2009) has shown that loss of *Fto* in mice leads to a significant reduction in adipose tissue and lean body mass, which was found to develop as a consequence of increased energy expenditure despite decreased spontaneous locomotor activity and relative hyperphagia. A peripheral role for *FTO* was proposed by a study in healthy women showing that FTO mRNA levels in adipose tissue increase with BMI, and carriers of the risk allele had reduced lipolytic activity, independent of BMI (Wahlen et al, 2008). For other loci, except *SH2B1* (Ren et al, 2007), *BDNF* (Nakagawa et al, 2003) and *MC4R* (Farooqi et al, 2003), the physiological role in relation to obesity risk is not or poorly understood.

Taken together, the three waves of high-density multistage genome-wide association scans, over the past 2 years, have identified 15 new loci convincingly associated with obesity traits, proving this approach more productive than any other gene-discovery methods previously applied for common traits. To date, of all identified loci, the genetic variation in the *FTO* has still the largest effect on obesity susceptibility.

Table 33.1 Obesity-susceptibility loci identified through genome-wide association studies

Chr. location	Gene symbol	Gene name	Potential function	Effect size (kg/m²)	Risk allele frequency (%)	Reference
1p31.1	NEGR1	Neuronal growth regulator 1	Regulation of neurite outgrowth in the developing brain	0.10–0.13	64	Willer et al. (2009) and Thorleifsson et al. (2009)
1q25.2	SEC16B, RASAL2	SEC16 homolog B (S.cerevisiae) RAS protein activator like 2	–	~0.11	25	Thorleifsson et al. (2009)
2p25.3	TMEM18	transmembrane protein 18	Neural development	0.19–0.26	85	Willer et al. (2009) and Thorleifsson et al. (2009)
3q27	ETV5	Ets variant gene 5	Spermatogonial stem cell self-renewal	~0.19	80	Thorleifsson et al. (2009)
4p13	GNPDA2	Glucosamine-6-phosphate deaminase 2	–	0.19	45	Willer et al. (2009)
10p12	PTER	Phosphotriesterase related protein	–	~0.07	91	Meyre et al. (2009)
11p13	BDNF	Brain-derived neurotrophic factor	BDNF expression is regulated by nutritional state and MC4R signaling	~0.19	77	Thorleifsson et al. (2009)
11p11.2	MTCH2	mitochondrial carrier homolog 2 (C. elegans)	A putative mitochondrial carrier protein – cellular apoptosis	0.07	36	Willer et al. (2009)
12q13	BCDIN3D, FAIM2	BCDIN3 domain containing Fas apoptotic inhibitory molecule 2	Adipocyte apoptosis	~0.09	35	Thorleifsson et al. (2009)
16p11.2	SH2B1, ATP2A1	SH2B adaptor protein 1 ATPase, Ca++ transporting, cardiac muscle, fast twitch 1	Neuronal role in energy homeostasis	0.15	38	Willer et al. (2009) and Thorleifsson et al. (2009)
16q22–q23	MAF	v-maf musculoaponeurotic fibrosarcoma oncogene homolog	Transcription factor involved in adipogenesis and insulin-glucagon regulation	~0.07	91	Meyre et al. (2009)
16q12.2	FTO	Fat mass- and obesity- associated gene	Neuronal function + control of appetite	0.26–0.66	46–48	Frayling et al. (2007), Scuteri et al. (2007), Loos et al. (2008), Willer et al. (2009), Thorleifsson et al. (2009), and Meyre et al. (2009)
18q11–q12	NPC1	Niemann-Pick disease, type C1	Intracellular lipid transport	~0.14	53	Meyre et al. (2009)
18q22	MC4R	Melanocortin 4 receptor	Hypothalamic signalling	0.19–0.32	27–28	Loos et al. (2008), Chambers et al. (2008), Willer et al. (2009), Thorleifsson et al. (2009), and Meyre et al. (2009)
19q13.11	KCTD15	potassium channel tetramerisation domain containing 15	–	~0.06–0.17	68–69	Willer et al. (2009) and Thorleifsson et al. (2009)

2.3 Obesity Susceptibility Genes, Food Intake and Energy Expenditure

The identification of the novel obesity suscepti-bility loci has instigated new studies exploring through which arm of the energy balance, i.e. food intake or energy expenditure, these loci lead to obesity.

In particular for the *FTO* locus, which was discovered as the first obesity susceptibility locus, new insights have begun to accumulate. Some studies have provided evidence for a role of the *FTO* locus in food intake. For example, two studies in a total of >8000 British children consistently showed that the BMI-increasing allele of the *FTO* locus was associated with increased energy intake, independent of body size (Cecil et al, 2008; Timpson et al, 2008). A third study in 3337 children showed that homozygotes for the *FTO* risk allele had a sig-nificantly reduced satiety responsiveness score (Wardle et al, 2008). This observation was con-firmed in a smaller study of 131 children with careful registration of the children's consump-tion of palatable food presented after having eaten a meal (Wardle et al, 2009). Homozygotes for the BMI-lowering *FTO*-allele ate signifi-cantly less than the heterozygotes or homozy-gotes of the BMI-increasing allele, suggesting that those with BMI-lowering allele are pro-tected against overeating by promoting respon-siveness to internal satiety signals (Wardle et al, 2009). However, not all studies have been able to support a role for the *FTO* locus in energy intake (Bauer et al, 2009; Hakanen et al, 2009; Johnson et al, 2009). While data from *fto*-deficient mice have suggested that *fto* might induce obesity through an effect on energy expenditure (Fischer et al, 2009), there is no evidence to support such role in humans (Berentzen et al, 2008; Cecil et al, 2008; Goossens et al, 2009; Hakanen et al, 2009; Haupt et al, 2009; Rampersaud et al, 2008; Speakman et al, 2008; Wardle et al, 2008).

For the locus identified in the second wave on genome-wide association studies (Chambers et al, 2008; Loos et al, 2008), the *MC4R* gene

is the nearest and most obvious candidate gene. Mutations in the *MC4R* gene are known to result in extreme obesity through hyperphagia (Farooqi et al, 2003). However, it is still unclear whether the near *MC4R* locus indeed reflects the func-tions of MC4R. A few studies, which were performed even before the genome-wide asso-ciation era, have examined the potential role of genetic variation near *MC4R* gene in contribut-ing to the physical activity energy expenditure based on evidence from studies of *Mc4r* knock-out mice (Butler et al, 2001; Ste Marie et al, 2000). A study in 669 individuals showed that homozygotes for a variant located downstream of the *MC4R* gene had the lowest moderate-to-strenuous activity scores ($p = 0.005$) and the highest inactivity scores (Loos et al, 2005). The same locus was found to be linked to physical activity levels in a genome-wide linkage study in 1030 siblings from 319 Hispanic families (Cai et al, 2006).

Little is known about the more recently dis-covered loci and genes. The neuron-specific over-expression of *SH2B1* has been shown to be protective against high-fat diet-induced obe-sity in mice (Ren et al, 2007), whereas the *BDNF* variant has been shown to be associated with eating behaviour in humans (Bauer et al, 2009; Shugart et al, 2009). A recent study in 1700 Dutch women (Bauer et al, 2009) exam-ined the majority of the newly discovered obesity loci found that the *SH2B1*, *KCTD15*, *MTCH2*, *NEGR1*, and *BDNF* loci were associated with dietary macronutrient intake.

Although the above-mentioned studies pro-vide some first evidence of association with energy intake and expenditure, replication of these observations in larger cohorts will be required to confirm the reported findings.

3 Type 2 Diabetes

3.1 Candidate Gene Studies

Candidate genes for type 2 diabetes are selected based on their involvement in pancreatic β-cell function, insulin action/glucose metabolism, or other metabolic conditions that increase type 2 diabetes risk (e.g. energy intake/expenditure and lipid metabolism) (Barroso et al, 2003). To date, more than 50 candidate genes for type 2 diabetes have been studied in various populations worldwide. However, most candidate gene studies for diabetes typically tested a limited number of genetic variants and often in only small samples or in cases and controls that were poorly matched or diagnosed, frequently resulting in lack of replication of the weak associations detected (Moore and Florez, 2008). In this section, we focus on a few of the most promising candidate genes (*PPARG*, *KCNJ11* and *WFS1*) for which the results are most convincing and the samples sizes are large.

The *PPARG* (peroxisome proliferatoractivated receptor-γ) gene has been widely studied because of its importance in adipocyte and lipid metabolism (Tontonoz and Spiegelman, 2008). In addition, it is a target for hypoglycemic drugs known as thiazolidinediones. A proline-to-alanine (Pro12Ala) change in codon 12 of *PPARG* was the first genetic variant to be definitively implicated in the common form of type 2 diabetes. The rare Ala allele is present in ~15% of white Europeans and was shown to be associated with increased insulin sensitivity. A study that combined data on a Finnish and a second generation Japanese cohort (Deeb et al, 1998) found that Pro allele homozygotes had 4.35 times higher risk for developing type 2 diabetes compared to those who do not carry the allele ($p = 0.028$). Although a number of subsequent small studies were not able to replicate this initial finding, a meta-analysis combining the results from 16 studies published before 2000 confirmed the association with type 2 diabetes (Altshuler et al, 2000). In addition, a meta-analysis of data from 57 studies comprising approximately 32,000 non-diabetic individuals further established the role of Pro12Ala variant in association with greater insulin sensitivity (standardized effect size 0.227, $P = 0.0067$) (Tönjes et al, 2006).

The beta-cell adenosine triphosphate-sensitive potassium (K_{ATP}) channel plays a critical role in insulin secretion. The channel is composed of two subunits: the sulfonylurea receptor-1 (SUR1) and an inward rectifying potassium channel (Kir6.2) that are encoded on chromosome lp15.1 by genes *ABCC8* and *KCNJ11*, respectively. SNP E23K of *KCNJ11* has been shown to be associated with type 2 diabetes. Although initial smaller studies failed to replicate the association of the E23K polymorphism with type 2 diabetes, large-scale studies and meta-analyses have consistently associated the lysine variant with type 2 diabetes, showing a 1.15 times higher risk for developing type 2 diabetes compared to those who do not carry this variant (Florez et al, 2004; Gloyn et al, 2003; Van Dam et al, 2005). Genome-wide association studies have further confirmed the association of *PPARG* and *KCNJ11* variants in association with type 2 diabetes (Diabetes Genetics Initiative of Broad Institute of Harvard and MIT et al, 2007; Scott et al, 2007; Zeggini et al, 2007).

WFS1 gene encodes wolframin, a protein that is defective in individuals with the Wolfram syndrome. This syndrome is characterized by diabetes insipidus, juvenile diabetes, optic atrophy and deafness. Disruption of *Wfs1* in mice causes overt diabetes or impaired glucose tolerance, depending on genetic background (Ishihara et al, 2004; Riggs et al, 2005). Both humans and mice deficient in Wolframin show pancreatic β-cell loss, possibly as a result of an enhanced endoplasmic reticulum stress response leading to increased β-cell apoptosis (Riggs et al, 2005; Yamada et al, 2006). Hence, WFS1 is critical for survival and function of insulin-producing pancreatic beta cells. The first evidence that variation in the *WFS1* gene influences susceptibility to type 2 diabetes was shown in a family-based association study (Minton et al, 2002). A study on 1,536 SNPs in 84 candidate genes using a gene-centric approach showed that only *WFS1* gene was associated with type 2 diabetes (Sandhu et al, 2007). This finding was further replicated in 9533 cases and 11,389 controls. Following this study, a meta-analysis of 11 studies (Franks et al, 2008), comprising up to 12,979 cases and 14,937 controls, further confirmed association between the *WFS1* gene variant, rs10010131 and type 2 diabetes (OR: 0.89, 95% CI 0.86–0.92; $p = 4.9 \times 10^{-11}$).

In summary, large-scale studies and meta-analyses have identified only three candidate genes to be robustly associated with type 2 diabetes traits.

3.2 Genome-Wide Studies

3.2.1 Genome-Wide Linkage Scans

So far, more than 20 genome-wide linkage studies have been carried out to localize type 2 diabetes predisposing variants (Huang et al, 2006; Guan et al, 2008). Although these genome-wide linkage scans have suggested that type 2 diabetes susceptibility loci reside across the whole genome, only one study has so far successfully pinpointed the gene underlying linkage with type 2 diabetes, with the discovery of the *TCF7L2* gene (Grant et al, 2006). The susceptibility effect was identified through a search for microsatellite associations across a large region of chromosome 10 that showed suggestive evidence of linkage with type 2 diabetes (Reynisdottir et al, 2003). Subsequent fine mapping of this region localized the variants associated with increased risk of type 2 diabetes to an intron in the *TCF7L2* gene. These findings were further replicated in two independent populations from the USA and Denmark (Grant et al, 2006). Overall, the effect was considerable, with each additional risk allele increasing the odds of type 2 diabetes 1.5-fold ($p = 10^{-18}$) (Grant et al, 2006).

TCF7L2, also known as TCF-4, is a transcription factor and forms part of the WNT signalling pathway, acting as a nuclear receptor for CTNNBL1 (β-catenin) (Florez, 2007; Jin and Liu, 2008). The evidence implicating variants within *TCF7L2* in type 2 diabetes susceptibility has instigated efforts to understand the mechanisms involved. It has been shown that the alteration of *TCF7L2* expression or function disrupts pancreatic islet function, possibly through dysregulation of proglucagon gene

expression, leading to reduced insulin secretion and enhanced risk of type 2 diabetes (Lyssenko et al, 2007).

To date, genetic variation in the *TCF7L2* gene has still the largest effect on type 2 diabetes susceptibility.

3.2.2 Genome-Wide Association Studies

The genome-wide association approach has led to the identification of at least 15 novel type 2 diabetes susceptibility loci (Frayling, 2007; Doria et al, 2008). Similar to obesity, the field of type 2 diabetes genetics has witnessed three waves of large-scale high-density genome-wide association studies so far. The three waves comprise six genome-wide association scans performed in European populations (Diabetes Genetics Initiative of Broad Institute of Harvard and MIT et al, 2007; Sladek et al, 2007; Steinthorsdottir et al, 2007; Scott et al, 2007; Wellcome trust case control consortium, 2007; Zeggini et al, 2007) and one in East Asians (Unoki et al, 2008).

The first wave of discoveries was based on a relatively small genome-wide association study (Sladek et al, 2007) including 661 cases and 614 controls from France identifying three novel loci, a non-synonymous polymorphism (rs13266634) in the zinc transporter *SLC30A8*, which is expressed exclusively in insulin-producing beta-cells and two loci that contain genes potentially involved in beta-cell development or function (*IDE–KIF11–HHEX* and *EXT2–ALX4*).

The second wave of discoveries involved three further scans performed by the WTCCC, DGI and FUSION (Diabetes Genetics Initiative of Broad Institute of Harvard and MIT et al, 2007; Scott et al, 2007; Wellcome trust case control consortium, 2007; Zeggini et al, 2007) that identified *CDKAL1* locus. These three studies collaborated by sharing data and co-ordinating replication studies and further identified *CDKN2A/2B*, *FTO* and *IGF2BP2*, in addition to other previously reported loci such as *PPARG*, *KCNJ11* and *TCF7L2*. Another genome-wide association study, which was conducted in 1399 cases and 5275 controls from Iceland, reported an intronic variant (rs7756992) in the *CDKAL1* gene as a novel type 2 diabetes locus (Steinthorsdottir et al, 2007). Furthermore, this study showed that the insulin response for homozygotes was approximately 20% lower than for heterozygotes or non-carriers, suggesting that this variant confers risk of type 2 diabetes through reduced insulin secretion. During the same time, a genome-wide association study for prostate cancer in 1501 cases and 11,290 controls identified two variants on chromosome 17. One of these was in the first intron of *TCF2* (*HNF1β*) gene, in which mutations are known to cause maturity-onset diabetes of the young type 5. As a follow-up, the *TCF2* variant, rs7501939, was examined in eight case–control groups comprising 9936 type 2 diabetic cases and 23,087 controls and the variant showed a significant protection against the development of type 2 diabetes (OR: 0.91, $p = 9.2 \times 10^{-7}$) (Gudmundsson et al, 2007).

In the third wave, a large-scale collaborative meta-analysis of genome-wide association scans for type 2 diabetes was performed as a three-stage study design by the Diabetes Genetics Replication and Meta-analysis (DIAGRAM) consortium (Zeggini et al, 2008). The DIAGRAM consortium combined data from the WTCCC, DGI and FUSION scans including 4549 cases and 5579 controls. A total of 69 genetic variants, showing the strongest associations in the genome-wide association meta-analysis, were taken forward for replication in a set of 22,426 individuals of which 11 variants were further replicated in an additional ~57,000 individuals. Eventually, six variants [Notch homologue 2, Drosophila (*NOTCH2*), ADAM metallopeptidase with thrombospondin type I motif 9 (*ADAMTS9*), calcium/calmodulin-dependent protein kinase 1D (*CAMK1D*), juxtaposed with another zinc finger gene 1 (*JAZF1*), tetraspanin 8 (*TSPAN8*)/leucine-rich repeat-containing G protein coupled (*LGR5*) and thyroid adenoma associated (*THADA*)] showed consistent association with the risk of type 2 diabetes. The putative functional mechanisms by

which they may affect type 2 diabetes risk are listed in Table 33.2. As part of the third wave, a study in 1561 cases and 2824 controls from Japan (Unoki et al, 2008) that genotyped over 200,000 tagSNPs, identified *KCNQ1* as a novel type 2 diabetes susceptibility locus and also confirmed the association of *CDKAL1* and *IGF2BP2* loci. *KCNQ1* locus was also identified by a second, smaller scan, again performed in a Japanese population (Yasuda et al, 2008). Another study (Wu et al, 2008) replicated the association of 17 common variants in the genes identified from previous genome-wide scans in 3210 unrelated Chinese Hans. This study showed that the common variants in *CDKAL1*, *CDKN2A/2B*, *IGF2BP2* and *SLC30A8* loci independently or additively contribute to type 2 diabetes risk. The risk alleles of the *CDKAL1* and *CDKN2A/2B* variants increased diabetes risk by ~1.4- and ~1.3-fold, respectively, which is higher than that observed in Europeans (Wellcome Trust Case Control Consortium, 2007; Zeggini et al, 2007). The risk allele frequencies of these variants were also higher in Chinese Hans compared to Europeans (Wu et al, 2008).

Besides the genome-wide scans for type 2 diabetes, scans for traits related to type 2 diabetes have also been performed. Two genome-wide association studies independently reported previously unknown genetic loci in association with fasting glucose concentrations. The first study (Prokopenko et al, 2009) showed that the variants in the gene encoding melatonin receptor 1B (*MTNR1B*) were consistently associated with fasting glucose across all the 10 genome-wide association studies ($n = 36,610$). The risk allele of the *MTNR1B* locus was associated with an increase of 0.07 (95% CI: 0.06–0.08) mmol/l in fasting glucose levels ($p = 3.2 \times 10^{-50}$) and with reduced beta-cell function as measured by homeostasis model assessment (HOMA-B, $p = 1.1 \times 10^{-15}$). The same allele was also associated with an increased risk of type 2 diabetes (odds ratio = 1.09 (1.05–1.12), per G allele $p = 3.3 \times 10^{-7}$) in a meta-analysis of 13 case–control studies (18,236 cases and 64,453 controls). This study also confirmed the previous associations of fasting glucose with variants

Table 33.2 Type 2 diabetes susceptibility loci identified through candidate gene, genome-wide linkage and genome-wide association studies

Chr. Location	Gene symbol	Gene name	Potential function	Effect size	Risk allele frequency	Reference
1p12	NOTCH2	Notch, Drosophila, homolog of, 2	Transmembrane receptor implicated in pancreatic organogenesis	1.13	0.10	Zeggini et al. (2008)
2p21	THADA	Thyroid adenoma associated gene	Thyroid adenoma; associates with PPARG	1.15	0.90	Zeggini et al. (2008)
3p14	ADAMTS9	Disintegrin-like and metalloproteinase with thrombospondin type 1 motif	Proteolytic enzyme regulating extracellular matrix	1.09	0.76	Zeggini et al. (2008)
3q25	PPARG[a]	Peroxisome proliferator activating receptor gamma	Transcription factor involved in adipocyte development	1.19	87	Altshuler et al. (2000)
3q28	IGF2BP2	Insulin-like growth factor 2 mRNA binding protein 2	Growth factor binding protein; pancreatic development	1.14	0.32	Zeggini et al. (2007), Diabetes Genetics Initiative of Broad Institute of Harvard and MIT et al. (2007), and Scott et al. (2007)
6p22.2	CDKAL1	CDK5 regulatory subunit associated protein 1-like 1	Presumed regulator of cyclin kinase; islet glucotoxicity sensor	1.14	0.32	Zeggini et al. (2007), Diabetes Genetics Initiative of Broad Institute of Harvard and MIT et al. (2007), and Scott et al. (2007)
7p15	JAZF1	Juxtaposed with another zinc finger gene 1	Transcriptional repressor; associated with prostate cancer	1.10	0.50	Zeggini et al. (2008)
8q24.11	SLC30A8	Solute carrier family 30 (zinc transporter), member 8	Beta-cell zinc transporter ZnT8; insulin storage and secretion	1.15	0.69	Sladek et al. (2007)
9p21	CDKN2A/ CDKAN2B	Cyclin-dependent kinase inhibitor 2a/2b	Cyclin-dependent kinase inhibitors 2A/2B and p15 tumour suppressor; islet development	1.20	0.83	Zeggini et al. (2007), Diabetes Genetics Initiative of Broad Institute of Harvard and MIT et al. (2007), and Scott et al. (2007)

Table 33.2 (Continued)

Chr. Location	Gene symbol	Gene name	Potential function	Effect size	Risk allele frequency	Reference
10p13-p14	CDC123/CAMK1D	Cell division cycle protein 123 homolog/ Calcium/calmodulin dependent protein kinase i-delta	CDC123: required for S phase entry of the cell cycle; CAMK1D: mediator of chemokine signal transduction in granulocytes	1.11	0.18	Zeggini et al. (2008)
10q23-q25	IDE/HHEX/KIF11	Insulin degrading enzyme/ Hematopoietically expressed homeobox/ Kinesin family member 11	IDE: neutral metallopeptidase that can degrade peptides; HHEX: transcription factor involved in pancreatic development; KIF11: kinesin related motor in microtubule and spindle function	1.13	0.65	Sladek et al. (2007)
10q25.3	TCF7L2[b]	Transcription factor 7-like 2	Transcription factor that transactivates proglucagon and insulin genes	1.37	31	Grant et al. (2006)
11p15.1	KCNJ11[a]	Potassium channel, inwardly rectifying, subfamily J, member 11	Kir 6.2 potassium channel; risk allele impairs insulin secretion	1.14	35	Florez et al. (2004)
11p15.5	KCNQ1	Potassium channel, voltage-gated, KQT-like subfamily, member 1	Beta-cell dysfunction	1.29	0.93	Unoki et al. (2008)
12q21	TSPAN8/LGR5	Tetraspanin 8/ Leucine-rich repeat containing G protein coupled	Cell surface glycoprotein implicated in gastrointestinal cancers	1.09	0.27	Zeggini et al. (2008)
4p16.1	WFS1[a]	Wolfram syndrome 1 (wolframin)	Critical for survival and function of insulin-producing pancreatic beta cells	1.12	0.60	Sandhu et al. (2007)
17q12	TCF2[a]	Transcription factor 2	transcription factor implicated in pancreatic islet development and function	0.91	0.55	Gudmundsson et al. (2007)
16q12.2	FTO	Fat mass and obesity associated	Altered BMI	1.17	0.40	Frayling et al. (2007)

Type 2 diabetes susceptibility loci marked with [a] were identified through the candidate gene approach, those marked with [b] were identified through genome-wide linkage, and all others were identified through genome-wide association studies.

at the *G6PC2* (rs560887, $p = 1.1 \times 10^{-57}$) and *GCK* (rs4607517, $p = 1.0 \times 10^{-25}$) loci. Another study (Bouatia-Naji et al, 2009) identified rs1387153, near *MTNR1B*, as a modulator of fasting plasma glucose ($p = 1.3 \times 10^{-7}$) in genome-wide association data from 2151 nondiabetic French individuals and also showed an association with the risk of developing type 2 diabetes (OR: 1.15, 95% CI = 1.08–1.22, $p = 6.3 \times 10^{-5}$). In addition, this study observed cumulative effects of the *MTNR1B* locus and the three previously identified genetic determinants of fasting plasma glucose (*G6PC2*, *GCK* and *GCKR*). Those carrying six or more high FPG alleles showed a mean 0.36 mmol/l increase in fasting plasma glucose compared to individuals with zero or one high fasting plasma glucose allele.

So far, 18 loci for type 2 diabetes (Table 33.2) and four loci for fasting glucose have been identified through genome-wide association scans. In comparison to the candidate gene and genome-wide linkage approaches, the genome-wide association studies have been extremely successful for both type 2 diabetes and BMI.

4 Genetic Prediction of Obesity and Diabetes

There is growing interest in the potential for the increasing numbers of genetic susceptibility variants to contribute towards individualized medical care. However, at this stage, the prospects for individual prediction seem limited.

In a recent study (Willer et al, 2009), the predictive value of eight validated obesity susceptibility loci (*TMEM18*, *KCTD15*, *SH2B1*, *MTCH2*, *NEGR1*, *GNPDA2*, *FTO* and *MC4R*) on obesity risk was examined in 14,409 men and women of the population-based EPIC-Norfolk cohort. A genetic predisposition score for each individual, summing the number of BMI-increasing alleles, was calculated. The average BMI of individuals carrying 13 or more risk alleles (<2% of the population) was 1.46 kg

m^{-2} (or 3.7–4.7 kg in body weight) higher compared to those carrying three or fewer risk alleles (<2% of the population). However, together, the eight variants explained less than 1% of the variation in BMI and had very limited power in prediction of obesity, contributing only 2–3% to the prediction on top of classical clinical predictors such as age and gender.

Similar results were observed for type 2 diabetes. Two studies examined the cumulative effects of 18 polymorphisms chosen from genome-wide association scans on type 2 diabetes (Lango et al, 2008; van Hoek et al, 2008). Both studies found a similar predictive value showing only a marginal improvement in the prediction of type 2 diabetes beyond classical clinical characteristics.

Thus, despite overwhelming significances and repeated replications, the explained variance and predictive value of the currently identified susceptibility loci is too low to be clinically useful.

5 Gene–Environment Interactions in Obesity and Diabetes

Susceptibility to obesity and diabetes is determined by both genetic and lifestyle factors. Suggestive evidence of gene–lifestyle interaction (Box 33.3) in the development of common diseases such as obesity and type 2 diabetes was first provided by descriptive epidemiological studies such as migration studies that compare the disease risk between genetically related populations who live different lifestyles. A classical example is the comparison of the risk of obesity and type 2 diabetes between Pima Indians living in the "obesogenic" environment of Arizona (69% of whom are obese and 55% have type 2 diabetes) and those living in the "restrictive" environment of the remote Mexican Sierra Madre Mountains (13% of whom are obese with only 6% having type 2 diabetes) (Esparza et al, 2000; Ravussin et al, 1994). These findings illustrate that despite a similar genetic predisposition, different lifestyles result in different prevalences of obesity and type 2 diabetes.

Box 33.3 – Gene–Environment Interaction

Seeing Gene–Environment Interaction from Different Perspectives

- **Genetic perspective:** The genetic perspective starts from a main-effect hypothesis that tests for association between a genetic variant and a disease or trait (e.g. whether a genotype is associated with BMI). Next, the interaction hypothesis tests whether the genotype disease association is different across different levels of environmental exposure (e.g. whether the genotype-BMI association is different in individuals on a low-fat diet compared with individuals on a high-fat diet). The gene–environment interaction would be statistically significant if the slopes of the two associations (low-fat diet vs. high-fat diet) differ significantly from each other.
- **Public health perspective:** The public health perspective first questions the association between an environmental factor and disease or trait (e.g. whether physical inactivity is associated with BMI/ diabetes). Subsequently, the interaction hypothesis tests whether carriers of a certain genotype are more susceptible to the influence that the environment has on disease than non-carriers (e.g. whether the detrimental effects of physical inactivity on BMI/ diabetes are more pronounced in the carriers of a specific allele than the non-carriers). Again, the gene–environment interaction will be statistically significant if the slopes of the two associations differ significantly from each other.

Besides descriptive epidemiological studies, genetic association studies have also identified gene–lifestyle interactions as can be seen in *TCF7L2* and *FTO* genes. The effect of the *TCF7L2* risk allele on the progression towards type 2 diabetes was abolished in the lifestyle intervention group, but evident in the placebo control group. This suggests an interaction between common variants in the *TCF7L2* gene and lifestyle in the risk of progression to type 2 diabetes (Florez et al, 2006; Wang et al, 2007). Studies in European populations have shown that the association between the *FTO* gene and the BMI was attenuated by physical activity levels (Andreasen et al, 2008b; Rampersaud et al, 2008; Vimaleswaran et al, 2009). However, others have failed to find such interaction (Tan et al, 2008; Lappalainen et al 2009), which could be due to insufficient power and differences in the physical activity measurements.

Unidentified gene–environment interaction may mask the presence of a genetic effect in a certain environment or it may mask the presence of an environmental effect for a given genotype. As an example, studies involving genome-wide associations (Loos et al, 2008; Zeggini et al, 2008) and large-scale meta-analyses of candidate genes (Kurokawa et al, 2008; Ludovico et al, 2007; Young et al, 2007) have shown that the overall effect size of a genetic polymorphism on the risk of a disease or on variation of a trait is generally very small. Often these meta-analyses show significant heterogeneity of effect sizes across studies, raising the possibility that the genetic contribution may be modified by unobserved environmental factors. Because of these reasons, association studies looking at main effects require data from tens of thousands of individuals to identify convincing and robust associations. In addition, gene–environment interaction studies may hold important public health messages. Individuals might be genetically susceptible to develop disease, but this does not mean that they are destined to become diseased. Changes in lifestyle can overcome genetic susceptibility, as illustrated by the *FTO*-physical activity example (Andreasen et al,

2008; Rampersaud et al, 2008; Vimaleswaran et al, 2009) or the *TCF7L2*-lifestyle intervention studies (Florez et al, 2006; Wang et al, 2007).

6 Future Directions

The next step forward will be the discovery of more susceptibility loci that are currently undetected and to explore the physiological mechanisms and pathways that underlie the observed association using various approaches.

One approach is to initiate a fourth wave of genome-wide association studies to further increase the sample size of the initial discovery stage. This will further improve the power to uncover common variants with even smaller effect sizes (Li and Loos, 2008). The power to reveal novel loci might vary across populations because of differences in effect sizes and allele frequencies; hence, the study of ethnicities other than white Europeans might also provide new gene-discovery opportunities. For example, a study in Asian Indians required only a small discovery sample to identify the near-*MC4R* because the frequency of the risk-allele was substantially higher than in Europeans (Chambers et al, 2008; Loos et al, 2008). Similarly, a relatively small study in Japanese individuals (Unoki et al, 2008) was sufficient to discover *KCNQ1* variants to be associated with type 2 diabetes.

Most of the studies, so far, have used BMI as a simple and inexpensive proxy measure of adiposity, which is easy to collect in large samples. More accurate measures of adiposity might further improve power, yet these are often more expensive and harder to collect. Genome-wide association studies for body fat percentage, waist circumference, extreme obesity risk and for mediating traits that underlie obesity, such as food intake and energy expenditure, may reveal new obesity susceptibility loci that are currently hidden in studies that use BMI as the main outcome. Similarly for type 2 diabetes, genome-wide association studies for fasting glucose, fasting insulin levels, HbA1C and other intermediary phenotypes for type 2 diabetes such as insulin resistance and impaired glucose tolerance might identify novel diabetes susceptibility loci.

Another strategy would be to examine the contribution of other sources of genetic variations such as copy number variants and rare variants to the predisposition to obesity and diabetes, which have so far been unexplored. Further advances in technology will be required before the analyses of copy number variants can be implemented at a larger scale. Yet, the observation that the *NEGR1* locus might represent a copy number variant indicates the potential importance of this source of variation (Willer et al., 2009).

Finally, follow-up of the established loci in molecular and physiological studies will be important to determine the mechanisms through which the loci confer disease susceptibility. A prime challenge before these loci can be passed on to physiologists is pinpointing the causal variant or gene. This will require high-throughput sequencing of the region of interest in extreme cases and controls from different ethnicities. It is only when the causal locus is identified and its modes of action are completely understood that this information can be translated into mainstream health care and clinical practice.

Genome-wide association studies have led to an era of gene discovery for common diseases such as obesity and type 2 diabetes. Although candidate gene studies have identified a few genetic variants convincingly associated with obesity and diabetes traits, genome-wide association studies have identified at least 15 loci in less than 3 years of time. This recent progress has also provided valuable insights into pathophysiological mechanisms and pathways that underlie the disease development. This offers great hopes for genetic risk profiling and therapeutic intervention; however, implementation of such strategies in health care remains in the future, as we need first to learn more about the causal variants and their functional implications in relation to obesity and type 2 diabetes.

References

Allison, D. B., Kaprio, J., Korkeila, M., Koskenvuo, M., Neale, M. C. et al (1996). The heritability of body mass index among an international sample of monozygotic twins reared apart. *Int J Obes Relat Metab Disord, 20*, 501–506.

Altshuler, D., Hirschhorn, J. N., Klannemark, M., Lindgren, C. M., Vohl, M. C. et al (2000). The common PPARγ Pro12Ala polymorphism is associated with decreased risk of type 2 diabetes. *Nat Genet, 26*, 76–80.

Andreasen, C. H., Mogensen, M. S., Borch-Johnsen, K., Sandbak, A., Lauritzen, T. et al (2008a). Non-replication of genome-wide based associations between common variants in INSIG2 and PFKP and obesity in studies of 18,014 Danes. *PLoS ONE, 3*, e2872.

Andreasen, C. H., Stender-Petersen, K. L., Mogensen, M. S., Torekov, S. S., Wegner, L. et al (2008b). Low physical activity accentuates the effect of the FTO rs9939609 polymorphism on body fat accumulation. *Diabetes, 57*, 95–101.

Barroso, I., Luan, J., Middelberg, R. P., Harding, A. H., Franks, P. W. et al (2003). Candidate gene association study in type 2 diabetes indicates a role for genes involved in beta-cell function as well as insulin action. *PLoS Biol, 1*, E20.

Bauer, F., Elbers, C. C., Adan, R. A., Loos, R. J., Onland-Moret, N. C. et al (2009). Obesity genes identified in genome-wide association studies are associated with adiposity measures and potentially with nutrient-specific food preference. *Am J Clin Nutr*, [Epub ahead of print].

Benzinou, M., Chèvre, J. C., Ward, K. J., Lecoeur, C., Dina, C. et al (2008a). Endocannabinoid receptor 1 gene variations increase risk for obesity and modulate body mass index in European populations. *Hum Mol Genet, 17*, 1916–1921.

Benzinou, M., Creemers, J. W., Choquet, H., Lobbens, S., Dina, C. et al (2008b). Common nonsynonymous variants in PCSK1 confer risk of obesity. *Nat Genet, 40*, 943–945.

Berentzen, T., Kring, S. I., Holst, C., Zimmermann, E., Jess, T. et al (2008). Lack of association of fatness-related FTO gene variants with energy expenditure or physical activity. *J Clin Endocrinol Metab, 93*, 2904–2908.

Butler, A. A., Marks, D. L., Fan, W., Kuhn, C. M., Bartolome, M. et al (2001). Melanocortin-4 receptor is required for acute homeostatic responses to increased dietary fat. *Nat Neuroscience, 4*, 605–611.

Bouatia-Naji, N., Bonnefond, A., Cavalcanti- Proença, C., Sparsø, T., Holmkvist, J. et al (2009). A variant near MTNR1B is associated with increased fasting plasma glucose levels and type 2 diabetes risk. *Nat Genet, 41*, 89–94.

Cai, G., Cole, S. A., Butte, N., Bacino, C., Diego, V. et al (2006). A quantitative trait locus on chromosome 18q for physical activity and dietary intake in Hispanic children. *Obesity, 14*, 1596–1604.

Cecil, J. E., Tavendale, R., Watt, P., Hetherington, M. M., Palmer, C. N. (2008). An obesity-associated FTO gene variant and increased energy intake in children. *N Engl J Med, 359*, 2558–2566.

Chambers, J. C., Elliott, P., Zabaneh, D., Zhang, W., Li, Y., Froguel, P. et al (2008). Common genetic variation near MC4R is associated with waist circumference and insulin resistance. *Nat Genet, 40*, 716–718.

Clement, K., Vaisse, C., Manning, B. S., Basdevant, A., Guy-Grand, B. et al (1995). Genetic variation in the β3-adrenergic receptor and an increased capacity to gain weight in patients with morbid obesity. *N Engl J Med, 333*, 352–354.

Dean, M. (2003). Approaches to identify genes for complex human diseases: lessons from Mendelian disorders. *Hum Mutat, 22*, 261–274.

Deeb, S. S., Fajas, L., Nemoto, M., Pihlajamäki, J., Mykkänen, L. et al (1998). A Pro12Ala substitution in *PPARγ2* associated with decreased receptor activity, lower body mass index and improved insulin sensitivity. *Nat Genet, 20*, 284–287.

Diabetes Genetics Initiative of Broad Institute of Harvard and MIT, Lund University, and Novartis Institutes of BioMedical Research, Saxena, R., Voight, B. F., Lyssenko, V., Burtt, N. P., de Bakker, P. I. et al (2007). Genome-wide association analysis identifies loci for type 2 diabetes and triglyceride levels. *Science, 316*, 1331–1336.

Doria, A., Patti, M. E., and Kahn, C. R. (2008). The emerging genetic architecture of type 2 diabetes. *Cell Metab, 8*, 186–200.

Esparza, J., Fox, C., Harper, I. T., Bennett, P. H., Schulz, L. O. et al (2000). Daily energy expenditure in Mexican and USA Pima Indians: low physical activity as a possible cause of obesity. *Int J Obes (Lond), 24*, 55–59.

Farooqi, I. S., Keogh, J. M., Yeo, G. S., Lank, E. J., Cheetham, T. et al (2003). Clinical spectrum of obesity and mutations in the melanocortin 4 receptor gene. *N Engl J Med, 348*, 1085–1095.

Farooqi, S., O'Rahilly, S. (2006). Genetics of obesity in humans. *Endocr Rev, 27*, 710–718.

Fischer, J., Koch, L., Emmerling, C., Vierkotten, J., Peters, T. et al (2009). Inactivation of the Fto gene protects from obesity. *Nature, 458*, 894–898.

Florez, J. C. (2007). The new type 2 diabetes gene TCF7L2. *Curr Opin Clin Nutr Metab Care, 10*, 391–396.

Florez, J. C., Burtt, N., de Bakker, P. I., Almgren, P., Tuomi, T. et al (2004). Haplotype structure and genotype-phenotype correlations of the sulfonylurea receptor and the islet ATP-sensitive potassium channel gene region. *Diabetes, 53*, 1360–1368.

Florez, J. C., Jablonski, K. A., Bayley, N., Pollin, T. I., de Bakker, P. I. et al (2006). *TCF7L2* polymorphisms and progression to diabetes in the Diabetes Prevention Program. *N Engl J Med, 355,* 241–250.

Franks, P. W., Rolandsson, O., Debenham, S. L., Fawcett, K. A., Payne, F. et al (2008). Replication of the association between variants in WFS1 and risk of type 2 diabetes in European populations. *Diabetologia, 51,* 458–463.

Frayling, T. M. (2007). Genome-wide association studies provide new insights into type 2 diabetes aetiology. *Nat Rev Genet, 8,* 657–662.

Frayling, T. M., Timpson, N. J., Weedon, M. N., Zeggini, E., Freathy, R. M. et al (2007). A common variant in the FTO gene is associated with body mass index and predisposes to childhood and adult obesity. *Science, 316,* 889–894.

Gerken, T., Girard, C. A., Tung, Y. C., Webby, C. J., Saudek, V. et al (2007). The obesity-associated FTO gene encodes a 2-oxoglutarate-dependent nucleic acid demethylase. *Science, 318,* 1469–1472.

Gloyn, A. L., Weedon, M. N., Owen, K. R., Turner, M. J., Knight, B. A. et al (2003). Large-scale association studies of variants in genes encoding the pancreatic β-cell KATP channel subunits Kir6.2 (*KCNJ11*) and SUR1 (*ABCC8*) confirm that the *KCNJ11* E23K variant is associated with type 2 diabetes. *Diabetes, 52,* 568–572.

Goossens, G. H., Petersen, L., Blaak, E. E., Hul, G., Arner, P. et al (2009). Several obesity-and nutrient-related gene polymorphisms but not FTO and UCP variants modulate postabsorptive resting energy expenditure and fat-induced thermogenesis in obese individuals: the NUGENOB study. *Int J Obes, 33,* 669–679.

Grant, S. F., Thorleifsson, G., Reynisdottir, I., Benediktsson, R., Manolescu, A. et al (2006). Variant of transcription factor 7-like 2 (TCF7L2) gene confers risk of type 2 diabetes. *Nat Genet, 38,* 320–323.

Grarup, N., Urhammer, S. A., Ek, J., Albrechtsen, A., Glumer, C. et al (2006). Studies of the relationship between the ENPP1 K121Q polymorphism and type 2 diabetes, insulin resistance and obesity in 7,333 Danish white subjects. *Diabetologia, 49,* 2097–104.

Gray, J., Yeo, G. S. H., Cox, J. J., Morton, J., Adlam, A. L. et al (2006). Hyperphagia, severe obesity, impaired cognitive function, and hyperactivity associated with functional loss of one copy of the brain-derived neurotrophic factor (BDNF) gene. *Diabetes, 55,* 3366–3371.

Guan, W., Pluzhnikov, A., Cox, N. J., Boehnke, M., International Type 2 Diabetes Linkage Analysis Consortium. (2008). Meta-analysis of 23 type 2 diabetes linkage studies from the International Type 2 Diabetes Linkage Analysis Consortium. *Hum Hered, 66,* 35–49.

Gudmundsson, J., Sulem, P., Steinthorsdottir, V., Bergthorsson, J. T., Thorleifsson, G. et al (2007). Two variants on chromosome 17 confer prostate cancer risk, and the one in TCF2 protects against type 2 diabetes. *Nat Genet, 39*(8):977–983.

Hakanen, M., Raitakari, O. T., Lehtimäki, T., Peltonen, N., Pahkala, K. et al (2009). FTO genotype is associated with body mass index after the age of seven years but not with energy intake or leisure-time physical activity. *J Clin Endocrinol Metab, 94,* 1281–1287.

Haupt, A., Thamer, C., Staiger, H., Tschritter, O., Kirchhoff, K. et al (2009). Variation in the FTO gene influences food intake but not energy expenditure. *Exp Clin Endocrinol Diabetes, 117,* 194–197.

Heid, I. M., Vollmert, C., Hinney, A., Döring, A., Geller, F. et al (2005). Association of the 103I MC4R allele with decreased body mass in 7937 participants of two population based surveys. *J Med Genet, 42,* e21.

Herskind, A. M., McGue, M., Sørensen, T. I., Harvald, B. (1996). Sex and age specific assessment of genetic and environmental influences on body mass index in twins. *Int J Obes Relat Metab Disord, 20,* 106–113.

Hill, J. O., Wyatt, H. R., Reed, G. W., Peters, J. C. (2003) Obesity and the environment: where do we go from here? *Science, 299,* 853–855.

Huang, Q. Y., Cheng, M. R., Ji, S. L. (2006). Linkage and association studies of the susceptibility genes for type 2 diabetes. *Yi Chuan Xue Bao, 33,* 573–589.

Huszar, D., Lynch, C. A., Fairchild-Huntress, V., Dunmore, J. H., Fang, Q. et al (1997). Targeted disruption of the melanocortin-4 receptor results in obesity in mice. *Cell, 88,* 131–141.

International Association for the Study of Obesity: (http://www.iotf.org/).

International HapMap Consortium, Frazer, K. A., Ballinger, D. G., Cox, D. R., Hinds, D. A. et al (2007). A second generation human haplotype map of over 3.1 million SNPs. *Nature, 449,* 851–861.

Ishihara, H., Takeda, S., Tamura, A., Takahashi, R., Yamaguchi, S. et al (2004). Disruption of the WFS1 gene in mice causes progressive beta-cell loss and impaired stimulus-secretion coupling in insulin secretion. *Hum Mol Genet, 13,* 1159–1170.

Jackson, R. S., Creemers, J. W., Ohagi, S., Raffin-Sanson, M. L., Sanders, L. et al (1997). Obesity and impaired prohormone processing associated with mutations in the human prohormone convertase 1 gene. *Nat Genet, 16,* 303–306.

Jalba M, S., Rhoads, G. G., and Demissie, K. (2008). Association of codon 16 and codon 27 beta 2-adrenergic receptor gene polymorphisms with obesity: a meta-analysis. *Obesity, 16,* 2096–2106.

Jin, T., and Liu, L. (2008). The Wnt signaling pathway effector TCF7L2 and type 2 diabetes mellitus. *Mol Endocrinol, 22,* 2383–2392.

Johnson, L., van Jaarsveld, C. H., Emmett, P. M., Rogers, I. S., Ness, A. R. et al (2009). Dietary energy density affects fat mass in early adolescence and is not modified by FTO variants. *PLoS One, 4,* e4594.

Kaprio, J., Tuomilehto, J., Koskenvuo, M., Romanov, K., Reunanen, A. et al (1992). Concordance for type 1 (insulin-dependent) and type 2 (non-insulin-dependent) diabetes mellitus in a population-based cohort of twins in Finland. *Diabetologia, 35,* 1060–1067.

Köbberling, J., and Tillil, H. (1982). Empirical risk figures for first degree relatives of non-insulin dependent diabetics. In J. Köbberling & R. Tattersall (Eds.), *The Genetics of Diabetes Mellitus* (pp. 201–209). London: Academic Press.

Kurokawa, N., Young, E. H., Oka, Y., Satoh, H., Wareham, N. J. et al (2008). The ADRB3 Trp64Arg variant and BMI: a meta-analysis of 44 833 individuals. *Int J Obes (Lond), 32,* 1240–1249.

Lango, H., UK Type 2 Diabetes Genetics Consortium, Palmer, C. N., Morris, A. D., Zeggini, E. et al (2008). Assessing the combined impact of 18 common genetic variants of modest effect sizes on type 2 diabetes risk. *Diabetes, 57,* 3129–3135.

Lappalainen, T. J., Tolppanen, A. M., Kolehmainen, M., Schwab, U., Lindström, J. et al (2009). The common variant in the FTO gene did not modify the effect of lifestyle changes on body weight: the Finnish Diabetes Prevention Study. *Obesity (Silver Spring), 17,* 832–836.

Li, S., and Loos, R. J. (2008). Progress in the genetics of common obesity: size matters. *Curr Opin Lipidol, 19,* 113–121.

Loos, R. J. (2009). Recent progress in the genetics of common obesity. *Br J Clin Pharmacol, 68,* 811–829.

Loos, R. J., Lindgren, C. M., Li, S., Wheeler, E., Zhao, J. H. et al (2008). Common variants near MC4R are associated with fat mass, weight and risk of obesity. *Nat Genet, 40,* 768–775.

Loos, R. J., Rankinen, T., Tremblay, A., Pérusse, L., Chagnon, Y. et al (2005). Melanocortin-4 receptor gene and physical activity in the Québec Family Study. *Int J Obes, 29,* 420–428.

Ludovico, O., Pellegrini, F., Di, P. R., Minenna, A., Mastroianno, S. et al (2007). Heterogeneous effect of peroxisome proliferator-activated receptor gamma2 Ala12 variant on type 2 diabetes risk. *Obesity (Silver Spring), 15,* 1076–1081.

Luke, A., Guo, X., Adeyemo, A. A., Wilks, R., Forrester, T. et al (2001). Heritability of obesity-related traits among Nigerians, Jamaicans and US black people. *Int J Obes Relat Metab Disord, 25,* 1034–1041.

Lyon, H. N., Florez, J. C., Bersaglieri, T., Saxena, R., Winckler, W. et al (2006). Common variants in the ENPP1 gene are not reproducibly associated with diabetes or obesity. *Diabetes, 55,* 3180–3184.

Lyssenko, V., Lupi, R., Marchetti, P., Del Guerra, S., Orho-Melander, M. et al (2007). Mechanisms by which common variants in the TCF7L2 gene increase risk of type 2 diabetes. *J Clin Invest, 117,* 2155–2163.

Maes, H. H., Neale, M. C., and Eaves, L. J. (1997). Genetic and environmental factors in relative body weight and human obesity. *Behav Genet, 27,* 325–351.

Magi, R., Pfeufer, A., Nelis, M., Montpetit, A., Metspalu, A. et al (2007). Evaluating the performance of commercial whole-genome marker sets for capturing common genetic variation. *BMC Genomics, 8,* 159.

Manolio, T. A., Brooks, L. D., and Collins, F. S. (2008). A HapMap harvest of insights into the genetics of common disease. *J Clin Invest, 118,* 1590–1605.

Meyre, D., Bouatia-Naji, N., Vatin, V., Veslot, J., Samson, C. et al (2007). ENPP1 K121Q polymorphism and obesity, hyperglycaemia and type 2 diabetes in the prospective DESIR Study. *Diabetologia, 50,* 2090–2096.

Meyre, D., Delplanque, J., Chèvre, J. C., Lecoeur, C., Lobbens, S. et al (2009). Genome-wide association study for early-onset and morbid adult obesity identifies three new risk loci in European populations. *Nat Genet, 41,* 157–159.

Minton, J. A., Hattersley, A. T., Owen, K., McCarthy, M. I., Walker, M. et al (2002). Association studies of genetic variation in the WFS1 gene and type 2 diabetes in U.K. populations. *Diabetes, 51,* 1287–1290.

Moore, A. F., and Florez, J. C. (2008). Genetic susceptibility to type 2 diabetes and implications for antidiabetic therapy. *Annu Rev Med, 59,* 95–111.

Nakagawa, T., Ogawa, Y., Ebihara, K., Yamanaka, M., Tsuchida, A. et al (2003). Anti-obesity and anti-diabetic effects of brain-derived neurotrophic factor in rodent models of leptin resistance. *Int J Obes Relat Metab Disord, 27,* 557–565.

Newman, B., Selby, J. V., King, M. C., Slemenda, C., Fabsitz, R. et al (1987). Concordance for type 2 (non-insulin-dependent) diabetes mellitus in male twins. *Diabetologia, 30,* 763–768.

Norman, R. A., Thompson, D. B., Foroud, T., Garvey, W. T., Bennett, P. H. et al (1997). Genomewide search for genes influencing percent body fat in Pima Indians: Suggestive linkage at chromosome 11q21–q22. *Am J Hum Genet, 60,* 166–173.

Pietri-Rouxel, F., Manning, B. S., Gros, J., and Strosberg, A. D. (1997). The biochemical effect of the naturally occurring Trp64 Arg mutation on human beta3-adrenoceptor activity. *Eur J Biochem, 247,* 1174–1179.

Permutt, M. A., Wasson, J., and Cox, N. (2005). Genetic epidemiology of diabetes. *J Clin Invest, 115,* 1431–1439.

Prokopenko, I., Langenberg, C., Florez, J. C., Saxena, R., Soranzo, N. et al (2009). Variants in MTNR1B influence fasting glucose levels. *Nat Genet, 41,* 77–81.

Qi, L., Zhang, C., van Dam, R. M., and Hu, F. B. (2007). Interleukin-6 genetic variability and adiposity: associations in two prospective cohorts and systematic review in 26,944 individuals. *J Clin Endocrinol Metab, 92,* 3618–3625.

Rampersaud, E., Mitchell, B. D., Pollin, T. I., Fu, M., Shen, H. et al (2008). Physical activity and the association of common FTO gene variants with body mass index and obesity. *Arch Intern Med, 168,* 1791–1797.

Rankinen, T., Zuberi, A., Chagnon, Y. C., Weisnagel, S. J., Argyropoulos, G. et al (2006). The human obesity gene map: The 2005 Update. *Obes Res, 14*, 529–644.

Ravussin, E., Valencia, M. E., Esparza, J., Bennett, P. H., and Schulz, O. (1994). Effects of a traditional lifestyle on obesity in Pima Indians. *Diabetes Care, 17*, 1067–1074.

Ren, D., Zhou, Y., Morris, D., Li, M., Li, Z. et al (2007). Neuronal SH2B1 is essential for controlling energy and glucose homeostasis. *J Clin Invest, 117*, 397–406.

Reynisdottir, I., Thorleifsson, G., Benediktsson, R., Sigurdsson, G., Emilsson, V., et al (2003). Localisation of a susceptibility gene for type diabetes to chromosome 5q34-q35.2. *Am J Hum Genet, 73*, 323–335.

Rice, T., Perusse, L., Bouchard, C., and Rao, D. C. (1999). Familial aggregation of body mass index and subcutaneous fat measures in the longitudinal Quebec Family Study. *Genet Epidemiol, 16*, 316–334.

Riggs, A. C., Bernal-Mizrachi, E., Ohsugi, M., Wasson, J., Fatrai, S. et al (2005). Mice conditionally lacking the Wolfram gene in pancreatic islet beta cells exhibit diabetes as a result of enhanced endoplasmic reticulum stress and apoptosis. *Diabetologia, 48*, 2313–2321.

Rios, M., Fan, G., Fekete, C., Kelly, J., Bates, B. et al (2001). Conditional deletion of brain-derived neurotrophic factor in the postnatal brain leads to obesity and hyperactivity. *Mol Endocrinol, 15*, 1748–1757.

Sanchez-Pulido, L., and Andrade-Navarro, M. A. (2007). The FTO (fat mass and obesity associated) gene codes for a novel member of the nonheme dioxygenase superfamily. *BMC Biochem, 8*, 23.

Sandhu, M. S., Weedon, M. N., Fawcett, K. A., Wasson, J., Debenham, S. L. et al (2007). Common variants in WFS1 confer risk of type 2 diabetes. *Nat Genet, 39*, 951–953.

Saunders, C. L., Chiodini, B. D., Sham, P., Lewis, C. M., Abkevich, V. et al (2007). Meta-analysis of genome-wide linkage studies in BMI and obesity. *Obesity, 15*, 2263–2275.

Scott, L. J., Mohlke, K. L., Bonnycastle, L. L., Willer, C. J., Li, Y. et al (2007). A genome-wide association study of type 2 diabetes in Finns detects multiple susceptibility variants. *Science, 316*, 1341–1345.

Scuteri, A., Sanna, S., Chen, W-M., Uda, M., Albai, G. et al (2007). Genome-wide association scan shows genetic variants in the FTO gene are associated with obesity-related traits. *PLos Genetics, 3*, e115.

Shugart, Y. Y., Chen, L., Day, I. N. M., Lewis, S. J., Timpson, N. J. et al (2009). Two British women studies replicated the association between the Val66Met polymorphism in the brain-derived neurotrophic factor (BDNF) and BMI. *Eur J Hum Genet, 17*, 1050–1055.

Sladek, R., Rocheleau, G., Rung, J., Dina, C., Shen, L. et al (2007). A genome-wide association study identifies novel risk loci for type 2 diabetes. *Nature, 445*, 881–885.

Speakman, J. R., Rance, K. A., and Johnstone, A. M. (2008). Polymorphisms of the FTO gene are associated with variation in energy intake, but not energy expenditure. *Obesity, 16*, 1961–1965.

Steinthorsdottir, V., Thorleifsson, G., Reynisdottir, I., Benediktsson, R., Jonsdottir, T. et al (2007). A variant in CDKAL1 influences insulin response and risk of type 2 diabetes. *Nat Genet, 39*, 770–775.

Ste Marie, L., Miura, G. I., Marsh, D. J., Yagaloff, K., and Palmiter, R. D. (2000). A metabolic defect promotes obesity in mice lacking melanocortin-4 receptors. *Proc Natl Acad Sci U S A, 97*, 12339–12344.

Stunkard, A. J., Foch, T. T., and Hrubec, Z. (1986). A twin study of human obesity. *JAMA, 256*, 51–54.

Stunkard, A. J., Sørensen, T. I., Hanis, C., Teasdale, T. W., Chakraborty, R. et al (1986). An adoption study of human obesity. *N Engl J Med, 314*, 193–198.

Stutzmann, F., Vatin, V., Cauchi, S., Morandi, A., Jouret, B. et al (2007). Nonsynonymous polymorphisms in melanocortin-4 receptor protect against obesity: the two facets of a Janus obesity gene. *Hum Mol Genet, 16*, 1837–1844.

Tan, J. T., Dorajoo, R., Seielstad, M., Sim, X. L., Ong, R. T. et al (2008). FTO variants are associated with obesity in the Chinese and Malay populations in Singapore. *Diabetes, 57*, 2851–2857.

Thorleifsson, G., Walters, G. B., Gudbjartsson, D. F., Steinthorsdottir, V., Sulem, P. et al (2009). Genome-wide association yields new sequence variants at seven loci that associate with measures of obesity. *Nat Genet, 41*, 18–24.

Timpson, N. J., Emmett, P. M., Frayling, T. M., Rogers, I., Hattersley, A. T. et al (2008). The fat mass- and obesity-associated locus and dietary intake in children. *Am J Clin Nutr, 88*, 971–978.

Tönjes, A., Scholz, M., Loeffler, M., and Stumvoll, M. (2006). Association of Pro12Ala polymorphism in peroxisome proliferator-activated receptor gamma with Pre-diabetic phenotypes: meta-analysis of 57 studies on nondiabetic individuals. *Diabetes Care, 29*, 2489–2497.

Tontonoz, P., and Spiegelman, B. M. (2008). Fat and beyond: the diverse biology of PPARgamma. *Annu Rev Biochem, 77*, 289–312.

Umekawa, T., Yoshida, T., Sakane, N., Kogure, A., Kondo, M. et al (1999). Trp64Arg mutation of beta3-adrenoceptor gene deteriorates lipolysis induced by beta3-adrenoceptor agonist in human omental adipocytes. *Diabetes, 48*, 117–120.

Unoki, H., Takahashi, A., Kawaguchi, T., Hara, K., Horikoshi, M. et al (2008). SNPs in KCNQ1 are associated with susceptibility to type 2 diabetes in East Asian and European populations. *Nat Genet, 40*, 1098–1102.

Van Dam, R. M., Hoebee, B., Seidel, J. C., Schaap, M. M., de Bruin, T. W. et al (2005). Common variants in the ATP-sensitive K+ channel genes KCNJ11 (Kir6.2) and ABCC8 (SUR1) in relation to glucose intolerance: population-based studies and meta-analyses. *Diabet Med, 22*, 590–598.

van Hoek, M., Dehghan, A., Witteman, J. C., van Duijn, C. M., Uitterlinden, A. G., Oostra, B. A. et al (2008). Predicting type 2 diabetes based on polymorphisms from genome-wide association studies: a population-based study. *Diabetes, 57*, 3122–3128.

Vimaleswaran, K. S., Li, S., Zhao, J. H., Luan, J., Bingham, S. A. et al (2009). Physical activity attenuates the body mass index-increasing influence of genetic variation in the FTO gene. *Am J Clin Nutr, 90*, 425–428.

Wahlen, K., Sjolin, E., and Hoffstedt, J. (2008). The common rs9939609 gene variant of the fat mass and obesity associated gene (FTO) is related to fat cell lipolysis. *J Lipid Res, 49*, 607–611.

Walston, J., Silver, K., Bogardus, C., Knowler, W. C., Celi, F. S. et al (1995). Time of onset of non-insulin-dependent diabetes mellitus and genetic variation in the {beta}3-adrenergic-receptor gene. *N Engl J Med, 333*, 343–347.

Wang, J., Kuusisto, J., Vanttinen, M., Kuulasmaa, T., and Lindstrom, J. (2007). Variants of transcription factor 7-like 2 (TCF7L2) gene predict conversion to type 2 diabetes in the Finnish Diabetes Prevention Study and are associated with impaired glucose regulation and impaired insulin secretion. *Diabetologia, 50*, 1192–1200.

Wardle, J., Carnell, S., Haworth, C. M., Farooqi, I. S., O'Rahilly, S. et al (2008). Obesity associated genetic variation in FTO is associated with diminished satiety. *J Clin Endocrinol Metab, 93*, 3640–3643.

Wardle, J., Llewellyn, C., Sanderson, S., and Plomin, R. (2009). The FTO gene and measured food intake in children. *Int J Obes, 33*, 42–45.

Weedon, M. N., Shields, B., Hitman, G., Walker, M., McCarthy, M. I. et al (2006). No evidence of association of ENPP1 variants with type 2 diabetes or obesity in a study of 8,089 U.K. Caucasians. *Diabetes, 55*, 3175–3179.

Wellcome Trust Case Control Consortium. (2007). Genome-wide association study of 14,000 cases of seven common diseases and 3,000 shared controls. *Nature, 447*, 661–678.

Widen, E., Lehto, M., Kanninen, T., Walston, J., Shuldiner, A. R., and Groop, L. C. (1995). Association of a polymorphism in the {beta}3-adrenergic-receptor gene with features of the insulin resistance syndrome in Finns. *N Engl J Med, 333*, 348–352.

Willer, C. J., Speliotes, E. K, Loos, R. J., Li, S., Lindgren, C. M. et al (2009). Six new loci associated with body mass index highlight a neuronal influence on body weight regulation. *Nat Genet, 41*, 25–34.

Wu, Y., Li, H., Loos, R. J., Yu, Z., Ye, X. et al (2008). Common variants in CDKAL1, CDKN2A/B, IGF2BP2, SLC30A8 and HHEX/IDE genes are associated with type 2 diabetes and impaired fasting glucose in a Chinese Han population. *Diabetes, 57*, 2834–2842.

Xiang, Z., Litherland, S. A., Sorensen, N. B., Proneth, B., Wood, M. S. et al (2006). Pharmacological characterization of 40 human melanocortin-4 receptor polymorphisms with the endogenous propriomelanocortin-derived agonists and the agouti-related protein (AGRP) antagonist. *Biochemistry, 45*, 7277–7288.

Yamada, T., Ishihara, H., Tamura, A., Takahashi, R., Yamaguchi, S. et al (2006). WFS1-deficiency increases endoplasmic reticulum stress, impairs cell cycle progression and triggers the apoptotic pathway specifically in pancreatic beta-cells. *Hum Mol Genet, 15*, 1600–1609.

Yasuda, K., Miyake, K., Horikawa, Y., Hara, K., Osawa, H. et al (2008). Variants in KCNQ1 are associated with susceptibility to type 2 diabetes mellitus. *Nat Genet, 40*, 1092–1097.

Young, E. H., Wareham, N. J., Farooqi, S., Hinney, A., Hebebrand, J. et al (2007). The V103I polymorphism of the MC4R gene and obesity: population based studies and meta-analysis of 29,563 individuals. *Int J Obes, 31*, 1437–1441.

Zeggini, E., Weedon, M. N., Lindgren, C. M., Frayling, T. M., Elliott, K. S. et al (2007). Replication of genome-wide association signals in UK samples reveals risk loci for type 2 diabetes. *Science, 316*, 1336–1341.

Zeggini, E., Scott, L. J., Saxena, R., Voight, B. F., Marchini, J. L. et al (2008). Meta-analysis of genome-wide association data and large-scale replication identifies additional susceptibility loci for type 2 diabetes. *Nat Genet, 40*, 638–645.

Chapter 34

A Life Course Approach to Health Behaviors: Theory and Methods

Gita D. Mishra, Yoav Ben-Shlomo, and Diana Kuh

1 Introduction

The second half of the 20th century saw a blossoming of the adult lifestyle model of chronic disease epidemiology as it was applied successfully to identify some key causes, such as smoking, on disease risk (Doll and Hill, 1950). Observational epidemiology has now linked a range of adult behaviors to later disease risk and can show that changes in these behaviors also change these risks. However, the limited effectiveness of interventions to change adult behavior led, in the last quarter of the 20th century, to studies of young people to understand better the origins and etiology of disease and of healthy lifestyles and so recognized the possibilities for early interventions.

At the same time, ideas were developed that adverse environments in utero (Barker, 1994) and during childhood (Forsdahl, 1977) played a potentially important role in the long-term development of chronic disease risk. Initially, the focus was on birth weight as a marker of prenatal exposure, and then on markers of postnatal growth, childhood cognition, and childhood social conditions (Kuh and Ben-Shlomo, 2004b). In these models adult health behaviors were seen by some as confounding variables that needed to be taken account of in order to reveal

the direct relationship between early exposures and later health, whereas by others they were treated as potential mediating or modifying variables on the causal pathway to disease. More recently, it has become clear that the cumulative and interactive effects of risk factors on later health outcomes are at least as important, and perhaps more important, than their independent effects (Kuh and Ben-Shlomo, 2004a).

Both of these developments in epidemiology have further increased the spotlight of research on the role of early life factors. A number of books on life course epidemiology have reviewed the increasing evidence of their associations (Kuh and Ben-Shlomo, 2004a; Kuh and Hardy, 2002); further effects and key associations can be found in recent systematic reviews, pooled analysis, and meta-analyses (dos Santos Silva et al, 2008; Harder et al, 2009; Nobili et al, 2008; Whincup et al, 2008). This has been accompanied by the development of life course models and the novel application of statistical techniques to test these models and elucidate pathways between early life factors and adult health (De Stavola et al, 2006; Mishra et al, 2009; Pickles et al, 2007). In the process life course epidemiology has become a field of study in its own right (see Section 2).

This chapter presents life course epidemiology as a highly complementary approach to the lifestyle model of disease etiology, since it recognizes the fundamental importance of health behaviors for chronic diseases (Schooling and Kuh, 2002). We begin by outlining theoretical models used in life course epidemiology (Section 2) and show how the approach

G.D. Mishra (✉)
MRC Unit for Lifelong Health and Ageing, Department of Epidemiology and Public Health, University College London, 33 Bedford Place, London WC1B 5JU, UK
e-mail: g.mishra@nshd.mrc.ac.uk

A. Steptoe (ed.), *Handbook of Behavioral Medicine*, DOI 10.1007/978-0-387-09488-5_34,
© Springer Science+Business Media, LLC 2010

integrates and enhances existing behavioral change theories (Section 3). We then set out a developmental framework (Section 4) as a way of delineating the pathways for social, psychological, biological, and environmental factors and the importance of timing for these factors in the initiation and continuation of health behaviors through life. The following Section 5 discusses the implications of this approach for health policies and interventions and we conclude with a brief outline of future directions for research in this area (Section 6).

2 Life Course Epidemiology

A life course approach to epidemiology is concerned with the effects on health and health-related outcomes of biological (including genetic), environmental, and social exposures during gestation, childhood, adolescence, young adulthood, and across generations (Kuh et al, 2003). It specifically investigates how risk and protective factors across life act independently, cumulatively, and interactively. Much of the interest in life course epidemiology has centered on chronic diseases (Kuh and Ben-Shlomo, 2004a), such as coronary heart disease, diabetes, and cancer, but its concepts can also be used to understand health behaviors (Schooling and Kuh, 2002). The life course approach to health behaviors can address a range of questions that are highly pertinent to the development of health policy. Does childhood socioeconomic environment influence the consumption of excessive alcohol or binge drinking and is this modified by education and adult socioeconomic position? Could the link between adverse health behaviors and chronic diseases be due to a common set of factors that affect them both and if so when should one intervene, and what are the best ways of avoiding adverse health behaviors? Do the methods and cost-effectiveness of different interventions differ for children and adults? Would family-based interventions, aimed at preventing adverse health behaviors in all family members (adults and children), provide the most

cost-effective means of preventing poor health behaviors and their health consequences (Lawlor and Mishra, 2009b), or should one go for a population approach that aims to shift the whole distribution of behaviors in a more favorable direction? (Rose, 1992).

At the heart of this life course perspective lies a unique theoretical framework that assumes and tests for a temporal ordering of exposure variables and their inter-relationships with the outcome measure, both directly and through intermediary (mediating or modifying) variables (Ben-Shlomo and Kuh, 2002; Kuh et al, 2003).

2.1 Life Course Epidemiology: Theoretical Models

The underlying purpose of life course epidemiology is to build and test theoretical models that postulate pathways linking exposures across the life course to later life health outcomes (Ben-Shlomo and Kuh, 2002). Given the wide range of exposures over the life span and the potential importance of timing and duration, exposures may affect disease risk in a variety of ways. Four broad hypothetical life course models that can operate for exposures acting at different points across the life course have been proposed (Fig. 34.1).

The critical period model pays attention to the timing of an exposure and assumes that the irreversible changes in body systems that occur during a particularly vulnerable phase of life, usually during early development, have implications on later health (Ben-Shlomo and Kuh, 2002; Kuh and Ben-Shlomo, 2004b). The basic critical period model, also known as biological programming or as a latency model, underlies the fetal origins of adult disease hypothesis (Ben-Shlomo and Kuh, 2002). An expanded version of this model includes the possibility of the exposures in early life interacting with later life exposures, thereby either enhancing or decreasing the risk of chronic disease in later life; this model can be described as the critical

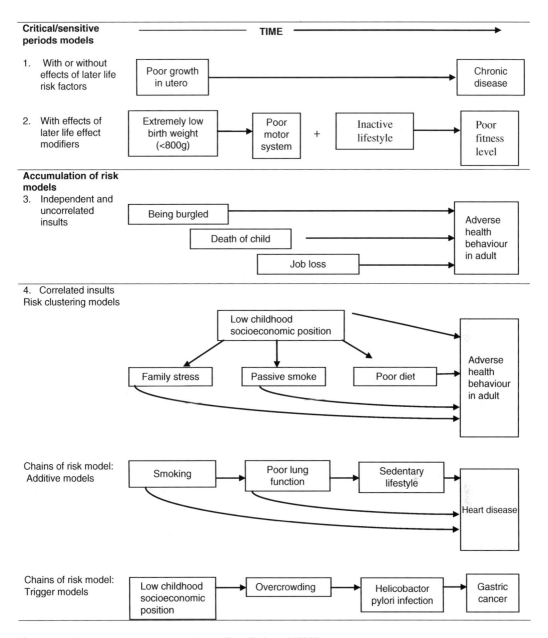

Fig. 34.1 Life course causal models. Adapted from Kuh et al (2003)

period with later effect modifiers (Ben-Shlomo and Kuh, 2002; Kuh et al, 2003). For instance, the low level of fitness in early adolescence of extremely low birth weight (<800 g) teenagers could be due to the interactive effects of premature birth on the motor system together with a more inactive lifestyle (Rogers et al, 2005; Whitfield and Grunau, 2006).

In contrast to the critical period models, the accumulation of risk model assumes that cumulative insults or exposures during the life course increase the risk of chronic disease irrespective of the timing. This idea corresponds to the notion of allostatic load (Ben-Shlomo and Kuh, 2002) so that as the number, duration, and severity of exposures increase, there is a cumulative damage to biological systems. Risk exposures may cause long-term, gradual damage to health in separate and independent ways (accumulation model with independent and uncorrelated insults). For example, an individual may experience a variety of unrelated exposures such as being burgled, subsequent death of a child, and finally being made redundant at work that cumulatively impact on their pattern of health behaviors.

It is far more common, however, for the environmental or behavioral insults to cluster together in socially patterned ways (accumulation model with risk clustering). For example, low childhood socioeconomic position is associated with low birth weight, fewer educational opportunities, more family stress, inadequate diet, and passive smoke exposure (Kuh and Ben-Shlomo, 2004a). Here, understanding the effects of childhood socioeconomic position by identifying the specific aspects of early physical or psychosocial environment or possible mechanisms (such as nutrition, infection, or stress) that are associated with adult disease/behaviors may provide further etiological insights (Ben-Shlomo and Kuh, 2002).

The chain of risk model is a special version of the accumulation model and refers to a sequence of linked events where one adverse (beneficial) exposure or experience tends to lead to another, and so on. For example, smoking will lead to poor lung function, which in turn will increase the likelihood of sedentary lifestyle and obesity leading to heart disease. Here, each exposure in a chain of risk may not only increase the risk of subsequent exposure in a probabilistic way, but they may also have an independent additive effect on later health. Alternatively, it may be that only the final link in the chain leads to the adverse outcome, for instance it is having the *Helicobacter Pylori* infection that leads to gastric cancer (trigger effect) (see Fig. 34.1).

2.2 Critical Period Versus Sensitive Periods

In life course epidemiology, a critical period is defined as a limited time window in which an exposure can have adverse or protective effects on development and subsequent disease outcomes (Ben-Shlomo and Kuh, 2002). Outside this window, there is no excess disease risk associated with the exposure. A sensitive period is a time period when an exposure has a stronger effect on development and hence disease risk than it would at other times. Critical periods may be more evident for chronic disease risk associated with developmental mechanisms in biological subsystems, whereas sensitive periods are likely to be more common in behavioral development (Ben-Shlomo and Kuh, 2002).

2.3 How Do We Disentangle the Different Life Course Models?

Recently we demonstrated that the critical period models, accumulation models, the effect modification models (such the critical period with later modifier) were each a special case of the saturated model, which contains the effects of all possible combinations of the exposure measures across the life course (Mishra et al, 2009). By comparing the model fit of a set of nested models – each corresponding to the accumulation, critical period, and effect modification hypotheses – to an all-inclusive (saturated) model, the model that best describes the data can be selected. As the life course models may operate simultaneously, this standard approach to model building can provide a more detailed understanding of the processes operating across the life course.

This framework was used on a prospective British cohort study to investigate life course models that best described the relationship between socioeconomic position measured once in childhood and twice in adulthood and adult BMI (Mishra et al, 2009). This nationally representative birth cohort study consists of a socially stratified sample of 2547 women and 2815 men born during 1 week in March 1946 (http://www.nshd.mrc.ac.uk/). There have been

22 follow-ups of the whole cohort from birth to the current day, with information about sociodemographic factors and medical, cognitive, and psychological functions being obtained by medical examination and postal questionnaire. We found that for men, the data supported the critical period model with those from manual background, regardless of their socioeconomic position in adult life, having higher BMI compared with those from non-manual background. For women, there was more evidence to support the accumulation model, with those spending more time in adverse social conditions having higher BMI (Mishra et al, 2009).

2.4 Methodological Challenges Encountered in Studying the Life Course

In recent years, there have been developments of new statistical approaches and epidemiological thinking in relation to causal models that can be usefully applied to etiological questions framed within life course paradigm (De Stavola et al, 2006; Pickles et al, 2007). However, it remains essential to have an understanding of the biological mechanisms underlying the effect of exposures on specific health outcomes upon which to base the statistical modeling. It is also important to consider the potential for confounding, such as due to exogenous events between time points and to consider the possibility for reverse causality, for instance a chronic condition associated with high BMI that leads to a lowering of socioeconomic position from childhood to adulthood. Regardless of which statistical methods have been selected – including structural equations models, path analysis, G-estimation, and multi-level models – issues of measurement errors, missing data, survival bias, and confounding factors are inevitable in life course studies and hence results may still be biased and caution is required in their interpretation (Ben-Shlomo and Kuh, 2002).

3 Life Course Perspective on Health Behavior Models

A number of behavioral change theories have emerged over recent decades that aim to understand the influences on health behaviors of both individuals and social groups; why people engage in unhealthy behaviors; and to inform the development of behavioral interventions (Murphy, 2005). Behavior change theories fall into one of the three broad categories according to the level of influence where the desired change is meant to occur, ranging from the theories of individual health to community-level and related models (US National Cancer Institute, 2005).

3.1 Individual-Level Models

While disciplines such as health psychology recognize that an individual's behavior does not occur in a vacuum, they tend to highlight the role of the individual in shaping their own behavior with their personal attitudes and feelings (see Chapter 2). Specifically, individual-level models, including the stages of change and health beliefs models, refer to the readiness and ability of an individual to adopt healthier behaviors according to their characteristics: level of knowledge, skills, perceptions, beliefs, values, motivation, levels of self-efficacy ('Can I do this?') and self-esteem ('Do I deserve to be healthy?'), and their need for approval from others (Murphy, 2005). Personality traits and genetic predisposition, such as reticence or a depressive nature, are also important factors. Although measures that concentrate on individuals are still the default mode for many health interventions, from the life course perspective the individual-level models should be seen as components embedded within a broader socioecological perspective for widespread and sustained behavior change to occur (Ben-Shlomo and Kuh, 2002). This approach also prompts the life course researcher to investigate the early origins of individual attitudes and feelings.

3.2 Interpersonal Models

These are reflected in the disciplines of sociology, anthropology, and social epidemiology
where the emphasis is placed on the role of social
context in shaping behavior. It recognizes that
an individual's health behaviors are informed
by the behavior of the other people, particularly family members and peers who can act
as role models. A recent sophisticated network
analysis has shown how mutual friends, spouse,
and siblings all contribute to a person-to-person
social transmission of obesity risk that was unrelated to geographic proximity (Christakis and
Fowler, 2007). Other individuals also provide
ideas, advice, assistance, and emotional support,
such as encouragement; equally they may disrupt, discourage, and withhold assistance. The
main interpersonal model is social learning theory that analyses psychosocial influences arising from the interactions of individual factors,
the social environment, and personal experience.
The life course approach embodies this model,
but in addition emphasizes the timing of factors
and their long-term influence, for instance the
effect of childhood socioeconomic environment
on adult health behaviors (Kuh et al, 2004c).

3.3 Community-Level Models

Public health messages are designed with the
intention of changing the health behaviors of
entire communities or specific groups, rather
than specific individuals. Regulatory and fiscal
measures also apply across society. Community-
level models provide a way to understand
how social systems function and therefore how
communities can be mobilized for change or
at least be supportive of health interventions
(Murphy, 2005). Societal change, such as the
widespread adoption of innovative technology
like the mobile phone, may alter not only the way
communities function but also the way health
messages can be delivered. Again a life course
perspective recognizes that cultural values held

by a community may shift over time or may
vary for community members at different stages
in life, for instance differences in attitudes
and social norms toward alcohol consumption
among young compared with older women and
how these may have altered over the time.

3.4 Ecological Perspective

This brings together the various behavioral disciplines and their behavioral change models by
recognizing explicitly that influences on health-
related behaviors occur across multiple levels:
individual and interpersonal factors, institutional
or organizational factors, community and societal characteristics, as well as the factors that
characterize public policy itself. The second key
idea is that *reciprocal causation* occurs between
individuals and the environment they inhabit:
that behavior both influences and is influenced
by the social environment in which it occurs. If
families spend considerable time watching television then it may alter their physical exercise
patterns; if enough families watch television,
then it can provide a medium to deliver targeted
public health messages about exercising more
(US National Cancer Institute, 2005). The ecological perspective captures the impossibility of
understanding an individual's behaviors without
also considering the social context in which they
live or analyzing group behaviors without appreciating differences among the individuals who
compose the group, and then considering how
these factors interrelate. In epidemiology this has
been referred to as the 'eco-social model' where
different levels of organization from the micro to
the macro operate embedded within each other
like Russian dolls or Chinese boxes (Susser and
Susser, 1996a, b). However, like many of the
behavioral change models, this approach does
not address the timing of factors on the development of an individual through life. Herein
lies the advantage of the life course perspective,
whereas we have seen the main emphasis is on
the timing and duration of factors and how this

varies their influence on health behavior in later life.

The integration of the behavioral change models within the life course approach can be illustrated as a series of socioecological contexts that change over time, as represented by ellipses at each level: national, community, and household (Ben-Shlomo and Kuh, 2002). Common genetic and/or social influences link grandparents, parents, and children across generations (see Fig. 34.2). The potential role of household, neighborhood, and national influences is illustrated acting across time and across individuals. For example, adverse neighboring conditions could affect a mother and her child (A). Similarly national exposures (e.g., wartime rationing) may be specific to a single population cohort (B) or period effects (e.g., economic recession) may be experienced by all individuals (C). When exploring patterns of health behaviors and their underlying mechanisms, the life course approach enables researchers to concentrate on factors involved with the

initiation and maintenance of health behaviors, as well as those that lead to their sustained change. Thus, it can inform policymakers not only of type and targeting of interventions but when their timing would be most effective (Kuh et al, 2004c; Schooling and Kuh, 2002).

4 Life Course Framework for Health Behavior

A developmental framework is inherent in the life course approach to health behaviors. Figure 34.3 shows the hypothesized pathways from childhood socioeconomic environment to health behaviors in adult life, influenced by the various factors at different stages through life (Kuh et al, 2004c; Schooling and Kuh, 2002). The life course models that underpin this diagram help to distinguish between variables acting through different pathways or

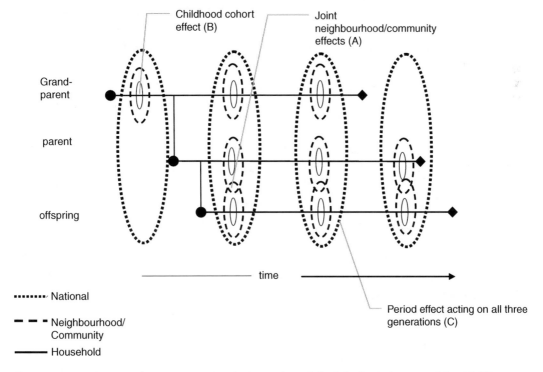

Fig. 34.2 Multi-factorial schema representing the integration of the behavioral change models with life course approach. Adapted from Ben-Sholmo and Kuh (2002)

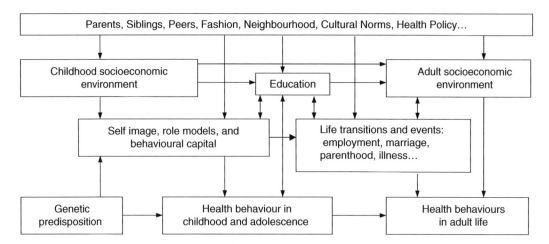

Fig. 34.3 Developmental life course framework showing the pathways between childhood socioeconomic environment and adult health behaviors

mechanisms and force one to consider the timing (*critical*), duration (*accumulation*), and temporal ordering (*chains of risk or interactions*) of exposures. These a priori visual box diagrams can assist with identifying the etiological pathways to be modeled and the need to distinguish confounders from mediators or modifiers (Ben-Shlomo and Kuh, 2002). The key elements of the life course framework on health behaviors are defined and discussed in the following sections.

It is worthwhile clarifying the definition of socioeconomic environment used here, since the different approaches to the role of social inequalities on health behaviors reflect the different traditions in social epidemiology (Kuh et al, 2004c). Socioeconomic position emphasizes the impact of economic resources and material conditions – it includes measures based on occupation, education, income, or wealth. The alternative approach studies health in relation to social integration and social roles and emphasizes psychosocial factors generated by human interaction (Kuh et al, 2004c). In this framework the term socioeconomic environment covers any measure of socioeconomic position or associated dimension of social inequality, including social integration and other psychosocial factors. In practice, we need to distinguish the different dimensions of socioeconomic environment

and that there are particular adverse or protective experiences which vary with social context and influence later health behaviors.

4.1 Socioeconomic Environment in Childhood and the Initiation and Maintenance of Health Behaviors

The framework illustrates the pathways from childhood to adult socioeconomic environment and from there the link to adult health behaviors. The socioeconomic environment in childhood directly constrains that of the adult through the availability of material wealth and social resources or via the accessibility to educational opportunities and other learning experiences. In addition to the 'health capital' (the accumulated biological resources inherited and acquired in early life that determine current health and future health potential) (Kuh et al, 2004c), childhood socioeconomic environment also shapes the development of health behaviors in adolescence, primarily through impacting on self-image and 'behavioral capital' (discussed in Section 4.6), that can endure and have long-term effects on adult health behaviors.

4.2 Initiation

Growing up in a disadvantaged socioeconomic environment, where there is poverty, unemployment, and low parental education, is associated with the initiation of some adverse health behaviors that may be carried through to adult life. In developed countries children from lower socioeconomic families have been found to have a higher consumption of unhealthy foods, including soft drinks, confectionary, and crisps; they have higher fat intakes and lower consumption of fruit, vegetables, and fiber (Neumark-Sztainer et al, 2003; Osler et al, 2008; Riediger et al, 2007; Sweeting et al, 1994; van Lenthe et al, 2001). Results for other health behaviors, such as physical activity, are less clear (Brodersen et al, 2007; Salmon and Timperio, 2007). This may be due to difficulties in obtaining accurate self-reported data for the type and duration of activities, which may vary widely for different socioeconomic groups. For instance, supervised sports have a considerably stronger socioeconomic differential than unsupervised activities (Offord et al, 1998). In a large-scale study of British adolescents, socioeconomic status (SES) differences in physical activity level were only seen in girls and not in boys, whereas SES differentials in sedentary behavior were found for everyone (Brodersen et al, 2007). Results from a longitudinal study of US children from ages 9 to 15 years, where accelerometers were used to measure physical activity levels, found that teenagers from low-income families had a greater rate of decline in moderate-to-vigorous physical activity (Nader et al, 2008).

For most of the developed world, teenage smoking is associated with lower parental socioeconomic status, though this relationship varies by gender and across culture. In the USA, although girls from minority groups are more likely to be less affluent than their white peers, they are less likely to take up smoking (2006; Johnson and Hoffmann, 2000). The relationship between parental socioeconomic status and alcohol consumption in adolescence is also not clear-cut (Hanson and Chen, 2007; Wiles et al, 2007).

4.3 Maintenance

With respect to the maintenance of health behaviors, a number of studies have examined the extent that childhood socioeconomic status has a long-term impact on adult behavior, independent of socioeconomic status in adulthood. For instance, after adjusting for current social class (at age 36), findings from the 1946 British birth cohort indicate that women from manual class in childhood were more likely to be a smoker, remain a smoker, be inactive, and have an unhealthy diet, but had lower alcohol consumption than women from non-manual backgrounds (Schooling and Kuh, 2002). However, findings from other studies are not consistent, possibly due to temporal trends, birth cohort effects, and eco-social differences between countries (Brunner et al, 1999; Leino et al, 1999).

4.4 Education

Childhood socioeconomic position greatly influences educational opportunities and other learning experiences (Kuh et al, 2004c), though the size of this effect may vary by culture, country, and location. Education can have an important role in shaping health behaviors, both in conjunction with and outside of the childhood socioeconomic status, and often provides an important setting for the delivery of targeted health messages. Findings from a number of studies indicate that the educational characteristics of students, such as having low aspirations, leaving school at an earlier age, and poor educational performance are associated with the uptake of smoking (McDermott et al, 2009; Tyas and Pederson, 1998), less healthy eating (Neumark-Sztainer et al, 2003; Sweeting et al, 1994), less physical activity, and more alcohol use and binge drinking (Crum et al, 2006, 1998; Sweeting et al, 1994). In contrast, other findings show that in adolescence the adoption of healthy lifestyle occurs prior to educational attainment and suggests that common factors may be behind the better outcomes in both these domains (Koivusilta et al, 2001, 2003) which we refer to as 'behavioral capital' and discuss in Section 4.6.

In addition, education characteristics have effects on some adult health behaviors independent of childhood and adult socioeconomic status. In the 1946 British birth cohort, after adjustment for socioeconomic effects, lower educational attainment remained strongly associated with smoking, less physical inactivity, and unhealthy diet (low fiber and vitamin C intake), but was not associated with alcohol consumption (Schooling and Kuh, 2002). Thus in addition to the influence of socioeconomic status in adulthood, the independent associations of childhood social class and educational characteristics with adult health behaviors suggest that attachments to cultural norms and the effects of psychosocial conditions first experienced in the home or classroom play a role in the maintenance of health behaviors into adult life. For example the ASSIST cluster randomized school-based trial found that informal peer support from influential role-model students was associated with a reduction of smoking (Campbell et al, 2008).

4.5 Tracking from Childhood and Adolescence into Adult Life

Tracking can be defined as the stability of health behavior over time or the 'preservation of relative position in rank of behavior over time' (Wardle, 1995) occurring from childhood to adulthood. Longitudinal studies have shown that smoking tracks strongly in adolescence and up until the late twenties (Twisk et al, 1997); findings from other studies indicate that alcohol use, dietary habits and preferences, and physical activity (Herman et al, 2008; Ovesen, 2006) do not track as strongly from adolescence into young adult life. During adolescence, individuals form identity, shaping their values, beliefs, and morals (Bissonnette and Contento, 2001). These processes, together with their past experiences in relation to the different health behaviors

and their individualized characteristics such as gender and socioeconomic position, contribute to their choice of behaviors. It is therefore not surprising that behaviors only track moderately from adolescence to young adulthood. Much research remains, however, to characterize tracking of health behaviors further over adult life.

4.6 Behavioral Capital

Behavioral capital has been defined as 'the accumulation of positive individual attributes such as social competence, decision making and problem-solving skills, coping strategies, personal efficacy, self-esteem, attitudes and values that help the individual remain resilient in times of adversity or take advantage of talents and opportunities' (Schooling and Kuh, 2002). It involves the kinds of adverse and protective childhood experiences with short- and possibly long-term effects on behavioral choices and the underlying mechanisms through which they may operate. Many of the attributes of behavioral capital are acquired more easily during child and adolescent development, and while they may be acquired later, it is often harder to do so (Hertzman and Wiens, 1996; Kuh et al, 2004c). Behavioral capital is likely to lead to healthy behavioral choices throughout life, either directly or indirectly by influencing many aspects of adult life that shape adult behaviors. Furthermore, as many aspects of behavioral capital affect educational aspirations and achievement as well as the adoption of health behaviors, the relationship found between educational achievements and health behaviors may reflect their common origins in behavioral capital (Kuh et al, 2004c)

4.7 Adult Transitions

There are many transitions in adult life that can greatly influence health behaviors, such as types of employment, partnership and marriage, and parenting. There is some evidence that spouses influence each other more with respect to health behaviors (Ellison et al, 1999; Pyke et al, 1997; Wood et al, 1997) than parents influence children or siblings influence each other (Mattocks et al, 2008). For example, in the Family Heart Health study from the National Heart, Lung and Blood Institute, familial associations for behaviors – alcohol consumption, exercise, and smoking – were strongest for spouses and notably weaker for parent–offspring and siblings correlations (Ellison et al, 1999).

5 Implications for Policy

The comprehensive nature of life course epidemiology which allows researchers to map pathways through life that lead to patterns of health behaviors has major implications for the development of health intervention policies. First, the time dimension of the life course approach highlights the progression of health behaviors from their initiation to their maintenance and their susceptibility to change at different life stages. As has been described in Section 2.2, sensitive time periods such as early in life can provide an opportunity to initiate beneficial health behaviors. For instance, introducing children to fruit and vegetables as part of their regular diet may influence their lifelong dietary choices. Alternatively many adverse health behaviors are taken up during adolescence, such as smoking, so leading up to this life stage represents a key period for behavior modification.

Equally important, a life course perspective identifies groups of people in their social context. It can identify the combination of characteristics in specific sectors of the population that leaves them at risk of adverse health behaviors, such as poor diet among people of low socioeconomic background. Furthermore, the social and environmental context in which those behaviors are more likely to occur may be identified. Thus it facilitates intervention policy not only to target at risk groups but to recognize the social context as an opportunity to change health behaviors, for instance in the use of role models in schools to influence adolescent smoking.

All these strands should inform an integrated approach to health intervention that spans education and economic and regulatory incentives. Policies should recognize that generic interventions have varying levels of effectiveness and relevance for different parts of the population, whereas policies targeting particular groups and in certain social contexts may be applied at key stages in life (Thomas and Perera, 2006; van Sluijs et al, 2007). Thus, health behavior policies should be developed as a systematic program of sustained interventions in multiple domains and across the life course. As Berkman notes, for successful health policies there need to be acknowledgment of the dynamic interplay between interventions and the social, economic, and environmental contexts in which they operate (Berkman, 2009).

6 Future Research

As the value of the life course approach to health is increasingly recognized, a number of areas have emerged as important directions for future research. With the proliferation of studies on health behaviors, the field would greatly benefit from more systematic reviews and meta-analyses of existing findings, particularly to explore the potential sources of differences in their results. Not only would this bring greater clarity to the understanding of established risk factors, but it is essential to inform the implementation of new and current cohort studies so that the right variables can be measured at the appropriate times through life (Baird et al, 2009; Flynn et al, 2006; Oldroyd et al, 2008).

Cross-cohort comparisons provide another way to add value to the research from existing studies. Recently there has been a rise in the numbers of multi-cohort collaborative programs, such as the Healthy Ageing across the Life Course (HALYCON) collaborative research program (www.halcyon.co.uk). This brings together nine UK cohort studies for meta- and pooled analysis to investigate how factors such as early development, lifetime health, and personality and nutrition influence indicators of healthy aging. By utilizing cross-cohort comparisons, one is able to detect whether determinants of health behaviors are replicated across cohorts and this may provide clues on the mechanisms at work. If applied to studies from different countries, it would either provide immediate cross-validation of research findings at an international level or establish which determinants vary according to factors such as country of residence, ethnicity, age, and cohort.

Family-based studies are also seen as another way of extending the range of data collected in life course research that can be used to investigate underlying mechanisms (Lawlor and Mishra, 2009a). Further to the previous sections, findings indicate that family can play a crucial role in determining health behaviors (Gilman et al, 2009; Simonen et al, 2002; Vink et al, 2003). Life course epidemiology is interested in three ways in which a family can influence health or health behaviors: (1) by the transfer or sharing of biological, environmental, and social factors across the generations; (2) detailed studies of family influences could help to understand the importance of timing of exposures as each family member may exert their impact on an individual's health in varying degrees at different times in the life course; and (3) comparing the relationships within and between different family members can help to clarify the mechanisms underlying associations in life course studies and help determine causality (Lawlor and Mishra, 2009b). The last decade has seen a rise in the number of studies that support evidence of genetic effects on smoking, drinking, and physical activity (Ginter and Simko, 2009; Maes et al, 2004; Warden and Fisler, 2008). Biologists suggest that the epigenetic alterations early in life due to stress can have a lifelong lasting impact on gene impression and thus on the phenotype, including susceptibility to disease (Szyf, 2009). The use of family-based studies such as the intergenerational studies, sibling studies, and twin studies can help to disentangle the role of genetic factors from shared and non-shared environments.

7 Conclusion

The life course epidemiology approach has many implications, both from current findings and from the possibilities embodied in future research, for the development of effective health policy that moves beyond considering the type of intervention to focus on their targeting and timing. It provides the evidence base that allows policymakers to move toward a systematic and comprehensive program of interventions that address the influences on health behavior and disease across the life span.

References

Baird, J., Cooper, C., Margetts, B. M., Barker, M., and Inskip, H. M. (2009). Changing health behaviour of young women from disadvantaged backgrounds: evidence from systematic reviews. *Proc Nutr Soc, 68,* 195–204.

Barker, D. J. P. (1994). *Mothers, babies, and disease in later life.* London: British Medical Journal Publishing Group.

Ben-Shlomo, Y. and Kuh, D. (2002). A life course approach to chronic disease epidemiology: conceptual models, empirical challenges, and interdisciplinary perspectives. *Int J Epidemiol, 31,* 285–293.

Berkman, L. F. (2009). Social epidemiology: social determinants of health in the United States: are we losing ground? *Annu Rev Public Health.*

Bissonnette, M. M. and Contento, I. R. (2001). Adolescents' perspectives and food choice behaviors in terms of the environmental impacts of food production practices: application of a psychosocial model. *J Nutr Educ, 33,* 72–82.

Brodersen, N. H., Steptoe, A., Boniface, D. R., and Wardle, J. (2007). Trend in physical activity and sedentary behaviour in adolescence: ethnic and socioeconomic difference. *Br J Sports Med, 41,* 140–44.

Brunner, E., Shipley, M. J., Blane, D., Davey Smith, G., and Marmot, M. G. (1999). When does cardiovascular risk start? Past and present socioeconomic circumstances and risk factors in adulthood. *J Epidemiol Commun Health, 53,* 757–764.

Campbell, R., Starkey, F., Holliday, J., Audrey, S., Bloor, M., Parry-Langdon, N. et al (2008). An informal school-based peer-led intervention for smoking prevention in adolescence (ASSIST): a cluster randomised trial. *Lancet, 371*, 1595–1602.

Christakis, N. A. and Fowler, J. H. (2007). The spread of obesity in a large social network over 32 years. *N Engl J Med, 357*, 370–379.

Crum, R. M., Ensminger, M. E., Ro, M. J., and McCord, J. (1998). The association of educational achievement and school dropout with risk of alcoholism: a twenty-five-year prospective study of inner-city children. *J Stud Alcohol, 59*, 318–326.

Crum, R. M., Juon, H. S., Green, K. M., Robertson, J., Fothergill, K. et al (2006). Educational achievement and early school behavior as predictors of alcohol-use disorders: 35-year follow-up of the Woodlawn Study. *J Stud Alcohol, 67*, 75–85.

De Stavola, B. L., Nitsch, D., dos, S. S., I, McCormack, V., Hardy, R. et al (2006). Statistical issues in life course epidemiology. *Am J Epidemiol, 163*, 84–96.

Doll, R. and Hill, A. B. (1950). Smoking and carcinoma of the lung. *Br Med J, ii*, 739–748.

dos Santos Silva, I. De Stavola, B., and McCormack, V. (2008). Birth size and breast cancer risk: re-analysis of individual participant data from 32 studies. *PLoS Med, 5*, e193.

Ellison, R. C., Myers, R. H., Zhang, Y., Djousse, L., Knox, S. et al (1999). Effects of similarities in lifestyle habits on familial aggregation of high density lipoprotein and low density lipoprotein cholesterol: the NHLBI Family Heart Study. *Am J Epidemiol, 150*, 910–918.

Flynn, M. A., McNeil, D. A., Maloff, B., Mutasingwa, D., Wu, M. et al (2006). Reducing obesity and related chronic disease risk in children and youth: a synthesis of evidence with 'best practice' recommendations. *Obes Rev, 7 Suppl 1*, 7–66.

Forsdahl, A. (1977). Are poor living conditions in childhood and adolescence an important risk factor for arteriosclerotic heart disease? *Br J Prev Soc Med, 31*, 91–95.

Gilman, S. E., Rende, R., Boergers, J., Abrams, D. B., Buka, S. L. et al (2009). Parental smoking and adolescent smoking initiation: an intergenerational perspective on tobacco control. *Pediatrics, 123*, e274–e281.

Ginter, E., and Simko, V. (2009). Alcoholism: recent advances in epidemiology, biochemistry and genetics. *Bratisl Lek Listy, 110*, 307–311.

Hanson, M. D., and Chen, E. (2007). Socioeconomic status and health behaviors in adolescence: a review of the literature. *J Behav Med, 30*, 263–285.

Harder, T., Roepke, K., Diller, N., Stechling, Y., Dudenhausen, J. W. et al (2009). Birth weight, early weight gain, and subsequent risk of type 1 diabetes: systematic review and meta-analysis. *Am J Epidemiol, 169*, 1428–1436.

Herman, K. M., Craig, C. L., Gauvin, L., and Katzmarzyk, P. T. (2008). Tracking of obesity and physical activity from childhood to adulthood: The Physical Activity Longitudinal Study. *Int J Pediatr Obes*, 1–8.

Hertzman, C., and Wiens, M. (1996). Child development and long-term outcomes: a population health perspective and summary of successful interventions. *Soc Sci Med, 43*, 1083–1095.

Johnson, R. A., and Hoffmann, J. P. (2000). Adolescent cigarette smoking in U.S. racial/ethnic subgroups: findings from the National Education Longitudinal Study. *J Health Soc Behav, 41*, 392–407.

Koivusilta, L., Rimpela, A., and Vikat, A. (2003). Health behaviours and health in adolescence as predictors of educational level in adulthood: a follow-up study from Finland. *Soc Sci Med, 57*, 577–593.

Koivusilta, L. K., Rimpela, A. H., Rimpela, M., and Vikat, A. (2001). Health behavior-based selection into educational tracks starts in early adolescence. *Health Educ Res, 16*, 201–214.

Kuh, D., and Ben-Shlomo, Y. (2004a). *A Life Course Approach to Chronic Disease Epidemiology*. Oxford: Oxford University Press.

Kuh, D. and Ben-Shlomo, Y. (2004b). Introduction. In D. Kuh and Y. Ben-Shlomo (Eds.), *A Life Course Approach to chronic Disease Epidemiology, 2nd Ed* (pp. 3–14). Oxford: Oxford University Press.

Kuh, D., Power, C., Blanc, D., and Bartley, M. (2004c). Socioeconomic pathways between childhood and adult health. In D. Kuh and Y. Ben-Shlomo (Eds.), *A Life Course Approach to Chronic Disease Epidemiology, 2nd Ed* (pp. 371–395). Oxford: Oxford University Press.

Kuh, D., Ben Shlomo, Y., Lynch, J., Hallqvist, J., and Power, C. (2003). Life course epidemiology. *J Epidemiol Commun Health, 57*, 778–783.

Kuh, D. and Hardy, R. (2002). *A Life Course Approach to Women's Health*. Oxford: Oxford University Press.

Lawlor, D. A., and Mishra, G. D. (2009a). *Family Matters: Designing, Analysing And Understanding Family-Based Studies in Life Course Epidemiology*. Oxford: Oxford University Press.

Lawlor, D. A., and Mishra, G. D. (2009b). Why family matters: an introduction. In D. A. Lawlor & G. D. Mishra (Eds.), *Family Matters: Designing, Analysing and Understanding Family-Based Studies in Life Course Epidemiology* (pp. 1–9). Oxford: Oxford University Press.

Leino, M., Raitakari, O. T., Porkka, K. V., Taimela, S., and Viikari, J. S. (1999). Associations of education with cardiovascular risk factors in young adults: the Cardiovascular Risk in Young Finns Study. *Int J Epidemiol, 28*, 667–675.

Maes, H. H., Sullivan, P. F., Bulik, C. M., Neale, M. C., Prescott, C. A. et al (2004). A twin study of genetic and environmental influences on tobacco initiation, regular tobacco use and nicotine dependence. *Psychol Med, 34*, 1251–1261.

Mattocks, C., Ness, A., Deere, K., Tilling, K., Leary, S. et al (2008). Early life determinants of physical activity in 11 to 12 year olds: cohort study. *BMJ, 336*, 26–29.

McDermott, L., Dobson, A., and Owen, N. (2009). Determinants of continuity and change over 10 years in young women's smoking. *Addiction, 104*, 478–487.

Mishra, G., Nitsch, D., Black, S., De Stavola, B., Kuh, D. et al (2009). A structured approach to modelling the effects of binary exposure variables over the life course. *Int J Epidemiol, 38*, 528–537.

Murphy, E. M. (2005). *Promoting Healthy Behaviour.* Washington, DC: Population Reference Bureau.

Nader, P. R., Bradley, R. H., Houts, R. M., McRitchie, S. L., and O'Brien, M. (2008). Moderate-to-vigorous physical activity from ages 9 to 15 years. *JAMA, 300*, 295–305.

Neumark-Sztainer, D., Wall, M., Perry, C., and Story, M. (2003). Correlates of fruit and vegetable intake among adolescents. Findings from Project EAT. *Prev Med, 37*, 198–208.

Nobili, V., Alisi, A., Panera, N., and Agostoni, C. (2008). Low birth weight and catch-up-growth associated with metabolic syndrome: a ten year systematic review. *Pediatr Endocrinol Rev, 6*, 241–247.

Offord, D. R., Lipman, E. L., and Duku, E. K. (1998). *Sports, the Arts and Community Programs: Rates and Correlated of Participation.* (Rep. No. Ottawa: report from the National Longitudinal Survey of Children and Youth, ˜W-98-18E.). Ottawa: Human Resources Development Canada.

Oldroyd, J., Burns, C., Lucas, P., Haikerwal, A., and Waters, E. (2008). The effectiveness of nutrition interventions on dietary outcomes by relative social disadvantage: a systematic review. *J Epidemiol Commun Health, 62*, 573–579.

Osler, M., Godtfredsen, N. S., and Prescott, E. (2008). Childhood social circumstances and health behaviour in midlife: the Metropolit 1953 Danish male birth cohort. *Int J Epidemiol, 37*, 1367–1374.

Ovesen, L. (2006). Adolescence: a critical period for long-term tracking of risk for coronary heart disease? *Ann Nutr Metab, 50*, 317–324.

Pickles, A., Maughan, B., and Wadsworth, M. (2007). *Epidemiological Methods in Life Course Research.* Oxford: Oxford University Press.

Pyke, S. D., Wood, D. A., Kinmonth, A. L., and Thompson, S. G. (1997). Change in coronary risk and coronary risk factor levels in couples following lifestyle intervention. The British Family Heart Study. *Arch Fam Med, 6*, 354–360.

Riediger, N. D., Shooshtari, S., and Moghadasian, M. H. (2007). The influence of sociodemographic factors on patterns of fruit and vegetable consumption in Canadian adolescents. *J Am Diet Assoc, 107*, 1511–1518.

Rogers, M., Fay, T. B., Whitfield, M. F., Tomlinson, J., and Grunau, R. E. (2005). Aerobic capacity, strength, flexibility, and activity level in unimpaired extremely low birth weight (<or=800 g) survivors at 17 years of age compared with term-born control subjects. *Pediatrics, 116*, e58–e65.

Rose, G. (1992). *The Strategy of Preventive Medicine.* New York: Oxford University Press.

Salmon, J., and Timperio, A. (2007). Prevalence, trends and environmental influences on child and youth physical activity. *Med Sport Sci, 50*, 183–199.

Schooling, M., and Kuh, D. (2002). A life course perspective on women's health behaviours. In D. Kuh & R. Hardy (Eds.), *A Life Course Approach to Women's Health* (pp. 279–303). Oxford: Oxford University Press.

Simonen, R. L., Perusse, L., Rankinen, T., Rice, T., Rao, D. C. et al (2002). Familial aggregation of physical activity levels in the Quebec Family Study. *Med Sci Sports Exerc, 34*, 1137–1142.

Susser, M,. and Susser, E. (1996a). Choosing a future for epidemiology: 1 Eras and paradigms. *Am J Pub Health, 86*, 668–673.

Susser, M., and Susser, E. (1996b). Choosing a future for epidemiology:II. From black box to Chinese boxes and eco-epidemiology. *Am J Public Health, 86*, 674–677.

Sweeting, H., Anderson, A., and West, P. (1994). Sociodemographic correlates of dietary habits in mid to late adolescence. *Eur J Clin Nutr, 48*, 736–748.

Szyf, M. (2009). The early life environment and the epigenome. *Biochim Biophys Acta, 1790*, 878–885.

Thomas, R. E., and Perera, R. (2006). Are school-based programmes for preventing smoking. *Cochrane Database Syst Rev*, CD001293.

Twisk, J. W., Kemper, H. C., van Mechelen, W., and Post, G. B. (1997). Tracking of risk factors for coronary heart disease over a 14-year period: a comparison between lifestyle and biologic risk factors with data from the Amsterdam Growth and Health Study. *Am J Epidemiol, 145*, 888–898.

Tyas, S. L., and Pederson, L. L. (1998). Psychosocial factors related to adolescent smoking: a critical review of the literature. *Tob Control, 7*, 409–420.

US National Cancer Institute (2005). *Theory at a Glance: A guide for Health Promotion Practice, 2nd Ed.* NIH Pub. No. 05-3896.

van Lenthe, F. J., Boreham, C. A., Twisk, J. W., Strain, J. J., Savage, J. M. et al (2001). Socioeconomic position and coronary heart disease risk factors in youth. Findings from the Young Hearts Project in Northern Ireland. *Eur J Public Health, 11*, 43–50.

van Sluijs, E. M., McMinn, A. M., and Griffin, S. J. (2007). Effectiveness of interventions to promote physical activity in children and adolescents: systematic review of controlled trials. *BMJ, 335*, 703.

Vink, J. M., Willemsen, G., Engels, R. C., and Boomsma, D. I. (2003). Smoking status of parents, siblings and friends: predictors of regular smoking? Findings from a longitudinal twin-family study. *Twin Res, 6*, 209–217.

Warden, C. H., and Fisler, J. S. (2008). Gene-nutrient and gene-physical activity summary--genetics viewpoint. *Obesity (Silver Spring), 16 Suppl 3*, S55–S59.

Wardle, J. (1995). Parental influences on children's diets. *Proc Nutr Soc, 54*, 747–758.

Whincup, P. H., Kaye, S. J., Owen, C. G., Huxley, R., Cook, D. G. et al (2008). Birth weight and risk of type 2 diabetes: a systematic review. *JAMA, 300*, 2886–2897.

Whitfield, M. F., and Grunau, R. E. (2006). Teenagers born at extremely low birth weight. *Paediatr Child Health, 11*, 275–277.

Wiles, N. J., Lingford-Hughes, A., Daniel, J., Hickman, M., Farrell, M. et al (2007). Socio-economic status in childhood and later alcohol use: a systematic review. *Addiction, 102*, 1546–1563.

Wood, D. A., Roberts, T. L., and Campbell, M. (1997). Women married to men with myocardial infarction are at increased risk of coronary heart disease. *J Cardiovasc Risk, 4*, 7–11.

Chapter 35

Prenatal Origins of Development Health

Christopher L. Coe

1 Introduction

> The difference between two radically different destinies often reflects disarmingly small variations in timing and circumstance.
>
> (Shaywitz and Melton, 2005)

A central tenet of behavioral medicine and health psychology is that stable features of an individual's personality, behavior, and physiology are important determinants of good health and can influence risk for disease. Assuming this view is correct, a logical corollary is that we need to learn more about the origins of these trait-like characteristics. For a long time we have looked to early rearing conditions as one means to explain how environmental conditions 'get under the skin' and begin to create physiological and behavioral biases. That large body of research on the persistent effects of 'early experience' has been very helpful in accounting for why one individual remains healthy and another deviates toward illness later in adulthood (Chen et al, 2007; Danese et al, 2007). Diet, pathogen exposure, and quality of parenting during childhood will always be very influential factors to take into consideration, but it has become increasingly evident that another significant part of the story starts earlier during the prenatal period. Today, there is substantial evidence from both human studies and animal models documenting that the antecedents of physiological regulation are laid down during fetal development (Bateson et al, 2004). At this immature stage, the developmental course of the fetus is also quite malleable and subject to considerable influence by maternal well-being and other conditions during pregnancy. As conveyed in the quotation above, seemingly small changes so early in development can result in large effects on later outcomes.

This new perspective on the far-reaching ramifications of the prenatal period is often captured by the shorthand 'prenatal programing' (Hodgson and Coe, 2006). That is a reasonable designation when it can be shown that there are lasting effects on the regulatory set points for a physiological system or behavioral process. In other instances, it may be more appropriate to use a different term, such as 'teratogenic,' to describe a specific pathogenic effect of a drug, environmental toxicant, infection, or hypoxic event during pregnancy (Rees et al, 2008). The myriad findings on teratogens that can perturb fetal development equally highlight the critical importance of in utero conditions for later health. There is another large category of more moderate influences on fetal development that should probably be grouped under a different heading, such as 'transformative.' These alterations do not push the young infant out of the normal range into the realm of developmental disabilities, nor do they result in a fundamental re-organization of the regulatory programs, but they still may change the

C.L. Coe (✉)
Department of Psychology, Harlow Center for Biological Psychology, University of Wisconsin, 22 N. Charter Street, Madison, WI 53715, USA
e-mail: ccoe@wisc.edu

A. Steptoe (ed.), *Handbook of Behavioral Medicine*, DOI 10.1007/978-0-387-09488-5_35,
© Springer Science+Business Media, LLC 2010

course of events. For example, in animal studies it is not uncommon to find that the offspring from experimentally manipulated pregnancies are more emotional and behaviorally reactive when tested under challenged conditions, while still appearing to be normal in the undisturbed state (Fortier et al, 2007; Shi et al, 2003). Here one sees a transactional effect – a synergistic interaction between genetic factors, maturational processes, and environmental context – serving to create unique individual propensities and foster population variation in behavior and physiology.

Tracing the beginnings of the developmental trajectory back into the prenatal period is not new. Researchers have known for nearly a century that many important steps involved in sexual differentiation are completed before birth. Certainly, the sculpting of reproductive anatomy has been achieved by term, accomplished to a large extent by mid-gestation in humans (Swain and Lovell-Badge, 1999). Extensive animal studies and clinical observations of people with endocrine anomalies have shown further that these processes are initially very susceptible to influence by the hormonal milieu in which the fetus develops (Abbott et al, 2005). In now classic studies with rodent and primate species, genetic female fetuses were exposed to androgenic hormones and thereby altered to look like male infants by birth (Goy et al, 1988a). More important for the take home message of this chapter, their behavior continued to be masculinized into adulthood (Goy et al, 1988b). In some species, even the menarcheal age for the androgen-exposed females was shifted toward the later pubertal age of males, suggesting that the neuroendocrine *zeitgebers* that will control adult reproduction are programed in utero (Whalen and Luttge, 1971; Wood et al, 1995). These prenatal influences on reproductive biology illustrate how long-term developmental trajectories can be set in motion, upon which the postnatal environment then acts (Wallen, 1996). With respect to gender differences in human behavior, the initial predispositions evident in childhood ultimately become substantiated via an overlay of familial values and cultural expectations about sex-typical norms (Berenbaum, 2006).

One can also look to the field of behavioral teratology for other compelling examples to demonstrate the significance of the fetal period. A widely known example is the fetal alcohol syndrome (FAS) (Jones and Smith, 1973). It has been definitively established that the normal development of the skeleton and brain can be compromised if a gravid female consumes high levels of alcohol during pregnancy (Guerri et al, 2009). Fetal exposure to alcohol can also result in irreversible deficits in emotionality, learning ability, and later school performance (Sampson et al, 1997). In addition, other aspects of a pregnant woman's behavior, such as poor diet, lack of exercise, and smoking, can affect fetal development, albeit not as severely as after exposure to a major teratogen (Fig. 35.1). In the case of smoking, the effects seem to be mediated primarily via alterations in blood flow to the placenta and a reduced delivery of oxygen (Spira et al, 1977), processes that are important in accounting for other challenges to pregnancy, including after stressful life events and emotional disturbance. FAS and the adverse effects of placental insufficiency and fetal hypoxia are just three of many examples supporting the general conclusion that maternal factors during pregnancy and the quality of the uterine environment matter

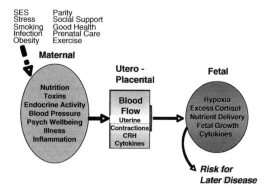

Fig. 35.1 To understand how positive and negative factors influence fetal development, one has to consider a three-compartment model, including maternal, uteroplacental, and fetal processes. The placenta is a key link because of its critical role in hormone synthesis and nutrient and oxygen delivery during pregnancy

(McFarlane et al, 1996; Yager and Ashwal, 2009).

Viewed collectively within the larger context of the many effects of maternal diet and environmental pollutants on the rapidly growing fetus, one can begin to appreciate the potential significance of these findings for behavioral medicine researchers (Birnbaum, 1995). Even in a study exclusively focused on adults, it is important to at least reflect on the possible origins of their behavior or illnesses much earlier in development. When trying to account for variation in health at the population level, the maternal–fetus relationship is an especially influential factor to consider. One just has to point to the strong associations found between low socioeconomic status and the prevalence of premature delivery and low birth weight infants (David and Collins, 1997; Kleinman and Kessel, 1987). In the United States over 12% of infants are born premature, and more than 8% are below 2500 g (Centers for Disease Control, 2000). An increased likelihood of adverse pregnancy outcomes and fetal growth restriction are major contributors to the health disparities that accompany poverty.

The surge of current research on prenatal programing was stimulated in large part by epidemiological studies that first implicated fetal growth patterns and birth weight as early risk factors for the later occurrence of several adult diseases. For every kilogram decrease in birth weight, there will be an increase in mean adult blood pressure (Huxley et al, 2002). But before discussing the relationship between birth weight and the likelihood of succumbing to diabetes and cardiovascular disease, let's consider the logic of such linkages from an evolutionary point of view.

2 Maternal Investment and Fetal Priming Within an Evolutionary Framework

To appreciate why it might be advantageous for the fetus to be responsive to maternal state, rather than to entirely buffer the fetus behind an impervious placental/uterine barrier, it is informative to discuss a few zoological examples. Our story did not begin with humans or even mammals and viviparity. We know from observations of egg-laying species that environmental conditions during incubation can be extremely influential. Ambient temperature affects not only the rate of development, but can even change the sex of the developing fetus in some oviparous fish and reptile species (Crews and Bull, 2008). Among birds, the egg-laying female will often vary nutrient and hormone concentrations across her clutch on the basis of the sequential order in which the eggs are laid (Cariello et al, 2006; Royle et al, 2001). Other important lessons about the extent of flexibility in fetal development can be garnered from the marsupial species. They have an extremely short gestation and a joey is born essentially midstream in the fetal state, continuing the rest of its maturation on the nipple within a pouch. These transitional animals include the wallabies and kangaroos with females that can have three offspring simultaneously, each in a different maturational stage. She can maintain one embryo in her reproductive tract in arrested diapause (or signal it to implant), while at the same time controlling the rate of the joey's growth within the pouch by varying the nutrient quality of her milk (Trott et al, 2003). She can further modify the lipid composition and caloric level in one nipple for this immature joey and in her second nipple for the larger infant already mobile and spending most of its time outside the pouch.

Given these examples from reptiles, birds, and marsupials, it is perhaps not too surprising to discover that uterine conditions continued to matter in the eutherian mammals, including ourselves. In fact, as the period of internal development became more extended, there was even greater opportunity for maternal factors and experiential events during pregnancy to shape the course of fetal maturation (Kaiser and Sachser, 2009). In addition, the placenta evolved to become more invasive and to facilitate more intimate support and communication with the fetus (Wildman et al, 2006). Among the species that have a hemochorial placenta, which includes the monkeys, apes, and humans, the barrier between maternal and fetal blood is considerably reduced, allowing for a ready exchange of proteins and even the periodic crossing of cells (in contrast to the greater separation that occurs with the epitheliochorial placenta of farm animals and prosimians).

To appreciate the implications of these types of evolutionary trends for pediatric health, one can look to the progressive changes in how antibody is transferred across the placenta from mother to the infant. Most mammalian species with altricial young provide maternal antibody primarily in breast milk postnatally. However, the higher primates including humans largely transfer immunoglobulin G (IgG) prenatally via the placenta before birth (Coe et al, 1994). This important immune process confers passive protection against bacteria and viruses encountered previously by the mother, enabling the infant to evade disease and to not have to produce substantial amounts of its own antibody for several months after birth. The immunoglobulin found in human milk is predominantly of the IgA class and functions instead to coat the mucosal surfaces of the baby's oral cavity and gut, very distinct from the prenatal bolus of IgG conveying a memory of prior pathogens encountered previously during the mother's life.

Along with the placental transfer of antibody, there is also a transmission of many antigenic proteins, a second process that becomes important to appreciate when trying to understand why some human babies are born already sensitized to food allergens and plant pollens (Liobichler et al, 2002). The fetal response to these proteins that become embedded in placental tissues or transfer into the fetal compartment helps one to predict which infants will go on to develop atopic dermatitis and asthma. Less frequently there may also be some problematic antibody from the mother transferred as well, which can result in maternal–fetal incompatibilities. One example is the maternal immune reaction against paternal antigens on fetal cells, such as to Rhesus factor. Another hypothesized problem is the transfer of maternal antibody that

reacts against the maturing brain tissue in the otherwise healthy fetus, which has been postulated as a putative cause of some types of autism (Braunschweig et al, 2009; Singer et al, 2009).

From the vantage point of evolutionary biology, one can argue further that some degree of maternal regulation over fetal development is for the most part beneficial, providing the mother with control over her investment and reproductive success. Under extreme conditions, including high levels of stress or following viral and bacterial infections, some species respond by embryo resorption, miscarrying, or even sacrificing a more mature fetus via premature delivery. Within the animal kingdom, even this fetal loss seems to serve an adaptive purpose, permitting the female to rear other viable offspring at optimal times when the chances of raising an infant to adulthood would be more successful. In fact, if one closely reads articles on pregnancy in mice and rats, it is not uncommon to see such compromises made within a single litter. After a stressful experimental manipulation or virulent infection, the gravid female often reduces her litter size (Fatemi et al, 2008). A vestige of this type of selection process may carry-over as a legacy to our own species, when one considers that bacterial infections during pregnancy or in the placental tissue (e.g., chorioamnionitis) are still major risk factors for premature delivery (Hiller et al, 1995). In fact, a rise in proinflammatory cytokines, especially tumor necrosis factor (TNF), in the third trimester is a major cause of prematurity (Rigo et al, 2004). In the clinical literature, high blood levels of TNF are one of the more sensitive diagnostic biomarkers of obstetrical risk (Menon et al, 2006).

It is important to emphasize that this communication between mother and fetus is bidirectional with an equivalent number of benefits from the fetal perspective. Many physiological changes that occur in a gravid female are actually induced by the placenta and fetus, such as the markedly increased estrogen and progesterone in maternal circulation that sustains the pregnancy. In the case of estrogen, the placenta is the primary source of the elevated hormone levels, not the mother's ovary, and the precursor of the placental estrogen in humans and other primate species is the dehydroepiandrosterone (DHEA) produced by the fetal adrenal (Rainey et al, 2004). Thus, it makes sense that the fetus should be responsive to feedback signals about hormone levels from the maternal compartment. Moreover, the fetus is not just a passive recipient of resources from the mother. Receptor levels on the placenta can be adjusted, as evinced by the placental Fc receptors for IgG, which increase during the final month of pregnancy and actively accelerate the transfer of maternal antibody (Coe et al, 1993). Even more dynamically, when a fetus is confronted with a low level of iron transfer during an anemic pregnancy, the transferrin receptors on the placental surface are upregulated, which serves to enhance the binding of iron in the mother's blood stream (Rao and Georgieff, 2002; see also Fig. 35.4). Finally, another benefit to the fetus of being responsive to environmental and maternal cues is that many of its maturing physiological systems, including the brain and immune system, require some priming to develop appropriately. In a real sense, they should already be thought of as 'learning systems,' even during the fetal period. The information crossing the placenta presages what will be experienced in short order when the neonate encounters the postnatal world. In this way, the infant has already taken important steps in preparing to appropriately pace its growth rate and regulate its energy expenditure in keeping with the likely acquisition of nutrients (Wintour et al, 2003).

3 The Link Between Birth Weight and Later Health

Any review of prenatal programing must begin with due recognition of the pioneering contributions of Dr. David Barker. He and his colleagues conducted the first large-scale epidemiological studies that systematically documented the strong associations between birth weight and adult disease (Barker, 1998). Their analyses showed that in both industrialized countries of northern Europe and rural regions of India, there is a high concordance between the geographic patterns and historic trends in birth weight and the prevalence of cardiovascular, respiratory disease, and type 2 diabetes. Infants born premature or very small had long been known to be at greater risk for many diseases, but the Barker papers provided compelling evidence for a more general association across the full continuum of weight in full-term babies and the extent of risk for adult disease later in life.

While evident at the population level for infants of all sizes, the influence of birth weight is certainly most pronounced in those born small-for-gestational age (SGA) (Dunger and Ong, 2005). Moreover, a number of researchers have argued further that there is added significance if a baby evinces signs of asymmetrical somatic growth, born with a relatively large head and a stunted body (Fergusson et al, 1997). The lack of proportionality in the lower body may connote an acute period of deprivation late in pregnancy, beyond just the slow growth sustained across the entire pregnancy, which would result in a small, but more symmetrical baby. A similar interpretation about the significance of asymmetry has been proposed when the placental size is relatively large with respect to a baby's low weight, suggesting a compensatory increase in response to a compromised pregnancy.

Analyses of neonatal appearance and fetal growth restriction following a period of undernutrition or placental insufficiency during pregnancy heralded what has become known today as the 'thrifty phenotype.' That is, when confronted with limited resources during pregnancy, the developing fetus re-programs its growth rate and metabolism in a manner that will facilitate adaptation to further nutrient shortages after birth. Assuming that the prenatal prophecy is correct, such a shift toward a slower growth rate could be advantageous for the baby presenting with a thrifty phenotype. Perhaps enabling it to survive in an adverse world by maximizing the uptake and efficient use of limited nutritional resources.

However, if subsequently there is a mismatch and the growing child now has abundant resources, the altered metabolism and coveting of nutrients can result in a propensity for obesity. Such a scenario sometimes occurs after adoption of a young infant from an impoverished setting to an affluent country. These children are then at greater risk for becoming overweight and developing the metabolic syndrome with glucose intolerance and atherogenic dyslipidemia and are more prone to cardiovascular disease. Clinical tests indicate that these individuals also have prothrombotic and proinflammatory profiles. In addition to the human studies supporting this line of reasoning, numerous reports on rodent and sheep models have begun to delineate the hormone mechanisms and metabolic pathways accounting for these long-term effects (Murphy et al, 2006; Wintour et al, 2003). These experiments indicate that the physiological programing includes changes in the kidney, with decreases in nephron number and/or size, which contribute to the later hypertension in adulthood (Moritz et al, 2009).

Beyond the obvious relevance for many regions of the world where food supplies are inadequate for pregnant women, these observations have proven to be germane to understanding long-lasting changes in population health after acute periods of deprivation during wars and environmental disasters. The best-documented example is certainly the decade-long effects of the Dutch Hunger famine in 1944 when the Netherlands was subjected to extreme food rationing during World War II (Ravelli et al, 1976). Food intake for many pregnant women was reduced to 500–800 calories per day for several months. When the deprivation occurred late in gestation, the neonates were of smaller size and grew up to be at greater risk for obesity and diabetes (Ravelli et al, 1998). For the pregnant women who experienced food restriction earlier in pregnancy and subsequently had access to a better diet, their babies were born at a larger size, but continued to be more likely to develop cardiovascular disease by 50 years of age (Roseboom et al, 2000).

Beyond the impact of stunted fetal growth during periods of social strife and turmoil, it is known that even under normal circumstances, infants who are born small and then undergo a period of rapid postnatal growth also have distinctive physiological profiles. This type of catch-up growth has the additional effect of placing high demands on iron reserves, increasing the likelihood of the infant becoming anemic during the first year of life (see Section 8 on risk factors for iron deficiency anemia).

While most clinical attention has been focused on premature and SGA babies, there is a complementary literature indicating that excessive fetal growth can present a different set of problems. With large-for-gestational age babies (LGA), there is a significant increase in obstetrical complications and need for caesarian delivery (Gregory et al, 1998). In addition, these infants are more likely to continue on the path toward obesity during childhood and adulthood, especially after diabetic pregnancies (Law et al, 1992). Longitudinal studies show they are predisposed to have poorer glucoregulation and to develop type 2 diabetes as adults. Here too, basic science studies in animals have provided considerable support for these associations and revealed several critical mediating pathways linking accentuated growth rates and later disease. For example, pregnant dams fed a high caloric diet will gestate offspring with a distinctive insulin response and altered pancreatic size and renal functioning. In addition, providing young rat pups with a period of overnutrition right after birth changes how their leptin and thyroid hormones are regulated in a manner that will permanently alter appetite and energy metabolism into adulthood (Rodrigues et al, 2009).

Obesity early in life thus seriously increases risk for many ailments, but especially for the Big Three: metabolic syndrome, diabetes, and cardiovascular disease. It is perhaps less well known that large babies and overweight children are also more likely to develop allergies and asthma (Pekkanen et al, 2001). In fact, if one were to compare the odds ratios of developing asthma in small neonates versus in large babies over 10 pounds, the greater pediatric concern would have to be for the bigger infants, especially in the heaviest ones gestated beyond 40 weeks postconception.

4 Prenatal Antecedents of Allergies and Asthma

While fetal growth is manifest clearly by infant size at birth, prenatal influences on other physiological systems are also occurring but are less overtly evident. For example, there is extensive evidence documenting the significance of prenatal priming for the developing immune system. It includes fetal exposure to allergens, which has a special relevance to pediatric medicine because it may contribute to the rising incidence of allergies and asthma worldwide. Although the placenta is usually an effective barrier that blocks the transfer of viruses and bacteria and keeps the fetal compartment sterile, the immune system actually starts to develop and become functional early in gestation. By 2 months after conception, the fetus has lymphocytes that can respond and proliferate. By mid-gestation, analyses of cell subsets in cord blood indicate the presence of activated T cells (Devereux et al, 2001; Warner et al, 2000). Some of this cellular activation is likely due to reactions to food proteins, such as ovalbumin and ß-lactoglobulin (Liobichler et al, 2002). Even some airborne allergens may reach the placenta via the mother. In addition, certain allergens, such as cat dander, can be pulled across the placenta as a conjugated complex with the IgG antibody (Casas and Brjorksten, 2001). In keeping with this evidence for fetal exposure to environmental allergens, analyses of cord blood from neonates across the year have documented that their cellular responses track seasonal variation in grass and tree pollen levels (Piccinni et al, 1993; Van Duren Schmidt et al, 1997).

As can be seen in Fig. 35.2, clinical allergists now believe that the initial biases toward atopic disorders and asthma begin before birth (Jones et al, 2000). Maternal exposure to allergens, tobacco smoke, and pollution increases the risk that infants will wheeze during the first year of life and subsequently develop asthma by 3–4 years of age. Early warning signs of being prone to atopy can often be detected in cord blood. Two neonatal indicators are (1) the presence of elevated levels of IgE, the antibody class associated with allergies and (2) a response bias toward Th2 cytokines when their mononuclear cells are stimulated in culture. If there is a high production of certain cytokines, such as interleukin-5 (IL-5), and relatively low levels of IL-12 and interferon-gamma, it is indicative of a Th2 cytokine or atopic profile. This type of infant is more likely to become asthmatic if subsequently exposed to a rearing environment with cockroaches, air pollution and second hand cigarette smoke, or opportunistically infected with rhinoviruses on a repeated basis, or subjected to chronic familial stressors (Chen et al, 2007). Yet one more example that in utero and maternal factors influence the propensity for allergies is that a woman's parity status also affects the levels of IgE found in the neonate. While the first child of a woman who has allergies herself will be born with high IgE, the antibody levels in her next infants will then decline progressively with each subsequent birth (Karmaus et al, 2004).

While these associations between prenatal conditions and pediatric allergies may suggest prenatal stimulation is mostly bad, we have also come to realize that the immune system must normally rely on early priming to mature correctly. A total absence of antigenic exposure would result in even more aberrant immune responses. The consequences of understimulation can be readily seen in animals reared in the unique conditions of the gnotobiotic laboratory, where they live in sterile conditions without bacteria. Not only does their lymphoid tissue develop abnormally, they fail to establish normal mucosal immune responses, which then undermine the competent maturation of systemic immunity. In addition, even the basic structure of their gut anatomy becomes abnormal in the absence of the resident gastrointestinal microbiota. Our awareness that some level of antigenic stimulation is critical during infancy has led to the formulation of an alternative idea that may seem counterintuitive: the 'hygiene hypothesis' of pediatric illness (Liu and Murphy, 2003). It proposes that there are some adverse unintended consequences of the modern rearing environment, which is now too clean and pathogen free.

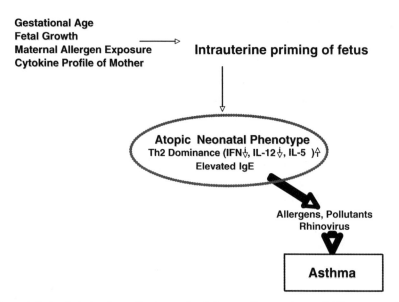

Fig. 35.2 Many infants that develop allergies and asthma are already predisposed toward atopic conditions at birth. Prenatal exposure to allergens, prematurity, and being small or very large at birth are among the many factors that affect how a neonate will respond to the rearing environment and to respiratory infections

If over the course of many millennia, the immune system had become selected to rely on antigenic priming, a child may not be able fully achieve normal immune competence without some exposure to viral and bacterial pathogens. Now that we have vanquished so many of the common parasites and infectious pathogens to which humans used to be exposed, our children today grow up in a more germ-free and hygienic world than ever before. It could help to explain why increasing numbers of people worldwide now seem to be over-reactive to formerly benign food antigens and plant pollens. Specifically, lymphoid cells such as the eosinophil, which are the ones that responded to microfilaria worms and protozoan parasites like malaria, now may be redirected toward other environmental stimuli.

We still have much to learn about how prenatal conditions set the stage for subsequent reactions during early encounters with the postnatal world (Salk et al, 1974). Our laboratory investigated some of these questions in a primate model and demonstrated that disturbances of pregnancy affected many immune responses in infant rhesus monkeys (Coe et al, 2007). Some immune abnormalities were evident already at birth; others emerged as the infant monkey developed across the first year of life. For example, the infants established atypical profiles of gut bacteria, with lower concentrations of beneficial Lactobacilli and Bifidobacteria, when generated from stressed pregnancies (Bailey et al, 2004). In turn, with reduced numbers of the protective microbiota, the infants were more vulnerable to enteric pathogens like Shigella and Campylobacter, two diarrhea-causing bacteria, especially during the subsequent stressful event of weaning (Bailey and Coe, 1999).

5 Challenges to Fetal Well-being: Maternal Stress

Much of the research on the prenatal origins of health emanates from an interest in investigating the long-term effects of maternal stress during pregnancy (Wadhwa et al, 1993). The concerns can be grouped in two related categories: (1) obstetrical ramifications, especially with regard to the likelihood of premature birth and delivery complications and (2) pediatric health issues with respect to the long-term physiological and behavioral functioning of the offspring (LaPlante et al, 2008; Reynolds et al, 2001). The worse case scenario is obviously fetal loss. In litter-bearing animals, it is not uncommon to see a reduction in fertility and fecundity, reflected in smaller litter sizes following stressful conditions, maternal infection, and sepsis. Even in humans, bacterial infections, including the relatively common diagnosis of bacterial vaginosis (BV), have been implicated as a major risk factor for premature delivery. In fact, maternal stress during pregnancy may aggravate a propensity for BV, which in turn becomes the specific gynecological factor contributing to a deleterious outcome (Culhane et al, 2001).

The likelihood that psychological stressors by themselves can result in premature delivery and obstetrical complications are less clear. Domestic violence, which sadly has been reported to occur in 4–8% of pregnancies, and up to 26% in some surveys, has been linked with increased morbidity, including a greater likelihood of hypertensive conditions like eclampsia and need for assisted deliveries (Cokkinides et al, 1999; Gazmararian et al, 1996; Newberger et al, 1992; Petersen et al, 1997). But the level of risk following other types of stressful events is more variable and nuanced (Hedegaard et al, 1996). For example, following an earthquake in southern California, a shortened gestation was more likely when the earthquake occurred during the first trimester, but it was less stress-inducing without deleterious consequences for women when they were further along in the pregnancy (Glynn et al, 2001). In contrast, pregnant women were found to have a slightly longer gestation if they lived or worked in proximity of the World Trade Center on September 11, 2001 (Berkowitz et al, 2003; Engel et al, 2005). Their babies were also born with smaller head circumferences, which might implicate a slowing of fetal growth as one contributing factor for the prolongation of pregnancy.

The literature on stress and pregnancy has been more consistent in animals and is replete with examples demonstrating that stressful events can definitely impede fetal development, with many long-lasting ramifications after birth (Weinstock, 1997). The experimental manipulations used to evoke stress range from immobilization or arousing sensory stimuli in rodent models to stressful husbandry conditions in farm animals and social aggression in primates. Even when gestation length and infant birth weight are not affected, many alterations in the infant's behavioral and physiological functioning have been described (Coe et al, 2007). The offspring from stressed pregnancies often appear to be more behaviorally and emotionally reactive. Thus, when challenged, they continue to manifest larger behavioral and hormonal responses to stressful events. In rats and mice, the secretion of hypothalamic–pituitary–adrenal hormones is typically greater, and increased HPA activity often persists into adulthood (Koehl et al, 1999). Basal levels of adrenal hormones are more typically reported to be normal in primates, but there may be alterations in the diurnal hormone rhythm or an altered negative feedback, which results in protracted cortisol responses once activated. Many effects of prenatal stress on brain development have also been described in animal studies (Welberg and Seckl, 2001). Brain regions sensitive to stress, such as the hippocampus, are often found to be smaller (Lemaire et al, 2000). Similarly, the monoamine neurotransmitter pathways are vulnerable. Baseline levels of norepinephrine and serotonin are frequently lower in offspring from stressed pregnancies. Disturbances of dopamine-related neurobiology have also been implicated as one reason for the greater emotional reactivity in animals generated from stressed pregnancies, especially with regard to explaining behavioral predilections to consume alcohol or to find addictive drugs more rewarding.

Figure 35.1 illustrated a number of the physiological pathways known to account for these effects of maternal stress and infection during pregnancy. Especially with regard to stress, it is not too surprising that most researchers have chosen to specifically investigate the glucocorticoids and have often concluded that it is the higher maternal level of adrenal hormones that overwhelms the fetus (Koehl et al, 1999). Much of the cortisol in fetal blood is derived from the mother, at least through mid-gestation (Gitau et al, 1998; Kajantie et al, 2003). Thus, it seems reasonable to postulate that the excessive transfer of adrenal corticosteroids is a major mediator of negative effects. It can hamper growth and protein synthesis, with many adverse effects on the immature brain and immune system (Munck et al, 1984). In rodent studies it is often possible to mitigate these effects of stress, and even to nutritional challenges during pregnancy, by removing the mother's adrenal glands or by pharmacological blockade of the actions of corticosteroids (Langley-Evans, 1997).

Nevertheless, there is some reason to temper the conclusion that increased HPA activity is the exclusive mediator of the effects of gestational stress. Under normal circumstances, the placenta has an excellent biochemical mechanism in place to limit the harmful effects of maternal cortisol, which is 11ß-HSD2, an enzyme that can convert cortisol to the less bioactive cortisone (Seckl, 1997). While the protection afforded by this barrier enzyme can be overwhelmed when cortisol levels get very high, it likely functions effectively when cortisol remains within the normal range (Campbell and Murphy, 1997). There is now considerable interest in what types of events or other hormones might lower 11ß-HSD2 and thereby reduce the buffering benefits it affords. On example is elevated catecholamine levels, which presumably would occur simultaneously in a stressed or hypoxic state.

Delineating all of the major pathways will always be challenging because three compartments must be taken into consideration: maternal, utero/placental, and fetal. Many physiological systems also function quite differently during pregnancy. One especially interesting hormone change is the dramatic rise in corticotrophin releasing hormone levels (CRH) (Wadhwa et al, 1997). In higher primates and humans, it is no longer secreted just from the hypothalamus, but is now released directly into circulation by the placenta. Placental CRH seems to have acquired a major role in determining the timing of parturition and rises progressively during the third trimester (Smith, 1999).

However, if elevated to high levels earlier in gestation, it is a warning sign that the pregnancy will not go to full term (Wadhwa et al, 2004). CRH levels can also increase as a consequence of maternal stress, probably because placental CRH activity does not have the typical negative feedback relationship with cortisol release. During pregnancy, placental CRH will actually be stimulated by cortisol. Thus, stressors that activate the mother's adrenocortical axis will augment the secretion of CRH.

6 The Mixed Blessing of Antenatal Corticosteroids

An additional reason for so much interest in the potentially adverse effects of corticosteroids on the fetus is its common use in clinical practice when babies are born premature (Merill and Ballard, 2001). Given the concerns about excess fetal exposure to maternal cortisol, it may seem paradoxical that one of the more important translational findings from animal research to clinical practice was the seminal finding that antenatal corticosteroid treatments are very beneficial in quickly advancing lung maturation (Liggins, 1969). Experiments in sheep showed that rising cortisol levels in the ewe signal the impending parturition and simultaneously accelerate the production of lung surfactant in the immature fetal lamb. The benefits for improving airway functioning in premature infants were soon extended to humans (Liggins and Howie, 1972). While these findings revolutionized the treatment of neonatal respiratory distress syndrome, reduced the likelihood of intraventricular hemorrhage and facilitated the management of very premature infants in the Neonatal Intensive Care Unit, there have continued to be some concerns about prolonged dosing and the use of multiple courses of dexamethasone or betamethasone (Kay et al, 2000). When prescribed in the standard manner as a 2-day course in the premature baby or to the gravid female prior to delivery, the safety of this regimen has been reasonably well established (Roberts and Dalziel, 2009), but for some expectant women threatening to deliver early, there have been up to 10 courses administered before birthing. When treatments are repeated or prolonged, studies in rodents, sheep, and monkeys have all found adverse effects, especially on sensitive brain regions like the hippocampus (Matthews, 2000; Uno et al, 1994). When extended over many days, antenatal corticosteroids can retard fetal growth, suppress both maternal and fetal adrenal activity, decrease thyroid activity, and affect kidney functioning in ways that would pose a long-term risk for later hypertension (Coe and Lubach, 2005; French et al, 1999; Seckl et al, 2000). One further reason for these concerns is that when administered directly to the mother before delivery, both dexamethasone and betamethasone can readily bypass the placental enzyme 11ß-HSD2 and then can become sequestered in fetal circulation. While examining the impact of a standard 2-day course of maternal dexamethasone in the rhesus monkey, we found fetal cortisol levels were still suppressed a full week later (Coe et al, 1993) see (Fig. 35.3).

If concerns about the potential long-term consequences of prolonged or multiple courses of

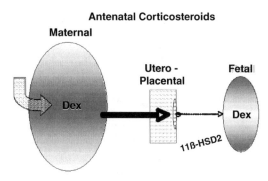

Antenatal Corticosteroids

Fig. 35.3 Synthetic corticosteroids, including dexamethasone and betamethasone, are routinely administered to pregnant women who may deliver early and to premature babies in order to stimulate lung maturation. As illustrated here, Dex readily bypasses the protective barrier enzyme 11 beta-hydroxysteroid dehydrogenase type 2 (11ß-HSD2), which normally limits fetal exposure to maternal cortisol by converting it to corticosterone, a less bioactive form. Some concerns linger about long-term effects of fetal exposure to high doses or sustained corticosteroid treatment

antenatal glucocorticoid therapies are warranted, it is of considerable significance. In the United States over 12% of infants are born premature, which means that each year up to 500,000 babies could experience a jolt of high levels of glucocorticoids, although most would receive only the standard 2-day treatment (Martin et al, 2009; Centers for Disease Control and Prevention, 2000).

7 The Risks Posed by Prenatal and Perinatal Infection

Maternal illness continues to be one of the more significant challenges to the maintenance of pregnancy and to fetal well-being (McGregor et al, 1995). In addition to concerns about miscarriage and premature delivery, many bacteria and viruses can pose a grave threat to the fetus if they are able to infect placental tissues or transfer across the placenta. Rubella, syphilis, and toxoplasma are among the pathogens that were once prominent health hazards. Even the common herpes viruses, such as cytomegalovirus, which are normally benign when restricted to the maternal compartment, can have devastating effects on brain development if they reach the fetal compartment or if there is exposure during delivery or the early postpartum period (Barry et al, 2006; Revello and Gerna, 2002).

There has also been a long-standing suspicion that prenatal infections and obstetrical complications may play a role in certain neurodevelopmental disorders and psychiatric conditions (Mednick et al, 1998). Viral infections have been implicated as possible causative agents for both autism and attention-deficit hyperactivity disorder (ADHD), although both of these pediatric conditions are obviously very complex and can be caused by other factors as well. Even more has been written about the possible involvement of prenatal infections as the reason for the brain dysfunction underlying schizophrenia (Brown, 2006; Byrne et al, 2007; Torrey and Torrey, 1979; Yolken et al, 1997). Concerns about exposure to influenza during pregnancy have been validated by support from animal models, at least after infection with more virulent strains (Shi et al, 2003, 2005; Fatemi et al, 2008; Fortier et al, 2007). In both rat and mouse models of maternal influenza infection during pregnancy, there have been effects found on brain size, structure, cortical thickness, and monoamine neurochemistry.

If infection with influenza during pregnancy can really be harmful to fetal brain development, it is a more serious concern when virulent strains circulate at pandemic levels (Harris, 1919). Even in a typical year, up to 11% of pregnant women are infected with influenza at some point during gestation (Irving et al, 2000). Moreover, the offspring of infected pregnant women who are asthmatic are at greater risk because they are more likely to progress on to bacterial pneumonia (Hartert et al, 2003). However, the jury is still out on whether the more benign strains of influenza that commonly circulate, which cause just a transient illness and fever, are of equivalent concern. One particularly active area of research right now is on the mediating role of the increased proinflammatory cytokine activity during infection, because it can adversely alter placental functioning (Dammann and Leviton, 1997). Some cytokines, such as interleukin-6, can also cross the placenta and reach the fetus or stimulate fetal tissues to synthesize their own cytokines. If cytokines in fetal circulation get high enough, they can disrupt the proliferation of neurons, formation of dendrites, and the establishment of synaptic connections in the maturing brain (Lowe et al, 2008; Saito et al, 2009).

8 Other Mediating Pathways of Importance: The Significance of Maternal Iron

The complexity of the physiological changes occurring during pregnancy challenge one to identify just one mediator of maternal influences on fetal development. Hormone levels rise dramatically, nutrients and oxygen must be transferred, and fetal brain maturation must be

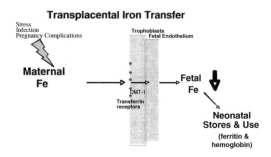

Fig. 35.4 Placental receptors facilitate the transfer of many proteins and micronutrients, including maternal iron. Inflammation, maternal stress, gestational hypertension, and diabetes can all compromise this process. When iron stores are low in the neonate, the high needs for growth and brain functions exceed the available iron in breast milk and predispose the infant to become anemic between 6 and 12 months of age

fostered. When the mother is taxed or threatened, more than one vital process will likely be perturbed. Notwithstanding the importance of the endocrine and vascular systems, one cannot overstate the significance of the nutritional support for the fetus.

This fact was made very clear to us while investigating the effects of prenatal stress in monkeys (Coe and Lubach, 2008). We inadvertently discovered that inducing stress in the pregnant monkey also compromised the placental transfer of maternal iron (Fig. 35.4). The clinical ramification of this reduced iron transfer later became very evident after the infant monkeys were born. The ones from prenatally stressed pregnancies became anemic by 4–8 months of age.

While effects on iron stores in the neonate had not been noticed previously by stress researchers, the significance of the prenatal iron transfer has been very prominent in the pediatric nutrition literature (Rao and Georgieff, 2002). About 50% of the iron needed to sustain physical growth and brain development during infancy must be acquired before birth. A rapidly growing baby cannot consume enough iron from breast milk alone. If iron levels are low at birth, human infants are destined to become anemic by 6–12 months of age. For the reader more concerned with population health, it should be highlighted that iron deficiency remains the most common micronutrient deficiency worldwide, believed to impact over 1–2 billion people. In some underdeveloped countries, up to 90% of children will become anemic, a statistic of concern given that iron is a required nutrient for many brain functions, including the synthesis of myelin and dopamine (Lozoff et al, 2006).

Three additional observations underscore the potential importance of this nutrient deficiency: (1) anemia during pregnancy is especially common in adolescent mothers, (2) impaired iron transfer is also seen in problematic pregnancies, including gestational hypertension and pregnancy-induced diabetes, and (3) virtually all premature infants have low iron. Thus, there would likely be a synergistic effect of maternal stress on iron homeostasis in all three of these more vulnerable populations. Despite the serious ramifications for pediatric health, fortunately there are therapeutic remedies readily available. Better prenatal care, iron supplementation during pregnancy, and nutritional interventions with iron-fortified food for the older infant are all effective ways to preemptively address these problems and thereby to promote child health.

9 Conclusion

The 13th century proverb that 'prevention is worth a pound of cure' can also be applied to several of the other issues discussed in this chapter. While many are apprehensive about immunization during pregnancy, the current recommendation to vaccinate against influenza seems to be the more prudent course (Mak et al, 2008). This public health policy is of particular relevance now as we face a growing pandemic of the 2009/H1N1 strain. It is exceedingly rare for influenza to change in a way that permits it to cross the placenta, but maternal immune and inflammatory responses could still impact placental and brain functioning (Dantzer et al, 2008). Concerns about fetal well-being should probably

be greatest after high fevers or following secondary infections with opportunistic bacterial pathogens. Even during the infamous 1918–1919 pandemic, bacterial pneumonias caused by *Streptococcus*, *Staphylococcus*, and *Haemophilus influenzae* were the greater concern for pregnant women (Harris, 1919). For pregnant women with a history of asthma, there is an additional risk of being more prone for respiratory complications after an infection (Hartert et al, 2003).

There are some other take home messages that are germane to a general understanding of the antecedents of both pediatric and adult health. We have come to appreciate that intrauterine conditions can leave an indelible stamp by affecting the regulatory set points for the endocrine system and for metabolic processes associated with growth. How our glucose and fat metabolism is regulated will determine whether we have a healthy physique of typical proportions or become overweight and obese. Especially after a brief period of undernutrition, there may be a re-setting of regulatory processes that influence the adult phenotype. We have cited only a few of the many epidemiological studies documenting how strongly fetal growth can be associated with a propensity for metabolic syndrome, type 2 diabetes and cardiovascular disease. These relationships also help us to understand why there are large disparities in adult health across different SES groups. Moreover, the 'prenatal origins' view offers a provocative way to account for the lingering consequences of societal perturbations across multiple generations (LaPlante et al, 2008; Yehuda et al, 2005).

It raises major policy issues for relief agencies to consider when intervening in parts of the world where strife has occurred. If we know that the well-being of an expectant mother will have an effect on the future health, immune competence, and cognitive abilities of her child, it is also essential to advocate for the universal provision of better prenatal care under normal circumstances. From these perspectives on maternal and child health, we know that a governmental policy of 'no child left behind' has to include comprehensive programs that begin earlier in development.

There is one final message that should be highlighted. The fetus is not just a passive recipient buffeted by extrinsic forces, it plays an active role in its own construction. Soon after implantation, the placental cells manipulate the endocrine physiology of the mother to sustain the pregnancy. They stimulate the initial angiogenesis to create the blood supply needed to nurture the baby. Throughout this chapter, the critical importance of the placenta as an integral factor has been emphasized. It is the conduit of a bidirectional communication, but fundamentally a tissue of fetal origin. Thus, early placental responses to uterine conditions are the first steps in what will become a complex and intricate dance with the surrounding environs. For most, this duet will establish the path to resiliency. For others, it can begin the trajectory toward ill health if the derailment is substantiated postnatally by the rearing environment.

Acknowledgments CLC is supported in part by grants from the National Institutes of Health, which have also supported the nonhuman primate studies on the developmental effects of maternal infection during pregnancy and iron deficiency anemia (AI067518, HD39386, HD057064).

References

Abbott, D. H., Barnett, D. K., Bruns, C. M., and Dumesic, D. A. (2005). Androgen excess fetal programming of female reproduction: a developmental aetiology for polycystic ovary syndrome? *Human Reprod Update, 11*, 357–374.

Bailey, M. T., and Coe, C. L. (1999). Maternal separation disrupts indigenous microflora of infant monkeys. *Devel Psychobio, 35*, 146–155.

Bailey, M. T., Lubach, G. R., and Coe, C. L. (2004). Prenatal conditions alter the bacterial colonization of the gut in the infant monkey. *J Pediatr Clin Gastroenterol, 38*, 414–421.

Barker, D. J. P. (1998). In utero programming of chronic disease. *Clin Sci, 95*, 115–128.

Barry, P. A., Lockridge, K. M., Salamat, S., Tinling, S. P., Yue, Y. et al (2006). Nonhuman primate models of intrauterine cytomegalovirus infection. *ILAR, 47*, 49–64.

Bateson, P., Barker, D. J. P., Clutton-Brock, T., Deb, D., D'Udine, B. et al (2004). Developmental plasticity and human health. *Nature, 430*, 419–421.

Berenbaum, S. A. (2006). Prenatal androgens and the ontogeny of behavior. In D. M. Hodgson & C. L. Coe (Eds.), *Perinatal Programming* (pp. 225–241). London: Taylor & Francis.

Berkowitz, G. S., Wolff, M. S., Janevic, T. M., Holzman, I. R., Yehuda, R. et al (2003). The World Trade Center disaster and intrauterine growth restriction. *JAMA, 290*, 595–596.

Birnbaum, L. S. (1995). Developmental effects of dioxins and related endocrine disrupting chemicals. *Toxicol Lett, 82–83*, 743–750.

Braunschweig, D., Ashwood, P., Krakowiak, P., Hertz-Picciotto, I., Hansen, R. et al (2009). Autism: maternally derived antibodies specific for fetal brain proteins. *Neurotoxicology, 29*, 226–231.

Brown, A. S. (2006). Prenatal infection as a risk factor for schizophrenia. *Schizophr Bull, 32*, 200–202.

Byrne, M., Agerbo, E., Benndese, B., Eaton, W., and Mortensen, P. (2007). Obstetric conditions and risk of first admission with schizophrenia: a Danish national register based study. *Schizophr Res, 97*, 51–59.

Campbell, A. L., and Murphy, B. E. P. (1977). The maternal-fetal cortisol gradient during pregnancy and at delivery. *J Clin Endocrinol Metab, 45*, 435–440.

Cariello, M. O., Macedo, R. H. F., and Schwabi, H. G. (2006) Maternal androgens in eggs of communally breeding guira cuckoos (Guira guira). *Horm Beh, 49*, 654–662.

Casas, R., and Brjorksten, B. (2001). Detection of Fel d-1-immunoglobulin G complexes in cord blood and sera from allergic and nonallergic mothers. *Pediat Allerg Immun, 12*, 59–64.

Centers for Disease Control and Prevention (2000). Racial and ethnic differences in infant mortality rates—60 largest US cities, 1995–1998. *MMWR Morb Mortal Wkly Rep, 51*, 329–343.

Chen, E. Chim, L. S., Strunk, R. C., and Miller, G. (2007). The role of the social environment in children and adolescents with asthma. *Am J Resp Crit Care Med, 176*, 644–649.

Cokkinides, V. E., Coker, A. L., Sanderson, M., Addy, C., and Bethea, L. (1999). Physical violence during pregnancy: maternal complications and birth outcomes. *Obstet Gynecol 93*, 661–666.

Coe, C. L., Kemnitz, J. W., and Schneider, M. L. (1993). Vulnerability of placental antibody transfer and fetal complement synthesis to disturbance of the pregnant monkey. *J Med Primatol, 22*, 294–300.

Coe, C. L., and Lubach, G. R. (2005). Developmental consequences of antenatal dexamethasone treatment in nonhuman primates. *Neurosci BioBehav Rev, 29*, 227–235.

Coe, C. L., and Lubach, G. R. (2008). Fetal programming: Prenatal origins of health and illness. *Cur Dir Psych Sci, 17*, 36–41.

Coe, C. L., Lubach, G. R. and Izard, K. M. (1994). Progressive improvement in the transfer of maternal antibody across the Order Primates. *Am J Primatol, 32*, 51–55.

Coe, C. L., Lubach, G. R., and Shirtcliff, E. (2007). Maternal stress during pregnancy increases risk for iron deficient infants impacting innate immunity. *Pediat Res, 61*, 520–524.

Crews, D., and Bull, J. J. (2008). Sex determination: some like it hot (and some don't). *Nature, 251*, 527–528.

Culhane, J. F., Rauh, V., and Farley-McCollum, K. (2001). Maternal stress is associated with bacterial vaginosis in human pregnancy. *Maternal Child Health J, 5*, 127–134.

Dammann, O., and Leviton, A. (1997). Maternal intrauterine infection, cytokines and brain damage in the preterm newborn. *Pediatr Res, 42*, 1–8.

Danese, A., Pariante, C. M., Caspi, A., Taylor, A., and Poulton, R. (2007). Childhood maltreatment predicts adult inflammation in a life-course study. *PNAS, 104*, 1319–1324.

Dantzer, R., O'Connor, J. C., Freund, G. G., Johnson, R. W., and Kelley, K. W. (2008). From inflammation to sickness and depression: when the immune system subjugates the brain. *Nature Rev Neurosci, 9*, 46–56.

David, R., and Collins, J. (1997). Differing birth weight among infants of US-born blacks, African-born blacks, and US-born whites. *N Engl J Med, 337*, 1209–1219.

Devereux, G., Seaton, A., and Barker, R. N. (2001). In utero priming of allergen specific helper T cells. *Clin Exp Allerg, 31*, 1686–1695.

Dunger, D. B., and Ong, K. K. (2005). Babies born small for gestational age: insulin sensitivity and growth hormone treatment. *Hormone Res, 64*, 58–65.

Engel, S. M., Berkowitz, G. S., Wolff, M., and Yehuda, Y. (2005). Psychological trauma associated with World Trade Center attacks and its effects on pregnancy outcome. *Paediat Perinatal Epidemiol, 19*, 334–341.

Fatemi, S. H., Reutiman, T. J., Folsom, T. D., Huang, H., Oishi, K. et al (2008). Maternal infection leads to abnormal gene regulation and brain atrophy in mouse offspring. *Schizophr Res, 99*, 56–70.

Fergusson, D. M., Crane, J., Beaseley, R., and Horwood, L. J. (1997). Perinatal factors and atopic disease in childhood. *Clin Exp Allerg, 27*, 1394–1401.

Fortier, M-. E., Luheshi, G. N., and Boksa, P. (2007). Effects of prenatal infection on PPI in rat depend upon nature of the infectious agent and stage of pregnancy. *Behav Brain Res, 181*, 270–277.

French, N. P., Hagan, R., Evans, S. F., Godfrey, M., and Newnham, J. P. (1999). Repeated antenatal corticosteroids: size at birth and subsequent development. *Am J Obstet Gynecol, 180*, 114–121.

Gazmararian, J. A., Lazorick, S., Spitz, A. M., Ballard, T. J., Saltzman, L. E. et al (1996). Prevalence of violence against pregnant women. *JAMA, 275*, 1915–1920.

Gitau, R., Cameron, A., Fisk, N. M., and Glover, V. (1998). Fetal exposure to maternal cortisol. *Lancet, 352*, 707–708.

Gregory, K. D., Henry, O. A., Ramicone, E., Chan, L. S., and Platt, L. D. (1998). Maternal and infant complications in high and normal weight infants by method of delivery. *Obstet Gynecol, 92*, 507–513.

Glynn, L. M., Wadhwa, P. D., Dunkel-Schetter, C., and Sandman, C. A. (2001). When stress happens matters: the effects of earthquake timing on stress responsivity in pregnancy. *Am J Obstet Gynecol, 184*, 637–642.

Goy, R. W., Uno, H., and Sholl, S. A. (1988a). Psychological and anatomical consequences of prenatal exposure to androgens in female rhesus. In T. Mori & H. Nagasawa (Eds.), *Toxicity of Hormones in Perinatal Life* (pp. 127–142). Boca Raton, Florida: CRC Press Inc..

Goy, R. W., Bercovitch, F. B., and McBrair, M. C. (1988b). Behavioral masculinization is independent of genital masculinization in prenatally androgenized female rhesus macaques. *Horm Behav 22*, 552–571.

Guerri, C., Bazinet, A., and Riley, E. P. (2009). Foetal alcohol spectrum disorders and alterations in brain and behavior. *Alcohol Alcoholism, 22*, 108–114.

Harris, J. W. (1919). Influenza occurring in pregnant women. A statistical study of 1350 cases. *JAMA, 72*, 978–980.

Hartert, T. V., Neuzil, K. M., Shintani, A. K., Mitchel, E. F., Snowden, M. S. et al (2003) Maternal morbidity and perinatal outcomes among pregnant women with respiratory hospitalizations during influenza season. *Am J Obstet Gyn, 189*, 1705–1712.

Hedegaard, M., Henriksen, T. B., Secher, N. J., Hatch, M. C., and Sabroe, S. (1996). Do stressful life events affect duration of gestation and risk of preterm delivery? *Epidemiology, 7*, 339–345.

Hiller, S. L., Nugent, R. P., Eschebach, D. A., Krohn, M. A., Gibbs, R. S. et al (1995). Association between bacterial vaginosis and preterm delivery of low-birth weight infants. *NEJM, 333*, 1737–1742.

Hodgson, D. M., and Coe, C. L. (2006). *Perinatal Programming: Early Life Determinants of Adult Health and Disease*. Abingdon: Taylor & Francis.

Huxley, R., Neil, A., and Collins, R. (2002). Unravelling the fetal origins hypothesis: is there really an inverse association between birthweight and subsequent blood pressure? *Lancet, 360*, 659–665.

Irving, W. L., James, D. K., Setphenson, T., Laing, P., Jameson, C. et al (2000). Influenza virus infection in second and third trimesters of pregnancy: a clinical and seroepidemiological study. *Br J Obstet Gynec, 107*, 1282–1289.

Jones, C. A., Holloway, J. A., and Warner, J. O. (2000). Does atopic disease start in foetal life? *Allergy, 55*, 2–10.

Jones, K. L., and Smith, D. W. (1973). Recognition of the fetal alcohol syndrome in early infancy. *Lancet, 2*, 999–1001.

Kaiser, S., and Sachser, N. (2009). Effects of prenatal social stress on offspring development: Pathology or adaptation *Cur Dir Psych Sci, 18*, 118–121.

Kajantie, E., Dunkel, L., Turpeinen, U., Stenman, U-. H., Wood, P. J. et al (2003). Placental 11ß- hydroxysteroid dehydrogenase-2 and fetal cortisol/cortisone shuttle in small preterm infants. *J Clin Endocrinol Metab, 88*, 493–500.

Karmaus, W., Arshad, S. H., Sadeghnejad, A., and Twiselton, R. (2004). Does maternal IgE decrease with increasing order of live offspring? *Clin Exp Allerg, 43*, 853–859.

Kay, H. H., Bird, I. M., Coe, C. L., and Dudley, D. J. (2000). Antenatal steroid treatment and adverse fetal effects: what is the evidence? *Soc Gynecol Invest, 7*, 269–278.

Kleinman, J., and Kessel, S. (1987). Racial differences in low birth weight. *N Engl J Med, 317*, 744–753.

Koehl, M., Darnaudery, M., Dulluc, J., Van Reeth, O., Le Moal, M. et al (1999). Prenatal stress alters circadian activity of hypothalamo-pituitary-adrenal axis and hippocampal corticosteroid receptors in adult rats of both gender. *J Neurobiol 40*, 302–315.

Langley-Evans, S. C. (1997). Hypertension induced by foetal exposure to a maternal low protein diet in the rat is prevented by pharmacological blockade of maternal glucocorticoid synthesis. *J Hypertens, 15*, 37–44.

LaPlante, D., Brunet, A., Schmitz, N., Ciampi, A., and King, S. (2008). Project Ice Storm: Prenatal maternal stress affects cognitive and linguistic functioning in 5 $1/2$ -year old children. J *Am Acad Child Adol Psychiat, 47*, 1063–1072.

Law, C. M., Barker, D. J. P., Osmond, C., Fall, C. H. D., and Simmonds, S. J. (1992). Early growth and abdominal fatness in adult life. *J Epidemiol Community Health, 46*, 184–186.

Lemaire, V., Koehl, M., Le Moal, M., and Abrous, D. N. (2000). Prenatal stress produces learning deficits associated with an inhibition of neurogenesis in the hippocampus. *PNAS, 97*, 11032–11037.

Liggins, G. C. (1969). Premature delivery of foetal lambs infused with glucocorticoids. *J Endocrinol, 45*, 515–523.

Liggins, C. G., and Howie, R. N. (1972). A controlled trial of antepartum glucocorticoid treatment for prevention of the respiratory distress syndrome in premature infants. *Pediatrics, 50*, 515–525.

Liobichler, C., Pichler, J., and Gestmayr, M. (2002). Materno-fetal passage of nutritive and inhalant allergens across placentas of term and preterm deliveries perfused in vitro *Clin Exp Allergy, 32*, 1546–1551.

Lowe, G. C., Luheshi, G. N., and Williams, S. (2008). Maternal infection and fever during late gestation are associated with altered synaptic transmission in the hippocampus of juvenile offspring rats. *Am J Physiol Regul Interg Comp Physiol, 295*, R1563–R1571.

Lozoff, B., Beard, J., Connor, J., Felt, B., Georgieff, M., and Schallert, T. (2006). Long-lasting neural and behavioral effects of iron deficiency in infancy. *Nutr Rev, 64*(Suppl 1), S34–S43.

Lui, A. H., and Murphy, J. R. (2003). Hygiene hypothesis: fact or fiction? *J Allergy Clin Immunol, 111*, 471–478.

Mak, T. K., Mangtani, P., Leese, J., Watson, J. M., and Pfeifer, D. (2008). Influenza vaccination in pregnancy: current evidence and selected national policies. *Lancet Infect Dis, 8*, 44–52.

Martin, J. A., Hamilton, B. E., Sutton, P. D., Ventura, S. J., Menacker, F. et al (2009). Births: final data for 2006. *National Vital Stat Rep, 57*, 3–104.

Matthews, S. G. (2000). Antenatal glucocorticoids and programming of the developing CNS. *Pediatr Res, 47*, 291–300.

McGregor, J. A., French, J. I., Parker, R., Draper, D., Patterson, E. et al (1995). Prevention of premature birth by screening and treatment for common genital tract infections: results of a prospective controlled evaluation. *Am J Obstet Gynecol, 173*, 157–167.

McFarlane, J., Parker, B., and Soeken, K. (1996). Physical abuse, smoking and substance use during pregnancy: prevalence, interrelationships and effects on birth weight. *J Obstet Gynecol Neonatal Nurse, 25*, 313–320.

Mednick, S. A., Machon, R. A., Huttunen, M. O., and Bonnet, D. (1988). Adult schizophrenia following prenatal exposure to an influenza epidemic. *Arch Gen Psychiat, 45*, 189–192.

Menon, R., Merialdi, M., Betran, A. P., Dolan, S., Jiang, L. et al (2006). Analysis of association between maternal tumor necrosis factor-alpha promoter polymorphism (-308), tumor necrosis factor concentration and preterm birth. *Am J Obstet Gynecol, 195*, 1240–1248.

Merill, J. D., and Ballard, R. A. (2001). Clinical use of antenatal corticosteroids: benefits and risks. *Pediat in Rev Neorev, 1*, E91–E98.

Moritz, K. M., Mazzuca, M. Q., Siebel, A. L, Mibus, A., Arena, D. et al (2009). Uteroplacental inusifficency causes a nephron deficit, modest renal insufficiency but no hypertension with aging in female rats. *J Physiol, 587*, 2635–2646.

Munck, A., Guyre, P. M., and Holbrook, N. J. (1984). Physiological functions of glucocorticoids in stress and their relation to pharmacological actions. *Endocrinol Rev, 5*, 25–44.

Murphy, V. E., Smith, R., Giles, W. B., and Clifton, V. L. (2006). Endocrine regulation of human fetal growth: the role of the mother, placenta, and fetus. *Endocr Rev, 27*, 141–169.

Newberger, E. H., Barkan, S. E., Lieberman, E. S., McCormick, M. C., Yllo, K. et al (1992). Abuse of pregnant women and adverse birth outcome: current knowledge and implications for practice. *JAMA, 267*, 2370–2372.

Pekkanen, J. et al (2001). Gestational age and occurrence of atopy at age 31 - a prospective birth cohort study in Finland. *Clin Exp Allerg, 31*, 95–102.

Petersen, R., Gazmararian, J. A., Spitz, A. M., Rowley, D. L., Goodwin, M. M. et al (1997). Violence and adverse pregnancy outcomes: a review of the literature and directions for future research *Am J Prev Med, 13,* 366–373.

Piccinni, M. P. et al (1993). Aeroallergen sensitization can occur during fetal life. *Int Arch Allergy Immun, 102,* 301–303.

Rao, R., and Georgieff, M. K. (2002). Perinatal aspects of iron metabolism. *Acta Paediatr Suppl, 91,* 124–129.

Rainey, W., Rehman, K., and Carr, B. R. (2004). The human fetal adrenal: making adrenal androgens for placental estrogens. *Semin Reprod Med, 22,* 327–366.

Ravelli, G. P., Stein, Z. A., and Susser, M. W. (1976). Obesity in young men after famine exposure in utero and early infancy. *N Engl J Med, 295,* 349–353.

Ravelli, A. C., van der Meulen, J. H. P., Michels, R. P. J., and Osmond, C. (1998). Glucose tolerance in adults after prenatal exposure to famine. *The Lancet, 351,* 173–177.

Revello, M. G., and Gerna, G. (2002). Diagnosis and management of human cytomegalovirus infection in the mother, fetus, and newborn infant. *Clin Microbiol Rev, 15,* 680–715.

Reynolds, R. M., Walker, B. R., Syddall, H. E., Andrew, R., Wood, P. J. et al (2001). Altered control of cortisol secretion in adult men with low birth weight and cardiovascular risk factors. *J Clin Endocr Metab, 86,* 245–250.

Rigo, J. J. R., Szelenyi, J., Selmeczy, Z., Papp, Z., and Vizi, E. S. (2004). Endotoxin-induced TNF production changes inversely to itsplasma level during pregnancy. *Eur J Obstet Gynec, 114,* 236–238.

Rees, S., Harding, R., and Walker, D. (2008). An adverse intrauterine environment: implications for injury and altered development of the brain. *Intern J Devel Neurosci, 26,* 3–11.

Roberts, D., and Dalziel, S. R. (2009). Antenatal corticosteroids for accelerating fetal lung maturation for women at risk of preterm birth. Cochrane Database of Systematic Reviews Issue 3, Art. No.: CD004454. DOI: 10.1002/14651858.CD004454.pub2.

Rodrigues, A. L., de Moura, E. G., Passos, M. C. F., Cristina, S., Durtra, P. et al (2009). Postnatal early overnutrition changes the leptin signaling pathway in the hypothalamic-pituitary-thyroid axis of young and adult rats. *J Physiol, 587.11,* 2647–2661.

Roseboom, T., van der Meulen, J. H. P., Osmond, C., Barker, D., Ravelli, A. et al (2000). Coronary heart disease after prenatal exposure to the Dutch famine, 1944–45. *Heart, 84,* 595–598.

Royle, N. J., Surai, P. F., and Hartley, I. R. (2001). Maternally derived androgens and antioxidants in bird eggs: complementary but opposing effects? *Behav Ecology, 12,* 381–385.

Saito, M., Matsuda, T., Okuyama, K., Kobayashi, Y., Kitanishi, R. et al (2009) Effect of intrauterine inflammation on fetal cerebral hemodynamics and white-matter injury in chronically instrumented fetal sheep. *Am J Obstet Gynecol, 200,* 663.e1–664.e11.

Salk, L., Grellong, B. A., Strauss, W., and Dietrich, J. (1974). Perinatal complications in the history of asthmatic children. *Am J Dis Child, 127,* 30–33.

Sampson, P. D., Streissguth, A. P., and Bookstein, F. L. (1997). Incidence of fetal alcohol syndrome and prevalence of alcohol-related neurodevelopmental disorder. *Teratology, 56,* 317–326.

Seckl, J. R. (1997). Glucocorticoids, feto-placental 11 beta-hydroxysteroid dehydrogenase type 2, and the early life origins of adult disease. *Steroids, 62,* 89–94.

Seckl, J. R., Cleasby, M., and Nyirenda, M. M. (2000). Glucocorticoids, 11beta-hydorxysteroid dehydrogenase and fetal programming. *Kidney International, 57,* 1412–1417.

Shaywitz, D. A., and Melton, D. A. (2005). The molecular biology of the cell. *Cell, 120,* 729–733.

Shi, L., Fatemi, S. H., Sidwell, R. W., and Patterson, P. H. (2003). Maternal influenza infection causes marked behavioral and pharmacological changes in the offspring. *J Neurosci 23,* 297–302.

Shi, L., Tu, N., and Patterson, P. H. (2005). Maternal influenza infection is likely to alter fetal development indirectly. *Int J Devel Neurosci, 23,* 299–305.

Singer, H. S., Morris, C., Gause, C., Pollard, M., Zimmerman, A. W. et al (2009). Prenatal exposure to antibodies from mothers of children with autism produces neurobehavioral alterations: a pregnant dam mouse model. *J Neuroimmunol, 211,* 39–48.

Smith, R. (1999). The timing of human birth. *Sci Amer, 3,* 68–75.

Spira, A., Phillipe, E., Spira, N., Dreyfus, J., and Schwartz, D. (1977). Smoking during pregnancy and placental pathology. *Biomed, 27,* 266–270.

Swain, A., and Lovell-Badge, R. (1999). Mammalian sex determination: a molecular drama. *Genes Dev, 13,* 755–767.

Torrey, E. F., and Torrey, B. B. (1979). A shifting seasonality of schizophrenic births. *Br J Psychiat, 134,* 183–186.

Trott, J. F., Simpson, K. J., Moyle, R. L. C., Hearn, C. M., Shaw, G. et al (2003). Maternal regulation of milk composition, milk production, and pouch young development during lactation in the tammar wallaby (Macropus eugenii). *Biol Reprod, 68,* 929–936.

Uno, H., Eisele, S., Sakai, A., Shelton, S., Baker, E. et al (1994). Neurotoxicity of glucocorticoids in the primate brain. *Horm Behav, 28,* 336–348.

Van Duren Schmidt, K., Pichler, J., Ebner, C., Bartmann, P., Forster, E. et al (1997). Prenatal contact with inhalant allergens. *Pediat Res, 41,* 128–131.

Wadhwa, P. D., Sandman, C. A., Porto, M., Dunkel-Schetter, C., and Garite, T. J. (1993). The association between prenatal stress and infant birthweight and gestational age at birth: a prospective investigation. *Am J Obstet Gynecol, 169,* 858–865.

Wadhwa, P. D., Sandman, C. A., Chicz-DeMet, A., and Porto, M. (1997). Placental CRH modulates maternal pituitary-adrenal function in human pregnancy. *Annals NY Acad Sci, 814,* 276–281.

Wadhwa, P. D., Garite, T. J., Porto, M., Chicz-DeMet, A., Dunkel-Schetter, C. et al (2004). Corticotropin-releasing hormone (CRH), preterm birth and fetal growth restriction: a prospective investigation. *Am J Obstet Gynecol, 191,* 1063–1069.

Warner, J. A., Jones, C. A., Jones, A. C., and Warner, J. O. (2000). Prenatal origins of allergic disease. *J Allerg Clin Immunol, 105,* 5493–5496.

Weinstock, M. (1997). Does prenatal stress impair coping and regulation of hypothalamic-pituitary-adrenal axis? *Neurosci Biobehav Rev, 21,* 1–10.

Welberg, L. A., and Seckl, J. R. (2001). Prenatal stress, glucocorticoids and the programming of the brain. *J Neuroendocrinol, 13,* 113–128.

Whalen, R. E., and Luttge, W. G. (1971). Perinatal administration of dihydrotestosterone to female rats and the development of reproductive function. *Endocrinol, 89,* 1320–1322.

Wallen, K. (1996). Nature needs nurture: the interaction of hormonal and social influences on the development of behavioral sex differences in rhesus monkeys. *Horm Behav 30,* 364–378.

Wildman, D. E., Chen, C., Erez, O., Grossman, L. I., Goodman, M. et al (2006). Evolution of the mammalian placenta revealed by phylogenetic analysis. *PNAS, 103,* 3203–3208.

Wintour, E. M., Johnson, K., Koukoulas, I., Moritz, K., Tersteeg, M. et al (2003). Programming the cardiovascular system, kidney and the brain: a review. *Placenta, 27*(Suppl. A), 65–71.

Wood, R. I., Mehta, V., Herbosa, C. G., and Foster, D. L. (1995). Prenatal testosterone differentially masculinizes tonic and surge modes of luteinizing hormone secretion in the developing sheep. *Neuroendocrinol, 62,* 238–247.

Yager, J. Y., and Ashwal, S. (2009). Animal models of perinatal hypoxic-ischemic brain damage. Pediatr Neruol, 40, 156–167.

Yehuda, R., Engel, S. M., Brand, S. R., Seckl, J., Marcus, S. M. et al (2005). Transgenerational effects of posttraumatic stress disorder in babies of mothers exposed to the World Trade Center attacks during pregnancy. *J Clin Endocr Metab, 90,* 4115–4118.

Yolken, R. H., and Fuller Torrey, E. (1997). Viruses as etiologic agents of schizophrenia. In A. E. Henneberg, & W. P. Kaschka (Eds.), *Immunological Alterations in Psychiatric Diseases, Vol 18* (pp. 1–12). *Adv Biol Psychiatry, 18,* 1–12. Karger, Basel.

Chapter 36

The Impact of Early Adversity on Health

Shelley E. Taylor

Good health begins early in life. Unfortunately, so does poor health. Low socioeconomic status (SES) in childhood and a harsh early family environment can adversely influence trajectories of health outcomes long into adulthood. It may come as no surprise that childhood physical and sexual abuse have negative mental and physical health consequences, both immediately and over the life span. These effects are well documented (e.g., Springer et al, 2003). What may be more surprising is that relatively modest family dysfunction that numerous people routinely experience can lead to adverse outcomes as well.

Both animal and human research conclusively documents that warm, nurturant contact early in life exerts permanent beneficial effects on the functioning of biological stress regulatory systems and on socioemotional skills that affect responses to stress across the life span (Francis et al, 1999; Liu et al, 1997; Repetti et al, 2002, 2007). When this contact is lacking, both biological stress regulatory systems and behavioral skills for managing stress are compromised. Adverse downstream consequences include problems in emotion regulation, social skills deficits, poor health habits, and exacerbation of biological stress responses prognostic for poor mental and physical health.

1 Early Family Environment

This review will be guided by the model pictured in Fig. 36.1. The model maintains that a stressful or harsh early environment, in conjunction with genetic or acquired risks, is linked to adverse health outcomes in adulthood via its impact on the (in)ability to develop effective socioemotional skills; through a propensity to experience chronic negative affect; by affecting health habits adversely; and by influencing the neural pathways that ultimately regulate neuroendocrine stress responses. Drawing on the concept of allostatic load (McEwen, 1998), we suggest that these pathways contribute to the experience of chronic or recurring stress which, in interaction with genetic predispositions and acquired risks such as poor health habits, lead to the accumulating damage to biological systems that ultimately results in risks for mental and physical health disorders.

2 Childhood Socioeconomic Status

The point of departure for the model is low childhood SES. Low childhood SES has been related to exposure to a broad array of early stressful events. These include neighborhood conflict, violence exposure, noise, poor housing, exposure to pathogens, and other chronic stressors (Adler et al, 1999). Substantial research also

S.E. Taylor (✉)
Department of Psychology, University of California, 1282A Franz Hall, Los Angeles, CA 90095, USA
e-mail: taylors@psych.ucla.edu

A. Steptoe (ed.), *Handbook of Behavioral Medicine*, DOI 10.1007/978-0-387-09488-5_36,

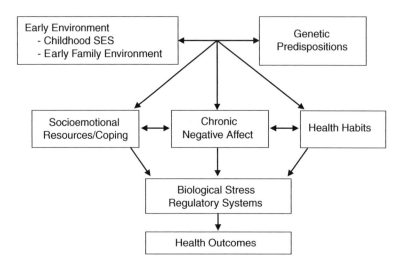

Fig. 36.1 A model of the impact of early environment on biological risk profiles and health outcomes

links economic adversity (low SES) early in life to mental and physical health disorders (Adler et al, 1999).

Research has consistently tied low childhood SES to all the downstream variables in the model (Fig. 36.1). It is associated with poor or deteriorating quality of parenting, including higher levels of family conflict, a harsh, restrictive parenting style, and chaotic or neglectful parenting (McLoyd, 1998). Low childhood SES has also been related to chronic negative affective states (Gallo and Matthews, 2003) and to problems in the development or use of socioemotional resources (Adler et al, 1999; Repetti et al, 2002; Taylor and Seeman, 2000). Low SES has been tied to unhealthful habits, including smoking (Winkleby et al, 1999), obesity (e.g., Wardle et al, 2002), poor sleep (Van Cauter and Spiegel, 1999), and drug abuse (Spooner, 1999). Low socioeconomic status has been tied to a broad array of diseases and all-cause mortality as well (e.g., Adler et al, 1999; Hemingway et al, 2003; Kivimäki et al, 2004; Lawlor, and Smith, 2005; Owen et al, 2003). In summary, there is substantial evidence that adverse health outcomes in adulthood have origins in SES, including SES in childhood, via pathways implicating socioemotional resources, chronic negative affect, and health behaviors.

3 Early Family Environment

Similar patterns are found when an early family environment is assessed directly. A harsh family upbringing has been related to poor health behaviors (Repetti et al, 2002); to high levels of depression, hostility, and anxiety (Repetti et al, 2002); to preclinical risk factors for physical health disorders, including elevated autonomic and cortisol responses to threatening circumstances (e.g., Roisman et al, 2009; Taylor et al, 2004); to risk factors for disease, including compromised metabolic functioning (Lehman et al, 2005) and C-reactive protein (Taylor et al, 2006b); and to diagnosed health disorders, including ischemic heart disease, some cancers, and depression (Felitti et al, 1998). Socioemotional resources that affect the ability to regulate emotional states effectively and to develop social competencies are implicated in these pathways. For example, offspring from harsh early environments experience difficulty in managing emotions in challenging circumstances (Repetti et al, 2002, 2007).

4 Genes and Gene–Environment Interactions

As the model indicates and as the theory of allostatic load maintains, a harsh early environment contributes to life span risk for health disorders, not only directly but also via gene–environment interactions (Repetti et al, 2002). Recently, what some of those genes may be has come to light.

One such gene is the serotonin transporter gene, certain alleles of which may predispose to anxiety and/or depression (see Chapter 31). People with two copies of the 5-HTTLPR short allele (short/short) who have experienced childhood maltreatment are more likely to be diagnosed with major depressive disorders than individuals with one or two copies of the long allele who have experienced similar harsh environments (Caspi et al, 2003; Kaufman et al, 2004). Taylor and colleagues (Taylor et al, 2006c) found that the short allele may function not only as a risk allele for depression in the face of an adverse early environment but as a general sensitivity allele, providing protection from symptoms of depression if the early environment is nurturant. Using a non-clinical sample of 118 adults, we found that people with two copies of the short allele had greater depressive symptomatology if they had experienced early familial adversity compared to people with the short/long or long/long genotypes, but significantly less depressive symptomatology if they reported a supportive early environment. Another gene whose functioning is affected by early environment is the gene that regulates monoamine oxidase (MAOA). Men with the low-expressing alleles of the MAOA-uVNTR are more likely to engage in aggressive and antisocial behavior than men with high expressing alleles; these outcomes appear to be especially likely if the men have also been exposed to maltreatment as children (Caspi et al, 2002; Kim-Cohen et al, 2006). Recent evidence suggests that the long allele of the DRD4 receptor gene, involved in the regulation of dopamine, may similarly interact with family environment; that is, the long allele may increase sensitivity to both negative and positive parental influences (e.g., Bakermans-Kranenburg and van IJzendoorn, 2007; Bakermans-Kranenburg et al, 2008).

Expression of the glucocorticoid receptor gene is also affected by the early environment. In animal studies, Meaney and colleagues have shown that rat pups exposed to highly nurturant mothering exhibit less emotionality in novel circumstances and more normative social behavior, including mothering in adulthood, compared to recipients of normal mothering (Francis et al, 1999; Weaver et al, 2004). These long-term effects of maternal care appear to be the result of epigenetic structural alteration (methylation) to the glucocorticoid receptor gene that affects its expression throughout the life span (Meaney and Szyf, 2005). This mechanism may help to explain why early family environment has such enduring effects on biological responses to stress and ultimately on long-term health outcomes, via altered glucocorticoid receptor expression that affects adult reactivity to stress.

Since the study of gene-by-environment interactions is in its early stages, especially those involving the early environment, these findings are more tantalizing than they are definitive. The coming decades will no doubt identify other genes and other ways in which early environment may interact to affect propensities for risk for illness.

5 Emotion Regulation

Problems in the regulation of emotional states are implicated in the pathways linking early adversity to adverse health outcomes. Emotion regulation is a broad term that includes skills for recognizing one's own and others' emotions, controlling one's emotional reactions to potentially stressful or challenging situations, and expressing one's emotions in socially appropriate ways (Eisenberg and Spinrad, 2004).

A variety of investigations have tied a harsh family environment to children's reactions to emotionally charged circumstances, understanding of emotions, and abilities to regulate their emotions (Repetti et al, 2002). Offspring from harsh family environments may overreact to threatening circumstances, responding aggressively to situations that are only modestly stressful (Reid and Crisafulli, 1990), but may also tune out or avoid stressful circumstances, as through behavioral escape/avoidance or substance abuse (Johnson and Pandina, 1991; O'Brien et al, 1991; Valentiner et al, 1994). Deficits in emotion regulation skills related to early family environment may appear in early childhood and compromise the development and use of socioemotional skills in adulthood (Repetti et al, 2002).

A harsh family environment also predicts an incomplete understanding of emotional experience in others. Investigations with young children have found that those who were maltreated or whose homes were marked by high levels of anger and distress are less accurate in their understanding of emotions compared to their peers (Camras et al, 1988; Dunn and Brown, 1994). Relatedly, Laible and Thompson (1998) found that children with insecure attachments showed less emotion understanding and less accurate appraisals of emotion in others.

In short, growing up in a risky family environment appears to interfere with the development of skills for processing emotional information in self and others.

6 Social Skills

A harsh family environment has been tied to fewer social skills for facilitating successful interactions with peers (Crockenberg and Lourie, 1996; Pettit et al, 1988). Children from risky families who evidence emotion regulation difficulties are more likely to behave in an aggressive or antisocial manner with their peers (Repetti et al, 2002), undermining their ability to develop friendships. Several studies attest to the peer rejection and even victimization experienced by children from harsh families (Dishion, 1990; Schwartz et al, 1997). Similarly, children whose

parents are unresponsive, cold, and insensitive are less likely to initiate social interactions, and they demonstrate more aggression and criticism in social relationships (see Repetti et al, 2007). Children of parents who are cold, unsupportive, or neglectful show deficits in social relationships throughout their lives, with more problematic and less supportive social networks (Repetti et al, 2007).

Inadequate social support networks may translate into some of the adverse health effects of a harsh early environment. More than 100 investigations have shown that social support reduces health risks of all kinds, affects the initial likelihood of illness, influences the course of recovery among people who are already ill, and affects mortality risk more generally (House et al, 1988; Seeman, 1996; see Taylor, 2009, for a review).

7 Chronic Negative Affect

Deficits in socioemotional skills may ultimately stabilize into enduring risks for emotional disorders, such as anxiety, depression, and other chronic negative emotional states. These states may act as predisposing factors for adverse physical health outcomes (Hemingway et al, 2003). For example, hostility has been tied to the development of metabolic syndrome among children and adolescents (Dembroski et al, 1985) and to an increased risk for coronary heart disease (CHD) and hypertension (Julkunen et al, 1994). Major depression, depressive symptoms, and history of depression have all been identified as predictors of cardiac events (Frasure-Smith et al, 1995), and depression is a risk factor for mortality following myocardial infarction, independent of cardiac disease severity (Frasure-Smith et al, 1995). State depression, as well as clinical depression, have been related to sustained suppressed immunity (Herbert and Cohen, 1993). Anger appears to play a significant role in the development of coronary artery disease and hypertension, at least among some individuals (e.g., Julkunen et al, 1994; Smith,

1992). Depression and anxiety are implicated in numerous health risks, including all-cause mortality (Martin et al, 1995), and evidence points to a dose–response relation between anxiety and coronary heart disease (Kubzansky et al, 1998).

Links between negative emotional states and health outcomes may result from chronic or recurring engagement of biological stress regulatory systems. Negative emotional states have been tied to heightened biological stress responses, including evidence of stronger autonomic response to stressful circumstances (e.g., Matthews et al, 1996) and stronger hypothalamic–pituitary–adrenocortical (HPA) responses to stress (e.g., Chorpita and Barlow, 1998; Flinn and England, 1997). Studies also suggest links between negative emotions and reduced heart rate variability (e.g., Kawachi et al, 1995), implicating potential compromises in parasympathetic functioning in these relations. Intense, chronic, or recurring biological responses to stress may, thus, represent one pathway by which a harsh early environment exerts adverse effects on adult health outcomes (McEwen, 1998; Repetti et al, 2002), effects that may be mediated, at least in part, by negative emotional states.

8 Health Habits

Health habits are also implicated in these pathways (e.g., Repetti et al, 2002). A harsh early environment has been tied to increased rates of smoking, alcohol abuse, drug use, and risky sexual behaviors in adolescence and adulthood (e.g., Wagner, 1997). Both cross-sectional and longitudinal investigations have found that neglect, abuse, and conflict in the early environment predict poor health habits in adulthood (Repetti et al, 2002). Prospective studies have found increased rates of substance abuse and risky sexual behaviors among offspring of families lacking cohesion or in offspring of parents who are neglectful and unsupportive (e.g., Baumrind, 1991; Shedler and Block, 1990), relations found in people who have been followed for many years after exposure to the initial environment (e.g., Repetti et al, 2002, 2007). Moreover, there is evidence for non-genomic intergenerational transfer of these and related adverse outcomes (e.g., Noll et al, 2009). By contrast, a nurturant early family environment is associated with beneficial health behaviors, including maintaining a good diet, a propensity to exercise, good dental care and flossing, and obtaining regular check-ups and immunizations (see Repetti et al, 2002, for a review).

The relation between a harsh early environment and poor health habits in adolescence may result from several factors. One is parental knowledge about and supervision of adolescent activities in homes. With less monitoring and more permissiveness, adolescents seek out more frequent sexual activity and are more likely to smoke and abuse other substances (see Repetti et al, 2002, for a review). Another potential route is the fact that substance abuse and risky sexual behavior may compensate for deficiencies in the social, emotional, and even biological functioning of offspring from risky families. That is, these adverse health-related behaviors may represent self-soothing behaviors that compensate for the absence of socioemotional resources that have been tied to a nurturant family environment (see Repetti et al, 2002, for a review). Unfortunately, poor health habits in adolescence can extend into adulthood and to future generations (Noll et al, 2009).

9 Neural Regulation of Stress Responses

The difficulties that offspring from harsh early environments have with developing effective socioemotional skills and self-regulatory behaviors may be evident in neural activity that affects downstream neuroendocrine stress responses. The socioemotional skills described earlier have reliable effects on neural responses to threat cues, which in turn regulate downstream biological responses to stress. Brain regions implicated in threat detection and responses to emotional stimuli may mediate the relation between a harsh early family environment and elevated biological responses to stress.

A region consistently associated with threat detection and affective processing is the amygdala (see Chapter 52). The amygdala responds to a variety of emotion-related stimuli, including pictures depicting physical threats (Hariri et al, 2002) and faces depicting fear and anger (Hariri et al, 2000). Once activated, the amygdala sets in motion a cascade of responses to threat via projections to the hypothalamus and prefrontal cortex (LeDoux, 1996). A neural region that is critical for regulating responses to emotional stimuli is the ventrolateral prefrontal cortex (VLPFC; Hariri et al, 2002). Studies have shown that the labeling of negative affective states activates the right VLPFC and that increased activity in right VLPFC is associated with decreased activity in the amygdala (Hariri et al, 2000, 2002; Lieberman et al, 2005). This pattern of increased right VLPFC activity and decreased amygdala activity may be implicated in emotion regulation.

To test these ideas, we (Taylor et al, 2006a) recruited participants who had previously completed assessments of family background. We conducted an fMRI investigation that examined amygdala reactivity to the observation of fearful and angry faces; amygdala and right VLPFC reactivity to labeling the emotions displayed in those faces; and the relation between right VLPFC and amygdala activity during the labeling task. We found that offspring from nurturant families showed expected amygdala activity in response to observing the fearful and angry faces and expected activation of right VLPFC while labeling the emotions. The relation between right VLPFC and amygdala reactivity was significantly negative, consistent with the idea that right VLPFC activity inhibits amygdala responses to the threatening faces. Offspring from harsh families, however, showed a different pattern. During the observation of fearful and angry faces, they showed little activation of the amygdala. During the labeling task, they showed expected activation of right VLPFC;

however, they also showed amygdala activation and a strong positive correlation between right VLPFC and amygdala activation, the opposite of what was seen in offspring from nurturant families. Thus, offspring from risky families exhibit atypical responses to emotional stimuli that are evident at the neural level (Taylor et al, 2006a). Of interest, this pattern of neural responses to threat cues maps onto behavioral research showing maladaptive coping among offspring from harsh families. That is, offspring from risky families may avoid threat-relevant stimuli with which they need not engage, but overreact to and demonstrate an inability to regulate emotional responses to emotional stimuli with which they must engage. These responses are evident at both the behavioral and the neural levels.

Socioemotional skills are themselves related to the neural regulation of threat responses and, thus, constitute an indirect route whereby early environment is implicated in the regulation of biological stress responses. In a recent study (Eisenberger et al, 2007), participants completed a signal-contingent daily diary experience sampling procedure over a 9-day period in which each time they were signaled, they rated how supportive their most recent social interaction had been. At the end of this period, participants took part in an fMRI investigation of neural responses to threat, specifically a virtual social rejection task (cyberball) that has previously been shown to evoke psychological distress (Eisenberger et al, 2003). At a third time point, participants experienced laboratory stress challenges (the Trier Social Stress Task (TSST), Kirschbaum et al, 1993) to assess autonomic and neuroendocrine reactivity to social stressors. People who reported frequent supportive interactions showed lower dorsal anterior cingulate cortex (dACC) and Brodmann's area 8 (BA 8) reactivity to social rejection. These are brain regions whose activity has previously been tied to social distress. They also showed lower cortisol reactivity to the laboratory challenges. Moreover, individual differences in dACC and BA 8 activity mediated the relationship between social support and cortisol reactivity. Thus, positive socioemotional contact may influence downstream biological stress responses by modulating neurocognitive reactivity to social stressors, which in turn attenuates neuroendocrine stress responses.

A second study (Taylor et al, 2008) also examined whether socioemotional resources modulate reactions to threat cues. We tested two hypotheses, namely, whether psychosocial resources, including optimism, a sense of control, and high self-esteem, are tied to decreasing sensitivity to threat or whether they are associated with enhanced prefrontal inhibition of threat responses during threat regulation. In an fMRI investigation, participants responded to the threatening faces task described earlier. Socioemotional resources were associated with greater right ventrolateral prefrontal cortex activity and less amygdala activity during a threat regulation task. Participants had also gone through laboratory stress tasks, and meditational analyses suggested that the relation of socioemotional resources to low cortisol reactivity was mediated by lower amygdala activity during threat regulation. These findings suggest that socioemotional resources downregulate biological stress responses by means of enhanced inhibition of threat responses during threat regulation, rather than by decreasing sensitivity to threat.

10 Impact of Early Environment on Biological Stress Responses

The neural regulation of responses to threat ultimately affects downstream biological stress regulatory systems. What are these systems? During times of stress, the body releases the catecholamines epinephrine and norepinephrine with concomitant sympathetic nervous system arousal. Stress may also engage the HPA (hypothalamic–pituitary–adrenocortical) axis, involving the release of corticosteroids including cortisol. These responses have short-term protective effects under stressful circumstances, because they mobilize the body to meet the demands of pressing situations. However, with

chronic or recurrent activation, they can be associated with deleterious long-term implications for health (e.g., Seeman and McEwen, 1996; Uchino et al, 1996, see Chapter 42). For example, excessive or repeated discharge of epinephrine or norepinephrine can lead to the suppression of cellular immune function, produce hemodynamic changes such as increases in blood pressure and heart rate, provoke abnormal heart rhythms such as ventricular arrhythmias, and produce neurochemical imbalances that may relate to psychiatric disorders. Intense, rapid, and/or long-lasting sympathetic responses to repeated stress or challenge have been implicated in the development of hypertension and coronary artery disease (McEwen and Stellar, 1993).

Stress can also suppress immune functioning in ways that leave a person vulnerable to opportunistic diseases and infections. Corticosteroids such as cortisol have immunosuppressive effects, and stress-related increases in cortisol have been tied to decreased lymphocyte responsivity to mitogenic stimulation and to decreased lymphocyte cytotoxicity. Such immunosuppressive changes may be associated with increased susceptibility to infectious disorders and to destruction of neurons in the hippocampus as well (McEwen and Sapolsky, 1995). Chronic stress can also diminish the immune system's sensitivity to glucocorticoid hormones that normally terminate the inflammatory cascade that occurs during stress (Miller et al, 2002).

Extensive evidence suggests that these systems – the HPA axis, the immune system, and the sympathetic nervous system – influence each other and thereby affect each other's functioning. To the extent, then, that early environment influences the affective states and socioemotional skills that can keep sympathetic nervous system and HPA axis responses to stress low, it may have a beneficial impact on other systems as well (Seeman and McEwen, 1996; Uchino et al, 1996). In turn, these may beneficially affect health.

Correspondingly, a lack of supportive contacts in early childhood has been tied to higher autonomic responses to stress in children (e.g.,

El-Sheikh et al, 1989) and to higher HPA axis responses to stressors in children (Gunnar et al, 1992). Studies of young adults reveal that a harsh early family environment is tied to elevated autonomic responses to a laboratory stressor and to an elevated flat cortisol response to laboratory stressors (Taylor et al, 2004). Thus, the existing literature provides a strong basis for pathways linking a stressful early childhood to high reactivity of biological stress regulatory systems.

11 Early Adversity and Health Outcomes: Tests of the Model

The association of early adversity with adverse health outcomes is clear. Not only does outright abuse impact health across the life span, but low SES in childhood and a harsh early family environment also affect health. To this point, we have identified socioemotional skills, chronic negative affective states, and health behaviors as among the mediators to health outcomes. As yet, however, no tests of the entire model have been presented to suggest that these are indeed the routes by which early environment has adverse health effects.

We accordingly undertook several collaborative studies with the Coronary Artery Risk Development in Young Adults Study (CARDIA), an ongoing, prospective, epidemiologic investigation of risk factors for coronary artery disease involving more than 3000 participants at four different recruitment sites (Lehman et al, 2005). The samples were approximately evenly balanced between African American and white participants and between men and women. At the initial examination, participants were between the ages of 18 and 25. There have been five follow-up studies since that time, most recently at year 15 (2000–2001). Our investigations with CARDIA used structural equation modeling to determine whether the model in Fig. 36.1 can account for individual differences in adult metabolic functioning, C-reactive protein (CRP), and blood pressure.

Metabolic functioning is a complex of risk factors for coronary artery disease and diabetes and is typically defined by fasting glucose, cholesterol, triglycerides, and abdominal obesity, among other indicators. High levels of these variables contribute to metabolic syndrome, which is prognostic for heart disease, diabetes, inflammatory disorders, and all-cause mortality (see Chapter 46). The prevalence of metabolic syndrome in the United States is approximately 22% (McEwen and Seeman, 1999), making it an important contributor to chronic illness.

We had included an assessment of early family environment during the year 15 CARDIA data collection and tested our model on this sample with a composite index of indicators of metabolic functioning as an outcome variable. Socioemotional functioning was assessed by depression/hostility and the positivity/negativity of social contacts. The model fit the data very well, with early family environment strongly related to socioemotional functioning, which in turn, was significantly related to metabolic functioning (Lehman et al, 2005). When each of the race–sex subgroups was examined separately, the model continued to be an acceptable fit. These findings suggest that early environment is significantly related to dysregulation in socioemotional functioning, which in turn leads to alterations in metabolic functioning.

A second investigation related the model to CRP (Taylor et al, 2006b). CRP is a biomarker of inflammatory processes which has been reliably related to depression (e.g., Suarez, 2004) and to enhanced risk for cardiovascular disease (King et al, 2004), among other diseases. As was true of metabolic functioning, the model was a good fit to the data, suggesting that the model helps to explain differences in CRP. Since CRP is related to risks for both mental and physical health disorders, it may be important for understanding the comorbidities observed between mental and physical health disorders (e.g., Martin et al, 1995).

In a third investigation (Lehman et al, 2009), we related the model to blood pressure and to changes in blood pressure across the longitudinal occasions with the CARDIA sample. We found that a harsh family environment was related to negative emotions and to obesity, which in turn predicted blood pressure as well as change in blood pressure. Low childhood SES directly predicted change in systolic blood pressure as well. The strength of these pathways did not vary by race or gender. Thus, the findings suggest that socioemotional factors contribute to biological mechanisms that may underlie the impact of early family environment on the development of elevated blood pressure.

Two important caveats deserve mention. First, the effects revealed in these tests of the model were modest in size. One reason is that genetic factors are strong contributors to these outcomes, and they could not be measured in this data set. Second, the fact that participants reconstructed their early family environment and that these studies were retrospective rather than prospective raises the possibility that negative emotions themselves color reconstruction of family environment. Accordingly, for all three of these investigations, we evaluated an alternative model that gave chronic negative affect causal priority in the model to see if it affected reconstruction of family environment. In all three cases, this model was a significantly poorer fit to the data. Moreover, there is parallel evidence from studies relating documented childhood maltreatment to adverse mental and physical health outcomes (Danese et al, 2007, 2008). As such, we conclude that although negative affect may color how people regard their families, reconstructive biases do not account for the relation of early family environment to adverse health outcomes.

12 Conclusions

Growing up in a stressful early environment marked by low SES and/or harsh parenting has effects on socioemotional skills, chronic negative affect, and health behaviors that are implicated in downstream adverse health outcomes. The evidence is, thus, consistent with our theoretical model, namely, that the failure to learn

emotion recognition and regulation skills in early childhood due to a harsh early environment may interfere with the ability to manage potentially threatening stimuli. Compromises in the regulation of stress responses may ultimately produce changes in biological stress regulatory systems, which, in turn, confer a broad array of mental and physical health risks. Findings such as these underscore the vital importance of developing methods for identifying children at risk for maltreatment early and for developing interventions to offset or attenuate adverse costs to socioemotional regulation incurred from maltreatment.

References

Adler, N. E., Marmot, M., McEwen, B. S., and Stewart, J. (1999). *Socioeconomic Status and Health in Industrial Nations: Social, Psychological, and Biological Pathways*. New York: New York Academy of Sciences.

Bakermans-Kranenburg, M. J., and van IJzendoorn, M. H. (2007). Research review: genetic vulnerability or differential susceptibility in child development: the case of attachment. *J Child Psychol Psychiatry, 48*, 1160–1173.

Bakermans-Kranenburg, M. J., van Ijzendoorn, M. H., Pijlman, F. T., Mesman, J., and Juffer, F. (2008). Experimental evidence for differential susceptibility: dopamine D4 receptor polymorphism (DRD4 VNTR) moderates intervention effects on toddlers' externalizing behavior in a randomized controlled trial. *Dev Psychol, 44*, 293–300.

Baumrind, D. (1991). The influence of parenting style on adolescent competence and substance use. *J Early Adolesc, 11*, 56–95.

Camras, L. A., Ribordy, S., Hill, J., Martino, S., Spaccarelli, S. et al (1988). Recognition and posing of emotional expression by abused children and their mothers. *Dev Psychol, 24*, 776–781.

Caspi, A., McClay, J., Moffitt, T. E., Mill, J., Martin, J. et al (2002). Role of genotype in the cycle of violence in maltreated children. *Science, 297*, 851–854.

Caspi, A., Sugden, K., Moffitt, T. E., Taylor, A., Craig, I. W. et al (2003). Influence of life stress on depression: Moderation by a polymorphism in the 5-HTT gene. *Science, 301*, 386–389.

Chorpita, B. F., and Barlow, D. H. (1998). The development of anxiety: the role of control in the early environment. *Psychol Bull, 124*, 3–21.

Crockenberg, S., and Lourie, A. (1996). Parents' conflict strategies with children and children's conflict strategies with peers. *Merrill Palmer Q, 42*, 495–518.

Danese, A., Moffitt, T. E., Pariante, C. M., Ambler, A., Poulton, R. et al (2008). Elevated inflammation levels in depressed adults with a history of childhood maltreatment. *Arch Gen Psychiat, 65*, 409–416.

Danese, A., Pariante, C. M., Caspi, A., Taylor, A., and Poulton, R. (2007). Childhood maltreatment predicts adult inflammation in a life-course study. *PNAS, 104*, 1319–1324.

Dembroski, T. M., MacDougall, J. M., Williams, R. B., Haney, T. L., and Blumenthal, J. A. (1985). Components of Type A, hostility, and angerin: relationship to angiographic findings. *Psychosom Med, 47*, 219–233.

Dishion, T. J. (1990). The family ecology of boys' peer relations in middle childhood. *Child Dev, 61*, 874–891.

Dunn, J., and Brown, J. (1994). Affect expression in the family, children's understanding of emotions, and their interactions with others. *Merrill-Palmer Quarterly, 40*, 120–137.

Eisenberg, N., and Spinrad, T. (2004). Emotion-related regulation: sharpening the definition. *Child Dev, 75*, 334–339.

Eisenberger, N. I., Lieberman, M. D., and Williams, K. D. (2003). Does rejection hurt? An fMRI study of social exclusion. *Science, 302*, 290–292.

Eisenberger, N. I., Taylor, S. E., Gable, S. L., Hilmert, C. J., and Lieberman, M. D. (2007). Neural pathways link social support to attenuated neuroendocrine stress responses. *NeuroImage, 35*, 1601–1612.

El-Sheikh, M., Cummings, E. M., and Goetsch, V. L. (1989). Coping with adults' angry behavior: behavioral, physiological, and verbal responses in preschoolers. *Dev Psychol, 25*, 490–498.

Felitti, V. J., Anda, R. F., Nordenberg, D., Williamson, D. F., Apitz, A. M. et al (1998). Relationship of childhood abuse and household dysfunction to many of the leading causes of death in adults. *Am J Prev Med, 14*, 245–258.

Flinn, M. V., and England, B. G. (1997). Social economics of childhood glucocorticoid stress responses and health. *Am J Phys Anthropol, 102*, 33–53.

Francis, D., Diorio, J., Liu, D., and Meaney, M. J. (1999). Nongenomic transmission across generations of maternal behavior and stress responses in the rat. *Science, 286*, 1155–1158.

Frasure-Smith, N., Lesperance, F., and Talajic, M. (1995). The impact of negative emotions on prognosis following myocardial infarction: is it more than depression? *Health Psychol, 14*, 388–398.

Gallo, L. C., and Matthews, K. A. (2003). Understanding the association between socioeconomic status and physical health: do negative emotions play a role? *Psychol Bull, 129*, 10–51.

Gunnar, M. R., Larson, M. C., Hertsgaard, L., Harris, M. L., and Brodersen, L. (1992). The stressfulness of separation among nine-month-old infants: effects of social context variables and infant temperament. *Child Dev, 63*, 290–303.

Hariri, A. R., Bookheimer, S. Y., and Mazziotta, J. C. (2000). Modulating emotional responses: effects of a neocortical network on the limbic system. *Neuroreport, 11*, 43–48.

Hariri, A. R., Tessitore, A., Mattay, V. S., Fera, F., and Weinberger, D. R. (2002) The amygdala response to emotional stimuli: a comparison of faces and scenes. *NeuroImage, 17*, 317–323.

Hemingway, H., Shipley, M., Mullen, M. J., Kumari, M., Brunner, E. et al (2003). Social and psychosocial influences on inflammatory markers and vascular function in civil servants (The Whitehall II Study). *Am J Cardiol, 92*, 984–987.

Herbert, T. B., and Cohen, S. (1993). Depression and immunity: a meta analytic review. *Psychol Bull, 113*, 1–15.

House, J. S., Umberson, D., and Landis, K. R. (1988). Structures and processes of social support. *Ann Rev Soc, 14*, 293–318.

Johnson, V., and Pandina, R. J. (1991). Effects of family environment on adolescent substance use, delinquency, and coping styles. *Am J Drug Alcohol Abuse, 17*, 71–88.

Julkunen, J., Salonen, R., Kaplan, G. A., Chesney, M. A., and Salonen, J. T. (1994). Hostility and the progression of carotid artherosclerosis. *Psychosom Med, 56*, 519–525.

Kaufman, J., Yang, B. Z., Douglas-Palumberi, H., Houshyar, S., Lipschitz, D. et al (2004). Social supports and serotonin transporter gene moderate depression in maltreated children. *Proc Natl Acad Sci U S A, 101*, 17316–17321.

Kawachi, I., Sparrow, D., Vokonas, P. S., and Weiss, S. T. (1995). Decreased heart rate variability in men with phobic anxiety (data from the Normative Aging Study). *Am J Cardiol, 75*, 882–885.

Kirschbaum, C., Pirke, K. M., and Hellhammer, D. H. (1993). The 'Trier Social Stress Test' - a tool for investigating psychobiological stress responses in a laboratory setting. *Neuropsychobiology, 28*, 76–81.

Kim-Cohen, J., Caspi, A., Taylor, A., Williams, B., Newcombe, R. et al (2006). MAOA, maltreatment, and gene-environment interaction predicting children's mental health: new evidence and a meta-analysis. *Mol Psychiatry, 11*, 903–913.

King, D. E., Mainous, A. G., and Taylor, M. L. (2004). Clinical use of C-reactive protein for cardiovascular disease. *South Med J, 97*, 985–988.

Kivimäki, M., Kinnunen, M. L., Pitkänen, T., Vahtera, J., Elovainio, M. et al (2004). Contribution of early and adult factors to socioeconomic variation in blood pressure: thirty-four-year follow-up study of school children. *Psychosom Med, 66*, 184–189.

Kubzansky, L. D., Kawachi, I., Weiss, S. T., and Sparrow, D. (1998). Anxiety and coronary heart disease: a synthesis of epidemiological, psychological, and experimental evidence. *Ann Behav Med, 20*, 47–58.

Laible, D. J., and Thompson, R. A. (1998). Attachment and emotional understanding in preschool children. *Dev Psychol, 34*, 1038–1045.

Lawlor, D. A. and Smith, G. D. (2005). Early life determinants of adult blood pressure. *Curr Opin Nephrol Hypertens, 14*, 259–264.

LeDoux, J. (1996). *The Emotional Brain: The Mysterious Underpinnings of Emotional Life.* New York: Simon & Schuster.

Lehman, B. J., Taylor, S. E., Kiefe, C. I., and Seeman, T. E. (2005). Relation of childhood socioeconomic status and family environment to adult metabolic functioning in the CARDIA study. *Psychosom Med, 67*, 846–854.

Lehman, B. J., Taylor, S. E., Kiefe, C. I., and Seeman, T. E. (2009). Relationship of early life stress and psychological functioning to blood pressure in the CARDIA Study. *Health Psychol, 28*, 338–346.

Lieberman, M. D., Hariri, A., Jarcho, J. M., Eisenberger, N. I., and Bookheimer, S. Y. (2005). An fMRI investigation of race-related amygdala activity in African-American and Caucasian-American individuals. *Nat Neurosci, 8*, 720–722.

Liu, D., Diorio, J., Tannenbaum, B., Caldji, C., Francis, D., Freedman, A. et al (1997). Maternal care, hippocampal glucocorticoid receptors, and hypothalamic-pituitary-adrenal responses to stress. *Science, 277*, 1659–1662.

Martin, L. R., Friedman, H. S., Tucker, J. S., Schwartz, J. E., Criqui, M. H. et al (1995). An archival prospective study of mental health and longevity. *Health Psychol, 14*, 381–387.

Matthews, K. A., Woodall, K. L., Kenyon, K., and Jacob, T. (1996). Negative family environment as a predictor of boys' future status on measures of hostile attitudes, interview behavior, and anger expression. *Health Psychol, 15*, 30–37.

McEwen, B. S. (1998). Protective and damaging effects of stress mediators. *N Engl J Med, 338*, 171–179.

McEwen, B. S., and Sapolsky, R. M. (1995). Stress and cognitive function. *Curr Opin Neurobiol, 5*, 205–216.

McEwen, B. S., and Seeman, T. (1999). Protective and damaging effects of mediators of stress: elaborating and testing the concepts of allostasis and allostatic load. *Ann N Y Acad Sci, 896*, 30–47.

McEwen, B. S., and Stellar, E. (1993). Stress and the individual: mechanisms leading to disease. *Arch Intern Med, 153*, 2093–2101.

McLoyd, V. C. (1998). Socioeconomic disadvantage and child development. *Am Psychol, 53*, 185–204.

Meaney, M. J., and Szyf, M. (2005). Environmental programming of stress responses through DNA methylation: life at the interface between a dynamic environment and a fixed genome. *Dialogues Clin Neurosci, 7*, 103–123.

Miller, G. E., Cohen, S., and Ritchey, A. K. (2002). Chronic psychological stress and the regulation of pro-inflammatory cytokines: a glucocorticoid-resistance model. *Health Psychol, 21*, 531–541.

Noll, J. G., Trickett, P. K., Harris, W. W., and Putnam, F. W. (2009). The cumulative burden borne by offspring whose mothers were sexually abused as children: descriptive results from a multigenerational study. *J Interperson Viol, 24*, 424–449.

O'Brien, M., Margolin, G., John, R. S., and Krueger, L. (1991). Mothers' and sons' cognitive and emotional reactions to simulated marital and family conflict. *J Consult Clin Psychol, 59*, 692–703.

Owen, N., Poulton, T., Hay, F. C., Mohamed-Ali, V., and Steptoe, A. (2003). Socioeconomic status, C-reactive protein, immune factors, and responses to acute mental stress. *Brain Behav Immun, 17*, 286–295.

Pettit, G. S., Dodge, K. A., and Brown, M. M. (1988). Early family experience, social problem solving patterns, and children's social competence. *Child Dev, 59*, 107–120.

Reid, R. J., and Crisafulli, A. (1990). Marital discord and child behavior problems: a meta-analysis. *J Abnorm Child Psychol, 18, 105–117.*

Repetti, R. L., Taylor, S. E., and Saxbe, D. (2007). The influence of early socialization experiences on the development of biological systems. In J. Grusec & P. Hastings (Eds.), *Handbook of Socialization* (pp. 124–152). New York, NY: Guilford.

Repetti, R. L., Taylor, S. E., and Seeman, T. E. (2002). Risky families: family social environments and the mental and physical health of offspring. *Psychol Bull, 128*, 330–366.

Roisman, G. L., Susman, E., Barnett-Walker, K., Booth-LaForce, C., Owen, M. T. et al (2009). Early family and child-care antecedents of awakening cortisol levels in adolescence. *Child Deve, 80*, 907–920.

Schwartz, D., Dodge, K. A., Pettit, G. S., and Bates, J. E. (1997). The early socialization of aggressive victims of bullying. *Child Dev, 68*, 665–675.

Seeman, T. E. (1996). Social ties and health. *Ann Epidemiol, 6*, 442–451.

Seeman, T. E., and McEwen, B. S. (1996). Impact of social environment characteristics on neuroendocrine regulation. *Psychosom Med, 58*, 459–471.

Shedler, J., and Block, J. (1990). Adolescent drug use and psychological health: a longitudinal inquiry. *Am Psychol, 45*, 612–630.

Smith, T. W. (1992). Hostility and health: current status of a psychosomatic hypothesis. *J Pers Soc Psychol, 48*, 813–838.

Springer, K. W., Sheridan, J., Kuo, D., and Carnes, M. (2003). The long-term health outcomes of childhood abuse: an overview and a call to action. *J Gen Intern Med, 18*, 864–870.

Spooner, C. (1999). Causes and correlates of adolescent drug abuse and implications of treatment. *Drug Alcohol Rev, 18*, 453–475.

Suarez, E. C. (2004). C-reactive protein is associated with psychological risk factors of cardiovascular disease in apparently healthy adults. *Psychosom Med, 66*, 684–691.

Taylor, S. E. (2009). Social support: a review. To appear in H. S. Friedman (Ed.), *Oxford Handbook of Health Psychology*. New York, NY: Oxford University Press.

Taylor, S. E., and Seeman, T. E. (2000). Psychosocial resources and the SES-health relationship. In N. Adler, M. Marmot, & B. McEwen (Eds.), *Socioeconomic Status and Health in Industrial Nations: Social, Psychological, and Biological Pathways* (pp. 210–225). New York: New York Academy of Sciences.

Taylor, S. E., Burklund, L. J., Eisenberger, N. I., Lehman, B. J., Hilmert, C. J. et al (2008). Neural bases of moderation of cortisol stress responses by psychosocial resources. *J Pers Soc Psychol, 95*, 197–211.

Taylor, S. E., Eisenberger, N. I., Saxbe, D., Lehman, B. J., and Lieberman, M. D. (2006a). Neural responses to emotional stimuli are associated with childhood family stress. *Biol Psychiatry, 60*, 296–301.

Taylor, S. E. Lehman, B. J., Kiefe, C. I., and Seeman, T. E. (2006b). Relationship of early life stress and psychological functioning to adult C-reactive protein in the Coronary Artery Risk Development in Young Adults Study. *Biol Psychiatry, 60*, 819–824.

Taylor, S. E., Lerner, J. S., Sage, R. M., Lehman, B. J., and Seeman, T. E. (2004). Early environment, emotions, responses to stress, and health. *J Pers, 72*, 1365–1393.

Taylor, S. E., Way, B. M., Welch, W. T., Hilmert, C. J., Lehman, B. J. et al (2006c). Early family environment, current adversity, the serotonin transporter polymorphism, and depressive symptomatology. *Biol Psychiatry, 60*, 671–676.

Uchino, B., Cacioppo, J., and Kiecolt-Glaser, J. (1996). The relationship between social support and physiological processes: a review with emphasis on underlying mechanisms and implications for health. *Psychol Bull, 119*, 488–531.

Valentiner, D. P., Holahan, C. J., and Moos, R. H. (1994). Social support, appraisals of event controllability, and coping: an integrative model. *J Pers Soc Psychol, 66*, 1094–1102.

Van Cauter, E., and Spiegel, K. (1999). Sleep as a mediator of the relationship between socioeconomic status and health: a hypothesis. In N. Adler, M. Marmot, B. McEwen, & J. Stewart (Eds.), *Socioeconomic Status and Health in Industrial Nations: Social, Psychological, and Biological Pathways* (pp. 254–261). New York: New York Academy of Sciences.

Wagner, B. M. (1997). Family risk factors for child and adolescent suicidal behavior. *Psychol Bull, 121*, 246–298.

Wardle, J., Waller, J., and Jarvis, M. J. (2002). Sex differences in the association of socioeconomic status with obesity. *Am J Public Health, 92*, 1299–1304.

Weaver, I. C., Cervoni, N., Champagne, F. A., D'Alessio, A. C., Sharma, S. et al (2004). Epigenetic programming by maternal behavior. *Nat Neurosci, 7*, 847–854.

Winkleby, M. A., Cubbin, C., Ahn, D. K., and Kraemer, H. C. (1999). Pathways by which SES and ethnicity influence cardiovascular disease risk factors. In N. Adler, M. Marmot, B. McEwen, & J. Stewart (Eds.), *Socioeconomic Status and Health in Industrial Nations: Social, Psychological, and Biological Pathways* (pp. 191–209). New York: New York Academy of Sciences.

Chapter 37

Health Disparities in Adolescence

Hannah M.C. Schreier and Edith Chen

1 Introduction

It is well established that there exists a gradient relationship between socioeconomic status (SES) and physical health (Adler and Newman, 2002; Adler et al, 1994, see Chapter 22). For example, individuals from lower SES environments are at an increased risk for morbidity and mortality due to a variety of causes (Mustard et al, 1997). While the majority of research has investigated SES–health relationships among adults and young children, until recently less research has focused on understanding these relationships during adolescence (although see Starfield et al (2002) and Chen et al (2002) for two reviews that highlight the impact that low SES may have on health outcomes in children and adolescents). However, as the adolescent years provide the basis for adult health, investigating health disparities among this age group is especially important.

The focus of this chapter is to review the nature of SES-based health disparities among adolescents. Adolescence is an important period in development that is marked by numerous transitions, both socially and biologically, and is generally viewed as the period between the beginning of puberty and adulthood. For the purpose of this chapter, studies are reviewed

that focus on youth in the 11- to 18-year-old age range, similar to approaches of other researchers studying adolescence (Leventhal and Brooks-Gunn, 2000; Starfield et al, 2002). In this chapter, we will also review several potential pathways through which SES may come to impact adolescent health. Understanding SES-based health disparities during this developmental period is important as adolescent health is likely to impact adult health, and because the beginnings of certain disease processes, such as atherosclerosis, emerge among adolescents (Strong et al, 1999).

2 Socioeconomic Disparities in Health Outcomes in Adolescence

A growing literature suggests that SES has a profound influence on a variety of health outcomes in adolescence, ranging from adolescents' perceptions of their own health to objective outcomes such as mortality.

Several large, cross-sectional studies have concluded that adolescents growing up in low SES environments generally experience greater mortality risks than their peers from higher SES families. For example, low SES youth are more likely to die from a number of causes, including pneumonia and influenza, fire, poisoning, and homicide (Nelson, 1992; Nersesian et al, 1985). In one of very few longitudinal studies, mothers were interviewed about SES at the time of their child's birth and families subsequently followed

H.M.C. Schreier (✉)
Department of Psychology, University of British Columbia, 2136 West Mall, Vancouver, BC V6T 1Z4, Canada
e-mail: hannahs@psych.ubc.ca

A. Steptoe (ed.), *Handbook of Behavioral Medicine*, DOI 10.1007/978-0-387-09488-5_37,
© Springer Science+Business Media, LLC 2010

until the children had reached age 20 (Oliveira et al, 2007). Low parental occupation at birth was predictive of greater adolescent mortality due to external causes, particularly among boys. Hence the existing data suggest that low SES environments increase adolescents' risk for premature mortality due to a wide range of causes across the adolescent years.

Most studies investigating health disparities in adolescence have focused on overall health status. Many of these studies draw from large, nationally representative samples. For example, two studies using large samples of US adolescents found that after accounting for other sociodemographic factors, low familial SES, measured through the family's income and parental education, was associated with below average self-rated physical health status and a greater likelihood of reporting fair to poor health (Caputo, 2003; Goodman, 1999). Similarly, in a British study (Emerson et al, 2005) lower household income was associated with lower health status as measured by a wide range of indicators, including overall health status, current physical illness, and disabilities, reported by parents and teachers. More recent research is beginning to indicate that adolescents' subjective perceptions of familial SES may be just as good, if not better, predictors of their health. Several studies have reported that adolescents' subjective perceptions and reports of family SES predicted self-reported health status and quality of life and did so even after objective and parent-reported indicators of family SES had been taken into account (Goodman et al, 2007; von Rueden et al, 2005; Piko and Keresztes, 2007). von Rueden and colleagues (2005) also demonstrated that the relationship between youth's perceptions of family wealth and health status as well as quality of life was much stronger among adolescents than children, suggesting that as youth become older their subjective perceptions of familial wealth may become increasingly important.

Symptom reports among adolescents also reveal SES disparities. Starfield et al (2002) found that lower SES, as measured by parents' income, was associated with a greater likelihood of adolescents reporting fair to poor health, physical activity limitations, bed-days, and restricted activity days. Huurre et al (2005) found that manual class origin was associated with higher rates of psychosomatic symptoms among adolescent females, but not males. Finally, one study found that low and high parental income is linked to different types of physical health symptoms (Rhee, 2005). Low SES youth's primary complaints included feeling hot, chest pain, urinary problems, and cold sweat, whereas high SES youth were more likely to complain about musculoskeletal pains.

Together, these studies suggest that SES influences not only symptom prevalence but also the types of symptoms that are reported. Overall, however, low SES adolescents tend to report greater symptoms, mirroring the findings for the relationship between SES and self-reported overall health.

We next provide examples using several specific types of health outcomes. For example, with respect to obesity, studies are fairly consistent in suggesting that low SES is associated with a greater likelihood of being obese among adolescents (e.g., Ahn et al, 2008; Goodman, 1999; Vieweg et al, 2007). For example, a longitudinal study (De Spiegelaere et al, 1998) followed adolescents from age 12 to 15 and tracked their obesity status. Consistent with other studies they found a relationship between low SES and increased risk of obesity. In addition, the gap between low and high SES youth also widened over time, indicating that existing SES differences may be further accentuated during adolescence. For a review on the negative impact of low SES on adolescent obesity, see Shrewsbury and Wardle (2008).

SES-based differences in adolescent sexual health have also been reported. For example, black adolescent females from low SES neighborhoods were more than twice as likely to report gonorrhea if their parents were unemployed, possibly indicating that youth from low SES neighborhoods are more likely to be part of high-risk sexual networks (Sionean et al, 2000). Similarly, Newbern et al (2004) reported data from a national sample in which lower and nonprofessional maternal education were related to higher rates of sexually transmitted infections (STIs) in adolescents, except for white females. Overall, higher rates of STIs were found among adolescents from one-parent homes. Note, however, that not all studies find relationships between SES and STIs (e.g., see Goodman, 1999; Santelli et al, 2000). Together these studies suggest some, although not definitive, evidence for a relationship between SES and adolescent sexual health.

Previous research furthermore points to SES differences in teenage pregnancy rates. US teenage women who become pregnant are more likely to come from low SES families (Boardman et al, 2006) and a British study examining teenage pregnancies in England across a 10-year period similarly reported higher mean conception rates in more deprived areas (Wilkinson et al, 2006). A study investigating teenage pregnancies among a sample of Scottish teenage women compared teenagers who gave birth with teenagers who also reported sexual intercourse but did not get pregnant and found that those who got pregnant were more likely to come from lower SES families (Buston et al, 2006). This suggests that the difference in teenage pregnancy rates between low and high SES teens may at least in part be explained by differences in contraceptive use and not simply differences in sexual activity. Finally, teenage women from low SES backgrounds also experience greater intended as well as unintended rapid repeat pregnancies, meaning they were more likely to become pregnant again within the 24 months following their first pregnancy (Boardman et al, 2006; Raneri and Wiemann, 2007).

SES has also been linked to chronic illness outcomes in adolescents. For example, adolescents from lower income families have overall poorer asthma control, even after taking into account controller medication use and primary care service utilization (Cope et al, 2008). Adolescents from low SES families are also more likely to live with undiagnosed frequent wheezing (Yeatts et al, 2003), experience less preventive care (fewer general check-ups and prescription fills; Kim et al, 2009), and are more likely to have been previously hospitalized because of their asthma (Dales et al, 2002). Hence, low SES affects not only the prevalence of health problems but also how illnesses are experienced and managed.

Finally, research has examined SES differences in adolescent rates of injuries. These studies seem inconclusive at first as they often fail to find differences by SES in the number of total injuries (e.g., Simpson et al, 2005; Williams et al, 1997) or find different directions of associations for different SES measures (Potter et al, 2005). Closer examination of the available data, however, suggests that differences in types of injuries may help explain different patterns within different SES groups. Rauscher and Myers (2008) for example found a dose–response relationship between SES and work-related injuries among adolescents. After controlling for hours worked per week, work history, and race, there was a 30% increase in injuries among adolescents whose mother had a low education as opposed to high education background. In addition, while Simpson et al (2005), using cross-sectional Canadian data, also did not find a clear direction for overall injury rates, adolescents from low SES environments were at greater risk for being hospitalized due to injury as well as for reporting fighting injuries. These patterns suggest that injuries among low SES adolescents may result in part from interpersonal conflict and unsafe physical environments, such as unsafe neighborhoods or work environments. In contrast, higher SES adolescents appear to be at greater risk for recreational and sports injuries (Simpson et al, 2005; Williams et al, 1997). This may be in part because low SES youth are less likely to be able to afford such activities. In sum, adolescents from different SES groups appear to be vulnerable to different types of injuries. In particular, youth from low SES environments are at an increased risk from work-related injuries, injuries resulting from interpersonal conflict, and road injuries, whereas youth from high SES environments are at increased risk for sports injuries.

3 Reasons for Why These Disparities Might Exist in Adolescence

SES is likely to impact factors at multiple levels, for example at the individual level, through health behaviors such as substance abuse, at the family level, for example through parenting behaviors, at the neighborhood level, such as through neighborhood violence, through the availability of health insurance and access to care, and finally, through physical environmental influences and a number of biological pathways. All of these, in turn, impact adolescent health. Below we describe some of the most well-studied pathways through which SES likely comes to impact child health in more detail.

3.1 Individual Level: Child Health Behaviors

One of the most well-studied pathways from SES to adolescent physical health is through adolescent health behaviors. For example, low SES adolescents are less likely to engage in physical activity (Abernathy et al, 2002; Janssen et al, 2006), thereby putting themselves at risk for overweight and related health problems. A recent study furthermore showed that adolescence is a period of significant decline in activity levels (Nader et al, 2009). Using accelerometers, the authors determined the time a sample of 9- to 15-year-old youth spent engaging in moderate-to-vigorous physical activity on a daily basis. While most 9-year olds showed evidence of healthy activity levels (about 3 h per day), 15-year-old study participants had dropped below the recommended time of 60 min of moderate-to-vigorous physical activity per day. Youth from low SES backgrounds also experienced somewhat faster decreases in physical activity over time. Sallis et al (1996) showed that one of the reasons for this lack of physical activity is the lack of resources low SES families have access to. Adolescents from more affluent school

districts had more frequent and active physical education classes at school and were twice as likely to take other exercise-related classes outside of school. Low-income families, on the other hand, did not have the financial resources to provide their children with comparable opportunities.

Other studies have further clarified that there is a distinction between physical activity and sedentary behaviors and that sedentary behaviors are also important to appreciate. While a lack of physical activity indicates that people are not engaging in regular structured exercise, this does not mean they also lead a very sedentary lifestyle, which includes behaviors such as watching TV and playing computer games. Two studies have found that sedentary behaviors, but not physical activity, mediated the low SES – overweight relationship among adolescents (Hanson and Chen, 2006; Lioret et al, 2007). Targeting sedentary health behaviors may be particularly important among adolescents as research suggests that as children move into adolescence their physical activity levels decline and sedentary behaviors become more common (Brodersen et al, 2007).

Finally, other studies suggest that lack of exercise and sedentary behaviors are also related to other negative health behaviors among adolescents. Wang et al (2006) found that low SES African American youth were not only more likely to not exercise and engage in sedentary behaviors, such as watching TV and playing video games, but were also more likely to consume fried foods and soft drinks, both of which would be particularly unhealthy in the context of an already sedentary lifestyle. Delva et al (2006) reported similar results based on a nationally representative sample of adolescents and found that in addition to being less likely to engage in good dietary and exercise habits, low SES adolescents were also less likely to eat breakfast on a regular basis.

Another set of health behaviors that has been proposed to vary by SES relates to substance use. However, evidence with regard to associations between SES and substance use is somewhat mixed. Soteriades and DiFranza (2003) report that adolescent cigarette smoking increases as parent income and education decrease and that this relationship may be partially mediated by parental smoking habits. These results are supported by a national longitudinal study which also found inverse SES gradients for cigarette smoking and alcohol use (Goodman and Huang, 2002). However, this study also reported that the nature of the relationships was not consistent across all SES indicators. Longitudinally, Harrell et al (1998) found that low SES children and adolescents were more likely to be experimental smokers and to start smoking earlier. In contrast, some evidence suggests that substance use may be more common among adolescents from high SES families (Hanson and Chen, 2007), perhaps because it is easier for high SES youth to acquire cigarettes, alcohol, and other drugs due to greater financial resources or because youth from affluent backgrounds are not exposed to the negative consequences of drug use on a regular basis which may provide a deterrent for engaging in substance use behaviors (see also Luthar and D'Avanzo, 1999). In addition, Georgiades et al (2006) found that immigrant youth were subject to greater economic hardship, but nonetheless were less likely to smoke. Overall, large-scale studies suggest that low SES youth are more likely to engage in substance use behaviors such as cigarette use, though there may be some subgroups that are less vulnerable to substance use and some circumstances under which higher SES youth have greater access to substances.

with lower education and income (Goodman, 1999; Goodman et al, 2003; Kubik et al, 2003; Mendelson et al, 2008). Depression among adolescents, in turn, is associated with a series of other outcomes. For example, Goodman and Huang (2001) report that depressed adolescents experience fewer routine physical examinations and utilize fewer medical and more mental health resources. Depression has also been linked to adolescent substance use (Kubik et al, 2003) and Goodman and Huang (2002) reported that depressive symptoms may be one mechanism through which SES affects cigarette smoking and cocaine use among adolescents.

Adolescents growing up in low SES environments also experience greater stress in their lives (Goodman et al, 2005a), which may predispose low SES youth to certain negative psychological and physical health outcomes. Chen et al (2004) and Chen and Matthews (2003) showed that youth from low SES environments more readily make interpretations of threat when presented with ambiguous, but not negative, events, perhaps as a result of having grown up in a more hostile environment where there was greater exposure to chronic as well as acute daily stressors. These psychological traits have also been linked to physiological health outcomes, such that these youth also showed evidence of greater diastolic blood pressure and heart rate reactivity (Chen et al, 2004), as well as heightened levels of inflammatory markers implicated in asthma (Chen et al, 2006).

3.2 Individual Level: Child Psychological Characteristics

Aside from youth's health behaviors, their psychological characteristics are also likely to be impacted by their environment and, in turn, to impact their health. One of the most common and most frequently studied mental health outcomes among adolescents is depression, which is more prevalent among youth from families

3.3 Family Factors

At the family level, a number of factors have also been identified as potential links between youth's low SES environment and physical health outcomes. Several studies have investigated the importance of family structure. Abernathy et al (2002) found that low SES adolescents were more likely to live in a one-parent household. In turn, girls (but not boys) living with one parent were more likely to be above the 85th percentile for weight (Delva et al, 2007), suggesting that there are health benefits to be gained from living in an intact household with both parents present. It may be easier for parents in a two-parent household to place a greater focus on active behaviors and away from sedentary behaviors, such as TV watching, and to enforce behaviors such as healthy eating.

In addition, the characteristics of low SES families have been shown to differ from those of high SES families in a number of ways. Low SES families are characterized by greater family violence (Emery and Laumann-Billings, 1998) and physical abuse within the family (Reid et al, 1999). In addition, family relationships in low SES families are less likely to be warm and supportive (Bradley et al, 2001), and parents are more likely to engage in hostile, punitive, and inconsistent behaviors (Wahler, 1990). In a recent review article, Repetti et al (2002) elaborated on this concept of 'risky families' and suggested that families marked by conflictual and cold interactions that fail to provide safe and warm environments for children and adolescents create vulnerabilities in these youth and increase their likelihood of experiencing a number of disruptions in daily life functioning and health behaviors. Repetti et al (2002) propose that risky family environments alter sympathetic-adrenomedullary (SAM) reactivity and hypothalamic–pituitary–adrenal (HPA) responses to stress, leading to negative mental and physical health outcomes among adolescents. Growing up in risky families has also been linked to disruptions in emotion processing and social competence as well as health behaviors such as substance abuse. Hence the family environment may have implications for health outcomes via a number of diverse pathways, both biological and behavioral.

3.4 Neighborhood Factors

An increasing number of studies have begun to investigate effects of SES on health at the neighborhood level, including whether neighborhoods provide a safe environment for youth and the types of resources and exposures that neighborhoods provide to youth (see Chapter 24).

In terms of social pathways, Cohen et al (2003) reported that neighborhood collective efficacy, meaning residents' willingness to help out for the common good, was lower in low SES neighborhoods in the Chicago area. This relationship mediated the association between low SES and all-cause premature mortality as well as mortality from cardiovascular disease and homicide among residents of these neighborhoods, such that lower collective efficacy was related to an increased likelihood of mortality. A recent review article (Leventhal and Brooks-Gunn, 2000) further supports this notion. Collective neighborhood efficacy is hypothesized to be one mediator through which low SES environments may come to impact adolescent health, for example, through increased supervision and monitoring by adults which could help to decrease the physical risk children and adolescents are exposed to in a neighborhood.

Neighborhoods may also be beneficial in terms of providing broader social networks allowing for greater access to informational resources. One laboratory study consistent with this explanation investigated whether being provided with informational resources from another person would affect physiological responses to stress. Chen (2007) investigated adolescents' physiological reactivity in response to a laboratory stressor over which participants received no intervention, were given control, or received social informational resources. Low SES (but not high SES) adolescents showed less reactivity when they received intervention. However, receiving social informational resources was more effective in reducing reactivity than having control over the stressor. This suggests that growing up in an environment that provides youth with increased access to informational resources may prove beneficial to their health.

Conversely, detrimental social characteristics at the neighborhood level can negatively impact health. Boynton-Jarrett et al (2008) studied a group of adolescents and found that cumulative violence exposure in their neighborhoods was associated with a graded increase in risk for poor health, such that youth who were exposed to more than five forms of cumulative exposure were almost five times more likely to report poor health.

Furthermore, the physical characteristics of neighborhoods carries its own implications for health. In the above-mentioned study on Chicago residents (Cohen et al, 2003), low SES neighborhoods were also more likely to score higher on an index of 'broken windows,' meaning physical indicators such as boarded up homes, litter, and graffiti. This in turn mediated the effect between low SES and all-cause premature mortality, mortality from cardiovascular disease, and homicide, such that greater physical disorder in the neighborhood was related to increased risk for mortality.

Moreover, the accessibility of facilities and the physical characteristics of neighborhoods, including the existence of sidewalks, influence the amount of time youth spend engaging in extracurricular activities and physical exercise. Romero (2005) reported a lack of adults who youth felt contributed to a safe environment, as well as a lack of good quality facilities as barriers to physical activity in a sample of adolescents living in low SES neighborhoods. Gordon-Larsen et al (2006) came to a similar conclusion and reported that physical activity facilities, including parks, schools, youth organizations, and instructional facilities, such as dance schools, were not distributed equally between low and high SES areas. This lack of facilities in low SES blocks in turn led to decreased activity among the adolescents living in those areas. Moore and Diez Roux (2008) furthermore found that access to healthy foods is also a concern in low SES neighborhoods. Low SES neighborhoods were shown to overall have fewer supermarkets, fruit and vegetable markets, and natural food stores, whereas liquor stores and small grocery stores were more common in these areas. Problems relating to the availability of institutional resources have also been discussed as a potential mediating pathway between low SES and negative health outcomes among adolescents in Leventhal and Brooks-Gunn (2000).

Levels of pollution are yet another neighborhood factor with relevance to adolescents' health. Lee et al (2006) reported that low SES youth growing up in a major Korean city were exposed to greater levels of small airborne particles, sulfur, and nitrogen dioxide. This greater ambient air pollution in low SES neighborhoods is particularly relevant for youth with and at risk of asthma, one of the most common chronic illnesses among children and adolescents. A recent review article suggests that the accumulation of environmental risk factors across early life such as more polluted air and water and more crowded and poorer quality housing negatively influences the health of youth (Evans, 2004).

In sum, youth's neighborhoods have a profound impact on their health, with neighborhood facilities, social cohesion, and the neighborhood physical environment affecting adolescent health by influencing the safety of their surroundings, the amount of exercise youth engage in, sexual risk behaviors, and exposure to pollutants.

3.5 Access to Care

Another structural factor at the societal level, access to health care and health insurance, relates to adolescents' health outcomes. Not surprisingly, in the USA low SES adolescents are less likely to have health-care coverage (Newacheck et al, 2003), which is problematic as a lack of health insurance has been linked to numerous undesirable outcomes among adolescents. The low SES adolescents in this study participated in the National Health Interview Survey and were on average disadvantaged on three of the four health status measures, six of the eight measures of access to and satisfaction with care, and six of the nine indicators of access to and use of medical care, dental care, and mental health coverage (Newacheck et al, 2003). In addition, Kim et al (2009) reported that youth without health insurance used fewer health services overall, and Haas et al (2003) reported a positive relationship between lacking health insurance or being insured publicly and the prevalence of being overweight.

3.6 Biological Pathways

A number of biological pathways are thought to link SES to adolescent health. In this section we provide a brief overview of the biological risk markers that are likely to impact adolescents' health into their adult life. Research has primarily focused on risk factors for cardiovascular health, such as blood pressure, cardiac reactivity, and hormonal profiles, for example, cortisol, which can provide information about the potential dysregulation of the hypothalamic–pituitary axis (HPA).

With respect to blood pressure in adolescence, Marin et al (2008) found that low early life family SES was associated with increased current blood pressure among adolescents. Similarly, McGrath et al (2006) reported that lower neighborhood income predicted increased systolic blood pressure during daily life.

SES has also been found to impact adolescents' cardiovascular reactivity. Chen et al (2004) demonstrated a relationship between low SES and greater cardiovascular reactivity during ambiguous (but not negative) videos of social situations that participants were presented with. Likewise, Gump et al (1999) reported that children and adolescents from low SES families showed increased cardiovascular reactivity in response to a laboratory stressor. These patterns linking low SES to greater cardiovascular reactivity may be particularly strong among youth from poor neighborhoods. Wilson et al (2000) found that among African American adolescents from poor neighborhoods those with less educated parents exhibited greater diastolic blood pressure in response to a competitive video game. Lastly, these associations may only be apparent in certain subgroups. Jackson et al (1999), for example, found a race by neighborhood SES interaction for systolic blood pressure reactivity such that both low SES whites and

high SES blacks had the greatest reactivity compared to their same race cohorts. The association between low SES and greater reactivity in whites is consistent with previous research. Jackson et al (1999) speculate that the reason for the relationship between high SES and increased reactivity among African American youth may be that these youth experience greater pressure to achieve and hence experience greater emotional stress in their everyday life. However, the exact mechanism underlying this phenomenon is still unclear.

Metabolic syndrome describes a cluster of risk factors for cardiovascular disease. Recent research linking SES to metabolic syndrome suggests that lower parent education is also associated with multiple metabolic risks among adolescents, including higher insulin and glucose, higher LDL cholesterol, waist circumference, and BMI, as well as cumulative risks (Goodman et al, 2005).

SES has also been linked to inflammatory markers related to coronary heart disease risk, such as fibrinogen, a coagulation protein, and C-reactive protein (CRP). Murasko (2008) reported that low SES adolescents had higher levels of CRP in a sample of US adolescents. However, there are conflicting results in this domain, as other studies have found no relationship between SES and fibrinogen among old children (Cook et al, 1999) or higher levels of fibrinogen and CRP among boys from high SES schools (Thomas et al, 2005).

In addition, some studies have found links between SES and hormonal profiles among adolescents. Results from a longitudinal study (Evans and Kim, 2007) showed that among 13-year olds, those who had been exposed to greater cumulative exposure to poverty over the course of their life span had higher levels of overnight urinary free cortisol at the follow-up assessment, after controlling for baseline values. Another study found evidence of increased daily salivary cortisol output among both healthy children and adolescents whose parents were less educated (Wolf et al, 2008). However, some studies have found that the association of low SES with higher salivary morning cortisol is stronger in younger children than in adolescents (Lupien et al, 2001).

Finally, SES has also been associated with biological markers within samples of adolescents with a chronic illness. For example, Chen et al (2003) examined immune and neuroendocrine markers of asthma in a group of adolescents with asthma. Living in a low neighborhood was associated with greater stimulated production of the asthma-relevant cytokine interleukin 5 (IL-5), and marginally lower morning cortisol (a hormone with anti-inflammatory effects) among these adolescents. Likewise, another study with children and adolescents with asthma showed that those coming from low SES environments had a heightened production of the asthma-relevant cytokines IL-5 and IL-13, as well as higher eosinophil counts, a type of white blood cell involved in the inflammatory process of asthma. Taken together, these findings suggest that SES can have biological effects that have implications for the progression of chronic diseases and that low SES among adolescents is associated with a differential profile of hormonal output that, over the long term, may have negative implications for health.

4 Conclusion

Health disparities among adolescents are common and have potentially far-reaching implications for adolescents' future health during adulthood. We have reviewed the recent literature and shown that SES disparities predispose adolescents to a wide range of physical health problems. Strong associations have been found in particular for the impact of SES on adolescent mortality, obesity, self-reported health, and cardiovascular reactivity. Other areas, for example, the impact of SES on sexual health, are in need of more research before conclusions about the strength and direction of these relationships can be drawn. But overall, low SES youth face a series of disadvantages. They live in neighborhoods that support unfavorable health behaviors and compromise their safety. They are less likely

to be adequately insured, receive the diagnosis, treatment, and prolonged care that they may be in need of. And they may come from families that may be unable to support them, both emotionally in times of distress and financially with respect to, for example, leisure time physical activity. Lastly, they are more likely to engage in unhealthy and unsafe behaviors, in addition to being more likely to experience psychological distress.

These patterns imply that interventions will need to address SES-related disparities on a number of levels, ranging from the individual to the societal. Consequently, no single intervention focusing only on the neighborhood, the family, or the individual will be enough. Multipronged interventions may be needed, with separate components targeting individual, family, and neighborhood contributors to health disparities in order to create meaningful reductions in adolescent health disparities. In addition, a number of methodological issues also require more attention in future research. For example, as adolescents typically still live at home with their parents but begin to be increasingly independent, at times already even earning their own money, it becomes more and more difficult to determine whether family, i.e., parental, SES is an acceptable indicator of adolescents' SES, and under what conditions adolescents' own SES should be accounted for. Second is the issue of age or pubertal stage. The issue of age/pubertal stage is that many studies look at combined samples of children and adolescents together, meaning that any disparity differences by age group or pubertal development will be masked. This is consistent with several studies that have found different influences of SES on health outcomes in children as opposed to adolescents (e.g., Cope et al, 2008; von Rueden et al, 2005). In addition, when biological outcomes are measured, puberty status becomes especially important given natural changes in, for example, hormones with puberty.

In sum, adolescents growing up in adverse, low SES environments, just like children and adults from low SES backgrounds, are more likely to experience a range of negative health outcomes. By better understanding and targeting the pathways between low SES and adolescent health, future research may be able to help place low SES youth on more positive trajectories leading to better health well into their adult years.

References

Abernathy, T. J., Webster, G., and Vermeulen, M. (2002). Relationship between poverty and health among adolescents. *Adolescence, 37*, 55–67.

Adler, N. E., and Newman, K. (2002). Socioeconomic disparities in health: pathways and policies. *Health Aff, 21*, 60–76.

Adler, N. E., Boyce, T., Chesney, M. A., Cohen, S., Folkman, S. et al (1994). Socioeconomic status: the challenge of the gradient. *Am Psychol, 49*, 15–24.

Ahn, M. K., Juon, H.-S., and Gittelsohn, J. (2008). Association of race/ethnicity, socioeconomic status, acculturation, and environmental factors with risk of overweight among adolescents in California, 2003. *Prev Chronic Dis, 5*, 1–10.

Boardman, L. A., Allsworth, J. A., Phipps, M. G., and Lapane, K. L. (2006). Risk factors for unintended versus intended rapid repeat pregnancies among adolescents. *J Adolesc Health, 39*, 597.e1-597.e8.

Boynton-Jarrett, R., Ryan, L. M., Berman, L. F., and Wright, R. J. (2008). Cumulative violence exposure and self-rated health: longitudinal study of adolescents in the United States. *Pediatrics, 122*, 961–970.

Bradley, R. H., Corwyn, R. F., McAdoo, H. P., and Coll, C. G. (2001). The home environments of children in the United States: I. Variations by age, ethnicity, and poverty status. *Child Dev, 72*, 1844–1867.

Brodersen, N. H., Steptoe, A., Boniface, D. R., and Wardle, J. (2007). Trends in physical activity and sedentary behaviors in adolescence: ethnic and socioeconomic differences. *Br J Sports Med, 41*, 140–144.

Buston, K., Williamson, L., and Hart, G. (2006). Young women under 16 years with experience of sexual intercourse: who becomes pregnant? *J Epidemiol Commun Health, 61*, 221–225.

Caputo, R. K. (2003). The effects of socioeconomic status, perceived discrimination and mastery on health status in a youth cohort. *Soc Work Health Care, 37*, 17–42.

Chen, E. (2007). Impact of socioeconomic status on physiological health in adolescents: an experimental manipulation of psychosocial factors. *Psychosom Med, 69*, 348–355.

Chen, E. and Matthews, K. A. (2003). Development of the cognitive appraisal and understanding of social events (CAUSE) videos. *Health Psychol, 22*, 106–110.

Chen, E., Fisher, E. B., Bacharier, L. B., and Strunk, R. C. (2003). Socioeconomic status, stress, and immune markers in adolescents with asthma. *Psychosom Med, 65*, 984–992.

Chen, E., Hanson, M. D., Paterson, L. Q., Griffin, M. J., Walker, H. A. et al (2006). Socioeconomic status and inflammatory processes in childhood asthma: the role of psychological stress. *J Allergy Clin Immunol, 117*, 1014–1020.

Chen, E., Langer, D. A., Raphaelson, Y. E., and Matthews, K. A. (2004). Socioeconomic status and health in adolescents: the role of stress interpretations. *Child Dev, 75*, 1039–1052.

Chen, E., Matthews, K. A., and Boyce, W. T. (2002). Socioeconomic differences in children's health: how and why do these relationships change with age? *Psych Bull, 128*, 295–329.

Cohen, D. A., Farley, T. A., and Mason, K. (2003). Why is poverty unhealthy? Social and physical mediators. *Soc Sci Med, 57*, 1631–1641.

Cook, D. G., Whincup, P. H., Miller, G., Carey, I. M., Adshead, F. J. et al (1999). Fibrinogen and factor VII levels are related to adiposity but not to fetal or social class in children aged 10–11 years. *Am J Epidemiol, 150*, 727–736.

Cope, S. F., Ungar, W. J., and Glazier, R. H. (2008). Socioeconomic factors and asthma control in children. *Pediatr Pulmonol, 43*, 745–752.

Dales, R. E., Choi, B., and Tang, M. (2002). Influence of family income on hospital visits for asthma among Canadian school children. *Thorax, 57*, 513–517.

Delva, J., Johnston, L. D., and O'Malley, P. O. (2007). The epidemiology of overweight and related lifestyle behaviors. *Am J Prev Med, 33*, 178–186.

Delva, J., O'Malley, P. M., and Johnston, L. D. (2006). Racial/ethnic and socioeconomic status differences in overweight and health-related behaviors among American students: national trends 1986–2003. *J Adolesc Health, 39*, 536–545.

De Spiegelaere, M., Dramaix, M., and Hennart, P. (1998). The influence of socioeconomic status on the incidence and evolution of obesity during early adolescence. *Int J Obes, 22*, 268–274.

Emerson, E., Graham, H., and Hatton, C. (2005). Household income and health status in children and adolescents in Britain. *Eur J Public Health, 16*, 354–360.

Emery, R. E., and Laumann-Billings, L. (1998). An overview of the nature, causes, and consequences of abusive family relationships. *Am Psychol, 53*, 121–135.

Evans, G. W. (2004). The environment of childhood poverty. *Am Psychol, 59*, 77–92.

Evans, G. W., and Kim, P. (2007). Childhood poverty and health: cumulative risk exposure and stress dysregulation. *Psychol Science, 18*, 953–957.

Georgiades, K., Boyle, M. H., Duku, E., and Racine, Y. (2006). Tobacco use among immigrant and nonimmigrant adolescents: individual and family level influences. *J Adolesc Health, 38*, 443e1–443e7.

Goodman, E. (1999). The role of socioeconomic gradients in explaining differences in US adolescents' health. *Am J Public Health, 89*, 1522–1528.

Goodman, E. and Huang, B. (2002). Socioeconomic status, depressive symptoms, and adolescent substance use. *Arch Pediatr Adolesc Med, 156*, 448–453.

Goodman, E., and Huang, B. (2001). Socioeconomic status, depression, and health service utilization among adolescent women. *Womens Health Issues, 11*, 416–426.

Goodman, E., Huang, B., Schafer-Kalkhoff, T., and Adler, N. E. (2007). Perceived socioeconomic status: a new type of identity that influences adolescents' self-rated health. *J Adolesc Health, 41*, 479–487.

Goodman, E., McEwen, B. S., Dolan, L. M., Schafer-Kalkhoff, T., and Adler, N. E. (2005a). Social disadvantage and adolescent stress. *J Adolesc Health, 37*, 484–492.

Goodman, E., McEwen, B. S., Huang, B., Dolan, L. M., and Adler, N. E. (2005b). Social inequalities in biomarkers of cardiovascular risk in adolescence. *Psychosom Med, 67*, 9–15.

Goodman, E., Slap, G. B., and Huang, B. (2003). The public health impact of socioeconomic status and adolescent depression and obesity. *Adolesc Health, 93*, 1844–1850.

Gordon-Larsen, P., Nelson, M. C., Page, P., and Popkin, B. M. (2006). Inequality in the built environment underlies key health disparities in physical activity and obesity. *Pediatrics, 117*, 417–424.

Gump, B. B., Matthews, K. A., and Raikkonen, K. (1999). Modeling relationships among socioeconomic status, hostility, cardiovascular reactivity, and left ventricular mass in African American and White children. *Health Psychol, 18*, 140–150.

Haas, J. S., Lee, L. B., Kaplan, C. P., Sonneborn, D., Phillips, K. A. et al (2003). The association of race, socioeconomic status, and health insurance status with the prevalence of overweight among children and adolescents. *Am J Public Health, 93*, 2105–2110.

Hanson, M. D., and Chen, E. (2007). Socioeconomic status and substance use behaviors in adolescents. *J Health Psych, 12*, 32–35.

Hanson, M. D., and Chen, E. (2006). Socioeconomic status, race, and body mass index: the mediating role of physical activity and sedentary behaviors during adolescence. *J Pediatr Psychol, 32*, 250–259.

Harrell, J. S., Faan, R. N., Bangdiwala, S. I., Deng, S., Webb, J. P. et al (1998). Smoking initiation in youth. *J Adolesc Health, 23*, 271–279.

Huurre, T., Rahkonen, O., and Aro, H. (2005). Socioeconomic status as a cause and consequence of psychosomatic symptoms from adolescence to adulthood. *Soc Psychiatry Psychiatr Epidemiol, 40*, 580–587.

Jackson, R. W., Treiber, F. A., Turner, J. R., Davis, H., and Strong, W. B. (1999). Effects of race, sex, and socioeconomic status upon cardiovascular stress responsivity and recovery in youth. *Int J Psychophysiol, 31*, 111–119.

Janssen, I., Boyce, W. F., Simpson, K., and Pickett, W. (2006). Influence of individual- and area-level measures of socioeconomic status on obesity, unhealthy eating, and physical inactivity in Canadian adolescents. *Am J Clin Nutr, 83*, 139–145.

Kim, H., Kieckhefer, G. M., Greek, A. A., Joesch, J. M., and Baydar, N. (2009). Health care utilization by children with asthma. *Prev Chronic Dis, 6*, 1–11.

Kubik, M. Y., Lytle, L. A., Birnbaum, A. S., Murray, D. M., Perry, C. L. et al (2003). Prevalence and correlates of depressive symptoms in young adolescents. *Am J Health Behav, 27*, 546–553.

Lee, J-. T., Son, J-Y., Kim, H., and Kim, S-Y. (2006). Effect of air-pollution on asthma-related hospital admissions for children by socioeconomic status associated with area of residence. *Arch Environ Occup Health, 61*, 123–130.

Leventhal, T. and Brooks-Gunn, J. (2000). The neighborhoods they live in: the effects of neighborhood residence on child and adolescent outcomes. *Psych Bull, 126*, 309–377.

Lioret, S., Maire, B., Volatier, J. -L., and Charles, M.-A. (2007). Child overweight in France and its relationship with physical activity, sedentary behavior and socioeconomic status. *Eur J Clin Nutr, 61*, 509–516.

Lupien, S. J., King, S., Meaney, M. J., and McEwen, B. S. (2001). Can poverty get under your skin? Basal cortisol levels and cognitive function in children from low and high socioeconomic status. *Dev Psychopathol, 13*, 653–676,

Luthar, S. S., and D'Avanzo, K. (1999). Contextual factors in substance use: a study of suburban and inner-city adolescents. *Dev Psychopathol, 11*, 845–867.

Marin, T. J., Chen, E., and Miller, G. E. (2008). What do trajectories of childhood socioeconomic status tell us about markers of cardiovascular health in adolescence? *Psychosom Med, 70*, 152–159.

McGrath, J. J., Matthews, K. A., and Brady, S. S. (2006). Individual versus neighborhood socioeconomic status and race as predictors of ambulatory blood pressure and heart rate. *Soc Sci Med, 63*, 1442–1453.

Mendelson, T., Kubzanksy, L. D., Datta, G. D., and Buka, S. L. (2008). Relation of female gender and low socioeconomic status to internalizing symptoms among adolescents: a case of double jeopardy. *Soc Sci Med, 66*, 1284–1296.

Moore, L. V. and Diez Roux, A. V. (2008). Associations of neighborhood characteristics with the location and type of food stores. *Am J Public Health, 96*, 325–331.

Murasko, J. E. (2008). Male-female differences in the association between socioeconomic status and atherosclerotic risk in adolescents. *Soc Sci Med, 67*, 1889–1897.

Mustard, C. A., Derksen, S., Berthelot, J. -M., Wolfson, M., and Roos, L. L. (1997). Age-specific education and income gradient in morbidity and mortality in a Canadian province. *Soc Sci Med, 45*, 383–397.

Nader, P. R., Bradley, R. H., Houts, R. M., McRitchie, S. L., and O'Brien, M. (2009). Moderate-to-vigorous physical activity from ages 9 to 15 years. *JAMA, 300*, 295–305.

Nelson, M. D. (1992). Socioeconomic status and childhood mortality in North Carolina. *Am J Public Health, 82*, 1131–1133.

Nersesian, W. S., Petit, M. R., Shaper, R., Lemieux, D., and Naor, E. (1985). Childhood death and poverty: a study of all childhood deaths in Maine, 1976 to 1980. *Pediatrics, 75*, 41–50.

Newacheck, P. W., Hung, Y. Y., Park, M. J., Brindis, C. D., and Irwin, C. E. (2003). Disparities in adolescent health and health care: does socioeconomic status matter? *Health Serv Res, 38*, 1235–1252.

Newbern, E. C., Miller, W. C., Schoenbach, V. J., and Kaufman, J. S. (2004). Family socioeconomic status and self-reported sexually transmitted diseases among black and white American adolescents. *Sex Transm Dis, 31*, 533–541.

Oliveira, Z. A. R., Bettiol, H., Gutierrez, M. R. P., Silva, A. A. M., and Barbieri, M. A. (2007). Factors associated with infant and adolescent mortality. *Braz J Med Biol Res, 40*, 1245–1255.

Piko, B. F., and Keresztes, N. (2007). Self-perceived health among early adolescents: role of psychosocial factors. *Pediatrics International, 49*, 577–583.

Potter, B. K., Speechley, K. N., Koval, J. J., Gutmanis, I. A., Campbell, M. K. et al (2005). Socioeconomic status and non-fatal injuries among Canadian adolescents: variations across SES and injury measures. *BMC Public Health, 5*, 132–143.

Rauscher, K. A., and Myers, D. J. (2008). Socioeconomic disparities in the prevalence of work-related injuries among adolescents in the United States. *J Adolesc Health, 42*, 50–57.

Raneri, L. G., and Wiemann, C. M. (2007). Social ecological predictors of repeat adolescent pregnancy. *Perspect Sex Reprod Health, 39*, 39–47.

Reid, J., Macchetto, P., and Foster, S. (1999). *No Safe Haven: Children of Substance-Abusing Parents.* New York: Center on Addiction and Substance Abuse.

Rhee, H. (2005). Racial/ethnic differences in adolescents' physical symptoms. *J Pediatr Nurs, 20*, 153–162.

Repetti, R. L., Taylor, S. E., and Seeman, T. E. (2002). Risky families: family social environments and the mental and physical health of offspring. *Psych Bull, 128*, 330–366.

Romero, A. J. (2005). Low-income neighborhood barriers and resources for adolescents' physical activity. *J Adolesc Health, 36*, 253–259.

Sallis, J. F., Zakarian, J. M., Hovell, M. F., and Hofstetter, C. R. (1996). Ethnic, socioeconomic, and sex differences in physical activity among adolescents. *J Clin Epidemiol, 49*, 125–134.

Santelli, J. S., Lowry, R., Brener, N. D., and Robin, L. (2000). The association of sexual behaviors

with socioeconomic status, family structure, and race/ethnicity among US adolescents. *Am J Public Health, 90*, 1582–1588.

Shrewsbury, V., and Wardle, J. (2008). Socioeconomic status and adiposity in childhood: a systematic review of cross-sectional studies 1990–2005. *Obesity, 16*, 275–284.

Simpson, K., Janssen, I., Craig, W. M., and Pickett, W. (2005). Multilevel analysis of associations between socioeconomic status and injury among Canadian adolescents. *J Epidemiol Community Health, 59*, 1072–1077.

Sionean, C., DiClemente, R. J., Wingood, G. M., Crosby, R., Cobb, B. K. et al (2000). Socioeconomic status and self-reported gonorrhea among African American female adolescents. *Sex Transm Dis, 28*, 236–239.

Soteriades, E. S. and DiFranza, J. R. (2003). Parent's socioeconomic status, adolescents' disposable income, and adolescents' smoking status in Massachusetts. *Am J Public Health, 93*, 1155–1160.

Starfield, B., Riley, A. W., Witt, W. P., and Robertson, J. (2002). Social class gradients in health among adolescence. *J Epidemiol Community Health, 56*, 354–361.

Strong, J. P., Malcom, G. T., McMahan, C. A., Tracy, R. E., Newman, W. P. et al (1999). Prevalence and extent of atherosclerosis in adolescents and young adults. *JAMA, 281*, 727–735.

Thomas, N. -E., Cooper, S. -M., Williams, S. R. P., Baker, J. S., and Davies, B. (2005). Fibrinogen, homocyst(e)ine, and c-reactive protein concentrations relative to sex and socioeconomic status in British young people. *Am J Human Biol, 17*, 809–813.

Vieweg, V. R., Johnston, C. H., Lanier, J. O., Fernandez, A., and Pandurangi, A. K. (2007). Correlation between high risk obesity groups and low socioeconomic status in school children. *South Med J, 100*, 8–13.

von Rueden, U., Gosch, A., Rajmil, L., Bisegger, C., Ravens-Sieberer, U. et al (2005). Socioeconomic determinants of health related quality of life in childhood and adolescence: results from a European study. *J Epidemiol Community Health, 60*, 130–135.

Wang, Y., Tussing, L., Odoms-Young, A., Braunschweig, C., Flay, B. et al (2006). Obesity prevention in low socioeconomic status urban African-American adolescents: study design and preliminary findings of the HEALTH-KIDS study. *Eur J Clin Nutr, 60*, 92–103.

Wahler, R. G. (1990). Some perceptual functions of social networks in coercive mother-interactions. *J Soc Clin Psychol, 9*, 43–53.

Williams, J. M., Currie, C. E., Wright, P., Elton, R. A., and Beattie, T. F. (1997). Socioeconomic status and adolescent injuries. *Soc Sci Med, 44*, 1881–1891.

Wilkinson, P., French, R., Kane, R., Lachowycz, K., Stephenson, J. Grundy, C. et al (2006). Teenage conceptions, abortions, and births in England, 1994–2003, and the national teenage pregnancy strategy. *Lancet, 368*, 1879–1886.

Wilson, D. K., Kliewer, W., Plybon, L., and Sica, D. A. (2000). Socioeconomic status and blood pressure reactivity in healthy black adolescents. *Hypertension, 35*, 496–500.

Wolf, J. M., Nicholls, E., and Chen, E. (2008). Chronic stress, salivary cortisol, and α-amylase in children with asthma and healthy children. *Biol Psychol, 78,* 20–28.

Yeatts, K., Davis, K. J., Sotir, M., Gerget, C., and Shy, C. (2003). Who gets diagnosed with asthma? Frequent wheeze among adolescents with and without a diagnosis of asthma. *Pediatrics, 111,* 1046–1054.

Chapter 38

Reproductive Hormones and Stages of Life in Women: Moderators of Mood and Cardiovascular Health

Susan S. Girdler and Kathleen C. Light

1 Menstrually Related Mood Disorders

1.1 Diagnosis and Prevalence

Since antiquity, medical professionals and lay people alike have been interested in the influence of reproductive hormones on mood. It was not until 1931, however, that Frank (1931) first documented in 15 of his patients the cyclical recurrence of a variety of emotional and behavioral symptoms that remitted shortly after the onset of menses. He termed this phenomenon "premenstrual tension syndrome." However, the term "PMS" (premenstrual syndrome) as commonly used is generic, imprecise, and usually incorporates normal physiologic, mood, and behavioral changes associated with the menstrual cycle. In this chapter our focus will be on women who meet criteria for more severe cyclical mood changes, including the most severe form of a menstrually related mood disorder, premenstrual dysphoric disorder (PMDD).

Briefly, the American Psychiatric Association (1994) criteria for PMDD require (1) that five or more symptoms are present during most of the last week of the luteal phase of the menstrual cycle and are absent in the week following the onset of menstruation; (2) at least one of these symptoms must be a major mood symptom; (3) symptoms must interfere with work, social activities, and/or relationships; (4) PMDD must be differentiated from the premenstrual exacerbation of a chronic mood disorder or general medical condition; and (5) criteria 1–4 must be confirmed with prospective daily ratings during at least two consecutive menstrual cycles. The requirement for prospective confirmation of PMDD is the cornerstone of the diagnosis since retrospective self-reports yield high false positive rates (Marvan and Cortes-Iniestra, 2001) and 50–75% of women who present with PMDD do not meet prospective criteria (e.g., Cohen et al, 2002). In the general population, PMDD afflicts 5–8% of reproductive age women, while an additional 20% of women have subsyndromal PMDD that results in impairment.

1.2 Pathogenesis of PMDD

1.2.1 Review of the Menstrual Cycle and Role of Gonadal Steroid Hormones in PMDD

The reproductive cycle can be divided into a follicular phase, an ovulatory phase, and a luteal phase. Day one of menses marks the beginning

S.S. Girdler (✉)
Department of Psychiatry, University of North Carolina at Chapel Hill, CB #7175, Medical School Wing D, Chapel Hill, NC 27599-7175, USA
e-mail: susan_girdler@med.unc.edu

A. Steptoe (ed.), *Handbook of Behavioral Medicine*, DOI 10.1007/978-0-387-09488-5_38,
© Springer Science+Business Media, LLC 2010

of the follicular phase, during the first half of which blood levels of estrogens and progesterone are low and stable. The second half of the follicular phase begins about 7–8 days before the preovulatory luteinizing hormone (LH) surge and is characterized by an increase in plasma estrogen levels (estradiol and estrone). Plasma progesterone levels do not increase during this period. During the ovulatory phase, there is a rapid rise in plasma LH levels which leads to the rupture of the mature follicle approximately 16–24 h later, marking the beginning of the luteal phase. The *sine qua non* of the luteal phase is the marked increase in progesterone secretion which reaches a maximum about 8 days after the mid-cycle LH peak. Estrone and estradiol plasma levels increase in parallel with that of progesterone.

Although early hypotheses about PMDD posited the presence during the luteal phase of a hormonal abnormality, women with PMDD do not reliably differ in ovarian function or steroid hormone levels across the cycle (e.g., Girdler et al, 1993). However, the importance of *changes* in gonadal steroids in PMDD was suggested by an early observational study (Halbreich et al, 1986) that showed the strongest predictor of premenstrual symptom severity in women with PMDD was the rate of change in luteal phase progesterone and estradiol, and not the absolute progesterone or estradiol levels. Subsequently, Schmidt and colleagues (1991) demonstrated that in those women in whom ovarian suppression with the gonadotropin-releasing hormone (GnRH) agonist leuprolide acetate (Depot Lupron) prevented the expression of PMDD symptoms, exogenous administration of either estradiol or progesterone (but not placebo) precipitated the return of symptoms. Notably, however, in the non-PMDD controls, neither the hypogonadal (Lupron alone) nor the hormone replacement (Lupron + estradiol or progesterone or placebo) conditions were associated with any perturbation of mood. Thus, PMDD women appear to be more sensitive to mood destabilization consequent to *changes* in normal ovarian steroid hormone levels across the menstrual cycle.

1.2.2 Assessing Menstrual Cycle Phase and Cardiovascular Stress Reactivity in PMDD

We have investigated evidence for dysregulation in cardiovascular stress responses in PMDD and the influence of menstrual cycle phase. Due to the significant between-subjects differences in absolute levels of gonadal steroid hormones over the menstrual cycle (Howards et al, 2009), a within-subjects design is methodologically important. In our studies, the timing of follicular phase test sessions is based on self-report of the first day of menses, defined as follicular cycle day 1. Timing of luteal phase test sessions is aided by the use of home urine ovulation test kits that detect the LH surge preceding ovulation. Because normal menstrual cycle lengths are variable (22–36 days) and there is a lack of correspondence between self-reported cycle length and actual cycle length (Howards et al, 2009), our subjects prospectively track their cycle length for two to three cycles, basing the start date for LH testing on the shortest cycle length documented. While blood hormone levels should be used to confirm phase and ovulation, the detection of the LH surge in urine is a reliable method with which to target luteal phase cycle days in compliant subjects.

In normally cycling non-PMDD women, the weight of the available evidence indicates that menstrual cycle phase does not influence blood pressure reactivity to laboratory stressors (e.g., Girdler et al, 1993, 1998, 2007; Hirshoren et al, 2002). However, in our studies that have employed impedance cardiography to assess myocardial versus vascular contributions to blood pressure increases, we have consistently found, both at rest and in response to stress, that the higher hormone luteal phase is associated with greater myocardial reactivity to stress, indexed by stroke volume, cardiac output, and/or heart rate, but lower vascular resistance levels relative to the lower hormone early follicular phase (Girdler et al, 1993, 1998, 2007), such that homeostasis of blood pressure levels is maintained across the menstrual cycle.

Regarding diagnosis-related differences in cardiovascular stress reactivity, although the menstrual cycle is obligatory to the expression of premenstrual symptoms, paradoxically we have obtained little evidence that the menstrual cycle influences PMDD-related differences in cardiovascular responses to stress. While PMDD women exhibit blunted heart rate, stroke volume, cardiac output, and blood pressure responses to a variety of laboratory stressors relative to non-PMDD controls, this is evident in both cycle phases (Girdler et al, 1993, 1998).

1.2.3 The Role of Historical Factors in the Pathogenesis of PMDD

In subsequent studies, using structured interview, we found that PMDD women are about twice as likely to have a history of physical and/or sexual abuse (Girdler et al, 2003, 2007). We also obtained evidence that the biological correlates of abuse may differ for PMDD women since only for PMDD women was prior abuse associated with increased β-adrenergic receptor responsivity relative to never abused PMDD women (assessed via the standardized isoproterenol sensitivity test) (Cleaveland et al, 1972). Abuse did not modify β-adrenergic receptor responsivity in non-PMDD controls (Girdler et al, 2003). In a placebo-controlled study involving a 2-month challenge with clonidine, a centrally acting presynaptic α2-adrenergic receptor agonist, we found that, when compared with pretreatment reactivity, clonidine was associated with greater reductions in blood pressure and heart rate reactivity to stress in abused PMDD women versus never abused PMDD women, indicating a greater contribution of α-adrenergic receptors to the stress responses of abused PMDD women (Bunevicius et al, 2005).

Given the high rate of depression in abused women, in our subsequent study (Girdler et al, 2007) we controlled for histories of depression in our analyses and found that both PMDD and non-PMDD women with prior abuse exhibited greater heart rate levels at rest and during stressors relative to never abused women. Again,

however, we found that the biological correlates of abuse differed in PMDD, since only the abused PMDD women had greater vascular resistance levels and blood pressure levels at rest and in response to stress relative to never abused PMDD women – effects not seen in non-PMDD women. Since the abused groups did not differ in heart rate or cardiac output, the greater blood pressure levels in abused PMDD women are likely due to their enhanced vascular tone, which is mediated, in part, by vascular α2-adrenergic receptors (Girdler et al, 1993). Thus, our work using pharmacologic adrenergic receptor challenges, together with impedance cardiography, indicates that PMDD women may be especially vulnerable to the effects of abuse on adrenergic function.

1.2.4 Progesterone-Derived GABAergic Neurosteroids in PMDD

In rodents, acute stress results in significant increases in both plasma and CNS concentrations of the 3α-hydroxy ring A-reduced steroid metabolite of progesterone, 3α,5α-THP (allopregnanolone) in physiologic ranges known to enhance GABA receptor-activated Cl^- currents (Purdy et al, 1991). Allopregnanolone is among the most potent allostatic modulator of the $GABA_A$ receptors (nanomolar concentrations), and it is through this mechanism that it exerts anxiolytic effects (e.g., Bitran et al, 2000). Allopregnanolone is synthesized in ovary, adrenals, and brain. Allopregnanolone is highly lipophilic. Animal studies have shown that the major proportion of brain allopregnanolone following stress is produced in periphery (Purdy et al, 1991), though the peripheral increase in allopregnanolone is delayed, peaking at 30–70 min following the onset of acute stress (Purdy et al, 1991).

Animal models provide consistent evidence that neurosteroids like allopregnanolone restore both normal GABAergic and hypothalamic–pituitary–adrenal (HPA) function following stress (e.g., Barbaccia et al, 1998; Guo et al, 1995). Thus, endogenous allopregnanolone represents a homeostatic mechanism in the context of adaptation to stress by limiting the extent and duration of reduction in GABAergic inhibitory transmission and activation of the HPA axis. It has been suggested that disruption in this homeostatic mechanism may play an etiopathogenic role in some psychiatric disorders related to stress and be associated with increased adrenal glucocorticoid output, such as depression.

We have had the opportunity to conduct some of the initial translational research on neurosteroid responses to mental stressors in humans. We initially reported that PMDD women had greater luteal phase allopregnanolone concentrations at rest, consistent with their lower cortisol concentrations, but blunted allopregnanolone stress reactivity relative to non-PMDD controls (Girdler et al, 2001). This is consistent with results from endocrine challenge studies showing a blunted allopregnanolone response to ACTH (Lombardi et al, 2004) and a GnRH challenge (Monteleone et al, 2000) in PMDD. However, the possibility existed that the blunted allopregnanolone reactivity in PMDD may have reflected the greater likelihood of lifetime depression in PMDD women (Cohen et al, 2002), since allopregnanolone concentrations are consistently lower in depressed patients (e.g., Strohle et al, 2000; Uzunova et al, 2006). In our next study (Klatzkin et al, 2006), we recruited PMDD and non-PMDD women with or without histories of clinical depression (>7 months in full remission) and sampled allopregnanolone immediately after venepuncture stress, again 25 min later after an extended baseline rest and at 30 and 60 min following the onset of the Trier Social Stress Test. By characterizing women based on prior depression and PMDD status, we demonstrated that all women with prior depression, regardless of PMDD, had blunted allopregnanolone reactivity to stress at both 30 and 60 min following stress relative to never depressed women. Thus, what our first study indicated was an effect of PMDD diagnosis on allopregnanolone stress reactivity may more parsimoniously be explained by histories of clinical depression. This is not to say,

however, that depression-related alterations in allopregnanolone reactivity to stress do not have special clinical relevance for PMDD, since allopregnanolone reactivity to challenge predicted greater premenstrual symptom severity, but only in PMDD women with histories of depression (Klatzkin et al, 2006).

1.3 Conclusions and Future Research Directions

The results of our recent studies indicate that histories of abuse and histories of depression are independently associated with persistent alterations in stress-responsive systems in women, and that these histories may have special biological relevance for women with PMDD. This suggests clinically distinct subgroups of PMDD women and may have treatment implications for many PMDD women since only 50–60% of PMDD women are responsive to current FDA approved treatments (Halbreich, 2008).

Our preliminary work on altered allopregnanolone reactivity to stress in women with depressive disorders suggests that investigations in the role of neuroactive steroid stress responsivity and the regulatory role of such responses with regard to the HPA axis in the pathophysiology of depressive disorders in humans may be indicated. While this represents an exciting new direction in behavioral medicine for understanding biobehavioral factors in depressive illness, it will be important to proceed cautiously by first establishing reliable studies in healthy human males and females on the time course of neurosteroid responses to stress, as has been done for the HPA axis response to social stress (Kirschbaum et al, 1993). Our prior work suggests that peak allopregnanolone stress levels in human females may occur at a different time point than in rodents.

It would also be important to investigate other neuroactive steroids that are detectable in human plasma, are stress responsive, and are potent modulators of the $GABA_A$ receptor.

Gas chromatography and mass spectrometry (GC–MS) allow for the simultaneous detection of low amounts of neuroactive steroids in brain, cerebrospinal fluid, and plasma. We have recently been involved with validating the biological application of this method using serum from healthy women tested in the follicular phase before and after a controlled oral dose of micronized progesterone. With GC–MS, we reported the ability to detect progesterone-induced elevations in all four GABAergic neuroactive steroids derived from progesterone and from deoxycorticosterone, while there was no effect of progesterone on any DHEA metabolite (Porcu et al, 2009). The simultaneous measurement of these neuroactive steroids is important not only to further explore their physiological roles but also to identify biomarkers of disease risk, treatment response, and more selective therapeutic targets.

2 Oxytocin and Vasopressin: Information from Animal Models

In addition to traditional reproductive hormones like estrogen and testosterone, two hypothalamic neuropeptides, oxytocin, and vasopressin that are shared across all mammalian species (including humans) have been shown to be central to reproductive success. These two neuropeptides are also of interest to behavioral medicine because they have major implications for physical and mental health, with effects on the cardiovascular system, wound healing, and pain sensitivity. Of these two, oxytocin has been much more studied in regard to reproduction while vasopressin, despite clear links to pair bonding in animal models, is much better known for its role in relation to blood pressure regulation through its effects on vasoconstriction and renal sodium excretion (hence its earlier common name as antidiuretic hormone).

Oxytocin plays a major role in a number of reproductive functions, beginning with sexual receptivity and mating in both genders,

ejaculation in males, and formation of long-term pair bonds in those species when monogamy is typical (for reviews, see Carter, 1998; Insel and Young, 2001). During and after pregnancy, oxytocin functions to advance labor and uterine contractions and is involved in initiation of most maternal behaviors including breast feeding, nest building, licking, and warm contact with offspring. Oxytocin is involved in many basic non-reproductive social behaviors as well, including the simple act of socially recognizing a familiar individual (Young, 2002). Oxytocin knockout mice, lacking the gene to produce oxytocin, are less able to recognize a formerly familiar conspecific despite having no deficits in underlying learning or sensory functions. This lack of social recognition disappears if oxytocin is administered to the animal's medial amygdala, while the behavioral deficit can be mimicked in normal mice by administering an oxytocin antagonist to the same region (Ferguson et al, 2000, 2001).

There appear to be long-term consequences of early life deficits in oxytocin activity. As infants, oxytocin knockout mice vocalize less during separations from their dams, eliciting less licking, close contact and other maternal behavior when separation ends. As adults, female oxytocin knockouts show less maternal behavior and the males show increased aggression (Winslow et al, 2003). Another maternal behavior enhanced by oxytocin is licking. Increased maternal pup licking (which increases oxytocin and decreases HPA activity in pups and dams) has diverse benefits that endure into adulthood: decreased stress behaviors, HPA activity, and blood pressure (Champagne et al, 2003). The oxytocin literature also indicates increased intergenerational maternal behavior in the female pups as adults; that is, pups that have experienced high maternal behavior by their dams tend to show high maternal behavior as adults (Pedersen and Boccia, 2002).

In addition to its effects on reproduction and maternal behaviors, oxytocin has much broader effects as a neuromodulator by potentiating or attenuating activity in other physiological systems. Its downstream effects influence the HPA and sympathetic-adrenomedullary "stress response" systems, the serotonin, dopamine, and GABA "mood and affect" responsive systems, and the opioidergic and other "pain regulating" systems. Uvnäs-Moberg (1998) has proposed that oxytocin is the central response system involved in what she has labeled the "relaxation and growth" response and the "calm and connection" response. This response is a complementary system to which behavioral medicine terms the "flight or fight" response, which involves activation of HPA and sympathetic stress-responsive systems. Not surprisingly, oxytocin activity can be enhanced after these systems are activated, as part of a negative feedback loop acting to turn off these systems and keep their activation to a short-term response. In the brain, the neural connections between the oxytocin tracts and the dopaminergic tracts, sometimes called the "reward system", are assumed to activate together and may partly explain why contact between mother and infant and even nonsexual contact between bonded partners and other family members is so rewarding. In rat dams, suckling by pups produced greater activation of dopaminergic pathways than cocaine did (Ferris et al, 2005). Interestingly, cocaine exposure during pregnancy appears to reduce oxytocin activity and maternal behaviors while increasing aggression in both the dams and in female offspring when adults and has been described as "highjacking" the pathways that make maternal behaviors rewarding (McMurray et al, 2008).

Centrally, oxytocin is produced in the paraventricular and supraoptic nuclei of the hypothalamus. From these nuclei, oxytocinergic magnocellular neurons project to the posterior pituitary, and secreted oxytocin of central nervous system origins then can travel via the circulation to the uterus, breasts, heart, and blood vessels, all of which have oxytocin receptors. The heart and larger vessels can themselves synthesize smaller additional amounts of oxytocin. Oxytocin administration to isolated heart and vessels (with and without oxytocin antagonist present) show that increased oxytocin-specific activity of local receptors can reduce heart rate and contractile force, thereby decreasing

cardiac output, and can enhance vasodilatation, all of which would decrease blood pressure (e.g., Petersson, 2002). Interestingly, the other social peptide, vasopressin, has the opposite effect on cardiovascular responses, increasing vasoconstriction, and sodium retention, and thereby increasing blood pressure. Chronic oxytocin administration in adult animals for five or more days leads to decreases in HPA activity as indexed by corticosterone lasting 10 days and long-lasting decreases in blood pressure, while postnatal oxytocin administration can lead to lower blood pressure into adulthood (e.g., Petersson, 2002). Persistent blood pressure reductions after oxytocin administration are presumed to be due to oxytocin's influence resetting other cardiovascular modulator pathways, including central alpha-2 adrenoceptor activity, parasympathetic activity, serotonergic activity, and atrial natriuretic peptide. Oxytocin may also reduce cardiovascular risk by inhibiting inflammatory processes implicated in atherogenesis. McCabe and colleagues have shown that social contact alters the progression of atherosclerotic changes in a susceptible rabbit strain: effects that appear related to oxytocin activity; using cultured human vascular cells, they further verified that oxytocin decreases both superoxide production and release of pro-inflammatory cytokines (e.g., Szeto et al, 2008). Oxytocin activity elicited by social contact also decreases acute inflammation and promotes wound healing (Detillion et al, 2004; DeVries et al, 2007).

The central oxytocin system exhibits unusual plasticity, remaining functional across the life span in both genders, but nevertheless is quite responsive to reproductive steroid hormone fluctuations. Although oxytocin receptors are distributed in the same brain regions of both males and females of the same species, social connection and anxiety effects are greater in females and/or enhanced by estrogen or hormonal variation during estrous cycles (Young, 2002). Choleris and colleagues (2003) demonstrated deficits in social recognition in three female genetic knockout mice models: oxytocin knockout, estrogen receptor-alpha knockout, and estrogen receptor-beta knockout. All three varieties of these knockout animals showed social recognition deficits compared with genetically normal mice, indicating that estrogen receptors directly contribute to OT-mediated social behaviors. Reduction of aggressive and anxiety behaviors associated with oxytocin activity has been documented in females of several species and appears to be influenced by estrogen (Harmon et al, 2002).

2.1 Oxytocin and Vasopressin: Information from Human Studies

Preliminary evidence from human mothers suggests that oxytocin helps modulate their affective state, and this may, in turn, influence their stress responses. In mothers who both breast and bottle feed their infants, the act of breast feeding (which typically elicits greater rises in plasma OT) is associated with less perceived stress, depression, and anxiety than bottle feeding (Mezzacappa and Katkin, 2002). Women who are breast feeders also report less anxiety than bottle-feeding women and show lower blood pressure before and during stress (Altemus et al, 2001). However, one randomized trial of intranasal oxytocin administration to enhance milk expression while using a breast pump in mothers of preterm infants found only faster initial let-down, but no other benefit (Fewtrell et al, 2006). In our research with mothers of infants, we found that high oxytocin responders to mother–infant interaction have lower overall blood pressure levels both in laboratory stress studies and during 24 h ambulatory monitoring at home (Light et al, 2000). Our most recent mother–infant studies have confirmed that oxytocin differences between breast and bottle feeders are evident during infant feeding, mother–infant interaction, and stressors (stressful speech and cold pressor test) using either salivary or plasma oxytocin samples (Grewen et al, 2010).

Early life experience in humans as well as animals (e.g., Pedersen and Boccia, 2002) may affect the function of the oxytocin and

vasopressin systems. Wismer Fries et al (2005) reported that children who had lived in orphanages with limited social contact for an average of 17 months before being adopted showed lower overall urinary vasopressin levels for 4 days and lower urinary oxytocin during a game involving lots of mother–child touching compared with age-matched children who had always lived with their parents. Adult men who experienced early parental separation have also failed to show normal inhibition of cortisol following intranasal oxytocin administration (Meinlschmidt and Heim, 2007), while adult women who had experienced childhood abuse or neglect had lower oxytocin levels in their cerebrospinal fluid (Heim et al, 2008). Together, these studies suggest that central oxytocin and vasopressin pathways may show long-term effects of early life events involving parental attachment. In young unmarried adults, higher plasma oxytocin levels were linked to stronger attachment to their parents and to lower levels of distress and depressive symptoms (Gordon et al, 2008). Stronger attachment was also associated with higher plasma oxytocin in premenopausal women, but in this case it was also linked to higher anxiety (Tops et al, 2007). The latter finding may reflect the role of oxytocin as part of the negative feedback loop for the HPA axis, since this pattern was also associated with higher cortisol. Guastella et al (2009) have recently observed significant benefits of intranasal oxytocin administration compared to placebo as adjunctive treatment in patients undergoing therapy for social anxiety disorder.

Our research group has also addressed the link between relationship characteristics, oxytocin response, and both sympathetic nervous system activity and blood pressure in married couples. We found that if even one of the spouses reports having strong, unambivalent support from the partner, both husband and wife will have high plasma oxytocin levels in anticipation of, as well as right after, a period of close contact with the their spouse when they cuddle and talk about a happy shared memory. In wives, higher partner support and more frequent partner hugs were also linked to lower resting blood pressure and sympathetic nervous system activity (indexed by plasma norepinephrine levels before and after partner cuddling), which appeared to be partly mediated by higher oxytocin (Grewen et al, 2005; Light et al, 2005a). Although wives with high oxytocin did not show reductions in blood pressure reactivity to stress, they did maintain lower absolute levels of blood pressure across both rest and stress compared with low oxytocin women (Light et al, 2005a). In a double-blind placebo-controlled study linking oxytocin activity to reproductive hormones, we found that oxytocin precursor activity was enhanced in postmenopausal women after 6 months of estrogen replacement therapy (ERT) compared to placebo (Light et al, 2005b). Also, this same study indicated that greater increases in oxytocin activity were related to greater decreases in blood pressure resulting from reduced vascular resistance, even after partialling out direct effects on the vasculature related to treatment condition or to changes in plasma estradiol. Furthermore, women with poorer partner relationships (indexed by divorced versus married status) were less likely to respond to ERT with high increases in oxytocin activity. This extends earlier work by Turner et al (1999) who reported oxytocin increases in response to positive emotion induction in some but not all premenopausal women, particularly those currently in couple relationships and those reporting fewer relationship problems. Furthermore, in parallel to animal model research, in a preliminary study, we observed that mothers who had used cocaine during pregnancy showed lesser oxytocin responses during our laboratory studies involving mother–infant interactions and higher blood pressure levels in the laboratory and at home, where they tended to spend less time holding their babies other than for feeding (Light et al, 2004). Our group has also obtained the first evidence in humans, to our knowledge, showing that high oxytocin activity is linked to altered pain tolerance (Grewen et al, 2008). Paralleling findings in animal models (Uvnäs-Moberg, 1998), we found that higher plasma oxytocin was correlated with

greater tolerance to ischemic and cold pressor pain tasks in a bi-racial sample of women. In this laboratory study of pain sensitivity, African American women showed both lower oxytocin and lower pain tolerance than other women.

Due to the powerful multisystem effects linked to oxytocin and vasopressin in regard to social phenomena, intervention research examining effects of increases in oxytocin in humans has recently burgeoned, including studies linking oxytocin to increased interpersonal trust, greater recognition of faces and decreased fear (Meyer-Lindenberg, 2008). For example, Ditzen and colleagues (2009) compared effects of intranasal oxytocin versus placebo in couples during conflict discussion, finding that oxytocin reduced cortisol and increased positive communication. Zak and colleagues observed that intranasal oxytocin increased experimentally assessed trust, reciprocity, and generosity behaviors (assessed by monetary transfer to strangers), and they also found that exposure to either deep massage or empathy-evoking film clips likewise increased both circulating oxytocin levels and such reciprocating or generous money sharing (Barrazza and Zak, 2009; Morhenn et al, 2008; Zak et al, 2007). As previously mentioned, intranasal oxytocin is also being used with some success in the treatment of social anxiety (Guastella et al, 2009) and is also being used with initially encouraging results in autism spectrum disorders (Bartz and Hollander, 2008). Another study using intranasal oxytocin to assess effects on male sexual function during a blinded cross-over protocol involving masturbation only obtained evidence that the men detected differences in arousal on oxytocin, but the authors acknowledged that future research should take into account that oxytocin should exert greater effects within the context of a bonded partner relationship. Finally, in a study of married couples (Holt-Lunstad et al, 2008), we obtained evidence supporting the hypothesis that endogenous oxytocin levels could be increased behaviorally. In this study, couples were randomized to intervention or monitoring only for 1 month, with intervention couples trained and instructed to practice Rosen listening touch together with head and neck massage four times/week. The intervention produced increases in salivary oxytocin and decreases in the sympathetic marker, salivary alpha amylase, in both husbands and wives, and husbands also showed lower post-intervention ambulatory blood pressure.

2.2 Conclusions and Future Directions

In summary, the function of physiological systems and behaviors influenced by oxytocin and vasopressin are important to major health outcomes. They are also important to some of the things that we as humans value most: attachment to family, friends, and other members of our social groups, desire for physical closeness, childbirth and parenting, and sexual response. We anticipate that in the next few years, there will be accelerating interest in human oxytocin and vasopressin research. In particular, we expect that there will be expanded research employing salivary and urinary oxytocin and vasopressin sampling, especially for studies in the home environment where obtaining blood for plasma measures is impractical. Although there is some skepticism about the validity of salivary oxytocin (Horvat-Gordon et al, 2005), a new study indicates that in mothers of infants, salivary and plasma oxytocin measures showed parallel increases and decreases during infant feeding, cuddling, rests, and stressors, and the two measures were reliably correlated during steady-state conditions (Grewen et al, 2010). Urinary oxytocin validation studies are in progress. We also believe that there will continue to be great interest in use of the intranasal administration of oxytocin both for laboratory research and for multi-session interventions. We especially look forward to human investigations examining potential benefits of enhanced oxytocin to rate of wound healing and to atherosclerosis.

3 The Menopause: Determining Female Reproductive Stage

Women do not start or end reproductive function at a particular chronological age. The menopause transition, like puberty, is a dynamic period with respect to the reproductive axis, and a multidimensional process because in addition to changes in hormonal factors, it represents a time of change associated with family and personal relationships, work status, and self-concept.

It was only recently that a staging system and nomenclature for healthy women who age spontaneously to a natural menopause was developed out of The Stages of Reproductive Aging Workshop (STRAW) (Soules et al, 2001). The relatively wide age range (42–58 years) for complete reproductive failure (menopause) in normal women underscores the importance of relying on criteria other than age to determine reproductive status. The STRAW criteria for reproductive staging are primarily based on the characteristics of the menstrual cycle and secondarily on follicle-stimulating hormone (FSH) levels. The anchor for the staging system is the final menstrual period. The STRAW system identifies seven stages: five precede and two follow the final menstrual period. Stages –5 to –3 encompass the reproductive interval, –2 to –1 are the menopausal transition, and +1 and +2 are the postmenopause. A woman's menstrual cycle remains regular in stage –2 (early menopausal transition), but the length changes by seven or more days. Stage –1 (late menopausal transition) is characterized by two or more skipped menstrual cycles and at least one intermenstrual interval of 60 days or more. A woman is postmenopausal when she has been amenorrheic for 12+ months, being in Stage +1 (early) for the first 5 years after the final menstrual period and in Stage +2 (late) until death. The term perimenopause literally means "about or around the menopause" and begins with Stage –2 and ends 12 months after the final menstrual period. The duration of the perimenopause is variable and can extend over many years (Schmidt et al, 2004).

3.1 Estrogen Deprivation Increases Risk for Depression and Medical Illness

While the most common symptoms associated with progressive ovarian failure and estrogen deprivation during the menopause transition are vasomotor (e.g., hot flushes), perimenopausal women are also at increased risk for clinical depression. While most women will *not* suffer from clinically significant depressive symptoms during the menopausal transition, longitudinal studies in community samples have consistently documented an increased risk for clinically significant depressive symptoms or major depressive episodes during the menopause transition, with odds ratios generally ranging from 1.3 to 4.0 (e.g., Cohen et al, 2006; Freeman et al, 2009). That the *fluctuations* in hormones during the menopause transition contribute to the development of depression in vulnerable women is supported by the work of Freeman (2006) who showed that greater variability in estradiol levels, and not the estradiol levels per se, was associated with both higher depressive symptoms and diagnosed major depressive disorder. Thus, vulnerability to the mood destabilizing effects of reproductive hormones may represent a pathophysiological mechanism contributing to the increased risk of new onset and recurrent depression during the perimenopause. Among the predictors of vulnerability to perimenopausal depression include longer duration of the menopause transition time, vasomotor symptoms, stressful life events proximate to the menopausal transition, and histories of depression (Bromberger et al, 2009; Cohen et al, 2006; Freeman et al, 2004, 2009; and see Deecher and Dorries, 2007 for review), though it must be emphasized that perimenopausal women are twice as likely to develop new onset depression relative to premenopausal women (Cohen et al, 2006; Freeman et al, 2006).

Depression is not only a major primary source of morbidity and mortality (Chen and Dilsaver, 1996), but as well it has been associated with an increased risk for cardiovascular disease morbidity and mortality in studies of both animals and humans (e.g., Shively et al, 2008). Transition into the postmenopausal years is also associated with a rapid increase in risk of cardiovascular disease for women, with rates in postmenopausal women surpassing those of men (e.g., Moller-Leimkubler, 2007). While age is the major determinant of increased cardiovascular risk, the importance of estrogen in cardiovascular risk is supported by observations among women undergoing early menopause or oophorectomy without estradiol replacement (e.g., Colditz et al, 1987), since these women show a substantial increase in cardiovascular disease risk, as do younger women with premature ovarian failure (Kalantaridou et al, 2006; Yildirir et al, 2006). Consequently, with 1.5 million U.S. women reaching menopause each year, a substantial number of women will be at increased risk for the comorbid expression of depression and cardiovascular disease, making the perimenopause an ideal window for studying the pathophysiology of cardiovascular risk and depression in women.

Not only is estrogen withdrawal associated with increased risk for depression and cardiovascular disease, but it is also associated with other negative health effects, the most notable of which may be osteoporosis. Osteoporosis is a disease characterized by the loss of bone mass and strength that leads to fragility fractures. That estrogen deficiency is critical to the pathogenesis of osteoporosis came initially from the evidence that postmenopausal women are at highest risk for the disease (see Raisz, 2005 for review). Bone remodeling is a dynamic process in which old bone is removed from the skeleton and new bone is added. It consists of two phases – resorption and formation – that involve activity of cells called osteoclasts and osteoblasts. Usually the removal and formation of bone are in balance and maintain skeletal strength and integrity. In postmenopausal women there is both an increase in bone resorption and a diminishment of the increased bone formation that normally occurs in response to mechanical loading, suggesting that estrogen is both anti-catabolic and anabolic (Lee et al, 2003; Raisz, 2005).

Osteoporosis is particularly common in white postmenopausal women and causes 1.5 million fractures per year in the United States (Cummings and Melton, 2002). Hip fracture is the most severe consequence of osteoporosis, and its incidence in women rises exponentially from approximately 100 to 1000 per 100,000 women per year from age 60 to 80 years (Cummings and Melton, 2002). Hip fractures are associated with significant impairment in quality of life, the most important of which may be loss of the ability to walk. Approximately half of individuals who are ambulatory prior to hip fracture are unable to walk independently following fracture (Miller, 1978); and among women who live independently before hip fracture, half remain in long-term care or need help with activities of daily living a year after the fracture (Cummings et al 1985). Thus, osteoporosis has a high morbidity rate for mid- and later-life women, is associated with increased mortality rates (primarily following hip fracture) (Cummings and Melton, 2002), and represents a significant public health problem.

3.2 Estrogen Replacement for Depression, Cardiovascular Disease, and Osteoporosis in Peri- and Postmenopausal Women

In recent controlled trials, a significant antidepressant effect of estrogen in moderately severe depression in perimenopausal (e.g., Cohen et al, 2003; Soares et al, 2001) but not postmenopausal (Morrison et al, 2004) women has been shown. In contrast to the beneficial effects seen with estrogen alone, a recent trial of estrogen plus a continuous progestin failed to observe antidepressant efficacy compared with an SSRI in

women with peri- and postmenopausal depression (Soares et al, 2006). Nonetheless, a meta-analysis from 26 controlled studies in peri- and postmenopausal women (Zweifel and O'Brien, 1997) reported that estrogen replacement with or without a progestin was associated with a substantial and significant reduction in depression symptoms. Thus, in peri- and postmenopausal women with moderate depression, estrogen therapy appears effective in reducing depression symptoms, with the antidepressant actions of estrogen especially apparent in studies using transdermal 17β-estradiol (see Frey et al, 2008 for review).

While the majority of cohort retrospective and prospective observational studies in peri- and postmenopausal women taking ERT or combined hormone replacement therapy (HRT) (estrogen plus a progestin) demonstrated a significant reduction in cardiovascular disease as well as all-cause mortality in hormone users (e.g., Bush, 1996; Stampfer et al, 1991), this substantial literature supporting the cardioprotective effects of ERT has been called in to question, if not repudiated, by several large secondary and primary prevention trials of ERT/HRT. The largest and most documented of the controlled trials for the prevention of cardiovascular disease is the Women's Health Initiative (WHI) that enrolled over 27,000 postmenopausal women, 50–79 years old (mean age – 63 years), and randomized each to either oral ERT (in those without a uterus), HRT (conjugated equine estrogen + medroxyprogesterone acetate [MPA]), or placebo. The HRT arm was terminated after 5 years due to an increased incidence of breast cancer; the results also suggested an increase in non-fatal MI and stroke (Rossouw et al, 2002).

Critical reviews subsequent to the initial WHI reports have argued that the discordant findings reflected problems in the design of the WHI, the most important of which may have been the age and condition of the study subjects (e.g., see Harman et al, 2005). Animal and human studies support the "timing hypothesis," – i.e., the effect of estrogen on cardiovascular disease risk depends on when therapy is started relative to the onset of ovarian failure: beneficial if started in the perimenopausal years (during the fatty streak to uncomplicated plaque stage of atherosclerosis) and neutral or adverse if started later (during the stage of plaque necrosis and inflammation) (Karas and Clarkson, 2003). A placebo-controlled 6-month trial of HRT from our laboratory supports the timing hypothesis since we observed significant reductions in resting and stress-induced blood pressure and vascular resistance with HRT in women who had been postmenopausal for less than 5 years, and no beneficial effects in women postmenopausal for more than 5 years (Brownley et al, 2004). Most women in the observational studies initiated HRT at or near the menopausal transition, while those enrolled into the WHI were, on average, 12 years postmenopausal, and thus, likely to be in the more advanced stages of atherosclerotic progression (Harman et al, 2005). Taken together, the animal and human data suggest that initiating HRT early in the perimenopause is a critical determinant of estradiol's beneficial effects regarding cardiovascular disease risk.

Given the age and conditions of its subjects, the International Menopause Society (IMS) concluded that "the WHI should not be considered a primary prevention trial of HRT to prevent cardiovascular disease . . . at present, the only valid studies of HRT for cardioprotection of women in the menopausal transition are the epidemiological and observational studies that generally agree with laboratory and animal studies, indicating cardioprotection by estrogen initiated in women during the menopausal transition" (Wright, 2004). The IMS report also indicates the need to study other routes of hormone administration since the WHI used only one formulation (oral conjugated equine estrogen and MPA) and differential effects of oral versus transdermal estradiol on measures of cardiovascular risk are well established. Moreover, the progestin used in the WHI, MPA, is particularly antagonistic (among progestins) to the beneficial cardiovascular effects of estradiol (Adams et al, 1997).

Although ERT and HRT have long been known to increase bone mineral density (North American Menopause Society, 2006), it is of interest here that the WHI was also the first large-scale controlled trial to demonstrate a significant reduction in hip fracture of about 35% associated with ERT and HRT use (Anderson et al, 2004; Cauley et al, 2003). While the controversy currently surrounding the use of ERT or HRT in postmenopausal women has limited its use in the prevention of osteoporosis, that estrogen can prevent bone loss in postmenopausal women at doses lower than those required to stimulate classic target tissues such as breast and uterus (Prestwood et al, 2003), suggests a more favorable cost/benefit ratio for estrogen in the treatment of osteoporosis. Controlled trials will be needed in order to confirm this. It should also be noted that there are a number of other available FDA approved pharmacotherapy options that have also proven to be efficacious in the treatment of osteoporosis, these include bisphosphonates, calcitonin, and parathyroid hormone medications (see Alexander, 2009 for review). Additionally, adequate calcium and vitamin D, appropriate physical activity, smoking cessation, and reduced alcohol intake may increase bone mass but also slow bone loss and reduce fracture risk throughout life (North American Menopause Society, 2006; Raisz, 2005).

3.3 Conclusions and Future Research Directions

With our greater understanding now of the factors that likely contributed to the findings in the WHI trial, any conclusions about the prophylactic benefit of ERT/HRT for cardiovascular risk in perimenopausal or healthy postmenopausal women are precluded. Consequently, with the appreciation in the field of behavioral medicine for identifying individual difference characteristics that predict both disease risk and response to intervention, we have reached a new dawn in research related to ERT/HRT in peri- and postmenopausal women. Future behavioral medicine research aimed at identifying behavioral phenotypes of perimenopausal women that would predict the beneficial effects of ERT on both cardiovascular and affective regulation could preserve and refine the use of a potentially valuable therapeutic option, with consequent enormous public health impact.

4 General Conclusions

It seems remarkable that not even two decades have passed since it was considered acceptable to exclude women from clinical research on the basis of "noise" that might be introduced into the data attributable to female reproductive hormones. Coincident with the 1993 National Institutes of Health (NIH) Revitalization Act directing the NIH to establish guidelines for inclusion of women and minorities in clinical research, we have had a burgeoning of research related to reproductive health in women. While there is a good deal of sobering information included in this chapter regarding the influence of reproductive hormones and reproductive stages on women's mental and physical health, the research summarized here clearly indicates that female reproductive hormones do not constitute "noise," but instead serve as important pathogenic triggers and mediators of mental and medical illness in vulnerable women. As such, however, they provide the potential for therapeutic targets for prevention and treatment of women's mental and medical disorders. As we move forward into the next two decades, the field of behavioral medicine is currently poised to lead the way in developing individualized approaches aimed at both the prevention and the treatment of women's mental and physical health impairments. This might come in the form of understanding the behavioral and historical context that increases vulnerability to reproductive hormone-related effects on mood or physical health. Certainly the context dependency of steroid action is well established in animal models (see Rubinow and Schmidt, 2006 for discussion). Or this might come in the form of

identifying behavioral phenotypes, such as stress reactivity profiles, that predict response to intervention. Thus, the "noise" has become a melody of hope that the next two decades will provide as much information about improving the lives of women's health as the prior two decades have provided about the causes of our illnesses.

Acknowledgments This research was supported by NIH grants R01 MH051246 and R01 MH081837 to Susan S. Girdler; NIH grants R01 HL084442 and P01 DA022446 (Project 2) to Kathleen C. Light; UNC GCRC support RR00046 and CTSA 1RR025747.

References

Adams, M. R., Register, T. C., Golden, L. L., Wagner, J. D., and Williams, J. K. (1997). Medroxyprogesterone acetate antagonizes inhibitory effects of conjugated equine estrogens on coronary artery atherosclerosis. *Arterioscler Thromb Vasc Biol, 17,* 217–221.

Alexander, I. M. (2009). Pharmacotherapeutic management of osteoprosis and osteopenia. *Nurse Pract, 34,* 30–40.

Altemus, M., Redwine, L., Leong, Y., Frye, C., Porges, S. et al (2001). Responses to laboratory psychosocial stress in postpartum women. *Psychosom Med, 63,* 814–821.

American Psychiatric Association (1994). Diagnostic and Statistical Manual of Mental Disorders, Fourth Edition (DSM-IV)

Anderson, G. L., Limacher, M., Assaf, A. R., Bassford, T., Beresford, S. A., et al (2004). Effects of conjugated equine estrogen in postmenopausal women with hysterectomy: the Women's Health Initiative randomized controlled trial. *JAMA, 291,* 1701–1712.

Bartz, J. A., and Hollander, E. (2008). Oxytocin and experimental therapeutics in autism spectrum disorders. *Prog Brain Res, 170,* 451–462.

Barbaccia, M. L., Concas, A., Serra, M., and Biggio, G. (1998). Stress and neurosteroids in adult and aged rats. *Exp Gerontol, 33,* 697–712.

Barrazza, J. A., and Zak, P. J. (2009). Empathy towards strangers triggers oxytocin release and subsequent generosity. *Ann NY Acad Sci, 1167,* 182–189.

Bitran, D., Klibansky, D. A., and Martin, G. A. (2000). The neurosteroid pregnanolone prevents the anxiogenic-like effect of inescapable shock in the rat. *Psychopharmacol (Berl), 151,* 31–37.

Bromberger, J. T., Kravitz, H. M., Matthews, K., Youk, A., Brown, C. et al (2009). Predictors of first lifetime episodes of major depression in midlife women. *Psychol Med, 29,* 55–64.

Brownley, K. A., Hinderliter, A. L., West, S. G., Grewen, K. M., Steege, J. F. et al (2004). Cardiovascular effects of six months of hormone replacement therapy vs. placebo: differences associated with years since menopause. *Am J Obstet Gynecol*, *190*, 1052–1058.

Bunevicius, R., Hinderliter, A. L., Leserman, J., Pedersen, C. A., Girdler, S. S. (2005). Histories of sexual abuse are associated with differential effects of clonidine on autonomic function in women with premenstrual dysphoric disorder. *Biol Psychol*, *69*, 281–96.

Bush, T. L. (1996). Evidence for primary and secondary prevention of coronary artery didease in women taking oestrogen replacement therapy. *Eur Heart J*, *17*(Suppl D), 9–14.

Carter, C. S. (1998). Neuroendocrine perspectives on social attachment and love. *Psychoneuroendocri nology*, 23, 779–818.

Cauley, J. A., Robbins, J., Chen, A., Cummings, S. R., Jackson, R. D., et al. (2003). Effects of estrogen plus progestin on risk of fracture and bone mineral density: the Women's Health Initiative randomized trial. *JAMA, 290*, 1729–1738.

Champagne, F. A., Weaver, I. C. G., Diorio, J,. Sharma, S., and Meaney, M. J. (2003). Natural variations in maternal care are associated with estrogen receptor-alpha expression and estrogen sensitivity in the medial preoptic area. *Endocrinology*, *144*, 4720–4724.

Chen, Y. W., and Dilsaver, S. C. (1996). Lifetime rates of suicide attempts among subjects with bipolar and unipolar disorders relative to subjects with other Axis I disorders. *Biol Psychiatry*, *39*, 896–899.

Choleris, E., Gustafsson, J.-A., Korach, K. S., Muglia, L. J., Pfaff, D. W. et al (2003). An estrogen-dependent four-gene micronet regulating social recognition: a study with oxytocin and estrogen receptor-alpha and –beta knockout mice. *Proc Natl Acad Sci USA*, *100*, 6192–6197.

Cleaveland, C. R., Rangno, R. E., and Shand, D. G. (1972). A standardized isoproterenol sensitivity test. The effects of sinus arrhythmia, atropine, and propranolol. *Arch Intern Med*, *130*, 47–52.

Cohen, L. S., Soares, C. N., Otto, M. W., Sweeney, B. H., Liberman, R. F. et al (2002). Prevalence and predictors of premenstrual dysphoric disorder (PMDD) in older premenopausal women – The Harvard Study of Moods and Cycles. *J Affect Disord*, *70*, 125–132.

Cohen, L. S., Soares, C. N., Poitras, J. R., Prouty, J., Alexandera, A. B. et al (2003). Short-term use of estradiol for depression in perimenopausal and postmenopausal women: a preliminary report. *Am J Psychiatry*, *160*, 1519–1522.

Cohen, L. S., Soares, C. N., Vitonis, A. F., Otto, M. W., and Harlow, B. L. (2006). Risk for new onset of depression during the menopausal transition: the Harvard study of moods and cycles. *Arch Gen Psychiatry*, *63*, 385–390.

Colditz, G. A., Willet, W. C., Stampfer, M. J., Rosner, B., Speizer, F. E. et al (1987). Menopause and the risk of coronary heart disease in women. *N Engl J Med*, *316*, 1105–1110.

Cummings, S.R., Kelsey, J. L., Nevitt, M., O'Dowd, K. (1985). Epidemiology of osteoporosis and osteoporotic fractures. *Epidemiol Rev*, *7*, 178–208.

Cummings, S. R., and Melton III, L. J. (2002). Epidemiology and outcomes of osteoporotic fractures. *Lancet*, *359*, 1761–1767.

Deecher, D. C., and Dorries, K. (2007). Understanding the pathophysiology of vasomotor symptoms (hot flushes and night sweats) that occur in perimenopause, menopause, and postmenopause life stages. *Arch Womens Ment Health*, *10*, 247–257.

Detillion, C. E., Craft, T. K., Glasper, E. R., Prendergast, B. J., and DeVries, A. C. (2004). Social facilitation of wound healing. *Psychoneuroendocrinology*, *29*, 1004–1011.

DeVries, A. C., Craft, T. K., Glasper, E. R., Neigh, G. N., and Alexander, J. K. (2007). Curt P. Richter award winner: social influences on stress responses and health. *Psychoneuroendocrinology*, *32*, 587–603.

Ditzen, B., Schaer, M., Gabriel, B., Bodenmann, G., Ehlert, U. et al (2009). Intranasal oxytocin increases positive communication and reduces cortisol levels during couple conflict. *Biol Psychiatry, 65*, 728–731.

Ferguson, J. N., Aldag, J. M., Insel, T. R., and Young, L. J. (2001). Oxytocin in the medial amygdala is essential for social recognition in the mouse. *J Neurosci*, *21*, 8278–8285.

Ferguson, J. N., Young, L. J., Hearn, E. F., Matzuk, M. M., Insel, T. R. et al (2000). Social amnesia in mice lacking the oxytocin gene. *Nat Genet*, *25*, 284–288.

Ferris, C. F., Kulkarni, P., Sullivan, J. M., Harder, J. A., Messenger, T. L. et al (2005). Pup suckling is more rewarding than cocaine: evidence from fMRI and three dimensional computational analysis. *J Neurosci*, *25*, 149–156.

Fewtrell, M. S., Loh, K. L., Blake, A., Ridout, D. A., and Hawdon, J. (2006). Randomised, double blind trial of oxytocin nasal spray in mothers expressing breast milk for preterm infants. *Arch Dis Child Fetal Neonatal Ed*, *91*, F169–F174.

Frank, R. T. (1931). The hormonal causes of premenstrual tension. *Arch Neurol Psychiatry*, *26*, 1053–1057.

Freeman, E. W., Sammel, M. D., Lin, H., and Nelson, D. B. (2006). Association of hormones and menopausal status with depressed mood in women with no history of depression. *Arch Gen Psychiatry*, *63*, 375–382.

Freeman, E. W., Sammel, M. D., Liu, L., Gracia, C. R., Nelson, D. B. et al (2004). Hormones and menopausal status as predictors of depression in women in transition to menopause. *Arch Gen Psychiatry*, *61*, 62–70.

Frey, B. N., Lord, C., and Soares, C. N. (2008). Depression during menopausal transition: a review of treatment strategies and pathophysiological correlates. *Menopause Int*, *14*, 123–128.

Girdler, S. S., Hinderliter, A., and Light, K. C. (1993). Peripheral adrenergic receptor contributions to cardiovascular reactivity: influence of race and gender. *J Psychosom Res, 37*, 177–193.

Girdler, S. S., Leserman, J., Bunevicius, R., Klatzkin, R., Pedersen, C. A. et al (2007). Persistent alterations in cardiovascular and neuroendocrine profiles in women with abuse histories: influence of premenstrual dysphoric disorder. *Health Psychol, 26*, 201–213.

Girdler, S. S., Pedersen, C. A., Stern R. A., and Light, K. C. (1993). Menstrual cycle and premenstrual syndrome: modifiers of cardiovascular reactivity in women. *Health Psychol, 12*, 180–192.

Girdler, S. S., Pedersen, C., Straneva, P. A., Leserman, J., Stanwyck, C. L. et al (1998). Dysregulation of cardiovascular and neuroendocrine responses to stress in premenstrual dysphoric disorder. *Psychiatry Res, 81*, 163–178.

Girdler, S. S., Sherwood, A., Hinderliter, A. L., Leserman, J., Costello, N. L. et al (2003). Biological correlates of abuse in women with premenstrual dysphoric disorder and healthy controls. *Psychosom Med, 65*, 849–856.

Girdler, S. S., Straneva, P. A., Light, K. C., Pedersen, C. A., and Morrow, A. L. (2001). Allopregnanolone levels and reactivity to mental stress in premenstrual dysphoric disorder. *Biol Psychiatry, 49*, 788–797.

Gordon, I., Zagoory-Sharon, O., Schneiderman, I., Leckman, J. F., Weller, A. et al (2008). Oxytocin and cortisol in romantically unattached young adults: associations with bonding and psychological distress. *Psychophysiology, 45*, 349–352.

Grewen, K., Davenport, R., and Light, K. (2010). An investigation of plasma and salivary oxytocin responses in breast- and formula-feeding mothers of infants. *Psychophysiology*, Jan 22. [Epub ahead of print], PMID: 20102537.

Grewen, K. M., Girdler, S. S., Amico, J. A., and Light, K. C. (2005). Effects of partner support on oxytocin, cortisol, norepinephrine and blood pressure before & after warm partner contact. *Psychosom Med, 67*, 531–538.

Grewen, K. M., Light, K. C., Mechlin, B., and Girdler, S. S. (2008). Ethnicity is associated with alterations in oxytocin relationships to pain sensitivity in women. *Ethn Health, 13*, 219–241.

Guastella, A. J., Howard, A. L, Dadds, M. R., Mitchell, P., and Carson, D. S. (2009). A randomized controlled trial of intranasal oxytocin as an adjunct to exposure therapy for social anxiety disorder. *Psychoneuroendocrinology, 34*, 917–923.

Guo, A. L., Petraglia, F., Criscuolo, M., Ficarra, G., Nappie, R. E. et al (1995). Evidence for a role of neurosteroids in modulation of diurnal changes and acute stress-induced corticosterone secretion in rats. *Gynecol Endocrinol, 9*, 1–7.

Halbreich, U. (2008). Selective serotonin reuptake inhibitors and initial oral contraceptives for the treatment of PMDD: effective but not enough. *CNS Spectr, 13*, 566–572.

Halbreich, U., Endicott, J., Goldstein, S., and Nee, J. (1986). Premenstrual changes and changes in gonadal hormones. *Acta Psychiatr Scand, 74*, 576–586.

Harmon, A. C., Huhman, K. L., Moore, T. O., and Albers, H. E. (2002). Oxytocin inhibits aggression in female Syrian hamsters. *J Neuroendocrinol, 14*, 963–969.

Harman, S. M., Naftolin, F., Brinton, E. A., and Judelson, D. R. (2005). Is the estrogen controversy over? Deconstructing the Women's Health Initiative study: a critical evaluation of the evidence. *Ann NY Acad Sci, 1052*, 43–56.

Heim, C, Young, L. J., Newport, D. J., Mletzko, T. Miller, A. H. et al (2008). Lower CSF oxytocin concentrations in women with a history of childhood abuse. *Mol Psychiatry* Epub; doi:10.1038/mp.2008.112.

Hirshoren, N., Tzoran, I., Makrienko, I., Edoute, Y., Plawner, M. M. et al (2002). Menstrual cycle effects on the neurohumoral and autonomic nervous systems regulating the cardiovascular system. *J Clin Endocrinol Metab, 87*, 1569–1575.

Holt-Lunstad, J., Birmingham, W. A., and Light, K. C. (2008). Influence of a "warm touch" support enhancement intervention among married couples on ambulatory blood pressure, oxytocin, alpha amylase, and cortisol. *Psychosom Med, 70*, 976–985.

Horvat-Gordon, M., Granger, D. A., Schwartz, E. B., Nelson, V. J., and Kivlighan, K. T. (2005). Oxytocin is not a valid biomarker when measured in saliva by immunoassay. *Physiol Behav, 84*, 445–448.

Howards, P. P., Schisterman, E. F., Wactawski-Wende, J., Reschke, J. E., Frazer, A. A. et al (2009). Timing clinic visits to phases of the menstrual cycle by using a fertility monitor: The BioCycle Study. *Am J Epidemiol, 169*, 105–112.

Insel, T. R., and Young, L. J. (2001). The neurobiology of attachment. *Nature Rev (Neurosci), 2*, 129–136.

Kalantaridou, S. N., Naka, K. K., Bechlioulis, A., Makrigiannakis, A., Michalis, L. et al (2006). Premature ovarian failure, endothelial dysfunction and estrogen-progestin replacement. *Trends Endocrinol Metab, 17*, 101–109.

Karas, R. H., and Clarkson, T. B. (2003). Considerations in interpreting the cardiovascular effects of hormone replacement therapy observed in the WHI: timing is everything. *Menopausal Med, 10*, 8–12.

Kirschbaum, C., Pirke, K. M., and Hellhammer, D. H. (1993). The Trier Social Stress Test – a tool for investigating psychobiological stress responses in a laboratory setting. *Neuropsychobiology, 28*, 76–81.

Klatzkin, R. R., Morrow, A. L., Light, K. C., Pedersen, C. A., and Girdler, S. S. (2006). Associations of histories of depression and PMDD diagnosis with allopregnanolone concentrations following the oral administration of micronized progesterone. *Psychoneuroendocrinology, 31*, 1208–1219.

Lee, K., Jessop, H., Suswillo, R., Zaman, G., and Lanyon, L. (2003). Endocrinology: bone adaptation requires oestrogen receptor-alpha. *Nature, 424*, 389.

Light, K. C., Grewen, K. M., and Amico, J. A. (2005a). More frequent partner hugs and higher oxytocin levels are linked to lower blood pressure and heart rate in premenopausal women. *Biol Psychol, 69*, 5–21.

Light, K. C., Grewen, K. M., Amico, J. A., Boccia, M., Brownley, K. et al (2004). Deficits in plasma oxytocin responses and increased negative affect, stress, and blood pressure in mothers with cocaine exposure during pregnancy. *Addict Behav, 29*, 1541–1564.

Light, K. C., Grewen, K. M., Amico, J. A., Brownley, K. A., West, S. G. et al (2005b). Oxytocinergic activity is linked to lower blood pressure and vascular resistance during stress in postmenopausal women on estrogen replacement. *Horm Behav, 47*, 540–548.

Light, K. C., Smith, T. E., Johns, J. M., Brownley, K. A., Hofheimer, J. A. et al (2000). Oxytocin responsivity in mothers of infants: a preliminary study of relationships with blood pressure during laboratory stress and normal ambulatory activity. *Health Psychol, 19*, 560–567.

Lombardi, I., Luisi, S., Quirici, B., Monteleone, P., Benardi, F. et al (2004). Adrenal response to adrenocorticotropic hormone stimulation in patients with premenstrual syndrome. *Gynecol Endocrinol, 18*, 79–87.

Marvan, M. L., and Cortes-Iniestra, S. (2001). Women's beliefs about the prevalence of premenstrual syndrome and biases in recall of premenstrual changes. *Health Psychol, 20*, 276–280.

McMurray, M. S., Joyner, P. W., Middleton, C. W., Jarrett, T. M., Elliott, D. L. et al (2008). Intergenerational effects of cocaine on maternal aggressive behavior and brain oxytocin in rat dams. *Stress, 11*, 398–410.

Meinlschmidt, G., and Heim, C. (2007). Sensitivity to intranasal oxytocin in adult men with early parental separation. *Biol Psychiatry, 61*, 1109–1111.

Meyer-Lindenberg, A. (2008). Impact of prosocial neuropeptides on human brain function. *Prog Brain Res, 170*, 463–470.

Mezzacappa, E. S., and Katkin, E. (2002). Breastfeeding is associated with reduced perceived stress and negative mood in mothers. *Health Psychol, 21*, 187–193.

Miller, W. (1978). Survival and ambulation following hip fracture. *J Bone Joint Surg, 60A*: 930–934.

Moller-Leimkuhler, A. M. (2007). Gender differences in cardiovascular disease and comorbid depression. *Dialogues Clin Neurosci, 9*, 71–83.

Monteleone, P., Luisi, S., Tonetti, A., Bernardi, F., Genazzani, A. D. et al (2000). Allopregnanolone concentrations and premenstrual syndrome. *Eur J Endocrinol, 142*, 269–273.

Morhenn, V. B., Park, J. W., Piper, E., and Zak, P. J. (2008). Monetary sacrifice among strangers is mediated by endogenous oxytocin release after physical contact. *Evol Human Behav, 29*, 375–383.

Morrison, M. F., Kallan, M. J., Ten Have, T., Katz, I., Tweedy, K. et al (2004). Lack of efficacy of

estradiol for depression in postmenopausal women: a randomized, controlled trial. *Biol Psychiatry, 55*, 406–412.

North American Menopause Society (2006). Management of osteoporosis in postmenopausal women: 2006 position statement of the North American Menopause Society. *Menopause, 13*, 340–367.

Pedersen, C. A., and Boccia, M. L. (2002). Oxytocin links mothering received, mothering bestowed and adult stress responses. *Stress, 5*, 259–267.

Petersson, M. (2002). Cardiovascular effects of oxytocin. *Prog Brain Res, 139*, 281–288.

Porcu, P., O'Buckley, T. K., Alward, S. E., Marx, C. E., Shampine, L. L. et al (2009). Simultaneous quantification of GABAergic $3\alpha,5\alpha/3\alpha,5\beta$ neuroactive steroids in human and rat serum. *Steroids, 74*, 463–473.

Prestwood, K.M., Kenny, A.M., Kleppinger, A., and Kulldorff, M. (2003). Ultralow-dose micronized 17beta-estradiol and bone density and bond metabolism in older women: a randomized controlled trial. *JAMA, 290*, 1042–1048.

Purdy, R. H., Morrow, A. L., Moore, P. H., Jr., and Paul, S. M. (1991). Stress-induced elevations of γ-aminobutyric acid type A receptor-active steroids in the rat brain. *Proc Natl Acad Sci, 88*, 4553–4557.

Raisz, L. G. (2005). Pathogenesis of osteoporosis: concepts, conflicts, and prospects. *J Clin Invest, 115*, 3318–3325.

Rossouw, J. E., Anderson, G. L., Prentice, R. L., LaCroix, A. Z., Kooperberg, C. (2002). Risks and benefits of estrogen plus progestin in healthy postmenopausal women: principal results from the Women's Health Initiative randomized controlled trial. *JAMA, 288*, 321–333.

Rubinow, D. R., and Schmidt, P. J. (2006). Gonadal steroid regulation of mood: the lessons of premenstrual syndrome. *Front Neuroendocrinol, 27*, 210–216.

Schmidt, P. J., Haq, N., and Rubinow, D. R. (2004). A longitudinal evaluation of the relationship between reproductive status and mood in perimenopausal women. *Am J Psychiatry, 161*, 2238–2244.

Schmidt, P. J., Nieman, L. K., Grover, G. N., Muller, K. L., Meriam, G. R. et al (1991). Lack of effect of induced menses on symptoms in women with premenstrual syndrome. *N Engl J Med, 324*, 1174–1179.

Shively, C. A., Register, T. C., Adams, M. R., Golden, D. L., Willard, S. L. et al (2008). Depressive behavior and coronary artery atherogenesis in adult female cynomolgus monkeys. *Psychosom Med, 70*, 637–645.

Soares, C. N., Almeida, O. P., Joffe, H., and Cohen, L. S. (2001). Efficacy of estradiol for the treatment of depressive disorders in premenopausal women: a double-blind, randomized, placebo-controlled trial. *Arch Gen Psychiatry, 58*, 529–534.

Soares, C. N., Arsenio H., Joffe, H., Bankier, B., Cassano, P. et al (2006). Escitalopram versus ethinyl estradiol and norethindrone acetate for symptomatic peri- and postmenopausal women: impact on depression, vasomotor symptoms, sleep, and quality of life. *Menopause, 13*, 780–786.

Soules, M. R., Sherman, S., Parrott, E., Rebar, R., Santoro, N. et al (2001). Stages of reproductive aging workshop (STRAW). *J Womens Health Gend Based Med, 10*, 843–848

Stampfer, M. J., Colditz, G. A., Willett, W. C., Manson, J. E., Rosner, B., et al. (1991). Postmenopausal estrogen therapy and cardiovascular disease. Ten-year follow-up from the nurses' health study. *N Engl J Med, 325*, 756–762.

Strohle, A., Pasini, A., Romeo, E., Hermann, B. Spalletta, G. et al (2000). Fluoxetine decreases concentrations of 3α,5α-tetrahydrodeoxycorticosterone (THDOC) in major depression. *J Psychiatry Res, 34*, 183–186.

Szeto, A., Nation, D. A., Mendez, A. J., Dominguez-Bendala, J., Brooks, L. G. et al (2008). Oxytocin attenuates NADPH-dependent superoxide activity and IL-6 secretion in macrophages and vascular cells. *Am J Physiol Endocrinol Metab, 295*, E1495-1501

Tops, M., van Peer, J. M., Korf, J., Wijers, A. A., and Tucker, D. M. (2007). Anxiety, cortisol, and attachment predict plasma oxytocin. *Psychophysiology, 44*, 444–449.

Turner, R., Altemus, M., Enos, T., Cooper, B., and McGuinness, T. (1999). Preliminary research on plasma oxytocin in healthy, normal cycling women: investigating emotion and interpersonal distress. *Psychiatry, 62*, 97–113.

Uvnäs-Moberg, K. (1998). Antistress pattern induced by oxytocin. *News Physiol Sci, 13*, 22–25.

Uzunova, V., Sampson, L., and Uzunov, D. P. (2006). Relevance of endogenous 3α-reduced neurosteroids to depression and antidepressant action. *Psychopharmacology, 186*, 351–361.

Winslow, J. T., Noble, P. L., Lyons, C. K., Sterk, S. M., and Insel, T. R. (2003). Rearing effects on cerebrospinal fluid oxytocin concentration and social buffering in rhesus monkeys. *Neuropsychopharmacology, 28*, 910–918.

Wismer Fries, A. B., Ziegler, T. E., Kurian, J. R., Jakoris, S., and Pollak, S. D. (2005). Early experience in humans is associated with changes in neuropeptides critical for regulating social behavior. *Proc Natl Acad Sci USA, 102*, 17237–17240.

Wright, J. (2004). Guidelines for the hormone treatment of women in the menopausal transition and beyond. Position Statement by the Executive Committee of the International Menopause Society. *Maturitas, 48*, 27–31.

Yildirir, A., Aybar, F., Kabakci, G., Yarali, H., and Oto, A. (2006). Heart rate variability in young women with polycystic ovary syndrome. *Ann Noninvasive Electrocardiol, 11*, 306–312.

Young, L. J. (2002). The neurobiology of social recognition, approach, and avoidance. *Biol Psychiatry, 51*, 18–26.

Zak, P. J., Stanton, A., and Ahmadi, S. (2007). Oxytocin increases generosity in humans. *PLoS One* 2: e1128. doi:10.1371/journal.pone.0001128.

Zweifel, J. E., and O'Brien, W. H. (1997). A meta-analysis of the effect of hormone replacement therapy upon depressed mood. *Psychoneuroendocrinology, 22*, 189–212.

Chapter 39

Aging and Behavioral Medicine

Brenda W.J.H. Penninx and Nicole Vogelzangs

1 The Importance of Aging

In the Western world, the old and especially the oldest of the old comprise the fastest growing segment of our population. This is due to a decreasing trend in the number of children born as well as to dramatic changes in mortality leading to increased life expectancy. Life expectancy has consistently been higher for women than for men. Consequently, the elderly population is composed of more women than men and, as a result, in absolute terms aging is affecting women more than men.

Aging has a profound impact on the individual. For the most part, individual aging is associated with many adverse changes in human anatomy and physiology. Consequences of these changes are, for instance, losses in the sense of balance and movement, poorer hearing and vision, slower reactions, and weaker muscles. For a large part of adult life, people are normally provided with "biological" reserves. In later life, these reserves are reduced, which can cause weakening of one or another biological function essential to life. As a result, conditions such as heart disease, cancer, respiratory infection, or osteoarthritis may arise. The biological age-related changes and the consequent development of degenerative and chronic conditions have a large impact on the physical functioning and behaviors of older persons. The number of older persons with difficulties in mobility and activities of daily living increases dramatically with increasing age.

In addition to the impact on biological and physical areas, other aspects of life are affected as well, not always in an unfavorable way. Individual aging is accompanied by a series of social and behavioral transitions, some entered into voluntarily, some imposed by circumstances. In the next sections, we will indicate for various domains of behavioral factors (social function, psychological function, and lifestyle behaviors) to what extent they are impacted by aging, and how these behavioral factors are associated with health outcomes in an older population. When describing the association between behavioral factors and health outcomes, we will place special emphasis on specific aging-related health outcomes, such as physical decline, frailty, and cognitive impairment. Finally, we will make several specific considerations that one has to keep in mind when examining or interpreting behavioral medicine in the older population.

B.W.J.H. Penninx (✉)
Department of Psychiatry, VU University Medical Center, AJ Ernststraat 887, 1081 HL, Amsterdam, The Netherlands
e-mail: b.penninx@vumc.nl

A. Steptoe (ed.), *Handbook of Behavioral Medicine*, DOI 10.1007/978-0-387-09488-5_39,
© Springer Science+Business Media, LLC 2010

2 Aging and Behavioral Aspects

2.1 Social Function in Old Age

Aging is generally associated with dramatic changes in social roles and personal relationships. Around the age of 65 most individuals retire. Irrespective of whether retirement is encountered as a welcome or an unpleasant life event, it involves two developmental challenges: adjustment to the loss of the work role and the social ties of work and the development of a satisfactory post-retirement lifestyle (van Solinge and Henkens, 2008). Besides possible adjustment problems this may bring about, the change from a working to a retired life evidently can be associated with large behavioral changes that influence social and physical activities, food intake, and alcohol consumption.

Another important element of aging is the loss by death of age-peers such as siblings and friends, but also of one's own partner. Some studies indicate that after the death of a spouse, the widowed on average report a reduction in social engagement (Bennett, 2005) and leisure activity (Janke et al, 2008). Furthermore, widowhood has systematically been shown to increase the risk of developing consequent depression and anxiety disorders (Onrust and Cuijpers, 2006), which might be especially true for men (van Grootheest et al, 1999). Increasing age also brings changes in relationship needs, for example, as the result of increasing impairment. Older adults may become more dependent on others when they lose the ability to fulfill certain social or instrumental tasks themselves. The existing balance in their relationships may be disrupted, introducing strain and discomfort. Widowhood, the need for instrumental support, and the loss of personal relationships might cause feelings of loneliness, dependency, and helplessness. Studies indeed show that loneliness increases with age due to increasing disability and decreasing social integration (Jylha, 2004). Although only a minority of older people experience severe loneliness, perhaps up to one-third may experience some degree of loneliness (Grenade

and Boldy, 2008). In general, when adjustment to the burdening circumstances related to aging is inadequate, an older person might experience substantial psychological stress and consequent symptoms of depression or anxiety (e.g., Cacioppo et al, 2006).

Table 39.1 shows some social aspects of aging in a community-based random sample of over 3000 older men and women aged 55 through 85 years who participated in the Longitudinal Aging Study Amsterdam (LASA) in the Netherlands. These results indeed show that as people are older, more persons are without a partner and network size and emotional support decrease, whereas loneliness increases. Interestingly, while at old age much more women are without a partner, changes in network size, social support, and loneliness show rather similar patterns for men and women. This is consistent with the finding that specifically men are affected by the loss of their spouse, possibly because their emotional well-being and social engagement is more centered around marriage, while women tend to have additional close relationships (Dykstra and de Jong Gierveld, 2004).

2.2 Psychological Function in Old Age

The most common psychological problems experienced in old age are depressive and anxiety symptoms. Prevalence rates of depressive and anxiety problems vary considerably depending on the sample studied and methods used. Studies in clinical settings generally find much higher prevalences than studies in community settings, and studies applying psychiatric diagnostic criteria for depression or anxiety disorders find much lower prevalences than studies using symptom checklists. It is possible to score relatively high on a symptom checklist without meeting diagnostic criteria for depressive or anxiety disorders. In fact, symptom checklists identify for the largest part persons who do not fulfill the diagnostic severity threshold

Table 39.1 Presence of social, psychological, and lifestyle factors in older men and women in different age groups in the Longitudinal Aging Study Amsterdam (LASA)

	Men			Women		
	55–65 years (n=490)	65–75 years (n=456)	75–85 years (n=560)	55–65 years (n=526)	65–75 years (n=517)	75–85 years (n=558)
Social function						
With partner (%)	88.6	86.0	70.0	76.0	57.6	28.0
Network size (mean no. of members)	15.1 (9.2)	13.6 (7.3)	12.6 (8.3)	15.6 (8.4)	14.1 (8.3)	12.0 (7.5)
Lack of emotional support (%)	39.3	40.1	44.2	21.4	29.4	38.4
Loneliness (0–11 scale)[a]	1.6 (2.1)	1.8 (2.3)	2.5 (2.7)	1.7 (2.4)	2.2 (2.7)	2.8 (2.8)
Psychological function						
Major depressive disorder[b] (%)	1.2	1.1	0.5	3.4	3.5	2.0
Subthreshold depression[c] (%)	8.2	8.1	13.2	9.7	14.1	21.0
Panic disorder[b] (%)	0.4	0.2	0.2	1.5	1.5	0.4
Social phobia[b] (%)	1.2	0.4	1.1	2.1	1.5	1.8
Generalized anxiety disorder[b] (%)	1.8	2.0	2.1	4.6	5.2	4.1
Subthreshold anxiety[d] (%)	5.3	4.2	4.5	6.7	7.7	7.2
Lifestyle behaviors						
Low physical activity (%)	13.2	11.9	27.1	6.2	15.3	32.2
Smoking						
Former (%)	54.4	60.2	62.7	32.6	30.5	24.5
Current (%)	37.6	33.6	30.3	23.5	16.7	10.2
Alcohol use						
Moderate (one or two drinks a day) (%)	78.9	76.4	74.3	77.0	69.7	63.8
Excessive (three or more drinks a day) (%)	12.5	7.8	4.2	1.7	1.1	0.2

[a]Measured by de Jong Gierveld loneliness scale
[b]1-Year prevalence rates based on diagnostic DSM criteria using the Diagnostic Interview Schedule
[c]Indicated by Center for Epidemiologic Studies Depression Scale ≥ 16, but no major depression diagnosis
[d]Indicated by Hospital Anxiety and Depression Scale – Anxiety subscale ≥ 8, but no anxiety disorder diagnosis.

of psychiatric depressive or anxiety disorders. This condition is often referred to as "subthreshold depression/anxiety." As confirmed in several aging studies, major depressive disorder and anxiety disorder (mainly comprised of panic disorder, social phobia, and generalized anxiety disorder) are affecting about 2–4% of the community-dwelling population (Beekman et al, 1999). Contrary to what some people might expect, psychiatrically defined depression and anxiety disorders appear to be less prevalent among older adults than among young and middle-aged adults. Table 39.1 shows the 1-year prevalence rates of depressive and anxiety disorders among participants of the community-based LASA study (see also Beekman et al, 1995; Beekman et al, 1998). These results confirm a prevalence of 1–4% for the main depression

and anxiety disorders in old age, and much higher prevalence rates of subthreshold depression and anxiety symptoms. Also, whereas the prevalence of psychiatric disorders does not clearly increase over time, the rates of subthreshold symptoms do. It is important to realize that a large proportion (at least 50%) of older persons with a depressive or anxiety disorder have had prior episodes during earlier phases of their lives. Thus, depression and anxiety disorders in old age most often represent recurring episodes of early-onset disorders. As in younger age groups, older women generally show higher rates of depression and anxiety disorders than older men. Whether the concepts of depressive and anxiety disorders and symptoms are entirely similar in an older population compared to a younger population has not been widely examined. Some studies indicate that the symptoms of moderate to severe depression presented to the clinician are rather similar across older persons and persons in midlife. However, some subtle differences in symptom experience across age groups have been described. Apathy (symptoms of non-interactiveness) appears to be a little more frequent in later age than in younger age, with psychomotor disturbances being more obvious in older persons (Mehta et al, 2008).

2.3 Lifestyle Behaviors in Old Age

Aging has generally rather profound effects on lifestyle behaviors as well, either due to changes in daytime activities (e.g., after retirement or widowhood) or as a result of the considerable increase in disabilities and chronic diseases associated with aging. Specifically, the degree of physical activity may decrease due to physical decline, acquired chronic conditions, and accompanying pain. But other lifestyle behaviors might also be affected. Smoking is an important accelerator of the aging process. In general, the percentage of persons smoking decreases with increasing age, but this may in large part be due to the selective survival of non-smokers, or due to the fact that certain older persons stop smoking because of health reasons. It is important to note, however, that those persons who smoke most probably have been smoking a large part of their lives. This accumulating effect of lifetime smoking might therefore be specifically detrimental in older persons. As with smoking, increasing morbidity in older adults may explain the age-related decline in alcohol consumption after the age of 65 (Ferreira and Weems, 2008). Lifestyle behaviors within the LASA population of community-dwelling older persons are presented in Table 39.1. In line with expectations, physical activity decreases with increasing age, the proportion of current smokers declines, while the relative proportion of former smokers increases, and both moderate and excessive alcohol consumption are reduced in the oldest age group.

3 Impact of Behavioral Factors on Health Outcomes in the Older Population

3.1 Mortality and Morbidity

Various other chapters in this book report on evidence that social, psychological, and lifestyle factors impact on overall health outcomes. Also, meta-analyses and systematic reviews suggest that lack of social support (Lett et al, 2005), depressive symptoms (Nicholson et al, 2006), and unhealthy lifestyle behaviors such as lack of physical exercise (Oguma et al, 2002) are associated with increased risk of developing cardiovascular disease and all-cause mortality. Although these reviews do not explicitly distinguish between studies using middle-aged and older populations, it is good to realize that in fact the majority of meta-analyzed studies examining the impact of behavioral factors on general health outcomes have been conducted among older persons, simply because morbidity and mortality most commonly occur in the oldest age groups. Therefore, there is no doubt that these behavioral factors continue to impact on general health outcomes such as mortality and (cardiovascular) morbidity patterns in the oldest population. It would be too much to provide a complete overview, but a few examples that unfavorable lifestyle, social, and psychological aspects remain important factors that increase the chance of poorer general health outcomes in old age are given below. Alcohol consumption shows a U- or J-shaped relationship with mortality, as in middle-aged populations (Ferreira and Weems, 2008), and older persons with light to moderate alcohol consumption show lower rates of cardiac events and longer survival (Maraldi et al, 2006). In a community-based sample of persons aged 70–79 years (Health Aging and Body Composition study), we found that psychological risk factors, especially negative life events and inadequate emotional support, were associated with the metabolic syndrome (Vogelzangs et al, 2007a). Also, in the Longitudinal Aging

Study Amsterdam, we described that older persons who reported high feelings of loneliness and low levels of emotional support had significantly higher risk of dying over the subsequent 4 years (Penninx et al, 1997). Furthermore, widowhood has been associated with an increased mortality risk, which likely goes beyond a correlational effect due to similarities in lifestyle, age, experience, and behaviors between a married couple (Espinosa and Evans, 2008). On the more positive side, favorable psychological characteristics in old age, such as a high sense of personal mastery and self-efficacy, are associated with a decrease in mortality risk (Penninx et al, 1997).

Nevertheless, although many behavioral factors have an impact on health in later life, the relative impact of social environment, affective state, and lifestyle behaviors on health might shift due to changes in behavioral factors during aging (as mentioned in Section 2), due to aging-related biological changes, or as a result of selective survival. There are some indications that in terms of psychological predisposition, older adults may be less vulnerable than younger adults. Although stressful life events still appear to increase the risk for adverse health outcomes in old age, the relationship between life events and health outcomes may actually be less strong in older than in younger adults. Older individuals have had the opportunity to learn how to cope with stressful circumstances and how to adjust their expectations so as to have fewer feelings of failure. On the basis of age and experience, older persons may have developed more effective skills with which to manage stressful life events and to reduce emotional distress. Specific stressors, such as loss of partner or other intimates, are more normative in old age and usual in that part of the life cycle than in younger age, and therefore potentially less disruptive. Indeed, evidence exists that recent life events, for example, do not relate very strongly to common mental disorders in persons above the age of 65 years (Jordanova et al, 2007).

On the other hand, there is some evidence to suggest that very disruptive events that occurred much earlier in life, such as childhood abuse, trauma, or severe negative life events, can have enduring effects and constitute significant risk factors for depression (Kasen et al, 2010; Ritchie et al, 2009) and poor physical health during later life (Draper et al, 2008). Intermediate pathways between childhood adversity and late-life poor health might include early-age smoking, alcohol or illicit drug use, difficulties in forming and maintaining social relationships, and lower educational attainment (Springer et al, 2003). Simultaneously (traumatic) childhood experiences might produce long-lasting psychobiological changes, such as disturbances in the hypothalamic–pituitary–adrenal (HPA) axis, which continue to impact health throughout life (Kendler et al, 2004; Lupien et al, 2009).

3.2 Aging-Related Outcome: Physical Decline and Disability

Especially in old age an individual often has multiple chronic conditions which vary in severity and may have synergistic effects on health status. This is why specifically in old age the full picture of the link between behavioral factors and health outcomes cannot be portrayed by looking at individual chronic diseases. Although individual diseases are important, and our system of modern medicine is often oriented toward the diagnosis and treatment of specific diseases, the consequences of single and multiple diseases can best be understood by an evaluation of the functional status of the patient. This is why, to date, functional assessment forms the hallmark of geriatric medicine and research. In line with this, functional status has been demonstrated to be one of the most potent of all health status indicators in predicting adverse outcomes such as mortality, hospitalization, and nursing home admission in older populations (Guralnik et al, 1996). Older adults themselves report that they worry about their risk of disability, often more than about disease itself, because function decline changes the scope of their daily life and threatens their ability to live independently.

Various assessments and concepts for functional status have been proposed and used over the last two decades. These various concepts generally fit into a conceptual model called the disablement process (Verbrugge and Jette, 1994). The disablement process model describes a pathway leading from pathology to impairment to functional limitations and ultimately to disability. In this model, pathology refers to biochemical and physiological abnormalities that are detected and medically labeled as disease, injury, or congenital or developmental conditions, whereas physical impairments are dysfunctions and structural abnormalities in specific body systems, for example, conceptualized in poor muscle strength, poor balance, or low walking speed. Functional limitations are experienced restrictions in performing fundamental physical actions used in daily life. Examples of functional limitations are the report of experiencing profound difficulty or inability with walking $\frac{1}{4}$ mile, climbing stairs, or lifting 10 pounds, which can be considered to be the building blocks of activities of daily life. Disability, the final stage of the disablement process, reflects how an individual's limitations interact with the demands of the environment. It indicates a restriction in or lack of ability to perform activities related to interpersonal relationships, work or school, or physical activities. Various disability types can be distinguished, ranging from disability in instrumental activities of daily living (IADLs, e.g., housekeeping tasks, grocery shopping) to disability in essential activities of daily living (ADLs, e.g., eating, dressing, and transferring from bed to chair).

The impact of behavioral factors on physical disability in the older population is undisputed. A meta-analysis by Lenze et al (2001) demonstrated that depressive symptoms are associated with physical disability. Not only is there a cross-sectional association, but among non-disabled persons depressive symptoms also increase the risk of disability development over time. In the Established Populations for Epidemiological Studies of the Elderly (EPESE) involving more than 6000 older adults, we described that persons with a high depression score (as defined by a high score on the Center of Epidemiologic Studies-Depression (CES-D) Scale) were 1.7 times more likely to develop new ADL disability or mobility disability during 6 years of follow-up. When risk estimates are adjusted for other variables that differed between depressed and non-depressed persons, such as age, gender, education, income, and medical conditions, the risk estimates decreased (to 1.4) but remained considerable and significant (Penninx et al, 1999). Also in various other studies, factors such as age, gender, education, and medical conditions could not explain the link between depression and incident disability risk. These observations have been confirmed for both the presence of significant depressive symptoms and depression that meets psychiatric criteria for major depressive disorder (Penninx et al, 2000). Using longitudinal data from the Dutch Longitudinal Aging Study Amsterdam we observed that depression is not only associated with physical impairments, but that the presence of depression also accelerates the transition from physical impairments to disability (Van Gool et al, 2005). In other words, these findings do indicate that depression appears to accelerate the disablement process in older persons.

In an extensive literature review by Stuck et al (1999), confirmative evidence for various other psychosocial determinants of physical function decline was described. Higher anxiety levels were associated with more physical decline in some studies, and a low level of social activity, low frequency of social contact, and high emotional support were associated with physical decline in at least ten studies (Stuck et al, 1999). For example, Moritz et al (1995) found that social isolation and lack of participation in social activities were associated with incident limitations in activities of daily living. Also, widowhood in elderly men was found to be a risk factor for dependence in instrumental activities of daily living and mobility (van den Brink et al, 2004).

Among lifestyle factors, low physical activity or a sedentary lifestyle form the most important factors for physical decline and the onset of disability in old age, especially when physical inactivity in midlife continues into old age (Ferrucci et al, 1999a; Pluijm et al, 2007). This is particularly an important observation, since the level of physical activity is potentially modifiable through exercise regimens. The latter is supported by evidence from exercise intervention studies, which have confirmed that older persons participating in an exercise intervention score better over time on self-reported physical function scales or objective physical assessments than peers in the control arm (Ettinger et al, 1997). Also, smoking and heavy alcohol consumption in old age – which likely reflect high life course exposure – have been consistently associated with increased physical function decline (Ferrucci et al, 1999a; Stuck et al, 1999; Wannamethee et al, 2005).

3.3 Aging-Related Outcome: Frailty

Frailty is an adverse, primarily gerontologic, health condition which is common in aging and identifies a state of vulnerability for adverse health outcomes such as falls, disability, hospitalization, and mortality. The definition of frailty was first proposed by Fried and colleagues (2001) and since then used and accepted in many aging studies. Fried and colleagues defined frailty as a clinical syndrome in which three or more of the following criteria are present: unintentional weight loss (10 lbs in past year), self-reported exhaustion, weakness (low grip strength), slow walking speed, and low physical activity. Although there is overlap in the co-occurrence of frailty and disability, the concepts are different. Frailty is considered a distinct clinical syndrome with a biological basis, which could (eventually) result in disability as an outcome. The frailty phenotype has been independently predictive of 3-year incident falls, worsening mobility or ADL disability, hospitalization, and death (Fried et al, 2001).

Although the impact of behavioral factors on functional status and disability have been widely examined (see Section 3.2), their impact on frailty has been examined to a much lesser extent. Low socioeconomic status, as assessed by either lower educational level or lower income level, has been associated with more frailty (Fried et al, 2001). Alvarado and colleagues (2008) indicated the importance of unfavorable life course social characteristics for the presence of frailty in older age. They found that social conditions in childhood (hunger, poor health, and poor socioeconomic conditions), in adulthood (little education and non-white-collar occupation), and in current older age (insufficient income) were associated with higher odds of frailty in both older men and women.

In addition, various cross-sectional reports have linked depressive symptoms to aspects of frailty. However, cross-sectional associations are hard to interpret since frailty status itself could result in increased feelings of depression and mood changes. For certain aspects of the frailty syndrome, longitudinal associations with depression have been confirmed as well. Persons with high depressive symptoms have shown a larger 4-year decline in walking speed (Penninx et al, 1998) and a larger decline in muscle strength (Rantanen et al, 2000). In addition to negative emotions, Ostir and colleagues (2004) found that positive affect could significantly reduce the onset of frailty, which adds to a growing positive psychology literature showing that positive affect is protective against the functional and physical decline associated with frailty (see Chapter 14).

3.4 Aging-Related Outcome: Cognitive Impairment

Another domain of functioning that becomes affected with aging is that of cognitive function. With normal aging, cognitive changes such as slowed speed of processing are common, and cognitive decline is clearly inevitable. However, there is substantial interindividual variability and in some older individuals cognitive decline is followed by severe cognitive impairment and eventually dementia. Consequently, aging studies generally not only focus on physical function and frailty as important health indicators but also consider the cognitive domain in order to reach a more integrative view of older individuals' function.

There is quite extensive evidence that behavioral factors can either progress or inhibit cognitive decline. Lifestyle behaviors, for instance, have been linked with cognitive decline. Certain nutritional indicators such as vitamin B_{12} and folate deficiency, but also an unfavorable cholesterol profile, have been associated with poorer cognition in old age (Solomon et al, 2007; Tangney et al, 2009). Smoking and excess alcohol intake have also been shown to contribute to cognitive decline and avoiding these activities may promote cognitive vitality in aging (Peters et al, 2008a, b). On the other hand, moderate alcohol consumption has been associated with better cognition (Bond et al, 2003; Ngandu et al, 2007). Finally, there is evidence from both animal and human studies to suggest that lifelong learning, mental and physical exercise, and continuing social engagement are important factors in promoting cognitive vitality in aging (Fillit et al, 2002).

Various studies have also linked unfavorable psychological and social factors to a more rapid cognitive decline. Depressive symptoms, for instance, have been found to speed up cognitive decline over time (Yaffe et al, 1999). Interpretation of such observations is not easy, since it could be that depressive symptoms impact on cognitive function through underlying physiological effects, or it could simply be that depressive symptoms pick up some early signs of deteriorating cognition and therefore are rather markers of an early stage of cognitive decline. Furthermore, widowhood has been shown to be associated with greater cognitive decline in older adults (Aartsen et al, 2005), which could partly be due to underlying loneliness, also shown to be linked with a more rapid cognitive decline and a doubled risk for Alzheimer's disease (Wilson et al, 2007).

4 Specific Considerations for Behavioral Medicine in the Aging Population

Studying behavioral medicine in older persons requires taking into account several considerations specific to the aging population, which we will briefly describe below.

4.1 Selective Survival

By definition, when recruiting a sample of older persons, those who have already died are not included in the cohort. This applies especially to the oldest old (85 years and older). It is certainly possible that for certain known behavioral risk factors, associations are no longer found to be predictive of diminished health, solely because those who were both exposed and affected by this risk factor are no longer alive. It is essential to take into account the possibility of selective survival for a comprehensive interpretation of causality between behavioral factors and health outcomes. Selective survival is not just a confounding factor for research, but can actually help in gaining insight into behavioral medicine. For instance, the finding that among centenarians cigarette smoking is extremely rare adds to the evidence that smoking is related to increased risk of mortality (Nicita-Mauro et al, 2008). There have been various reports where, for example, depression and life events have been found to be less predictive of mortality in the oldest (85 years and up) compared to the young old (70–84 years) (Jordanova et al, 2007; Rapp et al, 2008). Selective survival could partly explain some of these oldest age-specific findings. However, other issues could also explain these observations. As described in Section 3.1, some behavioral factors may simply have less effect on health outcomes in older age due to shifted impact of behavioral factors among the oldest old. In addition, competing (i.e., stronger) risk factors for general health outcomes in old age, for example, somatic conditions, could override the effects of behavioral factors. These specific issues are important to consider when interpreting behavioral medicine results in an older population.

4.2 Somatic Confounding

Another important issue in behavioral medicine among the oldest old is the increasing importance of somatic health aspects. Because in older age physical complaints and somatic conditions are very prevalent, the presence of these conditions should be considered since they can affect results of behavioral medicine studies. For instance, when examining psychosocial factors as predictors of cardiovascular disease, the presence of somatic comorbidities needs to be considered, as this may partly explain and/or confound the association of interest. One example of such potential confounding has been observed in studies linking social support to mortality. When social support assessments contain an instrumental support inventory, unexpected associations with mortality risk have been observed suggesting that more support is associated with a higher mortality risk (Penninx et al, 1997). Such a positive association likely illustrates the fact that underlying poor health status determines the receipt of more instrumental support. Another example of potential somatic confounding could appear when psychological inventories, such as depressive or anxiety symptom checklists, contain a considerable number of somatic symptoms. Older persons with many somatic health problems could then theoretically score high on depression or anxiety measures simply because of their somatic symptoms. This is a possibility that should be explored in behavioral medicine research among the oldest old, for instance, by checking for consistency of findings after exclusion of somatic items in checklists or by conducting subanalyses among the more healthy oldest old. In addition to confounding by somatic items, it is possible that somatic health has caused changes in behavioral factors that need to be specifically

considered in the older population. An example of this is "vascular depression," which reflects the hypothesis that vascular lesions in selected regions of the brain may contribute to a unique variety of late-life depression (Alexopoulos et al, 1997). Indeed, magnetic resonance imaging of older depressed patients has revealed structural abnormalities in areas related to the cortical–stratial–pallidal–thalamus–cortical pathway (de Groot et al, 2000), illustrating that concepts such as late-life depression could be partly influenced by underlying somatic health aspects.

4.3 Differential Role of Physiological Stress Mechanisms in the Oldest Old

As described in other chapters in this book, the biological mechanisms that could be responsible for effects of behavioral factors on health outcomes cover a range of mechanisms, including inflammation, and alterations in autonomic nervous system function and endocrine processes. Several of these biological mechanisms may play a role in both younger and older populations. However, for some mechanisms specific aging-related observations have been described.

Inflammation is characterized by a chronic mild elevated activity of the immune system which is illustrated by higher levels of, for example, C-reactive protein and interleukin (IL)-6. With aging, inflammation levels generally increase steadily over time, thereby reaching levels that are closer to critical levels at which health impacts could occur. IL-6 has been termed the "cytokine for gerontologists" (Ferrucci et al, 1999b). Although it has been linked with poor health in younger samples as well, its role in aging populations is eminent and striking. High levels of IL-6 have been linked to a large range of unfavorable health outcomes in older populations, varying from overall mortality, onset of cardiovascular disease, lung disease, cancer, frailty, and physical decline (Barzilay et al, 2007;

Cesari et al, 2004; Ferrucci et al, 2002; Gallucci et al, 2007; Heikkila et al, 2008; Kritchevsky et al, 2005; Leng et al, 2007; Yende et al, 2006). Consequently, inflammation is considered to be a very general biological risk factor that could be an interlinking mechanism between different disease processes and likely forms a central mechanism through which unfavorable social, psychological, and lifestyle characteristics impact on a range of unfavorable health outcomes in the oldest old.

Endocrine mechanisms are also considered to be important linking pathways through which behavioral factors exert their impact on health. With aging, and especially after menopause, levels of sex steroid hormones, such as testosterone, estradiol, and dehydroepiandrosterone sulfate (DHEA-S), decrease. Whereas in younger age groups, high levels of sex hormones have sometimes been shown to be unfavorably associated with behavioral factors such as depression, in aging populations low sex hormone levels have been linked with late-life depression (Morsink et al, 2007).

Other aging-specific observations have been found for the hypothalamus–pituitary–adrenal (HPA) axis which produces the stress hormone cortisol. Generally, high cortisol levels are hypothesized to be linking mechanisms between behavioral factors and adverse health outcomes. In an aged population, however, physical frailty could actually exhaust the body's responses to stress potentially resulting in hypoactivity of the HPA axis. This may explain why some studies among older frail persons have in fact observed not only hyperactivity but also hypoactivity of the HPA axis among depressed persons (Bremmer et al, 2007; Penninx et al, 2007). Consequently, not considering the possibility of reduced cortisol levels among depressed older persons might lead to erroneous conclusions. Results of the InCHIANTI study among 800 community-dwelling older persons showed that only hypercortisolemic depressed persons showed an increased prevalence of the metabolic syndrome (Vogelzangs et al, 2007b). Lastly, high cortisol levels are also considered a central mechanism in the effects of psychosocial

stressors on cognitive performance and cognitive decline among older persons (Lee et al, 2007; Lupien et al, 2007).

5 Concluding Remarks

This chapter first described the relative prevalence of behavioral factors in the older population, illustrating the commonality of certain social, psychological, and lifestyle changes that take place in old age. Although the effects of some of these changes may be relatively smaller at older compared with younger ages, there is no doubt that behavioral factors continue to impact on health among the oldest old. We described evidence for behavioral factors having an impact on general health outcomes such as mortality and morbidity patterns and also on specific aging-related health outcomes such as physical function decline, frailty, and cognitive decline. The chapter finished with emphasizing considerations – selective survival, somatic confounding, and the differential role of physiological stress mechanisms – that one has to keep in mind when examining and interpreting behavioral medicine in an older population.

Although this chapter has described many behavioral medicine studies in aging, there are various research questions that warrant more research. First, questions such as which behavioral factors have more impact and which behavioral factors have less impact in the aging population have mainly been addressed through indirect comparisons across different studies conducted in different age groups. There is an urgent need for comprehensive studies that directly compare and test the general health impact of behavioral factors in younger versus older age groups. Second, for certain specific aging-related health outcomes such as cognitive decline and physical decline and frailty, there remains a need for more detailed behavioral medicine research, since these are relatively underexamined research areas. Finally, most literature in the area of behavioral medicine and aging is based on a cross-sectional approach to classifying behavioral factors which generally only takes current or very recent exposure into account. A life course perspective (see also Chapter 34), in which the entire life span and the more cumulative exposure to behavioral risk factors are considered, is needed to further refine the quantification of behavioral factors in aging. Such a research perspective generally requires longitudinal assessments over an extensive period of time. This type of research can also help to identify the critical values for time of onset and duration of exposure to behavioral factors and can indicate to what extent negative health consequences are reversed when people change unfavorable health behaviors.

References

Aartsen, M. J., van Tilburg, T. T., Smits, C. H., Comijs, H. C., and Knipscheer, K. C. (2005). Does widowhood affect memory performance of older persons? *Psychol Med, 35*, 217–226.

Alexopoulos, G. S., Meyers, B. S., Young, R. C., Campbell, S., Silbersweig, D. et al (1997). 'Vascular depression' hypothesis.*Arch Gen Psychiatry, 54*, 915–922.

Alvarado, B. E., Zunzunegui, M. V., Beland, F., and Bamvita, J. M. (2008). Life course social and health conditions linked to frailty in Latin American older men and women. *J Gerontol A Biol Sci Med Sci, 63*, 1399–1406.

Barzilay, J. I., Blaum, C., Moore, T., Xue, Q. L., Hirsch, C. H. et al (2007). Insulin resistance and inflammation as precursors of frailty: the Cardiovascular Health Study. *Arch Intern Med, 167*, 635–641.

Beekman, A. T., Deeg, D. J., van Tilburg, T., Smit, J. H., Hooijer, C. et al (1995). Major and minor depression in later life: a study of prevalence and risk factors. *J Affect Disord, 36*, 65–75.

Beekman, A. T., Bremmer, M. A., Deeg, D. J., van Balkom, A. J., Smit, J. H. et al (1998). Anxiety disorders in later life: a report from the Longitudinal Aging Study Amsterdam. *Int J Geriatr Psychiatry, 13*, 717–726.

Beekman, A. T., Copeland, J. R., and Prince, M. J. (1999). Review of community prevalence of depression in later life. *Br J Psychiatry, 174*, 307–311.

Bennett, K. M. (2005). Psychological wellbeing in later life: the longitudinal effects of marriage, widowhood and marital status change. *Int J Geriatr Psychiatry, 20*, 280–284.

Bond, G. E., Burr, R., Rice, M. M., McCurry, S. M., Graves, A. B. et al (2003). Alcohol, aging, and cognitive performance: a cross-cultural comparison. *J Aging Health, 15*, 371–390.

Bremmer, M. A., Deeg, D. J., Beekman, A. T., Penninx, B. W., Lips, P. et al (2007). Major depression in late life is associated with both hypo- and hypercortisolemia. *Biol Psychiatry, 62*, 479–486.

Cacioppo, J. T., Hughes, M. E., Waite, L. J., Hawkley, L. C., and Thisted, R. A. (2006). Loneliness as a specific risk factor for depressive symptoms: cross-sectional and longitudinal analyses. *Psychol Aging, 21*, 140–151.

Cesari, M., Penninx, B. W., Pahor, M., Lauretani, F., Corsi, A. M. et al (2004). Inflammatory markers and physical performance in older persons: the InCHIANTI study. *J Gerontol A Biol Sci Med Sci, 59*, 242–248.

de Groot, J. C., de Leeuw, F. E., Oudkerk, M., Hofman, A., Jolles, J. et al (2000). Cerebral white matter lesions and depressive symptoms in elderly adults. *Arch Gen Psychiatry, 57*, 1071–1076.

Draper, B., Pfaff, J. J., Pirkis, J., Snowdon, J., Lautenschlager, N. T. et al (2008). Long-term effects of childhood abuse on the quality of life and health of older people: results from the Depression and Early Prevention of Suicide in General Practice Project. *J Am Geriatr Soc, 56*, 262–271.

Dykstra, P. A., and de Jong Gierveld, J. (2004). Gender and marital-history differences in emotional and social loneliness among Dutch older adults. *Can J Aging, 23*, 141–155.

Espinosa, J., and Evans, W. N. (2008). Heightened mortality after the death of a spouse: marriage protection or marriage selection? *J Health Econ, 27*, 1326–1342.

Ettinger, W. H., Jr., Burns, R., Messier, S. P., Applegate, W., Rejeski, W. J. et al (1997). A randomized trial comparing aerobic exercise and resistance exercise with a health education program in older adults with knee osteoarthritis. The Fitness Arthritis and Seniors Trial (FAST). *JAMA, 277*, 25–31.

Ferreira, M. P., and Weems, M. K. (2008). Alcohol consumption by aging adults in the United States: health benefits and detriments. *J Am Diet Assoc, 108*, 1668–1676.

Ferrucci, L., Izmirlian, G., Leveille, S., Phillips, C. L., Corti, M. C. et al (1999a). Smoking, physical activity, and active life expectancy. *Am J Epidemiol, 149*, 645–653.

Ferrucci, L., Harris, T. B., Guralnik, J. M., Tracy, R. P., Corti, M. C. et al (1999b). Serum IL-6 level and the development of disability in older persons. *J Am Geriatr Soc, 47*, 639–646.

Ferrucci, L., Penninx, B. W., Volpato, S., Harris, T. B., Bandeen-Roche, K. et al (2002). Change in muscle strength explains accelerated decline of physical function in older women with high interleukin-6 serum levels. *J Am Geriatr Soc, 50*, 1947–1954.

Fillit, H. M., Butler, R. N., O'Connell, A. W., Albert, M. S., Birren, J. E. et al (2002). Achieving and maintaining cognitive vitality with aging. *Mayo Clin Proc, 77,* 681–696.

Fried, L. P., Tangen, C. M., Walston, J., Newman, A. B., Hirsch, C. et al (2001). Frailty in older adults: evidence for a phenotype. *J Gerontol A Biol Sci Med Sc., 56,* M146–M156.

Gallucci, M., Amici, G. P., Ongaro, F., Gajo, G. B., De Angeli, S. et al (2007). Associations of the plasma interleukin 6 (IL-6) levels with disability and mortality in the elderly in the Treviso Longeva (Trelong) study. *Arch Gerontol Geriatr, 44 Suppl 1,* 193–198.

Grenade, L., and Boldy, D. (2008). Social isolation and loneliness among older people: issues and future challenges in community and residential settings. *Aust Health Rev, 32,* 468–478.

Guralnik, J. M., Fried, L. P., and Salive, M. E. (1996). Disability as a public health outcome in the aging population. *Annu Rev Public Health, 17,* 25–46.

Heikkila, K., Ebrahim, S., and Lawlor, D. A. (2008). Systematic review of the association between circulating interleukin-6 (IL-6) and cancer. *Eur J Cancer, 44,* 937–945.

Janke, M. C., Nimrod, G., and Kleiber, D. A. (2008). Reduction in leisure activity and well-being during the transition to widowhood. *J Women Aging, 20,* 83–98.

Jordanova, V., Stewart, R., Goldberg, D., Bebbington, P. E., Brugha, T. et al (2007). Age variation in life events and their relationship with common mental disorders in a national survey population. *Soc Psychiatry Psychiatr Epidemiol, 42,* 611–616.

Jylha, M. (2004). Old age and loneliness: cross-sectional and longitudinal analyses in the Tampere Longitudinal Study on Aging. *Can J Aging, 23,* 157–168.

Kasen, S., Chen, H., Sneed, J. R., and Cohen, P. (2010). Earlier stress exposure and subsequent major depression in aging women. *Int J Geriatr Psychiatry, 25,* 91–99.

Kendler, K. S., Kuhn, J. W., and Prescott, C. A. (2004). Childhood sexual abuse, stressful life events and risk for major depression in women. *Psychol Med, 34,* 1475–1482.

Kritchevsky, S. B., Cesari, M., and Pahor, M. (2005). Inflammatory markers and cardiovascular health in older adults. *Cardiovasc Res, 66,* 265–275.

Lee, B. K., Glass, T. A., McAtee, M. J., Wand, G. S., Bandeen-Roche, K. et al (2007). Associations of salivary cortisol with cognitive function in the Baltimore memory study. *Arch Gen Psychiatry, 64,* 810–818.

Leng, S. X., Xue, Q. L., Tian, J., Walston, J. D., and Fried, L. P. (2007). Inflammation and frailty in older women. *J Am Geriatr Soc, 55,* 864–871.

Lenze, E. J., Rogers, J. C., Martire, L. M., Mulsant, B. H., Rollman, B. L. et al (2001). The association of late-life depression and anxiety with physical disability: a review of the literature and prospectus for future research. *Am J Geriatr Psychiatry, 9,* 113–135.

Lett, H. S., Blumenthal, J. A., Babyak, M. A., Strauman, T. J., Robins, C. et al (2005). Social support and coronary heart disease: epidemiologic evidence and implications for treatment. *Psychosom Med, 67,* 869–878.

Lupien, S. J., Maheu, F., Tu, M., Fiocco, A., and Schramek, T. E. (2007). The effects of stress and stress hormones on human cognition: implications for the field of brain and cognition. *Brain Cogn, 65,* 209–237.

Lupien, S. J., McEwen, B. S., Gunnar, M. R., and Heim, C. (2009). Effects of stress throughout the lifespan on the brain, behaviour and cognition. *Nat Rev Neurosci, 10,* 434–445.

Maraldi, C., Volpato, S., Kritchevsky, S. B., Cesari, M., Andresen, E. et al (2006). Impact of inflammation on the relationship among alcohol consumption, mortality, and cardiac events: the health, aging, and body composition study. *Arch Intern Med, 166,* 1490–1497.

Mehta, M., Whyte, E., Lenze, E., Hardy, S., Roumani, Y. et al (2008). Depressive symptoms in late life: associations with apathy, resilience and disability vary between young-old and old-old. *Int J Geriatr Psychiatry, 23,* 238–243.

Moritz, D. J., Kasl, S. V., and Berkman, L. F. (1995). Cognitive functioning and the incidence of limitations in activities of daily living in an elderly community sample. *Am J Epidemiol., 141,* 41–49.

Morsink, L. F., Vogelzangs, N., Nicklas, B. J., Beekman, A. T., Satterfield, S. et al (2007). Associations between sex steroid hormone levels and depressive symptoms in elderly men and women: results from the Health ABC study. *Psychoneuroendocrinology, 32,* 874–883.

Ngandu, T., Helkala, E. L., Soininen, H., Winblad, B., Tuomilehto, J. et al (2007). Alcohol drinking and cognitive functions: findings from the Cardiovascular Risk Factors Aging and Dementia (CAIDE) Study. *Dement Geriatr Cogn Disord, 23,* 140–149.

Nicholson, A., Kuper, H., and Hemingway, H. (2006). Depression as an aetiologic and prognostic factor in coronary heart disease: a meta-analysis of 6362 events among 146 538 participants in 54 observational studies. *Eur Heart J, 27,* 2763–2774.

Nicita-Mauro, V., Lo, B. C., Mento, A., Nicita-Mauro, C., Maltese, G. et al (2008). Smoking, aging and the centenarians. *Exp Gerontol, 43,* 95–101.

Oguma, Y., Sesso, H. D., Paffenbarger, R. S., Jr., and Lee, I. M. (2002). Physical activity and all cause mortality in women: a review of the evidence. *Br J Sports Med, 36,* 162–172.

Onrust, S. A., and Cuijpers, P. (2006). Mood and anxiety disorders in widowhood: a systematic review. *Aging Ment Health, 10,* 327–334.

Ostir, G. V., Ottenbacher, K. J., and Markides, K. S. (2004). Onset of frailty in older adults and the protective role of positive affect. *Psychol Aging, 19,* 402–408.

Penninx, B. W., van Tilburg, T., Kriegsman, D. M., Deeg, D. J., Boeke, A. J. et al (1997). Effects of social support and personal coping resources on mortality in older age: the Longitudinal Aging Study Amsterdam. *Am J Epidemiol, 146*, 510–519.

Penninx, B. W., Guralnik, J. M., Ferrucci, L., Simonsick, E. M., Deeg, D. J. et al (1998). Depressive symptoms and physical decline in community-dwelling older persons. *JAMA, 279*, 1720–1726.

Penninx, B. W., Leveille, S., Ferrucci, L., van Eijk, J. T., and Guralnik, J. M. (1999). Exploring the effect of depression on physical disability: longitudinal evidence from the established populations for epidemiologic studies of the elderly. *Am J Public Health, 89*, 1346–1352.

Penninx, B. W., Deeg, D. J., van Eijk, J. T., Beekman, A. T., and Guralnik, J. M. (2000). Changes in depression and physical decline in older adults: a longitudinal perspective. *J Affect Disord, 61*, 1–12.

Penninx, B. W., Beekman, A. T., Bandinelli, S., Corsi, A. M., Bremmer, M. et al (2007). Late-life depressive symptoms are associated with both hyperactivity and hypoactivity of the hypothalamo-pituitary-adrenal axis. *Am J Geriatr Psychiatry, 15*, 522–529.

Peters, R., Poulter, R., Warner, J., Beckett, N., Burch, L. et al (2008a). Smoking, dementia and cognitive decline in the elderly, a systematic review. *BMC Geriatr, 8*, 36.

Peters, R., Peters, J., Warner, J., Beckett, N., and Bulpitt, C. (2008b). Alcohol, dementia and cognitive decline in the elderly: a systematic review. *Age Ageing, 37*, 505–512.

Pluijm, S. M., Visser, M., Puts, M. T., Dik, M. G., Schalk, B. W. et al (2007). Unhealthy lifestyles during the life course: association with physical decline in late life. *Aging Clin Exp Res, 19*, 75–83.

Rantanen, T., Penninx, B. W., Masaki, K., Lintunen, T., Foley, D. et al (2000). Depressed mood and body mass index as predictors of muscle strength decline in old men. *J Am Geriatr Soc, 48*, 613–617.

Rapp, M. A., Gerstorf, D., Helmchen, H., and Smith, J. (2008). Depression predicts mortality in the young old, but not in the oldest old: results from the Berlin Aging Study. *Am J Geriatr Psychiatry, 16*, 844–852.

Ritchie, K., Jaussent, I., Stewart, R., Dupuy, A. M., Courtet, P. et al (2009). Association of adverse childhood environment with late-life depression. *J Clin Psychiatry*, [Epub ahead of print].

Solomon, A., Kareholt, I., Ngandu, T., Wolozin, B., Macdonald, S. W. et al (2007). Serum total cholesterol, statins and cognition in non-demented elderly. *Neurobiol Aging*.

Springer, K. W., Sheridan, J., Kuo, D., and Carnes, M. (2003). The long-term health outcomes of childhood abuse. An overview and a call to action. *J Gen Intern Med, 18*, 864–870.

Stuck, A. E., Walthert, J. M., Nikolaus, T., Bula, C. J., Hohmann, C. et al (1999). Risk factors for functional status decline in community-living elderly people: a systematic literature review. *Soc Sci Med, 48*, 445–469.

Tangney, C. C., Tang, Y., Evans, D. A., and Morris, M. C. (2009). Biochemical indicators of vitamin B12 and folate insufficiency and cognitive decline. *Neurology, 72*, 361–367.

van den Brink, C. L., Tijhuis, M., van den Bos, G. A., Giampaoli, S., Kivinen, P. et al (2004). Effect of widowhood on disability onset in elderly men from three European countries. *J Am Geriatr Soc, 52*, 353–358.

van Gool, C. H., Kempen, G. I., Penninx, B. W., Deeg, D. J., Beekman, A. T. et al (2005). Impact of depression on disablement in late middle aged and older persons: results from the Longitudinal Aging Study Amsterdam. *Soc Sci Med, 60*, 25–36.

van Grootheest, D. S., Beekman, A. T., Broese van Groenou, M. I., and Deeg, D. J. (1999). Sex differences in depression after widowhood. Do men suffer more? *Soc Psychiatry Psychiatr Epidemiol, 34*, 391–398.

van Solinge, H., and Henkens, K. (2008). Adjustment to and satisfaction with retirement: two of a kind? *Psychol Aging, 23*, 422–434.

Verbrugge, L. M., and Jette, A. M. (1994). The disablement process. *Soc Sci Med, 38*, 1–14.

Vogelzangs, N., Beekman, A. T., Kritchevsky, S. B., Newman, A. B., Pahor, M. et al (2007a). Psychosocial risk factors and the metabolic syndrome in elderly persons: findings from the health, aging and body composition study. *J Gerontol A Biol Sci Med Sci, 62*, 563–569.

Vogelzangs, N., Suthers, K., Ferrucci, L., Simonsick, E. M., Ble, A. et al (2007b). Hypercortisolemic depression is associated with the metabolic syndrome in late-life. *Psychoneuroendocrinology, 32*, 151–159.

Wannamethee, S. G., Ebrahim, S., Papacosta, O., and Shaper, A. G. (2005). From a postal questionnaire of older men, healthy lifestyle factors reduced the onset of and may have increased recovery from mobility limitation. *J Clin Epidemiol, 58*, 831–840.

Wilson, R. S., Krueger, K. R., Arnold, S. E., Schneider, J. A., Kelly, J. F. et al (2007). Loneliness and risk of Alzheimer disease. *Arch Gen Psychiatry, 64*, 234–240.

Yaffe, K., Blackwell, T., Gore, R., Sands, L., Reus, V., and Browner, W. S. (1999). Depressive symptoms and cognitive decline in nondemented elderly women: a prospective study. *Arch Gen Psychiatry, 56*, 425–430.

Yende, S., Waterer, G. W., Tolley, E. A., Newman, A. B., Bauer, D. C., Taaffe, D. R. et al (2006). Inflammatory markers are associated with ventilatory limitation and muscle dysfunction in obstructive lung disease in well functioning elderly subjects. *Thorax, 61*, 10–16.

Part VII
Biological Measures and Biomarkers

Chapter 40

Use of Biological Measures in Behavioral Medicine

Andrew Steptoe and Lydia Poole

1 Introduction

The behavioral medicine approach has led researchers to seek ever more precise physiological measures in order to explore and quantify the multiple reciprocal pathways linking psychosocial and behavioral factors with biomedical outcomes. This in turn has resulted in significant progress in scientific techniques for the study, collection, and assessment of biological measures. Many of these advances have been made in the measurement of physiological and morphological features of the human phenotype, where self-reported health data have given way to anthropometric measures such as body weight and abdominal adiposity, physiological functions such as blood pressure and respiratory function, and biochemical markers such as cholesterol, C-reactive protein, and blood glucose. More recently, advances in the field of genetics have widened the arena of biomarkers into investigating genotypes (see Section 5), while brain imaging techniques are beginning to uncover the patterns of central nervous system activation underlying emotional states and systemic biological responses (see Section 8).

The application of different biological measurement systems to behavioral medicine is described in later chapters of Section 7 of the Handbook. The purpose of this chapter is to outline the use of biological measures more broadly, describing the strengths and limitations of their application in the diverse research paradigms of behavioral medicine. Four distinct fields of behavioral medicine that capitalize on the availability of biological measures are discussed: animal experiments, population-level surveys, psychophysiological stress testing in humans, and naturalistic/ambulatory monitoring. Our aim is not only to highlight the potential of biological measurement in each context, but also to point out the practical and interpretive pitfalls that need to be circumvented. The research literature on these topics is large, so the studies cited are for illustration only.

2 Biological Measures in Animal Experiments

Animal experiments are crucial to understanding the biology of stress and adaptation, the neurochemical systems underlying behaviorally driven physiological adjustments, and the factors contributing to behavioral influences on disease etiology and host resistance. There are many examples of animal research utilizing biological measures in other chapters of the handbook. One of the temptations that must be resisted in behavioral medicine is simplistic generalization to humans of the environmental or social contingencies affecting physical pathology in other species. A good example is the literature on social hierarchies. Animal studies have shown

A. Steptoe (✉)
Department of Epidemiology and Public Health, University College London, 1–19 Torrington Place, London WC1E 6BT, UK
e-mail: a.steptoe@ucl.ac.uk

A. Steptoe (ed.), *Handbook of Behavioral Medicine*, DOI 10.1007/978-0-387-09488-5_40,
© Springer Science+Business Media, LLC 2010

that physical pathology and psychobiological responses are associated with dominance hierarchies. Sapolsky's (1995) studies of wild olive baboons demonstrated that basal cortisol levels are higher in subordinate animals, while social subordination in female cynomolgus monkeys leads to stimulation of the hypothalamic–pituitary–adrenocortical (HPA) axis and is associated with increased coronary artery atherosclerosis and abdominal adiposity (Shively et al, 2009). These findings indicate that social status can be linked with neuroendocrine and metabolic factors and with cardiovascular disease outcomes. However, the analogy with social gradients in humans can be pursued only cautiously. A meta-analysis of the literature on cynomolgus monkeys has shown that the relationship between social hierarchies, social stress, and atherosclerosis is gender-specific (Kaplan et al, 2009); male dominant animals develop more rather than less coronary atherosclerosis than subordinates when exposed to unstable social conditions, while females show the reverse. Cortisol differences also vary across species and in relation to the animals' living conditions (Abbott et al, 2003), while in some rat strains blood pressure is higher in dominants than subordinates (Ely et al, 1997). There is nothing inherently pathogenic in either dominant or subordinate social status in animals, and it is unwise to draw parallels with humans just because in some cases there appear to be similarities with the social patterning of health and illness.

First, the recruitment of a large, preferably representative, population of individuals who are screened to ensure that they do not already suffer from the endpoint under investigation (e.g., diabetes, coronary heart disease). Second, the measurement of exposure to the risk factors or biological factors being tested (e.g., low social support, C-reactive protein, low physical activity), along with other factors known to influence the outcome. Third, the tracking of the population over time, monitoring the development of the health endpoints under investigation. Finally, multivariate analysis to test whether exposure to the putative risk factor is associated with the endpoint after the covariates have been controlled.

Biomarkers in population studies are important in behavioral medicine research for a number of reasons. First, they provide objective data about health and functioning. Much survey work is based on self-report and this may have limited accuracy in some (particularly older) individuals because of failures in recall or self-presentation bias. Second, biomarkers provide information about important health outcomes that may not have been clinically diagnosed and are therefore not effectively managed. Lastly, these measures help our understanding of the mechanisms and pathways through which psychosocial and economic factors influence health and well-being.

The different biological measures assessed in observational epidemiology fall into two broad groups. The first is related to specific disease outcomes and the second includes nonspecific biomarkers of health or resistance to disease.

3 Population-Level Epidemiological Studies

Epidemiological studies provide the core method for establishing the contribution of psychosocial factors to the development of disease and are also used to identify the biological mediators of these associations. Epidemiological studies take several forms, but perhaps the most fruitful in behavioral medicine has been the longitudinal observational epidemiological population study. Such studies have a number of components.

3.1 Biomarkers of Disease State

Biological indicators of disease states include markers such as blood pressure in hypertension and as a risk factor for coronary heart disease (CHD) and stroke, glycated hemoglobin or blood glucose for the assessment of diabetes, and airways resistance in bronchial asthma. These biological measures are direct markers of the physiological dysfunction constituting the disease and can be related to social, emotional, and economic experience. Observational epidemiology has been used to identify many risk factors for disease, including high blood pressure, elevated cholesterol levels, and excessive adiposity in CHD. In some cases, the information is valuable because it may help identify serious problems that have not been diagnosed clinically, so allowing researchers to estimate the "clinical iceberg." For example, results from the English Longitudinal Study of Ageing (ELSA) found that 77% of men and 84% of women had total cholesterol levels above the UK recommended level of 5.00 mmol/l (193 mg/dl), even though in many cases no medical advice or treatment had been given. A significant proportion of respondents (18% men, 16% women) had blood pressure levels in the hypertensive range even though hypertension had never been diagnosed (Pierce et al, 2006). These findings point to failures in primary prevention and unmet clinical needs.

Another use of observational epidemiology is to track changes in biological risk factors over time, so as to characterize the etiology of the disease. For example, recent data from the Whitehall II study of over 6500 British civil servants have shown the trajectories of fasting and post-load glucose, insulin sensitivity, and insulin secretion over a median follow-up period of 9.7 years (Tabák et al, 2009). All participants were non-diabetic at study entry, but by the time of follow-up, 505 diabetes cases had been diagnosed. Multilevel models adjusting for age, sex, and ethnicity showed that in the diabetic group, changes in glucose concentrations, insulin sensitivity, and insulin secretion occurred as much as 3–6 years before diagnosis of diabetes. Such data could contribute to more accurate risk prediction models that utilize the repeated measures available for patients through regular checkups and could allow for behavioral intervention in patients at an early stage.

3.2 Biological Indicators of Health or Resistance to Disease

Many of the more interesting associations between biological measures and well-being have emerged from analysis of the second group of biomarkers. This category is not disease specific, but instead relates to general indicators of health and resistance to disease, and also includes markers of stress reactivity. These indicators supply information about future risk but do not typically define a specific illness. Although elevations in some markers are associated with reduced risk, such as high density lipoprotein (HDL) cholesterol, most are related to increased risk of future disease. They include the inflammatory markers C-reactive protein and interleukin (IL)-6, the neuroendocrine parameter cortisol, and hemostatic markers such as fibrinogen and von Willebrand factor.

C-reactive protein is the commonest marker of inflammation measured in behavioral medicine. It is produced in the liver as part of the acute phase inflammatory hepatic response and can be activated by the cytokines IL-6 and tumor necrosis factor (TNF) α. C-reactive protein has been extensively studied as a novel cardiovascular risk factor, and meta-analysis of longitudinal observational studies indicates that both high C-reactive protein and IL-6 are independent risk factors for CHD (Helfand et al, 2009), although the causality of these associations is debated. These inflammatory markers are also related to other health problems in old age such as autoimmune conditions and type 2 diabetes and to psychosocial factors. For example, Kiecolt-Glaser and colleagues (2003) found that the chronic stress of spousal caregiving was associated with an accelerated increase in IL-6 over a 6-year period. An analysis of the Dunedin birth cohort study found that harsh treatment in childhood predicted elevated C-reactive protein when participants were aged 32 years, independently of demographic and behavioral confounders (Danese et al, 2007). In the MacArthur Study of Successful Aging, plasma IL-6 predicted speedier declines in cognitive function over a 2.5-year period (Weaver et al, 2002). Both C-reactive protein and IL-6 have also been related to depression (Howren et al, 2009).

Cortisol is involved in immune and metabolic regulation, and elevated levels are linked with abdominal adiposity, insulin resistance, diabetes,

CHD, and depression (Dekker et al, 2008; Herbert et al, 2006; Raison et al, 2006). Cortisol also contributes to memory function across the life span, with evidence that long-term exposure to high levels of glucocorticoids is associated with memory impairments and reduced hippocampal volume in the aging brain (Lupien et al, 2005). Until the advent of salivary assays, cortisol was primarily measured in blood or urine. Since cortisol secretion has a pronounced diurnal rhythm, this resulted in difficulty in accurately capturing representative cortisol levels in population studies, as the timing of data collection required standardization. Nevertheless, two studies showed that a single sample recorded early in the day was predictive of future clinical depression in adolescents or adults at high risk (Goodyer et al, 2000; Harris et al, 2000). A high cortisol/testosterone ratio was found to predict incident CHD in a longitudinal study in South Wales, UK, probably through influences on the metabolic syndrome (Davey Smith et al, 2005).

Hemostatic markers are another group of biological indicators that have received interest in behavioral medicine in recent years. These markers include fibrinogen and von Willebrand factor. Meta-analyses and reviews have consistently shown that increased levels of fibrinogen are associated with both the pathogenesis and presence of atherosclerosis (Feinbloom and Bauer, 2005; Fibrinogen Studies Collaboration, 2005). Both fibrinogen and von Willebrand factor are inversely related to socioeconomic status and have been associated with factors such as low job control, smoking, childhood adversity, and sedentary behavior (Brunner et al, 1996; Danese et al, 2007; Hamer and Steptoe, 2008; Kumari et al, 2000).

3.3 Interpretation of Biomarker Results in Population Studies

Cross-sectional studies associating biological measures with psychosocial or health outcomes of course suffer from the same limitations to

causal interpretation as any other correlations. It is not possible to determine which variable is cause and which is effect or whether both are determined by unmeasured confounding factors. This is not to dismiss cross-sectional studies, but rather to recognize their limitations. Take, for example, the association between inflammation and depression. The literature relating the two originated with small scale studies of patients with clinically defined depression (Maes, 1995), but rapidly progressed to larger scale population studies, and meta-analysis indicates that C-reactive protein and IL-6 are both consistently associated with depressed mood (Howren et al, 2009). Population studies are important, since they demonstrate that relationships between inflammation and depression are not limited to non-representative clinical samples. With large samples, it is possible not only to demonstrate a difference in levels of inflammatory markers between depressed and non-depressed people, but also to compute relative risks and "dose–response" effects. But does this mean that inflammation is a causal factor in depression, that depression leads to biological responses that include inflammation, that both pathways operate, or that both inflammation and depression are secondary to a third factor? Smoking, for instance, may stimulate inflammation and is also more common among depressed than non-depressed individuals. Fortunately, smoking can be measured and taken into account statistically, but other potential confounders are less easy to assess, and it is difficult to be completely certain that all possibilities have been taken into account.

A major benefit of longitudinal studies and repeated assessments of biological variables is that it is possible to begin to tease out the temporal sequence of such associations. In the case of depression and inflammation, the longitudinal biomarker data available within the Whitehall II study was used to examine the temporal relationship between depressive symptoms and both C-reactive protein and IL-6 (Gimeno et al, 2009). Just over 3000 participants completed measures of depression and had blood drawn for the analysis of inflammatory markers at a 12-year interval. It was found that baseline levels of C-reactive protein and IL-6 predicted the development of depressive symptoms at follow-up, independently of baseline depressive symptoms, age, gender, and ethnicity. The relationship remained significant after further adjustment for health behaviors (diet, physical activity, smoking, and alcohol consumption), other biomarkers (adiposity, blood pressure, and cholesterol), health status, and medication. By contrast, depression at baseline did not predict C-reactive protein or IL-6 at follow-up, suggesting that inflammation is a predictor of depressive mood and not vice versa. Findings such as these do not establish that inflammation causes depressed mood, since unmeasured third factors could be responsible, but do demonstrate temporal precedence.

Another limitation of population-level studies of biomarkers in behavioral medicine is that they provide little information about underlying mechanisms. Take the association between lower socioeconomic status and elevated plasma fibrinogen levels noted earlier. It is difficult to know whether this is due to central nervous system activation of pro-inflammatory and hemostatic processes, or if is it mediated by some of the numerous lifestyle factors that are related to fibrinogen and which are differentially distributed across the social gradient (Lee and Lip, 2003).

Many limitations to the interpretation of biological measurements in observational epidemiological studies in behavioral medicine can be attributed to the confounding effects of social, behavioral, and/or physiological factors that are hard to measure and, as a consequence, control. Epidemiological findings are not easily replicated by the use of randomized controlled trials because of ethical and practical constraints. New techniques derived from genetic epidemiology, notably Mendelian randomization, offer one way to circumvent some of these problems. A comprehensive introduction to Mendelian randomization and its limitations is provided by Lawlor and colleagues (2008a). Mendelian randomization refers to "studies that use genetic variants in observational epidemiology to make causal inferences about modifiable (non-genetic) risk factors for disease and health-related outcomes"

(Lawlor et al, 2008a, p. 1135). In other words, it is a method that allows researchers to establish causal risk factors by using genetic polymorphisms that are known to modify the disease endpoint via their effects on the exposure of interest (e.g., body mass index, alcohol consumption). Mendelian randomization is based on Mendel's second law which posits that the inheritance of one trait occurs independently of all other traits. This can be applied to populations in which the independent allocation of alleles from parents to offspring assures that the population genotype is unrelated to confounders (e.g., socioeconomic position, lifestyle factors). Because of this, Mendelian randomization studies have been termed "natural" randomized controlled trials (Hingorani and Humphries, 2005). In terms of statistics, Mendelian randomization is an application of the theory of "instrumental variable" analysis (see Didelez and Sheehan 2007), where an instrumental variable is a variable which is *only* associated with the outcome through its association with a mediating variable (i.e., the exposure of interest).

For example, one application of this method used the known relationship between the FTO polymorphism rs9939609 and body mass index to support the epidemiological evidence for the positive association between lifetime body mass index and atherosclerosis risk in a sample of over 2000 young adults (Kivimäki et al, 2008). In another study, Lawlor and colleagues (2008b) examined the relationship between C-reactive protein and CHD risk in 18,637 participants, using the known C-reactive protein genetic variant +1444C>T (rs1130864). Participants with one variant had higher C-reactive protein levels than others, but did not suffer more CHD. An instrumental variables analysis suggested that circulating C-reactive protein was not associated with CHD, thereby failing to support the hypothesis of a causal relationship, a result replicated by Elliott and colleagues (2009). However, it should be noted that there are exceptions to Mendel's second law, and the term "linkage disequilibrium" is used to describe instances where independent assortment of genes does not occur. Some studies may not have sufficient statistical power to disprove causal associations, since the sample sizes required can be daunting (Schatzkin et al, 2009). Nevertheless, this method promises to be valuable in unpicking the biological mediators of behavioral factors in health in the future.

4 Psychophysiological Stress Testing

The laboratory stress testing method involves monitoring biological responses to standardized psychological or social stimuli. A comprehensive discussion of laboratory stress testing methodology is provided in Chapter 41, so here we only highlight some aspects particularly salient to the measurement of biomarkers. A wide range of mental stress tests have been employed in behavioral medicine, including cognitive and problem solving tasks, simulated public speaking, upsetting films, and interpersonal conflict tasks. All these tasks elicit physiological reactions in participants that can be used to index stress reactivity. An important factor is that the absolute levels of biological measures are relatively unimportant – these can be measured better in a quiet, non-stimulating environment – since the focus is on changes over time: from pre-stressor through to recovery once the stressor has been removed (i.e., the task is completed). A typical stress testing session involves a period of rest so that baseline levels of physiological function can be established, followed by a challenge period that may last anything from 5 min to 3 h depending on the protocol in question. More than one stress task is sometimes used in the same session allowing comparisons to be made between responses to different challenges; for example, comparisons between actively controllable and passive stressors (Lovallo et al, 1985). However, such designs must be used very cautiously, since the time course of different biological responses varies widely. Blood pressure and heart rate respond rapidly, within 1–2 min after the onset of stress, while salivary and blood cortisol can take up to 30 min to peak, and inflammatory cytokines such as IL-6 continue to rise for up to 2 h post-stress. There is growing interest in variations in rate of post-stress recovery, since these may be indicative of chronic allostatic load (see Chapter 42). Protocols that are not sufficiently long to measure recovery processes lose data that are potentially significant to health. Recovery rates vary with psychosocial factors and with age. Blood pressure, for instance, may return to baseline within a few minutes of stress termination in young adults, but can remain elevated for more than 1 h in older individuals (Steptoe et al, 2002).

It is also important to recognize that stress tasks are not interchangeable, but have distinctive characteristics. Apart from well-known dimensions such as sensory intake/rejection, predictability/unpredictability, and controllabity/uncontrollability, the involvement of social challenges is relevant. Dickerson and Kemeny's (2004) meta-analysis of laboratory studies of cortisol responses clearly demonstrates that the largest cortisol increases are typically observed in reactions to social-evaluative challenges such as simulated public speaking, rather than during exposure to difficult tasks or aversive stimuli.

Perhaps the greatest value of psychophysiological stress testing in behavioral medicine is that the controlled conditions of the laboratory allow blood sampling and sophisticated physiological measures such as radionuclide ventriculography or whole body plethysmography that are impractical in other settings. Many of the advances in understanding the biological pathways through which environmental and psychosocial factors influence health have emerged because researchers have moved beyond monitoring blood pressure, heart rate, and skin conductance to investigate neuroendocrine and immune measures, many of which involve sophisticated processing of blood samples and to take advantage of newer functional imaging technologies of the brain, heart, and other organs. Additionally, biological responses to psychosocial stimuli can be monitored under standardized environmental conditions, reducing the many sources of bias and individual difference that may otherwise be present. Experimental designs can be used, with randomization to different conditions (such as low and high anger provocation), that is not feasible in population studies. There are, however, limitations to these methods, many of which are discussed in greater detail in Chapter 41. One important issue is that the stimuli applied are often arbitrary and bear little resemblance to those experienced in everyday life, threatening ecological validity. Second, the stimuli used are brief, so that only acute biological responses can be recorded. Chronic challenges may elicit different response patterns because of factors such as habituation, adaptation, and chronic allostatic load. The generalizability of findings is therefore uncertain in many cases. Because of this, psychophysiological testing has been increasingly complemented by naturalistic and ambulatory monitoring methods in behavioral medicine.

5 Naturalistic and Ambulatory Monitoring of Biological Variables

Naturalistic studies involve sampling biological variables during everyday life. This sampling method is known as ambulatory monitoring when the measurement instruments are carried on the person and operate automatically. Naturalistic studies take many forms, from recordings during challenging tasks such as parachuting or public speaking, to repeated measures of blood pressure or salivary cortisol over an ordinary day. Some of these techniques are extensions of methods used in clinical investigation, such as "Holter" monitoring of electrocardiogram in patients with coronary artery disease and the use of ambulatory blood pressure monitors for evaluating hypertension. The purpose of these methods in behavioral medicine research is to assess biological activity under natural conditions and thus to circumvent some of the problems with laboratory studies concerning ecological validity. In addition, these studies aim to examine the covariation between everyday activities, emotions, and biology. There are still technical limitations to the range of measures that can be obtained using naturalistic and ambulatory monitoring techniques; blood samples, for instance, are difficult to collect. Some of the primary biological measures used in behavioral medicine are detailed below, but are described in more detail in later chapters.

5.1 Cortisol

Salivary cortisol can easily be measured in naturalistic studies since samples can be readily collected and stored using Salivettes and other devices. Cortisol remains stable in saliva at room temperature and so can be kept for several days, allowing participants to return collection tubes by mail (Kirschbaum and Hellhammer, 2007). An immense advantage of assessing salivary cortisol is that repeated measures can be obtained, allowing the diurnal rhythm of the hormone to be recorded. The cortisol awakening response, the cortisol slope over the day, and total cortisol over the day have all received attention. For example, one study of 70 patients who had recently experienced an acute coronary syndrome (ACS) involved eight measures of salivary cortisol over a day at home (Molloy et al, 2008). Thirty-eight percent of the sample was identified as having type D personality. Type D personality was not related to the cortisol awakening response, but cortisol output during the day was higher in type D than non type D patients after adjustment for covariates.

Similar methods have also been applied in larger scale epidemiological studies, though these settings require stringent quality control and adherence to protocols (Adam and Kumari, 2009). For example, Kumari and colleagues (2009) reported that low waking salivary cortisol and a flat slope in cortisol secretion were associated with fatigue in a study of more than 4000 older men and women. Interestingly, these authors found that cortisol is associated with future onset of fatigue, which may suggest that changes in cortisol secretion are involved in the etiology or are part of the early stages of fatigue. In another study that used data from the Whitehall II cohort, cortisol output over the day was inversely related to adaptive coping styles such as seeking social support and problem engagement, independently of potential confounders (O'Donnell et al, 2008). This suggests that neuroendocrine pathways may partly mediate the relationship between psychological coping and health. Additional studies have investigated associations between cortisol output and low socioeconomic status, social isolation, and other psychosocial risk factors (Grant et al, 2009; Li et al, 2007).

A different design has been used to assess the concurrent and sequential associations between cortisol, mood, and daily experience. Multilevel modeling studies have demonstrated that negative affect is associated with rises in cortisol (Jacobs et al, 2007), while feelings of loneliness and sadness on 1 day are followed by greater cortisol awakening responses on the next (Adam et al, 2006). In studies of this type, accurate timing of saliva samples is essential, and most researchers remain dependent on participants reliably recording sampling times. Another limitation of such analyses is the need to take factors such as time of day, smoking, ingestive behaviors, and other confounders into account. These are largely assessed by self-report and may also not be entirely accurate.

5.2 Cardiovascular Measures

The cardiovascular measures primarily used in behavioral medicine ambulatory monitoring studies are blood pressure, heart rate, heart rate variability, and ST segment analysis. Devices for measuring ambulatory blood pressure consist of an arm cuff with inbuilt signal detection device, an air hose, and portable pump. They operate in the same way as standard blood pressure monitors, except that the equipment is miniaturized and portable, and can be worn beneath clothing.

The cuff is pre-programmed to inflate periodically, with intervals of 15–60 min being used depending on the protocol, so that a profile of blood pressure over the day can be built up. Ambulatory blood pressure monitors are often used at night as well and provide useful information about blood pressure "dipping" and subsequent morning surges (Kario et al, 2003). A recent meta-analysis has found that ambulatory monitoring of blood pressure provides clinically important information over and above that provided by conventional clinical measures and is consistently associated with stroke, cardiovascular mortality, total mortality, and cardiac events (Conen and Bamberg, 2008).

Perhaps the most common application of ambulatory blood pressure monitoring in behavioral medicine has been in studies of work stress. Job strain is more consistently related to ambulatory blood pressure than to measures taken in the clinic (Steenland et al, 2000). The reason is presumably that blood pressure is affected directly by the experience of work stress in the setting in which exposure occurs, although carry-over effects are also observed. For example, an investigation of around 200 men and women from the Whitehall II study involved ambulatory blood pressure monitoring every 20 min from early in the working day until going to bed (Steptoe and Willemsen, 2004). Systolic and diastolic blood pressure were greater in participants reporting low compared with high job control, and these effects were independent of gender, employment grade, body mass index, age, smoking status, and physical activity. Interestingly, differences were present both over the working day and the evening. Ambulatory blood pressure has been related to other psychosocial factors as well. For instance, it has been hypothesized that the impact of environmental stressors on blood pressure will increase with exposure to more than one challenge. Tobe and colleagues (2007) conducted a longitudinal study investigating the effects of job strain and marital cohesion on ambulatory blood pressure in a sample of more than 200 male and female volunteers. Over 1 year, the combination of high job strain and a low cohesive marriage was associated with a mean increase in ambulatory systolic BP of 3 mmHg, whereas participants with job strain who also had highly cohesive marriages showed a reduction of systolic BP of 3 mmHg. Barnett et al (2005) found that poor marital quality was associated with elevated ambulatory diastolic blood pressure but not with clinic measures, and these cardiovascular effects were coupled with elevated stress ratings over the day.

A variety of ambulatory heart rate monitors are now available that can be programmed either to record heart rate averaged into short epochs of 15–30 s or to complete beat by beat information. The latter is valuable, since it permits heart rate variability measures to be derived (see Chapter 47). Still more detail is provided by Holter monitors (named after their inventor) that record the complete electrocardiographic (EKG) signal; these can be analyzed for EKG markers of cardiac pathology such as ST segment changes and the long Q syndrome. Recent advances have led to the development of small wireless devices that require only two or three electrodes and can therefore be worn more comfortably under clothing (e.g., Actiheart, MetriSense Inc.). An example comes from a study by Pieper and colleagues (2007) who recorded ambulatory heart rate and heart rate variability in 73 male and female teachers for 4 days, during which time participants also kept an hourly computerized diary of worry and stressful events. Findings showed that worry episodes and stressful events were positively associated with heart rate and heart rate variability independently of psychological traits and biobehavioral variables. Effects were most pronounced for work-related worry and for worry about anticipated future stress.

Care has to be taken in the interpretation of ambulatory results, since smoking, consumption of caffeinated drinks and alcohol can all affect cardiovascular measures. Multilevel modeling has been used to analyze these ambulatory data in order to tease out the independent contribution of psychosocial factors (Schwartz et al, 1994). One of the most important determinants of cardiovascular function is physical activity and ongoing energy expenditure. This is illustrated in Fig. 40.1, which shows ambulatory data

obtained from 200 working women over two 24-h periods beginning at 5:00 pm. One period began on the evening of a working day and continued into the next working day, while the second was followed by a leisure day. For convenience, data are averaged into 2-h segments. The upper panel shows mean heart rate, where it can be seen that levels decreased in the night while participants were asleep and rose again in the morning. The morning rise took place 1–2 h earlier on the working day, because participants got up earlier. The lower panel shows physical activity recorded using an accelerometer. The pattern of change over day and night closely parallels that for heart rate, even down to the difference between work and leisure days.

5.3 Musculoskeletal Measures

Much research on musculoskeletal disorders relies on self-report or physical examination, but direct measurement of muscle tension using surface electromyography (EMG) has been used in behavioral medicine research to provide valuable additional information. Miniaturized transducers and telemetric equipment are available that allow readings to be obtained from free-moving individuals. Positive correlations have been reported between objectively assessed muscle tension and feelings of stress and exhaustion during work, and recently these findings have been correlated with lower pressure pain thresholds and higher pain intensity in people suffering from chronic neck and shoulder pain (Larsson et al, 2008). Surface EMG is also used extensively in headache research, with monitoring of muscles of the neck, back, and forehead. A meta-analysis of studies of frontal EMG indicated that patients with tension-type headache have higher muscle tension than controls on average, but with wide variability (Wittrock, 1997). This suggests that while EMG recordings in everyday life provide important data, they need to be interpreted in conjunction with self-report measures of pain and tension.

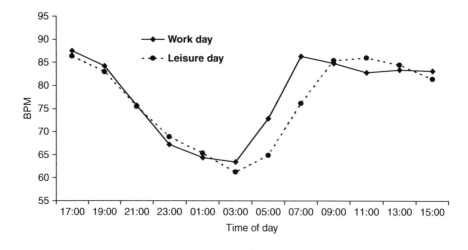

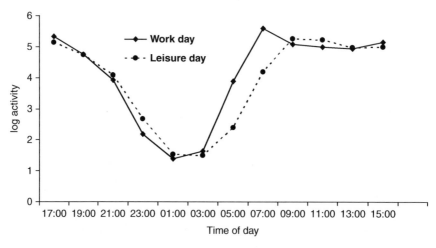

Fig. 40.1 Mean heart rate in bpm (*upper panel*) and log physical activity (*lower panel*) averaged into 2-h blocks over a working and leisure day in 200 working women in Budapest (Salavecz, Dockray, Kopp and Steptoe, unpublished)

5.4 New Developments in Ambulatory Monitoring Devices

Advances in technology have led to the expansion in the use of wireless ambulatory monitoring devices that are now capable of measuring ever greater numbers of biomarkers, including skin conductance, skin temperature, respiration rate, pulse rate, sleep/wake cycle, to name but a few. These devices have the advantages of being small, lightweight, and easy-to-wear, often in the form of a wristband (e.g., The SOMNOwatch, SOMNOmedics, DE) (for a review see Pantelopoulos and Bourbakis,

2008). Smart fabrics have also opened up new possibilities for monitoring biomarkers, and intelligent clothing can be used to detect respiration rate, the EKG, and motion (Lymberis and Paradiso, 2008). The cost of purchasing such equipment has led to little uptake in behavioral medicine research to date, but this situation is likely to change.

5.5 Summary and Limitations

Naturalistic and ambulatory monitoring methods have the advantage of improved ecological validity, evaluating biological activity in real life rather than under the artificial conditions of a laboratory or clinic. Associations between psychosocial factors and biological responses may be observed that are not detectable when single measures are taken under clinical or survey conditions. But naturalistic methods also have several drawbacks, in addition to the specific methodological issues described earlier. First, the range of biological markers that can be assessed is relatively small in comparison with the more sophisticated possibilities available in the laboratory setting. Second, the measurement techniques need to be relatively unobtrusive, so as not to interfere with ongoing activities. This is why some pioneering studies of repeated measurements over the day can now be questioned for their representativeness. For instance, much of the early data on circadian rhythms of cortisol secretion involved venepuncture every 1 or 2 h for 24 h or the periodic withdrawal of blood from an indwelling cannula. There is danger that such methods are so stressful in themselves that they will obscure any association between psychosocial factors and biological responses, and certainly they can cause sleep disturbance (Jarrett et al, 1984). Newer research using measures of hormones such as cortisol, dehydroepiandrosterone, testosterone, prolactin, and estrogen in saliva may overcome these problems. Third, there are several intrinsic and extrinsic factors that influence biological function that need to be taken into account, including cigarette smoking, food and caffeine intake, sleep, and physical activity. These factors need to be carefully monitored and recorded in naturalistic studies and controlled for statistically in data analysis. Multilevel modeling has become the method of choice in analyses of these data (see Chapter 56).

Another issue that has not been studied in sufficient detail is the impact of ambulatory or naturalistic monitoring on the behavior of the participant. The purpose of this type of assessment is to capture everyday experience, but it is possible that awareness that monitoring is being carried out might alter ongoing behavior. In one study, Costa and colleagues (1999) carried out ambulatory blood pressure and heart rate monitoring in 24 high school teachers over the working day and evening. The blood pressure monitors were programmed to record every 20 min, and the participant also completed a short log of their location, activity, and mood. Activity was measured on the same day using an accelerometer. On another day, the accelerometer was worn, but no cardiovascular monitoring was performed. It was found that energy expenditure was consistently lower on the blood pressure monitoring day, since participants were less active. Additionally, their range of activities was also more limited than when they just wore the accelerometer. This suggests that ambulatory monitoring may have led people to limit their usual activities. Further work is needed to evaluate the extent of this confounder of ambulatory monitoring data.

This issue is linked with another major concern in the literature on naturalistic and ambulatory monitoring, namely the relationship between measures in everyday life and those obtained in psychophysiological stress testing. "Lab–field" correlations are variable (Turner et al, 1994), and this has been taken to cast doubt on the validity of acute stress testing (Parati et al, 1991). This topic has been addressed most extensively in relation to blood pressure and heart rate. A factor that appears to be relevant is the situation in which ambulatory recordings are obtained. It can be argued that reactivity to behavioral stress in the laboratory will not be strongly correlated with blood pressure recorded in undemanding situations in everyday life, but only when people experience stressful episodes in their lives. Several studies have observed such effects (Johnston et al, 2008; Kamarck et al, 2003). This also appears to be the case in studies relating laboratory responses with everyday life experience for other physiological variables such as pulmonary function (Ritz et al, 2000). Other work has observed strong associations between post-stress recovery profiles of cardiovascular activity and ambulatory measures (Trivedi et al, 2008); this is logical, since the persistence of blood pressure changes after acute stress may be particularly relevant to levels in everyday life.

6 Conclusions

Developments in the use of biological measures in behavioral medicine are allowing researchers to ask ever more specific research questions: no longer are biomarkers merely used as measures of disease status but also as indicators of psychological, social, and economic experience. Moreover, the borrowing of techniques from other disciplines, especially genetics, may generate more detailed knowledge about the interaction between different biological systems and their impact on health in the future. A full understanding of the interplay between biological and behavioral factors in disease etiology, progression, and management does not depend on just one of the research paradigms outlined in this chapter. Rather, the field can only advance through the convergence and integration of knowledge acquired with different research methodologies. There is still much to be done, and the challenge for the coming decade will be to understand in greater detail the exact mechanisms underlying the pathway from biomarkers to illness, so that their full repercussions for sustained well-being can be delineated.

References

Abbott, D. H., Keverne, E. B., Bercovitch, F. B., Shively, C. A., Mendoza, S. P. et al (2003). Are subordinates always stressed? A comparative analysis of rank differences in cortisol levels among primates. *Horm Behav, 43*, 67–82.

Adam, E. K., and Kumari, M. (2009). Assessing salivary cortisol in large-scale, epidemiological research. *Psychoneuroendocrinology, 34*, 1423–1436.

Adam, E. K., Hawkley, L. C., Kudielka, B. M., and Cacioppo, J. T. (2006). Day-to-day dynamics of experience-cortisol associations in a population-based sample of older adults. *Proc Natl Acad Sci U S A, 103*, 17058–17063.

Barnett, R. C., Steptoe, A., and Gareis, K. C. (2005). Marital-role quality and stress-related psychobiological indicators. *Ann Behav Med, 30*, 36–43.

Brunner, E., Davey Smith, G., Marmot, M., Canner, R., Beksinska, M. et al (1996). Childhood social circumstances and psychosocial and behavioural factors as determinants of plasma fibrinogen. *Lancet, 347*, 1008–1013.

Conen, D., and Bamberg, F. (2008). Noninvasive 24-h ambulatory blood pressure and cardiovascular disease: a systematic review and meta-analysis. *J Hypertens, 26*, 1290–1299.

Costa, M., Cropley, M., Griffith, J., and Steptoe, A. (1999). Ambulatory blood pressure monitoring is associated with reduced physical activity during everyday life. *Psychosom Med, 61*, 806–811.

Danese, A., Pariante, C. M., Caspi, A., Taylor, A., and Poulton, R. (2007). Childhood maltreatment predicts adult inflammation in a life-course study. *Proc Natl Acad Sci U S A, 104*, 1319–1324.

Davey Smith, G., Ben-Shlomo, Y., Beswick, A., Yarnell, J., Lightman, S. et al. (2005). Cortisol, testosterone, and coronary heart disease: prospective evidence from the Caerphilly study. *Circulation, 112*, 332–340.

Dekker, M. J., Koper, J. W., van Aken, M. O., Pols, H. A., Hofman, A. et al (2008). Salivary cortisol is related to atherosclerosis of carotid arteries. *J Clin Endocrinol Metab, 93*, 3741–3747.

Dickerson, S. S., and Kemeny, M. E. (2004). Acute stressors and cortisol responses: a theoretical integration and synthesis of laboratory research. *Psychol Bull, 130*, 355–391.

Didelez, V., and Sheehan, N. 2007. Mendelian randomization as an instrumental variable approach to causal inference. *Stat Methods Med Res, 16*, 309–330.

Elliott, P., Chambers, J. C., Zhang, W., Clarke, R., Hopewell, J. C., et al (2009). Genetic Loci associated with C-reactive protein levels and risk of coronary heart disease. *J Am Med Assoc, 302*, 37–48.

Ely, D., Caplea, A., Dunphy, G., and Smith, D. (1997). Physiological and neuroendocrine correlates of social position in normotensive and hypertensive rat colonies. *Acta Physiol Scand Suppl, 640*, 92–95.

Feinbloom, D., and Bauer, K. (2005). Assessment of hemostatic risk factors in predicting arterial thrombotic events. *Arterioscler Thromb Vasc Bio, 25*, 2043–2053.

Fibrinogen Studies Collaboration. (2005). Plasma fibrinogen level and the risk of major cardiovascular diseases and nonvascular mortality: An individual participant meta-analysis. *JAMA, 294*, 1799–1809.

Gimeno, D., Kivimäki, M., Brunner, E. J., Elovainio, M., De Vogli, R. et al (2009). Associations of C-reactive protein and interleukin-6 with cognitive symptoms of depression: 12-year follow-up of the Whitehall II study. *Psychol Med, 39*, 413–423.

Goodyer, I. M., Herbert, J., Tamplin, A., and Altham, P. M. (2000). Recent life events, cortisol, dehydroepiandrosterone and the onset of major depression in high-risk adolescents. *Br J Psychiatry, 177*, 499–504.

Grant, N., Hamer, M., and Steptoe, A. (2009). Social isolation and stress-related cardiovascular, lipid, and cortisol responses. *Ann Behav Med, 37*, 29–37.

Hamer, M., and Steptoe, A. (2008). Walking, vigorous physical activity, and markers of hemostasis and inflammation in healthy men and women. *Scand J Med Sci Sports, 18,* 736–741.

Harris, T. O., Borsanyi, S., Messari, S., Stanford, K., Cleary, S. E. et al (2000). Morning cortisol as a risk factor for subsequent major depressive disorder in adult women. *Br J Psychiatry, 177,* 505–510.

Helfand, M., Buckley, D. I., Freeman, M., Fu, R., Rogers, K. et al (2009). Emerging risk factors for coronary heart disease: a summary of systematic reviews conducted for the U.S. Preventive Services Task Force. *Ann Intern Med, 151,* 496–507.

Herbert, J., Goodyer, I. M., Grossman, A. B., Hastings, M. H., de Kloet, E. R. et al (2006). Do corticosteroids damage the brain? *J Neuroendocrinol, 18,* 393–411.

Hingorani, A., and Humphries, S. (2005). Nature's randomized trials. *Lancet, 366,* 1906–1908.

Howren, M. B., Lamkin, D. M., and Suls, J. (2009). Associations of depression with C-reactive protein, IL-1, and IL-6: a meta-analysis. *Psychosom Med, 71,* 171–186.

Jacobs, N., Myin-Germeys, I., Derom, C., Delespaul, P., van Os, J. et al (2007). A momentary assessment study of the relationship between affective and adrenocortical stress responses in daily life. *Biol Psychol, 74,* 60–66.

Jarrett, D. B., Greenhouse, J. B., Thompson, S. B., McEachran, A., Coble, P., and Kupfer, D. J. (1984). Effect of nocturnal intravenous cannulation upon sleep-EEG measures. *Biol Psychiatry, 19,* 1537–1550.

Johnston, D. W., Tuomisto, M. T., and Patching, G. R. (2008). The relationship between cardiac reactivity in the laboratory and in real life. *Health Psychol, 27,* 34–42.

Kamarck, T. W., Schwartz, J. E., Janicki, D. L., Shiffman, S., and Raynor, D. A. (2003). Correspondence between laboratory and ambulatory measures of cardiovascular reactivity: a multilevel modeling approach. *Psychophysiology, 40,* 675–683.

Kaplan, J. R., Chen, H., and Manuck, S. B. (2009). The relationship between social status and atherosclerosis in male and female monkeys as revealed by meta-analysis. *Am J Primatol, 71,* 732–741.

Kario, K., Pickering, T. G., Umeda, Y., Hoshide, S., Hoshide, Y. et al (2003). Morning surge in blood pressure as a predictor of silent and clinical cerebrovascular disease in elderly hypertensives: a prospective study. *Circulation, 107,* 1401–1406.

Kiecolt-Glaser, J. K., Preacher, K. J., MacCallum, R. C., Atkinson, C., Malarkey, W. B. et al (2003). Chronic stress and age-related increases in the proinflammatory cytokine IL-6. *Proc Natl Acad Sci U S A, 100,* 9090–9095.

Kirschbaum, C., and Hellhammer, D. (2007). Salivary cortisol. In G. Fink (Ed.), *Encyclopedia of Stress, 2nd Ed, Vol 3* (pp. 405–409). Oxford: Academic Press.

Kivimäki, M., Smith, G. D., Timpson, N. J., Lawlor, D. A., Batty, G. D. et al (2008). Lifetime body mass index and later atherosclerosis risk in young adults: examining causal links using Mendelian randomization in the Cardiovascular Risk in Young Finns study. *Eur Heart J, 29,* 2552–2560.

Kumari, M., Badrick, E., Chandola, T., Adam, E. K., Stafford, M. et al (2009). Cortisol secretion and fatigue: associations in a community based cohort. *Psychoneuroendocrinology, 34,* 1476–1485.

Kumari, M., Marmot, M., and Brunner, E. (2000). Social determinants of von Willebrand factor: the Whitehall II study. *Arterioscler Thromb Vasc Biol, 20,* 1842–1847.

Larsson, B., Rosendal, L., Kristiansen, J., Sjøgaard, G., Søgaard, K. et al (2008). Responses of algesic and metabolic substances to 8 h of repetitive manual work in myalgic human trapezius muscle. *Pain, 140,* 479–490.

Lawlor, D. A., Harbord, R. M., Sterne, J. A., Timpson, N., and Davey Smith, G. (2008a). Mendelian randomization: using genes as instruments for making causal inferences in epidemiology. *Stat Med, 27,* 1133–1163.

Lawlor, D. A., Harbord, R. M., Timpson, N. J., Lowe, G. D., Rumley, A. et al (2008b). The association of C-reactive protein and CRP genotype with coronary heart disease: findings from five studies with 4,610 cases amongst 18,637 participants. *PLoS One, 3,* e3011.

Lee, K. W., and Lip, G. Y. (2003). Effects of lifestyle on hemostasis, fibrinolysis, and platelet reactivity: a systematic review. *Arch Intern Med, 163,* 2368–2392.

Li, L., Power, C., Kelly, S., Kirschbaum, C., and Hertzman, C. (2007). Life-time socio-economic position and cortisol patterns in mid-life. *Psychoneuroendocrinology, 32,* 824–833.

Lovallo, W. R., Wilson, M. F., Pincomb, G. A., Edwards, G. L., Tompkins, P. et al (1985). Activation patterns to aversive stimulation in man: passive exposure versus effort to control. *Psychophysiology, 22,* 283–291.

Lupien, S. J., Fiocco, A., Wan, N., Maheu, F., Lord, C. et al (2005). Stress hormones and human memory function across the lifespan. *Psychoneuroendocrinology, 30,* 225–242.

Lymberis, A., and Paradiso, R. (2008). Smart fabrics and interactive textile enabling wearable personal applications: R&D state of the art and future challenges. *Conf Proc IEEE Eng Med Biol Soc 2008,* 5270–5273.

Maes, M. (1995). Evidence for an immune response in major depression: a review and hypothesis. *Prog Neuro-Psychopharamcol Biol Psychiatry, 461,* 11–38.

Molloy, G. J., Perkins-Porras, L., Strike, P. C., and Steptoe, A. (2008). Type-D personality and cortisol in survivors of acute coronary syndrome. *Psychosom Med, 70,* 863–868.

O'Donnell, K., Badrick, E., Kumari, M., and Steptoe, A. (2008). Psychological coping styles and cortisol over the day in healthy older adults. *Psychoneuroendocrinology, 33,* 601–611.

Pantelopoulos, A., and Bourbakis, N. (2008). A survey on wearable biosensor systems for health monitoring. *Conf Proc IEEE Eng Med Biol Soc 2008*, 4887–4890.

Parati, G., Trazzi, S., Ravogli, A., Casadei, R., Omboni, S. et al (1991). Methodological problems in evaluation of cardiovascular effects of stress in humans. *Hypertension, 17*, III50–III5.

Pieper, S., Brosschot, J. F., van der Leeden, R., and Thayer, J. F. (2007). Cardiac effects of momentary assessed worry episodes and stressful events. *Psychosom Med, 60*, 901–909.

Pierce, M., Tabassum, F., Kumari, M., Zaninotto, P., and Steel, N. (2006). Measures of physical health. In J. Banks, E. Breeze, C. Lessof, & J. Nazroo (Eds.), *Retirement, Health and Relationships of the Older Population in England: The 2004 English Longitudinal Study of Ageing (Wave 2)* (pp. 127–163). London: Institute for Fiscal Studies.

Raison, C. L., Capuron, L., and Miller, A. H. (2006). Cytokines sing the blues: inflammation and the pathogenesis of depression. *Trends Immunol, 27*, 24–31.

Ritz, T., and Steptoe, A. (2000). Emotion and pulmonary function in asthma: reactivity in the field and relationship with laboratory induction of emotion. *Psychosom Med, 62*, 808–15.

Sapolsky, R. M. (1995). Social subordinance as a marker of hypercortisolism. Some unexpected subtleties. *Ann N Y Acad Sci, 771*, 626–639.

Schatzkin, A., Abnet, C. C., Cross, A. J., Gunter, M., Pfeiffer, R. et al (2009). Mendelian randomization: how it can--and cannot--help confirm causal relations between nutrition and cancer. *Cancer Prev Res (Phila Pa), 2*, 104–113.

Schwartz, J.E., Warren, K., and Pickering, T.G. (1994). Mood, location and physical position as predictors of ambulatory blood pressure and heart rate: application of a multi-level random effects model. *Ann Behav Med, 16*, 210–220.

Shively, C. A., Register, T. C., and Clarkson, T. B. (2009). Social stress, visceral obesity, and coronary artery atherosclerosis in female primates. *Obesity (Silver Spring), 17*, 1513–1520.

Steenland, K., Fine, L., Belkic, K., Landsbergis, P., Schnall, P. et al (2000). Research findings linking workplace factors to CVD outcomes. *Occup Med (Phil), 15*, 7–68.

Steptoe, A., and Willemsen, G. (2004). The influence of low job control on ambulatory blood pressure and perceived stress over the working day in men and women from the Whitehall II cohort. *J Hyperten, 22*, 915–920.

Steptoe, A., Feldman, P. M., Kunz, S., Owen, N., Willemsen, G. et al (2002). Stress responsivity and socioeconomic status: a mechanism for increased cardiovascular disease risk? *Euro Heart J, 23*, 1757–1763.

Tabák, A. G., Jokela, M., Akbaraly, T. N., Brunner, E. J., Kivimäki, M. et al (2009). Trajectories of glycaemia, insulin sensitivity, and insulin secretion before diagnosis of type 2 diabetes: an analysis from the Whitehall II study. *Lancet, 373*, 2215–2221.

Tobe, S. W., Kiss, A., Sainsbury, S., Jesin, M., Geerts, R. et al (2007). The impact of job strain and marital cohesion on ambulatory blood pressure during 1 year: the double exposure study. *Am J Hypertens, 20*, 148–153.

Trivedi, R., Sherwood, A., Strauman, T. J., and Blumenthal, J. A. (2008). Laboratory-based blood pressure recovery is a predictor of ambulatory blood pressure. *Biol Psychol, 77*, 317–323.

Turner, J., Ward, M., Gellman, M., Johnston, D., Light, K. et al (1994). The relationship between laboratory and ambulatory cardiovascular activity: current evidence and future directions. *Ann Behav Med, 16*, 12–23.

Weaver, J. D., Huang, M. H., Albert, M., Harris, T., Rowe, J. W. et al (2002). Interleukin-6 and risk of cognitive decline: MacArthur studies of successful aging. *Neurology, 59*, 371–378.

Wittrock, D.A. (1997). The comparison of individuals with tension-type headache and headache-free controls on frontal EMG levels: a meta-analysis. *Headache, 37*, 424–432.

Chapter 41

Laboratory Stress Testing Methodology

William Gerin

1 Introduction

Researchers in the health field are increasingly inclined to attribute the development of chronic disease in part to prolonged exposure to aspects of the environment that we find stressful or challenging. Epidemiological data unequivocally show that psychosocial factors have a substantial influence on the development of chronic illness, often as great or greater than traditional biological risk factors. However, the mediators of the stress–disease relationship remain poorly specified, though a clearer picture has emerged over the past few decades.

In the broadest sense, the perturbations in various biological measures, occasioned by chronic exposure to stressful situations, will ultimately lead to a dysregulation of those biological systems, and these, over time, may be implicated in the development of heart disease or cancer or rheumatoid arthritis, or any number of chronic illnesses. Given the need to cope with stress and to strive to overcome the barrage of obstacles and frustrations most of us encounter in the 21st century, the relevant biological systems may have little chance to shut off and give the vegetative systems a chance to perform their housekeeping chores.

One means of studying the mechanisms that underlie the stress–disease relationship is by examining the attributes of a particular stressor on the biological measures of interest. For example, were one interested in the acute effects of negative marital interactions on heart rate, he or she might compare dyads based on their levels of social support (a self-selected grouping) or couples exposed or not exposed to an anger management intervention (an experimental strategy). In this particular study one would measure heart rate – a continuous measure – throughout the baseline and stressor phases.

Most studies of the evaluation of the effects of stress on physiological responses are similar in structure. First, the biological parameter of interest – blood pressure, perhaps, or cortisol, or markers of inflammatory responses – is assessed while the subject is resting, to establish a baseline, or comparison, level. Next, the subject is exposed to a presumed stressor ("stressor" is an ambiguous and broad term that might include a challenging task, an arousal of anger, a foot placed in an ice-water bath, and many others) and the physiological parameter(s) of interest are assessed during the exposure. The difference between the baseline and stressor levels has been labeled the "reactivity" to the stimulus. Often, a third phase will be employed in which the subject is allowed to rest following the stressor to provide a measure of "recovery" of the parameter to pre-stress levels (Fig. 41.1).

The structure of the typical study is simple and straightforward. However, as is often the case, the devil is in the details. How should baseline best be measured? Should the subject be

W. Gerin (✉)
Department of Biobehavioral Health, The Pennsylvania
State University, 315 Health and Human Development
East, University Park, PA 16802, USA
e-mail: wxg17@psu.ed

A. Steptoe (ed.), *Handbook of Behavioral Medicine*, DOI 10.1007/978-0-387-09488-5_41,

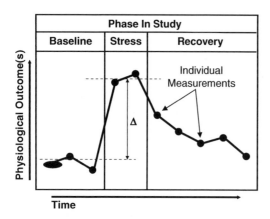

Fig. 41.1 Schematic representation of a typical psychophysiological stress study protocol

sitting up or prone? Allowed to read magazines, or even to fall asleep? Which stressor is going to be administered: Does it matter? If one is going to have the subject count backwards by 13s – a common laboratory task – should the experimenter harass the subject during the task? Should the task be made easier for subjects who cannot perform the arithmetic at all? Why mental arithmetic rather than a Stroop color-naming task, or an interpersonal stressor, or any number of other stimuli that can be used to provoke a physiological response?

For the most part, the stress-reactivity model was limited in earlier years to blood pressure, heart rate, and serum catecholamines. However, it is clear that several biological systems, including but not limited to the cardiovascular system, the hypothalamic–pituitary–adrenal axis, and the immune system, are implicated as mediators of stressor effects on chronic illness. An important advance over the past two or so decades has been the expansion of the stress-reactivity model to include a broader array of outcomes than heretofore tended to be assessed, illustrating the interdisciplinary nature of this research.

The aim of this chapter is to provide an introduction to the methodology by which the effects of stress on physiological outcomes are assessed. This chapter focuses on the independent variables rather than the outcomes; other chapters will go into detail concerning the specifics of various dependent measures.

However, the specifics of measurement of particular outcomes do not, as a rule, change the essential model. Rather, they call for adjustments in subtle aspects of the procedures. Reference to cardiovascular outcomes will be common in this chapter, as much of what we know in the laboratory was learned in studies of stressor effects on heart rate and blood pressure.

2 The Laboratory Setting May Have Powerful, Unintended Effects

Research participants arrive at the laboratory with a range of expectations, anxiety, hostility, excitement, and other characteristics that may have an effect on baseline measurements and possibly their task levels of the outcome measure(s). When these influences are not either manipulated or measured, they enter the statistical model as error, or unexplained variability, making it less likely that significant effects will be observed. Therefore, it is important to be aware of these influences and to control them when possible. Many researchers are careful to control the *physical* elements in the laboratory – temperature, ambient noise, the careful measurement of the target parameters – but ignore the social factors. Characteristics of the persons associated with the laboratory, and how they behave, may have a great effect on baseline measurements and possibly on stress responses.

2.1 Experimenter Characteristics

It is wise to be sensitive to the effect that constitutional characteristics of the experimenter or research assistants may have on the subject's psychological and biological states. For example, the results of a study that focuses on the effect of menstrual cycle on changes in inflammation may be different if a male rather than a female investigator is used. Resting affective and physiological variables may be affected, as well as physiological changes and recovery of the pre-stress baseline. It is a problem if such an effect exists consistently or randomly across conditions; if a male conducts sessions in one condition and a female in another, systematic bias may result, which is more of a problem than using a male for both conditions, in which Type II error may increased, which will obfuscate effects that might truly be present. Similarly, race may have an effect. This is an unfortunate fact of our times, but it must be addressed by the experimenter. Should same-race research assistants always be used? Or just in studies in which race is a factor? Should the issue be tested by including race (or sex) of experimenter as another factor in the study? That would go a way toward addressing the problem, but would also increase the number of groups that must be studied, and add a level of interaction that requires many more subjects and may be difficult to interpret in any case.

These possible effects are almost universally unmeasured; it would be a problem if bias was allowed to creep into the results, but it is also a problem if potential research assistants are excluded based on their gender or race, or other characteristics that cannot be controlled. This is a fine line that the experimenter must walk; at the least, she or he should discuss the issue openly with the laboratory staff and research assistants.

2.2 Experimenter Behavior

In contrast to constitutional factors, some sources of variability due to the experimenter or research assistants is more readily controllable. Mode of dress, for example, should be kept constant within and across conditions; even a shaven versus an unshaven research assistant might conceivably affect subjects in different ways, so it is up to the experimenter to use appropriate judgment as to which such factors need be controlled (cutoffs versus jacket and tie, for example, but not necessarily shoe color!). Then there are social factors that may contribute to the results in an unintended way. To address this problem, research assistants must be carefully trained in the *concepts*, not merely the specific

behaviors called for by the experimental protocol. Thus, it is important that the experimenter treats each subject as much like all the others as possible, not merely to mouth the same words to each. Moreover, the nature of these interactions should be as non-random as possible, and this can be accomplished by scripting, as much as possible, all the social interactions to which the subject will be exposed. The scripted lines should be recorded in the Manual of Operations for that study, and research assistants should learn the script (and the likely deviations). The researcher must develop a manual of operations for every study; it should detail every behavior (including the wording of instructions to the subjects and other relevant verbal behaviors) as they occur in sequence throughout the study. The manual should be revised at the outset of the study in pilot sessions and throughout the actual study based on the observations of the research assistants and experimenters; such observations should be recorded in a log. The scenarios should be thoroughly rehearsed using research assistants as sham subjects. It is not only the words, but the *tone*, that must be held constant; human beings are exquisitely sensitive to nuance. These assertions are based not only on commonsense but also on data that have tested the effects of various social phenomena in the laboratory. The following section will briefly describe some of the phenomena one may encounter.

2.3 Delivery of Instructions

One way to control differences between research assistants or between sessions is to use prerecorded instructions; thus, every subject hears exactly the same thing. The problem with this, however, concerns what it is the researcher wants to control: The objective reality (i.e., the words, the tone) or the subject's perception and understanding. It is more important that each subject *understands* the instructions in the same manner and that may require asking probe questions and allowing the subject to ask questions. Unless the instructions are so straightforward that they cannot be interpreted differently by different persons ("When you hear the tone, press the red button"), it is important to train the research assistant to give instructions verbally in a standardized manner, including probes to ensure that each subject understands the instructions in the same way.

2.4 The Social Context

In the 1990s, as the notion of "social-psychophysiological" research – studying the nature of social interactions in the psychophysiological laboratory – took hold, several studies addressed the question of the mechanisms by which "social support," which has been shown to have a substantive effect on morbidity and mortality, might operate to achieve this effect. The main thrust of the research was that the subject was exposed to stress, but in some conditions was alone and in others, was accompanied by a friend or a friendly research confederate. In general, the studies showed that when evaluation apprehension was not at issue (see next section), the presence of a supportive, friendly person had an attenuating effect on blood pressure and cortisol responsivity. In some of these studies, social support was manipulated by having the experimenter behave in a friendly manner – making appropriate eye contact, nodding in agreement as the subject spoke, murmuring "mm-hmm" at intervals; compared with a condition in which the experimenter was unresponsive, did not make eye contact, and gave little or no friendly feedback (Christenfeld et al, 1997). Again, these studies showed that the "support" condition reduced the cardiovascular response. Although blood pressure cannot be used as a simple measure of emotional or stress-induced activation, it certainly is an indicator; thus, although the outcomes might be different, the cardiovascular effects shown in these studies suggest that other outcome parameters may be similarly affected.

In many laboratories, such behaviors are now routinely scripted and controlled, and research assistants are carefully trained to act in a "clinical" manner, that is, one that is not overly friendly or sympathetic, nor hostile and unsympathetic. It is especially important to train research assistants to understand that their own likes and dislikes, prejudices, or bad or good moods must not be allowed to influence the manner of interaction with a particular research subject.

2.5 Evaluation Apprehension

The experiments that tested the effects of social support found, in general, that when compared with a control condition (in which no social support was provided), social supported led to decreased cardiovascular arousal. However, not all studies have found this pattern of results; indeed, under some conditions, the presence of even a friendly observer led to a *larger* cardiovascular stress response than the control condition. In an attempt to explain these inconsistencies, it has been argued that reduced cardiovascular reactivity as a function of social support was most consistently observed when the study protocols were designed to reduce the *evaluative* nature of the stressor. Researchers have noted that studies that showed greater cardiovascular responsivity as a function of social support shared the following characteristics: (a) The supportive observer was in a position of observing task performance and (b) The supportive observer provided no verbal feedback to the participant during task performance (Kamarck et al, 1995). These studies emphasized the *evaluative* nature of the manipulation.

The subtle differences between the effects of social support and evaluation apprehension point to the importance of considering the nature of the social interactions that are programmed to occur during the laboratory session. An observer or experimenter who appears unfriendly may cause greater sympathetic arousal (for example); however, a friendly observer may do the same, if he or she is in a position to evaluate the subject's performance on the stressor challenge.

2.6 Demand Characteristics

"Demand characteristics" of the situation constitute an unwanted influence in the experimental design that occurs when research subjects modify their behavior in response to subtle cues, such as a higher status researcher, such as a physician, compared to a student research assistant, for example, and in response to their own self-presentation styles and biases. One common cause of subjects responding to the demand characteristics of the situation concerns *evaluation apprehension* (see previous section) which may cause subjects to become over-concerned with achieving a good score (whatever that might be) rather than simply responding to the situation as presented. The researcher must also consider the context of the artificiality of the laboratory situation; it cannot be over-emphasized that research subjects tend to be acutely aware that they are participating in an experiment.

"Roles" have been observed on the part of the subjects, including

- The "good subject": The subject forms an opinion about what the experimenter wants, in terms of the results of the study, and tries to accommodate.
- The "bad subject": The subject forms an opinion about what the experimenter wants, in terms of the results of the study, and tries to behave in a way so as to *undermine* the study hypothesis. (Note: Subjects may come into the research laboratory with a degree of hostility, sometimes borne of anxiety, but also of other factors, such as "being forced" to participate for course credit, or even a general mistrust of the scientific enterprise).

2.7 Experimenter Expectancies

Perhaps the earliest to describe the effects of experimenter expectations concerning the behavior of the research subjects was Rosenthal (1994), who found evidence that when the experimenter or research assistant who was responsible for interacting with the subject was aware of the study hypothesis, or, of the condition to which a particular subject had been assigned, the results were stronger (in the predicted direction) than when a single or double "blind" was implemented, in which neither subjects nor experimenter was aware of assignment. It is often impractical, and sometimes impossible, to disguise the study hypothesis from the experimenter ("double blind"), but at least it helps if it is concealed from the subject ("single blind"). Upon further study, Rosenthal found expectancy effects in a broad range of experiments, including animal studies.

Blinding is now a staple of experimental design when it is feasible. In the laboratory, the experimenter will usually necessarily know which condition a subject is in because he or she conducts the study protocol, which presumably differs depending on condition. This may not be true, however, in studies in which person variables are the focus, and no manipulation occurs. In this case, all subjects are exposed to the identical protocol, and double blinding is a greater possibility.

Presumably, with experience with various protocols, the researcher will learn which factors matter and which do not; however, it is as wise to control these when possible and to be sensitive to others that may be missed. Note taking during the study to highlight protocol deviations and equipment failures that may occur – yet another potential source of Type II error – will allow better interpretation of data and can be crucial to the success of the experiment.

3 Methodological and Procedural Considerations

3.1 Between-Subjects and Within-Subjects Designs

Often, either of these designs will be appropriate for a particular research question. A within-subjects design may be deemed preferable, as it provides perfect control over within-subject factors that may influence the outcome (e.g., genetics, family history of illness, levels of personality measures, sex) and therefore increases the statistical power to detect effects. However, the benefits of the within-subjects design may be outweighed by the disadvantages. One important issue that often arises in such studies concerns the possibility of habituation to the stressor (and habituation to the laboratory situation in general, which may also mitigate the subject's stressor response). Pilot testing is crucial to assess this possibility, and the task may have to be tweaked to prevent it. This may be done by increasing the *dose* of the stressor (i.e., make the task more difficult at time 2) or by using a different form of the same stressor. In such an event, and in fact in most within-subject experiments, counterbalancing must be used (see following paragraph).

A second issue concerns the degree of *carryover* of the effects of the stressor administered at time 1 to the outcomes measured at time 2. It is often desirable that the outcomes at each session to be independent of each other, although carryover is an outcome of interest in some studies. Carryover may occur if one administers more than one task within a single session or it may occur across sessions. We can in theory control for carryover effects, and more generally to order effects, by counterbalancing – having half the subjects exposed to condition A at time 1 and condition B at time 2, and the reverse order for the other half of the subjects. If an order effect is suspected, the dummy-coded order variable is included in the model as a means of statistical control. This does not, however, provide a "pure" test of whichever condition comes second. It is desirable to avoid such effects altogether if possible. One way to do this is to separate the sessions in time as much as possible, which will mitigate potential carryover effects. In this event, however, the researcher must be concerned about confounding factors that may arise between sessions, such as changes in medication regimen, physical activity, developmental changes, disease progression, effects of aging. The longer apart the sessions, the more likely

that such factors will arise. One can estimate this by beginning with a cross-sectional comparison of the conditions, using only the first session, which will provide some insight into potential carryover effects.

Although it does cede something in terms of power, a between-subjects design may be more desirable, as it eliminates the carryover issue entirely.

3.2 Use of Multiple Stressors Within a Single Session

The preceding section discussed "within-subjects" designs in the context of the examination of changes that occur across more than one experimental session. However, a related issue concerns the administration of more than one stressor within a single session. For one thing, it may be more efficient by eliminating the need for the subject to come back for additional sessions. One may study a research question that calls for a comparison across more than one task (for example, testing the extent to which the physiological response to two different tasks are correlated, both tasks possibly tapping the same or a similar underlying dimension). One strategy is to have subjects engage in both tasks in the same laboratory session.

These can also be considered within-subjects designs, and the same cautions apply, especially regarding carryover effects. But, using more than one task within a single session brings other, specific issues that must be considered. For one: Is the parameter of interest subject to elevation over the duration of the session? If a resting blood pressure baseline before each new stressor is used, for example, the level tends to rise following the offset of each previous stressor. This is information that can be captured if one uses a post-stress resting or "recovery" phase. If measures tend to return to resting levels immediately following the termination of a stressor, the initial baseline measurement may be used as an index for the remaining stressors. However, if one suspects that the effect of the stressor may be sustained even after the stressor has ended, a new baseline period from which to assess the change for stressor 2 must be used.

As with within-subjects designs across sessions, these potential problems raise the issue of counterbalancing to avoid order effects. For example, if the protocol calls for a mental task (say, mental arithmetic) and a physical task (say, a handgrip task), one may want to present the mental task first in half the subjects and the physical task first in the other half. The effect of the ordering, if there is one, may be assessed. There may be occasions, however, on which one will wish to *not* counterbalance. For example, when using an anger-induction task, and using it effectively, the carryover of the anger might outlast the remainder of the session, and thereby affect the response to whatever task that followed. In such a situation, it is worth losing the advantage due to counterbalancing to avoid the systematic bias in one set of measurements. An alternative, which is often desirable, is to conduct each task in separate sessions. If the researcher does decide to forego counterbalancing, he or she must be careful when writing the manuscript to explain the reasoning.

There are two general frameworks in which to consider when using multiple stressors (whether within a single session or over more than one session). First, one may consider the individual stress tasks to each represent one facet of a broader construct – arousal of anger is an example. Both an anger provocation – for example, a (deliberately) annoying and offensive research assistant – and mental arithmetic with harassment will both arouse anger. In this instance, the results from the two tasks may be averaged to yield a more reliable measure. To the extent, however, that two different tasks are believed to elicit physiological changes that represent different psychosocial dimensions, one would not expect a high correlation between them; instead, he or she is probably looking for mean differences between rather than across them.

3.3 Inter-task Baseline

In the event that it is desired to use more than one task within a single session, one must decide whether or not to use a rest period to separate them. If using more than one task to increase exposure duration, it is not desirable to use an inter-task baseline between them. If, however, one plans to use multiple stressors for the unique information each may provide, it is preferable to use a baseline period for each of the tasks separately. Pains should be taken to separate them temporally as much as possible, within the limits of maximum duration of the session.

Returning to the question of whether to use multiple tasks within a single session. If there is concern over carryover or habituation effects from one to the other (it is useful to collect pilot data to find out), it would be useful to consider (1) having the subjects come for a separate laboratory visit for each task to be used or (2) going to a between-subjects design, in which subjects are randomly assigned to be exposed to one or the other of the tasks, which in this instance, would be thought of as "conditions."

3.4 Sampling Framework Is Specific to the Biological Outcomes

There is no correct sampling interval for physiological outcome measures; the sampling strategy will depend on the nature of the specific outcome parameter. Some measurements can be taken only once, usually at the end of each phase of the study, due to timing constraints or expense (e.g., echocardiogram). Other measures are assessed continuously (e.g., ECG) or intermittently (e.g., salivary cortisol, serum cholesterol) during phases of the study.

A second determinant of the frequency of the sampling interval concerns pre-planned events that occur during the session. An example may be the start of a stressor following a baseline period or a tone sounded to alert the subject that the shock grid has just been turned on. The measurement must be positioned, depending on what measure will be used, to capture the physiological changes occurring as a result of these events. Thus, if the stressor period is 5 min, and the researcher plans to sample blood pressure, one measurement every 3 min, he or she might prefer that the first measurement taken during the task phase occurs at 2 min into the task (by which time the stressor presumably would have had a chance to engage the subject) and again at 5 min. (It is important to maximize the number of such measurements to increase reliability.) Had the measurement been timed to occur at the third minute into the stressor, it would have only been possible to collect one measurement.

The measurement of salivary cortisol, for example, presents a specific challenge in terms of the proper sampling interval because there is a latency ($\sim$20 min) between the stressful event and the release of cortisol; therefore, the researcher has to map out the measurement intervals carefully. Thus, a saliva sample for assessment of cortisol might be obtained $\sim$20 min after stressor offset. If the interval is mis-specified, the effect of the manipulation may be missed entirely.

3.5 Pre-session Instructions and Controls

It is desirable that research participants to enter the laboratory in as "pure" a state as possible, that is, one free of unwanted influences that may affect the subject's behavior and physiological measures. It is obvious, for example, that it would be desirable for the subject to not have had a couple of beers while waiting for the session to begin. This might not occur to the subject, however, so pains must be taken to explain. What are the influences that one should be concerned with? Some generalize across most or all protocols and outcome measures, for example, alcohol or illicit drug use, prescription drug use depending on the nature of the drug (tranquilizers or mood elevators, for example). Some prohibitions

may be determined by the particular outcome; for example, caffeine use will have a substantial effect on resting heart rate and should be avoided if heart rate is a study outcome. Also, hemodynamic shifts may occur after meals and reach their peak at around 2 h post-meal. It is wise to schedule laboratory sessions at least 4 h after the subject has eaten. The researcher should be sure to provide the subject with a take-home list of items to avoid on the day – in some cases, on 1 or more days – prior to the experimental session. The specific time period should be noted; that is, if the experimenter wishes the subject to avoid food, caffeine, and nicotine use for 4 h prior to the session, the subject should be given (or mailed) an appointment form. If the appointment is for, say noon, the form should specify no caffeine (note on the form that tea and many carbonated beverages have caffeine in them) after 8 AM.

When the subject arrives at the laboratory, one of the first things to be done is to debrief them concerning these items. If it is important enough, and feasible, in some cases biological tests may be used to ascertain compliance with the instructions – use of cotinine to assess nicotine usage over the previous week or so is an example. One will, in the course of the debriefing, ask the subject if he or she did indeed comply with the instructions, but some subjects may lie about this had they not done so. To help elicit truthful statements, it is important not to appear punitive, but to explain to the subject beforehand that these substances will have a negative influence on the results, and that if the subject had been noncompliant, request that the he or she call and re-schedule (if this is permitted by the protocol), or, upon arrival at the laboratory, to let the experimenter know (again, offering to re-schedule, if the protocol permits it, will make it easier for the subject to admit the noncompliance).

Another aspect of the pre-session protocol concerns person factors that may affect the scheduling of the session. In women, for example, hormone fluctuations across the menstrual cycle have profound effects on systemic hemodynamics and neurohormonal reactivity to stress. In the absence of urine tests confirming ovulation, the best way to ensure that menstrual cycle phase is controlled is to use the "day counting" method. By asking a woman to schedule her lab session within 5–7 days of the start of her period, one can be reasonably sure that she is in the early follicular phase, when estrogen and progesterone are at their lowest levels. Day counting is not effective for targeting the peak hormone response in the late luteal phase because many cycles, particularly in young women, are anovulatory (Kirschbaum et al, 1999).

4 The Experimental Session

The following set of procedures are common to most laboratory stress studies, but is not meant to be exhaustive. Additional procedures may be called for depending on which particular outcome measures are to be used or the nature of the independent variable.

4.1 Adaptation

It is useful to allow the participant to acclimatize to the laboratory setting; simply being there may be highly stressful for some persons and may cause their baseline measurements to be elevated. During this period, the experimenter should take a few minutes putting the participant at ease. Like all parts of the protocol, this portion should be carefully scripted and piloted to ensure it has the desired effect. In some cases, it may be useful to have the subject come in on a day prior to the scheduled laboratory testing so he or she has a chance to get used to the experimental milieu.

4.2 Instructions

Next, the experimenter may describe the procedures and give instructions. This should be prior to the start of the baseline phase so the protocol

is not interrupted at a later point, when it may prove distracting. If necessary, the instructions should include instruction that the subject should be careful not to move during the measurements.

4.3 Instrumentation

For those measures that will be taken during each of the phases, participants are instrumented prior to the start of baseline. The researcher should explain what and why these are being done; it will help the participant relax.

4.4 Baseline

Most psychophysiological experiments begin with a baseline, or initial rest, period. This allows the examination of within-subject changes between baseline and task (and baseline and recovery). In most studies, the baseline involves resting quietly for a period of time appropriate to the target measure. The baseline period for blood pressure measurement, for example, ranges from about 5 min to half an hour, whereas a longer baseline may be necessary if, say, an IV line is used. Given the importance of the measures achieved during rest, a surprisingly scant literature has commented on specific procedures regarding the duration and content of the baseline period.

Obrist (1981) has suggested assessing subjects' baseline levels and stress responses on different days. In support of this notion, a recent study found that resting blood pressure and heart rate measures taken on the day of the study procedures were significantly higher than those taken on the preceding day (Gerin et al, 2006). However, while assessing baseline and task measures on different days may provide more accurate estimates of the true resting level, this may not be feasible in many cases.

Distracting materials, such as magazines or even a relaxing video (for example, of an aquatic scene; nothing that will arouse the subject), may be used to help the subject relax, unless there is a particular reason not to do this. Music, also, may help establish the baseline. Measurements are taken during or immediately following (depending on the specific measurement) the end of the baseline period and are thus considered reflective of the summary state of that phase on the dependent measure.

Finally, one must guard against reactivity to the measure itself. For example, insertion of an IV or the first couple of blood pressure measurements taken with an arm cuff may cause pain and fear or alerting or orienting responses. If measuring blood pressure, it is common to discard the first few readings (the rule must be established a priori) for this reason.

4.5 Exposure to Stress

A stressor (this term is used generically in this chapter, to refer to a challenging task, or a task designed to provoke an emotional response) is then presented. The duration of presentation tends to be brief, usually 2–5 min, although longer tasks (notably, the Trier Stress Task, described later in this chapter) have been used. As with baseline, measurements are taken during or immediately following (depending on the specific measurement) the end of the task period.

5 Selection of the Stressor

The question of which particular stressor is best for a particular study should be based on what the researcher hopes to accomplish. Virtually all stressors are intended to increase the activation of one or more physiological measures; however, each task carries with it other effects as well. For example, a serial subtraction task – one of the most commonly used stressors – may, depending on how it is presented, elicit anger and frustration. If it is desirable, given the purpose of the study, to arouse anger, then this may prove an appropriate stressor. To help with the decision, the general properties of laboratory stressors are

first discussed; then individual stressors will be classified on the basis of their psychological and physiological domains.

Several factors must be taken into account when deciding on a stressor.

5.1 Conceptuality

Does the task conceptually represent the "real-world" situation of interest, in terms of both psychological and physiological aspects? This is referred to as ecological validity. In decades past, social psychologists have referred to realism, defined as generalizability to other settings. They also distinguished between *Experimental Realism* (Are people involved/engaged in the same way as in the real world situation of interest?) and *Mundane Realism* (Does it merely look like the real world?). This is also referred to as "face validity." A third concept was that of *Functional Realism* (Does the process being studied function in the same manner as it does in the real world?). The researcher must ensure that the task takes account of experimental and functional realism, and does not get sidelined by mundane realism.

5.2 Feasibility

Is the task feasible in terms of the equipment, expertise, time, resources including research assistants, institutional support, financial constraints, and ability to obtain approval from the Institutional Review Board? No matter how scientifically appropriate the task, if the resources are not available, and/or the researcher cannot get the approvals, he or she should consider alternative designs.

5.3 Psychometric Properties

Is the task well supported in terms of its validity (e.g., does an anger provocation manipulation produce higher changes in a self-reported anger)? The entire experiment is based on the selection of the task. One must ensure that there is evidence that the task manipulates what it is supposed to manipulate (e.g., is the commonly used serial-subtraction task manipulating anger or evaluation apprehension or both?)

5.4 Usage

Has the task been used by others in the field for similar purposes? Note the pitfalls that may accompany a particular task, and in what sorts of studies the task has been used.

6 Stressor/Task Domains and Specific Tasks

Classification of stressors is complex and controversial. Any particular stimulus is likely to be classifiable in more than one domain, and very little has been published in this regard. A researcher may wish, for example, to manipulate the feedback the subject receives in regards to his or her performance on the task, and a variety of tasks would serve for that purpose. Serial subtraction, for example, could be used. However, serial subtraction also contains a social component: It is usually the subject performing, the experimenter observing; however, might the experimenter's performance be interpreted by the subject as evaluative? As sub-standard? In accordance with the subject's skin color or style of dress? One can see that the effects of the simple serial subtraction task may not be so simple to interpret.

The following sections are not intended to be an exhaustive listing of stressor tasks. Rather, it is intended to offer a broad guide to task selection based on conceptual characteristics of the study requirements.

6.1 Active Coping

Obrist described one model of the psychological properties of stress tasks, and the hemodynamic pathways by which a particular stressor may increase blood pressure. He hypothesized that some tasks may be thought of as "active coping" tasks, that is, challenges that can in theory be overcome by the subject's efforts and abilities. Mental arithmetic is an example of an active coping task. A "passive" task, alternatively, is one in which the subject perceives that exercising his or her efforts will have no affect on the outcome. Watching a frightening or shocking film is an example. What makes this typology significant is that there is some evidence that active coping tasks tend to be centrally mediated, via cardiac output, by beta-adrenergic receptors, in contrast to passive stressors that tend to be mediated in the periphery, via peripheral resistance, by alpha-adrenergic pathways.

6.2 Emotional Arousal

Many researchers focus on the arousal of an emotional state, as a means of examining the accompanying physiological arousal. The most common emotion to be manipulated in this way is anger, although some researchers have focused on anxiety. There are several ways to arouse anger. The anger-recall task is a relatively simple procedure in which the experimenter asks the subject to think about, and discuss, a situation in which he or she had become very angry (Ironson et al, 1992). The task has been shown to reliably raise blood pressure and heart rate, and self-reported anger and angry thoughts. A second means of anger arousal is through the use of the Type A Structured Interview, a measure that was originally devised by Rosenman (1978). The interview consists of a standardized series of questions posed to participants in a challenging and, at times, brisk manner aimed at eliciting Type A behavior and mild hostile reactions. Serial subtraction, or other forms of mental arithmetic, may be used to evoke anger as well. The task may be presented in a way that is harassing to the subject ("Can't you go any faster than that?") and that causes anger and resentment that outlast the task itself (Glynn et al, 2002). Other tasks that involve an evaluation component can be modified in a similar manner.

6.3 Social Interaction Tasks, Speech Tasks

Although social psychologists have been engaging in studies involving social interaction in the laboratory since the early 1900s, it is only within the past few decades that stress psychophysiologists have begun to make use of this tool. However, a great deal of the stress we tend to experience comes from our interactions with others. Many interesting questions can be asked using this paradigm, such as, what are the person dimensions – e.g., race, sex, emotional supportiveness, hostility – that affect physiological outcomes in social interactions? In addition, one may ask, what situational attributes, such as the presence of another person, the status difference between the subject and an observer, tend to exacerbate, or attenuate, the stressfulness of particular social interactions?

A relatively simple social interaction that may be modeled in the laboratory is public speaking, which is stressful for many people. For example, several researchers have examined the effects of the supportive versus non-supportive demeanor of the observer. A different type of design concerns structured, but real, interactions between persons; for example, Smith and Gallo (1999) have used a marital interaction situation, in which a married couple discusses their problems. This is a good example of a way to increase the external validity of the laboratory situation.

When one focuses on social interactions, which are unscripted, the researcher sacrifices a degree of experimental control, as not all interactions will take the same form. However, the tradeoff for additional external validity is often worth it.

6.3.1 The Trier Social Stress Test (TSST)

The TSST was initially developed to evaluate effects of psychosocial stress on cortisol activity

in a laboratory setting (Kirschbaum et al, 1993). Because the time course of cortisol is relatively slow – a measurement may reflect the state of the body 15–20 min earlier – the researcher has to pay particular attention to the timing of the task and the measurements. Moreover, for a stressor to have a substantial effect on cortisol, it must persist for a longer time than other measures require. The TSST was designed to address these concerns. The 20-min test comprises two stressors, conducted in front of a panel of judges: An impromptu speech (explaining why they had been caught shoplifting) and mental arithmetic (other variants of this task, however, are used).

6.4 The Cold Pressor

Historically, the cold pressor was the first task used in a published study of stressor effects (on cardiovascular reactivity) and was then used in virtually every such study until the late 1950s. The cold pressor is problematic, as it is not clear what processes mediate its effects. In hemodynamic terms, the task is "mixed," in that it produces both central (cardiac output) and peripheral (total peripheral resistance) effects. It has been used as a pain stimulus in some studies.

6.5 Duration of Stressor Exposure

A tradeoff exists between the advantages of a longer duration task, say one that goes on for 15 min, and the additional burden placed on the subject. In terms of measurement reliability, a longer duration allows more measurements to be taken. It also allows a greater ability to observe patterns of changes within the course of the stressor, something that would be difficult in a task that lasts only, say, 2 min. However, many standardized stressors do not lend themselves to extended durations. For example, the cold pressor cannot be longer than a few minutes for obvious reasons. Similarly, it would be difficult to have a subject engage in serial subtraction for longer than a few minutes.

7 Manipulation Checks/Probe Measures

Throughout the session, one may want to take measures – "probes" – that will help to interpret the data by serving as checks to see that the manipulation is indeed effective for its intended purpose. For example, if one is examining the effect of an anger-induction task, compared to a non-emotional control condition, on, say, platelet aggregation, it would be wise to ask the subject, at some point in the protocol, how angry he or she had become. This will help one to understand why null results may result and may provide the means for post hoc analyses that will at least serve as pilot data for the next study. For example, the researcher may want to separately analyze subjects who actually did report higher levels of anger. If that is done, however, the researcher must be careful about the conclusions drawn, and should anticipate the concerns that reviewers are likely to have when the data are written up for publication.

When and how to ask probe questions also is a delicate business. The report itself should be given as close to the relevant time period as possible (e.g., at the end of the stressor), and yet should not influence other measures. The wording of the question should be as neutral as possible and should not point to an expectation on the part of the researcher. For example, the phrasing "How angry do you feel at this moment?" differs only subtly from "Do you feel any anger at this moment?" but may produce a bias to report – or to avoid reporting – anger. It is best to keep such measures as brief as possible. For instance, if the researcher is interested in the degree of anxiety being experienced following the stressor, she or he might give a 1-question item with a Likert-type scale or might give a validated anxiety measure, such as Spielberger's. The former is probably less reliable and less valid, but the latter, comprising several questions, may simply be too intrusive for the purpose at hand.

8 Statistical/Measurement Issues

"Reactivity" refers to the change that occurs in a physiological or psychological parameter as a result of exposure to stress, in any of its various forms. As such, it has classically been measured as a simple change score: the mean of the measurements taken during the stressor less the mean of the measurements taken during baseline. A change score is easily interpretable; a change of zero means that the stressor had no effect on whatever was being measured; a change value of, say, +10 indicates that the subject responded to the stressor with a 10-point increase. However, change scores bring hidden perils, and it would be wise to study the basic statistical theory that explains the *why* of those perils (see, for example, Cronbach and Furby, 1970).

There are several other methods that are used, though less frequently than the simple change score: (1) repeated measures designs, in which baseline and stressor levels are treated as two levels of a single factor; (2) analysis of covariance, in which baseline levels are used as covariates; and (3) residualized change scores. Which of these is correct remains one of the controversial issues in this field.

8.1 Measurement Reliability

A particular measurement is useful only to the extent that it is reliable (does not change much from measurement to measurement) and valid (measures what it is supposed to measure). For physiological measurements, a major concern is the reliability – the stability – of the measurement over time. If the measurement varies a great deal from one occasion to the next without any intervention between measurements that indicates that a given score is a function more of environmental influences (which enter as measurement error), and less of the true score, than if the measurement were stable from time to time.

One may consider the following: A researcher, interested in the response of markers of immune function (C-reactive protein, intercellular adhesion molecule-1, interleukin-6, interleukin-10, etc.) takes a measurement following a 20-min baseline, then following a 5-min stressor, and computes the resulting change value between them. The researcher repeats this process under precisely the same conditions (even the same experimenter), 1 year later (long enough so that we may assume the stress of the first session has been forgotten) and finds a test–retest correlation of 0.8. (Test–retest reliability is usually assessed as a Pearson or intraclass correlation). Such a correlation would, for this dimension over this relatively long period of time, indicate fairly high stability over time. The greater the correlation, the more "true score" resides in the individual's score, and, therefore, the less error. Thus, a score with poor measurement reliability – whether used as an independent or dependent variable – will increase Type II error, and the resultant likelihood that an effect in the data will be missed.

Reliability may be increased using a variety of strategies. More measurements will usually increase the reliability of the measure; thus, one method by which the number of measurements may be increased during a particular phase is to lengthen the duration of the phase. This can usually be done more easily for the baseline period compared to the task period.

However, as discussed previously, not all measurements can be repeated during or following a particular phase. Some measures themselves are reactive; some are too expensive; some take too long, or are too distracting to the subject, or are (undesirably) invasive. However, the problem of insufficient reliability still exists. Therefore, another strategy must be considered. Some measurements can be repeated over days or sessions, rather than within the phase of a single session. For example, the assessment of vasodilation using brachial artery ultrasound cannot easily be performed more than once within an experimental phase. However, test–retest reliability for this method can be poor. One way to address the problem is to repeat the sessions on more than 1 day and take the mean of the measurements acquired during the same phase – for example, baseline – across the sessions. Other problems do arise, including the possibility of habituation, or stressor carryover, over sessions, but this may be the only way to increase the reliability of the measure.

8.2 Type I Error

Psychophysiological experiments provide many opportunities to take advantage of chance. Every additional outcome measured for which there is no strong, a priori hypothesis based on the literature and/or the researcher's own data adds to the experimentwise error rate. For example, blood pressure is often measured as both systolic and diastolic pressure, with each outcome treated in a separate analysis; the Type I error rate in that instance is almost *double* what is reported. However, there are few instances in which differential results are predicted for these two measures. It is not unusual to see published reports that provide data on 20 or more outcomes, most without the foundation of a strong hypothesis. In that event, the likelihood that some of the significant values have occurred by chance increases dramatically.

There are several methods that provide protection against Type I error. The strongest is to use only outcome measures that are based on specific hypotheses. However, often this is impractical, and it may be that different, albeit correlated, outcomes represent different aspects of the same construct and therefore must be considered simultaneously.

The use of a priori contrasts that test specific hypotheses may be used when appropriate. When specific hypotheses cannot be generated for each individual outcome measure (for example, systolic versus diastolic blood pressure or C-reactive protein versus interleukin-6), appropriate post hoc tests may be used, assuming the omnibus test is significant. Another method is to use a multivariate analysis in which more than one outcome measure that presumably tap the same dimension are included in the same model;

as with post hoc tests, if the omnibus test is significant, the analyses for the individual measures may be interpreted.

8.3 Assessment of Post-Stress Recovery

If the parameter of interest tends to return to its resting level immediately following the termination of the stressor, measurement of recovery becomes irrelevant. However, this is not true of many physiological measures; a degree of carryover of the effect of the stressor often exists. This was discussed previously as an obstacle to obtaining post-stress baselines used for a succeeding stressor; however, we now examine the same post-stress rest, but on its own merits as an independent predictor of other risk factors or disease endpoints. In this event, one may want to include a post-stress rest period in the protocol (Fig. 41.1) as a means of evaluating recovery of the parameter from the stress-induced levels. Assessment of recovery – a dynamic state – presents methodological and statistical challenges mostly avoided in the measurement of baseline and task levels, which are usually regarded as stable within state characteristics. For measurements that can only be taken a single time, at the end of the phase, assessment of recovery is fairly straightforward. However, when measurements that are taken during the recovery period are used, the correct measure to use is unclear. Unlike baseline and task phases, there is little agreement about how to assess recovery. A common method is to select a point during the recovery phase, and measure the parameter at that point; thus, one might say: "At 5 minutes into the recovery period, subjects in group A had recovered an average of 60% of their task values, compared to subjects in Group B, who had recovered only 30%." However, this method ignores a great deal of the information – it may be that it is the decline observed earlier or later in the period that is important, for example – and does not benefit from multiple measurements.

Alternatives to time to recovery include calculating area under the curve, obtaining post-stress measurements at arbitrary intervals, computing change scores from post-stress levels and baseline levels, and using curve-fitting estimates. The advantages and disadvantages of each of these approaches are discussed in detail with respect to blood pressure measurement in a review by Linden and colleagues (1997). In addition, Christenfeld et al (2000) and Llabre et al (2004) have published statistical models designed to assess recovery from stress.

9 Summary and Conclusion

An initial impression suggests that stress psychophysiological investigations are simple and straightforward: A resting baseline is measured, the subject is exposed to a stressor, another measurement (or measurements) is taken, the change computed, the results published. In fact, these studies truly are simple in design, but potential pitfalls abound. This chapter has provided a reference that points out the subtleties of the design of these experiments that will lead to interpretable data.

Acknowledgments I would like to thank my colleagues Christine Kapelewski, Gregg Solomon, Tanya Spruill, and Matthew Zawadzki who read versions of this chapter and contributed helpful comments and suggestions. I also wish to acknowledge the important influence on this work of my longtime friend, mentor, and colleague, Thomas G. Pickering, who recently passed away. Preparation of this chapter was supported by National Heart, Lung, and Blood Institute of the National Institutes of Health, Bethesda, MD, USA, Grant HL089402.

References

Christenfeld, N., Gerin, W., Linden, W., Sanders, M., Mathur, J. et al (1997). Social support effects on cardiovascular reactivity: is a stranger as effective as a friend? *Psychosom Med, 59,* 388–398.

Christenfeld, N., Glynn, L. M., and Gerin, W. (2000). On the reliable assessment of cardiovascular recovery: an application of curve-fitting techniques. *Psychophysiol, 37*, 543–550.

Cronbach, L. J., and Furby, L. (1970). How we should measure "change" — or should we?". *Psychol Bulletin, 74*, 68–80.

Gerin, W., Ogedegbe, G., Schwartz, J. E., Chaplin, W. F., Goyal, T. et al (2006). Assessment of the white coat effect. *J Hypertens, 24*, 67–74.

Glynn, L., Christenfeld, N., and Gerin, W. (2002). The role of rumination in recovery from reactivity: cardiovascular consequences of emotional States. *Psychosom Med, 64*, 714–726.

Ironson, G., Taylor, C. B., Boltwood, M., Bartzokis, T., Dennis, L. et al (1992). Effects of anger on left ventricular ejection fraction in coronary artery disease. *Amer J Cardiol, 70*, 281–285.

Kamarck, T. W., Annuziato, B., and Amateau, L. M. (1995). Affiliation moderates the effects of social threat on stress-related cardiovascular responses: boundary conditions for a laboratory model of social support. *Psychosom Med, 57*, 183–194.

Kirschbaum, C., Pirke, K. M., and Hellhammer, D. H. (1993). The Trier Social Stress Test: a tool for investigating psychobiological stress responses in a laboratory setting. *Neuropsychobiol, 28*, 76–81.

Kirschbaum, C., Kudielka, B. M., Gaab, J., Schommer, N. C., and Hellhammer, D. H. (1999). Impact of gender, menstrual cycle phase, and oral contraceptives on the activity of the hypothalamus-pituitary-adrenal axis. *Psychosom Med, 6*, 154–162.

Llabre, M. M., Spitzer, S., Siegel, S., Saab, P. G., and Schneiderman, N. (2004). Applying latent growth curve modeling to the investigation of individual differences in cardiovascular recovery from stress. *Psychosom Med, 66*, 29–41.

Linden, W., Earle, T. L., Gerin, W., and Christenfeld, N. (1997). Physiological stress reactivity and recovery: conceptual siblings separated at birth? *J Psychosom Res, 42*, 117–135.

Obrist, P. (1981). *Cardiovascular Psychophysiology: A Perspective*. New York: Plenum Press.

Rosenman, R. H. (1978). The interview method of assessment of the coronary-prone behavior pattern. In T. M. Dembroski, S. Weiss, J. Shields, S. G. Haynes, & M. Feinleib (Eds.), *Coronary-Prone Behavior* (pp. 55–70). New York: Springer.

Rosenthal, R. (1994). Interpersonal expectancy effects: a 30-year perspective. *Curr Direct Psychol Sci, 3*, 176–179.

Smith, T. W., and Gallo, L. C. (1999). Hostility and cardiovascular reactivity during marital interaction. *Psychosom Med, 61*, 436–445.

Chapter 42

Stress and Allostasis

Ilia N. Karatsoreos and Bruce S. McEwen

1 Introduction

"Stress!" Reading the term may actually set off the physiological processes which it describes. For decades, stress has had a negative connotation, and its usage in common parlance has fostered and nurtured the negative undertone of the term. However, when considered in its proper context, that is, in the context of regulation of homeostasis, stress and the stress axis are crucial for ensuring the survival of organisms.

The *stress response* is defined as the psychological, neural, and hormonal changes in response to a *stressor* or an environmental stimulus that impacts an organism's physiology. Evolutionarily, the stress response can be considered as a series of countermeasures the brain and body deploy in order to cope with changes in the environment that might otherwise mean death. Restated, stress responses promote adaptation to the environment, which is key to survival. This is true throughout the phylogenetic tree, from the simplest unicellular organism, all the way through to the complexity of *Homo sapiens*. The pressures of natural selection have resulted in organisms that possess regulatory systems that finely tune the processes of life. We can consider these homeostatic systems as being organized on a continuum of increasing complexity, spanning

a wide range from "simple" biochemical cascades (e.g., conversion of cholesterol to various steroid hormones) through to complex systems regulating the orchestration of multiple tissues and organs toward a singular result (e.g., the consumption of food, digestion, and metabolism). However, the proper functioning of these systems, regardless of their complexity, is crucial to the survival of the individual and is tuned to meet the specific demands of a given environmental niche.

Homeostasis is defined as maintaining the right conditions for various physiological and biochemical systems to operate within optimal parameters. When considered as an organismal process, this is no mean feat, since different biological systems may require different "optimal" conditions, and maintaining homeostasis may involve myriad physiological systems acting in concert. It is also important to consider that attempting to maintain homeostasis in a challenging environment is largely an active process. Maintaining body temperature within its optimal range (in humans, approximately $36.8°C \pm 0.7°C$), when threatened by either excessive heat or cold, is an excellent example of such a process. When body temperature begins to climb, we begin to perspire to increase heat loss from the skin, and blood vessels dilate to increase heat dissipation. When body temperature begins to fall, blood vessels constrict to reduce heat loss, we begin to shiver uncontrollably to generate more heat, and we form piloerections, raising the hair on the skin (goose bumps) to reduce heat dissipation. The body is maintained in its optimal range by a complex interplay between

I.N. Karatsoreos (✉)
Harold and Margaret Milliken Hatch Laboratory of Neuroendocrinology, The Rockefeller University, 1230 York Ave, New York, NY 10021, USA
e-mail: ikaratsore@mail.rockefeller.edu

A. Steptoe (ed.), *Handbook of Behavioral Medicine*, DOI 10.1007/978-0-387-09488-5_42,
© Springer Science+Business Media, LLC 2010

Normal Stress Response

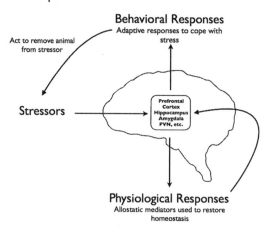

Chronic Stress and
Allostatic Overload

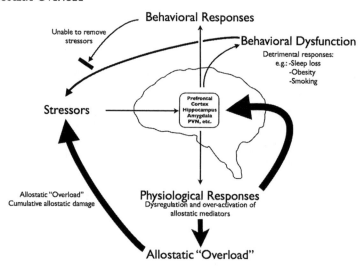

Fig. 42.1 Schematic representation of a normal stress response (*top*) and how the normal stress response is altered following chronic stress, resulting in allostatic overload (*bottom*). *Top:* In the normal stress response, stressors engage neural and neuroendocrine systems that result in a suite of behavioral and physiological responses. The behavioral responses are adaptive responses used to cope with the stressor, perhaps acting to remove the animal from the stress. The physiological responses (allostasis) make use of allostatic mediators that attempt to actively restore homeostasis. *Bottom:* If allostasis is repeatedly engaged or becomes poorly regulated, as can happen in chronic stress, allostatic overload can occur. This results in exaggerated physiological responses by allostatic mediators that now cause damage, rather than promote adaptation. These physiological responses can then exacerbate the environmental stressor, by becoming an "internal" stressor, adding to the already taxed system. To make matters worse, behavioral responses may no longer be adequate to cope with the stressor, and behavioral dysfunction may result in detrimental responses (e.g., insomnia, changes in appetite, increases in the use of alcohol, or tobacco), that further contribute to the stressors in the environment. Importantly, such responses may be sustained, *even if the initiating environmental stressor has been removed*, potentially setting up a "reverberating loop" that causes wear and tear on the brain and body and negative physical and mental health outcomes

neural, endocrine, and exocrine systems working together toward this single goal. Maintaining homeostasis in the face of environmental challenges is accomplished by a process referred to as *allostasis* or "the maintenance of stability through active intervention" (Boxes 42.1 and 42.2). Though the factors essential to an organism's survival (e.g., body temperature, pH, oxygen tension) are not themselves used for allostatic interventions, mediators of allostasis (e.g., epinephrine, cortisol, cytokines) are mobilized to maintain homeostasis in the face of environmental stressors (Box 42.1).

While the mediators of allostasis have a beneficial role to play in ensuring the survival of the organism during an environmental challenge, in situations of sustained external challenges or internal factors (e.g., chronic anxiety), they may become elevated and exceed the normal range (Box 42.2). Moreover, the mediators of allostasis each can have nonlinear, biphasic actions that are now designated by the term "hormesis" (Calabrese, 2008a, b), and these mediators regulate each other in a nonlinear (i.e., not a simple 1:1 or additive) fashion (McEwen, 2006). In such allostatic states, the interconnected, hormetic actions of the mediators of allostasis operating in a nonlinear network (McEwen, 2006) are also then forced to function outside of their optimal range. For example, elevated inflammatory cytokines can lead to elevated cortisol, which is then often accompanied by an imbalance in sympathetic and parasympathetic activity. At the same time, elevated parasympathetic activity can overcome inflammation in parallel with anti-inflammatory effects of glucocorticoids (Borovikova et al, 2000; Goldstein et al, 2007; Sloan et al, 2007a, b).

In the short-term, stress and the resulting allostatic responses help to overcome acute challenges and ensure survival of the organism by forcing systems to function outside of normal ranges. Conversely, long-term allostasis results in physiological difficulties resulting from "wear and tear." It is useful to consider an allostatic state as "borrowing" against a physiological system's integrity in the short-term, thus ensuring

Box 42.1 Defining Allostasis and Homeostasis

Allostasis – the active process of maintaining/re-establishing homeostasis, when one defines homeostasis as *those aspects of physiology (pH, oxygen tension, body temperature for homeotherms) that maintain life.*

Allostasis refers to *the ability of the body to produce hormones (like cortisol, epinephrine) and other mediators (e.g., cytokines)* that help an animal *adapt* to a new situation/challenge.

In contrast to the mediators (of allostasis) that actively promote adaptation, *those features that maintain life* (using the definition of homeostasis above) are ones that *operate in a narrower range and do not change in order to help us adapt, i.e., they are not the mediators of change.*

Box 42.2 Terminology

Homeostasis – the essential parameters of life
Allostasis – the active process of maintaining homeostasis
Allostatic state – elevated levels of allostatic mediators (e.g., increased blood pressure, hypercortisolemia)
Allostatic load – cumulative change due to allostatic mediators (e.g., body fat; remodeling of neuronal circuitry)
Allostatic overload – wear and tear, pathophysiology from prolonged allostatic load (e.g., atherosclerosis; neuronal damage, and cell loss)

long-term viability. For instance, small degrees of cumulative change (e.g., a bear putting on body fat for winter, prior to hibernation), referred to as allostatic load (Box 42.2), have adaptive advantages (McEwen and Wingfield, 2003). Such allostatic load states take place under the (somewhat anthropomorphic) notion that the state of indebtedness will be corrected quickly, as soon as the stressor subsides, and the environment returns to normal ranges. However, when the environment does not co-operate and return to baseline or, as can be the case with repeated activation of allostatic responses, the regulatory systems regulating allostasis fail to properly engage, a situation of "allostatic overload" may result. This overload state results in the wear and tear on body systems and eventually pathophysiology (e.g., atherosclerosis or obesity and type 2 diabetes).

In the brain, allostatic states occur in terms of neurotransmitter systems and the actions of elevated levels of external factors, such as circulating hormones that affect brain function and structure. In response to these internal and external factors, the brain responds with both structural and functional changes. Such plasticity is known as adaptive plasticity. These adaptive responses occur in the dendritic and synaptic structure of neurons in hippocampus, amygdala, and prefrontal cortex and are one of the consequences of prolonged, uncontrollable stress (McEwen, 2007). These responses are considered adaptive as they attempt to protect the brain from cumulative damage of the stressor. However, failure to reverse these plastic changes and/or the increased vulnerability to irreversible damage is an example of allostatic overload. Such consequences can be observed in states of chronic anxiety, depressed mood, and neural damage (e.g., after stroke, seizures, or neurodegenerative diseases). Restated, allostatic states allow physiological systems to adapt to stressors and exhibit plasticity when environmental pressures require. However, this added adaptability is accompanied by significant risk, in that allostatic overload can occur if the allostatic state is maintained for too long, forcing mediators normally promoting adaptation to become dysregulated and to operate outside of their optimal ranges for protracted periods of time. Such continued

drive results in damage to the very physiological systems that allostasis has attempted to protect.

2 Stress and Allostatic Overload-Related Illnesses

The costs of allostatic overload can be significant. As discussed previously, allostatic mediators are beneficial acutely, but if allostatic states are maintained for too long, improperly engaged, or unsuccessfully disengaged, the chronic allostatic state can lead to allostatic overload and cumulative wear and tear on the brain and body. In many cases, the balance between an adaptive stress response and maladaptive allostatic overload can be described using an inverted U-shaped curve heuristic. That is, a failure to engage the stress system can have just as detrimental effects on the survival and health of an organism as an overreaction or delayed shutdown of the response would. Restated plainly, an overly *hypo*active hypothalamic–pituitary–adrenal (HPA) axis can be just as bad as a *hyper*active HPA.

When it comes to metabolism, the effects of chronically high glucocorticoids are enigmatic. Food intake is inhibited by exposure to high levels of glucocorticoids. This effect may be mediated by the increase in corticotrophin releasing hormone (CRH) acting as a catabolic signal (Kellendonk et al, 2002). However, in other situations of high glucocorticoids, such as in hypercortisolemia, obesity can result (Marin et al, 1992; Nieuwenhuizen and Rutters, 2008; Pasquali et al, 1996; Rosmond et al, 1998). Hypercortisolism, such as is found in Cushing's disease, is also associated with increases in free fatty acids that contribute to insulin resistance. This then can exacerbate the increase in visceral fat accumulation, augment sympathetic activation, and can result in hypertension (Brindley and Rolland, 1989). However, in most animal models, chronic restraint or immobilization stress results in reduced weight gain (Lucas et al, 2007; Magarinos and McEwen, 1995a, b;

Watanabe et al, 1992), suggesting that the effects of stress on body composition and food intake may be different from the effects of glucocorticoids in the absence of a clear "stressor."

The interaction of stress and HPA function and immune function can also be described as an inverted U-shaped process (Calabrese, 2008b; McEwen et al, 1997). A hypoactive HPA can lead to a hyperinflammatory and even a hyperimmune state. Specifically, a hypoactive HPA is associated with an increase risk for chronic inflammation (Elenkov et al, 1999; Webster et al, 1997, 1998) and also vulnerability to autoimmunity (Sternberg and Wilder, 1989). This increased risk is thought to involve a shift from T-helper 2 (cellular) immunity to T-helper 1 (humoral) immunity (Elenkov and Chrousos, 1999). While acute stress and exposure to low levels of corticosterone actually improve aspects of immunity and reduce inflammation, chronic stress and exposure to high levels of corticosterone dramatically reduce the delayed-type hypersensitivity response (Dhabhar and McEwen, 1997, 1999). Sorrells and Sapolsky (2007) have provided a thought provoking recent review, contrasting the well-established anti-inflammatory aspect of glucocorticoids, with the mounting evidence for their pro-inflammatory effects both in the periphery and in the brain following chronic exposure. This pattern of results demonstrates that the acute stress response has clear beneficial components, while chronic exposure to allostatic mediators associated with chronic stress can have severe implications for immune function. Recently, there has been increased interest in inflammation and the balance between pro- and anti-inflammatory mediators in psychiatric disorders. The role of inflammation in depression and depressive syndromes is becoming increasingly obvious, and the specific mechanisms underlying this role are now being more fully elucidated (Anisman, 2009; Anisman and Merali, 2002; Raison et al, 2006).

The HPA is an essential mediator of allostatic responses to environmental stressors. The mediators of allostasis help to organize a body's response to environmental challenge and maintain stability in the face of homeostatic perturbations and threats (real or perceived) to homeostasis. Thus, any body systems that regulate overall homeostasis may be central players in allostatic responses. This leads us to the circadian (daily) timing system of the brain and body, a key biological system involved in timing of homeostatic events and changes in homeostasis that occur when an organism transits from a period of activity to a period of quiescence and back. As we will propose, the failure or improper functioning of this system may lead to increases in allostatic load and eventually allostatic overload.

3 Circadian Timing: Brain and Body Clocks

The alternation of dark and light that defines the solar day is perhaps the most salient environmental cue for terrestrial organisms. The rotation of the earth about its axis allows for a temporal framework to life and provides a level of predictability that organisms can use to anticipate daily recurring events and to adjust their physiology and behavior to meet these changes and challenges. For instance, daily rhythms in glucocorticoid secretion are tightly controlled by the circadian clock. In both nocturnal and diurnal animals, plasma corticoids reach their peak just before the onset of daily activity (i.e., just before dusk in a nocturnal species and just before dawn in a diurnal species). These rhythms are generated by a master circadian clock, which in mammals is located in the suprachiasmatic nucleus (SCN) of the hypothalamus. This brain region is comprised of cell-autonomous neuronal oscillators, in other words, individual cells that contain the genetic and molecular machinery to generate circadian rhythms. Intriguingly, the molecular "gears" of the clock are highly conserved throughout evolution, with the discovery of the *Period* gene in the fruit fly (*Drosophila melanogaster*) leading to the discovery and identification of the homologous mammalian *Period* gene. In the simplest of terms, and well-reviewed elsewhere (King and Takahashi, 2000), the molecular mechanism comprising the core circadian clockwork is based on a transcription–translation negative feedback loop. The positive elements BMAL1 and CLOCK act as transcription factors, and their binding to the DNA leads to the transcription of the negative elements *Period(1, 2, 3)* and *Cryptochrome(1, 2)*. These mRNAs then translocate to the cytoplasm of the cell, are translated into proteins, and form hetero- and homo-dimers with each other. The dimers then translocate back into the nucleus, where they inhibit their own transcription. This loop takes about 24 h to complete, with various other components, such as casein kinase 1, providing the necessary delays.

While this molecular machinery is essential for the ability of a cell to show a circadian oscillation, the unique tissue-level organization of the cells of the SCN into a complex network of different functional components ensures the SCN clock is able to maintain circadian rhythmicity, even in vitro. The neural network of the SCN is important to consider, as the molecular gears of the clock (clock genes, and clock controlled genes) are present in myriad cell types throughout the brain and body (Balsalobre, 2002). These "peripheral clocks" lose their synchronous rhythmicity rapidly when decoupled from the SCN (Yamazaki et al, 2000), in that while individual cells may remain rhythmic, the tissue itself no longer shows a coherent rhythm as individual oscillators have drifted out of phase with each other. Thus, timing in peripheral clocks seems to be an intrinsic property of these cells, but extrinsic synchrony must be imposed by the master clock in order for coherent tissue-level rhythms to be expressed.

Far from being oddities, or epiphenomenal, circadian oscillators in extra-SCN neural sites and peripheral organs seem to be crucial for the optimal functioning and mutual physiological cooperation between organ systems. Circadian rhythms allow for the separation of daily events, which on the cellular level may be reduced to ensuring that incompatible biochemical processes do not occur at the same time. In a sense, circadian rhythms can provide

a temporal partition in cases where anatomical partitioning may not be possible or desirable. These physiological effects are also transmitted to the behavioral level, manifesting as a balance between behaviors, physiological needs, and the realities of specific environmental and temporal niches. An example of such interlocking physiological systems in which timing is crucial is the awakening corticosterone (or cortisol, in humans) response. Before waking in the morning, body temperature gradually begins to rise, and neurons in the hypothalamus begin secreting CRH. In the anterior pituitary, CRH elicits the release of adrenocorticotrophin releasing hormone (ACTH), which travels through the bloodstream to the adrenal glands, signaling them to begin the release of corticosterone. At the same time, cells in the adrenal gland, which express clock genes, anticipate the arrival of the ACTH signal, so that the time between receipt of the "go" stimulus and the release of their hormone product is optimized and appropriately temporally gated (Oster et al, 2006). The released glucocorticoids then travel throughout the body, including returning to the brain, where they have myriad effects in different organ systems, especially in the regulation of glucose mobilization. The timing of these responses is important, as it serves to mobilize energy stores just before an individual awakes and needs to make use of this additional energy. Intriguingly, glucocorticoids seem to do double duty, as a hormonal signal generated by the SCN that can synchronize peripheral oscillators throughout the brain and body, largely by acting through the glucocorticoid receptor (GR), to which corticosterone binds (Balsalobre et al, 2000).

Given the relationship between the central clock and peripheral timing, and given that circulating glucocorticoids (whose rhythmic secretion is under control of the SCN clock) synchronize peripheral oscillators, it is easy to see how disruption of either or both of these systems could lead to potential problems for the rest of physiology. If one accepts that tight circadian control is essential to maintain the integrity of physiological systems and maintain them within optimal operating parameters, then one must also accept that disrupted circadian timing could lead to sub-optimal functioning of these systems and could potentially result in an internally generated "stressor" that would put animals under increased allostatic load. Importantly, these effects would apply not just to "vegetative" peripheral homeostatic systems but also to the brain, which clearly responds to allostatic states. Thus, disrupted circadian timing, manifested as altered phase relationships between cellular oscillators throughout the brain and body could lead to an allostatic state and eventually to allostatic overload.

3.1 Disruption of Circadian Rhythms as an Allostatic State

Anticipation of daily events is a key benefit of having an optimally functioning circadian system. The SCN regulates rhythms in myriad physiological systems through a combination of neural and humoral connections, and sometimes both. Moreover, at the level of the target brain region (or peripheral organ or gland), local clocks also contribute to the exquisite timing of the system. Such a wide reach through neural and diffusible signals places the SCN and the circadian system in a position to regulate multiple systems not just homeostatically but also in times of allostasis. As mentioned previously, allostatic overload can occur because of an improper and prolonged engagement of allostatic mediators or because of a lack of the proper termination of the response, once the stressor has been removed. In a sense, circadian rhythms may be one of the driving forces to restore normal homeostasis after a period of allostasis, and thus the circadian system may be central in terminating or reducing allostatic mediators.

Focusing on the HPA axis, the SCN and circadian timing play an intimate role in ensuring optimal functioning. The SCN projects directly to CRH containing cells of the paraventricular nucleus of the hypothalamus (Vrang et al,

1995a, b), the main hypothalamic component of the HPA. Rhythms in circulating ACTH and corticosterone are blunted or absent in animals with a lesioned SCN (Moore and Eichler, 1972) or with genetic ablations of normal SCN function (Dallmann et al, 2006; Loh et al, 2008). Moreover, the response of the HPA to endogenous releasing hormones and to stressors is dramatically altered, with a loss of time of day modulation of the adrenal responses to ACTH (Sage et al, 2002), and exaggerated corticosterone responses to stress observed in SCN-ablated animals (Buijs et al, 1993). In short, an intact SCN and circadian timing system are crucial for the optimal functioning of the HPA axis, a key component of the systems regulating the engagement and termination of the stress response.

3.2 Circadian Dysfunction Is a Hallmark of Many Physical and Neural Disorders

As discussed, disruption of circadian rhythms, be they environmentally, anatomically, or genetically triggered, can lead to many physiological problems. These effects are felt on a regular basis during transmeridian air travelers (i.e., jet-lag) and by shift workers. Fatigue and a general "malaise" are the usual reported symptoms. In many cases, this is also accompanied by physical complaints that may last for several days, such as digestive/gastrointestinal problems, as well as decreased immune function and increased susceptibility to illness. Usually, the psychological symptoms manifest as poor concentration, decreased attention, and problems remembering. While almost everyone has felt in some way the effects of acute circadian desynchrony, it is interesting to note that the number of studies looking at the effects of chronic disruption are still relatively small, though growing in number.

On more long-term timescales, circadian disruption seems to have a more insidious nature, and there is ample evidence in the literature that chronic circadian disruption may play a causal role in many disease states, including cancer (Boivin et al, 2007; Davis et al, 2001; Haus and Smolensky, 2006; Stevens, 2005). An interesting study by Cho (2001) showed that chronic jet lag (as investigated in flight crews) results in temporal lobe atrophy and spatial cognitive defects. In animal models, numerous studies present compelling data showing that chronic circadian dysfunction can lead to sub-syndromal mental and physical characteristics of "bad ageing," and even in some cases a decrease in life span (Costa, 2003; Davidson et al, 2006). In a study by Hurd and Ralph (1998), heterozygous *Tau* mutant hamsters, with an endogenous period of 22 h, die at a much faster rate when housed in a 24 h light–dark (LD) cycle, while those housed in constant dim light shows no such increased mortality. This same study also demonstrated that transplanting a fetal SCN into an old hamster increased life span by about 33%, while fetal grafts from other brain regions had no such effect (Hurd and Ralph, 1998). This pattern of results highlights the long-term effects of circadian disruption that may not be evident when one only considers the acute effects of disruption.

In addition to the physical effects resulting from circadian dysfunction, numerous psychiatric illnesses have circadian components. Depression is an interesting case study of a syndrome that presents with both circadian and HPA dysfunction symptomatology. Depressive disorders are characterized by multiple physiological and psychological symptoms. One of the most common physiological observations is disrupted circadian timing, which can manifest as changes in sleep wake cycles (Turek, 2007; Van Cauter and Turek, 1986) and a blunting of the daily rhythm of glucocorticoids (Deuschle et al, 1997). Circadian disruption is a characteristic of depression (Wirz-Justice, 2006), and shift workers often suffer from mood disturbances and an increased risk for depression. In addition, seasonal affective disorder (SAD) reflects dysfunctions in the circadian rhythms (Magnusson and Boivin, 2003). Thus, circadian disruption may be a consequence of experiences that lead to depression, and inability to cope with circadian perturbations may be a risk factor for depressive illness. How these various pathways interact and synergize remains unknown, though the allostatic load that results from a chronic circadian dysfunction may be a precipitating factor.

4 Concluding Remarks

In this chapter, we have attempted to explain stress and allostasis and have tried to clarify and demystify the term "stress." The stress response is essential for an organism's survival and allows the organism to adapt to a change in the environment. While homeostasis and homeostatic mechanisms are necessary for the functions of life, allostatic mechanisms and mediators allow an animal to maintain stability by changing various aspects of physiology, and eventually behavior. However, these allostatic responses need to be managed appropriately, by being turned on and off efficiently, and not being engaged improperly or out of context. Inefficient allostatic functioning or chronic exposure to stress can result in the mediators of allostasis becoming a burden, rather than a boon to the physiological system in which they are active. Such allostatic overload leads to increased wear and tear on bodily systems and can contribute to a wide range of physical and psychological dysfunction. We also present data about the central role circadian rhythms play in the maintenance of homeostasis, as well as a key system that may be able to regulate allostatic responses. We also propose that circadian dysfunction could lead to conditions of allostatic load and overload, by causing different body systems to function out of their normal phase relationships. This may also be extended to the brain, where circadian rhythms are robustly expressed in many nuclei, and where desynchronization can have important ramifications for optimal behavioral function, and homeostatic regulation. Our main hope is to highlight the importance of considering how interconnected physiological systems are with each other, and how these interconnections need not be purely physical or biochemical connections, but perhaps connections in terms of their temporal relationships. As is so often the case with many lines of scientific enquiry, most systems are investigated in relative isolation, whether to increase control over the preparation or to whittle down multiple hypotheses. However, sometimes it is useful to step back and examine how these different neural and endocrine systems can potentially interact with one another, and this added complexity might bring seemingly disparate findings into specific relief. It is important that in modern biology and medicine, with such tremendous focus on molecular and genetic mechanisms, we do not lose the ability to see the forest for the trees.

References

Anisman, H. (2009). Cascading effects of stressors and inflammatory immune system activation: implications for major depressive disorder. *J Psychiatry Neurosci*, *34*, 4–20.

Anisman, H., and Merali, Z. (2002). Cytokines, stress, and depressive illness. *Brain Behav Immun*, *16*, 513–524.

Balsalobre, A. (2002). Clock genes in mammalian peripheral tissues. *Cell Tissue Res*, *309*, 193–199.

Balsalobre, A., Brown, S. A., Marcacci, L., Tronche, F., Kellendonk, C. et al (2000). Resetting of circadian time in peripheral tissues by glucocorticoid signaling. *Science*, *289*, 2344–2347.

Boivin, D. B., Tremblay, G. M., and James, F. O. (2007). Working on atypical schedules. *Sleep Med*, *8*, 578–589.

Borovikova, L. V., Ivanova, S., Zhang, M., Yang, H., Botchkina, G. I. et al (2000). Vagus nerve stimulation attenuates the systemic inflammatory response to endotoxin. *Nature*, *405*, 458–462.

Brindley, D. N., and Rolland, Y. (1989). Possible connections between stress, diabetes, obesity, hypertension and altered lipoprotein metabolism that may result in atherosclerosis. *Clin Sci (Lond)*, *77*, 453–461.

Buijs, R. M., Kalsbeek, A., van der Woude, T. P., van Heerikhuize, J. J., and Shinn, S. (1993). Suprachiasmatic nucleus lesion increases corticosterone secretion. *Am J Physiol*, *264*, R1186–1192.

Calabrese, E. J. (2008a). Hormesis and medicine. *Br J Clin Pharmacol*, *66*, 594–617.

Calabrese, E. J. (2008b). Neuroscience and hormesis: overview and general findings. *Crit Rev Toxicol*, *38*, 249–252.

Cho, K. (2001). Chronic 'jet lag' produces temporal lobe atrophy and spatial cognitive deficits. *Nat Neurosci*, *4*, 567–568.

Costa, G. (2003). Shift work and occupational medicine: an overview. *Occup Med (Lond)*, *53*, 83–88.

Dallmann, R., Touma, C., Palme, R., Albrecht, U., and Steinlechner, S. (2006). Impaired daily glucocorticoid rhythm in Per1 (Brd) mice. *J Comp Physiol A Neuroethol Sens Neural Behav Physiol*, *192*, 769–775.

Davidson, A. J., Sellix, M. T., Daniel, J., Yamazaki, S., Menaker, M. et al (2006). Chronic jet-lag increases mortality in aged mice. *Curr Biol*, *16*, R914–916.

Davis, S., Mirick, D. K., and Stevens, R. G. (2001). Night shift work, light at night, and risk of breast cancer. *J Natl Cancer Inst*, *93*, 1557–1562.

Deuschle, M., Schweiger, U., Weber, B., Gotthardt, U., Korner, A. et al (1997). Diurnal activity and pulsatility of the hypothalamus-pituitary-adrenal system in male depressed patients and healthy controls. *J Clin Endocrinol Metab*, *82*, 234–238.

Dhabhar, F. S., and McEwen, B. S. (1997). Acute stress enhances while chronic stress suppresses cell-mediated immunity in vivo: a potential role for leukocyte trafficking. *Brain Behav Immun*, *11*, 286–306.

Dhabhar, F. S., and McEwen, B. S. (1999). Enhancing versus suppressive effects of stress hormones on skin immune function. *Proc Natl Acad Sci U S A*, *96*, 1059–1064.

Elenkov, I. J., and Chrousos, G. P. (1999). Stress Hormones, Th1/Th2 patterns, Pro/anti-inflammatory cytokines and susceptibility to disease. *Trends Endocrinol Metab*, *10*, 359–368.

Elenkov, I. J., Webster, E. L., Torpy, D. J., and Chrousos, G. P. (1999). Stress, corticotropin-releasing hormone, glucocorticoids, and the immune/inflammatory response: acute and chronic effects. *Ann N Y Acad Sci*, *876*, 1–11.

Goldstein, R. S., Bruchfeld, A., Yang, L., Qureshi, A. R., Gallowitsch-Puerta, M. et al. (2007). Cholinergic anti-inflammatory pathway activity and High Mobility Group Box-1 (HMGB1) serum levels in patients with rheumatoid arthritis. *Mol Med*, *13*, 210–215.

Haus, E., and Smolensky, M. (2006). Biological clocks and shift work: circadian dysregulation and potential long-term effects. *Cancer Causes Control*, *17*, 489–500.

Hurd, M. W., and Ralph, M. R. (1998). The significance of circadian organization for longevity in the golden hamster. *J Biol Rhythms*, *13*, 430–436.

Kellendonk, C., Eiden, S., Kretz, O., Schutz, G., Schmidt, I. et al. (2002). Inactivation of the GR in the nervous system affects energy accumulation. *Endocrinology*, *143*, 2333–2340.

King, D. P., and Takahashi, J. S. (2000). Molecular genetics of circadian rhythms in mammals. *Annu Rev Neurosci*, *23*, 713–742.

Loh, D. H., Abad, C., Colwell, C. S., and Waschek, J. A. (2008). Vasoactive intestinal peptide is critical for circadian regulation of glucocorticoids. *Neuroendocrinology*, *88*, 246–255.

Lucas, L. R., Wang, C. J., McCall, T. J., and McEwen, B. S. (2007). Effects of immobilization stress on neurochemical markers in the motivational system of the male rat. *Brain Res, 1155*, 108–115.

Magarinos, A. M., and McEwen, B. S. (1995a). Stress-induced atrophy of apical dendrites of hippocampal CA3c neurons: comparison of stressors. *Neuroscience, 69*, 83–88.

Magarinos, A. M., and McEwen, B. S. (1995b). Stress-induced atrophy of apical dendrites of hippocampal CA3c neurons: involvement of glucocorticoid secretion and excitatory amino acid receptors. *Neuroscience, 69*, 89–98.

Magnusson, A., and Boivin, D. (2003). Seasonal affective disorder: an overview. *Chronobiol Int, 20*, 189–207.

Marin, P., Darin, N., Amemiya, T., Andersson, B., Jern, S. et al. (1992). Cortisol secretion in relation to body fat distribution in obese premenopausal women. *Metabolism, 41*, 882–886.

McEwen, B. S. (2006). Protective and damaging effects of stress mediators: central role of the brain. *Dialogues Clin Neurosci, 8*, 367–381.

McEwen, B. S. (2007). Physiology and neurobiology of stress and adaptation: central role of the brain. *Physiol Rev, 87*, 873–904.

McEwen, B. S., Biron, C. A., Brunson, K. W., Bulloch, K., Chambers, W. H. et al. (1997). The role of adrenocorticoids as modulators of immune function in health and disease: neural, endocrine and immune interactions. *Brain Res Brain Res Rev, 23*, 79–133.

McEwen, B. S., and Wingfield, J. C. (2003). The concept of allostasis in biology and biomedicine. *Horm Behav, 43*, 2–15.

Moore, R. Y., and Eichler, V. B. (1972). Loss of a circadian adrenal corticosterone rhythm following suprachiasmatic lesions in the rat. *Brain Res, 42*, 201–206.

Nieuwenhuizen, A. G., and Rutters, F. (2008). The hypothalamic-pituitary-adrenal-axis in the regulation of energy balance. *Physiol Behav, 94*, 169–177.

Oster, H., Damerow, S., Kiessling, S., Jakubcakova, V., Abraham, D. et al. (2006). The circadian rhythm of glucocorticoids is regulated by a gating mechanism residing in the adrenal cortical clock. *Cell Metab, 4*, 163–173.

Pasquali, R., Anconetani, B., Chattat, R., Biscotti, M., Spinucci, G. et al (1996). Hypothalamic-pituitary-adrenal axis activity and its relationship to the autonomic nervous system in women with visceral and subcutaneous obesity: effects of the corticotropin-releasing factor/arginine-vasopressin test and of stress. *Metabolism, 45*, 351–356.

Raison, C. L., Capuron, L., and Miller, A. H. (2006). Cytokines sing the blues: inflammation and the pathogenesis of depression. *Trends Immunol, 27*, 24–31.

Rosmond, R., Dallman, M. F., and Bjorntorp, P. (1998). Stress-related cortisol secretion in men: relationships with abdominal obesity and endocrine, metabolic and hemodynamic abnormalities. *J Clin Endocrinol Metab, 83*, 1853–1859.

Sage, D., Maurel, D., and Bosler, O. (2002). Corticosterone-dependent driving influence of the suprachiasmatic nucleus on adrenal sensitivity to ACTH. *Am J Physiol Endocrinol Metab, 282*, E458–465.

Sloan, R. P., McCreath, H., Tracey, K. J., Sidney, S., Liu, K. et al (2007a). RR interval variability is inversely related to inflammatory markers: the CARDIA study. *Mol Med, 13*, 178–184.

Sloan, R. P., Shapiro, P. A., Demeersman, R. E., McKinley, P. S., Tracey, K. J. et al (2007b). Aerobic exercise attenuates inducible TNF production in humans. *J Appl Physiol, 103*, 1007–1011.

Sorrells, S. F., and Sapolsky, R. M. (2007). An inflammatory review of glucocorticoid actions in the CNS. *Brain Behav Immun, 21*, 259–272.

Sternberg, E. M., and Wilder, R. L. (1989). The role of the hypothalamic-pituitary-adrenal axis in an experimental model of arthritis. *Progress in Neuro-endocrine-immunology, 2*, 102–108.

Stevens, R. G. (2005). Circadian disruption and breast cancer: from melatonin to clock genes. *Epidemiology, 16*, 254–258.

Turek, F. W. (2007). From circadian rhythms to clock genes in depression. *Int Clin Psychopharmacol, 22*(Suppl 2), S1–S8.

Van Cauter, E., and Turek, F. W. (1986). Depression: a disorder of timekeeping? *Perspect Biol Med, 29*, 510–519.

Vrang, N., Larsen, P. J., and Mikkelsen, J. D. (1995a). Direct projection from the suprachiasmatic nucleus to hypophysiotrophic corticotropin-releasing factor immunoreactive cells in the paraventricular nucleus of the hypothalamus demonstrated by means of Phaseolus vulgaris-leucoagglutinin tract tracing. *Brain Res, 684*, 61–69.

Vrang, N., Larsen, P. J., Moller, M., and Mikkelsen, J. D. (1995b). Topographical organization of the rat suprachiasmatic-paraventricular projection. *J Comp Neurol, 353*, 585–603.

Watanabe, Y., Gould, E., and McEwen, B. S. (1992). Stress induces atrophy of apical dendrites of hippocampal CA3 pyramidal neurons. *Brain Res, 588*, 341–345.

Webster, E. L., Elenkov, I. J., and Chrousos, G. P. (1997). Corticotropin-releasing hormone acts on immune cells to elicit pro-inflammatory responses. *Mol Psychiatry, 2*, 345–346.

Webster, E. L., Torpy, D. J., Elenkov, I. J., and Chrousos, G. P. (1998). Corticotropin-releasing hormone and inflammation. *Ann N Y Acad Sci, 840*, 21–32.

Wirz-Justice, A. (2006). Biological rhythm disturbances in mood disorders. *Int Clin Psychopharmacol, 21*(Suppl 1), S11–S15.

Yamazaki, S., Numano, R., Abe, M., Hida, A., Takahashi, R. et al (2000). Resetting central and peripheral circadian oscillators in transgenic rats. *Science, 288*, 682–685.

Chapter 43

Neuroendocrine Measures in Behavioral Medicine

Petra Puetz, Silja Bellingrath, Andrea Gierens, and Dirk H. Hellhammer

Abbreviations

ACTH	Adrenocorticotropic hormone
AVP	Arginine vasopressin
CAR	Cortisol awakening rise
CRH	HCorticotropin releasing hormone
HPA axis	Hypothalamic–pituitary–adrenal axis
GH	Growth hormone
PTSD	Posttraumatic stress disorder
T3	Triiodothyronine
T4	Tetraiodothyronine (=thyroxine)
TSH	Thyroid-stimulating hormone
TRH	Thyrotropin-releasing hormone

1 Scope of Neuroendocrine Research

The endocrine system, acting in concert with the nervous and immune system, is one of three major regulatory systems in the body. Endocrine disorders potently alter mental states and basic body functions. In turn, a host of mental and medical disorders coincide with profound neuroendocrine perturbations. Psychoneuroendocrinology aims to describe, explain, and predict such interactions between psychological processes, the central nervous system, and the endocrine system. With this knowledge, medical disorders may finally be better diagnosed and treated.

1.1 Neuroendocrine Systems

Most neuroendocrine axes are regulated by the hypothalamic–pituitary unit, i.e., the hypothalamic–pituitary–adrenal (HPA) axis, the hypothalamic–pituitary–thyroid axis, the hypothalamic–pituitary–gonadal axis, the hypothalamic–pituitary–prolactin system, and the hypothalamic–pituitary–growth hormone axis. The sympatho-adrenal-medullary system with its hormones epinephrine and norepinephrine (see Section 5) and pancreatic insulin secretion (see Section 6) are further major neuroendocrine systems, while some tissues such as adipose tissues and the digestive tract also possess neuroendocrine properties (Druce et al, 2004; Kershaw and Flier, 2004).

1.1.1 The Hypothalamic–Pituitary Unit

The hypothalamic–pituitary unit forms the interface between brain and periphery, where incoming neural signals translate into hormonal messages. Both structures are connected via the pituitary stalk. The human pituitary consists of two ontogenetically and functionally different parts: the anterior pituitary lobe and the posterior pituitary lobe.

P. Puetz (✉)
Department of Clinical and Physiological Psychology, University of Trier, Johanniterufer 15, Trier, D-54290, Germany
e-mail: puet1301@uni-trier.de

A. Steptoe (ed.), *Handbook of Behavioral Medicine*, DOI 10.1007/978-0-387-09488-5_43,
© Springer Science+Business Media, LLC 2010

Anterior Lobe Endocrine Systems

Neurosecretory cells from specific nuclei of the hypothalamus deliver releasing factors and release-inhibiting factors into a portal blood system at the median eminence of the pituitary stalk, which carries them to a second portal blood sinusoid system in the anterior lobe from where endocrine cells are readily reached (for an overview, see Fink, 2000)

Corticotropin-releasing hormone (CRH), thyrotropin-releasing hormone (TRH), and gonadotropin-releasing hormone stimulate the release of a further set of glandotropic hormones (= hormones regulating a remote endocrine target gland) into the general circulation. Their binding to specific endocrine cells in the anterior pituitary induces the secretion of adrenocorticotropic hormone (ACTH), thyroid-stimulating hormone (TSH), and luteinizing hormone/follicle-stimulating hormone, respectively. These latter hormones, in turn, trigger the release of glucocorticoids, thyroid hormones, and sex hormones at their endocrine target glands, i.e., the adrenals, the thyroid gland, and the gonads. Hypothalamic neurons containing growth hormone (GH)-releasing factor or the GH-inhibiting hormone (also called somatostatin) regulate pituitary GH secretion. For prolactin, no releasing factor has been discovered, but TRH stimulates prolactin secretion as well. Dopamine secreted by the tuberoinfundibular system tonically inhibits prolactin.

Hypothalamic neurons may co-express other neuropeptides with synergistic functions (Renaud, 2007). For example, arginine-vasopressin (AVP) is co-expressed in CRH-containing neurons and potentiates ACTH release.

The regulation of hypothalamic neurons involves input of many different brain regions including the brain stem, midbrain, and higher brain areas, such as the limbic system. When secreted into the blood stream, most hormones are bound to plasma carrier proteins. Thus, only a minor unbound fraction is considered bioactive (Mendel, 1989).

Posterior Pituitary Lobe Systems

Axons from hypothalamic magnocellular neurons originating from supraoptic, paraventricular, and accessory magnocellular nuclei project to the posterior pituitary lobe, with their terminals ending at a bed of fenestrated capillaries. With incoming action potentials, they release the vesicle-stored nonapeptides AVP and oxytocin into the blood stream. Both substances are effector hormones, i.e., they directly affect their target tissues (Fink, 2000).

1.1.2 Inhibitory Feedback Regulation of Neuroendocrine Activity

Neuroendocrine systems self-regulate their activity via inhibitory feedback loops. Target hormones such as glucocorticoids, thyroid hormones, or sex hormones signal back to the central nervous system and the pituitary in order to dampen their own production. Feedback actions include rapid, intermediate, and long-term effects. Also positive feedback actions to several parts of the brain exist (Darlington and Dallman, 2001; Fink, 2000).

1.2 Methodological Aspects: What Sort of Biological Samples Are Useful?

Neuroendocrine markers may be measured in blood, saliva, urine, and cerebrospinal fluid. While assessing hormone levels in the blood still remains common, practical objections may speak against its use in behavioral medicine, e.g., need of medical assistance, invasiveness, and venipuncture-related endocrine stress reactions. This dilemma may be solved by the use of saliva samples: Lipophilic hormones, such as steroid hormones, quickly pass over from blood to saliva and reliably reflect the unbound, bioactive hormone fraction in the blood. The presence of non-lipophilic molecules such as protein hormones or conjugated steroids in saliva may be traced back to saliva contamination by gingival fluid or plasma exudates or depend on saliva flow rate (Hofman, 2001; Vining et al, 1983). Urine, usually collected over an extended period of time such as 24 h, may be analyzed as an integrative hormone measurement. Noteworthy, urinary hormone profiles including hormone metabolites may be more informative than assessing only one target substance (Shackleton, 1993). Cerebrospinal fluid can be obtained by lumbar puncture, but side effects of this invasive technique are rather high and the precise site of substance secretion remains vague (Wang and Schmidt, 1997).

1.3 Methodological Aspects: When to Measure Neuroendocrine Markers?

Apart from measuring unstimulated, i.e., basal hormone secretion, the reactivity of an endocrine axis may be tested by different challenge tests.

1.3.1 Basal Hormone Assessment and Endocrine Circadian/Ultradian Rhythms

For valid and reliable assessments of basal hormone levels, the circadian and ultradian nature of hormone secretion must be taken into consideration: Endocrine activity markedly changes during the course of the day-night shift and in accordance with food availability (Hastings et al, 2007). Time of day should therefore be standardized. Circadian variation itself, i.e., trough and peak hormone values may be of particular interest. In the same vein, diseases and symptoms accumulate at characteristic times of day (Manfredini et al, 2007) (see Chapter 42).

Single time point basal measurements in the individual case, however, may be strongly misleading, as hormones are secreted in a marked pulsatile fashion. For example, cortisol is released in hourly pulses with differing amplitudes across the day (Young et al, 2004).

1.3.2 Challenge Tests

Basal hormone assessments do not necessarily reveal information on the integrity and reactivity of neuroendocrine axes. Therefore, a variety of challenge tests have been developed, using either pharmacological agents or "real-life" stimuli. Pharmacological challenge tests either stimulate or suppress an endocrine axis. For stimulating hormone secretion, hypothalamic releasing hormones and pituitary hormones have been used. The feedback sensitivity of an axis may be estimated by the degree of axis suppression after administering a synthetic version of the natural hormone exerting inhibitory feedback actions (see also Section 2.2). Other physiological stimuli activating endocrine axes may be mimicked by the administration of pharmacological agents. For example, hypoglycemia, which stimulates the HPA axis, the hypothalamic–pituitary–gonadal axis and the prolactinergic system, can be induced by insulin administration (insulin tolerance test). Other pharmacological tests target brain regulatory systems (e.g., the naloxone test inhibiting opioidergic systems) or test effects of relative hormone deprivation through inhibiting hormone formation with an enzyme blockade (e.g., the metyrapone test inhibits cortisol conversion from its inactive form).

Apart from pharmacological challenges, psychological stimulation of endocrine axis under laboratory conditions includes public speaking and mental arithmetic as in the Trier Social Stress Test (Kudielka et al, 2007), emotion-inducing pictures, films, or role plays. Alternatively, 'real-life' situations, such as exams, effects of life events, or natural catastrophes may be studied (see also Sections 7.1 and 7.3).

1.4 Confounding Factors in Neuroendocrine Research

A proper study of hormones requires the consideration of a number of factors which may affect hormone levels itself: In terms of sample characteristics some of the most important factors are age, sex, pubertal stage (in adolescents), phase of the menstrual cycle/intake of oral contraceptives/menopause (in women), ethnicity, weight, smoking, caffeine/alcohol or drug intake, strenuous exercise, and history of endocrine/immune/hepatic or psychiatric disorders. In terms of the study setting, one may want to standardize time of day, food intake, and in case of multiple blood collections, allow for enough time between first venipuncture and subsequent hormone analysis, as an endocrine stress response may occur. Sleep disorders and shift working may distort circadian endocrine rhythms (for an overview, see Heim and Ehlert, 1999; Kudielka et al, 2007).

2 The Hypothalamic–Pituitary–Adrenal Axis

Cortisol, secreted by the adrenal gland, is a major stress hormone and exerts vital effects on the cardiovascular, immune, and metabolic systems. Cortisol stimulates hepatic gluconeogenesis, amino acid, and free fatty acid mobilization and inhibits glucose uptake by muscle and adipose tissues. It furthermore alters immune functions by upregulating the expression of anti-inflammatory proteins and dampening levels of pro-inflammatory substances. However, permanently enhanced HPA axis activity has been linked to health impairments (Charmandari et al, 2004; Puetz, 2008).

2.1 Cortisol Awakening Rise and Day Profiles

Activity of the HPA axis displays a pronounced circadian rhythm. Peak levels of cortisol and ACTH can be observed shortly after awakening, followed by decreasing concentrations throughout the day, a quiescent period of minimal secretory activity during the night and rising levels during late sleep. Superimposed on this circadian rhythm, a sharp increase (50–100%) in both free salivary cortisol levels and total plasma cortisol levels can be observed within the first hour after awakening in the majority of people (Dockray et al, 2008; Pruessner et al, 1997). Salivary cortisol levels are considered a reliable measure of HPA axis activity, due to the high correlation between salivary cortisol levels and free unbound cortisol levels in plasma and serum (Hellhammer et al, 2009). Thus, the CAR can be simply assessed by taking four saliva samples (directly after awakening, 30, 45, and 60 min after awakening), with strict reference to awakening time. A major advantage of this non-invasive measure is its utility at any place, e.g., home or workplace. However, compliance with saliva sampling procedures, especially their timing, is crucial to obtain valid data in such settings (Kudielka et al, 2003). Electronic monitoring devices (MEMS® Track Cap; AARDEX, Ltd., Switzerland) can be used to ensure accurate timing of saliva collection. Assessment of salivary cortisol measures also benefits from the high temporal stability of salivary cortisol at room temperature, with minimal changes demonstrable over periods of up to 1 month. Therefore, samples can be sent by post and do not require specialized storage (Kudielka and Wuest, 2008). The CAR has been shown to have a medium to high day-to-day stability (Wüst et al, 2000). However, a recent analysis by Hellhammer and colleagues (2007) demonstrated that the CAR on a given day is considerably influenced by situational factors. Thus, repeated daily measurements are almost certainly necessary in order to obtain reliable trait measures. The magnitude and time course of the CAR are influenced by a variety of factors, such as age, gender, socioeconomic status, and day of the week, while smoking, the female menstrual cycle and sleep length appear to be minor (for a review, see Fries et al, 2009).

Altered HPA axis regulation reflected in the CAR has been associated with various health outcomes (for a review, see Fries et al, 2009; Kudielka and Wuest, 2008). An increased CAR has been observed in subjects with visceral obesity, upper respiratory illness, borderline personality disorder, and depression. A blunted CAR on the contrary seems to be associated with systemic hypertension, chronic pain, functional gastrointestinal disorders, chronic fatigue syndrome, posttraumatic stress disorder (PTSD), and early loss experience. In patients with various forms of hippocampal damage and in a small sample of patients with global amnesia no CAR could be observed. However, the interpretation of individual differences in CAR levels is still under debate and whether positive health outcomes and well-being are consistently associated with a larger or smaller awakening responses remains unclear (Heim et al, 2000). Adam and colleagues (2006) suggest that day-to-day variations in psychosocial experience, such as loneliness, sadness, and feeling threatened, may moderate the CAR on the following day. Thus, one can speculate that the CAR is an adaptive response designed to provide the individual with the energy and resources needed to meet the anticipated demands of the upcoming day. In the case of chronic stress, this typically adaptive mechanism potentially gets exhausted over time and the CAR is no longer effectively modulated by anticipated daily demands, leading to long-term physiological costs.

Cortisol day profiles extend the cortisol sampling beyond the CAR and cover the peak waking level, the decrease over the course of the day and low evening levels. Alterations in rhythmicity of cortisol (typically flattened cortisol rhythms, often due to lower cortisol early in the day and higher cortisol in the evening) have been associated with negative health outcomes, including early mortality from cancer (Sephton et al, 2000), obesity and disrupted glucose metabolism (Rosmond et al, 1998), and depressive symptomatology (Bhattacharyya et al, 2008).

2.2 The HPA Axis Under Challenge

To investigate the functionality of the HPA axis, various ways to stimulate acute cortisol responses in the laboratory have been developed, including psychological stress protocols (e.g., cognitive tasks or public speaking paradigms (for an overview, see Kudielka et al, 2009) and a wide variety of pharmacological provocations, physical exercise, or intake of standardized meals. While psychological stressors are central stimuli that are processed at higher brain levels, pharmacological challenge tests are specifically tailored to act at certain levels of the HPA system and operate in a dose-dependent manner. The HPA axis is regulated by the negative feedback action of cortisol on receptors in the hippocampus, hypothalamus. and pituitary gland. The dexamethasone suppression test is used to test HPA axis negative feedback efficiency by determining the degree to which endogenous cortisol release is suppressed by intake of oral dexamethasone. This synthetic glucocorticoid acts primarily by binding to glucocorticoid receptors in the pituitary gland, mimicking the negative feedback effects of endogenous cortisol such that ACTH and cortisol release is reduced (de Kloet, 1997). The standard dose of 1 mg dexamethasone leads to an almost complete suppression of endogenous cortisol production in healthy subjects. Application of a low dose with concentrations of 0.5 mg or even 0.25 mg in adult humans is preferable in order to prevent complete suppression, allowing the detection of hypersuppression (strong suppression) or indications of non-suppression (less suppression, Huizenga et al, 1998). Virtually no side effects have been reported for this test. It has been demonstrated that patients with major depression show elevated cortisol levels after dexamethasone intake (Holsboer, 2001), while patients with PTSD and subjects with increased levels of exhaustion display enhanced cortisol suppression (Bellingrath et al, 2008; Yehuda et al, 1993).

The CRH stimulation test allows the assessment of pituitary as well as adrenal reactivity. When comparing different studies using the CRH stimulation test, the difference in the affinity of human CRH and ovine CRH to endogenous CRH-binding proteins, which leads to differential pharmacological effects, needs to be taken into account (Sutton et al, 1995). CRH injection will result in a marked increase in ACTH secretion from the pituitary after 15–30 min in healthy, unstressed humans, while cortisol peaks about 30–60 min after CRH administration. For depressed patients and patients with seasonal affective disorders, it was demonstrated that the CRH stimulation test triggers a blunted ACTH response, suggesting desensitized pituitary CRH receptors due to homologous down-regulation by hypersecreted CRH (Gold et al, 1986; Joseph-Vanderpool et al, 1991). In PTSD patients, CRH stimulation has led to conflicting results (Kellner et al, 2003).

Finally, the combined dexamethasone/CRH (DEX/CRH) test has proved to be most sensitive (above 80%) in detecting differences in HPA axis regulation, examining the stimulating effects of CRH on ACTH and cortisol under the suppressive action of dexamethasone. In contrast to healthy control subjects, patients with acute major depression show increased ACTH and cortisol responses to the combined DEX/CRH test, which can be explained by a central CRH hyperactivity as well as alterations in feedback sensitivity (Heuser et al, 1994). Elevated cortisol and ACTH responses have also been observed in patients with anxiety disorders (Schreiber et al, 1996). In PTSD, Stroehle and colleagues (2008) report that patients compared to healthy subjects showed a decreased ACTH response to the DEX/CRH test. In contrast, other studies have found no significant group differences between PTSD patients and controls in the DEX/CRH test (de Kloet et al, 2008; Muhtz et al, 2008). However, when considering the moderating effects of co-morbid major depression or history of childhood trauma, alterations in HPA regulation were observed. These results are in line with findings of Heim and colleagues (2001), who observed moderating effects of early life stress on HPA axis regulation in women with major depressive disorder.

A number of studies have administered the combined DEX/CRH test before as well as after the initiation of an antidepressant treatment, and normalization of the neuroendocrine response has been repeatedly observed (Ising et al, 2007). This effect can be explained with results from preclinical as well as animal studies, where it has been demonstrated that different types of antidepressants increase glucocorticoid receptor gene expression and restore the receptor's sensitivity (Holsboer, 2000).

3 The Hypothalamic–Pituitary–Gonadal Axis

The pituitary hormones, follicle-stimulating hormone, and luteinizing hormone regulate a variety of functions related to reproduction. In women, they stimulate sex hormone release (estrogens, gestagens, progesterone) from the ovaries and, in concert with these hormones, regulate the menstrual cycle. In men, luteinizing hormone stimulates testosterone secretion from Leydig cells in the testes. Follicle-stimulating hormone targets sertoli cells and, in concert with testosterone, regulates spermatogenesis.

Severe chronic stress and HPA axis activation results in suppression of the hypothalamic–pituitary–gonadal axis at all levels (hypothalamus, pituitary, gonads) and a decrease in reproductive activity in general. In women, stress-induced secondary hypothalamic amenorrhea due to glucocorticoid hypersecretion has been observed in melancholic depression, chronic alcoholism, and eating disorders (Chrousos and Gold, 1998; Kyrou et al, 2006). In men, severe stress in real life, i.e., exposure to war, to an earthquake or to a critical life event may lead to impaired sperm quality (Abu-Musa et al, 2008; Fukuda et al, 1996; Gollenberg et al, 2010). Interestingly, a psychological profile of being an active, competitive person may coincide with a low sperm count, possibly through activity-induced activation of the SNS and a deficiency of testicular blood flow. Behavioral therapy focusing on relaxation strategies appear to increase sperm counts and reproductive success in these men (Hellhammer and Gutberlet, 1988).

Women are much more likely to succumb to stress-related health impairments than men. Symptoms particularly aggravate during phases of estrogen withdrawal, i.e., the premenstrual, postpartum, or perimenopausal periods (see Chapter 38). Estrogens may exert protective effects through suppressing aversive glucocorticoid actions (Solomon and Herman, 2009).

4 Hypothalamic–Pituitary–Thyroid Axis

TSH-producing cells in the anterior pituitary are positively regulated by TRH, while TSH-inhibiting substances include dopamine, somatostatin, T3 (triiodothyronine), and cortisol. Given sufficient iodine levels, the biologically inactive form thyroxine (tetraiodothyronine, T4) is released through TSH binding at the thyroid gland. The conversion to bioactive T3 mostly happens in target tissue, such as the liver. T3 influences growth and development, oxygen consumption, and heat production (Joffe, 2002).

Hyperthyroidism, i.e., a functional hyperactivity of the thyroid gland marked by increased T3 and T4 levels, coincides with hypermetabolic activity, weight loss, increased heart rate, increased cold tolerance, tremulousness, fatigue, anxiety, restlessness, irritability, dysphoric mood, weakness, poor concentration, and cognitive deficits (Lesser and Flores, 2007). On the contrary, a deficient secretion of thyroid hormones in hypothyroidism is characterized by facial puffiness, dry skin, hair loss, myalgia, cold intolerance, constipation, fatigue, and manifest depression (Joffe, 2007).

Severe psychological or physiological stress such as fasting, severe illness, injury, and inflammation, coinciding with strong HPA axis activation, may lead to a reversible state of hypothyroidism manifesting in a decreased hepatic conversion of T4 to T3, altered binding of thyroid hormones to plasma proteins, altered tissue responsiveness, and altered thyroid metabolism, while a compensatory increase in TRH is lacking. This state, possibly an attempt to conserve energy, is known as "low T3 syndrome" or "euthyroid sick syndrome."

In critically ill patients, the low T3 syndrome has been considered a predictor for mortality (Chopra, 1997). In patients with anorexia nervosa, the low T3 syndrome as well as a smaller volume of the thyroid gland has been observed, which are both reversible after weight gain (Munoz and Argente, 2002). In PTSD and major depression, both hyper- and hypoactivity of the hypothalamic–pituitary–thyroid axis have been described (Boscarino, 2004; Newport and Nemeroff, 2000).

5 The Hypothalamic–Pituitary–Growth Hormone Axis

The release of GH (also referred to as somatotropin) is stimulated by neurons from the arcuate nucleus containing GH-releasing factor and inhibited by neurons from the periventricular nucleus containing GH-inhibiting factor. Further neurotransmitters, neuropeptides, and hormones affect GH release, such as dopamine, TRH, neuropeptide Y, sex hormones, glucocorticoid hormones, and thyroid hormones. Additionally, food-related substances such as free fatty acids, glucose, and amino acids alter GH regulation, as do alterations in caloric intake, physical activity, and stress. GH stimulates the production of hepatic insulin-like-growth factor -1 (IGF-1). In concert with IGF-1 both hormones regulate growth, somatic development, and cell metabolism (Laron, 2002). Gonadal steroids distinctively modulate GH-IGF-1 actions in a sex-specific way (Meinhardt and Ho, 2006).

Acute psychosocial stress, severe injury, hypoglycemia, pain or hemorrhage, increases plasma GH levels in humans, probably due to stimulating actions of glucocorticoids binding to a GH gene promoter. On the other hand, chronic stress or chronically increased glucocorticoid levels decrease GH secretion in humans and induce a state of IGF-1 resistance in peripheral tissues. This may occur because of CRH-induced increases in somatostatin secretion (Pacak and McCarthy, 2007). Severe psychosocial stress during childhood or adolescence may result in chronic GH suppression and subsequently, psychosocial short stature. However, with amelioration of environmental conditions during development, this may be reversed (Gohlke et al, 2004). Also Anorexia nervosa coincides with dysregulation in GH-IGF-1 functioning and, given a prepubertal disease onset, may result in diminished final body height (Munoz and Argente, 2002).

6 The Prolactinergic System

Prolactin exerts a variety of effects, i.e., it regulates mammary gland development, initiation and maintenance of lactation, modulates immune functions, and controls osmoregulation (Ben-Jonathan et al, 2002). Prolactin is secreted during orgasm and correlates with level of sexual satisfaction. Hyperprolactinemia during pregnancy and lactation causes anovulation. Hyperprolactinemia during non-pregnant states may be involved in some reproductive disorders (Bachelot and Binart, 2007).

7 The Oxytocinergic System

Oxytocin affects species-specific social and reproductive behaviors (for an overview, see Heinrichs and Domes, 2008, Heinrichs et al, 2009). Warm social contact with the partner, sexual arousal, orgasm, and attachment as well as regulation of parturition and lactation have been related to oxytocin actions in women. Oxytocin interacts with the HPA axis and has stress-reducing effects in both men and women: During laboratory stress, oxytocin was found to diminish cortisol responses, which is most likely due to a central inhibition of the HPA axis, involving reduced amygdala reactivity.

In men, vasopressin (see below) may be the analogue of oxytocin. Still, while central oxytocin appears to have anxiolytic effects, central AVP rather acts as an anxiogenic.

8 The Vasopressinergic System

Peripherally, AVP controls vasoconstriction, water homeostasis, and regulates antidiuresis in the kidney. Other AVP actions include promoting efficient blood platelet aggregation, the induction of liver glycogenolysis, and secretion of the hormones aldosterone and insulin. AVP secretion is strongly induced in response to dehydration, blood loss, and hypotension. In the central nervous system, AVP secretion modulates temperature regulation, cardiovascular functioning, and the regulation of circadian rhythms. In terms of behavior, rewarded behaviors, drug tolerance, social and reproductive behaviors as well as a role in feeding are ascribed to AVP secretion (Renaud, 2007).

Excess AVP plasma levels have been assessed in patients with head trauma, congestive heart failure, liver cirrhosis, and lung carcinomas, coinciding with inappropriate antidiuresis (Renaud, 2007). AVP has been considered to regulate male characteristic social behavior including aggression, territoriality, and stress reactivity (for an overview, see Heinrichs and Domes, 2008; Heinrichs et al, 2009).

9 The Sympatho-Adrenal-Medullary System

The adrenal medulla is an ontogenetic peculiarity: Being derived from the embryonic neural crest, it consists of modified postganglionic neurons belonging to the sympathetic branch of the autonomic nervous system. Its chromaffin cells, innervated by the splanchnic nerve, secrete the catecholamines epinephrine and norepinephrine directly into the blood stream. However, the major part of plasma norepinephrine, i.e., approx. 65%, is not of adrenal origin, but secreted by sympathetic nerve endings. As catecholamines do not cross the blood–brain barrier, their effects are mostly peripheral (Kvetnansky and McCarthy, 2007; Tentolouris et al, 2006).

The seminal role of adrenal hormones during stress was first reviewed by Cannon (1914), who summarized their actions as the "fight-or-flight reaction," with life-saving effects for the organism. Epinephrine and norepinephrine increase heart rate, the force of heart contraction and cardiac output, shift the blood supply to coronary arteries, skeletal muscle and the brain, while blood supply of skin, kidney, and mucosa is diminished. They reduce time for blood clotting through effects on blood platelets, reinforce glucagon-induced glycogenolysis, glucose production in the liver and lipolysis in adipose cells. Thus, through their actions, organ systems critical to survival are provided with energy and, via bronchodilatation, supplied with additional oxygen (Pollard, 2000).

Epinephrine and norepinephrine blood levels increase rapidly in response to challenge (<1 min). Epinephrine is furthermore very reactive to novelty, which should be considered when studying stress effects under laboratory conditions. In emergency medicine, epinephrine is administered in life-threatening conditions such as shock and cardiac arrest. On the other hand, increased catecholamine secretion during chronic stress may burden organ systems and may be involved in the pathogenesis of stress-related health impairments, such as atherosclerosis, myocardial ischemia, hypertension, and coronary heart disease (Lundberg, 2000). Of note, while cortisol responses habituate in the face of repeated stress exposure, catecholamine responses do not (Schommer et al, 2003).

In hypertension, a role for elevated norepinephrine levels has been established (DeQuattro and Feng, 2002). Epinephrine may furthermore interact with immune functions. In HIV, stress may be involved in disease progression partly due to epinephrine effects on HIV-infected leucocytes (Cole, 2008). In psoriasis and atopic dermatitis, a hyperresponsive plasma catecholamine response to psychosocial stress may be involved in dysregulations in Th1/Th2 mediated immune states (Buske-Kirschbaum et al, 2006). The sympatho-adrenal-medullary system may also play a role in the pathogenesis of obesity. Epinephrine

affects resting metabolic rate, lipolysis, and thermogenesis SNS overactivity is associated to visceral obesity (Tentolouris et al, 2006). Through actions on ascending vagal afferents, elevated systemic levels of epinephrine may possibly affect cognitive processes, such as memory and attention. An inverted U shape of catecholamine actions has been proposed, with moderate levels being beneficial, while low or high levels impairing cognitive performance (Lundberg, 2000; Roozendaal et al, 2009).

10 Insulin and the Pancreas

Insulin, a peptide hormone produced in β-cells of the islets of Langerhans in the pancreas, strongly modulates the metabolism, facilitating the uptake of glucose in the liver, muscle, and fat tissue. Insulin facilitates the storage of glucose as glycogen in the liver and muscle and inhibits the use of fat as an energy source. The HPA axis and the sympatho-adrenal-medullary system interact with insulin actions, and chronic stress exposure is associated with insulin resistance, diabetes mellitus 2, and the metabolic syndrome (Kyrou et al, 2006; for detail see also Chapter 46).

11 Summary and Outlook

In this chapter we treated the major neuroendocrine systems and their role in health and stress-related disorders, such as depression, PTSD, infertility, or eating disorders. It becomes evident that neuroendocrine systems are tightly intertwined with each other and perturbations in one system may cause multiple dysregulations in the others. Environmental events, and stress in particular, have profound effects on proper neuroendocrine functioning and may thus affect disease onset, maintenance, or progression.

The riddle of why environmental events, particularly during early development, may persistently alter the functioning of endocrine systems and lead to stress-related health impairments, may possibly be explained by modifications in the epigenome (see also Chapter 30). It has been shown in animals that the methylation of brain hormone receptor genes in response to experience alters complex behaviors such as parenting behavior or behavioral/endocrine responses to stress (for an overview, see Meaney et al, 2007). In the future, the study of epigenetics may help to understand how experience may be linked to persisting neuroendocrine alterations and ultimately, disease.

References

Abu-Musa, A. A., Kobeissi, L., Hannoun, A. B., and Inhorn, M. C. (2008). Effect of war on fertility: a review of the literature. *Reprod Biomed Online, 17 Suppl 1*, 43–53.

Adam, E. K., Hawkley, L. C., Kudielka, B. M., and Cacioppo, J. T. (2006). Day-to-day dynamics of experience--cortisol associations in a population-based sample of older adults. *Proc Natl Acad Sci U S A, 103*, 17058–17063.

Bachelot, A., and Binart, N. (2007). Reproductive role of prolactin. *Reproduction, 133*, 361–369.

Bhattacharyya, M. R., Molloy, G. J., and Steptoe, A. (2008). Depression is associated with flatter cortisol rhythms in patients with coronary artery disease. *J Psychosom Res 65*, 107–113.

Bellingrath, S., Weigl, T., and Kudielka, B. M. (2008). Cortisol dysregulation in school teachers in relation to burnout, vital exhaustion, and effort-reward-imbalance. *Biol Psychol, 78*, 104–113.

Ben-Jonathan, N., Khurana, S., and Hnasko, R. (2002). Brain Prolactin. In D. W. Pfaff (Ed.), *Hormones, Brain and Behavior Vol. 5* (pp. 97–121). Amsterdam: Academic Press.

Boscarino, J. A. (2004). Posttraumatic stress disorder and physical illness: results from clinical and epidemiologic studies. *Ann N Y Acad Sci, 1032*, 141–153.

Buske-Kirschbaum, A., Ebrecht, M., Kern, S., and Hellhammer, D. H. (2006). Endocrine stress responses in TH1-mediated chronic inflammatory skin disease (psoriasis vulgaris) - do they parallel stress-induced endocrine changes in TH2-mediated inflammatory dermatoses (atopic dermatitis)? *Psychoneuroendocrinology, 31*, 439–446.

Cannon, W. B. (1914). The emergency function of the adrenal medulla in pain and the major emotions. *Am J Physiol, 33*, 356–372.

Charmandari, E., Kino, T., and Chrousos, G. P. (2004). Glucocorticoids and their actions: an introduction. *Ann N Y Acad Sci, 1024*, 1–8.

Chopra, I. J. (1997). Clinical review 86: Euthyroid sick syndrome: is it a misnomer? *J Clin Endocrinol Metab, 82*, 329–334.

Chrousos, G. P., and Gold, P. W. (1998). A healthy body in a healthy mind--and vice versa--the damaging power of "uncontrollable" stress. *J Clin Endocrinol Metab, 83*, 1842–1845.

Cole, S. W. (2008). Psychosocial influences on HIV-1 disease progression: neural, endocrine, and virologic mechanisms. *Psychosom Med, 70*, 562–568.

Darlington, D. N., and Dallman, M. F. (2001). Feedback control in endocrine systems. In K. L. Becher (Ed.), *Principles and Practice of Endocrinology and Metabolism, 3rd Ed* (pp. 50–57). Philadelphia: Lippincott Williams & Wilkins.

de Kloet, E. R. (1997). Why dexamethasone poorly penetrates in brain. *Stress, 2*, 13–20.

de Kloet, C., Vermetten, E., Lentjes, E., Geuze, E., van Pelt, J. et al (2008). Differences in the response to the combined DEX-CRH test between PTSD patients with and without co-morbid depressive disorder. *Psychoneuroendocrinology, 33*, 313–320.

DeQuattro, V., and Feng, M. (2002). The sympathetic nervous system: the muse of primary hypertension. *J Hum Hypertens, 16* (Suppl 1), S64–69.

Dockray, S., Bhattacharyya, M. R., Molloy, G. J., and Steptoe, A. (2008). The cortisol awakening response in relation to objective and subjective measures of waking in the morning. *Psychoneuroendocrinology, 33*, 77–82.

Druce, M. R., Small, C. J., and Bloom, S. R. (2004). Minireview: gut peptides regulating satiety. *Endocrinology, 145*, 2660–2665.

Fink, G. (2000). Neuroendocrine systems. In G. Fink (Ed.), *Encyclopedia of Stress, Vol. 2* (pp. 851–864). Amsterdam: Academic Press.

Fries, E., Dettenborn, L., and Kirschbaum, C. (2009). The cortisol awakening response (CAR): facts and future directions. *Int J Psychophysiol, 72*(1), 67–73.

Fukuda, M., Fukuda, K., Shimizu, T., Yomura, W., and Shimizu, S. (1996). Kobe earthquake and reduced sperm motility. *Hum Reprod, 11*, 1244–1246.

Gohlke, B. C., Frazer, F. L., and Stanhope, R. (2004). Growth hormone secretion and long-term growth data in children with psychosocial short stature treated by different changes in environment. *J Pediatr Endocrinol Metab, 17*, 637–643.

Gold, P. W., Loriaux, D. L., Roy, A., Kling, M. A., Calabrese, J. R. et al (1986). Responses to corticotropin-releasing hormone in the hypercortisolism of depression and Cushing's disease. Pathophysiologic and diagnostic implications. *N Engl J Med, 314*, 1329–1335.

Gollenberg, A. L., Liu, F., Brazil, C., Drobnis, E. Z., Guzick, D., et al (2010). Semen quality in fertile men in relation to psychosocial stress. *Fertil Steril, 93*(4), 1104–1111.

Hastings, M., O'Neill, J. S., and Maywood, E. S. (2007). Circadian clocks: regulators of endocrine and metabolic rhythms. *J Endocrinol, 195*, 187–198.

Heim, C., and Ehlert, U. (1999). Pharmakologische Provokationstest zur Einschätzung der neuroendokrinen Funktionen. In C. Kirschbaum & D. Hellhammer (Eds.), *Enzyklopädie der Psychologie. Psychoendokrinologie und Psychoimmunologie.* (pp. 307–346). Göttingen: Hogrefe.

Heim, C., Ehlert, U., and Hellhammer, D. H. (2000). The potential role of hypocortisolism in the pathophysiology of stress-related bodily disorders. *Psychoneuroendocrinology, 25*(1), 1–35.

Heim, C., Newport, D. J., Bonsall, R., Miller, A. H., and Nemeroff, C. B. (2001). Altered pituitary-adrenal axis responses to provocative challenge tests in adult survivors of childhood abuse. *Am J Psychiatry, 158*, 575–581.

Heinrichs, M., and Domes, G. (2008). Neuropeptides and social behaviour: effects of oxytocin and vasopressin in humans. *Prog Brain Res, 170*, 337–350.

Heinrichs, M., von Dawans, B., and Domes, G. (2009). Oxytocin, vasopressin, and human social behavior. *Front Neuroendocrinol, 30*(4), 548–557.

Hellhammer, D., and Gutberlet, I. (1988). Male infertility: preliminary evidence for two neuroendocrine mediators of stress on gonadal function. In J. A. Ferrendelli, R. C. Collins, & E. M. Johnson (Eds.), *Neurobiology of Amino Acids, Peptides and Trophic Factors* (pp. 227–230). Boston, Dordrecht: Kluwer Academic.

Hellhammer, D. H., Wuest, S., and Kudielka, B. M. (2009). Salivary cortisol as a biomarker in stress research. *Psychoneuroendocrinology, 34*(2), 163–171.

Hellhammer, J., Fries, E., Schweisthal, O. W., Schlotz, W., Stone, A. A. et al (2007). Several daily measurements are necessary to reliably assess the cortisol rise after awakening: state- and trait components. *Psychoneuroendocrinology, 32*, 80–86.

Heuser, I., Yassouridis, A., and Holsboer, F. (1994). The combined dexamethasone/CRH test: a refined laboratory test for psychiatric disorders. *J Psychiatr Res, 28*, 341–356.

Hofman, L. F. (2001). Human saliva as a diagnostic specimen. *J Nutr, 131*, 1621S–1625S.

Holsboer, F. (2000). The corticosteroid receptor hypothesis of depression. *Neuropsychopharmacology, 23*, 477–501.

Holsboer, F. (2001). Stress, hypercortisolism and corticosteroid receptors in depression: implications for therapy. *J Affect Disord, 62*, 77–91.

Huizenga, N. A., Koper, J. W., De Lange, P., Pols, H. A., Stolk, R. P. et al (1998). A polymorphism in the glucocorticoid receptor gene may be associated with and increased sensitivity to glucocorticoids in vivo. *J Clin Endocrinol Metab, 83*, 144 151.

Ising, M., Horstmann, S., Kloiber, S., Lucae, S., Binder, E. B. et al (2007). Combined dexamethasone/corticotropin releasing hormone test predicts treatment response in major depression – a potential biomarker? *Biol Psychiatry, 62*, 47–54.

Joffe, R. T. (2002). Hypothalamic-pituitary-thyroid axis. In D. W. Pfaff (Ed.), *Hormones, Brain and Behavior, Vol. 4* (pp. 867–881). Amsterdam: Academic Press.

Joffe, R. T. (2007). Hypothyroidism. In G. Fink (Ed.), *Encyclopedia of Stress, Vol. 2* (pp. 439–441). Amsterdam: Academic Press.

Joseph-Vanderpool, J. R., Rosenthal, N. E., Chrousos, G. P., Wehr, T. A., Skwerer, R. et al (1991). Abnormal pituitary-adrenal responses to corticotropin-releasing hormone in patients with seasonal affective disorder: clinical and pathophysiological implications. *J Clin Endocrinol Metab, 72*, 1382–1387.

Kellner, M., Yassouridis, A., Hubner, R., Baker, D. G., and Wiedemann, K. (2003). Endocrine and cardiovascular responses to corticotropin-releasing hormone in patients with posttraumatic stress disorder: a role for atrial natriuretic peptide? *Neuropsychobiology, 47*, 102–108.

Kershaw, E. E., and Flier, J. S. (2004). Adipose tissue as an endocrine organ. *J Clin Endocrinol Metab, 89*, 2548–2556.

Kudielka, B. M., and Wuest, S. (2008). The cortisol awakening response (CAR): a useful tool for ambulant assessment of hypothalamic-pituitary-adrenal (HPA) axis activity. In A.-L. Leglise (Ed.), *Progress in Circadian Rhythm Research* (pp. 223–234). Hauppage, NY: Nova Science.

Kudielka, B. M., Broderick, J. E., and Kirschbaum, C. (2003). Compliance with saliva sampling protocols: electronic monitoring reveals invalid cortisol daytime profiles in noncompliant subjects. *Psychosom Med, 65*, 313–319.

Kudielka, B. M., Hellhammer, D. H., and Kirschbaum, C. (2007). Ten years of research with the Trier Social Stress Test – Revisited. . In E. Harmon-Jones & P. Winkielman (Eds.), *Social Neuroscience: Integrating Biological and Psychological Explanations of Social Behavior* (pp. 56–83). New York: Guilford Press.

Kudielka, B. M., Hellhammer, D. H., and Wüst, S. (2009). Why do we respond so differently? Reviewing determinants of human salivary cortisol responses to challenge. *Psychoneuroendocrinology 34*, 2–18.

Kvetnansky, R., and McCarthy, R. (2007). Adrenal medulla. In G. Fink (Ed.), *Encyclopedia of Stress, Vol. 1* (pp. 52–59). Amsterdam: Academic Press.

Kyrou, I., Chrousos, G. P., and Tsigos, C. (2006). Stress, visceral obesity, and metabolic complications. *Ann N Y Acad Sci, 1083*, 77–110.

Laron, Z. (2002). Growth hormone and insulin-like growth factor I: effects on the brain. In D. W. Pfaff (Ed.), *Hormones, Brain and Behavior, Vol. 5* (pp. 75–96). Amsterdam: Academic Press.

Lesser, I. M., and Flores, D. L. (2007). Hyperthyroidism. In G. Fink (Ed.), *Encyclopedia of Stress, Vol. 2* (pp. 388–390). Amsterdam: Academic Press.

Lundberg, U. (2000). Catecholamines. In G. Fink (Ed.), *Encyclopedia of Stress, Vol. 1* (pp. 419–423). Amsterdam: Academic Press.

Manfredini, R., Boari, B., Salmi, R., Malagoni, A. M., and Manfredini, F. (2007). Circadian variation of cardiovascular and other stress-related events. In G. Fink (Ed.), *Encyclopledia of Stress, 2nd Ed, Vol. 1* (pp. 500–504). Amsterdam: Academic.

Meaney, M. J., Szyf, M., and Seckl, J. R. (2007). Epigenetic mechanisms of perinatal programming of hypothalamic-pituitary-adrenal function and health. *Trends Mol Med, 13*, 269–277.

Meinhardt, U. J., and Ho, K. K. (2006). Modulation of growth hormone action by sex steroids. *Clin Endocrinol (Oxf), 65*, 413–422.

Mendel, C. M. (1989). The free hormone hypothesis: a physiologically based mathematical model. *Endocr Rev, 10*, 232–274.

Muhtz, C., Wester, M., Yassouridis, A., Wiedemann, K., and Kellner, M. (2008). A combined dexamethasone/corticotropin-releasing hormone test in patients with chronic PTSD--first preliminary results. *J Psychiatr Res, 42*, 689–693.

Munoz, M. T., and Argente, J. (2002). Anorexia nervosa in female adolescents: endocrine and bone mineral density disturbances. *Eur J Endocrinol, 147*, 275–286.

Newport, D. J., and Nemeroff, C. B. (2000). Neurobiology of posttraumatic stress disorder. *Curr Opin Neurobiol, 10*, 211–218.

Pacak, K., and McCarthy, R. (2007). Acute stress response: experimental. In G. Fink (Ed.), *Encyclopedia of Stress* (Vol. 1, pp. 7–14). Amsterdam: Academic Press.

Pollard, T. M. (2000). Adrenaline. In G. Fink (Ed.), *Encyclopedia of Stress, Vol. 1* (pp. 60–64). Amsterdam: Academic Press.

Pruessner, J. C., Wolf, O. T., Hellhammer, D. H., Buske-Kirschbaum, A., von Auer, K. et al (1997). Free cortisol levels after awakening: a reliable biological marker for the assessment of adrenocortical activity. *Life Sci, 61*, 2539–2549.

Puetz, P. (2008). Hypercortisolemic disorders. In D. H. Hellhammer & J. Hellhammer (Eds.), *Stress - The Brain-Body-Connection* (pp. 39–59). Basel: Karger.

Renaud, L. P. (2007). Vasopressin. In G. Fink (Ed.), *Encyclopedia of Stress, Vol. 3* (pp. 824–829). Amsterdam: Academic Press.

Roozendaal, B., McEwen, B. S., and Chattarji, S. (2009). Stress, memory and the amygdala. *Nat Rev Neurosci, 10*(6), 423–433.

Rosmond, R., Dallman, M. F., and Bjorntorp, P. (1998). Stress-related cortisol secretion in men: relationships with abdominal obesity and endocrine, metabolic and hemodynamic abnormalities. *J Clin Endocrinol Metab, 83*, 1853–1859.

Schommer, N. C., Hellhammer, D. H., and Kirschbaum, C. (2003). Dissociation between reactivity of the hypothalamus-pituitary-adrenal axis and the sympathetic-adrenal-medullary system to repeated psychosocial stress. *Psychosom Med, 65*, 450–460.

Schreiber, W., Lauer, C. J., Krumrey, K., Holsboer, F., and Krieg, J. C. (1996). Dysregulation of the hypothalamic-pituitary-adrenocortical system in panic disorder. *Neuropsychopharmacology, 15*, 7–15.

Sephton, S. E., Sapolsky, R. M., Kraemer, H. C., and Spiegel, D. (2000). Diurnal cortisol rhythm as a predictor of breast cancer survival. *J Natl Cancer Inst, 92*, 994–1000.

Shackleton, C. H. (1993). Mass spectrometry in the diagnosis of steroid-related disorders and in hypertension research. *J Steroid Biochem Mol Biol, 45*, 127–140.

Solomon, M. B., and Herman, J. P. (2009). Sex differences in psychopathology: of gonads, adrenals and mental illness. *Physiol Behav, 97*, 250–258.

Strohle, A., Scheel, M., Modell, S., and Holsboer, F. (2008). Blunted ACTH response to dexamethasone suppression-CRH stimulation in posttraumatic stress disorder. *J Psychiatr Res, 42*, 1185–1188.

Sutton, S. W., Behan, D. P., Lahrichi, S. L., Kaiser, R., Corrigan, A. et al (1995). Ligand requirements of the human corticotropin-releasing factor-binding protein. *Endocrinology, 136*, 1097–1102.

Tentolouris, N., Liatis, S., and Katsilambros, N. (2006). Sympathetic system activity in obesity and metabolic syndrome. *Ann N Y Acad Sci, 1083*, 129–152.

Vining, R. F., McGinley, R. A., Maksvytis, J. J., and Ho, K. Y. (1983). Salivary cortisol: a better measure of adrenal cortical function than serum cortisol. *Ann Clin Biochem, 20*, 329–335.

Wang, L. P., and Schmidt, J. F. (1997). Central nervous side effects after lumbar puncture. A review of the possible pathogenesis of the syndrome of postdural puncture headache and associated symptoms. *Dan Med Bull, 44*, 79–81.

Wüst, S., Wolf, J., Hellhammer, D. H., Federenko, I., Schommer, N. et al (2000). The cortisol awakening response - normal values and confounds. *Noise Health, 2*, 79–88.

Yehuda, R., Southwick, S. M., Krystal, J. H., Bremner, D., Charney, D. S. et al (1993). Enhanced suppression of cortisol following dexamethasone administration in posttraumatic stress disorder. *Am J Psychiatry, 150*, 83–86.

Young, E. A., Abelson, J., and Lightman, S. L. (2004). Cortisol pulsatility and its role in stress regulation and health. *Front Neuroendocrinol, 25*, 69–76.

Chapter 44

Immune Measures in Behavioral Medicine Research: Procedures and Implications

Michael T. Bailey and Ronald Glaser

1 Introduction

Over the past two decades, several immunological measures have been used to assess the physiological consequences of psychological stressors and different emotional states. In general, these immunological measures can be divided into two functional categories: circulatory measures and elicited measures. Both categories are informative, but will yield different types of information. In general, circulatory measures can provide information on the current physiological and immunological status of the individual and the potential of the immune system to react to dangerous stimuli. Elicited measures assess the actual immune response to a challenge. There is now an extensive literature demonstrating that these measures can be influenced by psychological stress and in individuals experiencing different emotional states. The purpose of this chapter is to provide an introduction to these immunological measures and how the assays are performed. Studies utilizing immunological measures will also be reviewed to illustrate the usefulness of these assays for studying mind–body interactions. The chapter will be concluded by discussing how animal models can help provide details of how psychosocial factors can influence the immune system.

2 Circulatory Measures

2.1 Natural Killer Cells

Natural killer (NK) cells are an immune cell subset that get their name from their ability to kill target cells that do not express major histocompatibility complex (MHC) class I (Biassoni, 2008). Most healthy cells in the periphery of the body express MHCI and when infected with a pathogenic microbe will present the microbial antigen in the context of MHCI. This MHCI-antigen complex helps antigen-specific cells recognize that this cell has been infected. A lack of any MHCI expression, however, can also be a cue that the host has been infected or is otherwise damaged. Many viruses cause cells to downregulate their expression of MHCI, and decreased MHCI expression often occurs in tumor cells. Natural killer cells recognize the missing MHCI, which in turn causes the NK cells to become activated and to kill the MHCI-lacking cells (Biassoni, 2008). Thus, NK cells can be very important in the initial stages of viral infection, by eradicating virally infected cells, and for certain types of cancers, by eradicating tumor cells.

The numbers of NK cells circulating in the blood, as well as the activity of these cells, can be easily measured using standard immunological techniques. Flow cytometry is routinely used to characterize and quantify cells circulating in the blood. This procedure involves staining the blood cells with fluorescently labeled antibodies that will bind to the cell of interest. The antibody

R. Glaser (✉)
Institute for Behavioral Medicine Research, The Ohio State University, 120 IBMR Building, 460 Medical Center Drive, Columbus, OH 43210, USA
e-mail: glaser.1@osu.edu; ronald.glaser@osumc.edu

A. Steptoe (ed.), *Handbook of Behavioral Medicine*, DOI 10.1007/978-0-387-09488-5_44,
© Springer Science+Business Media, LLC 2010

NK1.1 is widely used to stain for the presence of NK cells. Thus, one can count how many cells are in the blood, then use flow cytometery to determine the percentage of those cells that are NK cells to ultimately calculate the number of NK cells per milliliter of blood.

In addition to counting NK cells, NK cells can be isolated from peripheral blood and cultured to assess their ability to kill target cells. While there are many different mechanisms to enrich leukocyte populations from the blood, density gradient centrifugation is often used to enrich for different types of leukocytes, including NK cells. After enriching for the NK cells, the ability of the NK cells to kill target cells can be tested by co-culturing the NK cells with target cells such as MOLT-4 (human) or YAC-1 (rodent) cells. These cells lack expression of MHCI and thus are susceptible to NK-cell mediated lysis. The lysis of these target cells can be assessed using a standard chromium-51 (^{51}Cr) release cytotoxicity assay. In this type of assay, the target cells are radiolabeled with ^{51}Cr. Then, NK cells are added to the target cells at different effector-to-target-cell ratios (typically ranging from 100:1 to 10:1). After co-culture, the supernatants are collected and the amount of radioactivity in the supernatants is measured. Higher levels of radioactivity reflect an increased ability of the NK cells to lyse the target cells, causing the ^{51}Cr within those cells to be spilled into the medium.

2.1.1 Clinical Studies Involving Natural Killer Cells

Circulating NK cell numbers, as well as NK cell activity, are significantly changed by psychological stressors. Natural killer cell numbers, as assessed via flow cytometry, were shown to be significantly decreased in blood samples taken from medical students during their final examinations, in comparison to levels found in the blood 6 weeks prior to their examinations (i.e., during a low stress period) (Glaser et al, 1986). In addition, the percentage of target cells (i.e., cells lacking MHCI expression) that the NK cells were able to lyse was significantly

reduced during the examination period (Glaser et al, 1986; Kiecolt-Glaser et al, 1984a, 1986). This effect, however, was not consistently found in all the students. Students who were found to have higher scores on the stressful life events questionnaire (Glaser et al, 1986; Kiecolt-Glaser et al, 1986) or who were found to have higher levels of loneliness using the UCLA loneliness questionnaire also had the lowest levels of NK cell activity (Kiecolt-Glaser et al, 1984a). This relationship has been found in other subject populations; psychiatric patients with high scores on the UCLA loneliness questionnaire also had lower levels of NK cell activity as assessed by their ability to lyse target cells (Kiecolt-Glaser et al, 1984b). The decrease in NK cell activity was associated with a concomitant decrease in the ability of peripheral mononuclear cells to produce interferon-γ (IFN-γ) (Kiecolt-Glaser et al, 1984b). This finding was important since IFN-γ is a major regulator of NK cell activity. Moreover, in more prolonged stressors, such as caring for a spouse with Alzheimer's disease, NK cell activity, as induced by IFN-γ or IL-2, was significantly reduced (Esterling et al, 1994, 1996). These studies, as well as others, demonstrate that NK cell number and activity can be affected by psychosocial variables.

2.2 T Cells

T cells play an important role in combating infectious diseases and are a diverse group of cells that can be split into three general types based on their function. The primary function of helper T cells (also known as CD4+ T cells) is to produce cytokines. These cytokines help to drive and regulate the development of the immune response. Cytotoxic T cells (also known as CD8+ T cells) are effective at recognizing and destroying microbe-infected cells. The final category of T cells is the regulatory T cell (also called suppressor T cells) which generally function to suppress leukocyte activity and to further control the immune response (Schepers et al, 2005). Important characteristics of these T cells can be determined in the circulation by assessing their numbers and effector functions.

Perhaps the most reliable change in the T cells as a consequence of the stress response is a decrease in the percentage of CD4+ T helper cells in the blood and a corresponding decrease in the ratio of CD4/CD8 T cells (Biselli et al, 1993; Breznitz et al, 1998; Caggiula et al, 1995; Kiecolt-Glaser et al, 1986; Maes et al, 1999; Scanlan et al, 1998). This can be readily measured using flow cytometry and staining peripheral blood leukocytes with antibodies to CD3 (found on all T cell types), CD4 (found on helper T cells), CD8 (found on cytotoxic T cells), and CD25 (found on regulatory/suppressor T cells) (Schepers et al, 2005). By using flow cytometry, it is possible to determine the percentage of leukocytes in the blood that stain positively with each of these markers. Thus, one can determine the number of each type of T cell circulating in the blood at the time of the blood draw.

In addition to counting T cells, many assays have been developed to assess the function of these cells. In order to successfully combat an invading pathogen, T cells must rapidly proliferate early during the infectious process. This is because only a small percentage of circulating T lymphocytes has the necessary antigen specificity to respond to a given pathogen. Thus, the few antigen-specific T cells that do recognize a microbial infection must rapidly proliferate to produce additional effector cells that can respond to the infectious organism.

The ability of T cells to proliferate can be assessed in culture by stimulating the cells with mitogen lectins, such as concanavalin A (ConA) and phytohemagglutinin (PHA). These mitogens nonspecifically stimulate T lymphocyte proliferation by binding to cell surface glycoconjugates, which in turn triggers the cells to produce ribonucleic acid (RNA), proteins, and deoxyribonucleic acid (DNA), ultimately forming larger lymphoblasts that may then divide. The ability of the cells to divide is typically measured by the uptake and incorporation of radioactive thymidine (i.e., tritiated thymidine). The amount of radioactivity measured from the cells is directly related to cell division since the radiolabeled

thymidine is incorporated into newly synthesized DNA. Thus, this assay is considered a semi-quantitative assay and is often referred to as a thymidine incorporation assay.

The lectin mitogens are not the only way to induce T cell proliferation, and it is now recognized that stimulating T cells with antibodies to T cell receptors will result in cell activation. The most widely used antibodies are directed against the T cell marker CD3, which initiates the activation of T cells, and antibodies to CD28, which will induce proliferation. Again, this T cell proliferation is a nonspecific, polyclonal response that can be assessed with tritiated thymidine incorporation. Assessing monoclonal, or antigen specific, T cell proliferation is more involved because the number of antigen-specific T lymphocytes is very small (estimated to be about 1 in 10^5–10^6 cells). However, as discussed in the next section, antigen-specific T cell responses can be assessed in infected or vaccinated individuals.

The ability of T cells to produce cytokines is an important effector function of CD4+ T lymphocytes. In general, the types of cytokines that CD4+ T lymphocytes produce can be split into two functional categories: T helper type I (i.e., Th1) and T helper type 2 (i.e., Th2) cytokines (see also Chapter 45). The Th1 cytokines primarily function to facilitate cell-mediated, which consists of the differentiation of effector T cells from naïve T cells, which occurs in the peripheral lymph nodes, the migration of effector T cells (and other leukocytes) from the periphery to the site of infection, and the enhancement of microbial killing by either macrophages or antigen-specific CD8+ T cells. Th1 cytokines enhance each of these functions. For example, the Th1 cytokine IL-2 facilitates the differentiation and expansion of effector T cells within the lymph nodes, and TNF-α and IL-1 are important for allowing the migration of effector cells to the site of infection. Other Th1 cytokines, namely IL-12 and IFN-γ, are important for enhancing the phagocytic and microbicidal activity of macrophages (see Romagnani, 1995, 2000 for review). In contrast to Th1 cytokines, the Th2 cytokines primarily facilitate the humoral, i.e., antibody-centered immune response. For example, the Th2 cytokines, IL-4 and IL-13, promote the production of IgE, which plays an important role in neutralizing extracellular pathogens, such as parasites. Likewise, the Th2 cytokine IL-5 promotes the production of IgA, which can help to neutralize microbes at mucosal surfaces prior to their invasion of the body (Romagnani, 2000, 1995). The cytokine, IL-6 is important in the inflammatory response (making some classify it as a Th1 cytokine), but it also affects B cell production of antibodies (making others consider it a Th2 cytokine) (Diehl and Rincon, 2002; Romagnani, 2000). However, it is generally its stimulatory effect on the acute phase reaction, which can lead to systemic inflammation, and its ability to prolong inflammation by continuing to recruit monocytes/macrophages to sites of infection, that make it a useful marker of inflammation in human stress studies (Black, 2003; Gabay, 2006; Kaplanski et al, 2003).

Cytokine levels in circulation, or in culture supernatants from stimulated cells, are easily measured using commercially available assay kits. The most commonly used assay is an enzyme-linked immunosorbent assay (ELISA), which can detect a single cytokine at a time using antibodies directed toward the cytokine of interest. The resultant change in optical density of a colorimetric reaction that occurs when the antibodies are bound to the cytokine can be read on an ELISA plate reader. When compared to a standard curve, the optical density of the reaction can be calculated to give the concentration of the cytokine. Because circulating levels of cytokines are very low in the absence of overt infection, high sensitivity ELISAs are typically needed to measure circulatory cytokines in serum.

Newer technologies revolve around the basic principles of the ELISA, but have been developed to measure multiple cytokines in a single sample. These multiplex assays can save considerable time and can provide new insights into cytokine interactions during different emotional states. The primary limitation of this methodology is the large start up costs. However, after the initial investment, cytokine analyses can be run more efficiently using multiplex technology in comparison to running multiple traditional ELISAs.

2.2.1 Clinical Studies Involving T Lymphocytes

A variety of different stressors have been associated with significant changes in the number of T lymphocytes circulating in the blood. This was first evident in medical students during final examination week (Kiecolt-Glaser et al, 1986). As with the NK cells, the number of T lymphocytes was significantly decreased during final examinations as compared to numbers found 6 weeks prior to the exams. In this case, it was not a decrease in all subsets of T cells, but rather a specific decrease in helper and suppressor T lymphocytes (Kiecolt-Glaser et al, 1986). In addition, the stress of the examinations was sufficient to decrease the ratio of helper T lymphocytes to suppressor T lymphocytes (Kiecolt-Glaser et al, 1986). This finding was not unique to examinations and has also been described in men with low marital satisfaction (Kiecolt-Glaser et al, 1988).

In addition to changing the number of T lymphocytes found in the circulation, different types of stressors can also change the functioning of these cells. This is most evident in the ability of these lymphocytes to proliferate when stimulated with either PHA or ConA. For example, psychiatric patients scoring high on the UCLA loneliness scale had poorer T lymphocyte proliferative responses to PHA or ConA when compared with patients scoring lower on the loneliness scale (Kiecolt-Glaser et al, 1984b). Lower T cell proliferative responses were also found in patients diagnosed with, and having had surgery for, breast cancer (Andersen et al, 1998, 2004), in medical students taking final examinations (Glaser et al, 1985), in caregivers of Alzheimer's patients (Kiecolt-Glaser et al, 1991), and in women during marital discord (Kiecolt-Glaser et al, 1993). In general, a reduction in T cell proliferative responses to nonspecific mitogens is one of the most consistent ways in which immune functioning can be altered by psychosocial factors.

The ability of T lymphocytes to produce cytokines is also largely affected by psychosocial factors. In general, stressor exposure reduces the production of Th1 type cytokines. For example, peripheral blood leukocytes from medical students taking their final examinations produced significantly lower levels of IFN-γ, when the T cells were stimulated with Con A or with PHA (Glaser et al, 1986). In a similar study, the stress of the examination reduced the expression of IL-2 receptors on peripheral blood leukocytes (Glaser et al, 1990), and peripheral blood leukocytes from Alzheimer's caregivers produced less IL-2 when stimulated with influenza A viral proteins (Kiecolt-Glaser et al, 1996).

2.3 Reactivation of Latent Herpes Viruses

The adaptive immune response is an important factor in the control of herpes viruses. These viruses, which include herpes simplex virus type 1 and type 2 (HSV-1 and HSV-2), varicella zoster virus (VZV), cytomegalovirus (CMV), and Epstein–Barr virus (EBV) are the most ubiquitous viruses with very high prevalence rates in healthy adults. For example, greater than 90% of adults are seropositive for HSV-1 and EBV and therefore latently infected with the virus (Henle and Henle 1982; Pebody et al, 2004; Peter and Ray 1998; Xu et al, 2002). The initial encounter with HSV-1 (i.e., the causative agent of cold sores) typically occurs in childhood with few clinical symptoms, whereas infection with EBV, which commonly occurs in young adults, leads to mononucleosis in approximately 40% of those infected (Henle and Henle 1982). However, after the primary infection has been resolved, the herpes viruses are able to establish lifelong latent infections in host tissue. The site of latency is virus specific, and HSV-1, HSV-2, and VZV latently infect host sensory neurons; EBV latently infects host B lymphocytes. Under

certain conditions, such as suppression of the cellular immune response, the virus can be reactivated from the latent state. As the virus reactivates, the humoral immune system responds by producing higher levels of virus-specific antibodies (Glaser and Gottleib-Stematsky 1982). Thus, an increase in antibodies that are specific for latent viruses generally reflects a suppressed cellular immune response.

The cellular immune response to latent viruses can also be measured more directly. In this case, assays are aimed at assessing the ability of virus-specific memory cells to proliferate when exposed to the viral antigens. This assay involves separating mononuclear cells from whole blood using density gradient centrifugation, and then culturing the mononuclear cells with purified viral antigens for 5 days. During the last 8 h of incubation, tritiated thymidine is added to the cultures so that cell proliferation can be assessed by the incorporation of thymidine into proliferating cells.

2.3.1 Clinical Studies Involving the Reactivation of Latent Viruses

It was known anecdotally for many years that stressful periods were associated with increased recurrences of latent viral infections, such as HSV-1, HSV-2, as well as VZV (Cohen et al, 1999; Schmader et al, 1990). The mechanisms leading to reactivation during stressful situations were unknown, but it was known that for latent herpes virus infections, cellular immune competence was a critical factor in controlling the primary herpes virus infections and maintaining latency (Glaser and Gottleib-Stematsky 1982). Moreover, it was recognized that when cellular immunity was decreased, the humoral antibody response to the latent virus was significantly increased (Glaser and Gottleib-Stematsky 1982). Thus, the finding that many different types of stressors, such as academic stress in medical students and the stress of caring for a family member with Alzheimer's disease, resulted in significant elevations in antibody levels to EBV suggested that cellular immunity to the latent virus was significantly reduced. To test this hypothesis, the cellular immune response to EBV was measured in healthy medical students.

Peripheral blood leukocytes from medical students were taken during final examinations, and 1 month prior to exams, and assessed for their ability to proliferate when stimulated with purified proteins prepared from EBV (Glaser et al, 1993). When compared to the low stress time point, the examination period was associated with a significant decrease in EBV antigen-induced leukocyte proliferation. At the same time, medical students had higher antibody titers to the EBV (Glaser et al, 1993). Together these data demonstrated that this stressor could cause a significant reduction in cell-mediated immunity, thus allowing latent viruses, like EBV, to reactivate and stimulate the humoral immune response.

3 Elicited Functional Measures

3.1 Wound Healing

Wound repair progresses through a series of sequential stages, beginning with the inflammatory phase that involves vasoconstriction, blood coagulation, and the activation of platelets (Hubner et al, 1996; Lowry, 1993; Van de Kerkhof et al, 1994). This leads to the migration of macrophages and neutrophils into the wound during the proliferative phase. These cells protect against potential pathogens and also help to recruit additional leukocytes that are important for tissue regeneration and capillary growth. The final stage involves tissue remodeling of the collagen matrix and can last for several weeks. Successful completion of each stage is highly dependent upon successful completion of the previous stage, with the immune system playing an integral role in each of the stages (Lowry 1993; Van de Kerkhof et al, 1994). Psychosocial factors have the capacity to influence wound healing at any of these stages, but have been found to have the largest effects on wound healing by causing a dysregulation of cytokine production during the initial inflammatory phase.

Proinflammatory cytokines, like IL-1α/β, IL-8, and TNF-α, are important mediators in the early inflammatory phase of wound healing (Lowry, 1993). These cytokines help to recruit and activate phagocytes, such as macrophages and neutrophils, that can then defend against the invasion of microbes through the wound surface. These cytokines have additional affects that are important to wound healing, such as the production of metalloproteinases, that are important in the destruction and remodeling of the wound, and the recruitment of additional cells, like fibroblasts that produce collagen (Lowry, 1993). The regulation of this early inflammatory response is essential for optimal healing to occur, and if dysregulated, the early inflammatory stage can significantly change healing kinetics and success.

Wound healing and stress have been studied experimentally by using three general types of wound models: cutaneous biopsies, blister wounds, and mucosal wounds. Cutaneous biopsies are routinely used in dermatologic research (Nemeth et al, 1991) and consist of creating a 3.5 mm full-thickness wound on the forearm. In healthy adults, the rate at which this type of wound heals is quite consistent and can be assessed by simply measuring the diameter of the wound and determining the duration until complete closure (Grove, 1982). Complete closure can be determined by the absence of foaming when hydrogen peroxide is added to the wound. This type of wound, however, does not allow for an analysis of immunological factors that may be important for healing. Thus, additional wound models have been developed that allow an assessment of immune functioning.

Immune activity during wound healing can be assessed in blister wound fluids (Kuhns et al, 1992). Blister wounds are created by placing a plastic template on the forearm. Vacuum pressure (i.e., 350 mmHg) is then applied to the blister apparatus for approximately 1.5 h until blisters are formed. Through this methodology, the gentle suction creates fluid filled blisters that are 8 mm in diameter. The advantage of the blister wound is the ability to sample the wound fluid to measure the kinetics of the production of factors such as proinflammatory cytokines that are important for the healing wound. To do this, the blister fluid is drained immediately after creating the wound and the top layer of skin (i.e., the dermis) is removed from the blister. A new plastic template containing wells that are designed to cover each blister wound is placed over the wounds, and culture media containing autologous serum is added to the wells. The wells are then sealed with sterile tape so that cytokine production and cellular infiltrates can be measured in the sterile fluid over time (Kuhns et al, 1992).

Cutaneous wounds have different healing kinetics and properties in comparison to wounds at mucosal surfaces. When compared to cutaneous tissue, mucosal tissues heal much faster and with fewer cellular infiltrates and less inflammation (Szpaderska et al, 2003). Experimental wounds on most mucosal surfaces (e.g., the gastrointestinal, urogenital, and respiratory tracts) are not feasible, but experimental wounds have been created in the oral cavity to study mucosal wound healing. Oral wounds can be studied in a similar manner to cutaneous punch biopsy wounds, with a 3.5 mm tissue punch being used to create a wound on the hard palate in the area of the 2nd molar (Marucha et al, 1998). Most studies create duplicate wounds so that healing kinetics can be studied in one of the wounds, with tissue from the second wound being harvested during the course of healing to quantitate gene expression for inflammatory cytokines using semi-quantitative real-time PCR. The tissue can also be harvested to quantify cellular infiltration. The creation of either cutaneous or oral wounds is an intriguing way to test the impact of psychosocial factors on the immune system in a manner that is clearly biologically meaningful.

3.1.1 Clinical Studies of Wound Healing

Several human studies have now found an association between stressful periods and delayed wound healing. For example, in primary caregivers of a spouse with Alzheimer's disease (Kiecolt-Glaser et al, 1995), the complete healing of a 3.5 mm punch biopsy wound was delayed by 9 days when compared with controls. While the complete set of factors responsible for this delay are not completely understood, studies using blister wounds have demonstrated that the early inflammatory phase of wound healing can be significantly changed during psychological stress. For example, women with higher levels of perceived stress had lower levels of IL-1α and IL-8 in blister fluid (Glaser et al, 1999). Similar findings were obtained from couples with hostile marital interactions (Kiecolt-Glaser et al, 1995). Because these cytokines are important for recruiting additional leukocytes to the wound site and for helping to activate these leukocytes, the data indicate that delayed wound healing can occur in part through disruptions to the initial inflammatory phase of healing.

Delayed wound healing is not limited to cutaneous surfaces; wounds in the oral mucosa also heal more slowly in stressed individuals. Oral wounds created on the hard palate of dental students immediately before exam week healed 40% slower than wounds in the same individuals during vacation (Marucha et al, 1998). As with the cutaneous wounds, mucosal wounds from stressed individuals expressed significantly lower gene expression for the proinflammatory cytokine IL-1β, suggesting that the stressor disrupted the early inflammatory phase of mucosal wound healing (Marucha et al, 1998). As research progresses, it will be interesting to determine whether the stress response can influence other stages of wound healing or whether stressor effects are limited to the inflammatory stage.

3.2 Experimental Infection and Vaccination

While not feasible for many researchers, experimental infection with live, replicating pathogens can provide important information regarding the impact of emotions on the functioning of the immune system. Most of the studies assessing immune responses to viral infection in healthy volunteers have been conducted by Dr. Sheldon Cohen's group at Carnegie Mellon University. This group has challenged subjects with different types of respiratory viruses, including rhinovirus, respiratory synctial virus, corona virus, and influenza A virus (Cohen, 2005). To determine whether the viruses caused the subjects to become ill, cold symptoms, such as the production of nasal mucus, can be measured. Viral load in the nasal passages can be determined via standard virological methodology. In addition, immune measures, such as cytokine production, can be measured in circulation and in mucosal secretions (Cohen, 2005). While much can be learned from this type of study, this approach is not feasible to do for many investigators in the field of behavioral medicine, and determining links with subtle psychosocial factors are difficult due to the limited number of subjects that can be tested. An appropriate alternative to using live replicating viruses to study the impact of psychosocial factors on anti-viral immune responses is to study the immune response to viral vaccines.

Vaccines effectively mimic part of the immune response to viral infection. Designing vaccine-based studies of stress can be difficult, however, because in developed countries, most vaccines are given during childhood. Thus, most participants in laboratory studies already have preexisting immunity to existing vaccines, which makes experimental design and data interpretation difficult. Some vaccines, however, have only recently been recommended for children, such as the hepatitis B vaccine, while other vaccines vary from year to year based on the analysis of the latest antigenic characteristics of the virus determined by the Centers for Disease Control, e.g., influenza virus vaccine. This is important because many healthy adults have not been vaccinated against hepatitis B and thus are seronegative, and the antigen specificity of the previous year's influenza virus vaccine may be sufficiently different from the current year's vaccine to reliably detect immune responses to

the vaccine without influence from previous vaccinations.

The hepatitis B vaccine involves a three injection series, i.e., a booster injection 1 month after the initial injection followed by a third injection 5 months later. This paradigm allows for an analysis of the primary immune response to the vaccination (i.e., after the initial vaccination) and memory/recall responses to the vaccination (i.e., after the second and third injections). The vaccine against the influenza virus involves a single injection to initiate the immune response. For most vaccination studies, virus-specific antibody levels are measured since these antibodies confer resistance to subsequent infections. However, it should be noted that viral vaccines also need to generate a cell-mediated T cell response.

The cell-mediated (i.e., T cell) response to vaccines can be measured similarly to circulatory T cell function. The difference, however, is that the T cells assessed in vaccination-based studies are specific for the vaccine antigens because antigens from the vaccine can be purified and used to stimulate T cells from vaccinated individuals. For example, the hepatitis B surface antigen (HBsAg) is one of the components of the hepatitis B recombinant vaccine that will result in antibody formation and the generation of antigen-specific T cells. Thus, the HBsAg can be purified and used to stimulate HBsAg-specific T cells from the vaccinated individual to determine the ability of these T cells to recognize and respond to that component of the hepatitis B vaccine. Accordingly, the ability of the T cells to proliferate in response to the HBsAg can be measured via a tritiated thymidine incorporation assay and T cell cytokine production can be assessed with ELISA (Glaser et al, 1992). These measures can provide some idea of the responsiveness of a person's immune response to the original vaccine.

3.2.1 Clinical Studies Involving Experimental Infection and Vaccination

As already discussed, several studies have now been conducted in which participants have been experimentally infected with respiratory viruses (reviewed in Cohen, 2005). Overall, the studies show that symptom severity and the duration of illness tend to be strongest in individuals with higher levels of perceived stress. For example, persons with higher levels of perceived stress produced more nasal mucus after the experimental infection and had higher levels of IL-6 in the nasal secretions, which would reflect a more severe infection (Cohen, 2005). Interestingly, this effect was dependent upon social modifiers. Individuals that were more socially integrated were less likely to develop symptoms from the experimental viral challenge than were individuals that were less socially integrated (Cohen, 2005).

Immune responsiveness to microbial challenge can also be studied by administering vaccines to participants, and many studies have shown that cell-mediated and humoral immunity to vaccines can be significantly modified by psychosocial factors. This was first realized in medical students vaccinated with the recombinant hepatitis B vaccine series (Glaser et al, 1992). Approximately 21% of the students developed a protective antibody response to the vaccine after the initial exposure, with the remaining students producing a protective antibody response after the second exposure. Importantly, the 21% of the students that seroconverted 1 month after the primary exposure had lower Profile of Mood State (POMS) anxiety scores. Similarly, students with lower levels of anxiety also had stronger T lymphocyte proliferative responses to purified hepatitis B antigens (Glaser et al, 1992). This study suggested that mood could significantly change responsiveness to vaccination, with subsequent studies focusing more closely on populations undergoing stressful situations.

Caregivers of spouses with Alzheimer's disease were vaccinated against the influenza A virus using a trivalent vaccine composed of three different strains of influenza virus (Kiecolt-Glaser et al, 1996). In general, total and neutralizing antibody responses to influenza A virus were significantly lower in the caregivers when compared with appropriately matched control subjects. Moreover, the production of the Th1 cytokine IL-2 was significantly reduced when peripheral blood leukocytes from caregivers were stimulated with the influenza virus proteins (Kiecolt-Glaser et al, 1996). Similar results were evident when caregivers were given a pneumococcus bacterial vaccine. Caregivers produced significantly lower antibody levels to the pneumococcal vaccine (Glaser et al, 2000). These studies provide evidence from well-controlled studies that both the cellular and the humoral immune response to microbial challenge can be significantly affected during a stress response.

4 Importance of Animal Models

Studies involving human participants are the mainstay of behavioral medicine research. However, the use of animal models can greatly enhance understanding of the endocrine, behavioral, cellular, and molecular mechanisms through which psychosocial factors can affect the immune response. Many of the human studies performed by our group have been modeled in rodents to provide additional information on the mechanisms through which the stress-induced changes occur.

Wound healing has been studied in mice by creating the same 3.5 mm full-thickness skin wound that was used in the study with Alzheimer's caregivers. Exposing the wounded mice to a prolonged restraint stressor caused these cutaneous wounds to heal approximately 27% slower in comparison to wounds from the non-stressed control mice (Padgett et al, 1998). This delayed healing was associated with a significant decrease in leukocyte infiltration into wound sites, and lower cytokine levels in the wound site of the stressed animals (Padgett et al, 1998). This study confirmed the findings in humans indicating that the inflammatory stage of wound healing is dysregulated by psychological stress. These animal studies, however, extended this observation by demonstrating that blocking the stress-induced glucocorticoid response, using the glucocorticoid receptor antagonist RU4055, abolished the stress-induced delay in wound healing (Padgett et al, 1998). Glucocorticoids are known to decrease NF-κB activation. Thus, it is likely that the stressor-induced glucocorticoid response suppressed NF-κB activation, resulting in decreased inflammatory gene expression and delayed wound healing. Consistent with this premise, some stressors used in rodent studies, such as social disruption, do not affect wound healing in mice (Sheridan et al, 2004). Importantly, this stressor causes cytokine producing cells to become resistant to glucocorticoids (Bailey et al, 2004; Engler et al, 2005; Stark et al, 2001). Thus, glucocorticoids are unable to disrupt the inflammatory stage of wound healing in this paradigm. These data using animal models suggest that glucocorticoids play an important role in the stress-induced dysregulation of the inflammatory stage of wound healing.

In addition to providing important insights into the relationship between psychosocial stress and delayed wound healing, animal models have proven to be useful in determining how psychosocial factors influence the immune response to pathogens and to vaccines. As with human studies, studies in mice have shown that exposure to prolonged stressors significantly reduces immune reactivity to microbial pathogens. For example, prolonged restraint stress significantly reduces antibody production, proinflammatory cytokine responses, and NK cell activity during influenza viral infection (Sheridan et al, 1998; Tseng et al, 2005). In addition, the generation of CD8+ T lymphocytes was significantly reduced in restrained mice infected with HSV-1 (Bonneau et al, 1991). Because proinflammatory cytokines, NK cell cytotoxicity, and CD8+ lymphocytes are essential for defense against viral infections, the restraint stressor also increased viral titers and virus-induced mortality (Bonneau et al, 1991; Sheridan et al, 1998).

The neuroendocrine mechanisms through which this occurred were studied using pharmacological inhibitors of the stress response. In influenza A-infected mice, it was evident that blocking glucocorticoid receptors was ineffective at restoring all of the stress-induced changes of the immune system (Hermann et al, 1994).

In fact, blocking glucocorticoid receptors only reversed the stressor-induced decrease in leukocyte trafficking into draining lymph nodes and the lungs to combat the infection. Blocking glucocorticoid receptors did not, however, restore stressor-induced reductions in cell functioning. The stressor-induced reduction in CD8+ T lymphocyte activation was found to be due to activation of β-adrenergic receptors; blocking these receptors restored the activation of CD8+ T lymphocytes (Hermann et al, 1994). In contrast, NK cell cytotoxicity was not restored upon blockade of β-adrenergic receptors, but was restored when μ-opioid receptors were blocked (Tseng et al, 2005). These studies in rodents, as well as many other laboratory animal studies, demonstrate the many, and complex, ways through which psychological stressors affect the immune response.

5 Conclusion

The stress response has the ability to impact every cell in the body and thus has the potential to influence every function of the body. While many of these influences have been well described, the ramifications of such interactions on the functioning of the immune system are still only beginning to be realized. In a general sense, the impact of psychosocial factors on immune-mediated diseases or conditions is clear; the stress response will suppress our ability to fight a cold, generate an immune response to a vaccine, or heal a wound. But, the detailed mechanisms through which this occurs have not yet been fully delineated. Questions remain, such as why some stressors tend to suppress the immune response, whereas other stressors seem to leave the immune response intact. Other questions involve the mechanisms through which these psychosocial factors influence the immune response. Are these effects all mediated by traditional stress hormones or are other novel factors at play? Current evidence makes it clear that other immunomodulatory factors, like growth factors and cytokines themselves, can be induced during a stress response, but the extent of their impacts on the immune system are not clear. Well-designed clinical studies, and appropriate studies in animal models, as well as the methods outlined in this chapter, can provide a foundation on which to begin answering these existing questions.

Acknowledgments Work on this chapter was supported in part by NCI CA126857, NCI AG029562, NCI CA131029, and NIAID AI069097.

References

Andersen, B. L., Farrar, W. B., Golden-Kreutz, D., Kutz, L. A., MacCallum, R. et al (1998). Stress and immune responses after surgical treatment for regional breast cancer. *J Natl Cancer Inst, 90*, 30–36.

Andersen, B. L., Farrar, W. B., Golden-Kreutz, D. M., Glaser, R., Emery, C. F. et al (2004). Psychological, behavioral, and immune changes after a psychological intervention: a clinical trial. *J Clin Oncol, 22*, 3570–3580.

Bailey, M. T., Avitsur, R., Engler, H., Padgett, D. A., and Sheridan, J. F. (2004). Physical defeat reduces the sensitivity of murine splenocytes to the suppressive effects of corticosterone. *Brain Behav Immun, 18*, 416–424.

Biassoni, R. (2008). Natural killer cell receptors. *Adv Exp Med Biol, 640*, 35–52.

Biselli, R., Farrace, S., D'Amelio, R., and Fattorossi, A. (1993). Influence of stress on lymphocyte subset distribution--a flow cytometric study in young student pilots. *Aviat Space Environ Med, 64*, 116–120.

Black, P. H. (2003). The inflammatory response is an integral part of the stress response: implications for atherosclerosis, insulin resistance, type II diabetes and metabolic syndrome X. *Brain Behav Immun, 17*, 350–364.

Bonneau, R. H., Sheridan, J. F., Feng, N. G., and Glaser, R. (1991). Stress-induced suppression of herpes simplex virus (HSV)-specific cytotoxic T lymphocyte and natural killer cell activity and enhancement of acute pathogenesis following local HSV infection. *Brain Behav Immun, 5*, 170–192.

Breznitz, S., Ben-Zur, H., Berzon, Y., Weiss, D. W. et al (1998). Experimental induction and termination of acute psychological stress in human volunteers. effects on immunological, neuroendocrine, cardiovascular, and psychological parameters. *Brain Behav Immun, 12*, 34–52.

Caggiula, A. R., McAllister, C. G., Matthews, K. A., Berga, S. L., Owens, J. F. et al (1995). Psychological stress and immunological responsiveness in normally cycling, follicular-stage women. *J Neuroimmunol, 59*, 103–111.

Cohen, F., Kemeny, M. E., Kearney, K. A., Zegans, L. S., Neuhaus, J. M. et al (1999). Persistent stress as a predictor of genital herpes recurrence. *Arch Intern Med, 159*, 2430–2436.

Cohen, S. (2005). Keynote Presentation at the Eight International Congress of Behavioral Medicine: the Pittsburgh common cold studies: psychosocial predictors of susceptibility to respiratory infectious illness. *Int J Behav Med, 12*, 123–131.

Diehl, S., and Rincon, M. (2002). The two faces of IL-6 on Th1/Th2 differentiation. *Mol Immunol, 39*, 531–536.

Engler, H., Engler, A., Bailey, M. T., and Sheridan, J. F. (2005). Tissue-specific alterations in the glucocorticoid sensitivity of immune cells following repeated social defeat in mice. *J Neuroimmunol, 163*, 110–119.

Esterling, B. A., Kiecolt-Glaser, J. K., Bodnar, J. C., and Glaser, R. (1994). Chronic stress, social support, and persistent alterations in the natural killer cell response to cytokines in older adults. *Health Psychol, 13*, 291–298.

Esterling, B. A., Kiecolt-Glaser, J. K., and Glaser, R. (1996). Psychosocial modulation of cytokine-induced natural killer cell activity in older adults. *Psychosom Med, 58*, 264–272.

Gabay, C. (2006). Interleukin-6 and chronic inflammation. *Arthritis Res Ther, 8*(Suppl 2), S3.

Glaser, R., and Gottlieb-Stematsky, T. (1982). *Human herpesvirus Infections: Clinical Aspects*. New York: Marcel Dekker.

Glaser, R., Kennedy, S., Lafuse, W. P., Bonneau, R. H., Speicher, C. et al (1990). Psychological stress-induced modulation of interleukin 2 receptor gene expression and interleukin 2 production in peripheral blood leukocytes. *Arch Gen Psychiatry, 47*, 707–712.

Glaser, R., Kiecolt-Glaser, J. K., Bonneau, R. H., Malarkey, W., Kennedy, S. et al (1992). Stress-induced modulation of the immune response to recombinant hepatitis B vaccine. *Psychosom Med, 54*, 22–29.

Glaser, R., Kiecolt-Glaser, J. K., Marucha, P. T., MacCallum, R. C., Laskowski, B. F. et al (1999). Stress-related changes in proinflammatory cytokine production in wounds. *Arch Gen Psychiatry, 56*, 450–456.

Glaser, R., Kiecolt-Glaser, J. K., Stout, J. C., Tarr, K. L., Speicher, C. E. et al (1985). Stress-related impairments in cellular immunity. *Psychiatry Res, 16*, 233–239.

Glaser, R., Pearson, G. R., Bonneau, R. H., Esterling, B. A., Atkinson, C. et al (1993). Stress and the memory T-cell response to the Epstein-Barr virus in healthy medical students. *Health Psychol, 12*, 435–442.

Glaser, R., Rice, J., Speicher, C. E., Stout, J. C., and Kiecolt-Glaser, J. K. (1986). Stress depresses interferon production by leukocytes concomitant with a decrease in natural killer cell activity. *Behav Neurosci, 100,* 675–678.

Glaser, R., Sheridan, J., Malarkey, W. B., MacCallum, R. C., and Kiecolt-Glaser, J. K. (2000). Chronic stress modulates the immune response to a pneumococcal pneumonia vaccine. *Psychosom Med, 62,* 804–807.

Grove, G. L. (1982). Age-related differences in healing of superficial skin wounds in humans. *Arch Dermatol Res, 272,* 381–385.

Henle, W., and Henle, G. (1982). Epstein-Barr virus and infectious mononucleosis. In R. Glaser & T. Gottlieb-Stematsky (Eds.), *Human Herpesvirus Infections: Clinical Aspects* (pp. 151–162). New York: Marcel Dekker.

Hermann, G., Beck, F. M., Tovar, C. A., Malarkey, W. B., Allen, C. et al (1994). Stress-induced changes attributable to the sympathetic nervous system during experimental influenza viral infection in DBA/2 inbred mouse strain. *J Neuroimmunol, 53,* 173–180.

Hubner, G., Brauchle, M., Smola, H., Madlener, M., Fassler, R. et al (1996). Differential regulation of pro-inflammatory cytokines during wound healing in normal and glucocorticoid-treated mice. *Cytokine, 8,* 548–556.

Kaplanski, G., Marin, V., Montero-Julian, F., Mantovani, A., and Farnarier, C. (2003). IL-6: a regulator of the transition from neutrophil to monocyte recruitment during inflammation. *Trends Immunol, 24,* 25–29.

Kiecolt-Glaser, J. K., Dura, J. R., Speicher, C. E., Trask, O. J., and Glaser, R. (1991). Spousal caregivers of dementia victims: longitudinal changes in immunity and health. *Psychosom Med, 53,* 345–362.

Kiecolt-Glaser, J. K., Garner, W., Speicher, C., Penn, G. M., Holliday, J. et al (1984a). Psychosocial modifiers of immunocompetence in medical students. *Psychosom Med, 46,* 7–14.

Kiecolt-Glaser, J. K., Glaser, R., Gravenstein, S., Malarkey, W. B., and Sheridan, J. (1996). Chronic stress alters the immune response to influenza virus vaccine in older adults. *Proc Natl Acad Sci U S A, 93,* 3043–3047.

Kiecolt-Glaser, J. K., Glaser, R., Strain, E. C., Stout, J. C., Tarr, K. L. et al (1986). Modulation of cellular immunity in medical students. *J Behav Med, 9,* 5–21.

Kiecolt-Glaser, J. K., Kennedy, S., Malkoff, S., Fisher, L., Speicher, C. E. et al (1988). Marital discord and immunity in males. *Psychosom Med, 50,* 213–229.

Kiecolt-Glaser, J. K., Malarkey, W. B., Chee, M., Newton, T., Cacioppo, J. T. et al (1993). Negative behavior during marital conflict is associated with immunological down-regulation. *Psychosom Med, 55,* 395–409.

Kiecolt-Glaser, J. K., Marucha, P. T., Malarkey, W. B., Mercado, A. M., and Glaser, R. (1995). Slowing of wound healing by psychological stress. *Lancet, 346,* 1194–1196.

Kiecolt-Glaser, J. K., Ricker, D., George, J., Messick, G., Speicher, C. E. et al (1984b). Urinary cortisol levels, cellular immunocompetency, and loneliness in psychiatric inpatients. *Psychosom Med, 46,* 15–23.

Kuhns, D. B., DeCarlo, E., Hawk, D. M., and Gallin, J. I. (1992). Dynamics of the cellular and humoral components of the inflammatory response elicited in skin blisters in humans. *J Clin Invest, 89,* 1734–1740.

Lowry, S. F. (1993). Cytokine mediators of immunity and inflammation. *Arch Surg, 128,* 1235–1241.

Maes, M., Van Bockstaele, D. R., Gastel, A., Song, C., Schotte, C. et al (1999). The effects of psychological stress on leukocyte subset distribution in humans: evidence of immune activation. *Neuropsychobiology, 39,* 1–9.

Marucha, P. T., Kiecolt-Glaser, J. K., and Favagehi, M. (1998). Mucosal wound healing is impaired by examination stress. *Psychosom Med, 60,* 362–365.

Nemeth, A. J., Eaglstein, W. H., Taylor, J. R., Peerson, L. J., and Falanga, V. (1991). Faster healing and less pain in skin biopsy sites treated with an occlusive dressing. *Arch Dermatol, 127,* 1679–1683.

Padgett, D. A., Marucha, P. T., and Sheridan, J. F. (1998). Restraint stress slows cutaneous wound healing in mice. *Brain Behav Immun, 12,* 64–73.

Pebody, R. G., Andrews, N., Brown, D., Gopal, R., De, M. H. et al (2004). The seroepidemiology of herpes simplex virus type 1 and 2 in Europe. *Sex Transm Infect, 80,* 185–191.

Peter, J., and Ray, C. G. (1998). Infectious mononucleosis. *Pediatr Rev, 19,* 276–279.

Romagnani, S. (1995). Biology of human TH1 and TH2 cells. *J Clin Immunol, 15,* 121–129.

Romagnani, S. (2000). T-cell subsets (Th1 versus Th2). *Ann Allergy Asthma Immunol, 85,* 9–18.

Scanlan, J. M., Vitaliano, P. P., Ochs, H., Savage, M. V., and Borson, S. (1998). CD4 and CD8 counts are associated with interactions of gender and psychosocial stress. *Psychosom Med, 60,* 644–653.

Schepers, K., Arens, R., and Schumacher, T. N. (2005). Dissection of cytotoxic and helper T cell responses. *Cell Mol Life Sci, 62,* 2695–2710.

Schmader, K., Studenski, S., MacMillan, J., Grufferman, S., and Cohen, H. J. (1990). Are stressful life events risk factors for herpes zoster? *J Am Geriatr Soc, 38,* 1188–1194.

Sheridan, J. F., Dobbs, C., Jung, J., Chu, X., Konstantinos, A. et al (1998). Stress-induced neuroendocrine modulation of viral pathogenesis and immunity. *Ann N Y Acad Sci, 840,* 803–808.

Sheridan, J. F., Padgett, D. A., Avitsur, R., and Marucha, P. T. (2004). Experimental models of stress and wound healing. *World J Surg, 28,* 327–330.

Stark, J. L., Avitsur, R., Padgett, D. A., Campbell, K. A., Beck, F. M. et al (2001). Social stress induces glucocorticoid resistance in macrophages. *Am J Physiol Regul Integr Comp Physiol, 280,* R1799–R1805.

Szpaderska, A. M., Zuckerman, J. D., and DiPietro, L. A. (2003). Differential injury responses in oral mucosal and cutaneous wounds. *J Dent Res, 82*, 621–626.

Tseng, R. J., Padgett, D. A., Dhabhar, F. S., Engler, H., and Sheridan, J. F. (2005). Stress-induced modulation of NK activity during influenza viral infection: role of glucocorticoids and opioids. *Brain Behav Immun, 19*, 153–164.

Van de Kerkhof, P. C., Van, B. B., Spruijt, K., and Kuiper, J. P. (1994). Age-related changes in wound healing. *Clin Exp Dermatol, 19*, 369–374.

Xu, F., Schillinger, J. A., Sternberg, M. R., Johnson, R. E., Lee, F. K. et al (2002). Seroprevalence and coinfection with herpes simplex virus type 1 and type 2 in the United States, 1988–1994. *J Infect Dis, 185*, 1019–1024.

Chapter 45

Circulating Biomarkers of Inflammation, Adhesion, and Hemostasis in Behavioral Medicine

Paul J. Mills and Roland von Känel

1 Cytokines: Description and Classification

Cytokines are potent immunotransmitters that play a pivotal role in immune system response and communication with other physiological systems, both to maintain homeostasis and to respond appropriately to infection and injury (Dantzer et al, 2008). By definition, cytokines are a diverse group of potent, low molecular weight proteins and glycoproteins that mediate physiological processes within the immune system as well as the nervous and endocrine systems. Cytokines regulate and mediate immune and inflammatory responses. Major types of cytokines include the interleukins, tumor necrosis factors, and interferons. The functions of cytokines are diverse, assisting in the development and proliferation of immune cell subsets, promoting inflammatory as well as non-inflammatory processes, and alteration of neurochemical and neuroendocrine processes that affect overall physiology and behavior. Cytokines may be thought of as similar to neurotransmitters and hormones in that they are mediators of specific physiological responses; rely on receptor–ligand interactions; and have self (autocrine), local (paracrine), and distal (endocrine) effects (Elenkov, 2008).

The interleukins (IL) are a large class of cytokines that promote cell-to-cell interactions and stimulation of humoral or cell-mediated immune responses (Goshen and Yirmiya, 2009). The tumor necrosis factors (TNF) include a host of cytokines characterized by several molecules, including TNF-α and TNF-β, as well as soluble receptors TNF-RI and TNF-RII (Himmerich et al, 2006). Activation of the TNF family promotes a variety of cell functions related to inflammation as well as immune organ development and maintenance, including cell proliferation and adhesion, cell differentiation, apoptosis, and cell survival. The interferons (IFN) play an important role immunosurveillance, and antiviral and anti-tumor effects (Kobayashi et al, 2008). IFN-α and IFN-β inhibit virus replication in infected cells and IFN-γ stimulates major histocompatability complex (MHC) presentation on antigen-presenting cells, aiding in recognition and lysing of foreign cells. In addition, IFNs initiate cascades of cytokine responses which result in further immune activation (Miller et al, 2003).

Soluble cytokine receptors can function as *antagonists* (i.e., inhibiting the effects of a cytokine by binding to it and/or blocking it from attaching to a specific receptor) or *agonists* (i.e., promoting the effects of a cytokine by binding to it and forming a complex that binds to a different receptor subunit that initiates signal transduction) (Rose-John, 2003, Tracey et al, 2008). Soluble receptors of cytokines are formed by either cleavage of portions of transmembrane protein complexes – thereby becoming part of the extracellular matrix – or via translation from

P.J. Mills (✉)
Department of Psychiatry, Behavioral Medicine Program, University of California at San Diego, 9500 Gilman Drive, La Jolla, CA 92093-0804, USA
e-mail: pmills@ucsd.edu

A. Steptoe (ed.), *Handbook of Behavioral Medicine*, DOI 10.1007/978-0-387-09488-5_45,
© Springer Science+Business Media, LLC 2010

alternatively spliced mRNAs. Examples of soluble cytokine antagonists include IL-1 receptor antagonist (IL-1Ra) and TNF-receptor-1 antagonist (TNF-RI). Examples of soluble cytokine agonists include interleukin-6 receptor (IL-6-R). In certain situations, some cytokine receptors may function as agonists or antagonists, depending on the isoform.

Because of their notable variability in structure and function, there have been many attempts to classify cytokines. A classification system that has proven useful for behavioral medicine researchers is the classification of cytokines as either *pro-inflammatory* or *anti-inflammatory*. Pro-inflammatory cytokines, which include IL-1, IL-2, TNF-α, and IFN-γ, promote a variety of cell functions that stimulate and enhance inflammation through several mechanisms including promoting differentiation of cytotoxic T cells, enhancing increased vascular permeability and cellular adhesion and migration to tissues, and stimulating the release of acute-phase proteins from the liver (Schiller et al, 2006). These inflammatory immune responses are often described as *Th1 responses*, referring to the T-helper cell subset that generally produces cytokines that initiate inflammatory processes. Anti-inflammatory cytokines, which include IL-3, IL-4, IL-5, IL-10, and IL-13, are sometimes described as immunosuppressors due to their ability to inhibit the Th1-mediated inflammatory response (often via direct antagonism of Th1-secreted inflammatory cytokines) (Ganea et al, 2006). However, these cytokines can also promote certain increases in the immune response, most notably increased overall production of antibodies and increased eosinophil and mast cell production. Often called the *Th2 response*, these cascades of cytokine-induced immune activation support allergic reactions. It is important to note that some cytokines support both pro- and anti-inflammatory effects depending on the situation (e.g., IL-6 and IL-8), thus rendering the "pro-inflammatory" or "anti-inflammatory" nomenclature less than perfect. IL-6 is also classified as a *myokine* because it is produced by contracting skeletal muscle and plays an important role in the anti-inflammatory effects of acute exercise (Petersen and Pedersen, 2005).

1.1 Cytokines: Central Nervous System (CNS) Interactions

Cytokines have extensive bidirectional communication with the CNS and hypothalamic–pituitary–adrenal axis. Likely due to this communication, cytokines are correlated with a number of psychological states, including stress, fatigue, and depression. It is well-understood that cytokines are secreted by certain classes of brain cells, including microglial cells and astrocytes (Yang et al, 2007b). Endogenous expression of cytokines and their receptors have been found in the hypothalamus, basal ganglia, cerebellum, circumventricular sites, and brainstem nuclei. Included in the considerably large list of brain-active cytokines are IFN-α and IFN-γ; TNF-α and TNF-β; and IL-1, -2, -3, -4, -5, -6, -8, -10, and -12. Studies involving systematic administration of cytokines in some of the brain regions mentioned above indicate that cytokines promote the release of neurotransmitters, including norepinephrine, dopamine, and serotonin. Thus, in addition to their immunoprotective effects (such as regulation of infiltrating leukocytes during times of infection) within the brain, cytokines may promote neurochemical cascades that directly affect mood and behavior (Simmons and Broderick, 2005).

1.2 Cytokines: Hypothalamic–Pituitary–Adrenal Axis (HPA) Interactions

The HPA is part of the neuroendocrine system that is responsible for the cortical as well as adrenal release of hormones in response to stress. Considerable progress has been made in understanding the complex interactions between cytokines and the HPA (O'Brien et al, 2004).

Briefly, it is now well understood that complex and dynamic interactive communication exists between the cytokines and the HPA and that the regulation of cytokine release, as well as HPA responses to immune insults, is governed in part by positive and negative feedback loops between the two systems (Kariagina et al, 2004). In particular, pro-inflammatory cytokines have been shown to stimulate HPA stress responses, while Th2 cytokines can inhibit this activation. For example, pro-inflammatory cytokines appear to activate corticotropin releasing hormone (CRH) and arginine vasopressin neurons in the parvocellular paraventricular nucleus within the hypothalamus. This activation results in a downstream HPA cascade in which CRH is released from the hypothalamus, promoting release of corticotrophin (ACTH) from the anterior pituitary gland and resulting in release of the glucocorticoids corticosterone and cortisol from the adrenal cortex. There are several postulated mechanisms of action for how this cascade is initiated by pro-inflammatory cytokines, some of which involve mediating effects of cytokines on the HPA via afferent vagal fiber activity.

In addition to effects on the anterior pituitary and adrenal cortex via CRH release from the hypothalamus, pro-inflammatory cytokines also affect the anterior pituitary and adrenal cortex directly, resulting in similar end-organ effects (release of corticosterone from the adrenal cortex). For example, IL-6 is synthesized and released within the human adrenal gland itself, promoting glucocorticoid release (Path et al, 2000). The multitude of sites of action allows pro-inflammatory cytokines several pathways of promoting a similar end-organ response so that even if higher level actions of cytokines on hypothalamic or anterior pituitary structures are inhibited (for example, via antagonism by a Th2 cytokine such as IL-10), some level of glucocorticoid release into the circulation is preserved. In turn, glucocorticoid actions on cytokines help to maintain homeostasis via negative feedback loops. For example, cortisol inhibits cellular synthesis and release of pro-inflammatory cytokines, thus acting to preserve homeostasis in the system. However, the effects of glucocorticoids on maintaining this homeostasis are dampened in cases of chronic stress, possibly due to the ability of the pro-inflammatory cytokines to promote receptor desensitization, downregulation, or prevalence of negative isoforms of the glucocorticoid receptor, causing decreased glucocorticoid sensitivity or glucocorticoid resistance. Thus, cytokines are intimately intertwined with HPA responses, providing a potent influence on stress responses and appearing to play a very active role in HPA modulations during chronic stress and fatigue.

1.3 Cytokines, Stress, Negative Affect, and Sleep

1.3.1 Cytokines and Acute Stress

There is a relatively large literature in healthy individuals, and to some extent in individuals with chronic diseases, examining the effects of acute psychosocial stressors on levels of circulating cytokines. Several inflammatory cytokines do respond to acute stressors, but the response is typically delayed so a proper study design is needed to observe the effects. A recent meta-analysis of the literature synthesizing data from 30 studies showed robust effects for increased circulating levels of IL-6 and IL-1β following acute stress, but more marginal effects for C-reactive protein (CRP) (Steptoe et al, 2007). The effects of stressors on leukocyte-stimulated cytokine production were less consistent.

We investigated the IL-6 response to acute stress and whether the response would habituate to a repetitively applied stressor. As part of the mechanism of the response, we examined whether cortisol reactivity would show a relationship with IL-6 reactivity. Study participants underwent the Trier Social Stress Test three times with an interval of 1 week. Plasma IL-6 and free salivary cortisol were measured immediately before and after stress and at 45 and 105 min of recovery from stress. Cortisol samples were also obtained 15 and 30 min after

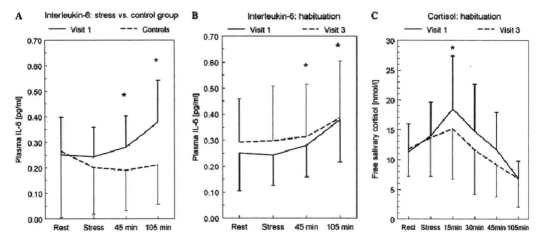

Fig. 45.1 IL-6 (**a** and **b**) and free salivary cortisol (**c**) measures. IL-6 was measured immediately before stress (rest), during mental arithmetic (stress), and 45 and 105 min after stress. Compared to the non-stressed control group, IL-6 had significantly increased (*) in the stress group 45 and 105 min after stress (**a**). In the stress group, IL-6 was significantly higher (*) 45 and 105 min after stress than at rest, but IL-6 showed no habituation between visit one and visit three (**b**). Mean peak response of cortisol occurred 15 min after stress and was significantly lower at visit three than at visit one (*) suggesting habituation (means ± SD) (von Känel et al, 2006b)

stress. Compared to non-stressed controls, IL-6 significantly increased between rest and 45 min post-stress and between rest and 105 min post-stress (Fig. 45.1). Peak cortisol responses to stress habituated between weeks 1 and 3. No adaptation occurred in the IL-6 responses to stress. The areas under the curve integrating the stress-induced changes in cortisol and IL-6 at week 3 were significantly negatively correlated @$r = -0.54$. The findings from this study suggest that the IL-6 response to acute mental stress occurs delayed and shows no adaptation to repeated moderate mental stress and that the HPA axis may attenuate stress reactivity of IL-6. The lack of habituation in IL-6 responses to daily stress could subject at-risk individuals to higher atherosclerotic morbidity and mortality (von Känel et al, 2006b).

Such responses have also been examined in patients with established cardiovascular disease. Kop et al, for example, examined the responses of IL-6 and CRP, as well as soluble intercellular adhesion molecule-1 (sICAM-1) in patients with coronary artery disease (CAD) as compared to healthy controls. Responses were examined to mental challenge tasks (anger recall and mental arithmetic) and to treadmill exercise. The results showed that CAD patients show greater responses than healthy individuals and that the increase in norepinephrine responses related to the CRP and IL-6 responses to the mental challenge tasks. The authors conclude that mental stress and exercise induce greater increased levels of inflammatory markers in patients with CAD and that the effect are related to the neurohormonal stress response (Kop et al, 2008).

1.3.2 Cytokines and Chronic Stress

Studies have examined the effects of chronic stressors on cytokines and many of them have been conducted with Alzheimer's disease caregivers. An early study examining chronic stress and wound healing in Alzheimer's disease caregivers compared to matched controls showed a decrease in IL-1 mRNA secretion in response to lipopolysaccharide (LPS) stimulation of peripheral blood leukocytes in the caregivers (Kiecolt-Glaser et al, 1995). Importantly, this effect might have contributed to slower wound healing in this group (see Chapter 44). Another study reported lower IL-1β and IL-2 responses to virus-specific stimulation for Alzheimer's caregivers versus controls. Alzheimer's caregivers have also shown increased intracellular IL-10 levels in T-helper and T-cytotoxic cells versus controls, with the difference between these groups being significantly greater for younger subjects (Glaser et al, 2001). A longitudinal study where IL-6 levels for Alzheimer's disease caregivers and matched controls were tracked over 6 years showed an almost fourfold rate of increase of IL-6 levels in caregivers (Kiecolt-Glaser et al, 2003). This result was consistent even for caregivers whose spouses had died during the 6-year period. Another study examining IL-6 associations with aging and chronic stress in women indicated that Alzheimer's caregivers show significantly higher levels of IL-6 compared to age-matched women who were experiencing moderate forms of stress, as well as compared to older and younger control subjects. These findings suggest that chronic stress associated with Alzheimer's caregiving in the elderly promotes increases in Th2 cytokines and inhibition of Th1 cytokines. We have reported that, independent of relevant covariates, Alzheimer's disease caregivers have higher levels of IL-6 and of the coagulatory biomarker D-dimer, suggesting the possibility that older caregivers could be at risk of a more rapid transition to the frailty syndrome and associated clinical manifestations of cardiovascular diseases (von Känel et al, 2006a). Together, findings suggest pathways by which caregiving in the elderly leads to significantly increased risk for deleterious health outcomes even well after the death of the spouse being cared for.

1.3.3 Cytokines and Fatigue

Fatigue is one of the most frequent complaints of cancer patients, with studies showing 40–75% of patients reporting feeling tired and weak and with rates up to 95% during chemotherapy and/or radiotherapy treatment (Kangas et al, 2008). Much of the fatigue that cancer patients experience may be attributed to cytokines that are elevated either by the cellular response to the cancer itself or by its treatment.

High levels of certain endogenous cytokines (e.g., TNF-α) are associated with tumor genesis and growth. Treatments such as chemotherapy and radiation therapy are associated with elevations in TNF-α, as well as other inflammatory cytokines including IL-1Ra and IL-6, which in turn are associated with elevations in fatigue.

We have shown that circulating levels of the cytokine vascular endothelial growth factor (VEGF) are elevated in response to chemotherapy for breast cancer and that these elevated levels are associated with the significantly increased feelings of fatigue and poorer quality of life that result from chemotherapy (Mills et al, 2004, 2005). Elevations in cytokines may also persist along with fatigue well after treatment. For example, significantly higher serum levels of IL-1Ra and sTNF-RII have been found among breast cancer survivors who report a high level of fatigue as compared to low-fatigued breast cancer patients, independent of depression (Bower et al, 2002). Higher levels of fatigue prior to the initiation of chemotherapy for breast cancer may predict poorer outcomes related to treatment. Our group has found that breast cancer patients with high fatigue prior to chemotherapy experience poorer sleep in response to chemotherapy (both subjectively and objectively), compared to those with lower fatigue prior to chemotherapy (Liu et al, 2009). Whether these alterations in sleep patterns for high-fatigued patients are associated with alterations in cytokine responses to chemotherapy remains to be elucidated.

1.3.4 Cytokines and Depression

It is well known that administration of inflammatory cytokines to treat medical diseases (such as the use of ILs to treat Hepatitis C) induces depressive symptoms (Patten, 2006). Inflammation found in many diseases has been implicated in the development of depressive symptoms and in the pathophysiology of depression itself, although this literature has not been consistent. Part of our work on depression and inflammation has focused on the role of generalized inflammation in the etiology of depression in heart failure (Rutledge et al, 2006). Studies of patients with other cardiovascular diseases, including coronary heart disease, report that patients with depressive mood have elevated IL-6 and C-reactive protein levels (Empana et al, 2005).

Other studies have looked at inflammation–depression links in otherwise non-ill populations. Unmedicated patients with major depression show elevated levels of IL-6 and TNF-α compared to normal controls (Yang et al, 2007a). Paradoxically, studies that have examined the number and activity of lymphocyte subsets, such as natural killer cells, typically show reduction in number and/or cytotoxicity. In addition to direct effects of cytokines on mood, including cytokine-induced sickness behavior, elevation of proinflammatory cytokines IL-2 and TNF-α can activate tryptophan- and serotonin-degrading enzymes, resulting in a decrease in brain serotonin, further supporting depressed mood (Muller and Schwarz, 2007).

1.3.5 Cytokines and Sleep

Cytokines can be both sleep inducing (e.g., IL-1β, TNF-α) and sleep inhibiting (e.g., IL-10 and IL-4), depending on the cytokine, the dose, and the circadian phase (Opp, 2005), although their sleep-associated effects are often less than straightforward. Sleep inhibiting cytokines may exert their effects through antagonizing somnogenic cytokines. IL-10 and IL-4, for example, may inhibit sleep by inhibiting the production of IL-1β and TNF-α (Kelley et al, 2003). Administration of TNF-α, IL-1β, or IL-18 increases the amount of non-rapid eye movement (NREM) sleep time and decreases the duration of REM sleep. TNF-α or IL-1β also increases the amplitude of slow-wave EEG, while administration of IL-10 and IL-4 on the other hand inhibits NREM. While circulating IL-2 levels increase during sleep, there is little evidence that there is a direct sleep promoting effect of IL-2. Although the precise mechanisms of the somnogenic or anti-somnogenic effects of cytokines have yet to be fully elucidated, growth hormone releasing hormone, corticotropin releasing hormone, prostaglandins, and molecular intermediates (e.g., activation of the DNA transcription binding protein NF-κB) have been implicated.

Like TNF-α, IL-6 is a somnogenic proinflammatory cytokine associated with disturbed sleep and with fatigue (Vgontzas et al, 2005). IL-6 negatively correlates with the amount of sleep as well as the depth of sleep. Better sleep is associated with decreased daytime secretion of IL-6, while nocturnal sleep disturbances are associated with increased daytime levels of IL-6, as well as TNF-α. In older adults, elevated IL-6 levels are associated with poor sleep and sleep disturbances, particularly when accompanied by elevations in cortisol levels (Vgontzas et al, 2003). We recently showed that disturbed sleep in spousal caregivers of Alzheimer's disease patients is associated with elevated levels of IL-6, as well as the coagulation marker D-dimer (Mills et al, 2008) (Fig. 45.2). Inflammation is common in the sleep disorder obstructive sleep apnea. Studies show that in addition to IL-6, TNF-α levels are elevated in OSA independent of obesity and the circadian rhythm of TNF-α is disrupted (Vgontzas et al, 2000).

1.4 Cytokine Measurement

When examining cytokines in biological fluids there are two broad categories for methods of measurement. *Immunoassays* measure the prevalence of cytokines or their soluble receptors by using either radioisotope-tagged antibodies (i.e., radioimmunoassays or RIA) or enzyme-linked antibodies (i.e., enzyme-linked immunosorbant assays, or ELISAs) that are specific for certain peptides that are part of the cytokine structure. Strengths of immunoassays in general are their ease in use and relatively low cost, combined with relatively high specificity due to the use of monoclonal antibodies. *Bioassays* measure cytokine functionality as indexed by specific biological responses such as chemotaxis (movement through a chemical diffusion gradient),

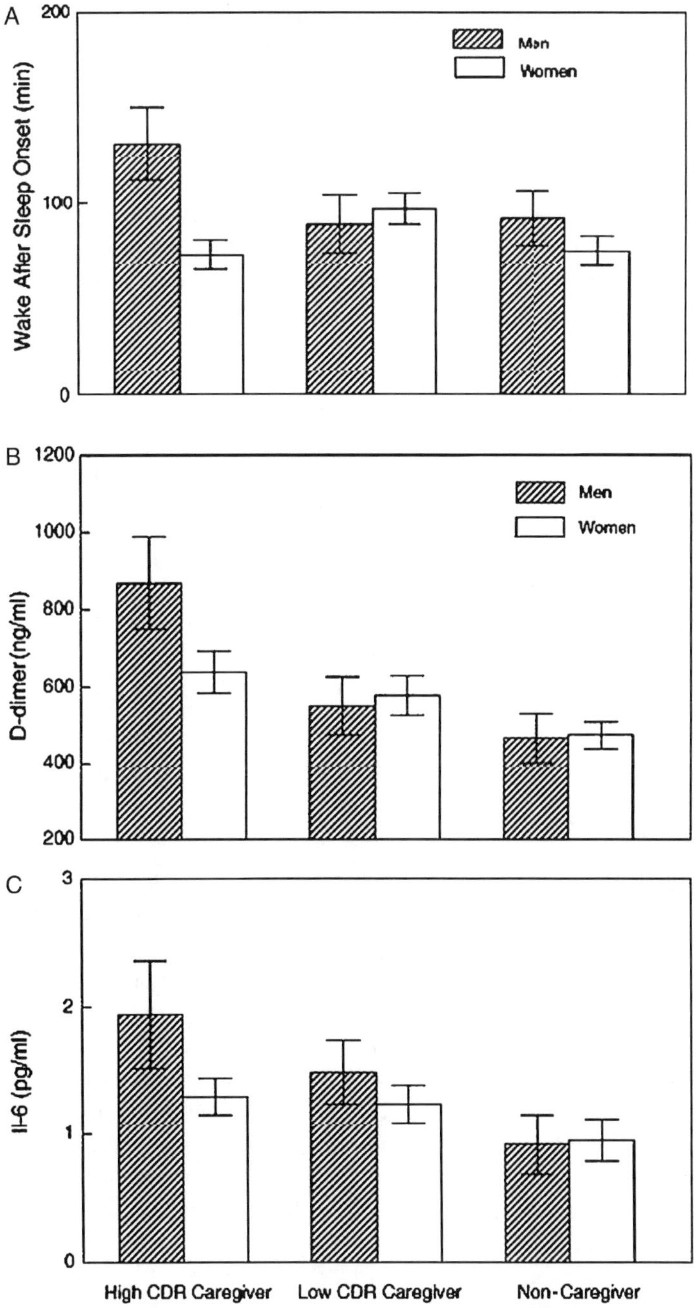

Fig. 45.2 Shown are minutes spent awake after sleep onset (**a**), circulating D-dimer levels (**b**), and circulating IL-6 levels (**c**) in spousal caregivers of Alzheimer's disease patients with high (high CDR) and low (low CDR) clinical dementia ratings (CDR) and non-caregiver controls. High CDR caregivers were those caring for moderate and severe dementia patients, while low CDR caregivers were those caring for questionable and mild dementia patients. Male caregivers caring for spouses with moderate and severe dementia (high CDR) spent more time awake after sleep onset than females caring for spouses with more severe dementia, and males caring for low dementia spouses and non-caregiving males ($p < 0.02$), and D-dimer levels and IL-6 were elevated ($p <0.05$). Independent of sleep, IL-6 levels were elevated ($p < 0.05$) in caregivers caring for spouses with more moderate to severe Alzheimer's disease (high CDR) compared to non-caregivers (Mills et al, 2008)

proliferation (increase in numbers of the particular cell line), cytotoxicity (ability of cells to kill pathogens), expression of cell surface molecules, or subsequent release of specific proteins. Bioassays thus give the researcher information simply not only about soluble cytokine levels but also about some aspect of their functionality. Although they are very sensitive tests, they are generally less specific, less reliable, and more time-consuming than immunoassays.

Other methods exist for examining whole cells' capacities to produce and release cytokines. Two such notable methods are flow cytometry and ELISPOT (enzyme-linked immunospot), both of which measure the abilities of single cells to produce or release cytokines, respectively. The majority of studies discussed in this chapter relied on ELISA methods for measuring circulating levels of cytokines in peripheral blood.

2 Leukocyte Trafficking and Cellular Adhesion Molecules

Circulation of immune cells throughout the body is a critical component of immunosurveillance. Even though only 2% of total leukocytes are in the peripheral circulation at any given time, they provide a diagnostic account of the functional status of the immune system. The majority is homed in lymphoid organs and the rest are diffusely distributed in other organs. Cellular adhesion molecules (CAMs) play a central role in mediating leukocyte migration and homing, as well as cell-to-cell interactions and adhesion.

Trafficking, rolling, and firm adhesion of leukocytes to sites of inflammation are mediated by diverse families of CAM ligand/receptor pairings (Radi et al, 2001). Inflammatory cytokines and chemokines (chemotactic cytokines) and antigen recognition by immune cells lead to the expression of CAMs on both immune cells and endothelial cells. Leukocytes then attach to endothelial cells lining the infected areas

("firm adhesion") and penetrate into the tissue ("transmigration"). The adhesion of leukocytes to the endothelium involves multiple processes, including the initial contact of leukocytes to the endothelium (mediated by selectins) and tethering loosely to carbohydrate ligands (like GlyCAM-1) as they roll along the surface. During leukocyte activation, chemokines are released by the endothelium and trigger integrin LFA-1 (CD11a) expression on the leukocyte surface to bind tightly to intercellular adhesion molecule ICAM-1 (CD54) on the endothelium. This event leads to eventual transendothelial migration (extravasation). CAMs such as L-selectin (CD62L), ICAM-1, and the vascular CAM VCAM-1 (CD106) are shed in a soluble form during the process and can further participate in biological processes.

2.1 CAMs and Behavioral Stressors

Numerous studies demonstrate mobilization of immune cells in response to acute and chronic psychological as well as physical stressors (Goebel and Mills, 2000). Evidence dates back to the 1930s when Farris described the relationship between emotional stress and increases in the number of circulating leukocytes. During the past two decades, with the more sophisticated research tools and techniques available, investigators have been actively examining the nuances of these phenomena, as well as researching the mechanisms that regulate them. Stress-induced leukocytosis is cell subset-specific and there is a dose–response-based on the intensity of the stressor.

2.1.1 CAMs and Acute Behavioral Stressors

Acute psychological stress leads to leukocytosis, with the magnitude depending on the type and duration of the stressor. A typical response shows a marked increase in the circulation of natural killer (NK) and CD8$^+$ T cell subsets, a decrease in the CD4$^+$/CD8$^+$ ratio, and possible small increases in B cells. Some types of NK subsets are more responsive to stressor than others. For example, the more cytotoxic $CD56^{Lo}$ expressing NK cells will triple in number in circulation while more immunoregulatory $CD56^{Hi}$ expressing NK cells will not change (Bosch et al, 2005). Part of the reason resides in the differences in CAM expression across these cell subtypes. It has been consistently shown, for example, that the phenomenon of lymphocyte subtype redistribution in response to acute stress can be differentiated according to L-selectin expression. It is primarily lymphocytes not expressing L-selectin ($CD62L^-$) that markedly increase in the circulation following acute stress (either psychological or physical). $CD8^+CD62L^-$ T cells, for example, show a two- to threefold increase in the circulation following acute stress as compared to $CD8^+CD62L^+$ T cells, which show either no change or a more moderate increase. A similar $CD62L^{-/+}$ response differentiation is shown for both $CD4^+$ and NK lymphocytes. This phenomenon most likely results from a combination of events, including a preferential release of $CD62L^-$ lymphocytes from the spleen and marginal pools, an increased rate of adhesion of $CD62L^+$ lymphocytes, and a possible downregulation or shedding of CD62L from the leukocyte's surface upon further activation.

2.1.2 CAMs and Chronic Behavioral Stressors

It is widely believed that more enduring stressors lead to downregulation of immune function and increased disease susceptibility. As with acute stress studies, CAMs appear to have an important role in mediating the effects of chronic stress on leukocytes. We conduced a study on CD62L expression on T lymphocytes among elderly (average age of 75 years) spousal caregivers of Alzheimer patients experiencing high stress levels due to increased caregiving burden (Mills et al, 1999). We compared them to a group of caregivers with a relatively low stress burden from caregiving. The highly stressed caregivers showed significantly lower numbers of

circulating $CD8^+CD62L^-$ and $CD4^+CD62L^-$ T cells at rest and following an acute psychological stressor but no differences in $CD62L^+$ T cells as compared to a control group (Fig. 45.3). Lower numbers of $CD62L^-$ T cells in the circulation indicate that there is decreased availability of activated/memory T cells. In addition, this "deficit" in activated/memory T lymphocytes, cells that are critical in mounting immune responses, may imply a stress-associated accelerated decline of immunity in these older individuals, which, in turn, might have adverse consequences for health. We have also reported that in otherwise healthy men and women, those individuals who report experiencing greater hassles in their lives have elevated circulating levels of soluble CAM sICAM-1 (Jain et al, 2007).

2.2 Underlying Mechanisms and Mediators: Sympathetic Nervous System (SNS) and Hypothalamic–Pituitary–Adrenal (HPA) Cortical Axis Activation

Both the SNS and the HPA axis help regulate immune cell responses to a variety of stressors. Adrenergic projections and sympathetic nerve terminals are found in many organs of the immune system, including the spleen. Sympathetic agonists (catecholamines) are rapidly released from nerve endings following acute SNS activation and act directly on α- and β-adrenergic receptors. β_2-adrenergic receptors are found on all white blood cells, including lymphocytes, neutrophils, and monocytes. Activation of these receptors leads to lymphocytosis. Adherence of NK cells to endothelial cells is decreased in a dose-dependent manner after adding β_2-adrenergic agonists in vitro. Catecholamines lead to increased recirculation of lymphocytes into the blood by decreasing the affinity of the lymphocyte to the vessel wall and possibly through a shedding of adhesion molecules such as CD62L and ICAM-1 from the cell surface.

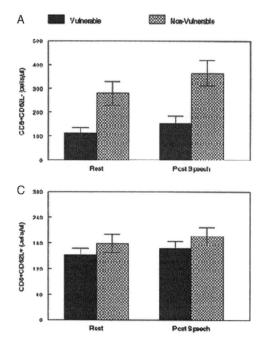

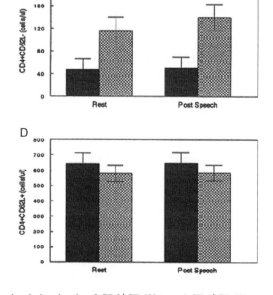

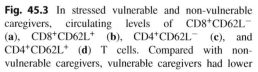

Fig. 45.3 In stressed vulnerable and non-vulnerable caregivers, circulating levels of CD8⁺CD62L⁻ (**a**), CD8⁺CD62L⁺ (**b**), CD4⁺CD62L⁻ (**c**), and CD4⁺CD62L⁺ (**d**) T cells. Compared with non-vulnerable caregivers, vulnerable caregivers had lower circulating levels of $CD8^+CD62L^-$ and $CD4^+CD62L^-$ T cells at rest ($p = 0.01$) and following a stressful speech task ($p = 0.01$). There were no differences in $CD8^+CD62L^+$ or $CD4^+CD62L^+$ cells (Mills et al, 1999)

Glucocorticoids induce immunosuppressive effects. Studies demonstrate that glucocorticoids reduce the number of circulating leukocytes and downregulate cytokine production and chemotaxis, as well as downregulation of CAMs including E-selectin (CD62E) and ICAM-1. In vivo studies demonstrate time-related effects of dexamethasone on ICAM-1 expression, in which prolonged treatment significantly reduces ICAM-1 expression on monocytes.

2.3 CAM Measurement

Assessment of soluble CAMs is typically done by enzyme linked immunosorbent assay (ELISA). Assessment of CAMs expressed on immune cells is typically done by flow cytometry.

3 Hemostasis

There are a number of hemostasis biomarkers that are highly relevant to behavioural medicine. The scheme in Fig. 45.4 simplifies complex and closely intertwined hemostasis pathways. Activation of hemostasis results in a sequential interaction between enzymes and inhibitors of the coagulation and fibrinolysis cascades, of platelets, and of the von Willebrand factor (VWF). Two pathways of blood coagulation are commonly distinguished. Whereas the intrinsic pathway is initiated by FXII, the extrinsic pathway is triggered when tissue factor becomes exposed to the blood stream at sites of tissue damage, e.g., on material of a ruptured atherosclerotic plaque. Tissue factor instantly binds to circulating FVII. Both pathways result in activation of several clotting factors in a sort of cascade, and eventually converge in a common activator complex. This complex

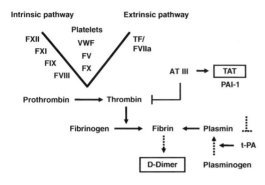

Fig. 45.4 Hemostasis pathways. The figure shows coagulation steps in *solid lines* and fibrinolysis steps in *dashed lines* with the symbol "→" meaning activation of a step and the symbol "⊣" meaning inhibition of a step. Hypercoagulability markers thrombin–antithrombin (AT) III complex (TAT) and D-dimer are depicted in boxes. Von Willebrand factor (VWF), platelets, clotting factor V and X are involved in both coagulation pathways. FXII, FXI, FIX, and FVIII are components of the intrinsic pathway, and tissue factor (TF) and FVII belong to the extrinsic pathway of blood coagulation. PAI-1, plasminogen activator inhibitor-1; t-PA, tissue-type plasminogen activator (cf. text for details in terms of activation steps)

converts prothrombin to thrombin, which, in turn, converts fibrinogen to fibrin. Together with platelet aggregates, fibrin forms a blood clot that, for example, may critically occlude a coronary artery to result in myocardial infarction. Circulating VWF mediates adherence of platelets to sites of blood vessel injury where platelets are activated and aggregate with each other through fibrinogen bridges. Negatively charged phospholipids on activated platelets catalyze activation of circulating clotting factors.

Termination of clot formation involves several anticoagulant steps, e.g., binding of antithrombin III to thrombin. This step neutralizes thrombin, a potent activator of several clotting factors and platelets, in a thrombin/antithrombin III (TAT) complex. Fibrinolysis is initiated by tissue-type plasminogen activator (t-PA) converting plasminogen into fibrin-cleaving plasmin. The breakdown of cross-linked fibrin chains yields soluble fibrin fragments such as D-dimer. The antifibrinolytic enzyme plasminogen activator inhibitor (PAI)-1 is the main inhibitor

of t-PA neutralizing t-PA in a t-PA/PAI-1-complex.

TAT and D-dimer are viewed as coagulation activation markers because they combine several coagulation steps leading to thrombin and fibrin formation, respectively. In addition, TAT and D-dimer are also hypercoagulability markers indicating exaggerated coagulation activity. It is important to note, that unlike individual clotting and fibrinolysis factors, D-dimer indicates activation of the entire hemostatic system, i.e., fibrin formation by the coagulation system and fibrin degradation by the fibrinolytic system.

3.1 Hemostasis Factors and Cardiovascular Disease

Numerous large-scale and prospectively designed epidemiologic studies suggest that hemostatic factors, for instance fibrinogen, D-dimer, VWF, and PAI-1, predict cardiovascular disease (CVD) in apparently healthy subjects as well as recurrent events in patients with established CVD (Lowe et al, 2002). These relationships have been shown to be independent of sociodemographic factors, lifestyle, and established cardiovascular risk factors smoking, diabetes, hypertension, and obesity, all of which may affect hemostasis. Altogether, this abundant epidemiologic research challenges the view that hemostasis factors are mere risk markers of CVD and do not actively contribute to atherosclerosis. It is assumed that a procoagulant milieu, as reflected by increased activity of clotting factors, coagulation activation markers, platelets, and the VWF on the one hand and impaired fibrinolysis on the other will gradually contribute to atherosclerosis progression over many decades by promoting fibrin deposits in the atherosclerotic vessel wall and inflammation (Falk and Fernandez-Ortiz, 1995). Moreover, a procoagulant milieu at the time of atherosclerotic plaque rupturing will accelerate coronary thrombus growth to determine myocardial ischemia and damage.

3.2 Effects of Behavioral Stressors and Negative Affect on Hemostasis

3.2.1 Acute Stressors

Different types of speech tasks, mental arithmetic, mirror star tracing task and the Stroop color-word conflict test, are regularly applied as mental stressors in studies. This research suggests that acute stress elicits a significant increase both in procoagulant factors (i.e., FXII, FVII, FVIII, fibrinogen, VWF, platelet activity) and in profibrinolytic t-PA (Table 45.1). However, findings of an increase in coagulation activation markers TAT and D-dimer suggests that the concomitant activation of virtually all hemostasis components with acute stress results in net hypercoagulability compatible with the evolution paradigm of Cannon (von Känel et al, 2001). We showed that, unlike changes in blood pressure and cortisol, changes in the coagulation system do not adapt in response to the same stressor (i.e., combined speech task and mental arithmetic) applied three times to healthy subjects with an interval of 1 week (von Känel et al, 2004a) (Fig. 45.5). Apparently, evolution empowered humans to mount the same hypercoagulability any time we might potentially be injured independent of whether or not we perceived this situation as threatening.

3.2.2 Modulators of the Acute Procoagulant Stress Response

Certain diseases and behavioral factors have been shown to exaggerate the acute procoagulant stress response. In particular, it has been shown that D-dimer formation is increased and fibrinolytic activation is attenuated in acutely stressed patients with CVD such as coronary artery disease and systemic hypertension partly because the endothelium has become dysfunctional and partially deprived of its anticoagulant properties in atherosclerotic vessels (von Känel et al, 2001). Also, recovery of platelet activity after stress is delayed in patients with atherosclerosis as compared to those without (Strike et al, 2004). Anxiety, depression, and poor coping strategies (e.g., low problem solving) were shown to be associated with greater D-dimer formation with acute stress in elderly subjects who were caregivers for a spouse with Alzheimer's disease (Aschbacher et al, 2005; von Känel et al, 2004b). These caregivers also experience greater acute procoagulability to stress when they experienced relatively more negative life events in the preceding months and if their spouse showed relatively more severe dementia. We also found that recovery of acute stress-induced increase in D-dimer was relatively prolonged in school teachers with higher levels of exhaustion and anhedonia, as well as in those who overcommitted to their job (von Känel et al, 2004a, b).

Table 45.1 Changes in hemostasis factors with behavioural stress

Hemostasis factor	Acute stress	Chronic stress
FVII	↑	↑
FXII	↑	
FVIII	↑	↑
Fibrinogen	↑	↑
Thrombin/antithrombin III complex	↑	—
D-dimer	↑	↑
Von Willebrand factor	↑	↑/—
Platelet activity markers	↑	
Plasminogen activator inhibitor-1	—	↑
Tissue-type plasminogen activator activity	↑	↓

↑: increase with stress; ↓: decrease with stress; —: no response to stress

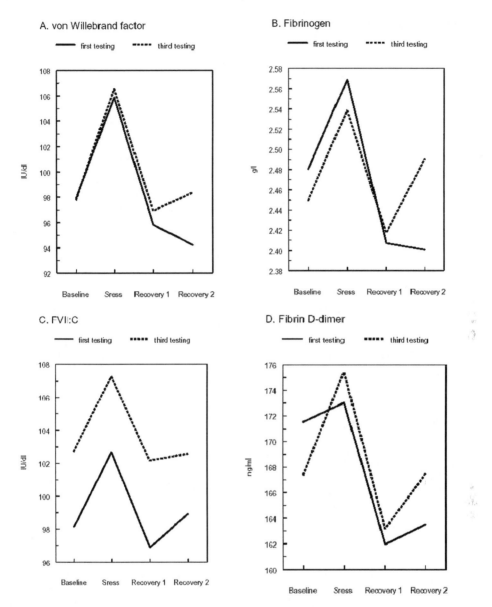

Fig. 45.5 Lack of habituation in the acute procoagulant stress response. Subjects underwent the same stressor three times with 1-week apart. Hemostatic factors were measured at week one and week three (but not at week two). While there was a significant increase in Willebrand factor (**a**), fibrinogen (**b**), clotting factor VII activity (FVII: **c**) and D-dimer (**d**) across the two sessions (all *p* values < 0.02), there was no significant difference in the magnitude of change from baseline to stress and 45 min (recovery 1) and 105 min (recovery 2) post-stress between testing sessions (von Känel et al, 2004a)

The latter findings may add to our mechanistic understanding about how job stress and related negative affect put workers at risk of developing CVD. In sum, a hyperactive procoagulant stress response might embed cardiovascular harm in certain individuals with certain diseases, and at certain times of their life as it might enhance thrombus formation at times of plaque rupture triggered by acute stress-induced blood pressure peaks.

3.2.3 Hemostasis and Chronic Stressors

As far as actual chronic stress effects, notably, the effects of chronic stress on fibrinolytic activity are distinctly different from those observed with acute stress (Table 45.1). Chronic stress impairs the fibrinolytic activity such that the balance between procoagulant factors and profibrinolytic factors is shifted toward hypercoagulability to an extent that exceeds the physiologic net hypercoagulable changes seen with acute stress in healthy individuals. Chronic stress has particularly been related to increases in plasma levels of fibrinogen, PAI-1, and D-dimer (von Känel and Dimsdale, 2003; von Känel et al, 2001). These findings derive from investigations on hemostasis factors in subjects with high job strain, low socioeconomic status, and caregivers of a demented spouse. In these studies, job strain is mainly defined as a mismatch between job demands and decision latitude and an imbalance between effort spent and reward obtained moderated by a personality trait of overcommitment to work. Whereas relationships between various job strain variables and elevated plasma levels of FVII, fibrinogen, and PAI-1 on the one hand and decreased activity of profibrinolytic t-PA on the other hand are independent, most of the association between low socioeconomic status and hypercoagulability becomes insignificant when statistics control for health habits (von Känel et al, 2001). We found that the number of negative life events in the preceding month correlate positively with plasma D-dimer levels in Alzheimer's caregivers (von Känel et al, 2003). In another study, chronically stressed dementia caregivers had higher D-dimer than age- and gender-equated non-caregiving controls, even when controlling for cardiovascular diseases and risk factors, life style, and medication (von Känel et al, 2006a).

3.2.4 Hemostasis and Negative Affect

Behavioral cardiology research has identified hemostatic perturbations in relation to different types of negative affect, particularly depression, anxiety, and exhaustion (von Känel et al,

2001). Depression has been associated with subtle platelet hyperactivity that was suggested to be greatest in depressed patients with coronary artery disease (von Känel, 2004). Depression is also shown to correlate with increased fibrinogen in a number of cross-sectional studies. In a prospective study over almost 2 years on healthy teachers, we found that increase in depressive symptoms and in fibrinogen levels are significantly correlated. Whereas controlling for baseline level of depressive mood yielded the association between changes in depression and fibrinogen nonsignificant, controlling for baseline fibrinogen levels maintained the predictive value of fibrinogen change for the change in depressive mood (von Känel et al, 2009c). Given that in addition to being a procoagulant factor, fibrinogen also exerts inflammatory properties; this dynamic relationship might advance our knowledge about psychophysiologic mechanisms underlying both atherosclerosis and sickness behavior. The literature on hemostasis and anxiety is comparably scant and less conclusive. For instance, there is hypercoagulability with a predominant activation of inhibitors in fibrinolysis in psychiatric patients with phobic anxiety (Geiser et al, 2008), whereas panic-like anxiety is associated with increased D-dimer but decreased fibrinogen in factory workers (von Känel et al, 2004c). A fairly consistent line of research suggests that a state of profound exhaustion ensuing from long-term psychological strain is associated with elevated PAI-1 (von Känel et al, 2004d). Such an antifibrinolytic effect might help explain the observation that excessive fatigue may precede an acute myocardial infarction.

3.3 Physiological Mechanisms of Acute and Chronic Stress Effects on Hemostasis

Molecular studies and in vivo studies in animals and humans convincingly demonstrate that the SNS regulates hemostatic activity. Much of this knowledge derives from human studies in which adrenergic compounds, particularly the stress hormones epinephrine and norepinephrine, had been infused together, with or without previous blockade of adrenergic receptors by various drugs (von Känel and Dimsdale, 2000). Via stimulation of vascular endothelial β2-adrenergic receptors, catecholamines release FVIII, VWF, and t-PA from endothelial storage pools into the circulation. This phenomenon takes place within minutes and shows dose dependency. Catecholamines also stimulate release of FVIII from the liver and affect hepatic clearance of t-PA. In addition, platelets are activated by stimulation of their α2-adrenergic receptors with platelet β2-adrenergic receptors likely exerting an inhibitory effect on platelet activation by catecholamines. Greater sensitivity of the β2-adrenergic receptor is associated with greater thrombin formation in response to acute stress. To date, there is little evidence for a significant effect of the HPA axis and cortisol activity on the acute stress procoagulant response. Conceivably, evolution wanted the blood to clot instantly after injury as mediated by the SNS. In contrast, the HPA axis peaks its activity only 15–30 min after stress and, therefore, is a system likely too slow to critically limit acute bleeding.

The pathophysiologic underpinnings of the link between hemostatic changes and chronic stress and negative affect are far from clear, though gene regulation, the autonomic nervous system, and the HPA axis could all be involved. In accordance with observed decrease in PAI-1 with chronic stress, restraint stress, and injection of non-selective β-adrenergic substances in animals (i.e., epinephrine, isoprenalin) both result in up-regulation of PAI-1 mRNA with a concomitant increase of PAI-1 activity in tissue homogenats. In factory workers we found relationships between overnight urinary excretion of cortisol and catecholamines on the one hand and morning plasma levels of PAI-1, fibrinogen, and D-dimer on the other (von Känel et al, 2004e). In women with stable coronary artery disease plasma levels of cortisol correlate directly with those in fibrinogen and VWF (von Känel et al, 2008). In terms of a potential parasympathetic

modulation of hemostasis, we find an inverse relationship between vagal indices of heart rate variability (i.e., high-frequency power, RMSSD) and FVII and fibrinogen in women with coronary artery disease and factory workers suggesting that vagal withdrawal might be associated with hypercoagulability (von Känel and Orth-Gomér, 2008; von Känel et al, 2009d).

3.4 Coagulation Measurement

Assessment of hemostasis factors in human plasma is typically done by ELISA or coagulometric methods using factor-deficient standard human plasma and reagents (von Känel et al, 2004a). Clotting factors, VWF, and fibrinolysis enzymes are either measured by immunological (i.e., antigen level) or functional (i.e., molecule activity) methods (von Känel et al, 2001). Several methods are available to assess platelet activity (von Känel, 2004). These include flow cytometry to assess expression and conformational change of glycoprotein receptors on the surface of (activated) platelets, measurement of platelet releasing factors in plasma (beta-thromboglobulin, platelet factor 4) using ELISA technique, and in vitro aggregation studies applying all sorts of platelet agonists (e.g., epinephrine, serotonin).

4 Inflammation, Adhesion, and Hemostasis: Clinical Relevance and Future Directions in Behavioral Medicine

Increases in rates of inflammation, cellular adhesion activity, and coagulation can initiate disease and/or influence the progression of already established disease. The effects of stressors on these physiological systems, while serving an earlier evolutionary need and beneficial effect for surviving in fight and flight, are essentially negative in our modern environment which is so often characterized by comparably long-lasting psychological stressors. Daily hassles experienced in a rapidly changing society, years of marital stress and job strain, and the fate of becoming a caregiver for a loved one can elicit repetitive and sustained inflammation and hypercoagulability that has lost its protective nature, thereby contributing to disease.

The good news is that some behavioral stressors can have beneficial effects. Recent studies provide insight into the immune-mediated positive effects of acute stressors. Edwards et al, for example, showed that exposure to brief psychological stress can enhance the antibody response to vaccination (Edwards et al, 2006). The application of such findings to clinical populations, including individuals with cancer, multiple sclerosis, and rheumatoid arthritis, merits investigation.

As far as behavioural interventions, if stressors do interact with inflammation, adhesion, and hypercoagulability in predicting disease such as cardiovascular disease, carefully conducted behavioural intervention studies on effects of stress management in its broadest sense on these endpoints seem warranted. For instance, increasing vagal nerve activity by behavioral modification, meditation, hypnosis, biofeedback, and cognitive and relaxation therapies might enhance the cholinergic anti-inflammatory pathway to curtail overshooting of inflammatory responses to stress (Tracey, 2007). In patients with coronary artery disease, stress management increases both vagal and endothelial function relative to usual care (Blumenthal et al, 2005). In early-stage breast cancer patients not receiving chemotherapy, mindfulness-based stress reduction re-establishes decreased natural killer cell activity and increases cytokine levels relative to a control condition (Witek-Janusek et al, 2008). While such investigations suggest that stress management may have positive effects on biomarkers of inflammation, adhesion, and hemostasis, studies on whether these effects will ultimately benefit health outcomes are sorely needed. This seems a fruitful field for future behavioral medicine research. For instance, it has been shown that meditation decreases

cardiovascular and all-cause mortality in patients with systemic hypertension (Schneider et al, 2005) and that cardiac rehabilitation particularly reduces recurrent events and mortality if it considers psychosocial treatment, including stress management (Linden et al, 1996). It is reasonable to hypothesize that positive effects on inflammation, adhesion, and/or hemostasis related to behavioral interventions are at least partially responsible for their positive outcomes.

Acknowledgment Funding/Support: This work was supported by grants HL-057265 and HL-073355 from the National Institutes of Health and by grants 81BE-056155 and 3200-068277 from the Swiss National Science Foundation.

References

Aschbacher, K., Patterson, T. L., von Känel, R., Dimsdale, J. E., Mills, P. J. et al (2005). Coping processes and hemostatic reactivity to acute stress in dementia caregivers. *Psychosom Med, 67*, 964–971.

Blumenthal, J. A., Sherwood, A., Babyak, M. A., Watkins, L. L., Waugh, R. et al (2005). Effects of exercise and stress management training on markers of cardiovascular risk in patients with ischemic heart disease: a randomized controlled trial. *JAMA, 293*, 1626–1634.

Bosch, J. A., Berntson, G. G., Cacioppo, J. T., and Marucha, P. T. (2005). Differential mobilization of functionally distinct natural killer subsets during acute psychologic stress. *Psychosom Med, 67*, 366–375.

Bower, J. E., Ganz, P. A., Aziz, N., and Fahey, J. L. (2002). Fatigue and proinflammatory cytokine activity in breast cancer survivors. *Psychosom Med, 64*, 604–611.

Dantzer, R., O'Connor, J. C., Freund, G. G., Johnson, R. W., and Kelley, K. W. (2008). From inflammation to sickness and depression: when the immune system subjugates the brain. *Nat Rev Neurosci, 9*, 46–56.

Edwards, K. M., Burns, V. E., Reynolds, T., Carroll, D., Drayson, M. et al (2006). Acute stress exposure prior to influenza vaccination enhances antibody response in women. *Brain Behav Immun, 20*, 159–168.

Elenkov, I. J. (2008). Neurohormonal-cytokine interactions: implications for inflammation, common human diseases and well-being. *Neurochem Int, 52*, 40–51.

Empana, J. P., Sykes, D. H., Luc, G., Juhan-Vague, I., Arveiler, D. et al (2005). Contributions of depressive mood and circulating inflammatory markers to coronary heart disease in healthy European men: the Prospective Epidemiological Study of

Myocardial Infarction (PRIME). *Circulation, 111*, 2299–2305.

Falk, E., and Fernández-Ortiz, A. (1995). Role of thrombosis in atherosclerosis and its complications. *Am J Cardiol, 75*, 3B–11B.

Ganea, D., Gonzalez-Rey, E., and Delgado, M. (2006). A novel mechanism for immunosuppression: from neuropeptides to regulatory T cells. *J Neuroimmune Pharmacol, 1*, 400–409.

Geiser, F., Meier, C., Wegener, I., Imbierowicz, K., Conrad, R. et al (2008). Association between anxiety and factors of coagulation and fibrinolysis. *Psychother Psychosom, 77*, 377–383.

Glaser, R., MacCallum, R. C., Laskowski, B. F., Malarkey, W. B., Sheridan, J. F. et al (2001). Evidence for a shift in the Th-1 to Th-2 cytokine response associated with chronic stress and aging. *J Gerontol A Biol Sci Med Sci, 56*, M477-M482.

Goebel, M. U., and Mills, P. J. (2000). Acute psychological stress and exercise and changes in peripheral leukocyte adhesion molecule expression and density. *Psychosom Med, 62*, 664–670.

Goshen, I., and Yirmiya, R. (2009). Interleukin-1 (IL-1): a central regulator of stress responses. *Front Neuroendocrinol, 30*, 30–45.

Himmerich, H., Fulda, S., Linseisen, J., Seiler, H., Wolfram, G. et al (2006). TNF-alpha, soluble TNF receptor and interleukin-6 plasma levels in the general population. *Eur Cytokine Netw, 17*, 196–201.

Jain, S., Mills, P. J., von Kanel, R., Hong, S., and Dimsdale, J. E. (2007). Effects of perceived stress and uplifts on inflammation and coagulability. *Psychophysiology, 44*, 154–160.

Kangas, M., Bovbjerg, D. H., and Montgomery, G. H. (2008). Cancer-related fatigue: a systematic and meta-analytic review of non-pharmacological therapies for cancer patients. *Psychol Bull, 134*, 700–741.

Kariagina, A., Romanenko, D., Ren, S. G., and Chesnokova, V. (2004). Hypothalamic-pituitary cytokine network. *Endocrinology, 145*, 104–112.

Kelley, K. W., Bluthe, R. M., Dantzer, R., Zhou, J. H., Shen, W. H. et al (2003). Cytokine-induced sickness behavior. *Brain Behav Immun 17*(Suppl 1), S112–S118.

Kiecolt-Glaser, J. K., Marucha, P. T., Malarkey, W. B., Mercado, A. M., and Glaser, R. (1995). Slowing of wound healing by psychological stress. *Lancet, 346*, 1194–1196.

Kiecolt-Glaser, J. K., Preacher, K. J., MacCallum, R. C., Atkinson, C., Malarkey, W. B. et al (2003). Chronic stress and age-related increases in the proinflammatory cytokine IL-6. *Proc Natl Acad Sci USA, 100*, 9090–9095.

Kobayashi, T., Takaku, Y., Yokote, A., Miyazawa, H., Soma, T. et al (2008). Interferon-beta augments eosinophil adhesion-inducing activity of endothelial cells. *Eur Respir J, 32*, 1540–1547.

Kop, W. J., Weissman, N. J., Zhu, J., Bonsall, R. W., Doyle, M. et al (2008). Effects of acute mental stress and exercise on inflammatory markers in patients with coronary artery disease and healthy controls. *Am J Cardiol, 101*, 767–773.

Liu, L., Fiorentino, L., Natarajan, L., Parker, B. A., Mills, P. J. et al (2009). Pre-treatment symptom cluster in breast cancer patients is associated with worse sleep, fatigue and depression during chemotherapy. *Psychooncology, 18*, 187–194.

Linden, W., Stossel, C., and Maurice, J. (1996). Psychosocial interventions for patients with coronary artery disease: a meta-analysis. *Arch Intern Med, 156*, 745–752.

Lowe, G. D., Rumley, A., Whincup, P. H., and Danesh, J. (2002). Hemostatic and rheological variables and risk of cardiovascular disease. *Semin Vasc Med, 2*, 429–439.

Miller, M. A., Skeen, M. J., Lavine, C. L., and Kirk Ziegler, H. (2003). IL-12-assisted immunization generates CD4+ T cell-mediated immunity to Listeria monocytogenes. *Cell Immunol, 222*, 1–14.

Mills, P. J., Ancoli-Israel, S., Kanel, R. V., Mausbach, B. T., Aschbacher, K. et al (2008). Effects of gender and dementia severity on Alzheimer's disease caregivers' sleep and biomarkers of coagulation and inflammation. *Brain Behav Immun.*

Mills, P. J., Parker, B., Dimsdale, J. E., Sadler, G. R., and Ancoli-Israel, S. (2005). The relationship between fatigue and quality of life and inflammation during anthracycline-based chemotherapy in breast cancer. *Biol Psychol, 69*, 85–96.

Mills, P. J., Parker, B., Jones, V., Adler, K. A., Perez, C. J. et al (2004). The effects of standard anthracycline-based chemotherapy on soluble ICAM-1 and vascular endothelial growth factor levels in breast cancer. *Clin Cancer Res, 10*, 4998–5003.

Mills, P. J., Yu, H., Ziegler, M. G., Patterson, T., and Grant, I. (1999). Vulnerable caregivers of patients with Alzheimer's disease have a deficit in circulating CD62L- T lymphocytes. *Psychosom Med, 61*, 168–174.

Muller, N., and Schwarz, M. J. (2007). The immune-mediated alteration of serotonin and glutamate: towards an integrated view of depression. *Mol Psychiatry, 12*, 988–1000.

O'Brien, S. M., Scott, L. V., and Dinan, T. G. (2004). Cytokines: abnormalities in major depression and implications for pharmacological treatment. *Hum Psychopharmacol, 19*, 397–403.

Opp, M. R. (2005). Cytokines and sleep. *Sleep Med Rev, 9*, 355–364.

Path, G., Scherbaum, W. A., and Bornstein, S. R. (2000). The role of interleukin-6 in the human adrenal gland. *Eur J Clin Invest 30*(Suppl 3), 91–95.

Patten, S. B. (2006). Psychiatric side effects of interferon treatment. *Curr Drug Saf, 1*, 143–150.

Petersen, A. M., and Pedersen, B. K. (2005). The anti-inflammatory effect of exercise. *J Appl Physiol, 98*, 1154–1162.

Radi, Z. A., Kehrli, M. E., Jr., and Ackermann, M. R. (2001). Cell adhesion molecules, leukocyte trafficking, and strategies to reduce leukocyte infiltration. *J Vet Intern Med*, 15, 516–529.

Rose-John, S. (2003). Interleukin-6 biology is coordinated by membrane bound and soluble receptors. *Acta Biochim Pol*, 50, 603–611.

Rutledge, T., Reis, V. A., Linke, S. E., Greenberg, B. H., and Mills, P. J. (2006). Depression in heart failure a meta-analytic review of prevalence, intervention effects, and associations with clinical outcomes. *J Am Coll Cardiol*, 48, 1527–1537.

Schiller, M., Metze, D., Luger, T. A., Grabbe, S., and Gunzer, M. (2006). Immune response modifiers – mode of action. *Exp Dermatol*, 15, 331–341.

Schneider, R. H., Alexander, C. N., Staggers, F., Rainforth, M., Salerno, J. W. et al (2005). Long-term effects of stress reduction on mortality in persons > or = 55 years of age with systemic hypertension. *Am J Cardiol*, 95, 1060–1064.

Simmons, D. A., and Broderick, P. A. (2005). Cytokines, stressors, and clinical depression: augmented adaptation responses underlie depression pathogenesis. *Prog Neuropsychopharmacol Biol Psychiatry*, 29, 793–807.

Steptoe, A., Hamer, M., and Chida, Y. (2007). The effects of acute psychological stress on circulating inflammatory factors in humans: a review and meta-analysis. *Brain Behav Immun*, 21, 901–912.

Strike, P. C., Magid, K., Brydon, L., Edwards, S., McEwan, J. R. et al (2004). Exaggerated platelet and hemodynamic reactivity to mental stress in men with coronary artery disease. *Psychosom Med*, 66, 492–500.

Tracey, D., Klareskog, L., Sasso, E. H., Salfeld, J. G., and Tak, P. P. (2008). Tumor necrosis factor antagonist mechanisms of action: a comprehensive review. *Pharmacol Ther*, 117, 244–279.

Tracey, K. J. (2007). Physiology and immunology of the cholinergic antiinflammatory pathway. *J Clin Invest*, 117, 289–296.

Vgontzas, A. N., Bixler, E. O., Lin, H. M., Prolo, P., Trakada, G. et al (2005). IL-6 and its circadian secretion in humans. *Neuroimmunomodulation*, 12, 131–140.

Vgontzas, A. N., Papanicolaou, D. A., Bixler, E. O., Hopper, K., Lotsikas, A. et al (2000). Sleep apnea and daytime sleepiness and fatigue: relation to visceral obesity, insulin resistance, and hypercytokinemia. *J Clin Endocrinol Metab*, 85, 1151–1158.

Vgontzas, A. N., Zoumakis, M., Bixler, E. O., Lin, H. M., Prolo, P. et al (2003). Impaired nighttime sleep in healthy old versus young adults is associated with elevated plasma interleukin-6 and cortisol levels: physiologic and therapeutic implications. *J Clin Endocrinol Metab*, 88, 2087–2095.

von Känel, R., and Dimsdale, J. E. (2000). Effects of sympathetic activation by adrenergic infusions on hemostasis in vivo. *Eur J Haematol*, 65, 357–369.

von Känel, R., Mills, P. J., Fainman, C., and Dimsdale, J. E. (2001). Effects of psychological stress and psychiatric disorders on blood coagulation and fibrinolysis: a biobehavioral pathway to coronary artery disease? *Psychosom Med*, 63, 531–544.

von Känel, R., and Dimsdale, J. E. (2003). Fibrin D-dimer: a marker of psychosocial distress and its implications for research in stress-related coronary artery disease. *Clin Cardiol*, 26, 164–168.

von Känel, R., Dimsdale, J. E., Patterson, T. L., and Grant, I. (2003) Association of negative life event stress with coagulation activity in elderly Alzheimer caregivers. *Psychosom Med*, 65, 145–150.

von Känel, R. (2004). Platelet hyperactivity in clinical depression and the beneficial effect of antidepressant drug treatment: how strong is the evidence? *Acta Psychiatr Scand*, 110, 163–177.

von Känel, R., Preckel, D., Zgraggen, L., Mischler, K., Kudielka, B. M. et al (2004a). The effect of natural habituation on coagulation responses to acute mental stress and recovery in men. *Thromb Haemost*, 92, 1327–1335.

von Känel, R., Dimsdale, J. E., Adler, K. A., Patterson, T. L., Mills, P. J. et al (2004b). Effects of depressive symptoms and anxiety on hemostatic responses to acute mental stress and recovery in the elderly. *Psychiatry Res*, 126, 253–264.

von Känel, R., Kudielka, B. M., Schulze, R., Gander, M. L., and Fischer, J. E. (2004c). Hypercoagulability in working men and women with high levels of panic-like anxiety. *Psychother Psychosom*, 73, 353–360.

von Känel, R., Frey, K., and Fischer, J. (2004d). Independent relation of vital exhaustion and inflammation to fibrinolysis in apparently healthy subjects. *Scand Cardiovasc J*, 38, 28–32.

von Känel, R., Kudielka, B. M., Abd-el-Razik, A., Gander, M. L., Frey, K., and Fischer, J. E. (2004e). Relationship between overnight neuroendocrine activity and morning haemostasis in working men. *Clin Sci*, 107, 89–95.

von Känel, R., Dimsdale, J. E., Mills, P. J., Ancoli-Israel, S., Patterson, T. L. et al (2006a). Effect of Alzheimer caregiving stress and age on frailty markers interleukin-6, C-reactive protein, and D-dimer. *J Gerontol A Biol Sci Med Sci*, 61, 963–969.

von Känel, R., Kudielka, B. M., Preckel, D., Hanebuth, D., and Fischer, J. E. (2006b). Delayed response and lack of habituation in plasma interleukin-6 to acute mental stress in men. *Brain Behav Immun*, 20, 40–48.

von Känel, R., and Orth-Gomèr, K. (2008). Autonomic function and prothrombotic activity in women after an acute coronary event. *J Womens Health*, 17, 1331–1337.

von Känel, R., Mausbach, B. T., Kudielka, B. M., and Orth-Gomèr, K. (2008) Relation of morning serum cortisol to prothrombotic activity in women with stable coronary artery disease. *J Thromb Thrombolysis, 25*, 165–172.

von Känel, R., Bellingrath, S., and Kudielka, B. M. (2009a). Association of vital exhaustion and depressive symptoms with changes in fibrin D-dimer to acute psychosocial stress. *J Psychosom Res* (in press).

von Känel, R., Bellingrath, S., and Kudielka, B. M. (2009b). Overcommitment but not effort-reward imbalance relates to stress-induced coagulation changes in teachers. *Ann Behav Med, 37*, 20–28.

von Känel, R., Bellingrath, S., and Kudielka, B. M. (2009c). Association between longitudinal changes in depressive symptoms and plasma fibrinogen levels in school teachers. *Psychophysiology* (in press).

von Känel, R., Thayer, J. F., and Fischer, J. E. (2009d). Night-time vagal cardiac control and plasma fibrinogen levels in a population of working men and women. *Ann Noninvasive Electrocardiol* (in press).

Witek-Janusek, L., Albuquerque, K., Chroniak, K. R., Chroniak, C., Durazo-Arvizu, R. et al (2008). Effect of mindfulness based stress reduction on immune function, quality of life and coping in women newly diagnosed with early stage breast cancer. *Brain Behav Immun, 22*, 969–981.

Yang, K., Xie, G., Zhang, Z., Wang, C., Li, W. et al (2007a). Levels of serum interleukin (IL)-6, IL-1beta, tumour necrosis factor-alpha and leptin and their correlation in depression. *Aust N Z J Psychiatry, 41*, 266–273.

Yang, M. S., Min, K. J., and Joe, E. (2007b). Multiple mechanisms that prevent excessive brain inflammation. *J Neurosci Res, 85*, 2298–2305.

Chapter 46

The Metabolic Syndrome, Obesity, and Insulin Resistance

Armando J. Mendez, Ronald B. Goldberg, and Philip M. McCabe

A major worldwide health issue is the dramatic increase in the prevalence of overweight and obese individuals. According to the World Health Organization (WHO, 2006), globally there are over 1.6 billion overweight adults, with approximately 400 million of them obese, and it is projected that by 2015 approximately 2.3 billion adults will be overweight and over 700 million obese. In the United States, the prevalence of obesity has more than doubled from 15% of the adult population in 1973–1976 to 34% in 2003–2006 (National Center for Health Statistics, 2008a), while the proportion of overweight individuals has remained relatively unchanged over the same period at approximately one-third of the population. During the same time period the incidence of overweight and obese children in the United States aged 2–5 years old has also more than doubled from 5 to 11%, but remained relatively constant in older children (approximately 17%). Increased ponderosity places individuals at risk for chronic diseases, including type 2 diabetes, cardiovascular disease (CVD), hypertension, stroke, and certain forms of cancer, which are morbidities that are likely to increase as individuals become overweight earlier in life.

It is thought that the major causes of the obesity epidemic are increased consumption of energy-dense foods high in saturated fats and sugars and reduced physical activity. Obesity is interrelated with a cluster of metabolic variables including insulin resistance, impaired glucose tolerance, dyslipidemia, and hypertension (Cornier et al, 2008) that when present together has been referred to as the metabolic syndrome. It has been shown that the metabolic syndrome can increase the risk of type 2 diabetes and CVD and that lifestyle interventions designed to reduce body weight, increase physical activity, and attenuate the metabolic syndrome components are associated with reductions in the incidence of disease.

1 Defining the Metabolic Syndrome

The first broadly utilized definition of the metabolic syndrome evolved from the work of Reaven (1988) who described a group or clustering of metabolic abnormalities associated with insulin resistance including glucose intolerance, hyperinsulinemia, dyslipidemia, and hypertension. Several refinements have been proposed in the definition of the metabolic syndrome, which has also been referred to as syndrome X, metabolic syndrome X, insulin resistance syndrome, and cardiometabolic syndrome. Although differences exist in the definitions used (see below), the major utility of the metabolic syndrome classification has been to identify persons with increased risk of future cardiovascular and/or diabetic complications. Diagnosis of

P.M. McCabe (✉)
Department of Psychology, University of Miami, P.O. Box 248185, Coral Gables, FL 33124, USA
e-mail: pmccabe@miami.edu

A. Steptoe (ed.), *Handbook of Behavioral Medicine*, DOI 10.1007/978-0-387-09488-5_46,
© Springer Science+Business Media, LLC 2010

the metabolic syndrome should initiate management of the condition, primarily through lifestyle interventions, to reduce future CVD and diabetes risk.

There are several published definitions of the metabolic syndrome, and while similar, each specifies distinct criteria. The WHO published its definition of the metabolic syndrome in 1998 (Alberti and Zimmet, 1998). In this report, impaired glucose tolerance (IGT), insulin resistance, or frank diabetes are required, in addition to two of the four other components that include increased body weight, elevated triglycerides, reduced HDL cholesterol (HDL-C), and hypertension or presence of microalbuminuria as a marker of vascular dysfunction (Table 46.1). Determination of insulin resistance, measured by the euglycemic clamp method, made this definition of the metabolic syndrome difficult to use in clinical practice or in epidemiological

studies. The WHO report identified the need for a clearer description of the essential components of the syndrome and further research to support the relative contribution of each component. Importantly, it was recognized that insulin resistance may be the common etiology affecting the other components defining the metabolic syndrome. Also noted was the increased risk of CVD imposed by the presence of multiple metabolic syndrome components. The report also discussed management of traditional CVD risk factors and hyperglycemia.

Subsequent to the WHO definition of the metabolic syndrome, the National Cholesterol Education Panel/Adult Treatment Panel III (ATP III) published its definition of the metabolic syndrome in 2001 (ATP III, 2001) and later modified this definition in 2004 after the National Heart, Lung, and Blood Institute (NHLBI) and the American Heart Association (AHA)

Table 46.1 Definitions and criteria of metabolic syndrome

	WHO (1998)	ATP III (2005)	IDF (2005)
Required criteria	IGT, IFG, type 2 diabetes, or insulin resistance plus any two additional components	Any three components	Increased waist circumference, plus any two additional components
Body weight/adiposity	Waist to hip ratio: Men >0.9 Women >0.85	Waist circumference Men ≥102 cm Women ≥88 cm	Gender and ethnicity-specific values for increased waist circumference
Blood pressure	≥ 140/90 mmHg	≥130 mmHg systolic ≥85 mmHg diastolic	≥130 mmHg systolic ≥85 mmHg diastolic
Hyperglycemia	IGT (fasting Glu < 126 and 2 h ≥ 140 and <200) or IFG (fasting Glu ≥ 110) or type 2 diabetes (fasting Glu ≥126 or insulin resistance	Fasting Glu ≥ 100 mg/dl or Rx for glucose or diabetes	Fasting Glu ≥100 mg/dl or diabetes
Triglycerides	>150 mg/dl	>150 mg/dl or TG lowering Rx	>150 mg/dl or TG lowering Rx
HDL cholesterol	Men <35 mg/dl Women <39 mg/dl	Men <40 mg/dl Women <50 mg/dl or HDL raising Rx	Men <40 mg/dl Women <50 mg/dl or HDL raising Rx
Other	Microalbuminuria	None	None

Adapted from Alberti and Zimmet (1998); Grundy et al (2004); Zimmet et al (2005)
Abbreviations: IGT, impaired glucose tolerance; IFG, impaired fasting glucose; Glu, glucose; TG, triglycerides; Rx, prescription

cosponsored a workshop to address issues raised by the cardiovascular and diabetes communities (Grundy et al, 2004a, b). In contrast to the WHO criteria, ATP III had no requirement that IGT or insulin resistance must exist for a subject to be classified as having the metabolic syndrome, but acknowledged the central role that insulin resistance holds in the syndrome. Instead, the diagnosis of the metabolic syndrome requires (see Table 46.1) that any three of the five identified risk components be present (increased waist circumference, elevated triglycerides, reduced HDL cholesterol, elevated blood pressure, or elevated fasting glucose). Another new approach offered in the ATP III definition was the incorporation of an abdominal index of obesity, rather than a generalized index because of data indicating greater predictive value of waist circumference over body mass index (BMI) for diabetes and CVD. The overall outcome of the 2004 workshop was to affirm the utility of the original ATP III guidelines with minor modification and clarifications. These included allowing for a lower waist circumference threshold for ethnic groups or individuals prone to insulin resistance and allowing for triglyceride, HDL cholesterol, and blood pressure to be counted as abnormal when an individual is on drug therapy for these conditions. Also, the threshold for elevated fasting glucose was lowered from ≥ 110 to ≥ 100, as recommended by the American Diabetes Association (but not WHO) revised definition of impaired fasting glucose (American Diabetes Association, 2002). Within the context of ATP III, the metabolic syndrome is considered a secondary target for treatment to reduce risk of CVD, with the recognition that the presence of any metabolic syndrome components increases CVD risk. The risk is even greater when three or more components are present (Klein et al, 2002; Knuiman et al, 2009; Sattar et al, 2003). It was also suggested in the ATP III guidelines that individual risk for CVD be assessed based on the Framingham Risk Assessment (Wilson et al, 1998).

The International Diabetes Federation (IDF) published its definition of the metabolic syndrome in 2005 (Zimmet et al, 2005). This definition emphasized central obesity, determined by gender and ethnic-specific values for waist circumference, as a required component. In addition, two other components were required for the metabolic syndrome diagnosis using similar criteria to ATP III (Table 46.1). While the role of insulin resistance was acknowledged as an important component associated with the metabolic syndrome, it was omitted as a criterion because of the difficulties in measuring insulin resistance accurately. The IDF consensus group also recommended additional metabolic criteria should be included in future research studies that might allow for future modification of the metabolic syndrome definition. These criteria include body fat distribution, atherogenic dyslipidemia, dysglycemia, direct measures of insulin resistance, vascular function, proinflammatory status, prothrombotic status, and hormonal factors.

The metabolic syndrome definitions described above are the most widely used in epidemiological studies, but others have been proposed. The European group on insulin resistance (EGIR) proposed a modified WHO definition of the metabolic syndrome (Balkau and Charles, 1999), but termed it insulin resistance syndrome (IRS), with the main assumption being that insulin resistance is the major cause of the metabolic dysregulation. By their criteria, IRS was defined as the presence of insulin resistance (measured as plasma insulin levels in the upper quartile of the population) and at least two other components (increased waist circumference, dyslipidemia, hypertension, or glycemia). The major purpose for developing these criteria was to identify risk factors for diabetes, and thus EGIR excluded subjects from the IRS diagnosis who already had type 2 diabetes.

The American Association of Clinical Endocrinologists (AACE) in 2003 used modified ATP III guidelines to define IRS (Einhorn et al, 2003). This diagnosis required the presence of insulin resistance (measured as impaired fasting glucose or impaired glucose tolerance) and additional components based on clinical judgment. The purpose of the AACE definition of insulin resistance syndrome was for identification of individuals at risk and to provide early and more aggressive lifestyle intervention for prevention of disease consequences. Similar to the EGIR, subjects with type 2 diabetes were excluded from the diagnosis.

Recently, the IDF, NHLBI, AHA, World Heart Federation, International Atherosclerosis Society, and International Association for the Study of Obesity proposed a common set of criteria for the clinical diagnosis of the metabolic syndrome (Alberti et al, 2009). This joint statement now recognizes that obesity (defined by waist circumference) should not be a prerequisite for the diagnosis, but that it represents one of five criteria, with the presence of any three criteria fulfilling the diagnosis of metabolic syndrome. This new consensus definition is very similar to the modified ATP III definition (Table 46.1) with the exception that the elevated waist circumference is both population and country specific.

Application of the metabolic syndrome criteria in children and adolescents requires modification of the adult criteria, and several studies have attempted to define childhood metabolic syndrome (e.g., Lambert et al, 2004; Rodriguez-Morín et al, 2004; Weiss et al, 2004). Reported prevalence of the metabolic syndrome in pediatric populations varies, and in general is low (below 10%); however, among obese children prevalence exceeds 30%. Recently, the IDF published its definition of the metabolic syndrome in children and adolescents (Zimmet et al, 2007). For children between the ages of 6 and 10 years old, the metabolic syndrome is defined as the presence of obesity (waist circumference $\geq$90th percentile). For children and adolescents between the ages of 10 and 16 years old, the metabolic syndrome is defined as the presence of obesity (waist circumference $\geq$90th percentile) and the adult criteria for triglycerides, HDL-C, blood pressure, and glucose. For youths over 16 years of age, the panel recommends using the existing IDF criteria for adults. More recently, the AHA published a scientific statement of childhood metabolic syndrome (Steinberger et al, 2009) that examines the issues related to metabolic and cardiovascular risk factors within a pediatric population. This statement identifies areas of research that require further investigation within this population so that lifestyle modification and medication may be used to reduce future CVD risk.

Although the metabolic syndrome has gained wide acceptance, there is some controversy concerning its diagnostic utility and its use for evaluating CVD and diabetes risk (Eckel et al, 2006; Greenland, 2005; Johnson and Weinstock, 2006; Kahn et al, 2005; Nilsson, 2007; Reaven, 2005, 2006, 2007; Service, 2003; Stern et al, 2004). It has been suggested that the cluster of metabolic components in the metabolic syndrome represents already known and established risk factors for CVD. Furthermore, it has been argued that the risk associated with the presence of the metabolic syndrome is no greater than the additive risk of any individual component. Regardless of the diagnosis, however, multiple CVD risk factors might still be present and therefore it is unlikely that clinical management would be affected. Questions have also arisen regarding the reliability and/or lack of data, especially from longitudinal studies, to support the cutoff values used for each of the metabolic syndrome components that are continuous variables. It was also noted that among the various definitions of the metabolic syndrome, there is inherent imprecision by which each of the criteria is defined. For example, there are no specific guidelines for how blood pressure measurements should be taken (sitting, supine, resting prior to measurement), and there are no clear criteria in determining cutoff values for waist circumference depending on ethnicity, as stated by the IDF (Zimmet et al, 2005) and commented on in the ATP III workshop (Grundy et al, 2004a).

Of central relevance to these arguments is the strong association of the metabolic syndrome components with insulin resistance. Evidence also suggests that insulin resistance per se can directly affect metabolic dysfunction and can significantly account for most of the CVD and type 2 diabetes risk attributed to the metabolic syndrome. For example, it has been shown that insulin resistance is strongly associated with hyperglycemia (Abdul-Ghani et al, 2008;

Godsland et al, 2004; Reaven et al, 1993), hypertension (Ferrannini et al, 1987; Kaplan, 1991), and dyslipidemia (Haffner et al, 1988; Orchard et al, 1983; Zavaroni et al, 1985). This debate is ongoing and beyond the scope of the current chapter; however, awareness of this ongoing discussion is essential to the evaluation and interpretation of data related to the metabolic syndrome.

2 Epidemiology of Obesity and the Metabolic Syndrome

Based on measures of BMI, it was reported (National Center for Health Statistics, 2008b; Steinberger et al, 2009) that 32.7% of US adults over the age of 20 are overweight (BMI 25.0–29.9), 34.3% are obese (BMI ≥ 30.0), and 5.9% are extremely obese (BMI ≥ 40.0). Although the prevalence of overweight Americans has remained stable since 1980, the prevalence of obesity in adults has more than doubled during that time period. Among ethnic groups, 45% of non-Hispanic black adults and 36.8% of Mexican Americans were obese, whereas approximately 30% of non-Hispanic white adults were obese. It was also reported that 17.1% of US children and adolescents are overweight; a figure that has tripled since 1980 (Ogden et al, 2006).

The prevalence of the metabolic syndrome is also increasing in the United States and throughout the world; however, the prevalence estimates depend upon the definition of the syndrome used. In addition, factors such as gender, ethnicity, and age greatly affect prevalence, as well as socioeconomic status and lifestyle habits (Cornier et al, 2008). Estimates of metabolic syndrome prevalence across all Americans have varied between 24 and 39% (Cornier et al, 2008), but it has been pointed out that this global statistic may not be useful because the prevalence of the metabolic syndrome increases dramatically with age (Cassells and Haffner, 2006; Ogden et al, 2006). The metabolic syndrome

prevalence increases with each decade of life, paralleling age-related increases in obesity and central adiposity and based on National Health and Nutrition Examination Survey (NHANES) data, reaches 50–60% by 60–69 years of age (Cornier et al, 2008). Metabolic syndrome prevalence is highest in Hispanics and lowest in African Americans, but the low prevalence in African Americans may be an artifact of the definition of the syndrome used (Cassells and Haffner, 2006).

Type 2 diabetes affects more than 7% of the population in the United States and is most prevalent in the elderly and in specific ethnic groups, such as Hispanics, African Americans, and American Indians (Crandall et al, 2008). Diabetes is often accompanied by many long-term health complications, and individuals with type 2 diabetes have a two- to fourfold increase in risk of developing CVD and stroke. The prevalence of the metabolic syndrome is high in individuals with type 2 diabetes, which is not surprising since glucose concentration is an important factor in the metabolic syndrome, and most diabetic individuals have waist circumferences that exceed the criterion for the metabolic syndrome (Cassells and Haffner, 2006). Based on NHANES data, it was reported that in diabetic patients over the age of 50, the prevalence of the metabolic syndrome is 85% (Alexander et al, 2003). It has been pointed out, however, that obesity, the metabolic syndrome, and insulin resistance do not always go hand-in-hand. Overweight/obese individuals can be insulin sensitive and normal weight subjects can be insulin resistant (Abbasi et al, 2002), which emphasizes the complex relationship among these variables.

3 Lifestyle Modification of the Metabolic Syndrome, Type 2 Diabetes, and CVD

Given the accumulating evidence that metabolic variables play an important role in type 2 diabetes, a number of randomized clinical trials (RCTs) have been conducted around the world to examine whether behavioral interventions can influence the progression of this disease. More specifically, it was hypothesized that weight loss and/or increased physical activity or exercise may favorably alter metabolic processes, thereby preventing type 2 diabetes. In addition, several follow-up studies have examined whether these lifestyle modifications also influence preclinical markers of morbidity and mortality due to CVD. Although there have also been long-term lifestyle intervention trials to treat hypertension, and shorter term trials directed at dyslipidemia, as yet there is no evidence that lifestyle interventions for the metabolic syndrome prevent CVD.

The first of these RCTs was conducted in China beginning in 1986 (Pan et al, 1997). Over 100,000 men and women from health clinics in the city of Daqing were screened for impaired glucose tolerance and type 2 diabetes. Using WHO criteria, 557 subjects were determined to have impaired glucose tolerance and subsequently were randomized into one of the four conditions: control, diet only, exercise only, or diet-plus-exercise. The goal of the diet intervention was to promote vegetable intake and lower alcohol and sugar consumption. Overweight subjects were encouraged to lose weight by reducing total caloric intake. The goal of the exercise intervention was to increase leisure time physical activity. Follow-up examinations were conducted every 2 years over a 6-year period to determine the incidence of type 2 diabetes. Over the 6-year follow-up period, the cumulative incidence of diabetes was 67.7% for the control group compared to 43.8% in the diet group, 41.1% in the exercise group, and 46.0% in the diet-plus-exercise group. A proportional hazards analysis, adjusted for differences in baseline body mass index and fasting glucose, revealed the three intervention groups were associated with 31% (diet), 46% (exercise), and 42% (diet-plus-exercise) reductions in risk of developing diabetes. It was concluded that all three lifestyle interventions were equally effective in preventing diabetes; however, the relationship between the amount of weight lost and the incidence of

diabetes was inconsistent. Recently, a 20-year follow-up study found that these interventions over a 6-year period prevented or delayed the onset of diabetes for up to 14 years after the active intervention (Li et al, 2008); however, the influence of the lifestyle modifications on first CVD events, CVD mortality, and all-cause mortality was inconclusive.

The Finnish Diabetes Prevention Study was an RCT conducted on 522 middle-aged, overweight men and women with impaired glucose tolerance (Tuomilehto et al, 2001). The intervention group received individualized counseling to reduce weight, total fat intake, and saturated fat intake, while increasing fiber consumption and physical activity. Annual follow-up exams included OGTT to assess the presence of diabetes, and the mean duration of follow-up was 3.2 years. The intervention group lost a significant amount of body weight compared to the control group over each of the first 2 years of the study, and the cumulative incidence of diabetes after 4 years in the intervention group was 11 and 23% in the control group. The risk of developing diabetes was reduced by 58% in the intervention group, which was directly associated with changes in lifestyle. A subsequent post hoc analysis focusing specifically on leisure time physical activity in these subjects found that increased physical activity reduced the incidence of type 2 diabetes in high-risk individuals (Laaksonen et al, 2005).

An extended follow-up of the Finnish Diabetes Prevention Study (Lindstrom et al, 2006) assessed the extent to which lifestyle changes and risk reduction persisted following the termination of the counseling intervention. Three years following the 4-year intervention, there was still a 43% reduction in the relative risk for diabetes in the intervention group. This reduction in risk was related to reaching intervention goals (i.e., weight loss, reduced intake of total and saturated fat, increased dietary fiber, and physical activity). A recent study (Herder et al, 2009) reported that the lifestyle intervention reduced subclinical inflammatory markers at the 1-year follow-up of the Finnish Diabetes Prevention Study; however, a separate follow-up study (Herder et al, 2009; Uusitupa et al, 2009) did not find a significant decrease in the 10-year mortality and CVD morbidity due to the lifestyle intervention.

The largest RCT to assess the potential benefits of lifestyle modification on diabetes was the US Diabetes Prevention Program (DPP; Knowler et al, 2002). In this RCT 3234 subjects who were non-diabetic but had elevated fasting glucose and impaired glucose tolerance were randomly assigned to placebo, lifestyle modification, or metformin (an antihyperglycemic drug) groups. The lifestyle intervention was designed to achieve a 7% weight loss across 24 weeks, and subjects in this group were instructed (and periodically counseled) to perform 150 min per week of moderate intensity physical activity and to consume a low-fat, reduced calorie diet. With an average follow-up time of 2.8 years, it was reported that the incidence of diabetes was 11.0% in the placebo group, 4.8% in the lifestyle modification group, and 7.8% in the metformin group. The lifestyle modification reduced the incidence of disease by 58% compared to placebo, whereas the metformin intervention only reduced diabetes by 31%. It was concluded that although both interventions reduced the incidence of diabetes, the lifestyle modification was significantly more effective than the pharmacological intervention.

A subsequent DPP follow-up study (Orchard et al, 2005) examined the prevalence of the metabolic syndrome at baseline and as a result of the lifestyle modification and metformin intervention. It was reported that at baseline 53% of study participants were determined to have had the metabolic syndrome (defined as three or more characteristics that met criteria from the ATP III). With a mean follow-up time of 3.2 years, the incidence of the metabolic syndrome was reduced by 41% in the lifestyle modification group and by 17% in the metformin treated group. Another DPP follow-up study (Hamman et al, 2006) determined that weight loss was the predominate predictor of the incidence of diabetes. For every kilogram of body weight loss there was a 16% reduction in risk. Increased physical activity helped to maintain weight loss,

and among the subjects who did not achieve the weight loss goal at the end of 1 year, those who met the exercise goal also had 44% less diabetes incidence. The DPP lifestyle intervention was equally effective in all ethnic groups and genders, but was greatest in older participants (Crandall et al, 2008). Lifestyle intervention also prevented increase in blood pressure, lowered triglycerides, LDL density, and CRP levels and raised HDL-C significantly compared to the placebo and metformin groups (Haffner et al, 2005; Ratner et al, 2005). The effectiveness of lifestyle modification on diabetes incidence has also been demonstrated in clinical trials in Japan (Kosaka et al, 2005) and India (Ramachandran et al, 2006), emphasizing the generalizability of these behavioral interventions across ethnic groups.

4 Pathophysiology of the Metabolic Syndrome

No specific etiology is known to account for the metabolic syndrome, nevertheless, subjects with the syndrome exhibit a variety of metabolic abnormalities associated with the individual components of the syndrome. Most notable are obesity and insulin dysregulation, which are the most frequently occurring metabolic syndrome components (Ervin, 2009). Multiple metabolic abnormalities could additively or synergistically influence the progression of CVD and diabetes.

Insulin resistance may be characterized by impaired glucose tolerance and elevated fasting glucose due to reduced insulin action. In the insulin-sensitive state, insulin not only affects glucose metabolism but also suppresses adipose tissue lipolysis. In overweight or obese individuals, increased adiposity results in elevated circulating free fatty acids (FFA) due to higher rates of triglyceride lipolysis, mediated primarily by the inability of insulin to suppress triglyceride lipolysis through the action of hormone sensitive lipase and reduced expression of adipose triglyceride lipase (Jocken et al, 2007).

Increased circulating FFA has been hypothesized to lead to tissue-specific lipotoxicity (Kusminski et al, 2009; Unger, 2003). Elevated FFA levels inhibit insulin-stimulated skeletal muscle glucose uptake and increase hepatic glucose production (Boden, 1999), thus contributing to peripheral insulin resistance. Further, the increase in FFA levels promotes increased hepatic triglyceride synthesis and storage, and the excess triglycerides are secreted as very low-density lipoproteins (VLDL) (Lewis, 1997), which lead to an increased production of LDL. Elevated plasma triglycerides are inversely correlated with HDL-C levels (Austin, 1989), which is thought to occur by the action of cholesteryl ester transfer protein (Sandhofer et al, 2006). This leads to smaller, triglyceride-rich HDL particles with higher catabolic rate due to increased renal clearance, which results in reduced HDL levels (Ji et al, 2006). In similar fashion, elevated triglyceride levels lead to formation of atherogenic small, dense LDL particles which are more slowly cleared by the LDL receptor and thus tend to accumulate (Kwiterovich, Jr., 2002). Therefore, increased adiposity through increased FFA flux, and compounded by insulin resistance, contributes to the dyslipidemia associated with metabolic syndrome. In muscle, increased FFA levels inhibit insulin-mediated glucose transport activity (McGarry, 2002), affecting peripheral glucose uptake (contributing to IGT) and eventually leading to hyperglycemia. Additionally, excess FFA levels result in an increase of myocyte triglyceride levels that have been shown to directly affect insulin resistance in the muscle (Krssak et al, 1999). Increased levels of FFA have also been shown to mediate vasoconstriction and activate the sympathetic nervous system (SNS), potentially contributing to hypertension and atherogenesis (Grekin et al, 1995; Tripathy et al, 2003). The consequences of increased adiposity can influence many of the metabolic syndrome components directly and contribute to, or exacerbate, the insulin-resistant state.

The SNS plays an important role in both etiology and pathogenesis of the metabolic syndrome and has been linked to an increased risk of CVD. Accumulating evidence suggests that human obesity is characterized by increased SNS activity and decreased cardiac vagal activity, which could contribute to the adverse consequences of the metabolic syndrome (Garruti et al, 2008; Straznicky et al, 2008; Tentolouris et al, 2008). Schneiderman and Skyler (1996) proposed a pathway for atherogenesis that is based on an interactive relation among insulin resistance, hyperinsulinemia, and sympathetic tone. According to this notion, social and emotional factors can interact with insulin-sensitive metabolic variables to promote the development of cardiovascular disease. Several studies have now shown that activation of the sympathoadrenal system inhibits glucose uptake by peripheral tissue and increases hepatic glucose uptake, thus directly impacting insulin resistance and hyperglycemia (Nonogaki, 2000). In hypertension, increased SNS activity may lead to CVD through modifications of heart rate, cardiac output, and renal sodium retention (Grassi, 2006). As mentioned above, stimulation of β-adrenergic receptors increases circulating FFA levels through increased adipose tissue triglyceride lipolysis, which contributes to the dyslipidemia associated with metabolic syndrome and to insulin resistance. Together, these observations suggest a direct role for SNS dysfunction in adverse outcomes associated with the metabolic syndrome. Still undetermined is whether sympathetic dysfunction is involved in the development of, or is a consequence of, the metabolic syndrome.

The metabolic syndrome condition has been described as a proinflammatory state characterized by an excessive release of inflammatory cytokines, accompanied by increased oxidant stress (Cornier et al, 2008). It has been reported that in subjects with the metabolic syndrome, plasma and tissue levels of inflammatory molecules are elevated, including C-reactive protein (CRP), tumor necrosis factor-α (TNF-α), interleukin (IL)-6, IL-1β, IL-18, and resistin (Espinola-Klein et al, 2008; Kowalska et al, 2008; Reilly et al, 2007; You et al, 2008). Increased adiposity contributes directly to cytokine levels by at least two mechanisms. The first involves increased numbers of adipose tissue resident macrophages, and the second direct cytokine production by the adipocytes (Weisberg et al, 2003; Xu et al, 2003). The adipocyte-derived cytokines can subsequently affect insulin action in other tissues and within the adipocyte (Kennedy et al, 2009). IL-6 is produced by both adipose tissue and skeletal muscle, has been shown to be associated with BMI and fasting insulin, and is elevated in subjects with type 2 diabetes (Ruge et al, 2009). IL-6 has been shown to affect insulin action by interfering with insulin receptor signaling, thus contributing to insulin resistance. Elevations of circulating cytokines, particularly TNF-α, can directly cause beta-cell dysfunction contributing to IGT, hyperlipidemia, and diabetes (LeRoith, 2002). Adiponectin, a cytokine released by adipose tissue, acts to sensitize tissues to insulin action and is reduced in individuals with the metabolic syndrome (Hung et al, 2008). Hepatic CRP production is induced by peripheral IL-6 (and other cytokines) and may serve as a relatively stable marker of inflammation and has been shown to be an independent predictor of CVD (Ridker et al, 2003). Population studies have shown that subjects with the metabolic syndrome and elevated CRP have increased risk of CVD relative to subjects with the syndrome and lower CRP levels.

Inflammation, oxidative stress, and dyslipidemia are all factors shown to promote CVD. Inflammatory cytokines induce endothelial dysfunction through expression of endothelial cell surface adhesion molecules, which leads to macrophage infiltration of the vessel wall and initiation of atherogenesis (Libby, 2006). Elevated plasma LDL results in increased transcytosis of LDL through the vessel wall. Intravascular oxidative stress leads to modification of LDL to an oxidized form readily taken up by macrophages and leading to formation of foam cells and fatty streaks, which are the earliest histologic manifestations of atherosclerosis (Ross, 1986). Decreased plasma HDL levels diminishe both the anti-inflammatory and the anti-oxidant properties attributed to this lipoprotein (Movva and Rader, 2008). Additionally, oxidant stress inhibits nitric oxide production,

which impairs vascular reactivity, further contributing to CVD.

5 Assessment of the Metabolic Syndrome and Insulin Resistance

Diagnosis of the metabolic syndrome requires the evaluation of each of the five defined components: insulin resistance and hyperglycemia, elevated triglycerides, reduced HDL-C, blood pressure, and obesity and waist circumference. The methods and considerations for the individual assessments are described in the following section.

5.1 Insulin Resistance and Hyperglycemia

The WHO definition of the metabolic syndrome is the only one that utilizes a measure of insulin resistance as a required component, although elevated fasting glucose levels, specified by the ATP III and IDF definitions, are often associated with an insulin-resistant state. Insulin resistance can be defined as the condition in which normal amounts of insulin are inadequate to produce a normal insulin response from fat, muscle, and liver cells. In mild cases of insulin resistance, increased insulin secretion by pancreatic β cells results in hyperinsulinemia to maintain euglycemia. As insulin resistance worsens, individuals whose increased pancreatic insulin secretion is unable to compensate for the reduced insulin action develop impaired glucose tolerance and hyperglycemia.

The "gold standard" for assessing insulin resistance is the euglycemic insulin clamp method (DeFronzo et al, 1979) and it remains the method to which all other tests of insulin sensitivity are compared. The method (Bergman et al, 1985; Del Prato s et al, 1985; Matsuda and DeFronzo , 1997) involves the administration of exogenous insulin to maintain a constant pre-set hyperinsulinemic level (typically 40–100 μIU/ml). Simultaneously, the plasma glucose concentration is "clamped" at the norm fasting levels by means of an exogenous glucose infusion. Since plasma glucose concentrations are held constant, the glucose infusion rate equals glucose uptake by all the tissues in the body and reflects the tissue sensitivity to exogenous insulin. Technically, the method requires that two intravenous lines be inserted in the subject, one for insulin and glucose infusions and the other for frequent blood sampling to measure glucose levels. Glucose is measured at approximately 5-min intervals and glucose infusion rates are adjusted throughout the study to maintain euglycemia. Infusions are typically maintained for 2 h and insulin sensitivity (or its inverse insulin resistance) is determined from the average glucose infusion rate during the final 40 min when steady-state conditions are assumed. Insulin sensitivity can then be calculated by published methods (Bergman et al, 1985; Del Prato et al, 1985; Matsuda and DeFronzo , 1997).

Because the euglycemic clamp method is expensive, time consuming, and labor intensive, it is mainly used in research settings and is not practical for large population-based studies. Several modifications aimed at simplifying the method and other surrogate assessments have been proposed. The Minimal Model, as described by Bergmann and colleagues (Bergman et al, 1987; Finegood et al, 1984), requires only intravenous administration of glucose. It is less labor intensive than clamp techniques, yet still requires as many as 25 blood samples over 3 h and a computer-assisted mathematical analysis. A later refinement of the Minimal Model utilizes a simplified 12 blood sample method, but still requires intravenous access and 3 h to complete (Steil et al, 1993). The Minimal Model has correlated well with the euglycemic clamp over a broad range of insulin sensitivities (Finegood et al, 1984; Bergman et al, 1987); however, the correlation was reported to be lower in subjects with elevated levels of insulin resistance (Saad et al, 1994).

The oral glucose tolerance test (OGTT), routinely used for the diagnosis of impaired glucose tolerance (IGT) and diabetes, has been used to assess insulin sensitivity as well. Because no intravenous access is needed, OGTT is more practical for assessment of large populations. In this procedure one typically uses a 75 g glucose load in the form of a drink, and glucose and insulin are measured at various intervals over 2 h. Using a variable number of OGTT measurement time points, several mathematical models have been used to assess insulin resistance, and in general, these models have provided values that are significantly correlated with data generated from the euglycemic clamp (e.g., Bergman et al, 1987; Mari et al, 2001; Matsuda and DeFronzo, 1999). An advantage of OGTT-based indices is that they incorporate an assessment of insulin resistance in both the fasting and the postprandial phases.

Several models have been proposed to assess insulin sensitivity using fasting (homeostatic) insulin and/or glucose levels (reviewed in Grundy, 1998a; Matthews et al, 1985a; Muniyappa et al, 2008). These measures assume that subjects are fasting and in a basal steady-state condition in which β-cell insulin secretion is relatively constant and glucose utilization matches glucose production. A limitation to all procedures that rely on insulin values is the lack of a standardized insulin assay (Sapin, 2007) which makes the results dependent on the assay chosen. Fasting serum insulin is a readily available measure, and elevated insulin levels can be indicative of insulin resistance; however, fasting insulin levels poorly correlate with insulin sensitivity as measured by the euglycemic clamp (Laakso, 1993).

The homeostasis model of insulin resistance (HOMA) (Matthews et al, 1985b) is calculated by the equation:

$$Homa = (Insulin_{fasting}(\mu IU/ml)$$
$$(\mu IU/ml) x Glucose_{fasting}(mg/dl)/405)$$

The denominator of 405 (22.5 if glucose is expresses as mmol/l) is a normalizing factor obtained for a "normal healthy individual" (fasting glucose 81 mg/dl and insulin 5 μIU/ml). Variants of the HOMA calculation (e.g., log(HOMA) and 1/(HOMA)) have been shown to correlate better with euglycemic clamp results (Wallace et al, 2004). An alternative model, the quantitative insulin sensitivity check index (QUICKI) (Katz et al, 2000), utilizes log transformed fasting insulin and glucose values:

$$QUICKI = 1 / \left[\log(\text{Insulin}_{fasting}) + \log(\text{Glucose}_{fasting}) \right]$$

QUICKI was shown to provide a better linear correlation with the euglycemic clamp method than other surrogate measures, including HOMA, and is superior to the other fasting measures of insulin resistance (Chen et al, 2005; Ferrannini and Mari, 2004; Muniyappa et al, 2008; Pacini and Mari, 2003).

5.2 Dyslipidemia

Common components to all definitions of the metabolic syndrome are elevated triglycerides and low HDL-C (Table 46.1). These measures are standardized (Myers et al, 1989), can be determined by most reference laboratories, and are directly comparable among most studies. The high triglyceride/low HDL-C phenotype is often associated with elevated levels of LDL-cholesterol, presence of atherogenic small dense LDL, and elevated postprandial hyperlipidemia. Each of these factors has been shown to independently elevate CVD risk (Grundy, 1998b).

5.3 Blood Pressure

Although none of the metabolic syndrome definitions provide explicit guidelines for accurate blood pressure measurement, it is clear that standardized methodology should be used. The AHA scientific statement for blood pressure measurement (Pickering et al, 2005) recommends the auscultatory technique utilizing a trained observer and mercury sphygmomanometer. While many variables can affect blood pressure readings, observer error accounts for the

majority of this variability (Beevers et al, 2001) and can be substantially reduced with appropriate training (Ostchega et al, 2003). For larger studies, it is strongly recommended that appropriate quality assurance and control procedures be included as an important component of study design (e.g., Kuznetsova et al, 2002).

Detailed descriptions for blood pressure assessment have been published (Beevers et al, 2001; National Health and Nutrition Examination Survey, 2009; Pickering et al, 2005). The subject should be seated with legs uncrossed, with back support and the arm at the level of the heart. It is recommended that the subject then rest for 5 min before the first reading is taken. The observer should ensure use of the appropriate cuff size for the arm circumference of the subject being tested. The cuff should be inflated to at least 30 mmHg above the pressure at which the radial pulse disappears and deflated at a rate of 2–3 mmHg per minute. A minimum of two readings at least 1 min apart should be taken and the average of the readings is then reported. If the two reading differ by more than 5 mmHg, then one or two additional readings should be taken and the average of all the readings reported.

5.4 Obesity and Waist Circumference

Each of the metabolic syndrome definitions includes a measure of increased body weight or adiposity using waist circumference as a surrogate measure. Decision points for waist circumference in ATP III have been standardized (≥ 102 cm for men and ≥ 88 cm for women), while the IDF criteria depend not only on gender but also on ethnicity to account for differences in stature and body type. In contrast, the WHO criteria utilize either the waist to hip ratio (0.9 for men and >0.85 for women) or a BMI greater than 30 kg/m^2. Each of the metabolic syndrome definitions utilizes slightly different locations for determination of the waist circumference. By ATP III guidelines, the waist circumference is measured immediately above the iliac crest. For

WHO and IDF criteria, the waist circumference is measured at the midpoint between the inferior margin of the last rib and the crest of the ileum. The difference in measurement sites has been evaluated in several studies, and although there is generally good agreement in defining increased waist circumference, differences do exist that can misclassify certain subjects (Mason and Katzmarzyk, 2009; Matsushita et al, 2009). For the WHO criteria, the hip circumference is also measured at the maximum extension of the buttocks, which allows for calculation of the waist to hip ratio.

Procedurally, the subject stands with their feet shoulder width apart, arms slightly away from the body or loosely crossed over the chest, and with clothing pulled down below the waist. Once the appropriate site is located, a measuring tape is placed around the trunk of the subject perpendicular to the body axis and parallel to the floor, and measurement is taken to the nearest 0.5 cm while the subject is exhaling. The procedure is usually repeated twice and the average of the two measures reported. While waist circumference measurements are easily obtained, reports of operator variability occur and can be reduced with proper training. Finally, the WHO criteria for increased body weight can also be satisfied by calculation of BMI, which is calculated by dividing body weight (kg) by height (in meters) squared.

6 Conclusion

The increasing prevalence of obesity is a major worldwide health issue. It is also clear that obesity, hyperglycemia, and dyslipidemia are important risk factors for type 2 diabetes and CVD. Furthermore, lifestyle interventions designed to reduce weight and body fat, as well as increasing physical activity, have been shown to reduce the risk of type 2 diabetes and CVD. Individuals at high risk for these diseases exhibited a cluster of interrelated risk factors, which has subsequently been termed the metabolic syndrome. Clinically,

the metabolic syndrome diagnosis was implemented to identify individuals at increased risk for CVD and type 2 diabetes who might benefit from early intervention. Unfortunately, ambiguities exist in the definition of the metabolic syndrome making it difficult to focus on the relative importance of each specific component of the syndrome. There is also an active debate among medical researchers and clinicians regarding the utility of the metabolic syndrome diagnosis.

The components of the metabolic syndrome are physiologically interrelated; however, the root cause of the syndrome has not yet been established. Clearly, obesity and insulin resistance are driving forces that produce an altered metabolic state. The pathophysiologic consequences of this metabolic dysregulation include systemic inflammation, oxidative stress, and dyslipidemia that affect disease burden. Further research is needed to better define the metabolic syndrome and to better understand its physiological origins and the contribution of the individual components to disease morbidity and mortality.

References

Abbasi, F., Brown, B. W., Jr., Lamendola, C., McLaughlin, T., and Reaven, G. M. (2002). Relationship between obesity, insulin resistance, and coronary heart disease risk. *J Am Coll Cardiol, 40*, 937–943.

Abdul-Ghani, M. A., Matsuda, M., Jani, R., Jenkinson, C. P., Coletta, D. K. et al (2008). The relationship between fasting hyperglycemia and insulin secretion in subjects with normal or impaired glucose tolerance. *Am J Physiol Endocrinol Metab, 295*, E401–E406.

Alberti, K. G., and Zimmet, P. Z. (1998). Definition, diagnosis and classification of diabetes mellitus and its complications. Part 1: diagnosis and classification of diabetes mellitus provisional report of a WHO consultation. *Diabet Med, 15*, 539–553.

Alberti, K. G. M. M., Eckel, R. H., Grundy, S. M., Zimmet, P. Z., Cleeman, J. I. et al (2009). Harmonizing the Metabolic Syndrome. A Joint Interim Statement of the International Diabetes Federation Task Force on Epidemiology and Prevention; National Heart, Lung, and Blood Institute; American Heart Association; World Heart Federation; International Atherosclerosis Society; and International Association for the Study of Obesity. *Circulation*, published online

Alexander, C. M., Landsman, P. B., Teutsch, S. M., and Haffner, S. M. (2003). NCEP-defined metabolic syndrome, diabetes, and prevalence of coronary heart disease among NHANES III participants age 50 years and older. *Diabetes, 52*, 1210–1214.

American Diabetes Association (2002). Report of the Expert Committee on the Diagnosis and Classification of Diabetes Mellitus. *Diabetes Care, 25*, s5–s20.

ATP III (2001). Executive Summary of the Third Report of the National Cholesterol Education Program (NCEP) Expert Panel on Detection, Evaluation, and Treatment of High Blood Cholesterol in Adults (Adult Treatment Panel III). *JAMA, 285*, 2486–2497.

Austin, M. A. (1989). Plasma triglyceride as a risk factor for coronary heart disease: the epidemiologic evidence and beyond. *Am J Epidemiol, 129*, 249–259.

Balkau, B., and Charles, M. A. (1999). Comment on the provisional report from the WHO consultation. European Group for the Study of Insulin Resistance (EGIR). *Diabet Med, 16*, 442–443.

Beevers, G., Lip, G. Y. H., and O'Brien, E. (2001). ABC of hypertension: blood pressure measurement Part II Conventional sphygmomanometry: technique of auscultatory blood pressure measurement. *BMJ, 322*, 981–985.

Bergman, R. N., Finegood, D. T., and Ader, M. (1985). Assessment of insulin sensitivity in vivo. *Endocr Rev, 6*, 45–86.

Bergman, R. N., Prager, R., Volund, A., and Olefsky, J. M. (1987). Equivalence of the insulin sensitivity index in man derived by the minimal model method and the euglycemic glucose clamp. *J Clin Invest, 79*, 790–800.

Boden, G. (1999). Free fatty acids, insulin resistance, and type 2 diabetes mellitus. *Proc Assoc Am Phys, 111*, 241–248.

Cassells, H. B., and Haffner, S. M. (2006). The metabolic syndrome: risk factors and management. *J Cardiovasc Nurs, 21*, 306–313.

Chen, H., Sullivan, G., and Quon, M. J. (2005). Assessing the predictive accuracy of QUICKI as a surrogate index for insulin sensitivity using a calibration model. *Diabetes, 54*, 1914–1925.

Cornier, M. A., Dabelea, D., Hernandez, T. L., Lindstrom, R. C., Steig, A. J. et al (2008). The metabolic syndrome. *Endocr Rev, 29*, 777–822.

Crandall, J. P., Knowler, W. C., Kahn, S. E., Marrero, D., Florez, J. C. et al (2008). The prevention of type 2 diabetes. *Nat Clin Pract Endocrinol Metab, 4*, 382–393.

DeFronzo, R. A., Tobin, J. D., and Andres, R. (1979). Glucose clamp technique: a method for quantifying insulin secretion and resistance. *AJP - Endocrinol Metabol, 237*, E214-E223.

Del Prato, S., Ferrannin, E., and DeFronzo, R. A. (1985). Evaluation of insulin sensitivity in man. In W. L. Clarke, J. Larner, & S. Pohl (Eds.), *Methods in diabetes research, volume II, clinical methods.* In *Methods in diabetes research, volume II, clinical methods* (pp. 36–76). New York: John Wiley.

Eckel, R. H., Kahn, R., Robertson, R. M., and Rizza, R. A. (2006). Preventing cardiovascular disease and diabetes. *Diabetes Care, 29*, 1697–1699.

Einhorn, D., Reaven, G. M., Cobin, R. H., Ford, E., Ganda, O. P. et al (2003). American College of Endocrinology position statement on the insulin resistance syndrome. *Endocr Pract, 9*, 237–252.

Ervin, R. B. (2009). Prevalence of metabolic syndrome among adults 20 years of age and over by sex, age, race and ethnicity, and body mass Index: United States, 2003–2006. *National Health Statistics Report, Hyattsville, MD National Center for Health Statistics, 13.*

Espinola-Klein, C., Rupprecht, H. J., Bickel, C., Lackner, K., Genth-Zotz, S. et al (2008). Impact of inflammatory markers on cardiovascular mortality in patients with metabolic syndrome. *Eur J Cardiovasc Prev Rehabil, 15*, 278–284.

Ferrannini, E., and Mari, A. (2004). Beta cell function and its relation to insulin action in humans: a critical appraisal. *Diabetologia, 47*, 943–956.

Ferrannini, E., Buzzigoli, G., Bonadonna, R., Giorico, M. A., Oleggini, M. et al (1987). Insulin resistance in essential hypertension. *N Engl J Med, 317*, 350–357.

Finegood, D. T., Pacini, G., and Bergman, R. N. (1984). The insulin sensitivity index. Correlation in dogs between values determined from the intravenous glucose tolerance test and the euglycemic glucose clamp. *Diabetes, 33*, 362–368.

Garruti, G., Cotecchia, S., Giampetruzzi, F., Giorgino, F., and Giorgino, R. (2008). Neuroendocrine deregulation of food intake, adipose tissue and the gastrointestinal system in obesity and metabolic syndrome. *J Gastrointestin Liver Dis, 17*, 193–198.

Godsland, I. F., Jeffs, J. A. R., and Johnston, D. G. (2004). Loss of beta cell function as fasting glucose increases in the non-diabetic range. *Diabetologia, 47*, 1157–1166.

Grassi, G. (2006). Sympathetic overdrive and cardiovascular risk in the metabolic syndrome. *Hypertens Res, 29*, 839–847.

Greenland, P. (2005). Critical questions about the metabolic syndrome. *Circulation, 112*, 3675–3676.

Grekin, R. J., Vollmer, A. P., and Sider, R. S. (1995). Pressor effects of portal venous oleate infusion: a proposed mechanism for obesity hypertension. *Hypertension, 26*, 193–198.

Grundy, S. M. (1998a). Hypertriglyceridemia, atherogenic dyslipidemia, and the metabolic syndrome. *Am J Cardiol, 81*, 18B–25B.

Grundy, S. M. (1998b). Hypertriglyceridemia, atherogenic dyslipidemia, and the metabolic syndrome. *Am J Cardiol, 81*, 18B–25B.

Grundy, S. M., Brewer, H. B., Jr., Cleeman, J. I., Smith, S. C., Jr., Lenfant, C., and for the Conference Participants (2004a). Definition of metabolic syndrome: report of the National Heart, Lung, and Blood Institute/American Heart Association Conference on Scientific Issues Related to Definition. *Circulation, 109*, 433–438.

Grundy, S. M., Hansen, B., Smith, S. C., Jr., Cleeman, J. I., Kahn, R. A., and for Conference (2004b). Clinical management of Metabolic Syndrome: Report of the American Heart Association/National Heart, Lung, and Blood Institute/American Diabetes Association Conference on Scientific Issues Related to Management. *Circulation, 109*, 551–556.

Haffner, S., Temprosa, M., Crandall, J., Fowler, S., Goldberg, R., Horton, E. et al (2005). Intensive lifestyle intervention or metformin on inflammation and coagulation in participants with impaired glucose tolerance. *Diabetes, 54*, 1566–1572.

Haffner, S. M., Fong, D., Hazuda, H. P., Pugh, J. A., and Patterson, J. K. (1988). Hyperinsulinemia, upper body adiposity, and cardiovascular risk factors in non-diabetics. *Metabolism, 37*, 338–345.

Hamman, R. F., Wing, R. R., Edelstein, S. L., Lachin, J. M., Bray, G. A. et al (2006). Effect of weight loss with lifestyle intervention on risk of diabetes. *Diabetes Care, 29*, 2102–2107.

Herder, C., Peltonen, M., Koenig, W., Sutfels, K., Lindstrom, J. et al (2009). Anti-inflammatory effect of lifestyle changes in the Finnish Diabetes Prevention Study. *Diabetologia, 52*, 433–442.

Hung, J., McQuillan, B. M., Thompson, P. L., and Beilby, J. P. (2008). Circulating adiponectin levels associate with inflammatory markers, insulin resistance and metabolic syndrome independent of obesity. *Int J Obes, 32*, 772–779.

Ji, J., Watts, G. F., Johnson, A. G., Chan, D. C., Ooi, E. M. M. et al (2006). High-Density Lipoprotein (HDL) Transport in the Metabolic Syndrome: application of a new model for HDL particle kinetics. *J Clin Endocrinol Metab, 91*, 973–979.

Jocken, J. W. E., Langin, D., Smit, E., Saris, W. H. M., Valle, C. et al (2007). Adipose triglyceride lipase and hormone-sensitive lipase protein expression is decreased in the obese insulin-resistant state. *J Clin Endocrinol Metab, 92*, 2292–2299.

Johnson, L. W., and Weinstock, R. S. (2006). The metabolic syndrome: concepts and controversy. *Mayo Clin Proc, 81*, 1615–1620.

Kahn, R., Buse, J., Ferrannini, E., and Stern, M. (2005). The metabolic syndrome: time for a critical appraisal. *Diabetes Care, 28*, 2289–2304.

Kaplan, N. M. (1991). Hyperinsulinemia in diabetes and hypertension. *Clin Diabetes, v9*, 1.

Katz, A., Nambi, S. S., Mather, K., Baron, A. D., Follmann, D. A. et al (2000). Quantitative insulin sensitivity check index: a simple, accurate method for assessing insulin sensitivity in humans. *J Clin Endocrinol Metab, 85*, 2402–2410.

Kennedy, A., Martinez, K., Chuang, C. C., LaPoint, K., and McIntosh, M. (2009). Saturated fatty acid-mediated inflammation and insulin resistance in

adipose tissue: mechanisms of action and implications. *J Nutr, 139*, 1–4.

Klein, B. E. K., Klein, R., and Lee, K. E. (2002). Components of the metabolic syndrome and risk of cardiovascular disease and diabetes in Beaver Dam. *Diabetes Care, 25*, 1790–1794.

Knowler, W. C., Barrett-Connor, E., Fowler, S. E., Hamman, R. F., Lachin, J. M. et al (2002). Reduction in the incidence of type 2 diabetes with lifestyle intervention or metformin. *N Engl J Med, 346*, 393–403.

Knuiman, M. W., Hung, J., Divitini, M. L., Davis, T. M., and Beilby, J. P. (2009). Utility of the metabolic syndrome and its components in the prediction of incident cardiovascular disease: a prospective cohort study. *Euro J Cardiovasc Prev Rehab, 16*, 235–241.

Kosaka, K., Noda, M., and Kuzuya, T. (2005). Prevention of type 2 diabetes by lifestyle intervention: a Japanese trial in IGT males. *Diabetes Res Clin Pract, 67*, 152–162.

Kowalska, I., Straczkowski, M., Nikolajuk, A., Adamska, A., Karczewska-Kupczewska, M. et al (2008). Insulin resistance, serum adiponectin, and proinflammatory markers in young subjects with the metabolic syndrome. *Metabolism, 57*, 1539–1544.

Krssak, M., Falk Petersen, K., Dresner, A., DiPietro, L., Vogel, S. M. et al (1999). Intramyocellular lipid concentrations are correlated with insulin sensitivity in humans: a 1H NMR spectroscopy study. *Diabetologia, 42*, 113–116.

Kusminski, C. M., Shetty, S., Orci, L., Unger, R. H., and Scherer, P. E. (2009). Diabetes and apoptosis: lipotoxicity. *Apoptosis, 14*, 1484–1495.

Kuznetsova, T., Staessen, J. A., Kawecka-Jaszcz, K., Babeanu, S., Casiglia, E. et al (2002). Quality control of the blood pressure phenotype in the European Project on Genes in Hypertension. *Blood Press Mon, 7*, 215–224.

Kwiterovich, P. O., Jr. (2002). Clinical relevance of the biochemical, metabolic, and genetic factors that influence low-density lipoprotein heterogeneity. *Am J Cardiol, 90*, 30i–47i.

Laakso, M. (1993). How good a marker is insulin level for insulin resistance? *Am J Epidemiol, 137*, 959–965.

Laaksonen, D. E., Lindstrom, J., Lakka, T. A., Eriksson, J. G., Niskanen, L. et al (2005). Physical activity in the prevention of type 2 diabetes: the Finnish diabetes prevention study. *Diabetes, 54*, 158–165.

Lambert, M., Paradis, G., O'Loughlin, J., Delvin, E. E., Hanley, J. A. et al (2004). Insulin resistance syndrome in a representative sample of children and adolescents from Quebec, Canada. *Int J Obes Relat Metab Disord, 28*, 833–841.

LeRoith, D. (2002). [beta]-cell dysfunction and insulin resistance in type 2 diabetes: role of metabolic and genetic abnormalities. *Am J Med, 113*, 3–11.

Lewis, G. F. (1997). Fatty acid regulation of very low density lipoprotein production. *Curr Opin Lipidol, 8*, 146–153.

Li, G., Zhang, P., Wang, J., Gregg, E. W., Yang, W. et al (2008). The long-term effect of lifestyle interventions to prevent diabetes in the China Da Qing Diabetes Prevention Study: a 20-year follow-up study. *Lancet, 371*, 1783–1789.

Libby, P. (2006). Inflammation and cardiovascular disease mechanisms. *Am J Clin Nutr, 83*, 456S–460.

Lindstrom, J., Ilanne-Parikka, P., Peltonen, M., Aunola, S., Eriksson, J. G. et al (2006). Sustained reduction in the incidence of type 2 diabetes by lifestyle intervention: follow-up of the Finnish Diabetes Prevention Study. *Lancet, 368*, 1673–1679.

Mari, A., Pacini, G., Murphy, E., Ludvik, B., and Nolan, J. J. (2001). A model-based method for assessing insulin sensitivity from the oral glucose tolerance test. *Diabetes Care, 24*, 539–548.

Mason, C., and Katzmarzyk, P. T. (2009). Effect of the site of measurement of waist circumference on the Prevalence of the Metabolic Syndrome. *Am J Cardiol, 103*, 1716–1720.

Matsuda, M., and DeFronzo, R. A. (1997). In vivo measurement of insulin sensitivity in humans. In B. Draznin & R. A. Rizza (Eds.), *Clinical Research in Diabetes and Obesity, Volume I, Methods, Assessment, and Metabolic Regulation* (pp. 23–65). Totowa, NJ: Humana Press.

Matsuda, M., and DeFronzo, R. A. (1999). Insulin sensitivity indices obtained from oral glucose tolerance testing: comparison with the euglycemic insulin clamp. *Diabetes Care, 22*, 1462–1470.

Matsushita, Y., Tomita, K., Yokoyama, T., and Mizoue, T. (2009). Optimal waist circumference measurement site for assessing the metabolic syndrome. *Diabetes Care, 32*, e70.

Matthews, D. R., Hosker, J. P., Rudenski, A. S., Naylor, B. A., Treacher, D. F. et al (1985b). Homeostasis model assessment: insulin resistance and +-cell function from fasting plasma glucose and insulin concentrations in man. *Diabetologia, 28*, 412–419.

Matthews, D. R., Hosker, J. P., Rudenski, A. S., Naylor, B. A., Treacher, D. F. et al (1985a). Homeostasis model assessment: insulin resistance and β-cell function from fasting plasma glucose and insulin concentrations in man. *Diabetologia, 28*, 412–419.

McGarry, J. D. (2002). Banting Lecture 2001: dysregulation of fatty acid metabolism in the etiology of type 2 diabetes. *Diabetes, 51*, 7–18.

Movva, R., and Rader, D. J. (2008). Laboratory assessment of HDL heterogeneity and function. *Clin Chem, 54*, 788–800.

Muniyappa, R., Lee, S., Chen, H., and Quon, M. J. (2008). Current approaches for assessing insulin sensitivity and resistance in vivo: advantages, limitations, and appropriate usage. *Am J Physiol Endocrinol Metab, 294*, E15–E26.

Myers, G. L., Cooper, G. R., Winn, C. L., and Smith, S. J. (1989). The Centers for Disease Control-National Heart, Lung and Blood Institute Lipid Standardization Program. An approach to accurate and precise lipid measurements. *Clin Lab Med, 9*, 105–135.

National Center for Health Statistics (2008a). *Prevalence of overweight, obesity and extreme obesity among adults: United States, trends 1976–80 through 2005–2006.*

National Center for Health Statistics (2008b). *Health, United States, 2008 With Chartbook.*

National Health and Nutrition Examination Survey (2009). National Health and Nutrition Examination Survey III Cycle 2. Pulse and Blood Pressure Procedures for Household Interviewers. http://www.cdc.gov/nchs/data/nhanes/nhanes3/cdrom/nchs/manuals/pressure.pdf.

Nilsson, P. M. (2007). Cardiovascular risk in the metabolic syndrome: fact or fiction? *Curr Cardiol Rep, 9*, 479–485.

Nonogaki, K. (2000). New insights into sympathetic regulation of glucose and fat metabolism. *Diabetologia, 43*, 533–549.

Ogden, C. L., Carroll, M. D., Curtin, L. R., McDowell, M. A., Tabak, C. J. et al (2006). Prevalence of overweight and obesity in the United States, 1999–2004. *JAMA, 295*, 1549–1555.

Orchard, T. J., Becker, D. J., and Bates, M. (1983). Plasma insulin and lipoprotein concentrations: An atherogenic association? *Am J Epidemiol, 118*, 326–337.

Orchard, T. J., Temprosa, M., Goldberg, R., Haffner, S., Ratner, R. et al (2005). The effect of metformin and intensive lifestyle intervention on the metabolic syndrome: the Diabetes Prevention Program randomized trial. *Ann Intern Med, 142*, 611–619.

Ostchega, Y., Prineas, R. J., Paulose-Ram, R., Grim, C. M., Willard, G. et al (2003). National health and nutrition examination survey 1999–2000: effect of observer training and protocol standardization on reducing blood pressure measurement error. *J Clin Epidemiol, 56*, 768–774.

Pacini, G., and Mari, A. (2003). Methods for clinical assessment of insulin sensitivity and [beta]-cell function. *Best Pract Res Clin Endocrinol Metab, 17*, 305–322.

Pan, X. R., Li, G. W., Hu, Y. H., Wang, J. X., Yang, W. Y. et al (1997). Effects of diet and exercise in preventing NIDDM in people with impaired glucose tolerance. The Da Qing IGT and Diabetes Study. *Diabetes Care, 20*, 537–544.

Pickering, T. G., Hall, J. E., Appel, L. J., Falkner, B. E., Graves, J. et al (2005). Recommendations for blood pressure measurement in humans and experimental animals: Part 1: blood pressure measurement in humans: a statement for professionals from the subcommittee of professional and public education of the American Heart Association Council on High Blood Pressure Research. *Hypertension, 45*, 142–161.

Ramachandran, A., Snehalatha, C., Mary, S., Mukesh, B., Bhaskar, A. D. et al (2006). The Indian Diabetes Prevention Programme shows that lifestyle modification and metformin prevent type 2 diabetes in Asian Indian subjects with impaired glucose tolerance (IDPP-1). *Diabetologia, 49*, 289–297.

Ratner, R., Goldberg, R., Haffner, S., Marcovina, S., Orchard, T. et al (2005). Impact of intensive lifestyle and metformin therapy on cardiovascular disease risk factors in the diabetes prevention program. *Diabetes Care, 28*, 888–894.

Reaven, G. M. (1988). Banting Lecture 1988. Role of insulin resistance in human disease. *Diabetes, 37*, 1595–1607.

Reaven, G. M., Brand, R. J., Chen, Y. D., Mathur, A. K., and Goldfine, I. (1993). Insulin resistance and insulin secretion are determinants of oral glucose tolerance in normal individuals. *Diabetes, 42*, 1324–1332.

Reaven, G. M. (2005). The metabolic syndrome: requiescat in pace. *Clin Chem, 51*, 931–938.

Reaven, G. M. (2006). The metabolic syndrome: is this diagnosis necessary? *Am J Clin Nutr, 83*, 1237–1247.

Reaven, G. M. (2007). The individual components of the metabolic syndrome: is there a raison d'etre? *J Am Coll Nutr, 26*, 191–195.

Reilly, M. P., Rohatgi, A., McMahon, K., Wolfe, M. L., Pinto, S. C. et al (2007). Plasma cytokines, metabolic syndrome, and atherosclerosis in humans. *J Investig Med, 55*, 26–35.

Ridker, P. M., Buring, J. E., Cook, N. R., and Rifai, N. (2003). C-reactive protein, the metabolic syndrome, and risk of incident cardiovascular events: an 8-Year follow-up of 14 719 initially healthy American women. *Circulation, 107*, 391–397.

Rodriguez-Morín, M., Salazar-Vízquez, B., Violante, R., and Guerrero-Romero, F. (2004). Metabolic syndrome among children and adolescents aged 10-18 years. *Diabetes Care, 27*, 2516–2517.

Ross, R. (1986). The pathogenesis of atherosclerosis--an update. *N Engl J Med, 314*, 488–500.

Ruge, T., Lockton, J. A., Renstrom, F., Lystig, T., Sukonina, V. et al (2009). Acute hyperinsulinemia raises plasma interleukin-6 in both nondiabetic and type 2 diabetes mellitus subjects, and this effect is inversely associated with body mass index. *Metabolism, 58*, 860–866.

Saad, M. F., Anderson, R. L., Laws, A., Watanabe, R. M., Kades, W. W. et al (1994). A comparison between the minimal model and the glucose clamp in the assessment of insulin sensitivity across the spectrum of glucose tolerance. Insulin Resistance Atherosclerosis Study. *Diabetes, 43*, 1114–1121.

Sandhofer, A., Kaser, S., Ritsch, A., Laimer, M., Engl, J. et al (2006). Cholesteryl ester transfer protein in metabolic syndrome. *Obesity, 14*, 812–818.

Sapin, R. (2007). Insulin immunoassays: fast approaching 50 years of existence and still calling for standardization. *Clin Chem, 53*, 810–812.

Sattar, N., Gaw, A., Scherbakova, O., Ford, I., O'Reilly, D. S. et al (2003). Metabolic syndrome with and without C-reactive protein as a predictor of coronary heart disease and diabetes in the West of Scotland coronary prevention study. *Circulation, 108*, 414–419.

Schneiderman, N., and Skyler, J. S. (1996). Insulin metabolism, sympathetic nervous system regulation, and coronary heart disease prevention. In K. Orth-Gomer & N. Schneiderman (Eds.), *Behavioral Medicine Approaches to Cardiovascular Disease Prevention* (pp. 105–134). Mahwah, NJ: Lawrence Erlbaum Associates.

Service, F. J. (2003). Mechanisms of metabolic mischief-meritorious or meretricious? *Endocr Pract, 9*, 101–102.

Steil, G. M., Volund, A., Kahn, S. E., and Bergman, R. N. (1993). Reduced sample number for calculation of insulin sensitivity and glucose effectiveness from the minimal model. Suitability for use in population studies. *Diabetes, 42*, 250–256.

Steinberger, J., Daniels, S. R., Eckel, R. H., Hayman, L., Lustig, R. H. et al (2009). Progress and challenges in metabolic syndrome in children and adolescents: a scientific statement from the American Heart Association Atherosclerosis, Hypertension, and Obesity in the Young Committee of the Council on Cardiovascular Disease in the Young. *Circulation, 119*, 628–0647.

Stern, M. P., Williams, K., Gonz+ílez-Villalpando, C., Hunt, K. J., and Haffner, S. M. (2004). Does the metabolic syndrome improve identification of individuals at risk of type 2 diabetes and/or cardiovascular disease? *Diabetes Care, 27*, 2676–2681.

Straznicky, N. E., Eikelis, N., Lambert, E. A., and Esler, M. D. (2008). Mediators of sympathetic activation in metabolic syndrome obesity. *Curr Hypertens Rep, 10*, 440–447.

Tentolouris, N., Argyrakopoulou, G., and Katsilambros, N. (2008). Perturbed autonomic nervous system function in metabolic syndrome. *Neuromolecular Med, 10*, 169–178.

Tripathy, D., Mohanty, P., Dhindsa, S., Syed, T., Ghanim, H. et al (2003). Elevation of free fatty acids induces inflammation and impairs vascular reactivity in healthy subjects. *Diabetes, 52*, 2882–2887.

Tuomilehto, J., Lindstrom, J., Eriksson, J. G., Valle, T. T., Hamalainen, H. et al (2001). Prevention of type 2 diabetes mellitus by changes in lifestyle among subjects with impaired glucose tolerance. *N Engl J Med, 344*, 1343–1350.

Unger, R. H. (2003). Minireview: weapons of lean body mass destruction: the role of ectopic lipids in the metabolic syndrome. *Endocrinology, 144*, 5159–5165.

Uusitupa, M., Peltonen, M., Lindstrom, J., Aunola, S., Ilanne-Parikka, P. et al (2009). Ten-year mortality and cardiovascular morbidity in the Finnish Diabetes Prevention Study--secondary analysis of the randomized trial. *PLoS One, 4*, e5656.

Wallace, T. M., Levy, J. C., and Matthews, D. R. (2004). Use and abuse of HOMA modeling. *Diabetes Care, 27*, 1487–1495.

Weisberg, S. P., McCann, D., Desai, M., Rosenbaum, M., Leibel, R. L. et al (2003). Obesity is associated with macrophage accumulation in adipose tissue. *J Clin Invest., 112*, 1796–1808.

Weiss, R., Dziura, J., Burgert, T. S., Tamborlane, W. V., Taksali, S. E. et al (2004). Obesity and the metabolic syndrome in children and adolescents. *N Engl J Med, 350*, 2362–2374.

Wilson, P. W. F., D'Agostino, R. B., Levy, D., Belanger, A. M., Silbershatz, H. et al (1998). Prediction of coronary heart disease using risk factor categories. *Circulation, 97*, 1837–1847.

World Health Organization. (2006). Obesity and overweight. WHO Fact Sheet 311.

Xu, H., Barnes, G. T., Yang, Q., Tan, G., Yang, D. et al (2003). Chronic inflammation in fat plays a crucial role in the development of obesity-related insulin resistance. *J Clin Invest, 112*, 1821–1830.

You, T., Nicklas, B. J., Ding, J., Penninx, B. W., Goodpaster, B. H. et al (2008). The metabolic syndrome is associated with circulating adipokines in older adults across a wide range of adiposity. *J Gerontol A Biol Sci Med Sci, 63*, 414–419.

Zavaroni, I., Dall'Aglio, E., Alpi, O., Bruschi, F., Bonora, E. et al (1985). Evidence for an independent relationship between plasma insulin and concentration of high density lipoprotein cholesterol and triglyceride. *Atherosclerosis, 55*, 259–266.

Zimmet, P., Alberti, G., Kaufman, F., Tajima, N., Silink, M. et al (2007). The metabolic syndrome in children and adolescents. *Lancet, 369*, 2059–2061.

Zimmet, P., Magliano, D., Matsuzawa, Y., Alberti, G., and Shaw, J. (2005). The metabolic syndrome: a global public health problem and a new definition. *J Atheroscl Thromb, 12*, 295–300.

Chapter 47

The Non-invasive Assessment of Autonomic Influences on the Heart Using Impedance Cardiography and Heart Rate Variability

Julian F. Thayer, Anita L. Hansen, and Bjorn Helge Johnsen

1 Autonomic Balance and Health

There is growing evidence for the role of the autonomic nervous system (ANS) in a wide range of somatic and mental diseases. The ANS is generally conceived to have two major branches – the sympathetic system, associated with energy mobilization, and the parasympathetic system, associated with vegetative and restorative functions. Normally, the activity of these branches is in dynamic balance. When this changes into a static imbalance, for example under environmental pressures, the organism becomes vulnerable to pathology.

The sympathetic nervous system is also further sub-divided into alpha-adrenergic and beta-adrenergic components. However, it is important to note that these distinctions, though based in anatomy and physiology, are largely for pedagogic purposes. That is, the body is a unified entity such that challenges energize the whole body in an attempt to produce a context appropriate response. This is similar, and of course related, to the idea that the whole brain is involved in generating responses and is also consistent with modern, parallel-distributed processing models. This is extremely important to remember as we search for measures that index different, specific aspects of function. Most measures will represent the confluence of a number of processes and in the context of the dynamics of a response where cascades are initiated and compensatory processes recruited, any outcome index that we generate will most likely be more complex than our current knowledge can accommodate. This will yield sometimes conflicting findings and will tax our ability to find universally consistent relationships.

Autonomic imbalance, in which one branch of the ANS dominates over the other, is associated with a lack of dynamic flexibility and health. Empirically, there is a large body of evidence to suggest that autonomic imbalance, in which typically the sympathetic system is hyperactive and the parasympathetic system is hypoactive, is associated with various pathological conditions (Sztajzel, 2004). In particular, when the sympathetic branch dominates for long periods of time, the energy demands on the system become excessive and ultimately cannot be met, eventuating in death. The prolonged state of alarm associated with negative emotions likewise places an excessive energy demand on the system. On the way to death, however, premature aging and disease characterize a system dominated by negative affect and autonomic imbalance.

Like many organs in the body, the heart is dually innervated. Although a wide range of physiologic factors determine cardiac functions

J.F. Thayer (✉)
Department of Psychology, The Ohio State University, 1835 Neil Avenue, Columbus, OH 43210, USA
e-mail: thayer.39@osu.edu

Note: This is an updated and expanded version of a previous chapter, Thayer JF, Hansen AL, Johnsen BH: Non-invasive assessment of autonomic influences on the heart: Impedance cardiography and heart rate variability. In Luecken LJ, Gallo LC (eds.), *Handbook of Physiological Research Methods in Health Psychology*. Newbury Park, CA: Sage Publications, 2008, 183-209.

A. Steptoe (ed.), *Handbook of Behavioral Medicine*, DOI 10.1007/978-0-387-09488-5_47,
© Springer Science+Business Media, LLC 2010

such as heart rate (HR), the ANS is the most prominent. Importantly, when both cardiac vagal (the primary parasympathetic nerve) and sympathetic inputs are blocked pharmacologically (for example, with atropine plus propranolol, the so-called double blockade), intrinsic HR is higher than the normal resting HR (Jose and Collison, 1970). This fact supports the idea that the heart is under tonic inhibitory control by parasympathetic influences. Thus, resting cardiac autonomic balance favors energy conservation by way of parasympathetic dominance over sympathetic influences. In addition, the HR time series is characterized by beat-to-beat variability over a wide range, which also implicates vagal dominance as the sympathetic influence on the heart is too slow to produce beat-to-beat changes (Saul, 1990). Low heart rate variability (HRV) is associated with increased risk of all-cause mortality, and low HRV has been proposed as a marker for disease (Task Force, 1996; Thayer and Lane, 2007).

2 Aspects of Cardiac Function: Chronotropy, Inotropy, and Dromotropy

With respect to autonomic influences on cardiac function it is useful to distinguish at least three types of functions, each with its own unique relationship with ANS activation including sympathetic–parasympathetic interactions (Berne and Levy, 2001, a highly recommended reference). For example, the heart is composed of a number of types of effector tissues such that, for example, the influence of ANS activation at the sinoatrial (SA) node is different from that at the atrioventricular (AV) node. In general the parasympathetic influences dominate the sympathetic influences on cardiac function. With respect to the control of heart rate (known as *chronotropy*) there have been numerous demonstrations of the predominance of the parasympathetic influences. In a classic paper, Levy and Zeiske (1969) showed that the effect of a given level of parasympathetic stimulation

varied as a function of the background level of sympathetic stimulation. Specifically, the decrease in HR associated with a given parasympathetic stimulus was greater the greater the level of background sympathetic activity. They termed this effect "accentuated antagonism." This effect represents the differential effect of sympathetic and parasympathetic influences at the sinoatrial node. Accentuated antagonism is thought to be due to both pre-junctional and post-junctional neurotransmitter effects (Levy, 1997; Uijtdehaage and Thayer, 2000).

The ANS effects are somewhat different at the atrioventricular node. In the absence of background sympathetic activity, the effect of parasympathetic stimulation on cardiac contractility (known as *inotropy*) is negligible. However, in the presence of sympathetic background activity the effect of parasympathetic activation produces a substantial (and non-algebraically additive) decrease in contractility (Levy, 1997).

Moreover, at the AV junction the conduction speed of the electrical impulse (known as *dromotropy*) increases with sympathetic activation and decreases with parasympathetic activation with an interaction that is algebraically additive such that simultaneous maximal stimulation leads to essentially a zero net effect (Levy and Martin, 1996). Thus in order to accurately interpret the effects of a given autonomic influence on the heart, knowledge of the level of activity of both branches is necessary.

In the service of the organism the individual measures that can be derived from non-invasive measurements such as impedance cardiography and HRV tend to cluster into patterns associated with regulatory functions. This patterning has been examined in the context of what has been called "cardiovascular activation components (CAC)" (Stemmler et al, 1991). These CAC's can be described in both functional and anatomical/physiological terms. For example, measures that index cholinergic activation tend to overlap with measures associated with cardiac chronotropy such as HR, various indices of HRV, and left-ventricular ejection time (LVET: a sympathetic chronotropic measure derived from impedance cardiography; Thayer and Uijtdehaage, 2001). Similarly, measures that index beta-adrenergic activation such as pre-ejection period (PEP), stroke volume (SV), cardiac output (CO), and the Heather Index of contractility (HI) are associated with cardiac inotropy. Total peripheral resistance (TPR), a measure that can be derived from the combination of impedance derived CO and blood pressure recordings, is associated with alpha-adrenergic activation.

One of the purposes to which impedance cardiography has been applied is in the characterization of individuals as either cardiac reactors or vascular reactors (Sherwood et al, 1990b). This is based upon the relationship between CO and TPR as components of blood pressure. Specifically, mean arterial pressure (MAP) = CO X TPR. Thus any given blood pressure is multiply determined and could arise from changes in either CO or TPR or both. Stevo Julius (Brook and Julius, 2000) has proposed a model of the development of hypertension which posits that the initial stages of the progression to hypertension are associated with increased CO but normal TPR. However, over time and with the establishment of the hypertensive state, CO returns to normal and TPR becomes elevated. Both Ring and colleagues (2002) and Miller and Ditto (1988) have shown that during an extended laboratory stress session a similar shift in hemodynamics takes place such that blood pressure elevations are initially due to increases in CO but over the course of the task (order of magnitude 10 min) there is a shift such that the same blood pressure is maintained by increased TPR. These distinctions are of more than academic interest. In particular, it has been shown that the deleterious effects of elevated blood pressure with respect to end-organ damage, morbidity, and mortality are due primarily to elevated TPR. For example, in both normotensive and hypertensive individuals it has been shown that elevated BP via TPR but not CO is associated with increased risk for cardiovascular events and death (Fagard et al, 1996; Mensah et al, 1993). Recent research (Ottaviani et al, 2006) has further refined the way in which individuals are characterized with respect to their hemodynamic

profile with Ottaviani and colleagues showing superior prediction of ambulatory blood pressure by this new approach compared to previous classification schemes.

3 The Baroreflex

A primary function of the cardiovascular system is to maintain optimal arterial blood pressure and to provide adequate blood flow to the brain and other vital organs. In response to environmental demands blood pressure and the distribution of blood flow throughout the body are finely tuned by an intricate system that includes the arterial baroreflex. Baroreceptors, which are stretch-sensitive nerve terminals mainly located in the central vascular tree and the heart, sense changes in blood pressure. These baroreceptors send afferent signals to the brain which reflexively adjust efferent outputs to regulate the changes in blood pressure. When blood pressure increases it elicits reflex decreases in heart rate, cardiac contractility, and vascular resistance via parasympathetic activation and sympathetic inhibition. Similarly, decreases in blood pressure elicit reflex increases in heart rate, cardiac contractility, and vascular resistance via parasympathetic inhibition and sympathetic activation (Benarroch, 2008).

This system serves to maintain optimal short-term blood pressure primarily through the regulation of heart rate and provides for the dynamic beat-to-beat regulation of blood pressure via negative feedback. It is important to understand that this dynamic system has many variables that can be indexed by ICG and HRV. Moreover, we typically capture only a snapshot of this continuously running movie. Thus our measures of heart rate, cardiac contractility such as PEP and CO, and vascular resistance such as TPR averaged over some time interval do not fully reflect the complex dynamic interplay of stimulus initiated cascades and compensatory responses.

Moreover, until recently it was thought that the major determinant of long-term blood pressure was fluid volume and that the baroreflex played little role in such long-term regulation (Coleman et al, 1977). However, recent research suggests a much more prominent role for the baroreflex in long-term blood pressure regulation and thus the baroreflex takes on even more importance in our understanding of autonomic influences on cardiovascular regulation (see Thrasher, 2006, for the history of this controversy and the recent evidence suggesting a role for the baroreceptors in long-term blood pressure regulation). Briefly, recent evidence suggests that baroreceptor afferent activity is chronically elevated in hypertension that prolonged afferent stimulation of the baroreceptors is associated with reductions in long-term blood pressure, and that baroreflex sensitivity is inversely related to ambulatory blood pressure in humans (Lohmeier, 2001; Lohmeier et al, 2004; Hesse et al, 2007).

Whereas a complete exposition about the baroreflex is beyond the scope of the present chapter, we will briefly summarize several key aspects of baroreflex function and measurement. Several indices of baroreflex function have been suggested and defined (Duschek and Reyes del Paso, 2007; Parati et al, 2000). Baroreflex *sensitivity* (BRS) refers to the extent of reflex changes in heart rate following fluctuations in blood pressure. The function of the baroreflex, though dually innervated, is largely under parasympathetic control and the various indices of baroreflex function correlate with vagally mediated HRV (Benarroch, 2008; Duschek and Reyes del Paso, 2007). As such baroreflex sensitivity is another index of parasympathetic activity that can be used to assess the autonomic influences on the cardiovascular system.

Parati and colleagues (2000) have provided an excellent review of the measurement of baroreflex sensitivity both in clinical medicine and in research. Two approaches are especially salient for the present discussion. Both methods rely on spontaneous fluctuations in HR and BP. The first method examines the sequence of changes in heart period (the inverse of heart rate) and BP in the time domain to find periods of spontaneous reflex adjustments and is called the "sequence" method.

Another method based on the spectral analysis of simultaneously recorded heart rate (IBI) and BP is called the spectral method and yields an index called the "alpha coefficient." Whereas the "sequence" method and the "spectral" method are correlated they are derived differently and have different characteristics. Most importantly, they have both been shown to be valid measures of baroreflex sensitivity and thus of autonomic influences on the cardiovascular system (Duschek and Reyes del Paso, 2007; Parati et al, 2000).

In summary, the use of non-invasive indices of autonomic control of the heart derived from impedance cardiography and HRV are useful and essential tools for behavioral medicine research. However, to fully utilize the wealth of data that can now be produced by turn-key systems a more comprehensive understanding of the complexities of the many factors that go into the outcome measures is necessary if we are to make reasonable inferences from our data. Hopefully the preceding discussion will aid in this endeavor. In the following, we will first discuss issues related to impedance cardiography and then address issues related to HRV.

4 Impedance Cardiography

Impedance cardiography (ICG) was introduced more than 40 years ago as a non-invasive technique to measure systolic time intervals and cardiac output (CO). The primary measures that can be derived from the ICG signal are systolic time intervals [total ejection time (ET), pre-ejection period (PEP), and left-ventricular ejection time (LVET); see Fig. 47.1] and stroke volume (SV). In combination with the electrocardiogram (ECG; and sometimes the phonocardiogram to measure the heart sounds) the ICG signal can be used to index the opening and closing of the left ventricle and thus can be used to calculate the systolic time intervals. However, the calculation of SV is the major variable derived from the ICG. ICG involves the application of a low voltage, high-frequency

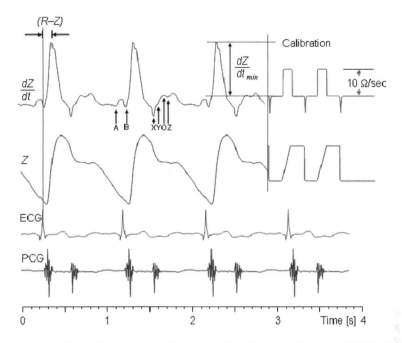

Fig. 47.1 The *top trace* is the firstderivative of the impedance (Z) signal. The *second trace* is the untransformed impedance signal. The *third trace* is the ECG and the *fourth trace* is the phonocardiogram signal. The time between A (which coincides with the R spike of the ECG) and B is the pre-ejection period (PEP), the time between B and X is the left-ventricular ejection time (LVET), and the time between A and X is the total ejection time. Adapted from the web version of Mamivuo and Plonsey (1995; Figure 25.4)

signal to the thoracic cavity. Because blood is a conductor of electricity, blood flow in the thorax can be calculated as the difference between the impedance associated with the blood flow during each heart beat. The most commonly used formula for the calculation of SV is due to Kubicek and uses the distance between the electrodes used to record the applied electrical current, the LVET, the resistivity of the blood, the baseline impedance, and the change in the slope of the first derivative of the ICG signal (Sherwood et al, 1990a). From these measures there are numerous indices that can be derived (see Sherwood et al, 1990a, for a complete description of the various indices). There is little debate in the literature about the ability of ICG to produce accurate absolute measures of the systolic time intervals (Cybulski et al, 2004). Furthermore, there is a general consensus on the ability of ICG to produce accurate *relative* levels of SV and thus to accurately track changes in SV and CO. However, there is a continuing controversy about the ability of ICG to produce accurate absolute levels of SV and thus CO. Part of this controversy stems from the fact that there is no truly agreed upon "gold standard" for the measurement of SV and CO (Jensen et al, 1995).

Both invasive and non-invasive methods for the assessment of SV and CO have relative advantages and disadvantages. Some methods such as the thermodilution method are not practical for use in behavioral medicine research. Others such as echocardiography require an experienced technician. Most importantly, recent technological advances have produced reliable and easy to use ambulatory devices for the measurement of ICG. The ability to record measures of cardiac dynamics in an ambulatory setting is a major advance for behavioral medicine research. In addition, recent studies suggest that such methods may yield measures of absolute levels of SV that are at least as reliable as measures derived from echocardiography in both supine and tilted postures (Cybulski et al, 2004). These authors noted that in the supine position there were no differences between SV measures via ICG compared to those measured by echocardiography. In the tilt position they noted that the ICG gave values that were 6 ml greater than echo-derived values but it was unclear if the ICG or the echo values were the source of the discrepancy.

Researchers have many questions about the use of impedance cardiography. One question concerns the use of ICG to obtain absolute values of SV and CO. As indicated above, this is an area of continuing controversy. Perhaps the safest answer is that ICG can be used to get good relative measures of SV and thus CO and TPR. Despite several studies suggesting that ICG can provide accurate absolute levels, caution should still be exercised when interpreting ICG-derived measures of SV and CO. Recently, other methods to assess SV and CO based upon pulse contour analysis have become available (Wesseling et al, 1993). Data suggest that the bias associated with the pulse contour method may be the least followed by ICG-based measures with thermodilution methods yielding the least reliable measures (Bogert and van Lieshout, 2005; Doerr et al, 2005).

Another question concerns the need to correct measures of SV, CO, and TPR for body size. Again there is a lack of consensus on this question. Men, due to their larger body and heart size, often have larger values for SV and CO than do women. Therefore, if one wants to make inferences about absolute levels of SV or CO between groups and the groups differ in their gender composition or body size, this may be problematic. Under such circumstances SV and CO values may be corrected for body size by an equation that weights SV and CO values by body surface area (see Sherwood et al, 1990a). This produces what are called SV index and CO index. By using this corrected value of CO in calculations of TPR one also gets a TPR index measure. On the other hand, differences in body size do contribute to absolute differences in SV and CO (and may affect changes in these measures as well). Therefore "correction" for body surface area may obscure "real" biological differences.

Issues about the use of spot electrodes versus band electrodes are another area that researchers have investigated. McGrath and colleagues (2005) recently revisited this topic with their own investigation as well as providing a detailed review and critique of five previous comparison studies. Despite various differences, inconsistencies, and shortcomings among the six studies, these authors concluded that given the better signal-to-noise ratio, validity, and participant comfort associated with spot electrodes as well as the increasing use of ambulatory devices, spot electrodes appear to be the better solution.

4.1 The Genetics of Impedance Derived Measures

There is surprisingly little research on the genetics of cardiac contractility (inotropy) and the associated measures derived from impedance cardiography. A recent study using an extended twin design reported that heritability estimates for PEP, PEP/LVET ratio, and HI ranged from 48 to 62% for PEP, 35 to 58% for PEP/LVET, and 38 to 50% for HI (Kupper et al, 2006). It was concluded that these impedance derived indices of cardiac contractility showed substantial evidence of heritability. In a bi-racial sample of youths, the heritabilities for CO and SV were reported as 50 and 56%, respectively. However, significant ethnic differences were found for TPR with a heritability of 51% for African Americans and a surprising 18% for European Americans (Snieder et al, 2003). In addition molecular genetic studies have linked indices of cardiac contractility to chromosome 11 of the human genome and the beta-2 adrenergic receptor gene has been associated with SV and TPR (Arnett et al, 2001; Snieder et al, 2002; Tang et al, 2002). Clearly additional research is needed in this area.

4.2 Summary

Impedance cardiography is a useful, albeit imperfect, technique for the measurement of cardiac hemodynamics. Measures of systolic time intervals and thus indices of the autonomic influences on certain indices of cardiac chronotropy (e.g., LVET) and inotropy (e.g, PEP) are relatively problem free from a measurement perspective. However, measures of SV and thus CO are more problematic. Absolute values of these measures must be treated with caution. Because of the lack of a clear "gold standard," there will always be some uncertainty associated with measures of SV and CO derived from *any* technology – impedance cardiography included.

5 Heart Rate Variability

The basic data for the calculation of all the measures of HRV is the sequence of time intervals between heart beats (see Fig. 47.2, top trace). This interbeat interval time series is used to calculate the variability in the timing of the heart beat. As mentioned earlier, the heart is dually innervated by the autonomic nervous system such that relative increases in sympathetic

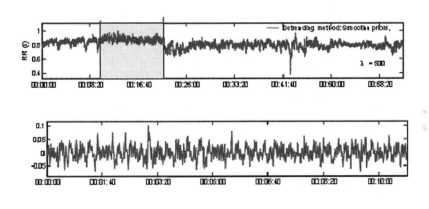

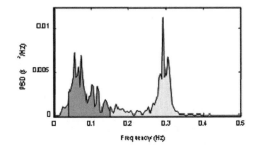
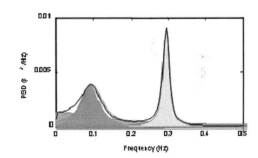

Frequency Band	Peak (Hz)	Power (ms^2)	Power (%)	Power (n.u.)
VLF (0-0.04 Hz)	0.0391	23	3.5	
LF (0.04-0.15 Hz)	0.0547	321	49.6	51.4
HF (0.15-0.4 Hz)	0.2930	304	46.9	48.6
Total		648		
LF/HF		1.058		

Frequency Band	Peak (Hz)	Power (ms^2)	Power (%)	Power (n.u.)
VLF (0-0.04 Hz)	0.0000	318	33.4	
LF (0.04-0.15 Hz)	0.0977	354	37.2	55.8
HF (0.15-0.4 Hz)	0.2930	281	29.4	44.2
Total		953		
LF/HF		1.263		

Fig. 47.2 The *top trace* shows an IBI time series. The *highlighted* portion is shown in more detail in the *second tracing*. The figure and values on the *left* are from a fast Fourier transform (FFT) analysis and those on the *right* are from an autoregressive analysis of the *highlighted* data. The tables show the frequency band, peak frequency, power, percentage power, and power in normalized units. Whereas the values from the two methods are similar they are not identical. Adapted from the output of free software provided by the Department of Applied Physics, University of Kuopio, Finland. See Niskanen et al. (2004)

activity are associated with heart rate increases and relative increases in parasympathetic activity are associated with heart rate decreases. The parasympathetic influences are pervasive over the frequency range of the heart rate power spectrum whereas the sympathetic influences "roll-off" at about 0.15 Hz (Saul, 1990; see Fig. 47.2 bottom panels). Therefore high-frequency HRV represents primarily parasympathetic influences, with lower frequencies (below about 0.15 Hz) having a mixture of sympathetic and parasympathetic autonomic influences. The differential effects of the ANS on the sinoatrial node, and thus the timing of the heart beats, are due to the differential effects of the neurotransmitters for the sympathetic and parasympathetic nervous systems. The sympathetic effects are on the time scale of seconds whereas the parasympathetic effects are on the time scale of milliseconds. Therefore the parasympathetic influences are the only ones capable of producing rapid changes in the beat-to-beat timing of the heart (see Fig. 47.2, middle trace). More detail concerning the various rhythms present in the interbeat interval time series is given below.

The number of publications on HRV has risen exponentially since the first clinical use of HRV in the assessment of fetal distress appeared in the late 1950s (Hon, 1958). However, the study of the various rhythms associated with the autonomic control of heart rate has a much longer history (see Berntson et al, 1997, for a nice historical review). HRV may be a particularly useful measure in behavioral medicine research. Reduced HRV is considered to be an index of diminished health. In addition, HRV has been associated with a number of psychological states and dispositions. Some of these relationships particularly relevant to behavioral medicine will be briefly summarized here but readers are referred to the above cited reviews for more extensive coverage of this topic.

5.1 Physiological Regulation

We have recently reviewed the literature on the relationship between vagal function and the risk for cardiovascular disease (CVD) and stroke (Thayer and Lane, 2007). The National Heart, Lung, and Blood Institute of the US National Institutes of Health list eight risk factors for heart disease and stroke (http://www.nhlbi.nih.gov/hbp/hbp/hdrf.htm). It is interesting to note that there is at least some data to suggest that each of these risk factors is associated with decreased vagal function as indexed by HRV. Furthermore, emerging risk factors for CVD and mortality such as inflammation and psychosocial factors are also associated with decreased HRV. In addition, several large epidemiological studies have shown that reduced HRV is a risk factor for all-cause mortality and morbidity (Thayer and Lane, 2007). Thus, HRV in part due to its relationship with physical health and physiological regulatory systems may be of special relevance to researchers in behavioral medicine. However, another area that will be of importance for behavioral medicine researchers is emotional regulation.

5.2 Emotional Regulation

We and others have recently reviewed the literature on the relationship between HRV and emotional regulation (Appelhans and Luecken, 2006). Emotional regulation is a valuable skill that has clear implications for health. Emotions represent a distillation of an individual's perception of personally relevant environmental interactions, including not only challenges and threats but also the ability to respond to them (Frijda, 1988). Viewed as such, emotions reflect the integrity of one's ongoing adjustment to constantly changing environmental demands. When the affective system works properly, it promotes flexible adaptation to shifting environmental demands. In another sense, an adequate emotional response represents a selection of an optimal response and the inhibition of less functional ones from a broad behavioral repertoire, in such a way that energy use is matched to fit situational requirements. Therefore, the relationship between HRV and emotional regulation will have important implications for those of us that study the link between emotional states and dispositions such as depression, anxiety, anger and hostility, alexithymia, and physical health. Yet another area of interest involves research on cognitive functioning and HRV.

5.3 Cognitive Regulation

We have also recently reviewed our research on the relationship between HRV and cognitive regulation (Thayer et al, 2009). Attentional regulation and the ability to inhibit prepotent but inappropriate responses are important for health in a complex environment. Many tasks important for survival in today's world involve cognitive functions such as working memory, sustained attention, behavioral inhibition, and general mental flexibility. These tasks are all associated with prefrontal cortical activity (Arnsten and Goldman-Rakic, 1998). Deficits in these cognitive functions tend to accompany aging and are also present in negative affective states and dispositions such as depression and anxiety. Stress can also impair cognitive function and may contribute to the cognitive deficits observed in various mental disorders. It is also possible that autonomic dysregulation contributes to decline in attention and cognitive performance. Importantly, we have shown that HRV is related to these important cognitive functions as well as to prefrontal cortical function.

5.4 Models of Neural Control of HRV

There are two major models of the neural control of HRV. They emphasize different aspects of the neural control of the heart but are by no means mutually exclusive. Whereas the Polyvagal Theory (Porges, 1995) is focused exclusively on the vagus, the neurovisceral integration model is concerned with autonomic influences on the viscera more generally but with an emphasis on the parasympathetic nervous system (Thayer and Lane, 2000, 2009). In addition, the neurovisceral integration model is based on nonlinear dynamical systems theory and emphasizes inhibitory processes (Thayer and Lane, 2009).

5.4.1 The Polyvagal Theory

Porges (1995) developed the "Polyvagal Theory," where he linked psychophysiological processes with neurophysiological processes and brain structures. Thus, Porges wanted to explain how vagal pathways regulated HR in response to novelty and a wide variety of stimulation (i.e., attention, motion, emotion, and communication). Porges (1995) emphasized the role of the vagus in the adaptation to external stimuli. Porges described vagal activity as functioning similar to a brake (Porges et al, 1996). The function of the vagal brake is to keep HR slow by increased vagal output and inhibition of sympathetic influences. Releasing the vagal brake reduces vagal inhibition on the cardiac pacemaker (sinoatrial node) and HR increases due to the intrinsic rate of the pacemaker, mechanical reflexes, and sympathetic influences.

Porges and colleagues (1999) extended the idea of the vagal brake as a tonic link between RSA and metabolic output such as HR in response to environmental challenge, to a state-dependent index of the dynamic regulation of brain stem function by cortical neurons. Thus, in this model, the cortex would monitor the visceral state of the organism and provide an immediate neural command to make instantaneous adjustment via dynamic shifts in the vagal control of the heart. The relation between the RSA and heart period would then be dependent on cortical activity (Porges et al, 1999). More recently, we have proposed another model of the neural control of the heart.

5.4.2 The Model of Neurovisceral Integration

The neurovisceral integration model has identified a flexible neural network associated with self-regulation and adaptability that might provide a unifying framework within which to view the diversity of observed responses across domains (Thayer and Lane, 2000, 2009). In this model a set of neural structures that regulate physiological, behavioral, emotional, and cognitive responses can be indexed via peripheral indices such as cortisol excretion, startle blink magnitude, inflammatory markers, and HRV. This model emphasized the role of HRV as an index of self-regulation and its ability to reflect neural feedback mechanisms between the central nervous system (CNS) and the autonomic nervous system (ANS).

At the core of this model is the central autonomic network (CAN; Benarroch, 1997). Importantly for the present discussion, the primary output of the CAN is mediated through the preganglionic sympathetic and parasympathetic neurons that innervate the heart via the stellate ganglia and the vagus nerve, respectively. The interplay of these inputs to the sinoatrial node of the heart generates the complex variability that characterizes the healthy HR time series (Saul, 1990). Furthermore, sensory information from the heart and other peripheral systems are fed back to the CAN. Thus, HRV can be used to index a set of neural structures associated with self-regulation and health.

In support of this model we have shown that HRV is associated with activity of the prefrontal cortex such that inactivation of the prefrontal cortex leads to increased HR, decreased HRV, and disinhibition of sub-cortical sympathoexcitatory circuits (Ahern et al, 2001). Thayer and Lane (2000, 2009) suggested that a common reciprocal inhibitory cortico-subcortical neural circuit serves as the structural link between psychological processes like emotion and cognition and health-related physiological processes, and that this circuit can be indexed with HRV. Thus, because of these reciprocally interconnected neural structures that allow prefrontal cortex to exert an inhibitory influence on sub-cortical structures, the organism is able to respond to demands from the environment and organize their behavior.

5.5 Measures of HRV

A variety of measures have been used to operationalize HRV. In the following we will briefly review some of the many measures available. However, readers should refer to the various guidelines for all the various measures available. In addition, Allen and colleagues (2007) have recently provided an extremely valuable primer and comparison of some of the metrics of cardiac chronotropy.

5.6 Time Domain Indices of HRV

Time domain indices may be based upon the interbeat intervals directly or on differences between successive interbeat intervals. In addition, there are both short-term and long-term indices. Short-term indices are based on recordings with a duration on the order of magnitude of minutes. Long-term indices are usually based on 24-h recordings. Those measures that are based on the interbeat intervals directly do not distinguish the autonomic sources of the variability. These indices include the standard deviation of all N–N (normal to normal) intervals (SDNN) and the standard deviation of the average of N–N intervals for each 5 min period over 24 h (SDANN).

The second type of indices is based on the differences between successive N–N intervals. These indices are based on the comparison of the lengths of adjacent cardiac cycles and include the percentage of adjacent cycles that are >50 ms apart (pNN50) and the root mean square successive differences in milliseconds (RMSSD). RMSSD is the most commonly used measure derived from interval differences. This index uses what is called first differencing in the econometrics literature and acts like a high pass filter thus removing long-term trends and slower frequency variability from the signal. Due to the frequency characteristics of the autonomic influences on the heart such that vagal influences cover the full frequency range and sympathetic influences are primarily restricted to the lower frequencies, RMSSD reflects primarily vagal influences (Saul, 1990).

5.7 Frequency Domain Indices of HRV

Frequency domain analysis gives information about the amount of variance or power in the heart rate or heart period time series explained by periodic oscillations at various frequencies. Power spectral analysis of the time series provides basic information on the amount of variance or power as a function of frequency (Task Force, 1996). Typically four frequency bands can be distinguished from 24-h recordings and two frequency bands can be reliably discerned in short-term recordings. These are high frequency (HF; 0.15–0.4 Hz), low frequency (LF; 0.04–0.15 Hz), very low frequency (VLF; 0.003–0.04 Hz), and ultra low frequency (ULF; ≤0.003 Hz). The HF and LF bands are prominent in short-term recordings with a VLF or direct current (DC) component being associated with aperiodic and artifactual variance (see Fig. 47.2). Thus the VLF and ULF bands are not usually interpretable in short-term recordings. It is important to note that the total spectral power is exactly equal to the time domain variance of the HR time series. This useful relationship can be helpful in troubleshooting spectral analysis algorithms. Moreover, this makes clear that spectral analysis is similar to analysis of variance in that both techniques are used to partition variance and attribute it to various sources.

The measurements of frequency power components described above are usually expressed as absolute values of power (milliseconds squared; Task Force, 1996). The absolute power measurements represent the variance of the measured signal about its mean value. The so-called normalized scores represent the relative value of each power component in proportion to the total power. In addition, the VLF or DC component is often subtracted from the total power in calculating the normalized values. The DC component is defined as the spectral components with a frequency <0.03 Hz (Pagani et al, 1986). The LF

to HF ratio (LF/HF) has been proposed to reflect the sympathovagal balance (but see below).

There are numerous algorithms for doing spectral analysis. Historically the fast Fourier transform (FFT) was used. However, there are several disadvantages to this approach including the necessity of specifying the boundaries of the frequency bands in advance. This is called "windowing" and can lead to serious misinterpretations of the data if they fail to capture the frequencies that one is interested in. For example, in doing spectral analysis on infants or other species such as rodents, the ranges of the frequency bands we have described will not apply. The frequency of respiration varies greatly from infancy to adulthood and across species so to capture respiratory modulated HRV one has to adjust the "windows" in an FFT. Whereas bioengineers have called the FFT the "classical" approach to spectral analysis, more modern approaches based on linear prediction analysis have been developed. The major algorithm in this approach is the autoregressive algorithm and overcomes the windowing problem by using a true components analysis in which the central frequency and width of the bands is determined empirically and on an individualized basis (Kay and Marple, 1981).

Still more recent developments include the use of wavelets and algorithms for what is called time–frequency analysis. These approaches go even further and do not make assumptions concerning stationarity and thus allow for relatively continuous estimates of spectral power (Akay, 1997). In addition, numerous indices based on nonlinear dynamical systems or "chaos" theory have proven useful in the analysis of HRV (Pincus, 2001; Snieder et al, 2007). However, detailed discussion of these techniques is beyond the scope of the present chapter. Below we give an overview on what is known about the various bands.

5.7.1 The Ultra low-Frequency Band: <0.003 Hz

The ULF band has shown strong relationships with mortality, and therefore an understanding of this band is important (Stein and Kleiger, 1999). Whereas, as noted earlier, all frequencies of HRV reflect autonomic, particularly parasympathetic, influences to some degree, the utility of the ULF band to predict morbidity and mortality appears to lie in its relationship to the functional capacity of the patient (Roach et al, 2004). Roach and colleagues in several studies have shown that SDNN and ULF power in 24-h recordings is related to the range of physical activity that patients engage in and not with differences in autonomic control of the heart per se. Given that approximately 1 h is needed to observe about 10 cycles at this frequency it is clear that this band cannot be resolved in short-term recordings and is thus not a meaningful index under such circumstances.

5.7.2 The Very Low-Frequency Band: 0.003–0.04 Hz

The physiological origins of the VLF band have remained elusive. This band has been variously linked to fluctuations in the renin–angiotensin system and to thermoregulation (Kitney, 1980). We undertook a study to investigate the relationship between ambient temperature and HRV with a special emphasis on the VLF band (Sollers et al, 2002). Compared to the hot and control conditions, the cold condition was associated with significantly greater VLF power. This increase in VLF power was accompanied by an increase in diastolic blood pressure (DBP). Moreover, this pattern of an increase in VLF power and DBP was unique to the cold condition. These results suggested that the VLF band responded, at least in part, to variations in ambient temperature and thus was associated with thermoregulation. Again because of the low frequency of these oscillations (approximately 2 per minute) this band is not resolved in short-term recordings.

5.7.3 The Low-Frequency Band: 0.04–0.15 Hz

There has been a great deal of controversy surrounding the meaning of variations in power in the LF band. Oscillations in this frequency band have been identified for over 100 years and are associated with baroreflex-mediated blood pressure variations (Penaz, 1978). In support of this idea, Moak and colleagues (2007) have recently shown in a very conclusive study that supine LF power reflects baroreflex function and is thus primarily of vagal origin. The empirical data support this analysis as LF power has been shown to correlate very highly with HF power (0.70 or higher) in numerous studies (Thayer and Lane, 2007). Therefore, raw LF power most likely reflects significant parasympathetic nervous system activity with varying degrees of sympathetic influence depending on various conditions. Given that approximately 2 min of data are necessary to provide adequate spectral resolution of this frequency (approximately 10 oscillations), LF power can be reliably assessed in short-term recordings.

5.7.4 The High-Frequency Band: 0.15–0.4 Hz

HF power is primarily parasympathetically mediated. The HF band primarily reflects the respiration-mediated HRV at 0.15–0.4 Hz (Saul, 1990). The defined frequency band for this parameter usually encompasses the frequency range corresponding to the frequency of normal respiration. Thus, the HF power predominantly measures the variability in HR induced by respiration (but see discussion about controlling for respiration below). This index of vagally mediated cardiac control correlates highly with the time domain-based measure of RMSSD.

Researchers have many questions about the use of HRV. One question that researchers often have is whether they can derive accurate measures of HRV from recording sources other than the ECG. Sometimes a researcher will have a HR or IBI time series derived from a photoplethysmograph or from a pulse wave such as might be derived from a blood pressure recording. Research has shown that while not ideal, the time series derived from these devices can under certain circumstances be used to provide reasonably accurate measures of HRV (Giardino et al, 2002; McKinley et al, 2003).

Another question that is frequently asked concerns the measurement of sympathetic nervous system activity using HRV. It would be very convenient if one could independently index both the parasympathetic *and* the sympathetic influences on the heart using HRV. Unfortunately the situation is not so simple. First, the notion of a unitary "sympathetic nervous system" is ill conceived. As noted above, there are many different types of adrenergic transmitters and receptors, and their distribution across the various cardiac effector tissues is neither completely segregated nor unique. For example, there are two major types of adrenergic receptors – alpha and beta. Using a gross oversimplification one could say that alpha-adrenergic receptors tend to dominate the vasculature and beta-adrenergic receptors tend to dominate the heart. Therefore, any discussion of an index of "sympathetic activity" must account for the local nature of sympathetic influences on effector tissues. This is highlighted by the fact that measures of sympathetic nerve activity derived from microneurography are highly location dependent (Wallin, 2006). Second, as noted above, with respect to the HRV power spectrum, the vagal influences cover a full range of frequencies whereas the sympathetic influences "roll-off" at about 0.15 Hz (Saul, 1990). Thus any measure derived from HRV analyses will have at least some parasympathetic influence. Thus, raw LF power has been empirically shown to be highly reflective of vagal influences under a wide range of situations.

It has been suggested that normalized LF power or the LF/HF ratio might be a better index of SNS influences. Again, the situation is not so simple. Empirically, "normalized" LF power and/or the LF/HF ratio in concert with HF power may provide some insight into the *relative* relationship among autonomic influences. However, it must be clearly stated that for various reasons noted above, these indices should never be taken to reflect "sympathetic" activity and therefore should be used with caution (Eckberg, 1997).

One of the most hotly debated issues in the use of HRV concerns the influence of respiration on indices of HRV. Allen and colleagues (2007) have recently proposed a multi-step strategy to deal with respiration which includes monitoring respiration rate to see if it differs between conditions and if it does, using analysis of covariance to ascertain if the HRV effects remain after statistical control. They argue that if the HRV effects are not accounted for by respiration then one can interpret the HRV effects with a certain degree of confidence. However, if the effects do not remain after accounting for respiration one is left in an interpretive bind. This is because some studies suggest that HRV indices adjusted for respiration parameters may in fact be less accurate indices of vagal influences than their unadjusted counterparts (Houtveen et al, 2002). Thus, the adjustment itself may do more harm than good. We also should note that not all indices of HRV are equally affected by respiration. For example, RMSSD has been recommended for ambulatory studies as it is less affected by changes in breathing frequency (Penttila et al, 2001). In addition, we have recently shown in a large sample that the nonlinear dynamical systems related measure of approximate entropy (ApEn) is uncorrelated with respiration and indeed may be a more sensitive indicator of cardiac autonomic effects than more traditional measures such as peak-to-trough RSA (Snieder et al, 2007). Finally, we have also shown that there may be individual differences in the degree of respiratory influences on different measures of HRV (Hill et al, 2009). Thus, great care must be exercised in using wholesale corrections of HRV indices for respiration.

An interesting aspect of the whole debate that has not been fully appreciated is that all of these arguments for the control of respiration assume that the direction of causality flows from respiration to the cardiac changes. That is, respiration causes the changes in the HRV. However, recent data in the respiratory physiology literature suggests that the heart beat might initiate the onset of inspiration. This has been known since the early 1920s when Walter Coleman observed that there was a marked tendency for there to be a fixed number of heart beats between inspirations (Coleman, 1921). That is, that the causal direction might flow from the cardiac change to respiration (Tzeng et al, 2003). If this is the case then controlling for respiration effects in HRV indices clearly may remove variability associated with neural influences on the control of the heart beat and thus at least partially remove variance that we are interested in studying. We raise this point here merely to show that the relationship between heart rate and respiration may be more complex than the arguments for the control of respiration might lead one to believe. The debate about the control of respiration will continue but the recommendations of Allen and colleagues (2007) seem like a reasonable approach to take at this time.

The recommendations of Allen and colleagues (2007) assume that one has a measure of respiratory rate available. If one does not have a direct measure of respiratory rate from a strain gauge or other device for the assessment of respiration one can derive an index of respiratory rate from the IBI time series (Thayer et al, 2002).

5.8 The Genetics of HRV

The investigation of the genetics of HRV is currently an area of very active exploration. Both behavioral and molecular genetic studies suggest that there is a significant genetic component to the individual differences in HRV including stress-induced HRV changes (Boomsma et al, 1990; Wang et al, 2009). Kupper and colleagues (2004) reported heritabilities for the time domain indices of SDNN (35–47%) and RMSSD (40–48%) in a large twin study of 772 participants across four time periods during the day. Wang and colleagues (2005) in a large study of African American and European American youth reported that SDNN, RMSSD, and HF were highly significant correlated ($r > 0.80$). Moreover, this combined factor had a heritability of 70%.

Several molecular genetic studies have also been reported with significant associations found with the angiotensin-converting enzyme insertion/deletion gene (Busjahn et al, 1998; Thayer et al, 2003) and the choline transporter gene (Neumann et al, 2005). Several research groups are continuing to explore possible candidate genes associated with HRV and much future work is needed.

5.9 Summary

HRV remains one of the best ways to measure cardiac autonomic control. It is clear that it has relationships with aspects of functioning including physiological, emotional, and cognitive regulation that are important for research in behavioral medicine. Given the pervasiveness of data collection and analysis systems the modern researcher now more than ever needs to know what to do with these data. Hopefully the preceding discussion will help researchers make better inferences from their data and help to guide them through some of the controversies and issues involved.

6 Conclusion

It has been more than 15 years since the publication of the Society for Psychophysiological Research's guidelines on impedance cardiography (ICG) and 10 years since their heart rate variability (HRV) guidelines (Sherwood et al, 1990a; Berntson et al, 1997). The Task Force of the European Society of Cardiology and the North American Society of Pacing and Electrophysiology guidelines on HRV were published simultaneously in Circulation and the European Heart Journal in 1996 (Task Force, 1996). Much has transpired in the areas of ICG and HRV since those seminal works. In this chapter we have tried to provide an update on the current state of affairs in the non-invasive assessment of autonomic control of the cardiovascular system as can be provided by ICG and HRV.

One extremely important development in the field has been the appearance of numerous turn-key systems for the measurement of both ICG and HRV. These systems range from inexpensive exercise watches for HRV and compact ambulatory devices for ICG to very elaborate laboratory-based systems. A particularly exciting development has been the appearance of several ambulatory systems for the recording of ICG and HRV. These systems allow researchers to collect large amounts of data with very little effort. With the advent of these turn-key systems for the collection of large amounts of high quality data the technological hurdles that once were obstacles to the widespread use of ICG and HRV have largely been surmounted. Thus the researcher must now be more prepared than ever to deal with the complexities of the data they are confronted with. Numerous future challenges still face us, however. The appropriate statistical analysis of the large amounts of data we collect particularly in the context of continuous recordings and time–frequency analytic techniques will require continued effort. The further explication of the neural concomitants of ICG and HRV measures also will be an area of active research. And perhaps one of the biggest challenges is the use of indices of HRV for risk assessment and stratification in clinical medicine. Given that numerous factors influence the values of spectral-derived indices, the use of time domain-based measures where a common and easily comprehended metric is available seems to be the most fruitful line of investigation (LaRover and the ATRAMI Investigators, 1998). The non-invasive assessment of autonomic control of the cardiovascular system has much to offer to the behavioral medicine researcher. It is hoped that the present chapter will aid in some small way those interested in this important topic.

References

Ahern, G. L., Sollers, J. J., Lane, R. D., Labiner, D. M., Herring, A. M. et al (2001). Heart rate and heart rate variability changes in the intracarotid sodium amobarbital (ISA) test. *Epilepsia, 42*, 912–921.

Akay, M. (1997). *Time Frequency and Wavelets in Biomedical Signal Processing*. New York: IEEE Press.

Allen, J. J. B., Chambers, A. S., and Towers, D. N. (2007). The many metrics of cardiac chronotropy: a pragmatic primer and a brief comparison of metrics. *Biol Psychol, 74*, 243–262.

Appelhans, B. M., and Luecken, L. J. (2006). Heart rate variability as an index of regulated emotional responding. *Rev Gen Psychol, 10*, 229–240.

Arnett, D. K., Devereux, R. B., Kitzman, D., Oberman, A., Hopkins, P. et al (2001). Linkage of left ventricular contractility to chromosome 11 in humans: The HyperGEN study. *Hypertension, 38*, 767–772.

Arnsten, A. F. T., and Goldman-Rakic, P. S. (1998). Noise stress impairs prefrontal cortical cognitive function in monkeys: evidence for a hyperdopaminergic mechanism. *Arch Gen Psychiatry, 55*, 362–369.

Benarroch, E. E. (1997). The central autonomic network. In P. A. Low (Ed.), *Clinical Autonomic Disorders, 2nd Ed* (pp. 17–23). Philadelphia, PA: Lippincott-Raven.

Benarroch, E. E. (2008). The arterial baroreflex: functional organization and involvement in neurologic disease. *Neurology, 71*, 1733–1738.

Berne, R. M., and Levy, M. N. (2001). *Cardiovascular Physiology*. London: Mosby Press.

Berntson, G. G., Bigger, J. T., Eckberg, D. L., Grossman, P., Kaufmann, P. G. et al (1997). Heart rate variability: origins, methods, and interpretive caveats. *Psychophysiology, 34*, 623–648.

Bogert, L. W. J., and van Lieshout, J. J. (2005). Non-invasive pulsatile arterial pressure and stroke volume changes from the human finger. *Exp Physiol, 90.4*, 437–446.

Boomsma, D. I., van Baal, G. C., and Orlebeke, J. F. (1990). Genetic influences on respiratory sinus arrhythmia across different task conditions. *Acta Genet Med Gemellol (Roma), 39*, 181–191.

Brook, R. D., and Julius, S. (2000). Autonomic imbalance, hypertension, and cardiovascular risk. *Am J Hypertens, 13*, 112S–122S.

Busjahn, A., Voss, A., Knoblauch, H., Knoblauch, M., Jeschke, E. et al (1998). Angiotensin-converting enzyme and angiotensinogen gene polymorphisms and heart rate variability in twins. *Am J Cardiol, 81*, 755–60.

Coleman, T. G., Guyton, A. C., Cowley, A. W. Jr, Bower, J. D. et al (1977). Feedback mechanisms of arterial pressure control. *Contrib Nephrol, 8*, 5–12.

Coleman, W. M. (1921). On the correlation of the rate of heart beat, breathing, bodily movement, and sensory stimuli. *J Physiol, 54*, 213–217.

Cybulski, G., Michalak, E., Kozluk, E., Piatkowska, A., and Niewiadomski, W. (2004). Stroke volume and systolic time intervals: beat-to-beat comparison between echocardiography and ambulatory impedance cardiography in supine and tilted positions. *Med Biol Eng Comput, 42*, 707–711.

Doerr, D. F., Ratliff, D. A., Sithole, J., and Convertino, V. A. (2005). Stroke volume during orthostatic challenge: comparison of two non-invasive methods. *Aviat, Space Environ Med, 76*, 935–939.

Duschek, S., and Reyes del Paso, G. A. (2007). Quantification of cardiac baroreflex function at rest and during autonomic stimulation. *J Physiol Sci, 57*, 259–268.

Eckberg, D. L. (1997). Sympathovagal balance—a critical appraisal. *Circulation, 96*, 3224–3232.

Fagard, R. H., Pardaens, K., Staessen, J. A., and Thijs, L. (1996). Prognostic value of invasive hemodynamic measurements at rest and during exercise in hypertensive men. *Hypertension, 28*, 31–36.

Frijda, N. H. (1988). The laws of emotion. *Am Psychol, 43*, 349–358.

Giardino, N. D., Lehrer, P. M., and Edelberg, R. (2002). Comparison of finger plethysmograph to ECG in the measurement of heart rate variability. *Psychophysiology, 35*, 246–253.

Hesse, C., Charkoudian, N., Liu, Z., Joyner, M. J., and Eisenach, J. H. (2007). Baroreflex sensitivity inversely correlates with ambulatory blood pressure in healthy normotensive humans. *Hypertension, 50*, 41–46.

Hill, L. K., Siebenbrock, A., Sollers, J. J., and Thayer, J. F. (2009). All are measures created equal? Heart rate variability and respiration. *Biomed Sci Instrum, 45*, 71–76.

Hon, E. H. (1958). The electronic evaluation of the fetal heart rate. *Am J Obstet Gynecol, 75*, 1215–1230.

Houtveen, J. H., Rietveld, S., and de Geus, E. J. (2002). Contribution of tonic vagal modulation of heart rate, central respiratory drive, respiratory depth, and respiratory frequency to respiratory sinus arrhythmia during mental stress and physical exercise. *Psychophysiology, 39*, 427–436.

Jensen, L., Yakimets, J., and Teo, K. K. (1995). A review of impedance cardiography. *Heart Lung, 24*, 183–193.

Jose, A. D., and Collison, D. (1970). The normal range and determinants of the intrinsic heart rate in man. *Cardiovasc Res, 4*, 160–167.

Kay, S. M., and Marple, S. L. (1981). Spectral analysis—a modern perspective. *Proc IEEE Inst Electr Electron Eng, 69*, 1380–1419.

Kitney, R. I. (1980). An analysis of thermoregulatory influences on heart-rate variability. In R. I. Kitney & O. Rompelman (Eds.), *The study of heart-rate variability* (pp. 81–106). Oxford: Clarendon Press.

Kupper, N., Willemsen, G., Boomsma, D., and De Geus, E. J. C. (2006). Heritability of indices of cardiac contractility in ambulatory recordings. *J Cardiovasc Electrophysiol, 17*, 877–883.

Kupper, N., Willemsen, G., van den Berg, M., de Boer, D., Posthuma, D., et al (2004). Heritability of ambulatory heart rate variability. *Circulation, 110*, 2792–2796.

LaRover, M. T., and the ATRAMI investigators (1998). Baroreflex sensitivity and heart rate variability in prediction of total mortality after myocardial infarction. *Lancet, 351*, 478–484.

Levy, M. N. (1997). Neural control of cardiac function. *Baillieres Clin Neurol, 6*, 227–244.

Levy, M. N., and Martin, P. J. (1996). Autonomic control of cardiac conduction and automaticity. In J. T. Shepard & S. J. Vatner (Eds.), *Nervous Control of the Heart* (pp. 201–225). Amsterdam: Harwood Academic Publishers .

Levy, M. N., and Zieske, H. (1969). Autonomic control of cardiac pacemaker activity and atrioventricular transmission. *J Appl Physiol, 27*, 465–470.

Lohmeier, T. E. (2001). The sympathetic nervous system and long-term blood pressure regulation. *Am J Hypertens, 14*, 147S–154S.

Lohmeier, T. E., Irwin, E. D., Rossing, M. A., Serdar, D. J., and Kieval, R. S. (2004). Prolonged activation of the baroreflex produces sustained hypotension. *Hypertension, 43*, 306–311.

Mamivuo, J., and Plonsey, R. (1995). *Bioelectromagnetism—Principles and Applications of Bioelectric and Biomagnetic Fields.* New York: Oxford University Press.

McGrath, J. J., O'Brien, W. H., Hassinger, H. J., and Shah, P. (2005). Comparability of spot versus band electrodes for impedance cardiography. *J Psychophysiol, 19*, 195–203.

McKinley, P. S., Shapiro, P. A., Bagiella, E., Myers, M. M., DeMeersman, R. E. et al (2003). Deriving heart rate variability from blood pressure waveforms. *J Appl Physiol, 95*, 1431–1438.

Mensah, G. A., Pappas, T. W., Koren, M. J., Ulin, R. J. et al (1993). Comparison of the classification of the severity of hypertension by blood pressure level and by WHO criteria in the prediction of concurrent cardiac abnormalities and subsequent complications in essential hypertension. *J Hypertens, 11*, 1429–1440.

Miller, S. B., and Ditto, B. (1988). Cardiovascular responses to an extended aversive video game task. *Psychophysiology, 25*, 200–208.

Moak, J. P., Goldstein, D. S., Eldadah, B. A., Saleem, A., Holmes, C. et al (2007). Supine low frequency power of heart rate variability reflects baroreflex function, not cardiac sympathetic innervation. *Heart Rhythm, 4*, 1523–1529.

Neumann, S. A., Lawrence, E. C., Jennings, J. R., Ferrell, R. E., and Manuck, S. B. (2005). Heart rate variability is associated with polymorphic variation in the choline transporter gene. *Psychosom Med, 67*, 168–171.

Niskanen, J. P., Tarvainen, M. P., Ranta-aho, P. O., and Karjalainen, P. A. (2004). Software for advanced HRV analysis. *Comput Methods Programs Biomed, 76*, 73–81

Ottaviani, C., Shapiro, D., Goldstein, I. B., James, J. E., and Weiss, R. (2006). Hemodynamic profile, compensation deficit, and ambulatory blood pressure. *Psychophysiology, 43,* 46–56.

Pagani, M. Lombardi, F., Guzzetti, S., Rimoldi, O., Furlan, R. et al (1986). Power spectral analysis of heart rate and arterial pressure variabilities as a marker of sympathovagal interaction in man and conscious dog. *Circ Res, 59,* 178–193.

Parati, G., Di Rienzo, M., and Mancia, G. (2000). How to measure baroreflex sensitivity: from the cardiovascular laboratory to daily life. *J Hypertens, 18,* 7–19.

Penaz, J. (1978). Mayer waves: history and methodology. *Automedica, 2,* 135–141.

Penttila, J., Helminen, A., Jartti,T., Kuusela, T., Huikuri, H. V. et al (2001). Time domain, geometrical and frequency domain analysis of cardiac vagal outflow: effects of various respiratory patterns. *Clin Physiol, 21,* 365–376.

Pincus, S. M. (2001). Assessing serial irregularity and its implications for health. *Ann New York Acad Sci, 954,* 245–267.

Porges, S. W. (1995). Orienting in a defensive world: mammalian modification of our evolutionary heritage. A Polyvagal Theory. *Psychophysiology, 32,* 301–318.

Porges, S. W., Doussard-Roosevelt, J. A., Portales, A. L., and Greenspan, S. I. (1996). Infant regulation of the vagal "brake" predicts child behavior problems: a psychobiological model of social. *Dev Psychobiol, 29,* 697–712.

Porges, S. W., Doussard-Roosevelt, J. A., Stifter, C. A., McClenny, B. D., and Riniolo, T. C.(1999). Sleep state and vagal regulation of heart period patterns in the human newborn: an extension of the polyvagal theory. *Psychophysiology, 36,* 14–21.

Ring, C., Burns, V. E., and Carroll, D. (2002). Shifting hemodynamics of blood pressure control during prolonged mental stress. *Psychophysiology, 39,* 585–590.

Roach, D., Wilson, W., Ricthie, D., and Sheldon, R. (2004) Dissection of long-range heart rate variability. *J Am Coll Cardiol, 43,* 2271–2277.

Saul, J. P. (1990). Beat-to beat variations of heart rate reflect modulation of cardiac autonomic outflow. *News Physiol Sci, 5,* 32–37.

Sherwood, A., Allen, M. T., Fahrenberg, J., Kelsey, R. M., Lovallo, W. R. et al (1990a). Methodological guidelines for impedance cardiography. *Psychophysiology, 27,* 1–23.

Sherwood, A., Dolan, C. A., and Light, K. C. (1990b). Hemodynamics of blood pressure responses during active and passive coping. *Psychophysiology, 27,* 656–668.

Snieder, H., Dong, Y., Barbeau, P., Harshfield, G. A., Dalageogou, C. et al (2002). Beta 2-adrenergic receptor gene and resting hemodynamics in European and African American youth. *Am J Hypertens, 15,* 973–979.

Snieder, H., Harshfield, G. A., and Treiber, F. A. (2003). Heritability of blood pressure and hemodynamics in African- and European-American youth. *Hypertension, 41,* 1196–1201.

Snieder, H., van Doornen, L. J. P., Boomsma, D., and Thayer, J. F. (2007). Sex differences and heritability of two indices of heart rate dynamics: a twin study. *Twin Res Hum Genet, 10,* 364–372.

Sollers, J. J., Sanford, T. A., Nabors-Oberg, R. E., Anderson, C. A., and Thayer, J. F. (2002). Examining changes in HRV in response to varying ambient temperature. *IEEE Eng Med Biol Mag, 21,* 30–34.

Stein, P. K., and Kleiger, R. E. (1999). Insights from the study of heart rate variability. *Annu Rev Med, 50,* 249–261.

Stemmler, G., Grossman, P., Schmid, H., and Foerster, F. (1991). A model of cardiovascular activation components for studies using autonomic receptor antagonists. *Psychophysiology, 28,* 367–382.

Sztajzel, J. (2004). Heart rate variability: a noninvasive electrocardiographic method to measure the autonomic nervous system. *Swiss Med Wkly, 134,* 514–522.

Tang, W., Arnett, D. K., Devereux, R. B., Province, M. A., Atwood, L. et al (2002). Sibling resemblance for left ventricular structure, contractility, and diastolic filling. *Hypertension, 40,* 233–238.

Task Force of the European Society of Cardiology and the North American Society of Pacing and Electrophysiology. (1996). Heart rate variability: Standards of measurement, physiological interpretation, and clinical use. *Circulation, 93,* 1043–1065.

Thayer, J. F., Hansen, A. L., Saus-Rose E., and Johnsen, B. H. (2009). Heart rate variability, prefrontal neural function and cognitive performance: the Neurovisceral Integration perspective on self-regulation, adapttion, and health. *Ann Behavl Med, 37,* 141–153.

Thayer, J. F., and Lane, R. D. (2000). A model of neurovisceral integration in emotion regulation and dysregulation. *J Affect Disord, 61,* 201–216.

Thayer, J. F., and Lane, R. D. (2007). The role of vagal function in the risk for cardiovascular disease and mortality. *Biol Psychol, 74,* 224–242.

Thayer, J. F., and Lane, R. D. (2009). Claude Bernard and the heart-brain connection: further elaboration of a model of Neurovisceral Integration. *Neurosci Biobehav Rev, 33,* 81–88.

Thayer, J. F., Merritt, M. M., Sollers, J. J., Zonderman, A. B., Evans, M. K. et al (2003). Effect of angiotensin-converting enzyme insertion/deletion polymorphism DD genotype on high-frequency heart rate variability in African Americans. *Am J Cardiol, 92,* 1487–1490.

Thayer, J. F., Sollers, J. J., Ruiz-Padial, E., and Vila, J. (2002). Estimating respiratory frequency from autoregressive spectral analysis of heart period. *IEEE Eng Med Biol Mag, 21,* 41–45.

Thayer, J. F., and Uijtdehaage, S. H. J. (2001). Derivation of chronotropic indices of autonomic nervous system activity using impedance cardiography. *Biomed Sci Instrum, 37*, 331–336.

Thrasher, T. N. (2006). Arterial baroreceptor input contributes to long-term control of blood pressure. *Curr Hypertens Rep, 8*, 249–254.

Tzeng, Y. C., Larsen, P. D., and Galletly, D. C. (2003). Cardioventilatory coupling in resting human subjects. *Exp Physiol, 88.6*, 775–782.

Uijtdehaage, S. B. H., and Thayer, J. F. (2000). Accentuated antagonism in the control of human heart rate. *Clin Auton Res, 10*, 107–110.

Wallin, B. G. (2006). Regulation of sympathetic nerve traffic to skeletal muscle in resting humans. *Clin Auton Res, 16*, 262–269.

Wang, X., Ding, X., Su, S., Li, Z., Riese, H. et al (2009). Genetic influences on heart rate variability at rest and during stress. *Psychophysiology, 46*, 458–465.

Wang, X., Thayer, J. F., Treiber, F., and Snieder, H. (2005) Ethnic differences and heritability of heart rate variability in African- and European American youth. *Am J Cardiol, 96*, 1166–1172.

Wesseling, K. H., Jansen, J. R., Settels, J. J., and Schreuder, J. J. (1993). Computation of aortic flow from pressure in humans using a nonlinear, three-element model. *J Appl Physiol, 74*, 2566–2573.

Chapter 48

Cardiac Measures

Gina T. Eubanks, Mustafa Hassan, and David S. Sheps

1 Myocardial Imaging

There are several techniques that can be used to perform myocardial imaging. This section of the chapter will cover the following five popular techniques: single photon emission computed tomography (SPECT), multigated acquisition (MUGA) scans, positron emission tomography (PET), computed tomography angiography (CTA), and cardiac magnetic resonance imaging (CMR).

1.1 SPECT Imaging

Single photon emission computed tomography (SPECT) is a nuclear imaging technique commonly used to measure myocardial perfusion, thickness, and contractility of the myocardium during various parts of the cardiac cycle in order to diagnose ischemic heart disease. Left ventricular ejection fraction (LVEF), stroke volume, and cardiac output can also be calculated with gated myocardial SPECT imaging. A cardiac-specific radionuclide, commonly ^{99m}Tc-tetrofosmin or ^{99m}Tc-sestamibi, is ideally injected during physical stress or, for those

who are unable to exercise, during pharmacologically induced stress. Approximately 1–2 h after the stressor, SPECT imaging is performed to depict the distribution of the radionuclide during stress. The images illustrate the relative blood flow to the different regions of the myocardium. The stress images are then compared to resting images in order to determine the presence of myocardial ischemia (the images obtained are also compared to normal databases using standardized software) (Fig. 48.1).

SPECT imaging has been used in behavioral studies in order to determine the effects that psychological stress has on the occurrence of myocardial ischemia in patients with coronary artery disease (CAD) (Hassan et al, 2007). Mental stress is induced in the laboratory setting, with the patients receiving an injection of the radioisotope during the stressor, and SPECT images are obtained after the stressor. The images from the mental stressor are compared to the resting images in order to determine the occurrence of myocardial ischemia due to psychological stress. Many studies have shown that psychological stress induces myocardial ischemia in CAD patients, even in the absence of ischemia during physical stress (Ramachandruni et al, 2006).

SPECT imaging is most commonly used as a non-invasive measure to diagnose ischemic heart disease and is of low risk. Use of SPECT imaging in behavioral studies is desirable because it allows more time between the stressor and the imaging, as compared to other imaging techniques that use radioisotopes with shorter

G.T. Eubanks (✉)
Division of Cardiovascular Medicine, Emory University, Atlanta, GA, USA; University of South Florida, 1717 W Hills Ave Unit 3, Tampa, FL 33606, USA
e-mail: geubank@emory.edu

A. Steptoe (ed.), *Handbook of Behavioral Medicine*, DOI 10.1007/978-0-387-09488-5_48,
© Springer Science+Business Media, LLC 2010

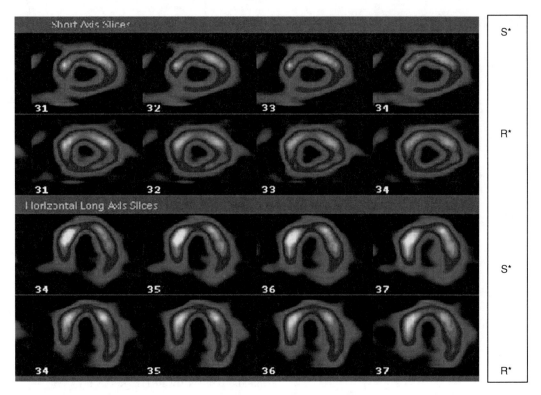

Fig. 48.1 Resting and Stress SPECT Images: this figure shows reversible ischemia in the inferior wall
*R = resting image, S = stress image

half-lives, such as positron emission tomography (PET). Additionally, SPECT imaging has become the more popular technique due to its greater sensitivity and specificity in women when compared to MUGA scans.

1.2 MUGA Imaging

A multigated acquisition (MUGA) scan is a nuclear cardiac measure used to evaluate the function of the heart ventricles at rest, during stress, or at both time points and provides movie-like, three-dimensional (3-D) images of the heart that show the wall motion of the heart allowing the identification of any wall motion abnormalities. During the test, a radioactive marker, Technetium-99m-pertechnetate, is injected intravenously after the introduction of

stannous (Tin) ions. The images obtained with a MUGA scan illustrate the circulation dynamics of the radioactive marker, therefore, the circulation of the blood in the chambers of the heart, and can be used to calculate the LVEF of the heart (Fig. 48.2) (Murphy and Lloyd, 2007). MUGA scans provide important information of the heart's function that allows doctors to determine the presence or extent of ischemic heart disease, congestive heart failure, as well as the cause for low cardiac output after open-heart

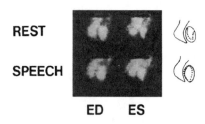

Fig. 48.2 MUGA: normal vs. abnormal wall motion

surgery, and to assess the effects of cardiotoxic drug agents and efficacy of procedures used for cardiac treatment (Murphy and Lloyd, 2007).

MUGA scans were predominantly the preferred nuclear cardiac measure for clinical diagnostic purposes and in behavioral cardiology studies, but have recently been replaced with SPECT imaging due to the time flexibility, sensitivity, and specificity offered with SPECT (Goldberg et al, 1996; Kim et al, 2003; Sheps et al, 2002).

1.3 PET Imaging

Positron emission tomography (PET) imaging is a nuclear medicine technique which allows the reader to examine certain bodily functions by targeting the injected radionuclide (Fleming, 2004). PET is used in many branches of medicine and research, such as oncology, neurology, cardiology, neuropsychology, psychiatry, and pharmacology. For cardiac purposes, PET studies are performed in order to identify atherosclerosis and vascular diseases (Murphy and Lloyd, 2007). However, as SPECT imaging is the most commonly used nuclear medicine technique for behavioral cardiology studies****. Still, there are potential advantages to the use of PET imaging in behavioral cardiology studies compared to SPECT, such as better spatial resolution and the ability to quantify blood flow.

1.4 CT Angiography

Computed tomography angiography (CTA) is an imaging technique that produces a 3-D image of the inside of an object using a series of two-dimensional (2-D) X-ray images taken around a single axis of rotation. CTA utilizes sub-second rotations in combination with multi-slice CT (up to 64-slice) to produce high-resolution and high-speed imaging with excellent quality. Cardiac CTA is used to capture images of the coronary arteries and can be coupled with retrospective

electrocardiogram (ECG) gating to produce better temporal resolution, which involves imaging each portion of the heart more than once while recording an ECG trace. This technique correlates the CT data with the corresponding phases of the cardiac cycle, and after ignoring the data collected during systole, images can be produced from the remaining data collected during diastole (Murphy and Lloyd, 2007).

Cardiac CTA is most commonly used to rule out coronary artery disease in order to avoid using the invasive catheterization procedure if possible. However, cardiac CTA has a less conclusive positive predictive value (i.e., is less accurate for diagnosing the severity of disease) and is, therefore, not commonly used for diagnosing CAD.

Cardiac CTA is not frequently used in behavioral cardiology studies due to cost and the high level of radiation exposure associated with this technique. Again, SPECT is the preferred imaging technique for research studies.

1.5 Cardiac MRI

Cardiac magnetic resonance imaging (CMR) is a non-invasive imaging technique that utilizes strong magnetic fields which align with hydrogen protons in various tissues. Radio frequency (RF) energy is then beamed through the tissues, temporarily exciting the protons. When the protons relax, the RF energy is released, creating the data to be measured (Fleming, 2004). Occasionally, MRIs are conducted using a contrast material, which alters the magnetic field and enhances or highlights the tissues seen in the images.

Clinically, CMR imaging provides a plethora of information that is used for diagnostic purposes. CMR images are able to capture vital clinical and diagnostic evidence for congenital heart disease, peripheral vascular disease, coronary artery disease, cardiomyopathy, acute and chronic rejection in heart transplant patients, pericardial disease, cardiac tumors, and valvular heart disease (Marcu et al, 2006; Pennell et al, 2004).

While CMR is able to provide a substantial amount of information for clinical purposes and has been utilized in cardiac research studies, it has not been adopted as an imaging technique in behavioral cardiology studies due to the high cost and the restrictions on the patient's movements during the study procedures.

2 Peripheral Arterial Tonometry (PAT)

Peripheral arterial tonometry (PAT) utilizes a device called the Endo-PAT2000 and measures endothelial function via signal changes in the fingertip of the patient. The test consists of placing a thimble-like probe on the patient's fingertip, which inflates and measures the digital pulsatile volume changes during testing procedures (Goor et al, 2004). Clinically, PAT is intended for use as a diagnostic aid in the detection of endothelial dysfunction or changes in sympathetic tone (Fig. 48.3).

PAT can be used in behavioral cardiology studies as a supplement to other cardiac measures for determining the presence of myocardial ischemia during exercise and psychological stressors; reproducibility of responses has not been well studied, but inter-observer agreement in measurements is greater than 95% (Goor et al, 2004; Hassan et al, 2009). Studies have shown that there is a significant correlation between the results obtained from nuclear imaging and the results obtained from PAT when measuring stress-induced myocardial ischemia in patients with CAD (Goor et al, 2004; Hassan et al, 2009).

3 Electrocardiogram (ECG) Measures

3.1 Standard 12 Lead and Ambulatory Monitoring

Standard 12 lead electrocardiograms (ECGs) measure the heart's rhythm, rate, and heart rate variability (HRV), in addition to providing evidence of ventricular irritability, such as ventricular premature contractions (PVCs), and manifest ischemia, illustrated by ST segment depression (Fig. 48.4) (Murphy and Lloyd, 2007).

Ambulatory monitoring is a technique that involves the use of a portable electrocardiographic device, usually the same size as a cassette-dictating recorder, which consists of electrodes attached to the person and is worn for 24 or 48 h. The electrocardiographic readings are correlated with personal diary recordings to examine the relationship between the ECG readings and the self-reported levels of emotional distress, physical distress, and/or other measurements which can be prompted by a palm pilot-type device and measured using a standardized scale, such as a visual analog scale (Francis et al, 2009; Murphy and Lloyd, 2007).

Both 12 lead ECGs and ambulatory monitoring are used in behavioral studies to assess HRV and changes in heart rate (HR) over time, as well as the relationship between the detection of arrhythmias and ischemia and/or the relationship between psychological stress and ischemia, indicated by ST segment depression (Krittayaphong et al, 1996).

Standard 12 lead ECGs are an advantageous cardiac measure to utilize because they have

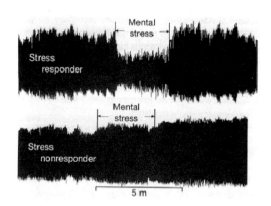

Fig. 48.3 PAT: mental stress responder vs. nonresponder.
Goor et al (2004)

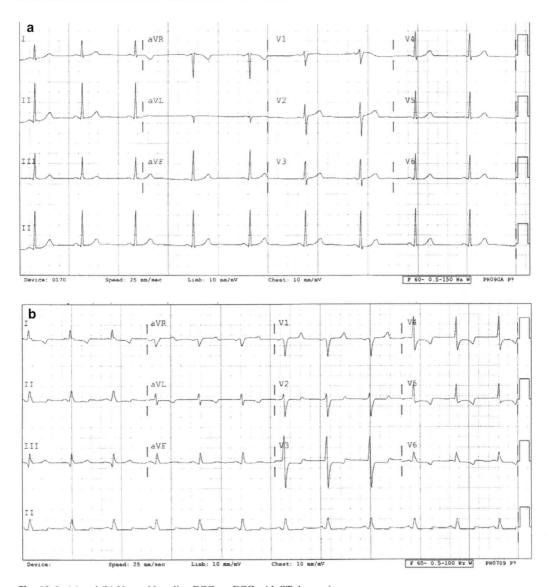

Fig. 48.4 (a) and (b) Normal baseline ECG vs. ECG with ST depression

been validated by years of experience as well as being inexpensive.

3.2 ECG Responses to Stress

Classically, HR, systolic blood pressure (SBP), and diastolic blood pressure (DBP) changes have been used to reflect the degree of physiological response to psychological stress (Krantz et al, 2000).

In addition to HR and BP responses, ST segment responses are examined during the interpretation of ECG responses to stress. ST segment depression is an indicator of ischemia to the heart and commonly occurs in patients with CAD who experience ischemia during exercise, but is a much less frequent occurrence (~15%) in patients with CAD during mental stress ischemia (Krantz et al, 2000).

ECG responses to stress can also be measured with QT measurements, which reflect the re-polarization of the ventricle. An abnormal response to stress can be measured by the difference between the shortest and the longest QT intervals on the standard 12 lead ECG, known as the QT dispersion (QTd). The more the QTd seen, the greater the disparity in the re-polarization of the ventricle, thereby, increasing the heart's vulnerability to subsequent arrhythmias. QTd is often used to evaluate the effect of stress on cardiac conduction or the propensity toward arrhythmias (Hassan et al, 2009).

4 ECHO Measurements

An echocardiogram (ECHO) is a technique using ultrasound, which allows accurate assessments of cardiac function and blood flow at rest and in response to stress. It uses ultrasound to obtain 2-D slices of the heart. However, recently, ultrasounds are utilizing 3-D real-time imaging, which allows for a better assessment of valvular defects and cardiomyopathies (Bharucha et al, 2008; Poh et al, 2008).

Clinically, ECHOs are able to assess the blood flow velocity and cardiac tissue by utilizing Doppler ultrasound in order to identify the size and shape of the heart, cardiac valve areas and functions, abnormal communications between the left and the right sides of the heart, and valvular regurgitation, in addition to allowing the calculation of cardiac output and ejection fraction (Murphy and Lloyd, 2007).

Echocardiography techniques have been used in some studies to assess ischemia (specifically, changes in wall motion and/or thickening of myocardium) (Kop et al, 2001; Murphy and Lloyd, 2007).

5 Differences Between Exercise and Psychological Stress-Induced Cardiac Responses

The greatest differences in exercise and psychological cardiac responses are seen in HR, SBP,

and DBP responses to stress. The HR increases to a greater extent during exercise vs. psychological stress. The SBP, however, changes much more quickly during psychological stress but reaches the same maximum point as during exercise stress. It is the DBP that illustrates the greatest difference in change between exercise and psychological stress. During psychological stress the DBP rises, but falls during exercise stress. This difference in reaction reflects the effect of peripheral vasodilation during exercise stress as opposed to vasoconstriction or increase in alpha tone during psychological stress (Goldberg et al, 1996; Krantz et al, 2000).

6 Summary

There are many different cardiac measures that can be used to assess cardiac responses in behavioral research. It is recommended that the design of studies should sometimes include the use of more than one technology in order to answer fundamental questions particularly related to physiologic mechanisms of responses to stress.

References

Bharucha, T., Roman, K. S., Anderson, R. H., and Vettukattil, J. J. (2008). Impact of multiplanar review of three-dimensional echocardiographic data on management of congenital heart disease. *Ann Thorac Surg*, *86*, 875–881.

Fleming, J. F. R. (2004). Traumatic Brain Injury: discussion paper prepared for the workplace safety and insurance appeals tribunal. http://www.wsiat.on.ca/tracITDocuments/MLODocuments/Discussions/traumatic.pdf

Francis, J. L., Weinstein, A. A., Krantz, D. S., Haigney, M. C., Stein, P. K. et al (2009). Association between symptoms of depression and anxiety with heart rate variability in patients with implantable cardioverter defibrillators. *Psychosom Med*, *71*, 821–827.

Goldberg, A. D., Becker, L. C., Bonsall, R., Cohen, J. D., Ketterer, M. W. et al (1996). Ischemic, hemodynamic, and neurohormonal responses to mental and exercise stress. Experience from the Psychophysiological Investigations of Myocardial Ischemia Study (PIMI). *Circulation*, *94*, 2402–2409.

Goor, D. A., Sheffy, J., Schnall, R. P., Arditti, A., Caspi, A. et al (2004). Peripheral Arterial tonometry: a diagnostic method for detection of myocardial ischemia induced during mental stress tests: a pilot study. *Clin. Cardiol, 27*, 1371–41.

Hassan, M., Mela, A., Li, Q., Brumback, B., Fillingim, R. B. et al (2009). The effect of acute psychological stress on QT dispersion in patients with coronary artery disease. *Pacing Clin Electrophysiol, 32*, 1178–1183.

Hassan, M., York, K. M., Li, H., Li, Q., and Sheps, D. S. (2007). Mental stress-induced myocardial ischemia in coronary artery disease patients with left ventricular dysfunction. *J Nucl Cardiol, 14*, 308–313.

Hassan, M., York, K. M., Li, H., Li, Q., Lucey, D. G. et al (2009). Usefulness of peripheral arterial tonometry in the detection of mental stress-induced myocardial ischemia. *Clin Cardiol, 32*, E1-E6.

Kim, C. K., Bartholomew, B. A., Mastin, S. T., Taasan, V. C., Carson, K. M. et al (2003). Detection and reproducibility of mental stress-induced myocardial ischemia with Tc-99m sestamibi SPECT in normal and coronary artery disease populations. *J Nucl Cardiol, 10*, 56–62.

Kop, W. J., Krantz, D. S., Howell, R. H., Ferguson, M. A., Papademetriou, V. et al (2001). Effects of mental stress on coronary epicardial vasomotion and flow velocity in coronary artery disease: relationship with hemodynamic stress responses. *J Am Coll Cardiol, 37*, 1359–1366.

Krantz, D. S., Sheps, D. S., Carney, R. M., and Natelson, B. H. (2000). Effects of mental stress in patients with coronary artery disease: evidence and clinical implications. *JAMA, 283*, 1800–1802.

Krittayaphong, R., Biles, P., Christy, C. G., and Sheps, D. S. (1996). Association between angina pectoris and ischemic indices during exercise testing and during ambulatory monitoring. *Am J Cardiol, 78*, 266–270.

Marcu, C. B., Beek, A. M., and Van Rossum, A. C. (2006). Clinical applications of cardiovascular magnetic resonance imaging. *Can Med Assoc J, 175*, 911–917.

Murphy, J. G., and Lloyd, M. A. (Eds.). (2007). *Mayo Clinic Cardiology Concise Textbook, 3rd Ed.* Rochesterd, Minnesota: Mayo Clinic Scientific Press.

Pennell, D. J., Sechtem, U. P., Higgins, C. B., Manning, W. J., Pohost, G. M. et al (2004). Clinical indications for cardiovascular magnetic resonance (CMR): consensus panel report. *Eur Heart J, 25*, 1940–1965.

Poh, K. K., Levine, R. A., Solis, J., Shen, L., Flaherty, M. et al (2008). Assessing aortic valve area in aortic stenosis by continuity equation: a novel approach using real-time three-dimensional echocardiography. *Eur Heart J, 29*, 2526–2535.

Ramachandruni, S., Fillingim, R. B., McGorray, S. P., Schmalfuss, C. M., Cooper, G. R. et al (2006). Mental stress provokes ischemia in coronary artery disease subjects without exercise- or adenosine-induced ischemia. *J Am Coll Cardiol, 47*, 987–991.

Sheps, D. S., McMahon, R. P., Becker, L., Carney, R. M., Freedland, K. E. et al (2002). Mental stress-induced ischemia and all-cause mortality in patients with coronary artery disease: results from the Pyschophysiological Investigations of Myocardial Ischemia study. *Circulation, 105*, 1780–1784.

Chapter 49

Behavioral Medicine and Sleep: Concepts, Measures, and Methods

Martica H. Hall

1 Introduction

Over the past 30 years, behavioral medicine researchers have identified important psychological, social, behavioral, and environmental risk factors for a variety of medical diseases, as reviewed in other chapters of this text. Researchers have also begun to identify biological mechanisms through which these psychological, social, behavioral, and environmental risk factors impact disease pathology such as autonomic, endocrine, immune, and neural pathways. At the other end of the spectrum, researchers have identified markers of resilience such as social networks and support, certain coping strategies and health behaviors, and positive affect which buffer or protect against the effects of adverse circumstances (e.g., psychological stress, low socioeconomic status) on health and functioning. Until recently, behavioral medicine research, including its conceptual models, measures, and clinical applications, has focused almost exclusively on psychological, social, behavioral, and environmental factors that occur or are measured during waking. Yet, humans spend 1/3 to 1/4 of their lives asleep, and there is strong evidence that sleep is essential to health and functioning (e.g., Tononi and Cirelli, 2006).

We know, for example, that experimental sleep deprivation or restriction protocols conducted in healthy young adults lead to profound changes in central and peripheral physiology as well as functional changes in cognition, affect, performance, and behavior (e.g., Irwin et al, 2006; Lim and Dinges, 2008; Sari et al, 2008; Spiegel et al, 1999, 2002, 2004; Stricker et al, 2006; Redwine et al, 2000; Vgontzas et al, 2004). If one takes a step back and considers the 24-h day, sleep is likely important to many of the psychological, social, behavioral, and environmental factors that are the focus of behavioral medicine research and its clinical applications.

The premise of this chapter is that behavioral medicine models that incorporate sleep, whether as a major variable of interest, a confounder, an effect modifier, or a therapeutic target, offer a more complete understanding of the processes through which psychological, social, behavioral, and environmental factors affect and are affected by health and functioning. Moreover, primary sleep disorders such as sleep apnea and insomnia, which are common, costly, and associated with considerable morbidity and decreased quality of life, may be also viewed by behavioral medicine researchers as significant health outcomes in their own right (Ancoli-Israel, 2006; Boivin, 2000; Somers, 2005; Tasali et al, 2008b). The goal of this chapter is to identify the dimensions of sleep that may be most relevant to behavioral medicine, describe how each may be assessed, and briefly summarize relevant evidence linking sleep to health and functioning. The chapter concludes by identifying important

M.H. Hall (✉)
Department of Psychiatry, University of Pittsburgh, Western Psychiatric Institute and Clinic, 3811 O'Hara St, Pittsburgh, PA 15213, USA
e-mail: hallmh@upmc.edu

A. Steptoe (ed.), *Handbook of Behavioral Medicine*, DOI 10.1007/978-0-387-09488-5_49,
© Springer Science+Business Media, LLC 2010

future directions related to the role of sleep in behavioral medicine research and its clinical applications.

2 Dimensions of Sleep Important to Health and Functioning

Sleep is a complex biobehavioral process that can be characterized along multiple dimensions (see Hall et al, 2007). This chapter is focused on four dimensions of sleep that have been most widely evaluated in relation to health and functioning; these include sleep *duration*, *continuity*, *architecture*, and *quality*. As described below, each of these dimensions of sleep may be measured along a continuum and each has been associated with indices of health and/or physiological processes known to contribute to disease pathology including central and peripheral endocrine, immune, autonomic, and metabolic mechanisms. Each of these dimensions of sleep changes across the life span, from infancy through old age, and may, additionally, be moderated by sex, race/ethnicity, and mental and physical health conditions (Carrier et al, 2001; Carskadon and Dement, 2005; Hall et al, 2009; Ohayon et al, 2004).

Not reviewed in this chapter are three dimensions of sleep that have been less studied in relation to health but may represent promising directions for future research; these include daytime naps, fatigue, and sleep debt. Daytime naps, which are difficult to accurately measure, may indirectly affect health through their impact on the duration, continuity, architecture, and quality of nocturnal sleep (Goldman et al, 2008). Fatigue is a common symptom of cardiovascular disease, diabetes, hepatitis, arthritis, and cancer and has been associated with disease course and treatment outcomes (e.g., Ancoli-Israel et al, 2001, 2006). Like daytime naps, fatigue is not easily measured and may affect and be affected by dimensions of nocturnal sleep important to health and functioning. Sleep debt refers to a biobehavioral state that is the result of obtaining too little sleep due to situational constraints

(Basner et al, 2007; Spiegel et al, 2005). At a conceptual level, sleep debt differs from measures of short sleep duration which do not take into account individual differences in sleep need, which may be genetically determined (Ying et al, 2009). Also not reviewed are sleep disorders and circadian rhythms which, although widely studied in relation to health and functioning, are beyond the scope of this chapter (see reviews by Ancoli-Israel, 2006; Boivin, 2000; Hall et al, 2007a; Somers, 2005; Tasali et al, 2008b).

2.1 Sleep Duration

2.1.1 Sleep Duration: Definitions and Measurement

The two most commonly assessed indices of sleep duration include "time in bed" and "total sleep time" (Hall et al, 2007a). Operationally, time in bed (TIB) may be defined as total hours elapsed between getting into bed to go to sleep at night ("good night time") and waking up in the morning ("good morning time"). Total sleep time (TST) may be operationalized as time in bed minus the amount of time needed to fall asleep ("sleep latency") and amount of time spent awake during the night ("wakefulness after sleep onset"). For example, if an individual gets in bed at 11:00 p.m., takes 30 min to fall asleep, is awake for a total of 30 min during the night, and gets out of bed at 6:00 a.m., their TIB and TST would equal 7 and 6 h, respectively.

Self-report measures of sleep duration may include retrospective questionnaires or diary-based measures, which are also sometimes referred to as sleep logs. As summarized below, the majority of studies that have evaluated relationships among sleep duration and indices of health and functioning are based on single, retrospective questions such as "How long do you sleep at night?" or "How much sleep do you usually get in a 24 h period?" In contrast to single items, questionnaires and diary-based measures may instruct participants to indicate sleep duration amounts (e.g., "8 h") or indicate clock times (11:00 p.m.) for later calculation of sleep duration variables. While questionnaires use retrospective referents (e.g., "last 2 weeks" or "past month") to calculate indices of sleep duration, sleep diary protocols typically instruct research participants to complete diary entries about the previous night's sleep each morning after awakening from sleep over a period of several days or weeks.

Objective measures of sleep duration may be derived from wrist actigraphy or polysomngraphy (PSG). Actigraphs are watch-sized devices (see Fig. 49.1), typically worn on the nondominant wrist, that use an internal accelerometer to record and store physical activity counts in pre-specified epoch lengths (e.g., each 30 s, each minute) over several days or weeks. Once actigraphy data are collected and uploaded into research computers, software programs may then be used to calculate TIB and TST, based on the participant's activity patterns (Kushida et al, 2001; Sadeh et al, 1994). Figure 49.2 shows activity counts derived from a mid-life female who wore a wrist actigraph for approximately 3 weeks. Her recording period began at approximately 9 p.m. on a Monday (21:00 h). Activity counts, starting with the first full day of recording (Tuesday), are "double-plotted" so that each full day appears first in the panel on the right (00:00 h to 00:00 h) and again on the next row down in the panel on the left (00:00 h to 00:00 h). Double-plotting provides a visual representation of the timing, duration, and variability of actigraphy-assessed sleep profiles across the study period.

In contrast to activity-based measures of sleep duration derived from wrist actigraphy, PSG may be used to calculate sleep duration based on electrophysiological signals derived from the electroencephalogram (EEG), electrooculogram (EOG), and electromyogram (EMG). These signals are recorded via surface electrodes during nocturnal sleep periods and/or daytime naps and then visually scored by trained polysomnographers, who "stage" each epoch of sleep (typically in 20- or 30-s epochs) based on EEG, EOG, and EMG waveforms, according to standardized criteria (Rechtschaffen and Kales, 1968). Epochs may be classified as awake, stages 1, 2, 3, or 4 of non-rapid eye movement (NREM) sleep or rapid eye movement (REM) sleep. Although the methods used by PSG and actigraphy to assess sleep and wakefulness differ, each may be used to quantify sleep duration using the same conceptual definitions applied to self-report measures of time in bed and total sleep time.

Advantages of self-report and actigraphy-based measures of sleep duration include their ease of administration and low cost. Sleep diaries and actigraphy, which can be measured over many days with relatively low participant burden, offer the additional advantage of being able to quantify day-to-day variability in sleep duration and timing and to distinguish between different types of days (e.g., work versus non-work days, school/weekday versus weekend days). Importantly, these characteristics of sleep duration may be affected by factors relevant to behavioral medicine research such as occupational differences related to the social gradient (e.g., shift work), health behaviors (e.g., caffeine and alcohol use), psychological stress, caregiving, and the quality of close personal relationships (Brummet et al, 2006; Capaldi et al, 2005; Dahlgren et al, 2005; Hall et al, 1997, 2000, 2008a; Sekine et al, 2006; Troxel et al, 2007a, 2007b; Walsh, 2004). The most significant disadvantages of self-report measures of sleep duration include measurement error and subjective bias. Individuals are not always aware of or

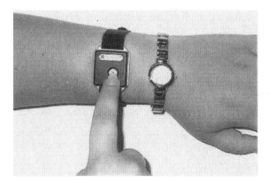

Fig. 49.1 Wrist actigraph

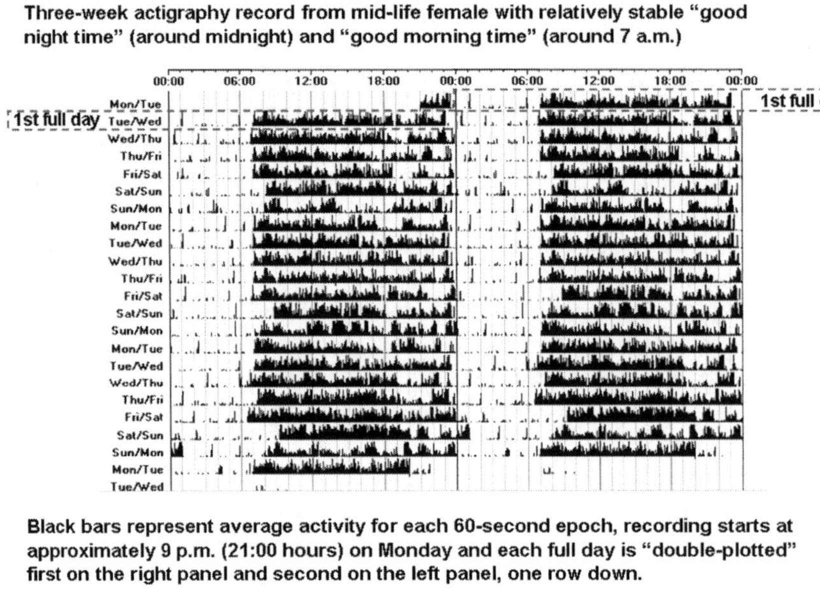
Three-week actigraphy record from mid-life female with relatively stable "good night time" (around midnight) and "good morning time" (around 7 a.m.)
00:00 06:00 12:00 18:00 00:00 06:00 12:00 18:00 00:00
1st full day
1st full day
Mon/Tue
Tue/Wed
Wed/Thu
Thu/Fri
Fri/Sat
Sat/Sun
Sun/Mon
Mon/Tue
Tue/Wed
Wed/Thu
Thu/Fri
Fri/Sat
Sat/Sun
Sun/Mon
Mon/Tue
Tue/Wed
Wed/Thu
Thu/Fri
Fri/Sat
Sat/Sun
Sun/Mon
Mon/Tue
Tue/Wed
Black bars represent average activity for each 60-second epoch, recording starts at approximately 9 p.m. (21:00 hours) on Monday and each full day is "double-plotted" first on the right panel and second on the left panel, one row down.

Fig. 49.2 Actigraphy output

able to recall brief awakenings from sleep and thus may overestimate sleep duration in comparison to actigraphy- or PSG-assessed indices of sleep duration (Hall et al, under review; Lauderdale et al, 2008; Owens et al, under review; Silva et al, 2007). Subjective bias can be especially evident in populations with significant sleep disturbances, including insomnia, sleep apnea, medical disorders involving pain, and psychiatric disorders (e.g., Rotenberg et al, 2000; Tang and Harvey, 2005). One of the limitations inherent with actigraphy is that the device cannot distinguish between sleep and immobility which reduces its accuracy, although several studies have reported non-significant differences between indices of sleep duration assessed by wrist actigraphy and polysomnography (Chae et al, 2009; Kushida et al, 2001; Hall et al, under review). Finally, it may be important to recognize that measures of sleep duration rarely account for or explicitly evaluate daytime napping.

While PSG uses physiology to quantify sleep and wakefulness and is often considered the "gold-standard" for measuring sleep, it is associated with greater participant burden and expense, including equipment and the need for expert personnel. Thus, PSG has not generally been used in epidemiological studies of sleep and health and is rarely used to evaluate variability in sleep duration and timing. An emerging trend in population- and community-based sleep studies relevant to behavioral medicine is the use of ambulatory PSG monitors, which use the same technology as laboratory-based monitors (Hall et al, 2009, 2008a; Iber et al, 2004; Matthews et al, 2008). Significant advantages of in-home ambulatory PSG, which allows participants to sleep in their own beds, under their usual circumstances, at their habitual sleep and wake times, include decreased participant burden associated with sleeping away from home and increased ecological validity of PSG-assessed sleep parameters, including the duration and timing of sleep.

2.1.2 Sleep Duration and Health: Evidence

Sleep duration is one of the most widely studied dimensions of sleep in relation to health and functioning due, in part, to a series of serendipitous findings based on secondary analyses of large epidemiologic studies of morbidity and mortality. In the first study of its kind, Kripke and colleagues reported a U-shaped relationship between self-reported sleep duration and all-cause mortality, after adjusting for demographics, health behaviors, co-morbidities, and medication use (Kripke et al, 2002). Since that time, numerous, but not all, studies have found similar relationships among extremes of sleep duration (generally, < 6 h or > 8 h) and mortality (Amagai et al, 2004; Ferrie et al, 2007; Ikehara et al, 2009; Knutson and Turek, 2006; Kripke et al, 2002; Patel et al, 2004; Tamakoshi and Ohno, 2004). A recent meta-analysis of 23 studies reported pooled relative risk (RR) values of 1.10 (95% CI = 1.06–1.15) and 1.23 (95% CI = 1.17–1.30) for all-cause mortality and short and long sleep duration, respectively (Gallechio and Kalesan, 2009).

Strong cross-sectional associations also have been observed for extremes of sleep duration and multiple indices of health and functioning, including increased blood pressure, elevated levels of inflammatory markers, and the metabolic syndrome (e.g., Hall et al, under review; Hall et al, 2008b; Knutson et al, 2009; Steptoe et al, 2006). With respect to temporal precedence, self-reported short and/or long sleep duration have been prospectively associated with weight gain, diabetes, hypertension, coronary artery disease, myocardial infarction, and stroke in several population-based studies (Ayas et al, 2003a, 2003b; Chen et al, 2008; Gangwisch et al, 2007; Hasler et al, 2004; Patel et al, 2006). For example, short sleep duration (<5 h) was associated with a nearly twofold increase in incident hypertension over an 8- to 10-year follow-up of mid-life National Health and Nutrition Examination (NHANES) participants (Gangwisch et al, 2006). With some exceptions, relationships among sleep duration, morbidity, and mortality in population-based studies have generally remained significant after adjusting for age, sex, race/ethnicity, health behaviors, and medical and psychiatric co-morbidities. In several recent studies, age and sex were found to moderate these relationships (Cappuccio et al, 2007; Gangwisch et al, 2008; van den Berg et al, 2008) while others failed to observe significant

associations among self-reported sleep duration and health outcomes after adjusting for relevant covariates (Bjorkelund et al, 2005; Lopez-Garcia et al, 2009; Taheri et al, 2007).

Fewer community- or population-based studies have used objective measures of sleep to assess relationships among sleep duration and indices of health and functioning. Analyses of actigraphy-assessed sleep duration in a subsample of the Coronary Artery Risk Development in Young Adults (CARDIA) cohort showed cross-sectional relationships between short sleep duration and increased body mass index (BMI) (Lauderdale et al, 2009). In the same sample, actigraphy-assessed short sleep duration was prospectively associated with incident hypertension [odds ratio (OR) = 1.37, 95% confidence interval (CI) = 1.05–1.78] and longer sleep duration was associated with lower incidence of coronary artery calcification (King et al, 2008; Knutson et al, 2009). Hall, Matthews and colleagues (under review) recently reported that decreased sleep duration, as measured by in-home PSG, was a significant cross-sectional correlate of the metabolic syndrome in a community-based sample of mid- to late-life adults. Increased sleep duration, as measured by total sleep time, was associated with lower odds of having the metabolic syndrome (OR = 0.70, 95% CI = 0.52–0.94) after adjusting for age, sex, race, exercise, smoking, symptoms of depression, and sleep disordered breathing. Relationships among PSG-assessed sleep duration and the metabolic syndrome did not differ by sex or race/ethnicity. In the only study of its kind conducted to date, time spent asleep as measured by laboratory-based PSG was unrelated to all-cause mortality in a sample of healthy elders without sleep or psychiatric disorders (Dew et al, 2003).

In summary, converging evidence suggests that extremes of sleep duration are associated with health and functioning, although prospective studies using objective measures (actigraphy, PSG) are lacking. The use of objective measures is especially important given discrepancies between self-reported and objective indices of sleep duration, which may be confounded by other risk factors for morbidity and mortality such as age, sex, race, BMI, and co-morbidities (Cappuccio et al, 2007; Gangwisch et al, 2008; Hall, Krafty et al, under review; Lauderdale et al, 2008; Owens et al, under review; van den Berg et al, 2008). Moreover, few studies (Hall, Matthews et al, under review) adjusted for sleep disordered breathing, including apnea–hypopnea index (AHI) or indices of intermittent hypoxia, which is a significant risk factor for increased morbidity and cardiovascular- and all-cause mortality (see review by Somers, 2005). A final limitation of the extant research linking sleep duration to indices of health and functioning is that these studies tell us little about how extremes of sleep duration might affect morbidity and mortality. Measures of sleep duration do not differentiate between sleep that is fragmented versus consolidated but of equivalent duration nor between sleep that is light (e.g., stages 1 or 2 of NREM sleep) versus deep (e.g., stages 3 or 4 of NREM sleep) but of equivalent duration. Nor do measures of sleep duration differentiate between individuals with or without primary sleep disorders such as sleep apnea and insomnia which have been widely linked to health and functioning (Ancoli-Israel, 2006; Boivin, 2000; Somers, 2005; Tasali et al, 2008b). As summarized in the following sections, emerging evidence suggests that sleep continuity, architecture, and quality are also linked to health and functioning.

2.2 Sleep Continuity

2.2.1 Sleep Continuity: Definitions and Measurement

Measures of sleep continuity focus on one's ability to initiate and maintain sleep and may be assessed by self-report, wrist actigraphy, or polysomnography (Hall et al, 2007a). *Sleep latency* refers to the amount of time it takes to fall asleep (e.g., minutes from "good night time" to onset of sleep), whereas *wakefulness after sleep onset* (WASO) refers to the total

amount of wakefulness during the sleep period (e.g., minutes of wakefulness between sleep onset and "good morning time"). *Sleep efficiency* is a proportional sleep continuity measure which refers to the percent of time in bed spent asleep. Although operational definitions may differ across laboratories, sleep efficiency is commonly calculated as (time spent asleep/time in bed) × 100. Using the example discussed above, an individual who spent 7 h in bed (420 min) and obtained a total of 6 h of sleep (360 min) would have a sleep efficiency value of 85.7%. *Arousal index*, which refers to the number of transient arousals from sleep as measured by changes in the EEG or EMG, has not been frequently evaluated in studies of sleep and health (American Sleep Disorders Association Task Force, 1992).

Retrospective questionnaires and diary-based measures of sleep continuity typically assess sleep latency and WASO. If time in bed is assessed, these data may also be used to calculate sleep efficiency. Wrist actigraphy uses activity-based algorithms to derive estimates of sleep latency, WASO, and sleep efficiency. Increasingly, researchers are also using actigraphy to quantify restlessness during sleep based on movement during the sleep period (e.g., Goldman et al, 2008). Visual sleep stage scoring and identification of transient arousals from sleep are used to quantify PSG-assessed indices of sleep latency, continuity, efficiency, and arousal (American Sleep Disorders Association Task Force, 1992; Rechtschaffen and Kales, 1968). While few studies have directly evaluated different modalities of sleep continuity, Hall and colleagues recently compared sleep latency, WASO, and sleep efficiency values derived from sleep diaries, actigraphy, and in-home PSG recorded over three consecutive nights in a community sample of 323 mid-life women (Hall, Krafty et al, under review). Overall, these analyses suggested that diary-based measures of sleep continuity underestimated sleep latency and WASO values derived from PSG and overestimated sleep efficiency compared to PSG. Although actigraphy similarly underestimated sleep latency and WASO compared to PSG, actigraphy- and PSG-assessed sleep efficiency values did not differ. Race/ethnicity and menopausal symptoms were significant effect modifiers in these analyses, which suggests that sample characteristics influence diary, actigraphy, and PSG-based estimates of sleep continuity.

The relative advantages and disadvantages of different measurement modalities for assessing sleep continuity are similar to those described for sleep duration. Compared to PSG, the decreased cost and participant burden associated with self-report and actigraphy-assessed measures of sleep continuity suggest these measurement modalities are well-suited for studies that include large numbers of participants as well as studies that require many nights of data. In these instances, actigraphy may be preferable to sleep diaries as actigraphy is less influenced by sample characteristics and may provide more accurate estimates of sleep efficiency. Although several reports have shown no differences between actigraphy- and PSG-assessed sleep efficiency, actigraphy does not generally provide accurate estimates of sleep latency and WASO (Hall, Krafty et al, under review; Kushida et al, 2001; Sadeh et al, 1994). Similar to measures of sleep duration, measurement error and subjective bias may influence self-report and/or actigraphy-assessed indices of sleep continuity, while PSG-derived measures provide more costly, yet precise and unbiased, estimates of this important dimension of sleep (Hall, Krafty et al, under review; Lauderdale et al, 2008; Owens et al, under review; Rotenberg et al, 2000). In-home ambulatory PSG may be used to decrease participant burden associated with laboratory-based sleep studies while simultaneously enhancing the ecological validity and precision of measures of sleep latency, WASO, and sleep efficiency.

2.2.2 Sleep Continuity and Health: Evidence

Compared to sleep duration, fewer population-based studies have evaluated relationships among sleep continuity and indices of health

and functioning. As reviewed by Mezick and colleagues (under review), five of seven longitudinal studies reported that poor sleep continuity, measured by self-report, was a significant predictor of incident cardiovascular disease after adjusting for symptoms of depression and other relevant covariates. Findings were similar for self-reported sleep continuity and incident diabetes in the two longitudinal studies published to date (as reviewed by Mezick et al, under review). Sleep efficiency may also protect against the common cold. In a study of 153 young to mid-life adults, diary-assessed sleep efficiency was a significant predictor of susceptibility to the common cold following experimental rhinovirus exposure (Cohen et al, 2009).

Fewer studies have used objective measures of sleep continuity to evaluate relationships among sleep and health. In two separate cross-sectional studies, Hall and colleagues reported that the metabolic syndrome was more prevalent in individuals with decreased sleep efficiency, as measured by in-home PSG and after adjusting for symptoms of depression, sleep disordered breathing, and other relevant covariates (Hall, Okun et al, under review; Hall, Matthews et al, under review). As shown in Fig. 49.3, the metabolic syndrome was more prevalent in mid-life women ($n = 340$; age range $= 46$–57 years) with PSG-assessed sleep efficiency values below 80%, compared with participants with sleep efficiency values of 80% or higher (Hall, Okun et al, under review). Similar results were observed in a sample of 219 mid- to late-life men and women (age range $= 46$–78 years); also shown in Fig. 49.3 (Hall, Matthews et al, under review) Other cross-sectional studies have reported significant associations among PSG- or actigraphy-assessed indices of poor sleep continuity and obesity, increased blood pressure, increased inflammation (e.g., interleukin-6, endothelin-1, soluble intercellular adhesion molecule), and decreased circulating natural killer cell numbers (Hall et al, 1998; Knutson et al, 2009; Mills et al, 2007; Motivala et al, 2005; van den Berg et al, 2008). Decreased sleep continuity has also been associated with increased autonomic arousal in experimental and

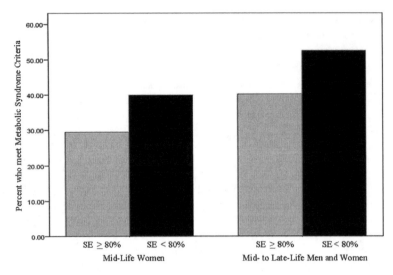

Fig. 49.3 Prevalence of participants who meet criteria for the metabolic syndrome based on PSG-assessed sleep efficiency

observational studies (Janackova and Sforza, 2008; Viola et al, 2002). In their longitudinal study of sleep and all-cause mortality in healthy older adults, Dew and colleagues reported that participants with PSG-assessed sleep latencies of greater than 30 min were at 2.14 times greater risk of death (95% CI = 1.25–3.6) compared to those who fell asleep in less than 30 min, after adjusting for age, medical burden, and other relevant covariates (Dew et al, 2003).

In summary, there is some evidence that sleep continuity is a significant correlate of morbidity and is prospectively linked with cardiovascular disease, diabetes, and all-cause mortality. Emerging evidence based on experimental models of sleep fragmentation suggests that endocrine, immune, metabolic, and autonomic mechanisms may be important mediators of these relationships (Bonnet et al, 1991; Janackova and Sforza, 2008; Redwine et al, 2003; Tartar et al, 2009). In terms of its relevance to behavioral medicine and health, sleep continuity appears to be exquisitely sensitive to psychological and social factors such as stress, loneliness, relationship quality, and socioeconomic status (Akerstedt et al, 2002, 2004; Cartwright and Wood, 1991; Cartwright et al, 1991; Cacioppo et al, 2002; Davidson et al, 1987; Friedman et al, 2005; Hall et al,

1997, 2008; Kecklund and Akerstedt, 2004; Ross et al, 1989). Although published data are limited at present, sleep continuity may represent an important pathway through which psychological and social factors influence health and functioning (Hall et al, 1998).

2.3 Sleep Architecture

2.3.1 Sleep Architecture: Definitions and Measurement

Sleep architecture refers to the pattern or distribution of visually scored NREM and REM sleep stages as well as quantitative measures derived from power spectral analysis of the EEG (Hall et al, 2007a). Within NREM sleep, measures of sleep architecture include stages 1–4, although stages 3 and 4 are often combined into one "slow-wave" or "delta sleep" measure. Measures specific to REM sleep including REM latency (minutes of sleep before the first appearance of REM) and REM density (total number of phasic REMs/time spent in REM sleep) are generally included in the sleep architecture domain as they, too, are structural measures of sleep; these measures are more strongly linked to major mood and anxiety disorders than to medical morbidity and mortality (see review by Benca, 2005). Lighter stages of sleep are characterized by low-amplitude, fast-frequency EEG activity, whereas deeper stages of sleep are characterized by high-amplitude, slow-frequency EEG activity generated by rhythmic oscillations of thalamic and cortical neurons (see Jones, 2005).

Visually scored and quantitative indices of sleep architecture may be measured using laboratory-based or in-home PSG studies. Sleep architecture cannot be assessed by self-report or actigraphy. In this context, it is important to remember that actigraphy measures rest/activity patterns and from these infers wakefulness or sleep; absence of movement during sleep as assessed by actigraphy cannot be used to infer that the individual was in deep or REM sleep. Studies focused on visually scored measures of sleep architecture generally include multiple nights of recording due to night-to-night variability in measures of NREM and REM sleep (Israel et al, under review; Merica and Gaillard, 1985). Due to adaptation effects, multi-night sleep studies typically discard the first night of data and average visually scored measures of sleep architecture across the remaining nights (Toussaint et al, 1995). In contrast, quantitative indices of sleep architecture are highly stable across nights and are often measured on a single night (Buckelmuller et al, 2006; Feinberg et al, 1978; Israel et al, under review; Tucker et al, 2007).

2.3.2 Sleep Architecture and Health: Evidence

Numerous studies have demonstrated that patients with medical disorders including cardiovascular and kidney disease, diabetes, and cancer exhibit lighter sleep architecture profiles, compared to healthy individuals (e.g., Jauch-Chara et al, 2008; Ranjbaran et al, 2007). Yet, these studies do not indicate whether sleep architecture profiles were a contributing cause or consequence of disease. Both possibilities are plausible given experimental evidence of

bi-directional relationships among components of sleep architecture and physiological processes important to health and functioning, including metabolic, endocrine, autonomic, and immune mechanisms (e.g., Hall et al, 2004; Opp, 2006; Rasch et al, 2007; Tasali et al, 2008a). In the only study of its kind conducted to date, Tasali and colleagues (2006) demonstrated that selective suppression of slow-wave sleep in healthy, lean adults resulted in marked decreases in insulin sensitivity. Changes in insulin sensitivity were strongly associated with EEG spectral power in the slow-wave delta band and were unaffected by sleep duration. These results are consistent with three observational studies that reported cross-sectional associations among the metabolic syndrome and decreased sleep depth, as measured by decreased visually scored slow-wave sleep or increased EEG spectral power in the fast-frequency "beta" band after adjusting for age, sleep apnea, and other relevant covariates (Hall, Okun et al, under review; Hall, Matthews et al, under review; Nock et al, 2009). The longitudinal study of sleep and mortality by Dew and colleagues (2003) is the only published study, to date, that has evaluated relationships among measures of sleep architecture and indices of morbidity or mortality. In that study, risk for mortality was significantly higher in individuals with extreme amounts of REM sleep (upper and lower 15th percentile of the sample distribution); visually scored slow-wave sleep percent was also modestly associated with survival time.

In summary, fewer studies have evaluated relationships among indices of sleep architecture and health. Experimental manipulation of sleep architecture, although technically complex, may be an especially promising approach to disentangling cause and effect and evaluating cellular and molecular mechanisms through which sleep architecture affects and is affected by health (e.g., Tasali et al, 2008a). Quantitative analysis of the EEG, which shows trait-like characteristics, may hold promise for identifying sleep phenotypes that confer vulnerability to or resilience against disease (e.g., Buckelmuller et al, 2006; Feinberg et al, 1980; Israel et al, under review;

Tucker et al, 2007). This latter point may be especially relevant to behavioral medicine models of disease given that decreased slow-wave sleep and increased EEG spectral power in the fast-frequency beta-band have been linked with symptoms of stress and a variety of chronic stressors including job strain, marital dissolution, and bereavement (Cartwright and Wood, 1991; Cartwright et al, 1991; Hall et al, 1997, 2000, 2007b, 2008a; Kecklund and Akerstedt, 2004). Experimental animal models have also demonstrated that pre-natal stress, early life experience, and acute stressors impact slow-wave and REM sleep characteristics (e.g., Lesku et al, 2008; Papale et al, 2005; Rabat et al, 2006; Rao et al, 1999).

2.4 Sleep Quality

2.4.1 Sleep Quality: Definitions and Measurement

Sleep quality generally refers to subjective perceptions about one's sleep and may be assessed using purely qualitative indicators (e.g., sleep that is "restful," "sound," "restorative," of "good quality") or a combination of qualitative and quantitative indicators. Sleep diaries often include one or more qualitative indicators about the previous night's sleep, which are assessed using visual analog or Likert-type scales (Monk et al, 1994). The Pittsburgh Sleep Quality Index (PSQI), which is the most widely used self-report sleep instrument and has been translated into over 30 languages, is an example of a "multiple-indicator" measure of sleep quality (Buysse et al, 1989). The PSQI includes 19 retrospective questions about one's sleep over the past month. These questions are used to derive seven subscales (sleep duration, sleep latency, sleep efficiency, sleep disturbance, daytime dysfunction, use of medications for sleep, overall sleep quality), each of which has a range of 0–3. These subscales may be summed to generate a global measure of subjective sleep quality with a range of 0–21; higher values reflect greater

subjective sleep complaints. Less frequently, researchers use multiple indicators assessed by actigraphy or PSG to characterize sleep quality, although the correspondence between self-report and objective measures of sleep quality has not been systematically evaluated. Subjective bias is the major disadvantage of self-report sleep quality measures. Moreover, single indicators such as "rested," "restorative," and "sound" have not been empirically validated, so it is unclear that participants are interpreting these indicators in the same way and responding in a reliable manner.

2.4.2 Sleep Quality and Health: Evidence

The majority of studies that have evaluated subjective sleep quality and indicators of health have been cross-sectional. For example, patients with hypertension, diabetes, kidney disease, polycystic ovary syndrome, and cancer report greater subjective sleep quality complaints than do age- and sex-matched healthy controls (e.g., Alebiosu et al, 2009; Haseli-Mashhadi et al, 2009; Knutson et al, 2006; Liu et al, 2009; Sabbatini et al, 2008; Tasali et al, 2006). In a community-based study of mid-life adults without clinical cardiovascular disease, Jennings and colleagues reported that higher PSQI-assessed sleep quality complaints were associated with increased prevalence of the metabolic syndrome (Jennings et al, 2007). Although these data preclude attributions of causality, sleep quality is likely related to health in complex and sometimes indirect ways. For example, evidence that sleep quality improves with treatment of the primary medical disease (e.g., allergic rhinitis, hypertension, heart failure) suggests that subjective sleep quality is more likely a consequence, rather than a cause, of these medical conditions (Mintz et al, 2004; Skobel et al, 2007; Yilmaz et al, 2008). Sleep quality may indirectly impact health via health behavior pathways. For instance, subjective perceptions that one's sleep is not sound or restorative may lead to increased daytime caffeine use and increased use of alcohol prior to sleep which, in turn, may negatively impact health and functioning.

3 Behavioral Medicine and Sleep: Future Directions

Research on sleep in behavioral medicine is in its infancy. A fair summary of the state-of-(this)-science is that converging evidence suggests numerous links between specific dimensions of sleep and health. As reviewed above, these relationships generally persist after adjusting for "traditional" risk and protective factors such as age, sex, co-morbidities, medication use, socioeconomic status, health behaviors, psychological stress, symptoms of depression, and the quality of close personal relationships. Here we address several methodological, conceptual, and empirical issues important to accelerating our understanding of sleep in relation to behavioral medicine models of health and disease.

The development of valid and reliable measures will play a critical role in our ability to evaluate relationships among sleep and health, including the translation of this knowledge to clinical applications. Epidemiologic studies, which play a key role in developing and refining conceptual models, are in need of validated and reliable, low-burden measures that assess traditional and emerging dimensions of sleep, including habitual sleep duration, daytime naps, fatigue, and sleep debt, as well as primary sleep disorders such as insomnia and sleep apnea. These measures may also prove important for reducing participant burden in studies that conduct multiple repeated assessments such as randomized clinical trials and experimental studies designed to probe mechanisms. Wrist actigraphy holds great promise for decreasing subjective bias associated with self-report measures and for providing "high-dimensional" data that may be used to probe temporal characteristics of dynamic relationships that unfold over time (i.e., To what extent does a bad night of sleep affect reactivity to stress and vice versa? Or, to

what extent does a bad night of sleep affect susceptibility to a viral infection and vice versa?). The greatest challenge facing actigraphy-based studies is the lack of standardized protocols for reliably identifying the beginning and end of sleep periods, including daytime naps and nocturnal sleep. This issue is far from trivial, as all actigraphy-assessed outcomes are calculated as a function of self-reported sleep start and stop times or algorithms based on movement. Although some have used event markers on wrist actigraphs to indicate "good night time" and "good morning time," this method, again, relies on the participant to use the event marker. Also sorely needed are experimental protocols that objectively quantify sleep quality, fatigue, and sleep debt, which may be especially sensitive to sample characteristics including expectations and negative affective biases.

At a conceptual level, behavioral medicine models that incorporate sleep need to think carefully about whether specific dimensions of sleep play different roles in health and disease. For instance, subjective sleep quality, which is adversely affected by medical and psychiatric disorders, may indirectly impact disease course and treatment outcomes via sleep-related health behaviors such as spending more time in bed or consuming alcohol to "help" sleep. In this case, sleep quality may be viewed as an outcome and well as a mediator. Moreover, sleep is likely to interact with other behavioral medicine risk factors (e.g., reactivity to stress, mood, quality of close personal relationships), so care must be taken to understand interrelationships among sleep and other psychological, behavioral, social, and environmental factors that affect and are affected by health. Practically speaking, it may prove fruitful to construct one or more multidimensional latent variable(s) to characterize sleep in relation to health and functioning.

Although individual dimensions of sleep have been related to various health outcomes, little is understood about *how* specific dimensions of sleep may confer vulnerability or resilience to disease. Identification of the cellular and molecular pathways through which sleep affects and is affected by health is critical to advancing our understanding of the sleep–health relationship in the context of behavioral medicine. Mechanism-oriented studies of the sleep–health relationship will benefit from basic sleep research which is a highly developed discipline. Our understanding of the neurobiology of sleep, the effects of experimental sleep deprivation or restriction on central and peripheral physiology, and emerging evidence regarding the genetic determinants of sleep and circadian rhythms are three examples of research that is ripe for translation into behavioral medicine studies of sleep and health.

In conclusion, sleep is a promising area of investigation in relation to behavioral models of health and disease although definitive, causal studies are lacking. The strength of the associations among sleep and indices of health and functioning suggest that, at minimum, it would be wise to consider sleep (including prevalent sleep disorders that impact health) as an important covariate when evaluating the pathways through which psychological, social, behavioral, and environmental factors contribute to or protect against disease. That sleep is a modifiable behavior suggests that it may represent an important therapeutic target for behavioral medicine research. The growing number of published studies of sleep in behavioral medicine suggests a receptive zeitgeist, which is certainly a step in the right direction.

Acknowledgments This chapter was supported in part by grants from the National Institutes of Health (AG019362; AG020677; HL076379; HL076852; MH024652; RR024153). Many thanks to Bonnee Wettlaufer for her administrative support on this chapter.

References

Alebiosu, O. C., Ogunsemi, O. O., Familoni, O. B., Kancir, P. B., Ayodele, O. E. (2009). Quality of sleep among hypertensive patients in a semi-urban Nigerian community: a prospective study. *Postgrad Med, 121*,166–172.

Akerstedt, T., Knutsson, A., Westerholm, P., Theorell, T., Alfredsson, L. et al (2002). Sleep disturbances, work stress and work hours: a cross-sectional study. *J Psychosom Res, 53*, 741–748.

Akerstedt, T., Knutsson, A., Westerholm, P., Theorell, T., Alfredsson, L. et al (2004). Mental fatigue, work and sleep. *J Psychosom Res, 57*, 427–433.

Amagai, Y., Ishikawa, S., Gotoh, T., Doi, Y., Kayaba, K. et al (2004). Sleep duration and mortality in Japan: the Jichi Medical School Cohort Study. *J Epidemiol, 14*, 24–128.

American Sleep Disorders Association Task Force. (1992). EEG arousals: scoring rules and examples. *Sleep, 15*, 174–184.

Ancoli-Israel, S., Moore, P. J., and Jones, V. (2001). The relationship between fatigue and sleep in cancer patients: a review. *Eur J Cancer Care, 10*, 245–255.

Ancoli-Israel, S. (2006). The impact and prevalence of chronic insomnia and other sleep disturbances associated with chronic illness. *Am J Manag Care, 12(Suppl)*, S221–S229.

Ancoli-Israel, S., Liu, L. Q., Marler, M., Parker, B. A., Jones, V. et al (2006). Fatigue, sleep, and circadian rhythms prior to chemotherapy for breast cancer. *Support Care Cancer, 14*, 201–209.

Ayas, N. T., White, D. P., Al Delaimy, W. K., Manson, J. E., Stampfer, M. J. et al (2003a). A prospective study of self-reported sleep duration and incident diabetes in women. *Diabetes Care, 26*, 380–384.

Ayas, N. T., White, D. P., Manson, J. E., Stampfer, M. J., Speizer, F. E. et al (2003b). A prospective study of sleep duration and coronary heart disease in women. *Arch Intern Med, 163*, 205–209.

Basner, M., Fomberstein, K. M., Razavi, F. M., Banks, S., William, J. H. et al (2007). American time use survey: sleep time and its relationship to waking activities. *Sleep, 30*, 1085–1095.

Benca, R. M. (2005). Mood disorders. In M. H. Kryger, T. Roth, & W. C. Dement (Eds.), *Principles and Practice of Sleep Medicine* (pp. 1311–1326). Philadelphia, PA: Elsevier Saunders.

Bjorkelund, C., Bondyr-Carlsson, D., Lapidus, L., Lissner, L., Mansson, J. et al (2005). Sleep disturbances in midlife unrelated to 32-year diabetes incidence: the prospective population of study of women in Gothenburg. *Diabetes Care, 28*, 2739–2744.

Boivin, D. B. (2000). Influence of sleep-wake and circadian rhythm disturbances in psychiatric disorders. *J Psychiatry Neurosci, 25*, 446–458.

Bonnet, M. H., Berry, R. B., and Arand, D. L. (1991). Metabolism during normal, fragmented and recovery sleep. *J Appl Physiol, 71*, 1112–1118.

Brummett, B. H., Babyak, M. A., Siegler, I. C., Vitaliano, P. P., Ballard, E. L. et al (2006). Associations among perceptions of social support, negative affect, and quality of sleep in caregivers and noncaregivers. *Health Psychol, 25*, 220–225.

Buckelmuller, J., Landolt, H. P., Stassen, H. H., Achermann, P. (2006). Trait-like individual differences in the human sleep electroencephalogram. *Neuroscience, 138*, 351–356.

Buysse, D. J., Reynolds, C. F., Monk, T. H., Berman, S. R., and Kupfer, D. J. (1989). The Pittsburgh Sleep

Quality Index: a new instrument for psychiatric practice and research. *Psychiat Res, 28*, 193–213.

Cacioppo, J. T., Hawkley, L. C., Berntson, G. G., Ernst, J. M., Gibbs, A. C. et al (2002). Do lonely days invade the nights? Potential social modulation of sleep efficiency. *Psychol Sci, 13*, 384–387.

Capaldi, I., Handwerger, K., Richardson, E., Stroud, L. R. (2005). Associations between sleep and cortisol responses to stress in children and adolescents: a pilot study. *Behav Sleep Med, 3*, 177–192.

Cappuccio, F. P., Stranges, S., Kandala, N. B., Miller, M. A., Taggart, F. M. et al (2007). Gender-specific associations of short sleep duration with prevalent and incident hypertension: the Whitehall II Study. *Hypertension, 50*, 693–700.

Carrier, J., Land, S., Buysse, D. J., Kupfer, D. J., Monk, T. H. (2001). The effects of age and gender on sleep EEG power spectral density in the middle years of life (aged 20-60 years old). *Psychophysiology, 38*, 232–242.

Carskadon, M. A., and Dement, W. C. (2005). Normal human sleep: an overview. In M. H. Kryger, T. Roth, & W. C. Dement (Eds.), *Principles and Practice of Sleep Medicine* (pp. 13–23). Philadelphia, PA: Elsevier Saunders.

Cartwright, R. D., and Wood, E. (1991). Adjustment disorders of sleep: the sleep effects of a major stressful event and its resolution. *Psychiat Res, 39*, 199–209.

Cartwright, R. D., Kravitz, H. M., Eastman, C. I., and Wood, E. (1991). REM latency and the recovery from depression: getting over divorce. *Am J Psychiatry, 148*, 1530–1535.

Chae, K. Y., Kripke, D. F., Poceta, J. S., Shadan, F., Jamil, S. M. et al (2009). Evaluation of immobility time for sleep latency in actigraphy. *Sleep Med, 10*, 621–625.

Chen, J. C., Brunner, R. L., Ren, H., Wassertheil-Smoller, S., Larson, J. C. et al (2008). Sleep duration and risk of ischemic stroke in postmenopausal women. *Stroke, 39*, 3185–3192.

Cohen, L., Warneke, C., Fouladi, R. T., Rodriguez, M. A., Chaoul-Reich, A. (2004). Psychological adjustment and sleep quality in a randomized trial of the effects of a Tibetan yoga intervention in patients with lymphoma. *Cancer, 100*, 2253–2260.

Cohen, S., Doyle, W. J., Alper, C. M., Janicki-Deverts, D., Turner, R. B. (2009). Sleep habits and susceptibility to the common cold. *Arch Intern Med, 169*, 62–67.

Dahlgren, A., Kecklund, G., and Akerstedt, T. (2005). Different levels of work-related stress and the effects on sleep, fatigue and cortisol. *Scand J Work Env Health, 31*, 277–285.

Davidson, L. M., Fleming, R., and Baum, A. (1987). Chronic stress, catecholamines, and sleep disturbance at Three Mile Island. *J Human Stress, Summer*, 75–83.

Dew, M. A., Reynolds, C. F., Monk, T. H., Buysse, D. J., Hoch, C. C. et al (1994). Psychosocial correlates and sequelae of electroencephalographic sleep in healthy elders. *J Gerontol, 49*, P8–P18.

Dew, M. A., Hoch, C. C., Buysse, D. J., Monk, T. H., Begley, A. E. et al (2003). Healthy older adults' sleep predicts all-cause mortality at 4 to 19 years of follow-up. *Psychosom Med, 65*, 63–73.

Feinberg, I., Fein, G., and Floyd, T. C. (1980). Period and amplitude analysis of NREM EEG in sleep: repeatability of results in young adults. *Electroencephalogr Clin Neurophysiol, 48*, 212–221.

Ferrie, J. E., Shipley, M. J., Cappuccio, F. P., Brunner, E., Miller, M. A. et al (2007). A prospective study of change in sleep duration: associations with mortality in the Whitehall II cohort. *Sleep, 30*, 1659–1666.

Friedman, E. M., Hayney, M. S., Love, G. D., Urry, H. L., Rosenkranz, M. A. et al (2005). Social relationships, sleep quality, and interleukin-6 in aging women. *Proc Nat Acad Sci USA, 102*, 18757–18762.

Gallicchio, L., and Kalesan, B. (2009). Sleep duration and mortality: a systematic review and meta-analysis. *J Sleep Res, 18*, 148–158.

Gangwisch, J. E., Heymsfield, S. B., Boden-Albala, B., Buijs, R. M., Kreier, F. et al (2006). Short sleep duration as a risk factor for hypertension: analyses of the first National Health and Nutrition Examination Survey. *Hypertension, 47*, 833–839.

Gangwisch, J. E., Heymsfield, S. B., Boden-Albala, B., Buijs, R. M., Kreier, F. et al (2007). Sleep duration as a risk factor for diabetes incidence in a large U.S. sample. *Sleep, 30*, 1667–1673.

Gangwisch, J. E., Heymsfield, S. B., Boden-Albala, B., Buijs, R. M., Kreier, F. et al (2008). Sleep duration associated with mortality in elderly, but not middle-aged, adults in a large US sample. *Sleep, 31*, 1087–1096.

Goldman, S. E., Hall, M., Boudreau, R., Matthews, K. A., Cauley, J. A. et al (2008). Association between night time sleep and napping in older adults. *Sleep, 31*, 733–740.

Hall, M., Buysse, D. J., Dew, M. A., Prigerson, H. G., Kupfer, D. J. et al (1997). Intrusive thoughts and avoidance behaviors are associated with sleep disturbances in bereavement-related depression. *Depress Anx, 6*, 106–112.

Hall, M., Baum, A., Buysse, D. J., Prigerson, H. G., Kupfer, D. J. et al (1998). Sleep as a mediator of the stress-immune relationship. *Psychosom Med, 60*, 48–51.

Hall, M., Buysse, D. J., Nowell, P. D., Nofzinger, E. A., Houck, P. et al (2000). Symptoms of stress and depression as correlates of sleep in primary insomnia. *Psychosom Med, 62*, 227–230.

Hall, M., Vasko, R., Buysse, D. J., Ombao, H., Chen, Q., et al (2004). Acute stress affects heart rate variability during sleep. *Psychosom Med, 66*, 56–62.

Hall, M., Okun, M. L., Atwood, C. W., Buysse, D. J., and Strollo, P. J. (2007a). Measurement of sleep by polysomnography. In L. L. Luecken & L. C. Gallo (Eds.), *Handbook of Physiological Research Methods in Health Psychology* (pp. 341–367). Thousand Oaks, CA: Sage Publications.

Hall, M., Thayer, J. F., Germain, A., Moul, D., Vasko, R. et al (2007b). Psychological stress is associated with heightened physiological arousal during NREM sleep in primary insomnia. *Behav Sleep Med, 5,* 178–193.

Hall, M., Buysse, D. J., Nofzinger, E. A., Reynolds, C. F., and Monk, T. H. (2008a). Financial strain is a significant correlate of sleep continuity disturbances in late-life. *Biol Psychol, 77,* 217–222.

Hall, M., Muldoon, M. F., Jennings, J. R., Buysse, D. J., Flory, J. D. et al (2008b). Self-reported sleep duration is associated with the metabolic syndrome in mid-life adults. *Sleep, 31,* 635–643.

Hall, M., Matthews, K. A., Kravitz, H. K., Gold, E. B., Buysse, D. J. et al (2009). Race and financial strain are independent correlates of sleep in mid-life women: The SWAN Sleep Study. *Sleep, 32,* 73–82.

Hall, M., Boudreau, R. M., Goldman, S. E., Stone, K. L., Visser, M. et al (Under Review). Association between sleep duration and mortality is mediated by markers of inflammation in older adults: The Health, Aging and Body Composition Study.

Hall, M., Krafty, R. T., Zhiang, Y., Campbell, I., Feinberg, I. et al (Under Review). Measuring sleep: how do different measurement modalities compare to one another?

Hall, M., Matthews, K. A., Kamarck, T. W., Buysse, D. J., Strollo, P. J. et al (Under Review). Sleep and the metabolic syndrome: looking beyond self-report measures and sleep disordered breathing.

Hall, M., Okun, M. L., Karpov, I., Sowers, M. F., Matthews, K. A. et al (Under Review). Sleep is associated with the metabolic syndrome in a multi-ethnic cohort of midlife women: The SWAN Sleep Study.

Haseli-Mashhadi, N., Dadd, T., Pan, A., Yu, Z., Lin, X., et al (2009). Sleep quality in middle-aged and elderly Chinese: distribution, associated factors and associations with cardio-metabolic risk factors. *BMC Public Health, 9,* 130.

Hasler, G., Buysse, D. J., Klaghofer, R., Gamma, A., Ajdacic, V. et al (2004). The association between short sleep duration and obesity in young adults: a 13-year prospective study. *Sleep, 27,* 661–666.

Iber, C., Redline, S., Kaplan Gilpin, A. M., Quan, S. F., Zhang, L. et al (2004). Polysomnography performed in the unattended home versus the attended laboratory setting--Sleep Heart Health Study methodology. *Sleep, 27,* 536–540.

Ikehara, S., Iso, H., Date, C., Kikuchi, S., Watanabe, Y. et al (2009). Association of sleep duration with mortality from cardiovascular disease and other causes for Japanese men and women: the JACC study. *Sleep, 32,* 295–301.

Israel, B., Buysse, D. J., Begley, A., Cheng, Y., and Hall, M. (Under Review). Night-to-night stability in visually-scored and quantitative measures of sleep and nocturnal physiology.

Irwin, M. R., Wang, M., Campomayor, C. O., Collado-Hidalgo, A., and Cole, S. (2006). Sleep deprivation and activation of morning levels of cellular and genomic markers of inflammation. *Arch Intern Med, 166,* 1756–1762.

Janackova, S., and Sforza, E. (2008). Neurobiology of sleep fragmentation: cortical and autonomic markers of sleep disorders. *Current Pharmaceutical Design, 14,* 3474–3480.

Jauch-Chara, K., Schmid, S. M., Hallschmid, M., Born, J., and Schultes, B. (2008). Altered neuroendocrine sleep architecture in patients with type 1 diabetes. *Diabetes Care, 31,* 1183–1188.

Jennings, J. R., Muldoon, M., Hall, M., Buysse, D. J., and Manuck, S. B. (2007). Self-reported sleep quality is associated with the metabolic syndrome. *Sleep, 30,* 219–223.

Jones, B. E. (2005). Basic mechanisms of sleep-wake states. In M. H. Kryger, T. Roth, & W. C. Dement (Eds.), *Principles and Practice of Sleep Medicine* (pp. 136–153). Philadelphia, PA: Elsevier Saunders.

Kecklund, G., and Akerstedt, T. (2004). Apprehension of the subsequent working day is associated with a low amount of slow wave sleep. *Biol Psychol, 66,* 169–176.

King, C. R., Knutson, K. L., Rathouz, P. J., Sidney, S., Liu, K. et al (2008). Short sleep duration and incident coronary artery calcification. *JAMA, 300,* 2859–2866.

Knutson, K. L., and Turek, F. W. (2006). The U-shaped association between sleep and health: the 2 peaks do not mean the same thing. *Sleep, 29,* 878–879.

Knutson, K. L., Ryden, A. M., Mander, B. A., and Van Cauter, E. (2006). Role of sleep duration and quality in the risk and severity of type 2 diabetes mellitus. *Arch Intern Med, 166,* 1768–1774.

Knutson, K. L., Van Cauter, E., Rathouz, P. J., Yan, L. L., Hulley, S. B. et al (2009). Association between sleep and blood pressure in midlife: the CARDIA sleep study. *Arch Intern Med, 169,* 1055–1061.

Kripke, D. F., Garfinkel, L., Wingard, D. L., Klauber, M. R., and Marler, M. R. (2002). Mortality associated with sleep duration and insomnia. *Arch Gen Psychiatry, 59,* 131–136.

Kushida, D. A., Chang, A., Gadkary, C., Guilleminault, C., Carrillo, O. et al (2001). Comparison of actigraphic, polysomnographic and subjective assessment of sleep parameters in sleep-disordered breathing patients. *Sleep Med, 2,* 389–396.

Lauderdale, D. S., Knutson, K. L., Yan, L. L., Liu, K., and Rathouz, P. J. (2008). Self-reported and measured sleep duration: How similar are they? *Epidemiology, 19,* 838–845.

Lauderdale, D. S., Knutson, K. L., Rathouz, P. J., Yan, L. L., Hulley, S. B. et al (2009). Cross-sectional and longitudinal associations between objectively measured sleep duration and body mass index: the CARDIA Sleep Study. *Am J Epidemiol, 170,* 805–813.

Lesku, J. A., Bark, R. J., Martinez-Gonzalez, D., Rattenborg, N. C., Amlaner, C. J. et al (2008). Predator-induced plasticity in sleep architecture in wild-caught Norway rats (Rattus norvegicus). *Behav Brain Res*, *189*, 298–305.

Lim, J., and Dinges, D. F. (2008). Sleep deprivation and vigilant attention. *Ann NY Acad Sci*, *1129*, 305–322.

Liu, L., Fiorentino, L., Natarajan, L., Parker, B. A., Mills, P. J. et al (2009). Pre-treatment symptom cluster in breast cancer patients is associated with worse sleep, fatigue and depression during chemotherapy. *Psycho-Oncology*, *18*, 187–194.

Lopez-Garcia, E., Faubel, R., Guallar-Castillon, P., Leon-Munoz, L., Banegas, J. R. et al (2009). Self-reported sleep duration and hypertension in older Spanish adults. *J Amer Ger Soc*, 57, 663–668.

Matthews, K. A., Kamarck, T. W., Hall, M., Strollo, P. J., Owens, J. F. et al (2008). Blood pressure dipping and sleep disturbance in African American and Caucasian men and women. *Am J Hypertens*, *21*, 826–831.

Merica, H., and Gaillard, J. M. (1985). Statistical description and evaluation of the interrelationships of standard sleep variables for normal subjects. *Sleep*, *8*, 261–273.

Mezick, E. J., Hall, M., and Matthews, K. A. (Under Review). Are sleep and depression independent or overlapping risk factors for cardiometabolic disease?

Mills, P. J., von Kanel, R., Norman, D., Natarajan, L., Ziegler, M. G. et al (2007). Inflammation and sleep in healthy individuals. *Sleep*, *30*, 729–735.

Mintz, M., Garcia, J., Diener, P., Liao, Y., Dupclay, L. et al (2004). Triamcinolone acetonide aqueous nasal spray improves nocturnal rhinitis-related quality of life in patients treated in a primary care setting: the Quality of Sleep in Allergic Rhinitis study. *Ann Allerg Asthma Immunol*, *92*, 255–261.

Monk, T. H., Reynolds, C. F., Kupfer, D. J., Buysse, D. J., Coble, P. A. et al (1994). The Pittsburgh sleep diary. *J Sleep Res*, *3*, 111–120.

Motivala, S. J., Sarfatti, A., Olmos, L., and Irwin, M. R. (2005). Inflammatory markers and sleep disturbance in major depression. *Psychosom Med*, *67*, 187–194.

Nock, N. L., Li, L., Larkin, E. K., Patel, S. R., and Redline, S. (2009). Empirical evidence for "Syndrome Z": a hierarchical 5-factor model of the metabolic syndrome incorporating sleep disturbance measures. *Sleep*, *32*, 615–622.

Ohayon, M. M., Carskadon, M. A., Guilleminault, C., and Vitiello, M. V. (2004). Meta analysis of quantitative sleep parameters from childhood to old age in healthy individuals: developing normative sleep values across the human lifespan. *Sleep*, *27*, 1255–1273.

Opp, M. R. (2006). Sleep and psychoneuroimmunology. *Neurol Clin*, *24*, 493–506.

Owens, J. F., Mezick, E. J., Buysse, D. J., Hall, M., Kamarck, T. W. et al What factors account for differences in estimates of sleep duration by self-report, polysomnography and actigraphy? Under review.

Papale, L. A., Andersen, M. L., Antunes, I. B., Alvarenga, T. A. F., and Tufik, S. (2005). Sleep pattern in rats under different stress modalities. *Brain Res*, *1060*, 47–54.

Patel, S. R., Ayas, N. T., Malhotra, M. R., White, D. P., and Schernhammer, E. S. (2004). A prospective study of sleep duration and mortality risk in women. *Sleep*, *27*, 440–444.

Patel, S. R., Malhotra, A., White, D. P., Gottlieb, D. J., and Hu, F. B. (2006). Association between reduced sleep and weight gain in women. *Am J Epidemiol*, *164*, 947–954.

Prather, A. A., Marsland, A. L., Hall, M., Neumann, S. A., Muldoon, M. F. et al (2009). Normative variation in self-reported sleep quality and sleep debt is associated with stimulated pro-inflammatory cytokine production. *Biol Psychol*, *82*, 12–17.

Rabat, A. Bouyer, J. J., George, O., Le Moal, M., and Mayo, W. (2006). Chronic exposure of rats to noise: relationship between long-term memory deficits and slow wave sleep disturbances. *Behav Brain Res*, *171*, 303–312.

Ranjbaran, Z., Keefer, L., Stepanski, E., Farhadi, A., and Keshavarzian, A. (2007). The relevance of sleep abnormalities to chronic inflammatory conditions. *Inflamm Res*, *56*, 1–7.

Rao, U., McGinty, D. J., Shinde, A., McCracken, J. T., and Poland, R. E. (1999). Prenatal stress is associated with depression-related electroencephalographic sleep changes in adult male rats: a preliminary report. *Prog Neuro-Psychopharm Biol Psychiatry*, *23*, 929–939.

Rasch, B., Dodt, C., Moelle, M., and Born, J. (2007). Sleep-stage-specific regulation of plasma catecholamine concentration. *Psychoneuroendocrinology*, *32*, 884–891.

Rechtschaffen, A., and Kales, A. (1968.). *A Manual of Standardized Terminology, Techniques and Scoring System for Sleep Stages of Human Subjects NIH Publication 204*. Washington, D.C.: U.S. Government Printing Office, Department of Health Education and Welfare.

Redwine, L., Dang, J., Hall, M., and Irwin, M. (2003). Disordered sleep, nocturnal cytokines and immunity in alcoholics. *Psychosom Med*, *65*, 75–85.

Redwine, L., Hauger, R. L., Gillin, J. C., and Irwin, M. (2000). Effects of sleep and sleep deprivation on interleukin-6, growth hormone, cortisol, and melatonin levels in humans. *J Clin Endocrinol Metab*, *85*, 3597–3603.

Ross, R. J., Ball, W. A., Sullivan, K. A., and Caroff, S. N. (1989). Sleep disturbance as the hallmark of post-traumatic stress disorder. *Am J Psychiatry*, *146*, 697–707.

Rotenberg, V. S., Indursky, P., Kayumov, L., Sirota, P., and Melamed, Y. (2000). The relationship between subjective sleep estimation and objective sleep variables in depressed patients. *Int J Psychophysiol, 37*, 291–297.

Sadeh, A., Sharkey, K. M., and Carskadon, M. A. (1994). Activity-based sleep-wake identification: an empirical test of methodological issues. *Sleep, 17*, 201–207.

Sabbatini, M., Pisani, A., Crispo, A., Nappi, R., Gallo, R. et al (2008). Renal transplantation and sleep: a new life is not enough. *J Nephrol, 21 Suppl, 13*, S97–101.

Sari, I., Davutoglu, V., Ozbala, B., Ozer, O., Baltaci, Y. et al (2008). Acute sleep deprivation is associated with increased electrocardiographic P-wave dispersion in healthy young men and women. *Pacing Clin Electrophysiol, 31*, 438–442.

Sekine, M., Chandola, T., Martikainen, P., McGeoghegan, D., Marmot, M. et al (2006). Explaining social inequalities in health by sleep: the Japanese civil servants study. *J Public Health (Oxf), 28*, 63–70.

Silva, G. E., Goodwin, J. L., Sherrill, D. L., Arnold, J. L., Bootzin, R. R. et al (2007). Relationship between reported and measured sleep times: the sleep heart health study (SHHS). *J Clin Sleep Med, 3*, 622–630.

Somers, V. K. (2005). Sleep: a new cardiovascular frontier. *N Engl J Med, 353*, 2070–2073.

Spiegel, K., Leproult, R., and Van Cauter, E. (1999). Impact of sleep debt on metabolic and endocrine function. *Lancet, 354*, 1435–1439.

Spiegel, K., Sheridan, J. F., and Van Cauter, E. (2002). Effect of sleep deprivation on response to immunization. *J Am Med Assoc, 288(12)*, 1471–1472.

Spiegel, K., Leproult, R., L'Hermite-Baleriaux, M., Copinschi, G., Penev, P. D. et al (2004). Leptin levels are dependent on sleep duration: relationships with sympathovagal balance, carbohydrate regulation, cortisol, and thyrotropin. *J Clin Endocrinol Metab, 89*, 5762–5771.

Spiegel, K., Knutson, K., Leproult, R., Tasali, E., and Van Cauter, E. (2005). Sleep loss: a novel risk factor for insulin resistance and Type 2 diabetes. *J Appl Physiol, 99*, 2008–2019.

Skobel, E. C., Sinha, A., Norra, C., Randerath, W., Breithardt, O. et al (2005). Effect of cardiac resynchronization therapy on sleep quality, quality of life, and symptomatic depression in patients with chronic heart failure and Cheyne-Stokes respiration. *Sleep Breath, 9*, 159–166.

Steptoe, A., Peacey, V., and Wardle, J. (2006). Sleep duration and health in young adults. *Arch Intern Med, 166*, 1689–1692.

Stricker, J. L., Brown, G. G., Wetherell, L. A., and Drummond, S. P. (2006). The impact of sleep deprivation and task difficulty on networks of fMRI brain response. *J Int Neuropsychol Soc, 12*, 591–597.

Suarez, E. C. (2008). Self-reported symptoms of sleep disturbance and inflammation, coagulation, insulin resistance and psychosocial distress: evidence for gender disparity. *Brain Behav Immun, 22*, 960–968.

Taheri, S., Austin, D., Lin, L., Nieto, F. J., Young, T. et al Correlates of serum C-reactive protein (CRP): no association with sleep duration or sleep disordered breathing. *Sleep, 30*, 991–996.

Tamakoshi, A., and Ohno, Y. (2004). Self-reported sleep duration as a predictor of all-cause mortality: results from the JACC study, Japan. *Sleep, 27*, 51–54.

Tang, N. K., and Harvey, A. G. (2005). Time estimation ability and distorted perception of sleep in insomnia. *Behav Sleep Med, 3*, 134–150.

Tartar, J. L., Ward, C. P., Cordeira, J. W., Legare, S. L., Blanchette, A. J. et al (2009). Experimental sleep fragmentation and sleep deprivation in rats increases exploration in an open field test of anxiety while increasing plasma corticosterone levels. *Behav Brain Res, 97*, 450–453.

Tasali, E., Van Cauter, E., and Ehrmann, D. A. (2006). Relationships between sleep disordered breathing and glucose metabolism in polycystic ovary syndrome. *J Clin Endocrinol Metab, 91*, 36–42.

Tasali, E., Leproult, R., Ehrmann, D. A., and Van Cauter, E. (2008a). Slow-wave sleep and the risk of type 2 diabetes in humans. *Proc Nat Acad Sci USA, 105*, 1044–1049.

Tasali, E., Mokhlesi, B., and Van Cauter, E. (2008b). Obstructive sleep apnea and type 2 diabetes: interacting epidemics. *Chest, 133*, 496–506.

Tononi, G., and Cirelli, C. (2006). Sleep function and synaptic homeostasis. *Sleep Med Rev, 10*, 49–62.

Toussaint, M., Luthringer, R., Schaltenbrand, N., Carelli, G., Lainey, E. et al (1995). First-night effect in normal subjects and psychiatric inpatients. *Sleep, 18*, 463–469.

Troxel, W. M., Robles, T., Hall, M., and Buysse, D. J. (2007a). Marital quality and the marital bed: Examining the covariation between relationship quality and sleep. *Sleep Med Rev, 11*, 389–404.

Troxel, W. M., Cyranowski, J. M., Hall, M., Frank, E., Buysse, D. J. (2007b). Attachment anxiety, relationship context, and sleep in women with recurrent major depression. *Psychosom Med, 69*, 692–699.

Tucker, A. M., Dinges, D. F., and Van Dongen, H. P. (2007). Trait interindividual differences in the sleep physiology of healthy young adults. *J Sleep Res, 16*, 170–180.

van den Berg, J. F., Miedema, H. M., Tulen, J. H., Neven, A. K., Hofman, A. et al (2008). Long sleep duration is associated with serum cholesterol in the elderly: the Rotterdam Study. *Psychosom Med, 70*, 1005–1011.

Vgontzas, A. N., Zoumakis, E., Bixler, E. O., Lin, H. M., Follett, H. et al (2004). Adverse effects of modest sleep restriction on sleepiness, performance, and inflammatory cytokines. *J Clin Endocrinol Metab, 89*, 2119–2126.

Viola, A. U., Simon, C., and Ehrhart, J. et al (2002). Sleep processes exert a predominant influence on the 24-h profile of heart rate variability. *J Biol Rhythms*, *17*, 539–547.

Yilmaz, M. B., Erdem, A., Yalta, K., Turgut, O. O., Yilmaz, A. et al (2008). Impact of beta-blockers on sleep in patients with mild hypertension: a randomized trial between nebivolol and metoprolol. *Adv Therapy*, *25*, 871–883.

Ying, H., Jones, C. R., Fujiki, N., Xu, Y., Buo, B. et al (2009). The transcriptional repressor DEC2 regulates sleep length in mammals. *Science*, *325*, 866–870.

Part VIII
Brain Function and Neuroimaging

Chapter 50

Neuroimaging Methods in Behavioral Medicine

Peter J. Gianaros, Marcus A. Gray, Ikechukwu Onyewuenyi, and Hugo D. Critchley

1 Overview of Neuroimaging Methods

Neuroimaging permits the in vivo (and largely non-invasive) study of the human brain through quantification of functional neurochemical, metabolic, and micro- (e.g., white matter tracts) and macro-structural (localized volume and density of gray and white matter) features. In particular, using magnetic resonance imaging (MRI), the same scanner can generate a range of quantifiable biological measurements within the same individual to give convergent multivariate information about functional and structural integrity of brain processes. Among MRI methods, functional MRI (fMRI) of brain (measuring regional hemodynamic changes contingent on local neural activity) now represents a leading human neuroscientific tool, having developed rapidly from positron emission tomography (PET) techniques for measuring regional cerebral blood flow and metabolism. By labeling specific molecules with radioisotopes, PET uses the source localization of radioactive decay to provide three-dimensional, absolute rather than relative, measures of metabolic activity

(e.g., glucose uptake and utilization) or blood flow (e.g. using ^{15}O-labeled water). PET is also the unrivalled technique for quantifying in vivo in humans the distribution of neurotransmitter/neuromodulator and receptor activity and the presence of pathological proteins, such as amyloid. These approaches are complemented by electrical and magnetic imaging methodologies that provide information on synchronization of neural (primarily cortical) function with exceptional temporal resolution. Finally, newer optical imaging techniques increasingly offer the potential to image localized blood flow within the cortex at a temporal resolution equal to electrical and magnetic techniques. Below we outline each of these imaging techniques, with attention to the basic principles which underlie their generation and common utilization techniques in neuroscientific research.

2 Functional Neuroimaging Methods

There are several functional neuroimaging methods available for behavioral medicine research. Of these, the most widely employed and most likely relevant to questions in our field include PET and fMRI. Broadly stated, PET and fMRI differ in their invasiveness, in their ability to localize ongoing changes in neural activity to particular brain areas (referred to as *spatial resolution*), and in their ability to resolve the timing of changes in neural activity in relation to a given psychological, behavioral, or

P.J. Gianaros (✉)
Department of Psychiatry, University of Pittsburgh, Western Psychiatric Institute and Clinic, 3811 O'Hara Street, Pittsburgh, PA 15213, USA
Clinical Imaging Sciences Center, Brighton Sussex Medical School, University of Sussex, Brighton, East Sussex, BN19RR, UK
e-mail: gianarospj@upmc.edu

A. Steptoe (ed.), *Handbook of Behavioral Medicine*, DOI 10.1007/978-0-387-09488-5_50,
© Springer Science+Business Media, LLC 2010

physiological process (referred to as *temporal resolution*). Both methods quantify changes in and interactions between neural activity patterns from distributed brain areas over short time periods. Hence, PET and fMRI can reveal dynamic changes in the activity of brain *networks*, as opposed to isolated patterns of activity from disparate brain areas. Importantly, these co-occurring functional changes in brain networks can be linked to wide-ranging and time-varying cognitive, emotional, behavioral, physiological, and interpersonal response processes important for understanding the neurobiological bases of aspects of health and well-being in behavioral medicine research. Here, we focus on key issues involved in PET and fMRI studies, referring readers to in-depth resources where relevant. Throughout, we will emphasize the use of PET and fMRI to indirectly measure regional *increases* and *decreases* in brain activity, conventionally referred to as patterns of brain "activation" and "deactivation," which are complexly determined by changes in regional blood flow, oxygen concentration, and metabolism in areas of neural activity. For more detailed treatments of the PET and fMRI methods reviewed next, we refer the reader to several informative texts (Buxton, 2002; Cabeza and Kingstone, 2006; Frackowiak et al, 2003; Huettel et al, 2004; Jezzard et al, 2001; Toga and Mazziotta, 2002).

2.1 Positron Emission Tomography

Both PET and fMRI quantify regional changes in hemodynamic and metabolic activity that are *correlated* with changes in neural activity (Raichle, 2006; Savoy, 2001). Neuroimaging methods employing PET provide three-dimensional images of the brain corresponding to quantitative levels of glucose metabolism, oxygen consumption, regional cerebral blood flow (rCBF), and neurotransmitter receptor-binding potentials during passive (resting or baseline) or active (task-related) behavioral states. This is achieved by localizing emitted positrons from radioactive tracers injected into the bloodstream. With PET, these tracers can be distributed and concentrated differentially throughout the blood vessels supplying brain tissue. Specifically, in PET, radioactive decay releases a proton, which is annihilated after colliding with an oppositely charged free electron, releasing two gamma rays in opposite directions. Co-incident scintillation detectors arranged in a ring around the decaying radio nucleotide can detect these paired gamma rays and calculate a vector along which this annihilation must have occurred. By measuring many thousand annihilation events, the spatial location of these emissions can be determined. Biologically active radiotracer molecules with rapid decay rates (short half lives) are administered into the body. These radiotracers accumulate in active regions where their decay can be localized, and three-dimensional images can be constructed to identify blood flow or active metabolism with a spatial resolution of approximately $3 \ mm^2$. Hence, PET methods capitalize on these distributional and concentration characteristics to assess levels of brain activity because of the close relationship between cellular (neural) activity, blood flow, and metabolism. The most common PET methods rely on ^{18}FDG and $H_2^{15}O$ as injected tracers to measure regional cerebral glucose metabolism and cerebral blood flow, respectively. To localize brain activity patterns, PET data are analyzed using kinetic modeling procedures, which estimate the spatial concentration of a particular radioactive tracer. The resulting PET images can then be examined within individuals across experimental periods or between individuals at rest or during task performance as a function of another variable of interest (e.g., as a function of stressor-evoked changes in a measure of peripheral physiological reactivity). As discussed by Gray and colleagues (this volume), for example, stressor-evoked changes in cardiovascular (Critchley et al, 2000; Gianaros et al, 2004; Lane et al, 2001) and neuroendocrine activity (Dedovic et al, 2005; Pruessner et al, 2007) have been linked to changes in rCBF using PET imaging.

The particular development of PET spans an appreciably long methodological history, with over 50 years between the French physicist Paul Villard's discovery of gamma rays in 1900 to the first published study of positron counting with medical possibilities (Wrenn et al, 1951). Twenty more years followed before Phelps and colleagues (1975) published the methods underlying the PET techniques used today. Further refinement of scintillation technology (Weber and Monchamp, 1973) and the synthesis of radiolabeled deoxyglucose (Sokoloff et al, 1977) provided the necessary basis for the massive increases in detector elements and computing found in modern commercial PET imaging systems. In the context of this historical development, the neuroimaging applications of PET are being increased rapidly by the more recent development of radioligands, such as carbon 11-labeled raclopride, which selectively antagonizes and binds to the D2 dopamine receptor, allowing investigation of psychiatric disorders associated with disturbance of dopamine transmission. PET radioligands have also been developed with specificity for a range of other neuromodulators and neurotransmitter receptor subtypes including GABA, serotonin, norepinephrine, with the potential to provide fundamental insight into a range of psychiatric and central nervous system disorders (Zipursky et al, 2007). Development of radiolabeled ligands to identify discrete neuopathological processes promises much for "biomarking" neurodegenerative diseases. A ligand for quantifying beta amyloid deposition in Alzheimer disease (Pittsburgh compound B) represents the most developed of these approaches and may emerge as a diagnostic marker and means of monitoring interventions (Klunk et al, 2004). PET is also commonly used in conjunction with computed tomography (CT), where many two-dimensional x-ray images are combined to provide detailed three-dimensional images of the body. Combining PET and CT allows for detailed structural images which also contain information about metabolism.

2.2 Functional Magnetic Resonance Imaging

The biophysical basis of fMRI differs from PET in several ways. With fMRI, short-term changes in neural activity (e.g., on the order of seconds) can be localized without ionizing radiation or radioactive tracers. As detailed below, fMRI localizes neural activity by exploiting the blood oxygenation level-dependent (BOLD) effect, a phenomenon discovered in the field of nuclear magnetic resonance physics (Ogawa et al, 1990a, b; for review, see Raichle, 2006). The BOLD effect is based on the concentration of oxygen in the blood that flows to brain areas where there is a change in neural activity. Specifically, when the activity of neural tissue increases, blood flow to that tissue increases to provide a metabolic substrate for cellular activity (Buxton, 2002; Huettel et al, 2004; Logothetis, 2002). However, in areas of neural activity, blood flow changes disproportionately to oxygen consumption. In consequence, there is a change in the oxygen concentration within blood vessels supplying that tissue. This change in oxygen concentration can be detected with MRI because the oxygen level in hemoglobin (the protein molecule in red blood cells) changes the extent to which hemoglobin disturbs a local magnetic field. Hence, changes in fMRI BOLD signal intensity reflect changes in the ratio of deoxygenated to oxygenated hemoglobin in the blood supplying particular brain areas. Given that the BOLD effect is dependent on measuring *relative changes* in oxygen concentration, fMRI studies routinely employ task paradigms involving a comparison of brain activity during two or more conditions (see below). These comparisons are used to quantify functional neural changes, which have been labeled as patterns of BOLD "activation" and "deactivation."

To elaborate on the biophysical basis of this imaging modality, magnetic resonance imaging (MRI) exploits the physical magnetic properties of the nuclei of the atoms which make up our bodies. In the 1940s it was discovered that atomic nuclei when placed within a magnetic field absorb radiofrequency (RF) energy and later emit this energy at a resonant RF frequency (Bloch, 1946; Purcell et al, 1946). This insight (nuclear magnetic resonance, NMR) was applied initially to identify chemical components of complex molecules or mixtures. Imaging of biological tissues (MRI) emerged with techniques for measuring and localizing the density of hydrogen atoms in large three-dimensional samples such as the body. The signals from resonant hydrogen nuclei (mostly in water molecules) are modulated by proximate and neighboring tissue classes and fluids, enabling images to provide detailed information about the internal structure of organs including the brain. Placing the head in the magnetic field generated by an MRI scanner aligns the spinning nuclei of hydrogen atoms within the brain and skull. By applying repeated tailored pulses of RF energy, these nuclei can be made to emit RF resonances that can be recorded and measured. The position of these nuclei can be determined with the addition of a magnetic gradient which is stronger at the top of the head and grows weaker toward the chin and neck, and as a result the nuclei at the strongest end of the magnetic field spin faster than those within the weaker field. Applying RF energy will only evoke a resonant signal within atoms that spin at the frequency of the RF pulse, allowing individual slices within the head to be separately excited and measured. Additional gradients (phase-encoding gradient and frequency-encoding gradient) further alter the speed of procession within a slice, allowing the identification of resonant signals from precise locations within each slice.

Resonant signals from tissue excited during MRI naturally decay rapidly for a variety of reasons. By using differently timed sequences of RF and gradient pulses (pulse sequences) the signal measured during MRI can be made more or less sensitive to different sources of decay. Two critical features of a pulse sequence which determine the sensitivity to differential sources of signal decay are the echo time (TE) and the volume repetition time (TR). Most MRI sequences make use of a gradient field or secondary radiofrequency pulse (gradient recalled echo sequence or spin echo sequence, respectively) to refocus nuclei spins. The signal measured during this echo form the basis of the images generated during MRI. By varying the lengths of the TE and TR, MRI images can be made more or less sensitive to T1-or T2-weighted effects. Structural or T1-weighted MRI imaging utilizes differences

in the longitudinal relaxation of various tissue classes. After a slice of tissue is excited by RF energy, the alignment of spinning protons within the slice gradually returns to alignment with the magnetic field, and as a result the resonant signal decays smoothly. The speed at which this signal decays (longitudinal relaxation time or T1) depends on the ability of the surrounding tissue lattice to efficiently absorb resonant energy, and this varies according to tissue type. Fat, for example, is more efficient at absorbing energy, therefore resonant signals from fat decay more quickly than neural tissue or water. Structural MRI uses a pulse sequence which maximizes the differences in signal decay as different tissues realign themselves with the static magnetic field.

As noted earlier, functional MRI (fMRI) is now commonly used to investigate dynamic activity within the brain or rather the changes in regional blood flow and perfusion consequent upon neural activity. fMRI is tuned to be sensitive to BOLD signal changes. More precisely, this is achieved by using a pulse sequence which maximizes signal sensitivity to $T2^*$ effects. $T2^*$ refers to the loss of signal due to interactions with nearby nuclei and by inhomogeneities in the local magnetic field, causing variation in local precession rates. The interaction of nuclei procession with nearby nuclei and unevenness in the magnetic field results in a rapid de-coherence and resulting loss of signal intensity in the transverse plane. The rate at which energy is released is dependent on the biology of the tissue, and it is this feature which makes it possible to index neural activity. When a region of neural tissue becomes active, its metabolic needs increase and a neurovascular coupling mechanism results in increased localized blood flow, increasing the level of oxygenated blood locally. Again, even after accounting for the increased metabolic demands of active neural tissue, this causes an increase in the ratio of oxygenated to deoxygenated blood in the vicinity of functionally active neural tissue. Oxygenated and deoxygenated hemoglobin have different magnetic susceptibilities and as a result differing $T2^*$ decay time courses. It was this observation which led to optimization of BOLD-sensitive pulse sequences. Like T1-weighted imaging, this is typically achieved with a gradient-recalled echo sequence, however, unlike T1 imaging where the echo (TE) and repetition (TR) times are short, BOLD T2*-weighted imaging typically uses a long TR (greater than 1500 ms) and a long TE (greater than 60 ms) (Ogawa et al, 1990a, b).

It is important to emphasize here that the fMRI BOLD signal is subject to numerous confounding factors, including the dramatic effects of even slight (millimeter) head movements on signal quality, the compromising impact of cerebrovascular insults, lesions, and atherosclerotic disease on the vessels supplying brain tissue, the appreciable decrease in the signal-to-noise ratio within particular areas of the brain that abut air–tissue interfaces (i.e., sinus areas near the ventral orbitofrontal cortex), and the physical movement of the brain that occurs with breathing and each beat of the heart. Further, one disadvantage of fMRI relative to PET is that it poses challenges to recording concurrent changes in peripheral (e.g., stressor-evoked) physiology, which is often a major goal in behavioral medicine and stress research. This disadvantage stems from several sources. One includes the radiofrequency and electrical artifacts introduced into peripheral recordings (e.g., the electrocardiogram) by the changing magnetic gradients imposed by fMRI scanning. Another disadvantage reflects the fact that the metallic instrumentation often used for peripheral physiological recording is not safe in the MRI environment (see http://www.mrisafety.com/). However, instrumentation for recording concurrent changes in peripheral physiology in the MRI environment is becoming increasingly available, and this instrumentation will better allow for the assessment of electroencephalographic, electrocardiographic, blood pressure, respiratory, and other physiological measures during fMRI protocols (Gray et al, 2009; Lane et al, 2009a, b). If such instrumentation is not available to the behavioral medicine researcher, then an alternative approach to integrating assessments of peripheral physiological activity into fMRI studies is to have participants perform the same task in an fMRI scanner and in a laboratory setting or plastic replica of the scanner to emulate the same experimental environment. Notably, many of these methodological challenges are not an issue for fMRI and imaging studies of neuroendocrine function discussed by Gray et al in this volume, where measurements commonly rely on salivary sampling procedures (for review, see Dedovic et al, 2009).

Notwithstanding these issues, fMRI has several advantages over PET, including the ability to scan the same person over multiple sessions within a short period of time (because of the lack of radiation exposure), the higher spatial and temporal resolution of the BOLD signal, and the relatively lower cost and wider availability of fMRI at most research institutions. Indeed, the increasing availability of MRI scanners with higher magnetic field strengths (measured in Tesla units, where 1 Tesla = 10,000 Gauss) is expected to provide unprecedented opportunities for localizing functional and structural aspects of the brain at increasingly precise levels of spatial resolution.

2.3 Arterial Spin Labeling

As noted above, the fMRI BOLD signal indirectly reflects relative changes in neural activity because it is based on interacting changes in neurovascular function and oxygen concentration. In this way, measuring the BOLD signal has at least one disadvantage compared with PET; namely, it provides a surrogate and *non-quantitative* parameter of neurophysiological activity. However, using specialized MRI scanning parameters (referred to as pulse sequences), the quantitative parameter, rCBF, can be estimated with a technique called perfusion imaging, which relies on arterial spin labeling (Detre and Wang, 2002). This technique is gaining increasing use in the field of neuroimaging, and as reviewed by the complementary chapter on neuroimaging in this volume, it has been applied recently in behavioral medicine studies of cardiovascular and neuroendocrine stress reactivity (Gianaros et al, 2009; Wang et al, 2005, 2007). Hence, perfusion MRI is an emerging non-invasive method that may better capture quantitative changes in cerebral blood flow that are more closely related to neural activity and metabolism patterns.

3 Structural MRI Methods

3.1 Volumetric MRI

T1-weighted MRI scans can provide exceptionally detailed high-resolution images of the physical structure of the brain through enhanced contrast between gray and white matter compartments, with suppression of cerebrospinal fluid signal. Quantitative methods have been applied to T1-weighted brain scans to examine the relative density and volume of the different neural tissue classes, particularly gray and white matter, on a region-by-region basis. The most common approach is termed voxel-based morphometry, or VBM (Ashburner and Friston, 2000). This is an automated technique to analyze the amount of gray and white matter density or volume on a voxel-wise basis and allows examination and comparison of differences within specific brain regions that are the consequence of maturational or neurodegenerative processes that include genetic, constitutional, neurodevelopmental, experience-driven, and atrophic process associated with disease or aging that may lead to inter-group or cross individual variation in regional brain structure.

3.2 Diffusion MRI

By utilizing a bipolar gradient pulse sequence, MRI data can be made sensitive to movement of water molecules in a specific direction, producing phase-shift data which is sensitive to the velocity of water movement. The laws of molecular diffusion, or Brownian motion, can be applied to this phase-shift MRI acquired in multiple planes data to characterize a diffusion tensor, a representation of the local restrictions on the movement of water molecules at a specific brain location (Hagmann et al, 2006). Diffusion tensor data can be used to infer the directionality of local fiber tracts, as water molecules are freer to move along nerve fibers within the brain, than to travel across them. Diffusion tensor imaging (DTI) can be used to investigate tractography, the shape, density, and integrity of white matter fiber tracts within the brain and for examining the effects of neurostructural pathology such as subcortical lesions on brain connectivity (Burgel et al, 2006).

4 Neurochemical Imaging

4.1 Magnetization Transfer MRI

MRI pulse sequences can also be specified so as to reduce the signal sensitivity to both T1 and T2 effects by specifying a long TR (to minimize T1 signal differences) and a short TE (to minimize T2 signal differences). The resulting images are sensitive to differences in the overall density of protons within different brain locations. Proton density images can contain information about proton density within fluid relative to macromolecular brain structure (i.e., neural tissue/membranes) through the application of an RF pulse which saturates protons in macromolecular brain structures. Magnetization transfer imaging (MTR) then compares sequential proton density images with and without the additional saturating RF pulse to identify alterations in neurochemical (macromolecular) integrity within hard neural tissue, such as white matter plaques in multiple sclerosis or prolactin-secreting tumors versus non-secreting adenomas (Argyropoulou et al, 2003; Zackowski et al, 2009).

4.2 Magnetic Resonance Spectroscopy

Magnetic resonance spectroscopy (MRS) can be used to quantify chemical features of neural tissues. Most commonly, ^{1}H-MRS (proton MRS) has been used in human studies, though MRS can be applied to other atomic nuclei, notably phosphorus. The key insight in ^{1}H-MRS is that electrons surrounding the protons in an atom shield the resonant energy emitted from the proton during MRI. This induces a chemical shift in the resonant frequency emitted from protons, and as there are different numbers of electrons in different elements, the chemical shift differs between different chemical compounds and molecular isotopes. When applied in a research context MRS combines the structural information obtainable from MRI and spectroscopy to assess the relative concentrations of biological metabolites at a specific brain location. The major signals of interest obtainable using ^{1}H-MRS reflect the amount of choline (Cho), creatine/phosphocreatine (Cr), and *N*-acetylaspartate (NAA). These can be quantified relative to each other and to the most prominent "water peak." Interpretation of relative differences in concentrations of these chemicals has been heuristic; consensus suggests Cho concentration reflects membrane integrity and turnover, Cr a measure of metabolic activity, and NAA a marker of neural integrity and density (Gujar et al, 2005; McKnight, 2004). With higher field MRI scanners other metabolite peaks are becoming reliably quantifiable from brain tissue including lactate (Lac), glutamate/glutamine (Glx), myo-inositol (MyoI), and alanine (Ala). "Incidental" information from MRS studies of brain can also include measures of brain temperature and pH.

5 Electrophysiological and Optical Imaging

5.1 Electroencephalograph (EEG)

The first published reported measures of electrical brain activity were made by Richard Caton who after placing two unipolar electrodes attached to a galvanometer on the scalp reported responses to light, head rotation and chewing (Caton, 1875). Interest in electrical measures of brain function became widespread following publication of Hans Berger's papers "On the EEG in humans," in 1929 (Berger, 1929). Today EEG measures are used routinely in clinical investigations of sleep and seizures and in neuropsychiatric research. Electroencephalographic (EEG) measures of neural function provide excellent temporal resolution of activity within the cortex. Within patients groups, notably epilepsy, delirium, and types of dementia, EEG abnormalities (e.g., spikes and slow waves) are apparent as diagnostic signatures on the raw trace and may also provide insight into the location of abnormal brain function. In an experimental context EEG analytic methods include both analyses of frequency components (reflecting synchronized activity) evoked event-related potentials. The applications of EEG to behavioral medicine are covered in detail in the chapter by Jennings, Zanstra, and Egizio in this volume.

5.2 Magnetoencephalography (MEG)

MEG developed out of predictions based on superconductivity made by Brian Josephson in 1962. He predicted that when two superconductive metal plates are separated by a tiny gap or junction, tunneling electrons produce a current flow between the physically insulated superconductors (Josephson, 1962). Further, increasing the conductive current beyond a critical threshold should induce the tunneling current to alternate over time in the tetrahertz range (approximately 500 GHz) current (AC). These predictions were confirmed the following year by experimental work (Anderson and Rowell, 1963). One key feature of the quantum tunneling AC current induced across a Josephson junction is exquisitely sensitivity interference from even minute magnetic fields and as a result can be used to make precise measurements of extremely weak magnetic activity. This feature has been exploited to construct superconducting quantum interference devices (SQUID), which are magnetometers sensitive to exceptionally small changes in magnetism. Electrical currents by necessity also generate magnetic currents. As a result, electrical activity generated by the synchronized firing of pyramidal neurons generates tangential magnetic waves. Unlike electrical potentials originating from the cortex, magnetic potentials are not impeded by the skull and scalp. This may offer some advantages in the reconstruction of source density models for MEG activity. As in EEG, new developments in source localization and parametric mathematical models allow increasing precision in the identification of localized cortical activity underlying the generation of MEG waveforms. Current MEG systems have over 100 squid sensors, which can provide very high (millisecond) temporal resolution and can be cortically resolved with high spatial resolution 2 mm^2.

5.3 Optical Imaging

Finally, optical imaging provides another alternative to electrical, magnetic, metabolic, and MRI methods for imaging the brain. A widely recognized feature of living tissue in medicine, and particularly the development and manufacture of medical monitoring equipment, is the influence of functional status on a tissue's optical properties (Villringer and Chance, 1997). Light in the near infrared range (approximately 700–1000 nm) is able to pass relatively easily through living tissue. Light passing through tissue may be affected in three basic ways (1) by scattering of photons, (2) by absorption, and (3) by birefringence or double refraction (Foust and Rector, 2007). Brain function may be explored via optical means by one or a number of these features. Techniques for optically imaging the brain are currently not widely used within neuroscience, however their adoption is increasing and this may be expected to expand significantly during the coming decade. Currently, two basic methods of optically imaging brain function are being used, and these are outlined briefly below.

5.3.1 Near InfraRed Spectroscopy (NIRS)

Near infrared spectroscopy (NIRS) is the most established optical method for investigating brain function, emerging from studies in neonates. NIRS is a spectroscopic method; i.e., it derives information on brain function by exploring the absorption of light as it passes through the body (brain). In NIRS imaging, light within the near infrared spectrum is directed toward the brain at the surface of the scalp. Most biological material within the head has a high scattering influence on near infrared light (NIR) light, and as a result, NIR is not able to pass completely through the head, but is instead randomly diffused over a distance of few centimeters from the NIR source. NIR detectors placed near the emitter will receive light which has been reflected along an elliptical- or banana-shaped path; the further apart the emitter and receiver, the deeper this ellipse must travel until at a distance of 7–10 cm very little light is detected (Okada and Delpy, 2003a, b). By carefully separating the NIR emitters and detectors, it is possible to ensure the elliptical light path passes through cortical gray matter, allowing assessment of cortical activity (Huppert et al, 2009). As the specific frequencies of light which are absorbed by oxy- and deoxy-hemoglobin are known, spectroscopy can be applied to provide a measure of the BOLD signal and hence the functional status of localized gray matter. While the characterization of BOLD activity in NIRS is restricted to cortical regions close to the scalp and therefore is unsuitable for assessing many midbrain, limbic, or brainstem regions, the temporal resolution of NIRS data is extremely high. It is not difficult to sample NIRS data thousands of times more rapidly than typical fMRI data, allowing for smoothing to increase signal-to-noise features of these measures (Koh et al, 2007).

5.3.2 Event-Related Optical Signal (EROS)

In addition to spectroscopic optical imaging methods, other techniques characterize the influence that neuronal firing has on NIR transmission. It has been recognized since at least the 1940s that the transmission of light through a neuron is altered by neuronal firing (Hill and Keynes, 1949). This influence is not dependent on the delayed alterations in hemoglobin ratios which follow 4–6 s after neuronal firing, but is instead associated with changes in the refractivity of neuronal membranes within a millisecond of neuronal firing (Stepnoski et al, 1991; Villringer and Chance, 1997). Current research with event-related optical signal (EROS) methods makes use of these "fast" optical signals, and as a consequence can identify cortical activity with a much great temporal resolution than measures based on the BOLD response; e.g., NIRS, fMRI (Gratton and Fabiani, 2001a, b). Despite the restriction to shallow cortical regions, the exceptionally high temporal and good spatial resolution makes EROS methods a likely area for future development.

6 Some Basic Design Principles in Functional Neuroimaging

Of the methods reviewed above, it is most likely that researchers in behavioral medicine will most likely employ methods of functional neuroimaing, particularly those of fMRI and PET. Accordingly, this section highlights salient design and inferential issues associated with these modalities. As noted above, in most functional neuroimaging studies, the goal is to characterize relative changes in neural activity in specific brain areas when a person performs a behavioral task. A long-standing supposition is that achieving this goal will help define the role of specific brain areas in cognitive, emotional, and behavioral processes (Raichle, 2006; Savoy, 2001). For most PET and fMRI studies, this goal is achieved with a canonical 'subtraction paradigm' derived from the early work of Donders (1969). Employing this paradigm in functional neuroimaging studies involves requiring people to engage in a behavioral task with

two or more conditions. One (or more) of the conditions will serve as an active condition of interest, whereas another (or more) will serve as a control condition. In a common approach to the analysis of the neuroimaging data, brain "activation" will be determined by subtracting the control condition from the active condition to compute a so-called contrast or difference image of neural activity. Conversely, brain "deactivation" could be similarly determined by subtracting the active condition from the control condition, which may be of relevance to those interested in decreased or task-suppressed neural activity. For behavioral medicine researchers interested in stress reactivity processes, the active condition of interest will generally require the participant to engage in a stressful or challenging task that evokes peripheral physiological changes, whereas the control condition will involve a minimally stressful task or relaxing baseline. In this way, physiological reactivity and brain activation measures can both be computed by taking the difference between task and baseline levels.

Importantly, there are a range of experimental designs in which the canonical subtraction paradigm can be implemented. The most common are *blocked* and *event-related* designs (Aguirre and D'Esposito, 2000; Culham, 2006; Rosen et al, 1998). In a typical blocked design, two or more task conditions will be alternated in blocks or epochs for predefined time periods (e.g., ~15 s to ~2 min, depending on the neuroimaging modality). For each alternating block, only one task condition will be administered. According to the subtraction paradigm logic described above, if the task conditions in a blocked design differ only in the process of interest engaged, then the fMRI or PET signal changes in particular brain areas that differentiate the conditions will presumably reveal patterns of neural activity associated with the process of interest.

While blocked designs are common, one of their disadvantages is that they present challenges to assessing short-term changes in neural activity (e.g., those occurring within a few seconds after a stimulus is presented or after a behavioral response is made). This has led to the development of event-related designs, particularly in fMRI research (at this time, the temporal resolution in PET imaging precludes event-related designs). In event-related fMRI designs, aspects of brief changes in the BOLD signal can be quantified following a single stimulus or a behavioral response. In this way, the onset, peak latency, length, and other short-term changes in the BOLD signal waveform relative to (subtracted) pre-stimulus (control) levels can be assessed and associated with individual difference factors or stimulus or response variables (Donaldson and Buckner, 2001; Rosen et al, 1998). Importantly, these short-term changes in the BOLD signal can reveal considerably more information than the aggregate difference in fMRI or PET activity between two or more conditions, as determined in blocked designs. However, it is important to note that BOLD signal changes are small in comparison to the noise inherent to the signal, resulting in reduced statistical power for event-related designs (Donaldson and Buckner, 2001). Hence, an increasing number of studies are employing mixed designs blending both blocked and event-related features (Visscher et al, 2003).

As discussed above, neuroimaging methods offer several approaches to studying patterns of brain activity of interest to behavioral medicine researchers. Unfortunately, however, there are no universally agreed upon ways to design, analyze, and interpret all types of functional and structural neuroimaging studies. Nevertheless, there are some standards of practice that should be considered. First, neuroimaging studies should be driven by focused hypotheses targeting *specific* brain areas or networks of interest. This focus could be based on prior animal or human research on the process(es) presumably supported by the brain area(s) of interest. Second, careful attempts should be made to control for salient confounds in functional neuroimaging studies. This often involves matching control and active conditions (or stimuli) of interest along as many dimensions as possible. Importantly, this will support stronger inferences using the subtraction procedure described above. Such control could involve matching conditions (e.g., stressor and non-stressor conditions) in terms of the number of motor responses that are made during task performance, the perceptual and cognitive aspects of the stimuli presented, and the peripheral physiological recording procedures if they are employed [e.g., inflating a blood pressure cuff during both control (non-stress) and active (stress) conditions]. Other inferential issues in functional neuroimaging research have been detailed elsewhere (Logothetis, 2008).

Finally, for functional neuroimaging studies, there are a number of statistical procedures available to (i) make simple comparisons between task conditions or event types, (ii) assess neural activity patterns that vary according to interactions between task conditions and events, and (iii) compute correlations between changes in neural activity to determine connectivity patterns expressed between brain areas. For all of these procedures, it is important to account for the inflated likelihood of observing statistically significant effects by chance alone, given that (i) the brain is a three-dimensional structure necessitating multiple (often univariate) statistical tests and (ii) multiple (correlated) measures are often derived from repeated observations of the same person over time, as in the case of functional neuroimaging studies and longitudinal structural neuroimaging studies (Genovese et al, 2002; Nichols and Hayasaka, 2003). Hence, it is routine in neuroimaging studies to employ random or mixed effects statistical analyses to permit appropriate generalizations to the population and to apply some form of correction for performing multiple statistical tests across the brain (Friston et al, 1995; Worsley et al, 1992). Most recently, there has also been much debate and recommendations offered for the appropriate analysis of correlations in neuroimaging studies of individual differences, which are particularly relevant for studies of stress reactivity (see Lieberman et al, 2009; Vul et al, 2009).

7 Summary

Only recently have neuroimaging methods and neurobiological theoretical frameworks been directed at understanding the "brain–body" pathways linking cognitive, emotional, social, behavioral, and physiological processes to aspects of health and well-being. As reviewed here, there are a number of available neuroimaging and related methods that can be applied in behavioral medicine research. The complementary chapter by Gray and colleagues in this volume illustrates several of these methodological applications, and it highlights future research directions incorporating these methods into behavioral medicine research.

Acknowledgements Preparation of this chapter was supported by National Institutes of Health Grants K01-MH070616 and R01-HL089850 (P.J.G.) and by a Programme Grant from the Wellcome Trust (H.D.C).

References

Aguirre, G. K., and D'Esposito, M. (2000). Experimental design for brain fMRI. In C. T. W. Moonen & P. A. Bandettini (Eds.), *Functional MRI* (pp. 369–380). Heidelberg: Springer-Verlag Berlin.

Anderson, P. W., and Rowell, J. M. (1963). Probable observation of the Josephson superconducting tunneling effect. *Phys Rev Lett, 10*, 230–232.

Argyropoulou, M. I., Xydis, V., Drougia, A., Argyropoulou, P. I., Tzoufi, M. et al (2003). MRI measurements of the pons and cerebellum in children born preterm; associations with the severity of periventricular leukomalacia and perinatal risk factors. *Neuroradiology, 45*, 730–734.

Ashburner, J., and Friston, K. J. (2000). Voxel-based morphometry: the methods. *NeuroImage, 11*, 805–821.

Berger, H. (1929). Über das Elektrenkephalogramm des Menschen. *Arch Psychiat Nervenkr, 87*, 527–570.

Bloch, F. (1946). Nuclear induction. *Phys Rev, 70*, 460.

Burgel, U., Amunts, K., Hoemke, L., Mohlberg, H., Gilsbach, J. M. et al (2006). White matter fiber tracts of the human brain: three-dimensional mapping at microscopic resolution, topography and intersubject variability. *Neuroimage, 29*, 1092–1105.

Buxton, R. B. (2002). *Introduction to Functional Magnetic Resonance Imaging: Principles and Techniques*. Cambridge, MA: Cambridge University Press.

Cabeza, R., and Kingstone, A. (Eds.). (2006). *Handbook of Functional Neuroimaging of Cognition, 2nd Ed.* Cambridge, MA: MIT Press.

Caton, R. (1875). The electric currents of the brain. *Br Med J, 2*, 278.

Critchley, H. D., Corfield, D. R., Chandler, M. P., Mathias, C. J., and Dolan, R. J. (2000). Cerebral correlates of autonomic cardiovascular arousal: a functional neuroimaging investigation in humans. *J Physiol, 523*, 259–270.

Culham, J. C. (2006). Functional neuroimaging: experimental design and analysis. In R. Cabeza & A. Kingstone (Eds.), *Handbook of Functional Neuroimaging of Cognition, 2nd Ed.* Cambridge, MA: MIT Press.

Dedovic, K., D'Aguiar, C., and Pruessner, J. C. (2009). What stress does to your brain: a review of neuroimaging studies. *Can J Psychiatry, 54*, 6–15.

Dedovic, K., Renwick, R., Mahani, N. K., Engert, V., Lupien, S. J. et al (2005). The Montreal Imaging Stress Task: using functional imaging to investigate the effects of perceiving and processing psychosocial stress in the human brain. *J Psychiatry Neurosci, 30*, 319–325.

Detre, J. A., and Wang, J. (2002). Technical aspects and utility of fMRI using BOLD and ASL. *Clin Neurophysiol, 113*, 621–634.

Donaldson, D. L., and Buckner, R. L. (2001). Effective paradigm design. In P. Jezzard, P. M. Matthews, & S. M. Smith (Eds.), *Functional MRI: An Introduction to Methods*. New York: Oxford University Press.

Donders, F. C. (1969). On the speed of mental processes. *Acta Psychologica, 30*, 412–431.

Foust, A. J., and Rector, D. M. (2007). Optically teasing apart neural swelling and depolarization. *Neuroscience, 145*, 887–899.

Frackowiak, R. S. J., Friston, K. J., Frith, C., Dolan, R., Price, C. J. et al (Eds.). (2003). *Human Brain Function, 2nd Ed.* San Diego, CA: Academic Press.

Friston, K. J., Holmes, A. P., Worsley, K. J., Poline, J. P., Frith, C. D. et al (1995). Statistical parametric maps in functional imaging: a general approach. *Hum Brain Mapp, 2*, 189–210.

Genovese, C. R., Lazar, N. A., and Nichols, T. (2002). Thresholding of statistical maps in functional neuroimaging using the false discovery rate. *NeuroImage, 15*, 870–878.

Gianaros, P. J., Sheu, L. K., Remo, A. M., Christie, I. C., Crtichley, H. D. et al (2009). Heightened resting neural activity predicts exaggerated stressor-evoked blood pressure reactivity. *Hypertension, 53*(5):819–825.

Gianaros, P. J., Van Der Veen, F. M., and Jennings, J. R. (2004). Regional cerebral blood flow correlates with heart period and high-frequency heart period variability during working-memory tasks: Implications for the cortical and subcortical regulation of cardiac autonomic activity. *Psychophysiology, 41*, 521–530.

Gratton, G., and Fabiani, M. (2001a). Shedding light on brain function: the event-related optical signal. *Trends Cogn Sci, 5*, 357–363.

Gratton, G., and Fabiani, M. (2001b). The event-related optical signal: a new tool for studying brain function. *Int J Psychophysiol, 42*, 109–121.

Gray, M. A., Minati, L., Harrison, N. A., Gianaros, P. J., Napadow, V. et al (2009). Physiological recordings: basic concepts and implementation in the fMRI scanner. *NeuroImage*.

Gujar, S. K., Maheshwari, S., Bjorkman-Burtscher, I., and Sundgren, P. C. (2005). Magnetic resonance spectroscopy. *J Neuroophthalmol, 25*, 217–226.

Hagmann, P., Jonasson, L., Maeder, P., Thiran, J. P., Wedeen, V. J. et al (2006). Understanding diffusion MR imaging techniques: from scalar diffusion-weighted imaging to diffusion tensor imaging and beyond. *Radiographics, 26 Suppl 1*, S205–223.

Hill, D. K., and Keynes, R. D. (1949). Opacity changes in stimulated nerve. *J Physiol, 108*(3), 278–281.

Huettel, S. A., Song, A. S., and McCarthy, G. (2004). *Functional Magnetic Resonance Imaging*. Sunderland, M: Sinauer Associates.

Huppert, T. J., Diamond, S. G., Franceschini, M. A., and Boas, D. A. (2009). HomER: a review of time-series analysis methods for near-infrared spectroscopy of the brain. *Appl Opt, 48*, D280–298.

Jezzard, P., Matthews, P. M., and Smith, S. M. (Eds.). (2001). *Functional MRI: An Introduction to Methods*. New York: Oxford University Press.

Josephson, B. D. (1962). Possible new effects in superconductive tunneling. *Phys Lett, 1*, 251.

Klunk, W. E., Engler, H., Nordberg, A., Wang, Y., Blomqvist, G. et al (2004). Imaging brain amyloid in Alzheimer's disease with Pittsburgh Compound-B. *Ann Neurol, 55*, 306–319.

Koh, P. H., Glaser, D. E., Flandin, G., Kiebel, S., Butterworth, B. et al (2007). Functional optical signal analysis: a software tool for near-infrared spectroscopy data processing incorporating statistical parametric mapping. *J Biomed Opt, 12*, 064010.

Lane, R. D., Reiman, E. M., Ahern, G. L., and Thayer, J. F. (2001). Activity in the medial prefrontal cortex correlates with vagal component of heart rate variability. *Brain Cogn, 47*, 97–100.

Lane, R. D., Waldstein, S. R., Chesney, M. A., Jennings, J. R., Lovallo, W. R. et al (2009a). The rebirth of neuroscience in psychosomatic medicine, part I: historical context, methods and relevant basic science. *Psychosom Med, 71*, 117–134.

Lane, R. D., Waldstein, S. R., Critchley, H. D., Derbyshire, S. W., Drossman, D. A. et al (2009b). The rebirth of neuroscience in psychosomatic medicine, part II: clinical applications and implications for research. *Psychosom Med, 71*, 135–151.

Lieberman, M. D., Berkman, E. T., and Wager, T. D. (2009). Correlations in social neuroscience aren't voodoo: a reply to Vul et al. *Persp Psychol Sci, 4*, 299–307.

Logothetis, N. K. (2002). The neural basis of the blood-oxygen-level-dependent functional magnetic resonance imaging signal. *Philos Trans R Soc Lond B Biol Sci, 357*, 1003–1037.

Logothetis, N. K. (2008). What we can do and what we cannot do with fMRI. *Nature, 453*, 869–878.

McKnight, T. R. (2004). Proton magnetic resonance spectroscopic evaluation of brain tumor metabolism. *Semin Oncol, 31*, 605–617.

Nichols, T. E., and Hayasaka, S. (2003). Controlling the familywise error rate in functional neuroimaging: a comparative review. *Stat Meth Med Res, 12*, 419–446.

Ogawa, S., Lee, T. M., Kay, A. R., and Tank, D. W. (1990a). Brain magnetic resonance imaging with contrast dependent on blood oxygenation. *Proc Nat Acad Sci USA, 87*, 9868–9872.

Ogawa, S., Lee, T. M., Nayak, A. S., and Glynn, P. (1990b). Oxygenation sensitive contrast in magnetic resonance imaging of rodent brain at high magnetic fields. *Magn Res Med, 14*, 68–78.

Okada, E., and Delpy, D. T. (2003a). Near-infrared light propagation in an adult head model. I. Modeling of low-level scattering in the cerebrospinal fluid layer. *Appl Opt, 42*, 2906–2914.

Okada, E., and Delpy, D. T. (2003b). Near-infrared light propagation in an adult head model. II. Effect of superficial tissue thickness on the sensitivity of the near-infrared spectroscopy signal. *Appl Opt, 42*, 2915–2922.

Phelps, M. E., Hoffman, E. J., Mullani, N. A., and Ter-Pogossian, M. M. (1975). Application of annihilation coincidence detection to transaxial reconstruction tomography. *J Nucl Med, 16*(3), 210–224.

Pruessner, J. C., Dedovic, K., Khalili-Mahani, N., Engert, V., Pruessner, M. et al (2007). Deactivation of the limbic system during acute psychosocial stress: evidence from positron emission tomography and functional magnetic resonance imaging studies. *Biol Psychiatry, 63*, 234–240.

Purcell, E. M., Torrey, H. C., and Pound, R. V., (1946). Resonance absorption by nuclear magnetic moments in a solid. *Phys Rev, 69*, 37.

Raichle, M. E. (2006). Functional neuroimaging: a historical and physiological perspective. In R. Cabeza & A. Kingstone (Eds.), *Handbook of Functional Neuroimaging of Cognition, 2nd Ed.* (pp. 3–20). Cambridge, MA: MIT Press.

Rosen, B. R., Buckner, R. L., and Dale, A. M. (1998). Event-related functional MRI: past, present, and future. *Proc Natl Acad Sci U S A, 95*, 773–780.

Savoy, R. L. (2001). History and future directions of human brain mapping and functional neuroimaging. *Acta Psychol, 107*, 9–42.

Sokoloff, L., Reivich, M., Kennedy, C., Des Rosiers, M. H., Patlak, C. S. et al (1977). The [14C]deoxyglucose method for the measurement of local cerebral glucose utilization: theory, procedure, and normal values in the conscious and anesthetized albino rat. *J Neurochem, 28*, 897–916.

Stepnoski, R. A., LaPorta, A., Raccuia-Behling, F., Blonder, G. E., Slusher, R. E. et al (1991). Noninvasive detection of changes in membrane potential in cultured neurons by light scattering. *Proc Natl Acad Sci U S A, 88*, 9382–9386.

Toga, A. W., and Mazziotta, J. C. (Eds.). (2002). *Brain Mapping: The Methods*. San Diego, CA: Academic Press.

Villringer, A., and Chance, B. (1997). Non-invasive optical spectroscopy and imaging of human brain function. *Trends Neurosci, 20*, 435–442.

Visscher, K. M., Miezin, F. M., Kelly, J. E., Buckner, R. L., Donaldson, D. I. et al (2003). Mixed blocked/event-related designs separate transient and sustained activity in fMRI. *Neuroimage, 19*, 1694–1708.

Vul, E., Harris, C., Winkielman, P., and Pashler, H. (2009). Puzzlingly high correlations in fMRI studies of emotion, personality, and social cognition. *Persp Psychol Sci, 4*, 274–290.

Wang, J. J., Korczykowski, M., Rao, H., Fan, Y., Pluta, J. et al (2007). Gender difference in neural response to psychological stress. *Soc Cogn Affect Neurosci, 2*, 227–239.

Wang, J. J., Rao, H., Wetmore, G. S., Furlan, P. M., Korczykowski, M. et al (2005). Perfusion functional MRI reveals cerebral blood flow pattern under psychological stress. *Proc Natl Acad Sci U S A, 102*, 17804–17809.

Weber, M. J., and Monchamp, R. R. (1973). Luminescence of Bi4 Ge3 O12 spectral and decay properties. *J Appl Phys, 44*, 5495–5499.

Worsley, K. J., Evans, A. C., Marrett, S., and Neelin, P. (1992). A three-dimensional statistical analysis for CBF activation studies in human brain. *J Cereb Blood Flow Metab, 12*, 900–918.

Wrenn, F. R., Jr., Good, M. L., and Handler, P. (1951). The use of positron-emitting radioisotopes for the localization of brain tumors. *Science, 113*, 525–527.

Zackowski, K. M., Smith, S. A., Reich, D. S., Gordon-Lipkin, E., Chodkowski, B. A. et al (2009). Sensorimotor dysfunction in multiple sclerosis and column-specific magnetization transfer-imaging abnormalities in the spinal cord. *Brain, 132*, 1200–1209.

Zipursky, R. B., Meyer, J. H., and Verhoeff, N. P. (2007). PET and SPECT imaging in psychiatric disorders. *Can J Psychiatry, 52*, 146–157.

Chapter 51

Applications of Neuroimaging in Behavioral Medicine

Marcus A. Gray, Peter J. Gianaros, and Hugo D. Critchley

1 Value of Neuroimaging Applications in Medicine

Over the past few decades there has been an exponential increase in the use of these neuroimaging techniques in neuroscience research. Medical imaging of the brain has not to date been used primarily for diagnostic purposes, unlike for example medical imaging of the heart or lungs, in these cases identification of structural functional or metabolic differences (tumor, stenosis, aneurysm, calcification, etc.). Neuroimaging on the other hand is not typically for clinically diagnostic processes, with the exception of identifying stroke or lesions. The value of modern neuroimaging applications lies in their ability to investigate brain structure and neurochemistry in healthy and disease populations. Functional neuroimaging adds to this, allowing investigation of how activity within circumscribed neural structures and circuits may differentiate clinical and healthy populations, both at rest and while performing specific experimental tasks which tap relevant psychological functions. The applications of neuroimaging methods in behavioral medicine are broad, and include psychological processes, social and interpersonal processes,

genetic processes, the identification of biomarkers, development and the life course, epidemiology, behavioral and psychosocial interventions, and treatment. In addition to these specific applications, neuroimaging has made valuable contributions in understanding how mental states are instantiated in the brain, associated with information processing systems and integrated with the ongoing physiological function of the body (Lane et al, 2009a). Neuroimaging investigation of these mind–body linkages offers the potential of significant advances in understanding the physical/physiological basis of human thoughts, feelings, and behavior. In the sections below we highlight how specific applications of neuroimaging have valuably contributed to behavioral medicine, including with specific examples. We then focus in detail on an emerging application within behavioral medicine; the application of neuroimaging to stress reactivity and characterize in detail findings which suggest corticolimbic brain areas are jointly involved in processing stressors and regulating the cardiovascular system.

2 Behavioral Medicine Applications

2.1 Psychological Processes

Human anxiety represents a domain where neuroimaging has informed understanding of psychological processes relevant to behavioral medicine. Anxiety serves an adaptive role in directing attention to real or potential sources

M.A. Gray (✉)
Trafford Centre/Clinical Imaging Sciences Centre,
University of Sussex, Falmer, Brighton, BN1 9PX, UK
e-mail: m.gray@bsms.ac.uk

A. Steptoe (ed.), *Handbook of Behavioral Medicine*, DOI 10.1007/978-0-387-09488-5_51,
© Springer Science+Business Media, LLC 2010

of threat and to mobilize both cognitive and behavioral and physiological resources toward successful resolution of the threatening situation. Anxiety reactions may also cross into the spectrum of clinical disorders when situationally inappropriate, excessive, or prolonged. A key neural structure emerging from animal and human neuroscience research into anxiety is the amygdala (LeDoux, 2000; Vuilleumier, 2005). Originally identified in animal models of fear conditioning (Davis and Whalen, 2001; LeDoux, 1996), recent functional neuroimaging research has identified its engagement by a variety of biologically and motivationally salient stimuli. One class of stimuli in particular, robustly engages the amygdala: human faces (Adolphs, 2008). Facial expressions convey a rich variety of information vital for hyper-social animals such as human beings and are potent social cues of potential or actual threat, a feature particularly relevant for fearful facial expressions (Anderson et al, 2003). Interestingly, the amygdala responds to the content of facial expression, even when presented outside of conscious awareness (Williams et al, 2004; Whalen et al, 1998) or when attention is directed elsewhere (Vuilleumier et al, 2001). These findings illustrate that amygdala function contributes to the psychological processing of social emotional information encoded in facial expressions and has particular relevance for the psychology of anxiety responses.

The importance of the amygdala to anxiety-related psychological processes in behavioral medicine is highlighted by neuroimaging studies of patients with damage to the amygdala. Anderson et al (2002) investigated trait and day-to-day emotional experience within ten left, ten right, and one bilaterally amygdala-damaged patient(s). Despite localized damage to the amygdala, patients did not differ from a sample of 20 control participants in the magnitude and frequency of self-reported positive or negative affect including anxiety. Further insight into these intriguing findings is provided by Anderson and colleagues' (2000) findings from a female bilaterally amygdala-damaged patient whose ability to express emotions including

fear remained intact, while the ability to recognize these emotions from facial expressions was severely impaired. Adolphs and colleagues (2005) also reported findings from a different female patient with bilateral amygdala damage who displayed a similarly severe impairment in fear recognition with facial stimuli. They show that this deficit is associated with impairments in eye direction while assessing facial expressions. This patient failed to make the spontaneous fixations on the eyes while assessing facial expressions, fixations which characterize normal evaluation of others facial expressions observed in healthy adults. These findings suggest that the perception of fear and anxiety cues is heavily dependent on the guidance of attentional processes subserved by the functional activity of the amygdala (see Fig. 51.1).

In healthy adults, functional imaging also demonstrates a positive association between the degree of amygdala engagement during experimental tasks and trait measures of anxiety. During assessment of facial emotional

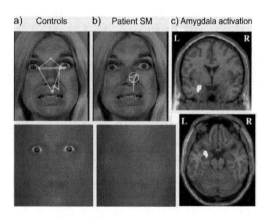

Fig. 51.1 Perception of facial expressions of fear and the amygdale. Neuroimaging research highlights the role of the amygdala in processing of face stimuli. (**a**) Healthy people perceive fear in facial expressions by examining the eyes in fearful expressions (above) more than other facial features (in the image below facial features are weighted by inspection time). (**b**) In a patient with amygdala lesions, the eyes are not preferred and fear is not recognized. (**c**) In healthy controls, fearful faces activate the amygdala regardless of spatial attention. (**a**) and (**b**) reproduced with permission from Adolphs et al (2008). (**c**) reproduced with permission from Vuilleumier et al (2001)

expressions individuals differ in their degree of amygdala reactivity, differences which appear stable over time (Johnstone et al, 2005; Manuck et al, 2007; see Hariri, 2009). Further, functional neuroimaging reveals that individual differences in amygdala reactivity during the processing of emotional stimuli predict both trait (Dickie and Armony, 2008; Etkin et al, 2004; Haas et al, 2007; Killgore and Yurgelun-Todd, 2005; Most et al, 2006; Ohrmann et al, 2007; Ray et al, 2005) and state anxiety (Bishop et al, 2004; Ewbank et al, 2009; Somerville et al, 2004; again see Hariri, 2009). Moreover, amygdala reactivity is accentuated across clinically anxious groups including post-traumatic stress disorder (Bryant et al, 2005; Liberzon et al, 1999), obsessive compulsive disorder (Van der Heuvel et al, 2005a, b), specific phobia (e.g., Wik et al, 1996), and social phobia (e.g., Birbaumer et al, 1998).

Amygdala activity in the context of threat (Critchley et al, 2002; Williams et al, 2004), processing of social stimuli including faces (e.g., Critchley et al, 2005a), and mental effort (Gianaros et al, 2008a) is directly coupled to peripheral autonomic sympathetic activity, which in turn is implicated in the negative physical health consequences of chronic stress and anxiety (Gianaros et al, 2009) (see below).

2.2 Social and Interpersonal Processes

Social relationships are intimately tied to well-being and mental health (Sullivan, 1953). The close association between mental health and social/interpersonal processes is highlighted by the pervasiveness of severely impoverished social networks and deficits in social skills of persons with schizophrenia, depression, social anxiety, and eating disorders for example. Primary assumptions embedded in social and interpersonal perspectives in behavioral medicine are that interpersonal disturbances may function as (1) causally disruptive phenomena in the development of mental illness, (2)

stressors within a diathesis-stress model of illness, and (3) a frequent consequence of, and maintaining factor in, mental illness (see Segrin, 2001). Animal research demonstrates how positive social bonds underlie well-being, reducing stress-related neuroendocrine activity (Carter, 1998), while human research shows well-being and satisfaction are associated with perceived social support (Kafetsios and Sideridis, 2006). As a consequence, insights gained within social cognitive neuroscience and the study of social cognition have wide applicability to the field of behavioral medicine (Cacioppo and Berntson, 2005; Ochsner and Lieberman, 2001).

Neuroimaging research contributes to understandings of the importance of social and interpersonal processes in a variety of ways, including investigating the neural processes which underlie effective social/interpersonal interactions and facilitate identification, attachment, and social bonding. Simple social interactions reveal a surprising complexity of coordinated responses, many of which occur outside of conscious awareness (Lakin and Chartrand, 2008). Study of effective social interactions reveals a high degree of moment by moment symmetry between participants in terms of emotional expression, posture, and general levels of autonomic arousal. As strong bonds form over time, people increasingly resemble each others' emotional styles (Anderson et al, 2003). During interaction, our expressions posture and arousal levels become social responses. These in turn evoke social responses in others which we perceive as social stimuli, in turn evoking further responses (Frith, 2008; Frith and Singer, 2008). Understanding the neural correlates of these symmetries was strongly influenced by the discovery of mirror neurons within monkeys. While it is unsurprising that specific motor neurons fire during specific behaviors, such as grasping an object, mirror neurons intriguingly fire both when an action is performed and when one watches another performing that action (Rizzolatti and Luppino, 2001). Mirror neurons therefore are important in mediating rapid nonconscious imitation (see Jeannerod, 1994) and are now believed to play a critical role in inferring and understanding the meaning of observed actions (Cattaneo and Rizzolatti, 2009). Mirror neuron systems then may form a critical social/interpersonal function, in that they underlie shared feelings and understandings. This is demonstrated in the work of Tania Singer on empathy. Singer et al (2004) investigated neural activity both when people received painful experimental stimuli and when they watched a loved one receive painful stimuli. While each condition was associated with specific patterns of activity, activity within the anterior insula (AI) and anterior cingulate cortex (ACC) responded in a similar way to receiving pain and watching a loved one receive pain. Further, individual levels of empathy correlated with the activation within these structures, suggesting that the degree to which AI and ACC neurons mirrored others pain reflected how empathic these people were. Singer went on to examine how empathy is modified by affection or its absence. In a money-making game, males and females learnt to trust and distrust specific game players. They then watched these players receive painful experimental stimuli. "Empathic mirror neuron activity" was again observed within the AI and ACC, but only if these were "fair players." Conversely, males displayed activity in reward circuitry when "unfair players" received pain which correlated with expressed desire for revenge (Singer et al, 2006). By mirroring others we care about, empathy allows for shared emotions and facilitates social bonding. Neuroimaging research within social cognitive neuroscience furthers understandings of the neural underpinnings of trust (Vuilleumier and Sander, 2008) and effective social bonding, and of how these processes may be compromised during fraught interpersonal interactions, with direct relevance to social and interpersonal processes in behavioral medicine.

2.3 Genetic Processes

A new era in medical science was marked by the draft sequencing of the human genome in 2001 (Lander et al, 2001) and the completion of DNA mapping of each human chromosome (Gregory et al, 2006). The focus on individual disease processes perhaps overrides the integrative agenda of behavioral medicine, but nevertheless represents a significant opportunity for new discoveries and treatments. Alzheimer's disease is one area where genetic information, utilized within neuroimaging studies, is contributing to behavioral medicine. Alzheimer's disease (AD), the single most common cause of dementia in the elderly, is characterized by the presence of beta-amyloid plaques and hyperphosphorylated tau tangles (Blennow et al, 2006). In addition, post-mortem examinations reveal widespread reductions in gray and white matter volume associated with cortical thinning and demyelination and enlargement of the ventricles. A range of genetic features have been identified which confer increased risk for development of AD. These include inherited autosomal dominant conditions such as presenilin mutations (PS1 or PS2) or the amyloid precursor protein gene, however, these familial mutations only account for around 5% of AD cases (Bookheimer and Burggren, 2009). Conversely, a diagnosis of AD in both parents confers a 40% risk for AD, suggesting further progress in identifying the genetic risk factors is possible (Jayadev et al, 2008). To date, the best genetic risk factors in the development of AD are polymorphisms of the apolipoprotein E gene on chromosome 19.

Apolipoprotein E (ApoE) is one of six apolipoproteins which combine into lipoprotein assemblies in order to transport lipids, including triglycerides and cholesterol, through the blood. Within the brain cholesterol is an essential component of myelin and membranes and after secretion by astrocytes promotes healthy synapse formation (Mauch et al, 2001). Each of the paired ApoE alleles are expressed as the E2, E3, or E4 variants, allowing six potential ApoE genotypes (Bu et al, 2009). In the general population, the frequency of the E4 allele is approximately 15%, however, within patients with AD this allele is considerably more frequent (approximately 40%). Further, relative to those without the E4 allele, possession of a single

E4 allele increases the risk of AD (particularly late onset AD) between three and four times (Bu et al, 2009). Research exploring the mechanisms through which the ApoE E4 allele confers increased risk for AD suggests effects via multiple pathways involving both beta-amyloid (Aβ) and tau (see Fig. 51.2i).

Neuroimaging research is increasingly utilizing genetic information. One important

development in the neuroimaging of AD has been the development of Pittsburgh compound B (PiB), PiB combines a radioactive isotype of carbon (11C) with an analogue of the histology stain thioflavin T which selectively binds to fibrillar aggregates of Aβ (Klunk et al, 2004). Reiman and colleagues (2009) investigated the presence of fibrillar Aβ in healthy adults (mean age 64 years). While all subjects were normal

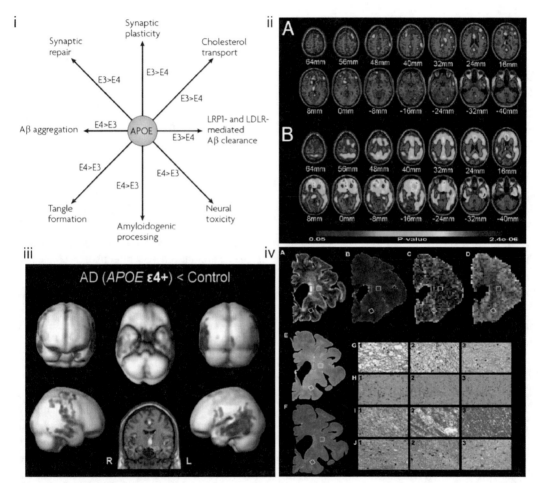

Fig. 51.2 Neuroimaging of Alzheimer's disease. (i) Summary of apolipoprotein E (ApoE) functions in normal brain function and the pathogenic processes of Alzheimer's disease (AD). (ii) Brain maps showing greater PiB binding in (A) eight cognitively normal ApoE 4 heterozygotes subjects and (B) eight cognitively normal homozygotes (B) compared with 12 cognitively normal non carriers. Figure reproduced with permission from Reiman et al (2009). (iii) Gray matter decrease in patients with AD who carry the ApoE 4 allele compared to healthy controls. Reproduced with permission from Drzezga et al (2009). (iv) Multiple neuroimaging explorations of pathophysiological changes within AD disease are displayed for a single 88-year-old subject. Images include (A) FLAIR image, (B) T1-map, (C) fractional anisotropy map, and (D) apparent diffusion coefficient map. Additionally, sections are displayed after histochemical staining with (E) Bodian Silver, and (F) Luxol-Fast-Blue/Cresyl-Violet. Finally microscopic sections (G–J) illustrate white matter hyperintensities. Reproduced with permission from Gouw et al (2008)

cognitively and did not differ on the mini mental status exam, ApoE testing revealed subjects carried either two, one, or no ApoE E4 alleles. Despite being otherwise closely matched, PET imaging of fibrillar Aβ aggregates with PiB clearly differentiated the ApoE E4 allele (see Fig. 51.2ii). Subjects with either one (see Fig. 51.2iiA) or two (see Fig. 51.2iiB) copies of the E4 allele displayed significantly greater PiB binding than subjects without this ApoE allele, clearly identifying increased fibrilliar Aβ risk, even within cognitively normal adults. Neuroimaging research is also investigating differences in how gene markers differentiate functional activity within the brain. Filippini et al (2009a) examined healthy young adults either with or without the ApoE E4 genotype, looking at memory encoding and spontaneous activity when subjects were simply waiting quietly (i.e., "default network" activity, see Rachile et al, 2001). They report increased activity at rest within default brain networks and, conversely, increased hippocampal activity during memory encoding within E4 carriers. Additionally, a growing body of research has investigated functional brain activity in elderly adults, either with or without mild cognitive impairment to explore the impact of the ApoE E4 allele on brain activity and cognitive function, and extending similar observations from older adults carrying ApoE E4 (Bondi et al, 2005; Bookheimer et al, 2000; Buggren et al, 2002; Johnson et al, 2006a, 2006b; Lind et al, 2006; Smith et al, 1999; Trivedi et al, 2008, 2006; Wishart et al, 2006a; Woodard et al, 2009).

In addition to functional MRI research and PET imaging of fibrilliar amyloid binding, a range of structural/anatomical papers are increasing understanding of AD. Regional brain volume can be quantified with T1-weighted MRI scans, allowing examination of vulnerable regions including the entorhinal cortex and hippocampus. Blennow and colleagues (2006) present volumetric measures of hippocampal and entorhinal volume within a single AD patient over a period of 10 years, clearly demonstrating progressive decline in regional brain volume.

Additionally, automated techniques such as volumetric brain mapping (VBM) are increasingly being applied in AD (Cherbuin et al, 2008; Filippini et al, 2009b; Thomann et al, 2008; Wishart et al, 2006b; Xie et al, 2006). Increasingly neuroimaging research is combining imaging methodologies. Drzega et al (2009) for example combined Aβ imaging in PET and automated VBM measures from MRI scanning in AD patients, examining differences associated with the ApoE genotype. Increased PiB uptake within E4-positive AD patients indicated a greater fibillary amyloid load, however, while both E4-positive and negative AD patients displayed greater cortical atrophy in VBM measures relative to healthy controls (see Fig. 51.2iii), E4 expression within AD patients did not significantly increase cortical atrophy. The impact of functional neuroimaging methods in investigating the neuropathological genetic processes is considerable. Previously, including histological analysis at autopsy represented the only objective method of quantifying the impact of neuropathological processes in AD patients. An area of active investigation in AD is the examination of white matter connectivity in vivo via MRI diffusion tensor imaging (DTI) (e.g., Damoiseaux et al, 2009; Medina et al, 2008; Stricker et al, 2009; Ringman et al, 2007). Additionally, a range of measures may be examined in combination. Gouw and colleagues (2008) examined eleven AD patients and presented a direct comparison of stained brain slices at autopsy with a range of functional imaging measures including T1 white matter mapping, DTI tractography, and apparent diffusion coefficient mapping (see Fig. 51.2iv), identifying AD specific neuropathological processes including differences in microglial activation, axonal, and myelin density.

Beyond neurodegenerative conditions there has been increasing interest in understanding the mechanisms through which genetic processes interact with emotional traits and vulnerabilities to psychological stress. Thus genetic variation affecting (by fourfold) the activity of catechol-O-methyltransferase (COMT; the enzyme that breaks down monoamine neuromodulators dopamine and norepinephrine) is associated with a range of differences in the processing of emotional stimuli within brain regions such as amygdala (Smolka et al, 2005). Similarly genetic variants affecting the function of serotonin (5HT) via receptor transporter or gene promoter molecules are also linked to differential amygdala reactivity and emotional traits and vulnerabilities (e.g., Fakra et al, 2009; Friedel et al, 2009).

2.4 Development and the Life Course

Behavioral medicine broadens traditional organismic disease models to include wider social, cultural, and developmental contributions to health and disease. Just as cognitive and emotional development is embedded in, and dependent upon, an immediate social context (Vygotsky, 1930), so the normal maturational stages of cognitive development (Piaget, 1971) occur within the context of a developing brain. Neuroimaging methods have been applied to investigate both the development of cognitive capacities (functional development) and physical alterations in brain structure during the life course (structural development). For example, Dubois and colleagues (2008) explored the influence of inter-uterine environment on the functional and anatomical development of brain in premature newborns, observing abnormal and delayed gyrification within growth restricted, but not other infants, including twins. Figure 51.3a illustrates the minimal gyral and sulcal development in the normal premature infant brain. Longitudinal studies of healthy children highlight the different growth phases during brain maturation, an important consideration when seeking a neurobiological correlate of environmental influences across the lifespan. Thus Gogtay et al (2008) scanned children who returned every 2 years for MRI scanning. Periods of reducing gray matter corresponded to known times of selective pruning of neuronal synapses and the study also highlighted gradual myelination within the developing brain (see

Fig. 51.3b). Synaptic pruning occurs at a nonlinear rate, with significant reductions during childhood and adolescence acting to streamline "inefficient" neuronal circuits (Huttenlocher, 1994; Somogyi et al, 1998). Similarly myelination also occurs non-linearly (Bartzokis et al, 2009) and continues into middle age, achieving peak volume at approximately 44 years in the frontal lobes and 47 years in the temporal lobes. Tractography with DTI in combination with other MRI techniques permitted more detailed understanding of these maturational processes. Figure 51.3c presents age associated increases in fractional and decreases in mean diffusivity in 168 healthy participants aged between 8 and 30 years (Tamnes et al, 2010). These findings are also consistent with Sowell and colleagues' (2003) findings in 176 adults aged between 8 and 87 years (see Fig. 51.3d) and Lu et al's (2009) findings, where improved cognition functionally activated regions which also displayed maturational changes of structure (see Fig. 51.3e). By understanding normal developmental brain trajectories, the impact of lived experience on health can be interpreted more confidently.

2.5 Biomarkers

Both structural and functional neuroimaging data may serve as biomarkers for disease processes, increased disease risk, and treatment response. As noted above, certain signatures, for example amygdala reactivity, may have particular biomarker status in the context of behavioral medicine. Within bipolar disorder Kruger and colleagues (2006) explored neural responses during sadness induction within nine euthymic bipolar patients and their healthy siblings (i.e., increased bipolar risk). As with previous bipolar patients who responded to sodium valproate (but not healthy controls without increased genetic risk) reductions in inferior temporal and orbitofrontal cortex activity and increases in dorsal/rostral cingulate and anterior insula were observed (see Phillips and Vietta, 2007). This pattern of activity during emotional

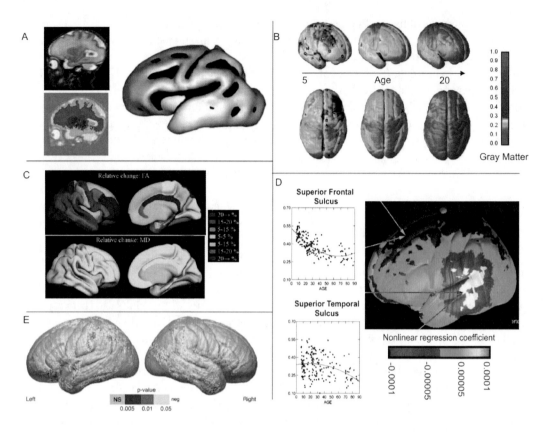

Fig. 51.3 Brain development over the life course. (**a**) Cortical folding and volume of the brain at birth identified using T2-weighted MRI images (*top left*) and segmented (*bottom left*) into cortex (*green*), unmyelinated/myelinated white matter (*red/orange*), and basal ganglia/thalamiregions (*maroon*). From this data, a sulcation index was computed (right). Reproduced with permission from Dubois et al (2008). (**b**) Dynamics of GM maturation over the cortical surface. The *side bar* shows a color representation in units of GM volume. Modified from original in Gogtay et al (2004). (**c**)

Relative magnitude of developmental changes over the age span 8–30 years. Illustrated are percentage changes in white matter (WM) volume and mean diffusivity (MD). Figure reproduced with permission from Tamnes et al (2010). (**d**) Gray matter volume within the superior frontal and superior temporal sulci changes as a nonlinear function of age. Reproduced with permission from Sowell et al (2003). (**e**) Regions of the cortical surface which display a significant linear association between age and gray matter thickness. Reproduced with permission from Lu et al (2009)

challenge, if reproduced within other patients and healthy first degree relatives may represent a functional biomarker for bipolar disorder, indicative of affective instability, and potential for emotional dysregulation (Phillips and Vietta, 2007). Functional biomarkers observed with neuroimaging methodologies may offer advantages over purely genetic biomarkers, as it is understood that in many cases simple gene–disease associations are unlikely to exist. Rather, in line with the diathesis-stress model, genetics, environment and life events frequently interact

in determining disease susceptibility. Functional biomarkers may be sensitive to a range of genetic, environmental, and psychosocial influences, and therefore better reflect vulnerability arising from a variety of sources.

2.6 Behavioral and Psychosocial Intervention

Epidemiological perspectives within behavioral medicine are also informing interventional approaches. A range of psychosocial factors including low socioeconomic status (SES), psychosocial stress, social isolation, and personality factors increase risk for medical and psychiatric conditions and cluster together within groups and individuals (Sobel, 1995). Greater understanding of psychosocial risks in disease processes can inform development of effective interventions, and neuroimaging can contribute by exploring how psychosocial risks influences brain structure and function.

For example, Farah et al (2006) examined the impact of significant alcohol exposure on fetal brain development using MRI. They explored cognitive, verbal, and visuospatial function within people with heavy prenatal alcohol exposure. These participants people displayed poorer performance on measures including verbal and visuospatial functioning. Interestingly, like previous findings (Sowell et al, 2001, 2002) they also exhibited increased gray matter thickness, particularly over regions of the temporal cortex which may reflect a retardation of normal maturational reduction in gray matter volume during childhood (see Fig. 51.4a) (Sowell et al, 2008).

Similar research has examined the association of socioeconomic status (SES), parental social standing, and perceived life stress with brain circuitry supporting cognitive or mood disorders and vulnerabilities to physical illness (Gianaros et al, 2008b, 2009). Low SES increases risk for medical and psychiatric disorders and is also associated with deficits in working memory and cognitive control and language (see Fig. 51.4B). Further, language ability (i.e., phonological awareness) of low, but not high, SES children was observed by Noble and colleagues (2006) to correlate strongly with activity within the left fusiform cortex during a listening task (see Fig. 51.4c), suggesting poor language abilities within lower SES children was associated with a failure of neural activity underlying phonological processing. Similar results are reported by Raizada and colleagues (2008) who observed greater hemispheric specialization within Broca's area with higher SES. Interventions informed by this type of research involve tailored education for at-risk low SES children in letter recognition, decoding print, and increased overall print exposure (see Noble et al, 2006). Overall, better understanding of the

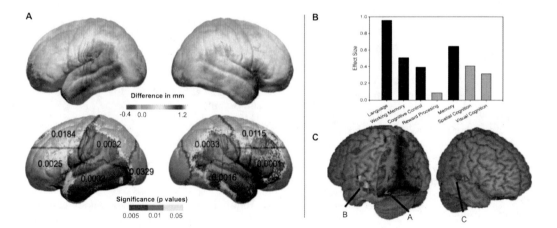

Fig. 51.4 Prenatal alcohol and social effects on brain maturation and function. (a) Differences in cortical thickness within fetal alcohol spectrum disordered children versus control children. (Ai) Group differences expressed in millimeters. (Aii) Uncorrected P maps representing significant group differences in cortical thickness. Reproduced with permission from Sowell et al (2008). (**b**) Performance on the composite of seven different measures of neurocognitive function between low and middle SES children. Effect sizes are illustrated; *black bars* represent statistically significant differences. Reproduced with permission from Farah et al (2006). (**c**) Correlations between phonological awareness and activity in (A) left fusiform, (B) left perisylvian cortex, and (C) right perisylvian cortex. Reproduced with permission from Noble et al (2006)

neural correlates of deficits associated with psychosocial risk factors can improve the ability to target vulnerabilities with behavioral medicine treatment interventions.

2.7 Neuroimaging and Treatment

Neuroimaging techniques may also develop into treatment tools. Medical investigations, including brain scans, may have intrinsic therapeutic value imparted by a reduction in diagnostic uncertainty or in educating the patient with respect to the absence or likely consequences of neuropathology (something that can be repeated over time). Beyond this though there has been a concerted effort to apply brain imaging technology to behavioral interventions. In the last few years real-time (rt) imaging with functional (f)MRI is being developed as a means to train the modulation of brain activity for therapeutic benefit (deCharms, 2008; Weiskopf et al, 2003). A second wave of research papers on this topic, and brain computer interfaces more generally, is anticipated to emerge very soon, but technical obstacles are now largely overcome and proof-of-principle studies using rtfMRI for pain (deCharms et al, 2005) and emotion regulation (Caria et al, 2007) have been well received by the neuroscience community. Other related imaging methods may follow, for example near-infrared spectroscopy which may provide similar feedback information about brain activity for self-regulatory training, but at lower equipment costs and in more naturalistic settings than fMRI (Abdelnour and Huppert, 2009; Coyle et al, 2007). The value of these techniques to clinical populations in comparison to the circumscribed applications of neurofeedback with EEG needs to be established.

2.8 Epidemiology and Population

Neuroimaging research may also contribute to informing epidemiological and population-based approaches within behavioral medicine.

Population medicine approaches reflect the insight that specific features within a population may be associated with increased risk for certain disease processes, whereas at an individual level these associations may not be as easy to identify. For example, psychosocial and social factors are increasingly recognized as differentiating risk factors to a wide range of disease states. Depression, stress, and social isolation are, at the population level, strongly associated with a range of illnesses including cardiovascular disease and weakened immune responses. Emotional stress including anxiety and depression is associated with increased rates of cardiovascular disease occurrence (Wulsin and Singal, 2003) and cardiovascular disease mortality rates can precipitate cardiac arrhythmia and sudden death in patients with heart disease (Lampert et al, 2005; Oppenheimer et al, 1990; van Melle et al, 2004). Exploring these associations has revealed that mood, trauma, and stress directly influence cardiac function (Lampert et al, 2005; Wulsin and Singal, 2003; van Melle et al, 2004). Further, poorly regulated physiological reactions may initiate or exacerbate ill health among vulnerable individuals. Understandings of epidemiology and disease risk gained at the level of population medicine motivate neuroimaging research. In turn neuroscience furthers understandings of how population risks may be mediated within the body. In the following section we consider in more detail the applications of neuroimaging to investigating links between stress reactivity and the brain.

3 Stress Reactivity

As highlighted above, an individual's tendency to show exaggerated or otherwise dysregulated cardiovascular reactions to acute stressors is associated with increased risk for clinical and preclinical endpoints of coronary heart disease (CHD) (Krantz and Manuck, 1984; Obrist, 1981; Schwartz et al, 2003; Treiber et al, 2003). Specifically, there are several lines of evidence suggesting that exaggerated stressor-evoked cardiovascular reactions may predict (1) an accelerated progression of atherosclerosis in humans and nonhuman primates; (2) the premature development of high blood pressure (hypertension) and other precursors to CHD; and (3) the likelihood of having a future coronary event (e.g., myocardial infarction) (Schwartz et al, 2003; Treiber et al, 2003). Consequently, identifying "brain–body" mechanisms linking central nervous system activity during acute stress with cardiovascular reactions implicated in CHD risk is essential (Lane et al, 2009b; Lovallo, 2005). Below, we focus more closely on specific applications of neuroimaging research, which links individual differences in stressor-evoked reactions (primarily blood pressure or cortisol reactivity) with activation of, and covariation between, corticolimbic (including cingulate cortex, insula, and amygdala) and brain stem (pons, periaqueductal gray [PAG]) areas involved in mobilizing hemodynamic and metabolic support for stress-related behavioral responding.

In a PET study of six men (mean age 35 years), Critchley and colleagues (2000) tested whether changes in mean arterial pressure correlated with concurrent changes in functional neural activation evoked by two reliable stressors; mental arithmetic and isometric handgrip. An explicit aim of this study was to isolate neural activity patterns that covaried directly with stressor-evoked blood pressure changes irrespective of task. Increased stressor-evoked mean arterial pressure correlated on a within-individual basis with increased cerebral blood flow to the perigenual and mid-anterior areas of the cingulate cortex, the orbitofrontal cortex, postcentral gyrus, insula, and cerebellum (see Table 2 in Critchley et al, 2000) – providing the first human neuroimaging evidence in support of the view that these brain regions may initiate or represent increases in blood pressure to behavioral stressors (see Fig. 51.5a). Critchley et al (2005b) followed this by examining myocardial function during these acute stress tasks in 10 cardiology outpatients (mean age 57 years), patients in whom stress increases the likelihood of uneven or dysregulated heart contraction (i.e., is pro-arrhythmic; Lown et al,

1977). Electrocardiogram (ECG) derived measures revealed that acute stress increased the unevenness of global ventricular wall motion and the variability of ventricular repolarization between small localized regions of the heart. The degree to which vulnerable cardiac outpatients displayed these pro-arrhythmic alterations was reflected by lateralized brain stem activity, suggesting that unbalanced cardiac drive was reflected by disturbances in coordinated cardiac function. Gray et al (2007) explored these associations further, examining EEG measures of cortical function in tandem with clinical ECG within 10 similarly vulnerable cardiac outpatients (mean age 59 years) during induced stress. While stressor tasks induced sympathetic arousal and demand on the heart, the effectiveness of cardiac responses to stress within these patients was mixed. Interestingly, activity overlying the dorsolateral prefrontal cortex and insula reflected the functional activity of the heart, suggesting that these neural regions supported an ongoing representation of cardiac function at a beat-by-beat level, consistent with cardiac afferent (baroreceptor generated) activation during each cardiac cycle. Gray and colleagues (2009) further explored the influence of baroreceptor generated signals from the heart during acute cardiovascular stress reactions. Acute cardiovascular reflexes were induced via electrical skin stimuli in 11 healthy controls (mean age 27 years). By delivering electric shocks during differing phases of the cardiac cycle, the influence of baroreceptor activation (a vagal signal with generally inhibitory actions) on shock-induced cardiovascular reflexes was explored. Blood pressure reactions were markedly attenuated when electrical stimulation was delivered during baroreceptor firing. In addition activity in the amygdala, anterior insula, and brain stem which regulated mean arterial pressure (MAP) reactions also differed when electrical stimuli were presented during baroreceptor discharge. Neural activity within the amygdala, insula, and PAG also reflected between subject differences in heart rate variability, suggesting baroreceptor influences on cardiovascular reflexes depends on vagal reactivity (see Fig. 51.5b).

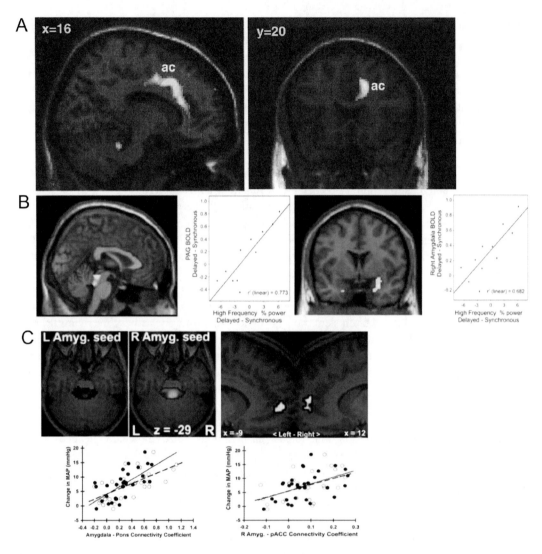

Fig. 51.5 Neural activity associated with acute alterations in cardiovascular function. (**a**) Anterior cingulate activity showing positive covariance with mean arterial pressure in exercise and mental arithmetic tasks. Adapted with permission from Critchley et al (2000). (**b**) Neural activity associated with different mean arterial pressure reactions to cardiac timed stimuli. Within the amygdala (*left*) and PAG (*right*) changes in neural activity were significantly associated with changes in high-frequency heart rate variability flowing baroreceptor synchronous shocks. (**c**) During an acute stress task, increased connectivity between the amygdala and pons was associated with greater mean arterial pressure reactivity (*left*). Similarly, increased connectivity between the amygdala and perigenual anterior cingulate cortex was associated with greater mean arterial pressure reactivity. Reproduced with permission from Gianaros et al (2008)

Gianaros and colleges have also examined neural correlates of stressor-evoked blood pressure reactivity. In an fMRI study, 20 adults (mean age 64 years) completed a performance-titrated Stroop color-word interference task, specifically adapted from previous epidemiological studies of stressor-evoked blood pressure reactivity and CHD risk. Increased stressor-evoked MAP correlated (within-subjects) with greater activation in the perigenual and mid-anterior cingulate cortex (areas 24 and 32), insula, medial and lateral prefrontal cortex, supplementary motor area, and regions of the temporal, inferior parietal, and occipital cortex. Subcortical regions in which greater activation correlated with increased MAP included the basal ganglia, lentiform area bordering the extended amygdala and caudate, thalamus, cerebellum, and PAG (see Table 2 of Gianaros et al, 2005).

In an fMRI study of individual differences in stressor-evoked blood pressure reactivity, 46 postmenopausal women (mean age 68 years) performed a similar version of the Stroop task described above (Gianaros et al, 2007). Across individuals, a larger rise in systolic and diastolic blood pressure covaried with heightened activation of the perigenual anterior cingulate cortex (pACC) (extending into Brodmann areas 10 and 31), insula, the lateral prefrontal cortex, and cerebellum (see Table 2 in Gianaros et al, 2007). Moreover, Stroop-evoked blood pressure reactivity during the fMRI recordings correlated with those evoked in subsequent laboratory session, illustrating that the individual differences in stressor-evoked blood pressure reactivity were stable across individuals and testing settings. In this study, however, no associations were observed between blood pressure reactivity and activation in amygdala, midbrain, and brain stem areas, regions thought to be involved in cardiovascular regulation. These null findings, however, were attributed to the scanning sequence and field of view coverage used in this particular study.

As a consequence, Gianaros et al (2008) employed a region of interest approach to directly examine amygdala activity and covariation within corticolimbic and subcortical areas during stressor processing and cardiovascular regulation. Thirty-two young adults (mean age 20 years) again completed the Stroop task described above while blood pressure and fMRI data were acquired. Using this targeted approach, individuals who exhibited greater MAP reactivity showed greater stressor-evoked pACC, pCC, insula, and amygdala activation and a stronger positive functional connectivity between the amygdala and pACC and between the amygdala and pons (see Fig. 51.5c).

Collectively, these neuroimaging findings support the notion that individual differences in stressor-evoked blood pressure reactivity are correlated not only with patterns of co-activation in corticolimbic systems, but also with the functional interactions between these systems.

The amygdala expresses reciprocal connections with pontine cell groups critical for cardiovascular control (Dampney, 1994; Hopkins and Holstege, 1978; Miller et al, 1991). In view of this circuitry the above results suggest that the pons may represent a relay area that specifically links individual differences in stressor-evoked amygdala activity with the peripheral expression of blood pressure reactions. Hence, stronger efferent amygdala pre-autonomic signaling could reflect stronger descending commands for rises in blood pressure during acute stressful experiences, whereas stronger afferent pre-autonomic amygdala signaling could reflect stronger ascending negative feedback to the amygdala, curtailing excessive blood pressure rises (i.e., greater negative amygdala-pons connectivity was associated with reduced blood pressure reactivity). In addition to the pons, areas of the anterior cingulate cortex, such as the pACC, are also reciprocally connected to the amygdala, and both fear-conditioning and emotion-regulation research suggest that the anterior cingulate cortex (particularly the perigenual area) may regulate amygdala activity (Etkin et al, 2006; Ochsner and Gross, 2005; Quirk and Beer, 2006). Indeed the pACC and the amygdala are recognized as components of a corticolimbic circuit orchestrating integrated behavioral and visceromotor stress responses (cf., Bush et al, 2000; Critchley et al, 2005a; Devinsky et al, 1995; Paus, 2001; Vogt, 2005). Hence, differential coupling between these areas may also influence individual differences in stressor-evoked blood pressure reactivity (i.e., greater negative amygdala–pACC connectivity was also associated with reduced blood pressure reactivity). Future research employing effective connectivity procedures (Friston, 1994) and continuous (beat-by-beat) blood pressure monitoring (Gray et al, 2009) may help to more clearly distinguish directionality by parsing efferent from afferent signals in cardio-vascular control networks including corticolimbic and pre-autonomic brain stem nuclei. Such research may also prove useful in understanding the pathophysiological processes underling CHD risk. For example, heightened amygdala activation to threatening emotional stimuli has been associated with increased intima-media vessel wall thickness in the carotid arteries, indicating preclinical atherosclerosis and potential clinical endpoints of CHD (Gianaros et al, 2009). As above, increased functional connectivity between the pACC and amygdala was associated with increased pathophysiological changes, suggesting alterations in co-activation and connectivity may impact atherosclerotic disease processes and consequent CHD risk via stress-related processes such as blood pressure reactivity.

Finally, in addition to the cardiovascular system, the hypothalamic–pituitary–adrenal (HPA) axis is also increasingly studied in neuroimaging research on stress reactivity (Dedovic et al, 2005, 2009; Eisenberger et al, 2007; Pruessner et al, 2007; Taylor et al, 2008; Wang et al, 2005). As detailed by Puetz and colleagues (Chapter 43), several endpoints of the HPA axis can be measured reliably. Cortisol in particular can be measured as it changes from pre- to post-stressor periods and as it varies over the course of the day. Urry and colleagues (2006) measured diurnal cortisol changes and fMRI activity as participants were instructed to increase or decrease their experienced negative affect while viewing emotionally evocative pictures. Intentionally increasing negative affect increased prefrontal (ventrolateral, dorsolateral, and dorsomedial cortex) and amygdala activity. Further, while decreasing negative affect, greater prefrontal (dorsolateral and dorsomedial cortex) and lower amygdala activity was associated with a steeper decline in cortisol over the day. Considering that a flatter diurnal cortisol slope predicts greater mortality risk among cancer patients (Abercrombie et al, 2004) and subclinical atherosclerosis in the coronary arteries (Matthews et al, 2006), a greater capacity to regulate negative emotions (via prefrontal

control mechanisms) may protect against potentially adverse HPA stress reactions. Similarly, cortisol elevations elicited by the Trier Social Stress Task (TSST) correlated with increased dACC and dorsal medial prefrontal activation during a subsequent social rejection task performed during fMRI scanning (Eisenberger et al, 2007). Moreover, individual differences in perceived social support mediated this association, again highlighting the importance of interpersonal processes in brain–body reactions to stress. As illustrated above, individual differences in the functionality of key cortical, limbic, and brain stem systems have been linked to both acute (stressor-evoked) and circadian (diurnal) changes in cardiovascular and HPA axis function. Neuroimaging methodologies have proved valuable in this context to elucidate how individual differences in stress reactivity are associated not only with regional brain activity, but also with patterns of covariation between cortical, limbic, and brain stem nuclei.

4 Conclusions

This chapter has reviewed the widespread application of neuroimaging techniques within behavioral medicine. Neuroimaging techniques enabled considerable advances in understanding how the mind and the body interact within both health and disease. A wide range of neuroimaging methods, reviewed in the previous chapter, are routinely used to elucidate structural, functional, metabolic, and neurochemical features of the brain. These techniques have applications in understanding psychological processes such as normal and abnormal anxiety reactions. Social and interpersonal processes are intimately tied to human behavior in both health and disease both statically and across the lifespan, and neuroimaging furthers understandings of how these processes are related to neural function. Further, advances in genetics are increasingly integrated with neuroimaging research, highlighting their specific neural consequences and also how genetic features may interact with social and environmental factors to predict disease. Epidemiological approaches are also being integrated with neuroimaging in identifying how population-based risk may translate into specific brain–body disturbances within the individual. Neuroimaging of cardiovascular stress reactivity offers a good example of how cognitive or emotional stress, which increases the risk of adverse cardiovascular events, is closely associated with coordinated functional changes within corticolimbic and mesencephalic regions of the brain. Further and more generally, these neuroscientific approaches are increasingly providing insight into brain–body interactions which promote broader understandings of health and disease, considering not only the biology and functions of the body, but also their interaction with mind, behavior, and the environment.

Acknowledgment HDC is supported by a Program Grant from the Wellcome Trust. PJG is supported by National Institutes of Health Grants K01-MH070616 and R01-HL089850.

References

Abercrombie, H. C., Giese-Davis, J., Sephton, S., Epel, E. S., Turner-Cobb, J. M. et al (2004) Flattened cortisol rhythms in metastatic breast cancer patients. *Psychoneuroendocrinology, 29*, 1082–1092.

Abdelnour, A. F., and Huppert, T. (2009). Real-time imaging of human brain function by near-infrared spectroscopy using an adaptive general linear model. *NeuroImage, 46*, 133–143

Adolphs, R. (2008). Fear, faces, and the human amygdala, *Curr Opin Neurobiol, 18*, 166–172.

Adolphs, R., Gosselin, F., Buchanan, T. W., Tranel, D., Schyns, P. et al (2005). A mechanism for impaired fear recognition after amygdala damage, *Nature, 433*, 68–72.

Anderson, A. K., and Phelps, E. A. (2002). Is the human amygdala critical for the subjective experience of emotion? Evidence of intact dispositional affect in patients with amygdala lesions, *J Cogn Neurosci, 14*, 709–720.

Anderson, A. K., Christoff, K., Panitz, D., De Rosa, E., and Gabrieli, J. D. (2003). Neural correlates of the automatic processing of threat facial signals. *J. Neurosci, 23*, 5627–5633.

Bartzokis, G., Lu, P. H., Tingus, K., Mendez, M. F., Richard, A. et al (2009). Lifespan trajectory of myelin integrity and maximum motor speed, *Neurobiol Aging.* doi:10.1016/j.neurobiolaging.2008.08.015

Birbaumer, N., Grodd, W., Diedrich, O., Klose, U., Erb, M. et al (1998). fMRI reveals amygdala activation to human faces in social phobics. *Neuroreport, 9*, 1223–1226.

Bishop, S. J., Duncan, J., and Lawrence, A. D. (2004). State anxiety modulation of the amygdala response to unattended threat-related stimuli. *J Neurosci, 24*, 10364–10368.

Blennow, K., de Leon, M. J., and Zetterberg, H. (2006). Alzheimer's disease, *Lancet, 368*, 387–403.

Bondi, M. W., Houston, W. S., Eyler, L. T., and Brown, G. G. (2005). fMRI evidence of compensatory mechanisms in older adults at genetic risk for Alzheimer disease, *Neurology, 64*, 501–508.

Bookheimer, S., and Burggren, A. (2009). APOE-4 genotype and neurophysiological vulnerability to Alzheimer's and cognitive aging, *Annu Rev Clin Psychol, 5*, 343–362.

Bookheimer, S. Y., Strojwas, M. H., Cohen, M. S., Saunders, A. M., Pericak- Vance, M. A. et al (2000). Patterns of brain activation in people at risk for Alzheimer's Disease. *N Engl J Med, 343*, 450–456.

Bryant, R. A., Felmingham, K. L., Kemp, A. H., Barton, M., Peduto, A. S. et al (2005). Neural networks of information processing in posttraumatic stress disorder: a functional magnetic resonance imaging study, *Biol Psychiatry, 58*, 111–118.

Bu, G. (2009). Apolipoprotein E and its receptors in Alzheimer's disease: pathways, pathogenesis and therapy, *Nat Rev Neurosci, 10*, 333–344.

Burggren, A. C., Small, G.,W., Sabb, F.,W. and Bookheimer, S. Y. (2002). Specificity of brain activation patterns in people at genetic risk for Alzheimer disease, *Am J Geriatr Psychiatry, 10*, 44–51.

Bush, G., Luu, P., and Posner, M. I. (2000) Cognitive and emotional influences in anterior cingulate cortex. *Trends Cog Sci, 4*, 215–222.

Cacioppo, J. T., and Berntson, G. C. (2005). Analysis of the social brain through the lens of human brain imaging. In J. T. Cacioppo & G. G. Berntson (Eds.). *Social Neuroscience: Key readings* (pp. 1–19). New York and Hove: Psychology Press.

Caria, A., Veit, R., Sitaram, R., Lotze, M., Weiskopf, N. et al (2007). Regulation of anterior insular cortex activity using real-time fMRI. *NeuroImage, 35*, 1238–1246.

Carter, C. S. (1998). Neuroendocrine perspectives on social attachment and love, *Psychoneuroendocrinology, 23*, 779–818.

Cattaneo, L., and Rizzolatti, G. (2009). The mirror neuron system. *Arch Neurol, 66*, 557–560.

Cherbuin, N., Anstey, K. J., Sachdev, P. S., Maller, J. J., Meslin, C. et al (2008). Total and regional gray matter volume is not related to APOE*E4 status in a community sample of middle-aged individuals. *J Gerontol A Biol Sci Med Sci, 63*, 501–504.

Coyle, S. M., Ward, T. E. and Markham, C. M. (2007). Brain-computer interface using a simplified functional near-infrared spectroscopy system. *J Neural Eng. 4*, 219–226.

Critchley, H. D., Corfield, D. R., Chandler, M. P., Mathias, C. J., and Dolan, R. J. (2000). Cerebral correlates of autonomic cardiovascular arousal: a functional neuroimaging investigation in humans. *J Physiol, 523*, 259–270.

Critchley, H. D., Rotshtein, P., Nagai, Y., O'Doherty, J., Mathias, C. J. et al (2005a). Activity in the human brain predicting differential heart rate responses to emotional facial expressions. *NeuroImage, 24*, 751–762.

Critchley, H. D., Taggart, P., Sutton, P. M., Holdright, D. R., Batchvarov, V. (2005b). Mental stress and sudden cardiac death: asymmetric midbrain activity as a linking mechanism. *Brain, 128*, 75–85.

Critchley, H. D., Mathias, C. J., and Dolan, R. J. (2002). Fear conditioning in humans: the influence of awareness and autonomic arousal on functional neuroanatomy. *Neuron, 33*, 653–663.

Damoiseaux, J. S., Smith, S. M., Witter, M. P., Sanz-Arigita, E. J., Barkhof, F. et al (2009). White matter tract integrity in aging and Alzheimer's disease. *Hum Brain Mapp. 30*, 1051–1059.

Dampney, R. A. (1994) Functional organization of central pathways regulating the cardiovascular system. *Physiol Rev 74*, 323–364.

Davis, M., and Whalen, P. J. (2001). The amygdala: vigilance and emotion. *Mol Psychiatry, 6*, 13–34.

deCharms, R. C., Maeda, F., Glover, G. H., Ludlow, D., Pauly, J. M. et al (2005) Control over brain activation and pain learned by using real-time functional MRI. *Proc Natl Acad Sci U S A 102*, 18626–18631.

deCharms, R. C. (2008). Applications of real-time fMRI. *Nat Rev Neurosci, 9*, 720–729.

Dedovic, K., Renwick, R., Mahani, N. K., Engert, V., Lupien, S. J. et al (2005). The Montreal Imaging Stress Task: using functional imaging to investigate the effects of perceiving and processing psychosocial stress in the human brain. *J Psychiatry Neurosci, 30*, 319–325.

Dedovic, K., D'Aguiar, C., and Pruessner, J. C. (2009). What stress does to your brain: a review of neuroimaging studies. *Can J Psychiatry, 54*, 6–15.

Devinsky, O., Morrell, M. J., and Vogt, B. A. (1995). Contributions of anterior cingulate cortex to behaviour. *Brain, 118*, 279–306.

Dickie, E. W., and Armony, J. L. (2008). Amygdala responses to unattended fearful faces: interaction between sex and trait anxiety. *Psychiatry Res, 162*, 51–57.

Drzezga, A., Grimmer, T., Henriksen, G., Mühlau, M., Perneczky, R. et al (2009). Effect of APOE genotype on amyloid plaque load and gray matter volume in Alzheimer disease. *Neurology, 72*, 1487–1494.

Dubois, J., Benders, M., Borradori-Tolsa, C., Cachia, A., Lazeyras, F. et al (2008). Primary cortical folding in the human newborn: an early marker of later functional development. *Brain, 131*, 2028–2041.

Eisenberger, N. I., Taylor, S. E., Gable, S. L., Hilmert, C. J., and Lieberman, M. D. (2007). Neural pathways link social support to attenuated neuroendocrine stress responses. *NeuroImage, 35*, 1601–1612.

Etkin, A., Egner, T., Peraza, D. M., Kandel, E. R., and Hirsch, J. (2006). Resolving emotional conflict: a role for the rostral anterior cingulate cortex in modulating activity in the amygdala. *Neuron, 51*, 871–882.

Etkin, A., Klemenhagen, K. C., Dudman, J. T., Rogan, M. T., Hen, R. et al (2004). Individual differences in trait anxiety predict the response of the basolateral amygdala to unconsciously processed fearful faces, *Neuron, 44*, 1043–1055.

Ewbank, M. P., Lawrence, A. D., Passamonti, L., Keane, J., Peers, P. V. et al (2009). Anxiety predicts a differential neural response to attended and unattended facial signals of anger and fear, *NeuroImage, 44*, 1144–1151.

Fakra, E., Hyde, L. W., Gorka, A., Fisher, P. M., Muñoz, K. E. et al (2009). Effects of HTR1A C(-1019)G on amygdala reactivity and trait anxiety. *Arch Gen Psychiatry, 66*, 33–40.

Farah, M. J., Shera, D. M., Savage, J. H., Betancourt, L., Giannetta, J. M. et al (2006). Childhood poverty: specific associations with neurocognitive development. *Brain Res, 1110*, 166–174.

Filippini, N., Raom, A., Wetten, S., Gibson, R. A., Borrie, M. et al (2009a). Anatomically-distinct genetic associations of APOE epsilon4 allele load with regional cortical atrophy in Alzheimer's disease. *NeuroImage, 44*, 724–728.

Filippini, N., Scassellati, C., Boccardi, M., Pievani, M., Testa, C. et al (2009b). Influence of serotonin receptor 2A His452Tyr polymorphism on brain temporal structures: a volumetric MR study. *Eur J Hum Genet, 14*, 443–449.

Friedel, E., Schlagenhauf, F., Sterzer, P., Park, S. Q., Bermpohl, F. et al (2009) 5-HTT genotype effect on prefrontal-amygdala coupling differs between major depression and controls. *Psychopharmacology (Berl), 205*, 261–271.

Friston, K. (1994). Functional and effective connectivity in neuroimaging: a synthesis. *Hum Brain Mapp, 2*, 56–78.

Frith, C. D., and Singer, T. (2008). The role of social cognition in decision making. *Philos Trans R Soc Lond B Biol Sci, 363*, 3875–3886.

Frith, C. D. (2008). Social cognition. *Philos Trans R Soc Lond B Biol Sci, 363*, 2033–2039.

Gianaros, P. J., Derbyshire, S. W., May, J. C., Siegle, G. J., Gamalo, M. A. et al (2005). Anterior cingulate activity correlates with blood pressure during stress. *Psychophysiology, 42*, 627–635.

Gianaros, P. J., Hariri, A. R., Sheu, L. K., Muldoon, M. F., Sutton-Tyrrell, K. et al (2009). Preclinical atherosclerosis covaries with individual differences in reactivity and functional connectivity of the amygdala. *Biol Psychiatry, 65,* 943–950.

Gianaros, P. J., Sheu, L. K., Matthews, K. A., Jennings, J. R., Manuck, S. B. et al (2008a). Individual differences in stressor-evoked blood pressure reactivity vary with activation, volume, and functional connectivity of the amygdala. *J Neurosci, 28,* 990–999.

Gianaros, P. J., Horenstein, J. A., Hariri, A. R., Sheu, L. K., Manuck, S. B. et al (2008b). Potential neural embedding of parental social standing. *Soc Cogn Affect Neurosci, 3,* 91–96.

Gianaros, P. J., Jennings, J. R., Sheu, L. K., Greer, P. J., Kuller, L. H. et al (2007). Prospective reports of chronic life stress predict decreased grey matter volume in the hippocampus. *NeuroImage, 35,* 795–803.

Gogtay, N., Lu, A., Leow, A. D., Klunder, A. D., Lee, A. D. et al (2008). Three-dimensional brain growth abnormalities in childhood-onset schizophrenia visualized by using tensor-based morphometry. *Proc Natl Acad Sci U S A, 105,* 15979–15984.

Gouw, A. A., Seewann, A., Vrenken, H., van der Flier, W. M., Rozemuller, J. M. et al (2008). Heterogeneity of white matter hyperintensities in Alzheimer's disease: post-mortem quantitative MRI and neuropathology. *Brain, 131,* 3286–3298.

Gray, M. A., Rylander, K., Harrison, N. A., Wallin, B. G., and Critchley, H. D. (2009) Following one's heart: cardiac rhythms gate central initiation of sympathetic reflexes. *J Neurosci, 29,* 1817–1825.

Gray, M. A., Taggart, P., Sutton, P. M., Groves, D., Holdright, D. R. et al (2007). A cortical potential reflecting cardiac function. *Proc Natl Acad Sci U S A, 104,* 6818–6823.

Gregory, S. G., Barlow, K. F., McLay, K. E., Kaul, R., Swarbreck, D. et al (2006). The DNA sequence and biological annotation of human chromosome 1. *Nature, 441,* 315–321.

Haas, B. W., Omura, K., Constable, R. T., and Canli, T. (2007). Emotional conflict and neuroticism: personality-dependent activation in the amygdala and subgenual anterior cingulate. *Behav Neurosci, 121,* 249–256.

Hariri, A. R. (2009). The neurobiology of individual differences in complex behavioral Traits. *Annu Rev Neurosci, 32,* 225–247.

Hopkins, D. A., and Holstege, G. (1978). Amygdaloid projections to the mesencephalon, pons and medulla oblongata in the cat. *Exp Brain Res 32,* 529–547.

Huttenlocher, P. R. (1994). Synaptogenesis in human cerebral cortex. In G. Dawson & K. W. Fischer (Eds.). *Human Behavior and the Developing Brain* (pp. 137–152). New York: Guilford Press.

Jayadev, S., Steinbart, E. J., Chi, Y. Y., Kukull, W. A., Schellenberg, G. D. et al (2008). Conjugal Alzheimer disease: risk in children when both parents have Alzheimer disease. *Arch Neurol, 65,* 373–378.

Jeannerod, M., (1994). The representing brain: neural correlates of motor intention and imagery. *Behav Brain Res, 17,* 187–245.

Johnson, S. C., Schmitz, T. W., Moritz, C. H., Meyerand, M. E., Rowley, H. A. et al (2006a). Activation of brain regions vulnerable to Alzheimer's disease: the effect of mild cognitive impairment. *Neurobiol Aging, 27,* 1604–1612.

Johnson, S. C., Schmitz, T. W., Trivedi, M. A., Ries, M. L., Torgerson, B. M. et al (2006b). The influence of Alzheimer disease family history and apolipoprotein E epsilon4 on mesial temporal lobe activation. *J Neurosci, 26,* 6069–6076.

Johnstone, T., Somerville, L. H., Alexander, A. L., Oakes, T. R., Davidson, R. J. et al (2005). Stability of amygdala BOLD response to fearful faces over multiple scan sessions. *NeuroImage, 25,* 1112–1123.

Kafetsios, K., and Sideridis, G. (2006). Attachment, social support, and well being in younger and older adults. *J Health Psychol, 11,* 867–879.

Killgore, W. D., and Yurgelun-Todd, D. A. (2005). Social anxiety predicts amygdala activation in adolescents viewing fearful faces. *Neuroreport, 16,* 1671–1675.

Klunk, W. E., Engler, H., Nordberg, A., Wang, Y., Blomqvist, G. et al (2004). Imaging brain amyloid in Alzheimer's disease with Pittsburgh Compound-B. *Ann Neurol, 55,* 306–319.

Krantz, D. S., and Manuck, S. B. (1984) Acute psychophysiologic reactivity and risk of cardiovascular disease: a review and methodologic critique. *Psychol Bull, 96,* 435–464.

Kruger, S., Alda, M., Young, T., Goldapple, K., Parikh, S. et al (2006). Risk and resilience markers in bipolar disorder, brain responses to emotional challenge in bipolar patients and their healthy siblings. *Am J Psychiatry, 163,* 257–264.

Lakin, J. L., Chartrand, T. L., and Arkin, R. M. (2008). I am too just like you: nonconscious mimicry as an automatic behavioral response to social exclusion. *Psychol Sci, 19,* 816–822.

Lampert, R., Shusterman, V., Burg, M. M., Lee, F. A., Earley, C. et al (2005) Effects of psychologic stress on repolarization and relationship to autonomic and hemodynamic factors, *J Cardiovasc Electrophysiol, 16,* 372–377.

Lander, E. S., Linton, L. M., Birren, B., Nusbaum, C., Zody, M. C. et al (2001). Initial sequencing and analysis of the human genome. *Nature, 409,* 860–921.

Lane, R. D., Waldstein, S. R., Chesney, M. A., Jennings, J. R., Lovallo, W. R. et al (2009a). The rebirth of neuroscience in psychosomatic medicine. Part I: historical context, methods, and relevant basic science. *Psychosom Med, 71,* 117–134.

Lane, R. D., McRae, K., Reiman, E. M., Chen, K., Ahern, G. L. et al (2009b). Neural correlates of heart rate variability during emotion. *NeuroImage, 44,* 213–222.

LeDoux, J. E. (1996). *The Emotional Brain.* New York: Simon and Schuster.

LeDoux, J. E. (2000). Emotion circuits in the brain. *Annu Rev Neurosci, 23,* 155–184.

Liberzon, I., Taylor, S. F., Amdur, R., Jung, T. D., Chamberlain, K. R. et al (1999). Brain activation in PTSD in response to trauma-related stimuli. *Biol Psychiatry, 45,* 817–826.

Lind, J., Persson, J., Ingvar, M., Larsson, A., Cruts, M. et al (2006). Reduced functional brain activity response in cognitively intact apolipoprotein E epsilon4 carriers. *Brain, 129,* 1240–1248.

Lovallo, W. R. (2005). Cardiovascular reactivity: mechanisms and pathways to cardiovascular disease. *Int J Psychophysiol, 58,* 119–132.

Lown, B., Verrier, R. L., and Rabinowitz, S. H. (1977). Neural and psychologic mechanisms and the problem of sudden death. *Am J Cardiol, 39,* 890–902.

Lu, L. H., Dapretto, M., O'Hare, E. D., Kan, E., McCourt, S. T. et al (2009). Relationships between brain activation and brain structure in normally developing children. *Cereb Cortex, 19,* 2595–2604.

Manuck, S. B., Brown, S. M., Forbes, E. E., and Hariri, A. R. (2007). Temporal stability of individual differences in amygdala reactivity. *Am J Psychiatry, 164,* 1613–1614.

Matthews, K., Schwartz, J., Cohen, S., and Seeman, T. (2006). Diurnal cortisol decline is related to coronary calcification: CARDIA study. *Psychosom Med, 68,* 657–661.

Mauch, D. H., Nägler, K., Schumacher, S., Göritz, C., Müller, E. C. et al (2001). CNS synaptogenesis promoted by glia-derived cholesterol. *Science, 294,* 1354–1357.

Medina, D. A., and Gaviria, M. (2008). Diffusion tensor imaging investigations in Alzheimer's disease: the resurgence of white matter compromise in the cortical dysfunction of the aging brain, *Neuropsychiatr Dis Treat, 4,* 737–742.

Miller, F. J., Jr., Marcus, M. L., Brody, M. J., and Gutterman, D. D. (1991). Activation in the region of parabrachial nucleus elicits neurogenically mediated coronary vasoconstriction. *Am J Physiol, 261,* H1585–1596.

Most, S. B., Chun, M. M., Johnson, M. R., and Kiehl, K. A. (2006). Attentional modulation of the amygdala varies with personality, *NeuroImage, 31,* 934–944.

Noble, K. G., Wolmetz, M. E., Ochs, L. G., Farah, M. J., and McCandliss, B. D. (2006). Brain-behavior relationships in reading acquisition are modulated by socioeconomic factors. *Dev Sci, 9,* 642–654.

Obrist, P. A. (1981) *Cardiovascular Psychophysiology: A Perspective.* New York: Plenum Press.

Ochsner, K. N., and Lieberman, M. D. (2001). The emergence of social cognitive neuroscience. *Am Psychol, 56,* 717–734.

Ochsner, K. N., and Gross, J. J. (2005). The cognitive control of emotion. *Trends Cogn Sci, 9,* 242–249.

Ohrmann, P., Rauch, A. V., Bauer, J., Kugel, H., Arolt, V. et al (2007). Threat sensitivity as assessed by automatic amygdala response to fearful faces predicts speed of visual search for facial expression. *Exp Brain Res, 183,* 51–59.

Oppenheimer, S. M., Cechetto, D. F., and Hachinski, V. C. (1990). Cerebrogenic cardiac arrhythmias.

Cerebral electrocardiographic influences and their role in sudden death. *Arch Neurol, 47,* 513–519.

Paus, T. (2001) Primate anterior cingulate cortex, where motor control, drive, and cognition interface. *Nat Neurosci Rev, 2,* 417–424.

Phillips, M. L., and Vieta, E. (2007). Identifying functional neuroimaging biomarkers of bipolar disorder: toward DSM-V, *Schizophr Bull, 33,* 893–904.

Piaget, J. (1971). *Biology and Knowledge.* Chicago: University of Chicago Press.

Pruessner, J. C., Dedovic, K., Khalili-Mahani, N., Engert, V., Pruessner, M. et al (2007). Deactivation of the limbic system during acute psychosocial stress: evidence from positron emission tomography and functional magnetic resonance imaging studies. *Biol Psychiatry, 63,* 234–240.

Quirk, G. J., and Beer, J. S. (2006). Prefrontal involvement in the regulation of emotion: convergence of rat and human studies. *Curr Opin Neurobiol, 16,* 723–727.

Raichle, M. E., MacLeod, A. M., Snyder, A. Z., Powers, W. J., Gusnard, D. A. et al (2001). A default mode of brain function. *Proc Natl Acad Sci U S A, 98,* 676–682.

Raizada, R. D., Richards, T. L., Meltzoff, A., and Kuhl, P. K. (2008) Socioeconomic status predicts hemispheric specialisation of the left inferior frontal gyrus in young children. *NeuroImage, 40,* 1392–1401.

Ray, R. D., Ochsner, K. N., Cooper, J. C., Robertson, E. R., Gabrieli, J. D. et al (2005). Individual differences in trait rumination and the neural systems supporting cognitive reappraisal. *Cogn Affect Behav Neurosci, 5,* 156–168.

Reiman, E. M., Chen, K., Liu, X., Bandy, D., Yu, M. et al (2009). Fibrillar amyloid-beta burden in cognitively normal people at 3 levels of genetic risk for Alzheimer's disease. *Proc Natl Acad Sci U S A, 106,* 6820–6825.

Ringman, J. M., O'Neill, J., Geschwind, D., Medina, L., Apostolova, L. G. et al (2007). Diffusion tensor imaging in preclinical and presymptomatic carriers of familial Alzheimer's disease mutations. *Brain, 130,* 1767–1776.

Rizzolatti, G., and Luppino, G. (2001). The cortical motor system. *Neuron, 31,* 889–901.

Cattaneo, L., and Rizzolatti, G. (2009). The mirror neuron system. *Arch Neurol, 66,* 557–560.

Schwartz, A. R., Gerin, W., Davidson, K. W., Pickering, T. G., Brosschot, J. F. et al (2003). Toward a causal model of cardiovascular responses to stress and the development of cardiovascular disease. *Psychosom Med, 65,* 22–35.

Segrin, C. (2001). *Interpersonal Processes in Psychological Problems.* New York: The Guilford Press.

Singer, T., Seymour, B., O'Doherty, J., Kaube, H., Dolan, R. J. et al (2004). Empathy for pain involves the affective but not sensory components of pain. *Science, 303,* 1157–1162.

Singer, T., Seymour, B., O'Doherty, J. P., Stephan, K. E., Dolan, R. J. et al (2006). Empathic neural responses are modulated by the perceived fairness of others. *Nature, 439,* 466–469.

Smith, C. D., Andersen, A. H., Kryscio, R.,J., Schmitt, F. A., Kindy, M. S. et al (1999). Altered brain activation in cognitively intact individuals at high risk for Alzheimer's disease. *Neurology, 53,* 1391–1416.

Smolka, M. N., Schumann, G., Wrase, J., Grüsser, S. M., Flor, H. et al (2005). Catechol-O-methyltransferase val158met genotype affects processing of emotional stimuli in the amygdala and prefrontal cortex. *J Neurosci, 25,* 836–842.

Sobel, D. S. (1995). Rethinking medicine: improving health outcomes with cost-effective psychosocial interventions. *Psychosom Med, 57,* 234–244.

Somerville, L. H., Kim, H., Johnstone, T., Alexander, A. L., and Whalen, P. J. (2004). Human amygdala responses during presentation of happy and neutral faces: correlations with state anxiety. *Biol Psychiatry, 55,* 897–903.

Somogyi, P., Tamás, G., Lujan, R., and Buhl, E. H. (1998). Salient features of synaptic organisation in the cerebral cortex. *Brain Res Brain Res Rev, 26,* 113–135.

Sowell, E. R., Mattson, S. N., Kan, E., Thompson, P. M., Riley, E. P. et al (2008). Abnormal cortical thickness and brain-behavior correlation patterns in individuals with heavy prenatal alcohol exposure. *Cereb Cortex, 18,* 136–144.

Sowell, E. R., Delis, D., Stiles, J., and Jernigan, T. L. (2001). Improved memory functioning and frontal lobe maturation between childhood and adolescence: a structural MRI study. *J Int Neuropsychol Soc, 7,* 312–322.

Sowell, E. R., Peterson, B. S., Thompson, P. M., Welcome, S. E., Henkenius, A. L. et al (2003). Mapping cortical change across the human life span. *Nat Neurosci, 6,* 309–315.

Sowell, E. R., Thompson, P. M., Rex, D., Kornsand, D., Tessner, K. D. et al (2002). Mapping sulcal pattern asymmetry and local cortical surface gray matter distribution in vivo: maturation in perisylvian cortices. *Cereb Cortex, 12,* 17–26.

Stricker, N. H., Schweinsburg, B. C., Delano-Wood, L., Wierenga, C. E., Bangen, K. J. et al (2009). Decreased white matter integrity in late-myelinating fiber pathways in Alzheimer's disease supports retrogenesis. *NeuroImage, 45,* 10–16.

Sullivan, H. S. (1953). Infancy: interpersonal situations. In H. S. Perry & M. L. Gawel (Eds.), *The Interpersonal Theory of Psychiatry* (pp. 110–134) New York, NY: W. W. Norton and Company.

Tamnes, C. K., Ostby, Y., Fjell, A. M., Westlye, L. T., Due-Tønnessen, P. et al (2010). Brain maturation in adolescence and young adulthood: regional age-related changes in cortical thickness and white matter volume and microstructure. *Cereb Cortex, 20,* 534–548.

Taylor, S. E., Burklund, L. J., Eisenberger, N. I., Lehman, B. J., Hilmert, C. J. et al (2008) Neural bases of moderation of cortisol stress responses by psychosocial resources. *J Pers Soc Psychol, 95,* 197–211.

Thomann, P. A., Roth, A. S., Dos Santos, V., Toro, P., Essig, M. et al (2008). Apolipoprotein E polymorphism and brain morphology in mild cognitive impairment. *Dement Geriatr Cogn Disord, 26,* 300–305.

Treiber, F. A., Kamarck, T., Schneiderman, N., Sheffield, D., Kapuku, G. et al (2003). Cardiovascular reactivity and development of preclinical and clinical disease states. *Psychosom Med, 65,* 46–62.

Trivedi, M. A., Schmitz, T. W., Ries, M. L., Hess, T. M., Fitzgerald, M. E. et al (2008). fMRI activation during episodic encoding and metacognitive appraisal across the lifespan: risk factors for Alzheimer's disease. *Neuropsychologia, 46,* 1667–1678.

Trivedi, M. A., Schmitz, T. W., Ries, M. L., Torgerson, B. M., Sager, M. A. et al (2006). Reduced hippocampal activation during episodic encoding in middle-aged individuals at genetic risk of Alzheimer's disease: a cross-sectional study. *BMC Med, 4,* 1.

Urry, H. L., van Reekum, C. M., Johnstone, T., Kalin, N. H., Thurow, M. E. et al (2006). Amygdala and ventromedial prefrontal cortex are inversely coupled during regulation of negative affect and predict the diurnal pattern of cortisol secretion among older adults. *J Neurosci, 26,* 4415–4425.

Van den Heuvel, O. A., Veltman, D. J., Groenewegen, H. J., Cath, D. C., van Balkom, A. J. et al (2005a). Frontal-striatal dysfunction during planning in obsessive-compulsive disorder. *Arch Gen Psychiatry, 62,* 301–309.

van den Heuvel, O. A., Veltman, D. J., Groenewegen, H. J., Witter, M. P., Merkelbach, J. et al (2005b). Disorder-specific neuroanatomical correlates of attentional bias in obsessive-compulsive disorder, panic disorder, and hypochondriasis. *Arch Gen Psychiatry, 62,* 922–933.

van Melle, J. P., de Jonge, P., Spijkerman, T. A., Tijssen, J. G., Ormel, J. et al (2004). Prognostic association of depression following myocardial infarction with mortality and cardiovascular events: a meta-analysis, *Psychosomat Med, 66,* 814–822.

Vogt, B. A. (2005). Pain and emotion interactions in subregions of the cingulate gyrus. *Nat Rev Neurosci, 6,* 533–544.

Vuilleumier, P., and Sander, D. (2008). Trust and valence processing in the amygdala. *Soc Cogn Affect Neurosci, 3,* 299–302.

Vuilleumier, P. (2005). Cognitive science: staring fear in the face. *Nature, 433,* 22–23.

Vuilleumier, P., Armony, J. L., Driver, J., and Dolan, R. J. (2001). Effects of attention and emotion on face processing in the human brain: an event-related fMRI study. *Neuron, 30,* 829–841.

Vygotsky, L. (1930). The problem of the cultural development of the child and the socialist alteration of man.

In R. van der Veer & J. Valsiner (Eds.). *The Vygotsky Reader* (1994). Oxford: Blackwell Publishers.

Wang, J. J., Rao, H., Wetmore, G. S., Furlan, P. M., Korczykowski, M. et al (2005). Perfusion functional MRI reveals cerebral blood flow pattern under psychological stress. *Proc Natl Acad Sci U S A, 102,* 17804–17809.

Weiskopf, N., Veit, R., Erb, M., Mathiak, K., Grodd, W. et al (2003). Physiological self-regulation of regional brain activity using real-time functional magnetic resonance imaging (fMRI): methodology and exemplary data. *NeuroImage, 19,* 577–586.

Whalen, P. J., Rauch, S. L., Etcoff, N. L., McInerney, S. C., Lee, M. B. et al (1998). Masked presentations of emotional facial expressions modulate amygdala activity without explicit knowledge. *J Neurosci, 18,* 411–418.

Wik, G., Fredrikson, M., and Fischer, H. (1996). Cerebral correlates of anticipated fear: a PET study of specific phobia. *Int J Neurosci, 87,* 267–276.

Williams, M. A., Morris, A. P., McGlone, F., Abbott, D. F., and Mattingley, J. B. (2004). Amygdala responses to fearful and happy facial expressions under conditions of binocular suppression. *J. Neurosci, 24,* 2898–2904.

Wishart, H. A., Saykin, A. J., McAllister, T. W., Rabin, L. A., McDonald, B. C. (2006b). Regional brain atrophy in cognitively intact adults with a single APOE epsilon4 allele. *Neurology, 67,* 1221–1224.

Wishart, H. A., Saykin, A. J., Rabin, L. A., Santulli, R. B., Flashman, L. A. et al (2006a). Increased brain activation during working memory in cognitively intact adults with the APOE epsilon4 allele. *Am J Psychiatr, 163,* 1603–1610.

Woodard, J. L., Seidenberg, M., Nielson, K. A., Antuono, P., Guidotti, L. et al (2009). Semantic memory activation in amnestic mild cognitive impairment. *Brain, 132,* 2068–2078.

Wulsin, L. R., and Singal, B. M. (2003). Do depressive symptoms increase the risk for the onset of coronary disease? A systematic quantitative review. *Psychosom Med, 65,* 201–210.

Xie, S., Xiao, J. X., Gong, G. L., Zang, Y. F., Wang, Y. H. et al (2006). Voxel-based detection of white matter abnormalities in mild Alzheimer disease, *Neurology, 66,* 1845–1849.

Chapter 52

Neuroimaging of Depression and Other Emotional States

Scott C. Matthews and Richard D. Lane

1 Introduction

Depression is increasingly being recognized as an important predictor of adverse medical outcomes. Depression is associated with increased mortality rates in the context of coronary artery disease (Frasure-Smith and Lesperance, 2005), diabetes (Katon et al, 2005), stroke (Jorge et al, 2003), and breast cancer (Onitilo et al, 2006). Multiple mechanisms likely play a role across these various disorders, including increased sympathetic and decreased parasympathetic activity, altered inflammatory and other immune mechanisms, blood hypercoagulability, reduced adherence to treatment regimens, etc. It is likely that depression influences each of these processes through altered brain function. Although the way that altered brain mechanisms contribute to each of these processes is not known, our understanding of how brain structure and function is altered in clinical depression is growing. The purpose of this chapter is to selectively review brain imaging findings in depression and interpret these alterations in light of current understanding of how these brain structures function in normative contexts.

In behavioral medicine self-report measures, such as the Beck Depression Inventory (Beck et al, 1961), are often used as continuous measures of depression severity. In post-myocardial infarction patients, for example, the mortality risk associated with depression increases linearly with scores on the Beck Depression Inventory (Lesperance et al, 2002) and, relatedly, the relative risk of mortality is greater with major depressive disorder (MDD) compared to subclinical symptoms of depression (Ruguiles, 2002). It is therefore important to note that much of what we know about the neural substrates of depression are derived from imaging studies of MDD as a category, rather than studies using depressive symptoms as a continuous variable. It is not yet known with certainty whether the brain changes that occur with MDD vary continuously with increasing symptom severity, although there are some indications that this is the case based on evidence from studies of patients with MDD (Drevets et al, 1999; Matthews et al, 2008; Strigo et al, 2008).

Another challenge in this area of investigation is the heterogeneity of MDD. This heterogeneity is manifested in the lack of consistency across neuroimaging laboratories in reaching definitive conclusions about the neural substrates of MDD. This is a complex problem that gets to the heart of the challenges in this area of investigation and there is no immediate solution available. The challenges can roughly be divided into "known unknowns" and "unknown unknowns."

In the former category, we know from clinical experience (or believe that we know) that several factors contribute to heterogeneity among patients with MDD: (1) family history of the disorder; (2) number of previous episodes of

S.C. Matthews (✉)
University of California San Diego, 3350 La Jolla
Village Drive (Mail Code 116-A), San Diego, CA
92161, USA
e-mail: scmatthews@ucsd.edu

A. Steptoe (ed.), *Handbook of Behavioral Medicine*, DOI 10.1007/978-0-387-09488-5_52,
© Springer Science+Business Media, LLC 2010

depression; (3) severity and duration of the current episode; (4) life events that may trigger depressive episode; (5) presence of psychosis (e.g., major depression with psychotic features such as delusions); (6) cumulative lifetime duration of illness (number of days of untreated depression); (7) age and gender mix of the samples (e.g., males and females have different levels of risk for depression); (8) presence of early life trauma, (9) co-morbid psychiatric disorders such as anxiety or substance abuse; (10) inter-current medical illness; (11) use of antidepressant medication, (12) use of non-pharmacologic antidepressant treatments such as electroconvulsive therapy or psychotherapy. We also know that common genetic variants such as allelic variation in the serotonin transporter promoter region or the val/met variants of the catechol-O-methyltransferase gene (involved in dopamine and other catecholamine metabolism) contribute to variation in the activity of key brain regions such as the amygdala (Hariri et al, 2002) and dorsolateral prefrontal cortex (PFC) (Egan et al, 2001), respectively. These different factors can potentially influence brain structure, brain function, or both. However, the specific ways in which these "known" factors influence the neural basis of depression are incompletely understood.

Among the "unknown unknowns," there are likely sources of variation among patients with MDD that we have not yet been able to define. For example, our reliance on self-report measures of depression in behavioral medicine research, and in psychiatric diagnosis more generally, may have inherent limitations when attempting to use such findings to uncover the neural basis of MDD. This general topic has been eloquently addressed by Nancy Andreasen (1997), who points out that when trying to identify the neurobiological basis of a psychiatric disorder (i.e., the so-called biotype) we are constrained by the requirement to use the existing definitions of a disorder. In our current nosology, which is based on symptoms or syndromes, the so-called phenomenotype is largely based on self-report occasionally augmented by a few observations such as psychomotor retardation.

Since the phenomenotype and the yet-to-be discovered biotype are incongruent, as evidenced by inconsistent neuroimaging findings across laboratories, one must somehow work iteratively to refine the phenotype in search of a better-matching biotype.

One way of refining the search is to select subsets of individuals who share certain features of the larger syndrome and to determine if they are more homogeneous from a neurobiological perspective. For example, some studies have been conducted that aim to identify the neural correlates of anhedonia (Tremblay et al, 2005; Wacker et al, 2009). However, this may not be an adequate solution, as patients with the same symptoms may have a different neurobiology. Moreover, this still leaves the problem of matching (or mismatching) other depressive symptoms needed to make the diagnosis of MDD. In fact, there are several hundred different symptom combinations that will yield the diagnosis of MDD. An alternative approach is illustrated by the work of Drevets and colleagues (1992), who used family history (a proxy for genetic loading) to compare "pure familial depressive disorder" patients to healthy controls. While promising, such an approach does not typically define the actual genetic substrates or account for gene–environment interactions. Unfortunately, there is no simple way to address the problem of heterogeneity among MDD individuals.

Given the challenges of recruiting an adequate number of depressed subjects who otherwise meet criteria for an imaging study (no implanted devices or extensive dental work, no claustrophobia, no brain lesions, no centrally acting medications except those under study, restrictions on weight and size, etc.), it is customary to study patients who meet criteria for MDD, even though the specific constellation of symptoms used to define MDD are typically quite different across patients. Currently, there are no standards in the field for selecting subsets. Should the neurobiology of a subgroup of MDD patients be found, it would certainly constitute a significant advance, but it would still fail to identify the neurobiology of the remaining patients with MDD.

Thus, conclusions about the brain basis of depression must be offered cautiously, and wherever possible we will focus on findings that have been replicated across laboratories. One consequence of this variability is that brain imaging findings in MDD do not yet have sufficient reliability to be used for clinical decision making in the care of individual patients. Once this heterogeneity is fully understood it will be possible to use functional and structural neuroimaging in individual patients for the purpose of diagnosis, treatment selection, and the monitoring of treatment effectiveness. Given the importance of depression as a world-wide health problem, and the challenges involved, this is likely to remain an area of active investigation in the decades ahead.

2 Normative Emotional States

Emotional responses are initiated by an automatic (often implicit, unconscious) assessment about the extent to which goals, values, or needs are being met in interaction with the environment (Clore and Ortony, 2000). Emotional responses also involve a concomitant automatic resetting of physiology (e.g., heart rate increase), behavior (e.g., avoidance behavior), thought (e.g., more alert), and feeling (e.g., fear) to enable the organism to adapt to changing circumstances (Levenson, 1994). Given the complexity of functions involved, it is not surprising that multiple brain structures participate as components of a coordinated network in generating emotional responses. This brief review will highlight the functions of the amygdala, the insula, and the ventral striatum including nucleus accumbens, hippocampus, anterior cingulate cortex (ACC), posterior cingulate cortex (PCC), and ventromedial PFC including orbitofrontal cortex as structures that participate in this network (Figs. 52.1 and 52.2).

The amygdala is a prototypical emotion-related structure that can be activated through either interoceptive processes or exteroceptive sensory stimuli. Often associated with fear and anxiety (Davis, 2000; LeDoux, 2000), the amygdala functions as a "salience detector" by evaluating the emotional significance of internal and external events (Amaral et al, 1992). It is essential for aversive conditioning and preferentially participates in negative emotional states, although it also participates in positive emotional states (Zald, 2003). The amygdala orchestrates the somatomotor, visceral, and cognitive responses to threats by virtue of its connections with cortical brain structures above and hypothalamic and brainstem structures below it (LeDoux et al, 1990). The nucleus accumbens and ventral striatum participate in reward responses and positive emotional states. Other structures that are involved in generating both positive and negative emotional responses include the thalamus, hypothalamus, basal ganglia, and ventromedial PFC (Phan et al, 2002).

The hippocampus lies adjacent to the amygdala in the medial temporal lobe. Although originally thought to be a key component of the limbic system, it is now thought to have a primarily cognitive function and plays a major role in organizing memory mechanisms such as the ability to consciously recall facts and autobiographical events (Gazzaniga et al, 2008). The hippocampus participates in emotional responding in an adjunctive way by assessing the contextual significance of incoming information (Fanselow, 2000). The hippocampus is also an important feedback site for circulating cortisol and has an important influence on regulation of the hypothalamic–pituitary–adrenal axis (Sapolsky, 2000).

The posterior insular cortex is the primary projection area for visceral sensation, while the anterior insula, particularly on the right side (Craig, 2003), is a higher association area for these bodily signals (Critchley et al, 2001) and is involved in remapping these signals into conscious bodily feelings. In addition to perceiving and modulating the physiological condition of the body, the insula participates in anticipation of aversive stimuli such as physical pain (Craig, 2002; Strigo et al, 2008b). In some ways the insula functions as a high level *sensory* structure.

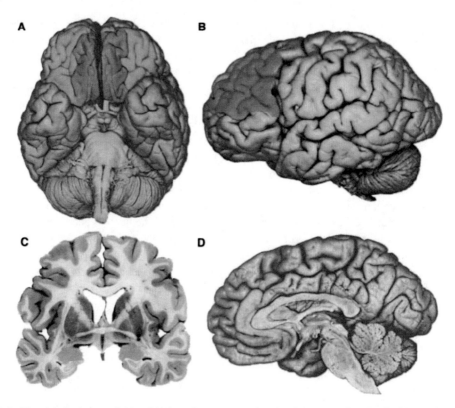

Fig. 52.1 Pictorial depiction of (**a**) orbitofrontal cortex (*green*) and ventromedial prefrontal cortex (*brown*); (**b**) dorsolateral prefrontal cortex; (**c**) amygdala; and (**d**) anterior cingulate cortex. Reprinted with permission from Davidson, et al (2000)

The ACC, by contrast, is primarily a *motor* structure situated in the medial frontal lobe that is considered a paralimbic structure in part because it has fewer cell layers than neocortex (Paus, 2001). The ACC is highly interconnected with other paralimbic structures, such as the insula, as well as limbic and other subcortical structures. The ACC has several divisions. The subgenual ACC, also called Brodmann's area 25, is the principal site of autonomic regulation in the frontal lobe and has important bidirectional connections with the amygdala, periaqueductal gray, nucleus accumbens, hypothalamus, anterior insula, and orbitofrontal cortex, all of which are involved in different aspects of the generation and processing of emotional responses (Vogt, 2009; Price, 1999). The rostral (pregenual) ACC has strong bidirectional connections with the amygdala. It is activated in a variety of emotional states and participates both in conscious processing of emotional feeling states as well as performing related cognitive operations, such as thinking about feelings, reflecting upon feelings (Lane, 1997, 2000), and resolving emotional conflicts (Etkin et al, 2006). The supragenual ACC is the area of the limbic lobe between the pregenual ACC and the mid-cingulate cortex. The mid-cingulate cortex (also called the dorsal ACC) plays a major role in the executive control of attention and is predominantly connected to the lateral PFC, parietal cortex, and pre- and supplementary motor areas. Dysfunction in this area in depression is thought to contribute to cognitive changes associated with the disorder, such as difficulties in concentration (Mayberg et al, 1999). More generally, the ACC is an interface for cognition and affect and is a higher level brain area where the physiological adjustments

Coronal view

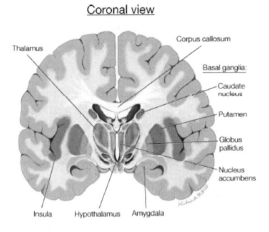

Limbic Structures

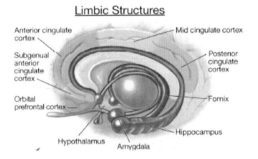

Fig. 52.2 The coronal view depicts the insula (*purple*), hypothalamus, thalamus, amygdala, and basal ganglia. The "limbic structures" figure depicts the anterior, mid, and posterior cingulate cortices, orbitofrontal cortex, hippocampus, amygdala, and hypothalamus. Reprinted with permission from Lane et al (2009)

necessary for supporting adaptive cognitive and affective responses (Lane, 2009) are generated.

The orbitofrontal cortex is also a paralimbic structure that participates in the evaluation of the emotional significance of stimuli from the internal and external environments and is densely interconnected with the amygdala (Zald and Rauch, 2006). By contrast, the medial PFC is a neocortical structure adjacent to the ACC and orbitofrontal cortex that is involved in representing states of the self and monitoring and regulating the internal milieu (Lane, 2008). The medial PFC is a critical node in the medial visceromotor network given its direct connections to the hypothalamus and periaqueductal gray (Kober et al, 2008). The medial PFC is also reciprocally

connected to the PCC, an area involved in evaluating the personal significance of information from the external environment given its close proximity to the parietal cortex and hippocampus (O'Connor et al, 2007). The ACC and PCC are key nodes in the so-called default network that is active "at baseline" (Raichle et al, 2001; Gusnard et al, 2001). This network is activated when subjects are not engaged in specific tasks and may be related to daydreaming or related types of self-related cognitions.

The dorsolateral PFC is a neocortical structure involved in mediating working memory and setting goals for behavioral responses (Goldman-Rakic, 1996). It is densely connected to the motor cortex and the hippocampus and plays a key role in integrating behavior with existing circumstances in the external environment, including the regulation of emotional behavior. Imaging studies have shown that the dorsolateral PFC is activated during performance of reappraisal tasks that require regulation of emotion (Ochsner and Gross, 2005).

3 Overview of Brain Changes in MDD

The cognitive model of depression (Beck, 1961) posits that stressful life events activate cognitive vulnerability and the depressive state develops, resulting in the depressive phenotype that is characterized by increased negative emotion processing (i.e., negative bias) and impaired emotional control (e.g., emotional responses that are too intense or prolonged). Extensive behavioral evidence supports this model, revealing that depressed individuals (1) focus more on negative stimuli and less on positive stimuli (Mogg et al, 1995; Scher et al, 2005), (2) are less easily distracted from negative emotion processing (Ellenbogen et al, 2002; Lyubomirsky et al, 1998; Siegle et al, 2002; Wenzlaff and Bates, 1998), (3) show heightened stress hormone levels such as cortisol that may have deleterious effects on the brain (Sapolsky, 2000), and (4) experience nonpainful physical stimuli as emotionally aversive (Strigo et al, 2008a).

Functional neuroimaging studies have identified the brain structures that process negative emotions (Adolphs, 2002) and a neural network that is involved in emotional control (Ochsner and Gross, 2005). Several positron emission tomography (PET) and functional magnetic resonance imaging (fMRI) studies indicate that neural substrates such as the amygdala, subgenual ACC, and insula, which are critical for emotion processing, are hyperactive in individuals with MDD, both at rest (Mayberg et al, 1999) and during performance of emotional tasks (Drevets et al, 1997; Sheline et al, 2001; Siegle et al, 2007). Related studies show that the response in this network is sustained in depressed individuals (Siegle et al, 2002) and that increased activity of this network is related to increased severity of depression (Drevets et al, 1992). These brain imaging findings suggest a neural correlate of negative emotion processing in depression.

Conversely, brain structures in the lateral PFC and supragenual ACC, which are involved in the cognitive control of behavior (Aron, 2007) and emotion (Ochsner and Gross, 2005), are hypoactive in individuals with MDD both at rest (Mayberg et al, 1999) and during performance of interference processing tasks that require cognitive control (George et al, 1997). These findings suggest a brain basis for the impaired emotional control observed in depression. For more extensive reviews the reader is referred to Mayberg (1997) and Drevets (2001).

4 Structural Brain Changes in MDD

Psychiatric disorders have traditionally been distinguished from neurological disorders by the absence of identifiable brain lesions. However, with the advent of modern high-resolution brain imaging techniques, and the ability to quantitatively aggregate data across subjects, abnormalities in brain structure are being identified in a variety of psychiatric disorders. As we review below, a variety of structural changes have been observed in patients with MDD. These are significant in at least two major respects. First, structural brain differences between patients and controls are suggestive of either a factor predisposing to the development of the disorder or a consequence of the disorder or its treatment. Second, structural brain changes must be taken into account when comparing functional brain activity in patients and controls. For example, functional brain activity in ventromedial PFC reveals decreased activity in MDD patients compared to controls in unadjusted comparisons, but when structural volume loss in this area in depressed patients is taken into account, activity in ventromedial PFC is actually hyperactive in depression (Drevets et al, 1997).

Recent reviews (Konarski et al, 2008; Lorenzetti et al, 2009) describe the volumetric changes associated with major affective disorders. Studies investigating ventricle to brain ratios, an index of possible brain atrophy, reveal relative increases in ventricular size in heterogeneous samples of individuals with MDD (Morys et al, 2003; Salokangas et al, 2002). Related studies have shown an association between more severe depressive symptoms and smaller PFC volumes (Bremner et al, 2002; Lacerda et al, 2004; Shah 2002). As noted above, several related studies show that the subgenual cingulate is small but hyperactive in MDD (Botteron et al, 2002; Drevets et al, 1997). There are also accumulating reports of decreased volume of the supragenual ACC (Ballmaier et al, 2004; Hastings et al, 2004), orbitofrontal cortex (Ballmaier et al, 2004; Bremner et al, 2002; Lacerda et al, 2004; Lai et al, 2000; Lee et al, 2003; Lavretsky et al, 2004; Steffens et al, 2003; Taylor et al, 2003), and dorsolateral PFC (Coffey et al, 1993; Krishnan et al, 1992) in MDD. Therefore, although discrepant reports exist (Axelson et al, 1993; Ashtari et al, 1999; Bremner et al, 2000; Hastings et al, 2004; Husain et al, 1991; Krishnan et al, 1992; Kumar et al, 1998; Pillay et al, 1997; Rosso et al, 2005; Sheline et al, 1996), there is some convergence of evidence showing that MDD is associated with volume reduction in several regions of the PFC and ACC.

Alterations in limbic and paralimbic structures have also been frequently observed in MDD. Numerous studies have shown that MDD is associated with decreased volume of the hippocampus (Bremner et al, 2000; Caetano et al, 2004; Frodl et al, 2004b; Hickie et al, 2005; Janssen et al, 2004; MacMaster and Kusumakar, 2004a; MacQueen et al, 2003; Shah et al, 1998; Sheline et al, 1996, 1999; Taylor et al, 2005). In several studies, decreased hippocampal volume has been related to a greater number of depressive episodes (Bell-McGinty et al, 2002; Caetano et al, 2004; Frodl et al, 2004a; MacQueen et al, 2003) and to increased severity of depressive symptoms (Caetano et al, 2004; MacQueen et al, 2003; Vakili et al, 2000), suggesting that decreased volume of the hippocampus may be a marker of increased severity and chronicity of MDD. Additionally, although further research is needed, there is accumulating evidence that hippocampal volume may be related to clinical manifestations of MDD, such as a different response to antidepressant medication in men and women (Vakili et al, 2000).

Although the preponderance of data suggests smaller amygdala volumes in MDD (Caetano et al, 2004; Hastings et al, 2004; Sheline et al, 1998; Siegle et al, 2003; Rosso et al, 2005), several discrepant studies reveal larger amygdala volumes (Bremner et al, 2000; Frodl et al, 2002; MacMillan et al, 2003). A recent meta-analysis of 13 relevant studies (Hamilton et al, 2008) indicates that amygdala volume is significantly decreased in unmedicated depressed individuals and significantly increased in medicated depressed individuals. In addition, there is evidence that duration of illness may also affect amygdala volumes, such that MDD individuals earlier in the course of illness may show increased amygdala volume (Frodl et al, 2002), whereas MDD individuals with a more chronic and recurrent history of MDD may show decreased amygdala volume (Bremner et al, 2000; Caetano et al, 2004; Hastings et al, 2004).

Further research is needed to clarify whether MDD is associated with decreased amygdala volumes primarily on the right side (Bremner et al, 2000) and/or whether females are more likely than males to show decreased amygdala volume (Hastings et al, 2004).

Finally, although limited data are available, there is evidence that MDD is associated with a decreased volume of the basal ganglia, particularly the striatum (i.e., caudate nucleus and putamen) (Greenwald et al, 1997; Husain et al, 1991; Kim et al, 2008; Krishnan et al, 1992) and a larger pituitary (MacMaster and Kusumakar, 2004b).

Taken together, these studies suggest that MDD is associated with anatomical alterations in a widely distributed cortico-limbic-striatal circuit. Although a lack of consistency among these studies has prevented the formulation of a parsimonious mechanistic model of mood disorders, evidence from animal and human studies suggests that anatomical brain changes may occur as a result of ongoing depressive episodes. In a recent prospective study (Frodl et al, 2008), healthy controls and MDD individuals underwent high-resolution structural MRI magnetic resonance imaging at baseline and again after 3 years. Results from a voxel-based morphometry analysis, an automated structural brain imaging analysis technique that permits separate measurement of gray and white matter volumes, revealed that over time MDD individuals relative to healthy controls showed a significantly greater decrease in gray matter density in the ACC and dorsomedial PFC as well as the hippocampus and amygdala. Additionally, greater volume decreases in gray matter density in these regions were observed in individuals who did not remit compared to remitters. In future studies, it will be important to replicate these findings to confirm that ongoing depressive symptoms cause the anatomical brain abnormalities observed in MDD, to determine whether successful treatment of MDD stops volume loss, and to explore whether pre-existing anatomical abnormalities may lead to depressive symptomatology.

5 Functional Brain Changes in MDD

Functional neuroimaging studies have contributed greatly to the widely held view that MDD is a brain disorder affecting an integrated system of cortical, subcortical, and limbic structures (Mayberg, 1997). To fully appreciate the complexity of the functional neuroanatomy of MDD, it is useful to consider at least two types of studies. The first are studies in which functional activity in specific brain regions at one point in time differs in MDD relative to nondepressed control subjects. The second are fMRI studies of antidepressant treatment response. Studies using different methodologies provide converging results, which support the conceptualization of MDD as a disorder associated with increased functional activity in reciprocally connected (Mesulam and Mufson, 1982) structures such as the amygdala, subgenual ACC, and insula, which are critically involved in emotion processing, and with decreased activity in the PFC and ACC, which are involved in emotion regulation. Debate remains regarding whether MDD symptoms are driven primarily by excessive activity in emotion processing structures, which "overwhelms" control circuits in the PFC and ACC (i.e., bottom-up dysfunction), or rather primarily from a failure of structures in the PFC and ACC to appropriately modulate emotion processing structures such as the amygdala (i.e., top-down dysfunction). Recent evidence suggests that both mechanisms may be at play (Fales et al, 2008).

The negative bias in MDD has been demonstrated in studies showing that MDD individuals are more likely to classify ambiguous facial expressions as negative (Bouhuys et al, 1999; Gur et al, 1992; Surguladze et al, 2004), and that this bias for negative facial expressions predicts clinical variables such as relapse (Bouhuys et al, 1999). Therefore, because they provide an ecologically valid stimulus for probing emotion processing, emotional face tasks have been implemented frequently in imaging studies of depression. In such tasks, individuals are typically instructed to identify the emotion of a face or match the emotions of faces within a group of faces, and activation during face processing is contrasted with activation during a control condition such as shape matching. Hyperactivity of the amygdala and adjacent structures in the medial temporal lobe has been observed repeatedly both at rest (Mayberg et al, 1999), and in response to face processing and related emotionally evocative tasks (Drevets et al, 1997; Matthews et al, 2008; Sheline et al, 2001; Siegle et al, 2007) in individuals with MDD.

The subgenual ACC (Brodmann's area 25) is another critical node of the cortico-limbic network that is involved in mood regulation and emotion processing. On the basis of functional imaging results and its pattern of connectivity, this structure was selected as the site for deep brain stimulation of treatment refractory depression (Mayberg et al, 2005; see below). The subgenual ACC is part of the "default mode network," i.e., the neural circuit that is engaged during non-task related behavior and is centrally involved in self-awareness, emotion processing, and conscious experience (Mazoyer et al, 2001; Raichle et al, 2001). Accumulating evidence suggests that the subgenual ACC is deactivated during performance of demanding cognitive tasks that require an external focus of attention (Kennedy et al, 2006; Marsh et al, 2006). Such deactivation may be an indicator of the degree to which affective processing is inhibited (Gusnard et al, 2001). Given this evidence, it is not surprising that increased subgenual ACC activity has been observed in MDD, a disorder that is characterized by an impaired ability to disengage from negative self-referential emotion processing. Consistent with this formulation, recent evidence indicates that an impaired ability to deactivate this structure during a demanding cognitive task appears to relate to increased depressive symptom severity (Matthews et al, 2009). This evidence suggests that MDD symptom severity may relate to the ability to "turn off" the subgenual ACC, an effect induced by deep brain stimulation.

Compelling evidence shows that insula activity related to emotion processing and homeostatic control is also dysregulated in MDD

(Nagai et al, 2007). Recent fMRI research reveals that unmedicated individuals with current MDD show hyperactivity of the anterior insula during emotional tasks (Grimm et al, 2008), and that pretreatment activation in anterior insula predicts antidepressant treatment response (Langenecker et al, 2007). In accordance with the cognitive model, depressive symptoms often result from excessive focus and worry about anticipated events that may or may not come to fruition. Based on this evidence, a recent study used a pain processing task during fMRI to examine the neurobiological basis of pain anticipation in MDD (Strigo et al, 2008b). In that study, MDD was associated with increased activation in the amygdala, insula, and ACC during pain anticipation, suggesting that MDD individuals experience increased affective processing even before they actually experience pain. Additionally, greater right amygdala activation during pain anticipation was associated with greater levels of perceived helplessness in MDD individuals, suggesting that greater amygdala activity may represent a neural correlate of a passive coping style in MDD. A third finding from this study was that, for the same perceived intensity of painful stimulation, MDD subjects showed decreased activation of a neural network that is involved in the modulation of pain and emotion. This is an observation that is consistent with a large body of converging studies showing that MDD is associated with decreased activity of a fronto-cingulate network that participates in behavioral and emotional control.

As indicated above, prior evidence implicates prefrontal brain structures in emotional control. Research in healthy non-depressed volunteers shows that during the voluntary suppression of negative affect, the PFC exerts an inhibitory influence on the amygdala (Urry et al, 2006), both through direct anatomical connections and through indirect connections with the ventromedial PFC (Ongur and Price, 2000). This research further shows that stronger coupling between the ventromedial PFC and amygdala during the down-regulation of negative affect is related to more adaptive diurnal fluctuations in circulating free cortisol (Urry et al, 2006). Consistent

research in healthy volunteers shows that distraction by negative pictures during performance of a working memory task is associated with increased activity in the inferior frontal gyrus (IFG), and that less IFG activity to emotional distracters is observed in subjects who rate emotional distracters as less distracting (Dolcos and McCarthy, 2006).

In MDD, activity in the PFC-amygdala circuit during emotional control is dysregulated. Specifically, prior evidence suggests that MDD individuals do not show the inverse relationship between the ventromedial PFC and amygdala during affect regulation, but rather the opposite relationship whereby greater ventromedial PFC activation is associated with greater amygdala activation, perhaps due to greater right lateralized PFC activity (Johnstone et al, 2007). Recent studies indicate that MDD individuals show decreased activity in a network of structures that includes the IFG during error trials of a validated inhibitory task (Matthews et al, 2009) and during performance of an oddball detection task (Wang et al, 2008). These findings suggest that MDD is associated with an inability to appropriately activate a neural network that is involved in emotional control, and that these brain abnormalities may underlie important bodily changes that occur in MDD.

Related studies indicate that resting connectivity of default mode network structures such as the subgenual ACC is increased in MDD, and that increased subgenual ACC connectivity is related to a greater length of depressive episodes (Greicius et al, 2007). Converging evidence reveals that default mode connectivity in MDD is increased during performance of emotionally evocative tasks (Chen et al, 2007; Pezawas et al, 2005). This evidence suggests that MDD is associated with dysregulated default mode network activity.

6 Changes in Brain Function due to Antidepressant Treatment

A series of studies has identified neural systems that are involved in the antidepressant treatment response. Importantly, antidepressant medication and psychotherapy may affect different neural nodes in unique ways that are consistent with the cognitive model of depression. These findings add a neuroanatomical perspective to the robust observation that the combination of antidepressant medication and psychotherapy is more effective in the treatment of depression than either treatment alone (Pampallona et al, 2004).

In one study (Kennedy et al, 2007), response to venlafaxine relative to response to cognitive behavior therapy was associated with larger decreases in subgenual ACC activity, consistent with the notion that antidepressant medications may primarily affect the regions of the cortico-limbic network that are involved in automatic emotional responses. This evidence is reinforced by studies in healthy volunteers, which indicate that depletion of tryptophan, a precursor to serotonin, is associated with increased amygdala responses to fearful stimuli (van der Veen et al, 2007). Conversely, in the Kennedy study response to cognitive behavior therapy relative to response to venlafaxine was associated with larger increases in structures such as the supragenual ACC, suggesting that cognitive behavior therapy may act primarily to modify activity in brain regions involved in emotion regulation. This evidence is consistent with studies showing that MDD is associated with decreased functional coupling between the amygdala and supragenual ACC (Chen et al, 2007; Matthews et al, 2008), and with findings that decreased amygdala–supragenual cingulate functional coupling is related both to increased depressive symptom severity (Matthews et al, 2008) and to a poorer antidepressant treatment response in the ACC (Chen et al, 2007).

Related evidence shows that increased baseline metabolic activity in pregenual ACC during PET (Mayberg, 1997) and increased error-related activity in the rostral ACC as well as increased inhibition-related activity in the IFG, amygdala, insula, and nucleus accumbens during fMRI (Langenecker et al, 2007) predict a positive response to pharmacological treatments.

7 Brain-Based Treatments of Depression

Despite the growing knowledge about its biological basis, it is estimated that 10–20% of individuals who suffer from MDD continue to be severely disabled despite adequate trials of psychopharmacologic or psychotherapeutic treatments and/or electroconvulsive therapy (Judd et al, 2008). Improved antidepressant treatments are needed. An exciting development is the emerging evidence of the relatively safe and effective methods of brain stimulation in the treatment of depression.

A landmark advance in psychiatry occurred in 2005 when it was demonstrated that deep brain stimulation of subgenual ACC was an effective treatment for depression (Mayberg et al, 2005). The decision to stimulate this brain structure was based on a network analysis of functional changes in the brain in depression and a determination of which loci were most important. In the largest study to date, 20 patients with treatment-resistant depression received subgenual ACC deep brain stimulation and were assessed at multiple time points before and after deep brain stimulation (Lozano et al, 2008). Additionally, PET was used to measure changes in brain metabolism associated with the antidepressant response to deep brain stimulation. Significant reductions in depressive symptoms were observed 1 week after deep brain stimulation, and a progressive increase in the proportion of treatment-resistant depression patients that showed a clinically significant reduction in depressive symptoms increased from 2 weeks to 6 months following deep brain stimulation. Importantly, PET data from eight deep brain stimulation responders revealed that deep brain stimulation was associated with decreased metabolism in the subgenual ACC gray matter immediately adjacent to the deep brain stimulation electrodes, as well as altered metabolism in several frontal, cortical, subcortical, and limbic structures of the cortico-limbic network. These findings suggest that there are immediate and longer term beneficial effects of deep brain stimulation for individuals with treatment-resistant depression and provide further mechanistic evidence of the brain abnormalities in MDD.

Vagus nerve stimulation (VNS) has received Food and Drug Administration approval for the treatment of epilepsy and more recently for treatment-resistant depression (George et al, 2007). The use of VNS in depression is consistent with evidence that vagal tone is reduced in depression: a meta-analysis of 13 studies in medically healthy individuals found a small-to-medium reduction in vagal tone associated with depression (effect size of $d= .332$) and comparable reductions in vagal tone in six studies of depressed patients with cardiovascular disease (effect size of $d = 0.280$) (Rottenberg, 2007). During VNS, the left vagus nerve is stimulated in the neck. Such stimulation leads to direct effects on the brain, which is consistent with evidence that 80% of vagal fibers are afferent (from the periphery to the brain). Functional brain imaging evidence suggests that VNS influences the brain through afferent vagal fibers, which are known to enter the midbrain at the nucleus tractus soli tarius and then connect to the reticular activating system, the parabrachial nucleus, raphe nucleus, locus ceruleus, thalamus, and then limbic, paralimbic, and cortical regions including the anterior insula and ACC. In general, VNS initially activates brain structures but then deactivates them over time with repeated stimulation, which may explain its antidepressant effects. A recent fMRI study in treatment-resistant depression, for example, found that VNS was associated with decreased activity in right medial prefrontal, subgenual ACC, left anterior temporal pole, and right somatosensory cortex, as well as increases in right superior temporal cortex (Nahas et al, 2007).

Another nonpharmacological treatment of depression is transcranial magnetic stimulation. Repetitive transcranial magnetic stimulation of the left dorsolateral PFC is an effective treatment for depression (Gross et al, 2007), and slow transcranial magnetic stimulation of the right dorsolateral PFC may also have utility in some contexts. Although functional imaging studies of transcranial magnetic stimulation are quite limited, there is evidence that repetitive transcranial magnetic stimulation of the left dorsolateral PFC is associated with increased activity in the mid-cingulate cortex (Paus et al, 2001), a structure that is hypoactive in depression.

8 Conclusions

Brain imaging can advance the behavioral medicine research agenda by contributing to the delineation of mechanisms that mediate established relationships between psychosocial variables on the one hand and medical outcome on the other (Lane et al, 2009a). Some of the most compelling evidence in the field of behavioral medicine concerns the effects of depression on early mortality (Steptoe, 2006). Progress has been made in identifying some of the autonomic, neuroendocrine, and immune effects of depression that can affect disease pathophysiology. Yet, there is considerable variability in the effects of depression on health that are still poorly understood. Elucidation of the brain basis of depression can potentially contribute to a greater understanding of the sources of such variability. This review has demonstrated that modern brain imaging has begun to define the key brain structures that are altered either structurally or functionally in depression. Much remains to be done, however, to identify the origins of individual variation in the peripheral manifestations of depression. Doing so will require a research strategy that includes assessment of psychosocial, brain, peripheral mediators, and end-organ variables within the same individuals (Lane et al, 2009b). This research strategy promises to improve our ability to identify those at risk and to provide new methods for primary and secondary prevention.

References

Adolphs, R. (2002). Neural systems for recognizing emotion. *Curr Opin Neurobiol, 12,* 169–177.

Alexopoulos, G. S., Kiosses, D. N., Choi, S. J., Murphy, C. F., and Lim, K. O. (2002). Frontal white matter microstructure and treatment response in late-life depression: a preliminary study. *Am J Psychiatry, 159*, 1929–1932.

Alexopoulos, G. S., Murphy, C. F., Gunning-Dixon, F. M., Latoussakis, V., Kanellopoulos, D. et al (2008). Microstructural white matter abnormalities and remission of geriatric depression. *Am J Psychiatry, 165*, 238–244.

Amaral, D. G., Price, J. L., Pitkanen, A., and Carmichael, S. T. (1992). Anatomical organization of the primate amygdaloid complex. In J. Aggleton (Ed.), *The Amygdala* (pp. 143–165). New York: Wiley-Liss.

Andreasen, N. C. (1997). Linking mind and brain in the study of mental illnesses: A project for a scientific psychopathology. *Science, 275*, 1586–1593.

Aron, A. R. (2007). The neural basis of inhibition in cognitive control. *Neuroscientist, 13*, 214–228.

Ashtari, M., Greenwald, B. S., Kramer-Ginsberg, E., Hu, J., Wu, H. et al (1999). Hippocampal/amygdala volumes in geriatric depression. *Psychol Med, 29*, 629–638.

Axelson, D. A., Doraiswamy, P. M., McDonald, W. M., Boyko, O. B., Tupler, L. A. et al (1993). Hypercortisolemia and hippocampal changes in depression. *Psychiatry Res, 47*, 163–173.

Ballmaier, M., Sowell, E. R., Thompson, P. M. Kumar, A., Narr, K. L. et al (2004). Mapping brain size and cortical gray matter changes in elderly depression. *Biol Psychiatry, 55*, 382–389.

Ballmaier, M., Toga, A. W., Blanton, R. E., Sowell, E. R., Lavretsky, H. et al (2004). Anterior cingulate, gyrus rectus, and orbitofrontal abnormalities in elderly depressed patients: an MRI-based parcellation of the prefrontal cortex. *Am J Psychiatry, 161*, 99–108.

Beck, A. T., Ward, C. H., Mendelson, M., Mock, J., Erbaugh, J. (1961). An inventory for measuring depression. *Arch Gen Psychiatry, 4*, 561–571.

Beck, A. T., Rush, A. J., Shaw, B. F., and Emery, G. (1979). *Cognitive Therapy of Depression*. New York: Guilford Press.

Bell-McGinty, S., Butters, M. A., Meltzer, C. C., Greer, P. J., Reynolds, C. F. et al (2002). Brain morphometric abnormalities in geriatric depression: long-term neurobiological effects of illness duration. *Am J Psychiatry, 159*, 1424–1427.

Botteron, K. N., Raichle, M. E., Drevets, W. C., Heath, A. C., and Todd, R. D. (2002). Volumetric reduction in left subgenual prefrontal cortex in early onset depression. *Biol Psychiatry, 51*, 342–344.

Bouhuys, A. L., Geerts, E., and Gordijn, M. C. (1999). Depressed patients' perceptions of facial emotions in depressed and remitted states are associated with relapse: a longitudinal study. *J Nerv Ment Dis, 187*, 595–602.

Bremner, J. D., Narayan, M., Anderson, E. R., Staib, L. H., Miller, H. L. et al (2000). Hippocampal volume reduction in major depression. *Am J Psychiatry, 157*, 115–118.

Bremner, J. D., Vythilingam, M., Vermetten, E., Nazeer, A., Adil, J. et al (2002). Reduced volume of orbitofrontal cortex in major depression. *Biol Psychiatry, 5*, 273–279.

Caetano, S. C., Hatch, J. P., Brambilla, P., Sassi, R. B., Nicoletti, M. et al (2004). Anatomical MRI study of hippocampus and amygdala in patients with current and remitted major depression. *Psychiatry Res, 132*, 141–147.

Chen, C. H., Ridler, K., Suckling, J., Williams, S., Fu, C. H. et al (2007). Brain imaging correlates of depressive symptom severity and predictors of symptom improvement after antidepressant treatment. *Biol Psychiatry, 62*, 407–414.

Clore, G., and Ortony, A. (2000). Cognition in emotion: always, sometimes or never? In R. Lane & L. Nadel (Eds.), *Cognitive Neuroscience of Emotion*. New York: Oxford University Press.

Coffey, C. E., Wilkinson, W. E., Weiner, R. D., Parashos, I. A., Djang, W. T. et al (1993). Quantitative cerebral anatomy in depression. A controlled magnetic resonance imaging study. *Arch Gen Psychiatry, 50*, 7–16.

Craig, A. D. (2002). How do you feel? Interoception: the sense of the physiological condition of the body. *Nat Rev Neurosci, 3*, 655–666.

Craig, A. D. (2003). Interoception: the sense of the physiological condition of the body. *Curr Opin Neurobiol, 13*, 500–505.

Critchley, H. D., Mathias, C. J., and Dolan, R. J. (2001). Neural correlates of first and second-order representation of bodily states. *Nature Neurosci, 4*, 207–212.

Davidson, R. J., Putnam, K. M., and Larson, C. L. (2000). Dysfunction in the neural circuitry of emotion regulation – a possible prelude to violence. *Science, 289*, 591–594

Davis, M. (2000). The role of the amygdala in conditioned and unconditioned fear and anxiety. In J. Aggleton (Ed.), *The Amygdala: A Functional Analysis* (pp. 213–287). Oxford: Oxford University Press.

Dolcos, F., and McCarthy, G. (2006). Brain systems mediating cognitive interference by emotional distraction. *J Neurosci, 26*, 2072–2079.

Drevets, W. C. (2001). Neuroimaging and neuropathological studies of depression: implications for the cognitive-emotional features of mood disorders. *Curr Opin Neurobiol, 11*, 240–249.

Drevets, W. C., Price, J. L., Simpson, J. R. Jr., Todd, R. D., Reich, T. et al (1997). Subgenual prefrontal cortex abnormalities in mood disorders. *Nature, 386*, 824–827.

Drevets, W. C., Videen, T. O., Price, J. L., Preskorn, S. H., Carmichael, S. T. et al (1992). A functional anatomical study of unipolar depression. *J Neurosci, 12*, 3628–3641.

Egan, M. F., Goldberg, T. E., Kolachana, B. S., Callicott, J. H., Mazzanti, C. M. et al (2001). Effect of COMT Val108/158 Met genotype on frontal lobe function and risk for schizophrenia. *Proc Natl Acad Sci U S A*, 98, 6917–22.

Ellenbogen, M. A., Schwartzman, A. E., Stewart, J., and Walker, C. D. (2002). Stress and selective attention: the interplay of mood, cortisol levels, and emotional information processing. *Psychophysiology, 39*, 723–732.

Etkin, A., Egner, T., Peraza, D. M., Kandel, E. R., and Hirsch, J. (2006). Resolving emotional conflict: a role for the rostral anterior cingulate cortex in modulating activity in the amygdala. *Neuron, 51*, 871–882.

Fales, C. L., Barch, D. M., Rundle, M. M., Mintun, M. A., Snyder, A. Z. et al (2008). Altered emotional interference processing in affective and cognitive-control brain circuitry in major depression. *Biol Psychiatry, 63*, 377–384.

Fanselow, M. S. (2000). Contextual fear, gestalt memories, and the hippocampus. *Behav Brain Res, 110*, 273–281.

Frasure-Smith, N., and Lesperance, F. (2005). Reflections on depression as a cardiac risk factor. *Psychosom Med, 67*, S19–25.

Frodl, T., Meisenzahl, E., Zetzsche, T., Bottlender, R., Born, C. et al (2002). Enlargement of the amygdala in patients with a first episode of major depression. *Biol Psychiatry, 51*, 708–714.

Frodl, T., Meisenzahl, E. M., Zetzsche, T., Hohne, T., Banac, S. et al (2004a). Hippocampal and amygdala changes in patients with major depressive disorder and healthy controls during a 1-year follow-up. *J Clin Psychiatry, 65*, 492–499.

Frodl, T., Meisenzahl, E. M., Zill, P., Baghai, T., Rujescu, D. et al (2004b). Reduced hippocampal volumes associated with the long variant of the serotonin transporter polymorphism in major depression. *Arch Gen Psychiatry, 61*, 177–183.

Frodl, T. S., Koutsouleris, N., Bottlender, R., Born, C., Jäger, M. et al (2008). Depression-related variation in brain morphology over 3 years: effects of stress? *Arch Gen Psychiatry, 65*, 1156–1165.

Gazzaniga, M., Ivry, R. B., and Mangun, G. R. (2008). *Cognitive Neuroscience -- The Biology of the Mind, 3rd Ed.* New York: Norton.

George, M. S., Ketter, T. A., Parekh, P. I., Rosinsky, N., Ring, H. A. et al (1997). Blunted left cingulate activation in mood disorder subjects during a response interference task (the Stroop). *J Neuropsychiatry Clin Neurosci, 9*, 55–63.

George, M. S., Nahas, Z., Borckardt, J. J., Anderson, B., Foust, M. J. et al (2007). Brain stimulation for the treatment of psychiatric disorders. *Curr Opin Psychiatry, 20*, 250–254.

Goldman-Rakic, P. S. (1996). Regional and cellular fractionation of working memory. *Proc Natl Acad Sci, 93*, 13473–13480.

Greenwald, B. S., Kramer-Ginsberg, E., Bogerts, B., Ashtari, M., Aupperle, P. et al (1997). Qualitative magnetic resonance imaging findings in geriatric depression. Possible link between later-onset depression and Alzheimer's disease? *Psychol Med, 27*, 421–431.

Greicius, M. D., Flores, B. H., Menon, V., Glover, G. H., Solvason, H. B. et al (2007). Resting-state functional connectivity in major depression: abnormally increased contributions from subgenual cingulate cortex and thalamus. *Biol Psychiatry, 62*, 429–437.

Grimm, S., Beck, J., Schuepbach, D., Hell, D., Boesiger, P. et al (2008). Imbalance between left and right dorsolateral prefrontal cortex in major depression is linked to negative emotional judgment: an fMRI study in severe major depressive disorder. *Biol Psychiatry, 63*, 369–376.

Gross, M., Nakamura, L., Pascual-Leone, A., and Fregni, F. (2007). Has repetitive transcranial magnetic stimulation (rTMS) treatment for depression improved? A systematic review and meta-analysis comparing the recent vs. the earlier rTMS studies. *Acta Psychiatr Scand, 116*, 165–173.

Gur, R. C., Erwin, R. J., Gur, R. E., Zwil, A. S., Heimberg, C. et al (1992). Facial emotion discrimination: II. Behavioral findings in depression. *Psychiatry Res, 42*, 241–251.

Gusnard, D. A., Raichle, M. E., and Raichle, M. E. (2001). Searching for a baseline: functional imaging and the resting human brain. *Nat Rev Neurosci, 2*, 685–694.

Hamilton, J. P., Siemer, M., and Gotlib, I. H. (2008). Amygdala volume in major depressive disorder: a meta-analysis of magnetic resonance imaging studies. *Mol Psychiatry, 13*, 993–1000.

Hariri, A. R., Mattay, V. S., Tessitore, A., Kolachana, B., Fera, F. et al (2002). Serotonin transporter genetic variation and the response of the human amygdala. *Science, 297*, 400–403.

Hastings, R. S., Parsey, R.V., Oquendo, M. A., Arango, V., and Mann, J. J. (2004). Volumetric analysis of the prefrontal cortex, amygdala, and hippocampus in major depression. *Neuropsychopharmacology, 29*, 952–959.

Hickie, I., Naismith, S., Ward, P. B., Turner, K., Scott, E. et al (2005). Reduced hippocampal volumes and memory loss in patients with early and late-onset depression. *Br J Psychiatry, 186*, 197–202.

Husain, M. M., McDonald, W. M., Doraiswamy, P. M., Figiel, G.S., Na, C. et al (1991). A magnetic resonance imaging study of putamen nuclei in major depression. *Psychiatry Res, 40*, 95–99.

Janssen, J., Hulshoff Pol, H. E., Lampe, I. K., Schnack, H. G., de Leeuw, F. E. et al (2004). Hippocampal changes and white matter lesions in early-onset depression. *Biol Psychiatry, 56*, 825–831.

Johnstone, T., van Reekum, C. M., Urry, H. L., Kalin, N. H., and Davidson, R. J. (2007). Failure to regulate: counterproductive recruitment of top-down prefrontal-subcortical circuitry in major depression. *J Neurosci, 27*, 8877–8884.

Jorge, R. E., Robinson, R. G., Arndt, S., and Starkstein, S. (2003). Mortality and poststroke depression: a placebo-controlled trial of antidepressants. *Am J Psychiatry, 160*, 1823–1829.

Judd, L. L., Schettler, P. J., Solomon, D. A., Maser, J. D., Coryell, W. et al (2008). Psychosocial disability and work role function compared across the long-term course of bipolar I, bipolar II and unipolar major depressive disorders. *J Affect Disord, 108(1–2)*, 49–58.

Katon, W., Rutter, C., Simon, G., Lin, E., Ludman, E. et al (2005). The association of comorbid depression with mortality in patients with Type 2 diabetes. *Diabetes Care, 28*, 2668–2672.

Kennedy, S. E., Koeppe, R. A., Young, E. A., and Zubieta, J. K. (2006). Dysregulation of endogenous opioid emotion regulation circuitry in major depression in women. *Arch Gen Psychiatry, 63*, 1199–1208.

Kennedy, S. H., Konarski, J. Z., Segal, Z. V., Lau, M. A., Bieling, P. J. et al (2007). Differences in brain glucose metabolism between responders to CBT and venlafaxine in a 16-week randomized controlled trial. *Am J Psychiatry, 164*, 778–788.

Kim, M. J., Hamilton, J. P., and Gotlib, I. H. (2008). Reduced caudate gray matter volume in women with major depressive disorder. *Psychiatry Res, 164*, 114–122.

Kober, H., Barrett, L. F., Joseph, J., Bliss-Moreau, E., Lindquist, K. et al (2008). Functional grouping and cortical-subcortical interactions in emotion: a meta-analysis of neuroimaging studies. *Neuroimage, 42*, 998–1031.

Konarski, J. Z., McIntyre, R. S., Kennedy, S. H., Rafi-Tari, S., Soczynska, J. K. et al (2008). Volumetric neuroimaging investigations in mood disorders: bipolar disorder versus major depressive disorder. *Bipolar Disord, 10*, 1-37.

Krishnan, K. R., McDonald, W. M., Escalona, P. R., Doraiswamy, P. M., Na, C. et al (1992). Magnetic resonance imaging of the caudate nuclei in depression. Preliminary observations. *Arch Gen Psychiatry, 49*, 553–557.

Kumar, A., Jin, Z., Bilker, W., Udupa, J., and Gottlieb, G. (1998). Lateonset minor and major depression: early evidence for common neuroanatomical substrates detected by using MRI. *Proc Natl Acad Sci U S A, 95*, 7654–7658.

Lacerda, A. L., Keshavan, M. S., Hardan, A. Y., Yorbik, O., Brambilla, P. et al (2004). Anatomic evaluation of the orbitofrontal cortex in major depressive disorder. *Biol Psychiatry, 55*, 353–358.

Lai, T., Payne, M. E., Byrum, C. E., Steffens, D. C., and Krishnan, K. R. (2000). Reduction of orbital frontal cortex volume in geriatric depression. *Biol Psychiatry, 48*, 971–975.

Lane, R. (2000). Neural correlates of conscious emotional experience. In R. Lane, L. Nadel, G. Ahern., J. Allen, A. Kaszniak, S. Rapcsak, & G. Schwartz (Eds.), *Cognitive Neuroscience of Emotion* (pp. 345–370). New York: Oxford University Press.

Lane, R. (2008). Neural substrates of implicit and explicit emotional processes: a unifying framework for psychosomatic medicine. *Psychosom Med, 70*, 213–230.

Lane, R. (2009). Anterior cingulate cortex. In D. Sander & K. Scherer (Eds.), *Oxford Companion to the Affective Sciences* (pp. 38–39). New York, NY: Oxford University Press.

Lane, R. D., Fink, G. R., Chau, P. M., and Dolan, R. J. (1997). Neural activation during selective attention to subjective emotional responses. *Neuroreport, 8*, 3969–3972.

Lane, R., Waldstein, S., Jennings, R., Lovallo, W., Rose, R. et al (2009a). The rebirth of neuroscience in psychosomatic medicine, part I: historical context, methods and relevant basic science. *Psychosom Med, 71*, 117–134.

Lane, R., Waldstein, S., Jennings, R., Lovallo, W., Rose, R., et al (2009). The rebirth of neuroscience in psychosomatic medicine, part I: historical context, methods and relevant basic science. *Psychosomat Med, 71*, 117–134.

Lane, R., Waldstein, S., Critchley, H., Derbyshire, S., Drossman, D. et al (2009b). The rebirth of neuroscience in psychosomatic medicine, part II: clinical applications and implications for research. *Psychosom Med, 71*, 135–151.

Langenecker, S. A., Kennedy, S. E., Guidotti, L. M., Briceno, E. M., Own, L. S. et al (2007). Frontal and limbic activation during inhibitory control predicts treatment response in major depressive disorder. *Biol Psychiatry, 62*, 1272–1280.

Lavretsky, H., Kurbanyan, K., Ballmaier, M., Mintz, J., Toga, A. et al (2004). Sex differences in brain structure in geriatric depression. *Am J Geriatr Psychiatry, 12*, 653–657.

LeDoux, J. E. (2000). Emotion circuits in the brain. *Annu Rev Neurosci, 23*, 155–184.

LeDoux, J. E., Cicchetti, P., Xagoraris, A., and Romanski, L. M. (1990). The lateral amygdaloid nucleus: sensory interface of the amygdala in fear conditioning. *J Neurosci, 10*, 1062–1069.

Lee, S. H., Payne, M. E., Steffens, D. C., McQuoid, D. R., Lai, T. J. et al (2003). Subcortical lesion severity and orbitofrontal cortex volume in geriatric depression. *Biol Psychiatry, 54*, 529–533.

Lespérance, F., Frasure-Smith, N., Talajic, M., and Bourassa, M. G. (2002). Five-year risk of cardiac mortality in relation to initial severity and one-year changes in depression symptoms after myocardial infarction. *Circulation, 105*, 1049–1053.

Levenson, R. W. (1994). Human emotion: a functional view. In P. Ekman & R. Irwin (Eds.), *The Nature of Emotion – Fundamental Questions* (pp. 123–126). New York: Oxford University Press.

Lorenzetti, V., Allen, N. B., Fornito, A., and Yücel, M. (2009). Structural brain abnormalities in major depressive disorder: a selective review of recent MRI studies. *J Affect Disord, 117(1–2)*, 1–17.

Lozano, A. M., Mayberg, H. S., Giacobbe, P., Hamani, C., Craddock, R. C. et al (2008). Subcallosal cingulate gyrus deep brain stimulation for treatment-resistant depression. *Biol Psychiatry, 64(6)*, 461–7.

Lyubomirsky, S., Caldwell, N. D., and Nolen-Hoeksema, S. (1998). Effects of ruminative and distracting responses to depressed mood on retrieval of autobiographical memories. *J Pers Soc Psychol, 75*, 166–177.

MacMaster, F. P., and Kusumakar, V. (2004a). Hippocampal volume in early onset depression. *BMC Med, 2*, 2.

MacMaster, F. P., and Kusumakar, V. (2004b). MRI study of the pituitary gland in adolescent depression. *J Psychiatr Res, 38*, 231–236.

MacMillan, S., Szeszko, P. R., Moore, G. J., Madden, R., Lorch, E. et al (2003). Increased amygdala: hippocampal volume ratios associated with severity of anxiety in pediatric major depression. *J Child Adolesc Psychopharmacol, 13*, 65–73.

MacQueen, G. M., Campbell, S., McEwen, B. S., Macdonald, K., Amano, S. et al (2003). Course of illness, hippocampal function, and hippocampal volume in major depression. *Proc Natl Acad Sci U S A, 100*, 1387–1392.

Marsh, R., Zhu, H., Schultz, R. T., Quackenbush, G., Royal, J. et al (2006). A developmental fMRI study of self-regulatory control. *Hum Brain Mapp, 27*, 848–863.

Matthews, S. C., Strigo, I. A., Simmons, A. N., Yang, T. T., and Paulus, M. P. (2008). Decreased functional coupling of the amygdala and supragenual cingulate is related to increased depression in unmedicated individuals with current major depressive disorder. *J Affect Disord, 111*, 13–20.

Matthews, S. C., Simmons, A. N., Strigo, I. A., Gianaros, P. J., Yang, T. T. et al (2009). Inhibition-related activity in subgenual cingulate is associated with symptom severity in major depression. *Psychiatry Res, 172(1)*, 1–6.

Mayberg, H. S. (1997). Limbic-cortical dysregulation: a proposed model of depression. *J Neuropsychiatry Clin Neurosci, 9*, 471–481.

Mayberg, H. S., Liotti, M., Brannan, S. K., McGinnis, S., Mahurin, R. K. et al (1999). Reciprocal limbic-cortical function and negative mood: converging PET findings in depression and normal sadness. *Am J Psychiatry, 156*, 675–682.

Mayberg, H. S., Lozano, A. M., Voon, V., McNeely, H. E., Seminowicz, D. et al (2005). Deep brain stimulation for treatment-resistant depression. *Neuron 45*, 651–660.

Mazoyer, B., Zago, L., Mellet, E., Bricogne, S., Etard, O. et al (2001). Cortical networks for working memory and executive functions sustain the conscious resting state in man. *Brain Res Bull, 54*, 287–298.

Mesulam, M. M., and Mufson, E. J. (1982). Insula of the old world monkey. I. Architectonics in the insuloorbito-temporal component of the paralimbic brain. *J Comp Neurol, 212*, 1–22.

Mogg, K., Bradley, B. P., and Williams, R. (1995). Attentional bias in anxiety and depression: the role of awareness. *Br J Clin Psychol, 34*, 17–36.

Morys, J. M., Bobek-Billewicz, B., Dziewiatkowski, J., Ratajczak, I., Pankiewicz, P. et al (2003). A magnetic resonance volumetric study of the temporal lobe structures in depression. *Folia Morphol Warsz, 62*, 347–352.

Nagai, M., Kishi, K., and Kato, S. (2007). Insular cortex and neuropsychiatric disorders: a review of recent literature. *Eur Psychiatry, 22(6)*, 387–394.

Nahas, Z., Teneback, C., Chae, J. H., Mu, Q., Molnar, C. et al (2007). Serial vagus nerve stimulation functional MRI in treatment-resistant depression. *Neuropsychopharmacology, 32*, 1649–1660.

Ochsner, K. N., and Gross, J. J. (2005). The cognitive control of emotion. *Trends Cogn Sci, 9*, 242–249.

O'Connor, M. F., Guendel, H., McRae, K., and Lane, R. (2007). Baseline vagal tone predicts BOLD response during elicitation of grief. *Neuropsychopharmacology, 32*, 2184–2189.

Ongur, D., and Price, J. L. (2000). The organization of networks within the orbital and medial prefrontal cortex of rats, monkeys and humans. *Cereb Cortex, 10*, 206–219.

Onitilo, A., Nietert, P., and Egede, L. (2006). Effect of depression on all-cause mortality in adults with cancer and differential effects by cancer site. *Gen Hosp Psychiatry, 28*, 396–402.

Pampallona, S., Bollini, P., Tibaldi, G., Kupelnick, B., and Munizza, C. (2004). Combined pharmacotherapy and psychological treatment for depression - a systematic review. *Arch Gen Psychiatry*, 61, 714–719.

Paus, T. (2001). Primate anterior cingulate cortex: where motor control, drive and cognition interface. *Nat Rev Neurosci, 2*, 417–424.

Paus, T., Castro-Alamancos, M. A., and Petrides, M. (2001). Cortico-cortical connectivity of the human mid-dorsolateral frontal cortex and its modulation by repetitive transcranial magnetic stimulation. *Eur J Neuroscience, 14*, 1405–1411

Pezawas, L., Meyer-Lindenberg, A., Drabant, E. M., Verchinski, B. A., Munoz, K. E. et al (2005). 5-HTTLPR polymorphism impacts human cingulate-amygdala interactions: a genetic susceptibility mechanism for depression. *Nat Neurosci, 8*, 828–834.

Phan, K., Wager, T., Taylor, S., and Liberzon, I. (2002). Functional neuroanatomy of emotion: a meta-analysis of emotion activation studies in PET and fMRI. *Neuroimage, 16*, 331–348.

Pillay, S. S., Yurgelun-Todd, D. A., Bonello, C. M., Lafer, B., Fava, M. et al (1997). A quantitative magnetic resonance imaging study of cerebral and cerebellar gray matter volume in primary unipolar major depression: relationship to treatment response and clinical severity. *Biol Psychiatry, 42*, 79–84.

Price, J. L. (1999). Prefrontal cortical networks related to visceral function and mood. *Ann NY Acad Sci, 877*, 383–396.

Raichle, M. E., and Gusnard, D. A. (2005). Intrinsic brain activity sets the stage for expression of motivated behavior. *J Comp Neurol, 493,* 167–176.

Raichle, M. E., MacLeod, A. M., Snyder, A. Z., Powers, W. J., Gusnard, D. A. et al (2001). A default mode of brain function. *Proc Natl Acad Sci U S A, 98,* 676–682.

Rosso, I. M., Cintron, C. M., Steingard, R. J., Renshaw, P. F., Young, A. D. et al (2005). Amygdala and hippocampus volumes in pediatric major depression. *Biol Psychiatry, 57,* 21–26.

Rottenberg, J. (2007). Cardiac vagal control in depression: a critical analysis. *Biol Psychol, 74,* 200–211.

Rugulies, R. (2002). Depression as a predictor for coronary heart disease. *Am J Prev Med, 23,* 51–61.

Salokangas, R. K., Cannon, T., Van Erp, T., Ilonen, T., Taiminen, T. et al (2002). Structural magnetic resonance imaging in patients with first-episode schizophrenia, psychotic and severe non-psychotic depression and healthy controls. Results of the schizophrenia and affective psychoses SAP project. *Br J Psychiatry Suppl, 43,* S58-S65.

Sapolsky, R. M. (2000). Glucocorticoids and hippocampal atrophy in neuropsychiatric disorders. *Arch Gen Psychiatry, 57,* 925–935.

Sapolsky, R. M. (2000). The possibility of neurotoxicity in the hippocampus in major depression: a primer on neuron death. *Biol Psychiatry, 48,* 755–765.

Scher, C. D., Ingram, R. E., and Segal, Z. V. (2005). Cognitive reactivity and vulnerability: empirical evaluation of construct activation and cognitive diatheses in unipolar depression. *Clin Psychol Rev, 25,* 487–510.

Shah, P. J., Ebmeier, K. P., Glabus, M. F., and Goodwin, G. M. (1998). Cortical grey matter reductions associated with treatment-resistant chronic unipolar depression. Controlled magnetic resonance imaging study. *Br J Psychiatry, 172,* 527–532.

Sheline, Y. I., Barch, D. M., Donnelly, J. M., Ollinger, J. M., Snyder, A. Z. et al (2001). Increased amygdala response to masked emotional faces in depressed subjects resolves with antidepressant treatment: an fMRI study. *Biol Psychiatry, 50,* 651–658.

Sheline, Y. I., Gado, M. H., and Price, J. L. (1998). Amygdala core nuclei volumes are decreased in recurrent major depression. *Neuroreport, 9,* 2023–2028.

Sheline, Y. I., Sanghavi, M., Mintun, M. A., and Gado, M. H. (1999). Depression duration but not age predicts hippocampal volume loss in medically healthy women with recurrent major depression. *J Neurosci, 19,* 5034–5043.

Sheline, Y. I., Wang, P. W., Gado, M. H., Csernansky, J. G., and Vannier, M. W. (1996). Hippocampal atrophy in recurrent major depression. *Proc Natl Acad Sci U S A, 93,* 3908–3913.

Siegle, G. J., Konecky, R. O., Thase, M. E., and Carter, C. S. (2003). Relationships between amygdala volume and activity during emotional information processing tasks in depressed and never-depressed individuals: an fMRI investigation. *Ann NY Acad Sci, 985,* 481–484.

Siegle, G. J., Steinhauer, S. R., Thase, M. E., Stenger, V. A., and Carter, C. S. (2002). Can't shake that feeling: event-related fMRI assessment of sustained amygdala activity in response to emotional information in depressed individuals. *Biol Psychiatry, 51,* 693–707.

Siegle, G. J., Thompson, W., Carter, C. S., Steinhauer, S. R., and Thase, M. E. (2007). Increased amygdala and decreased dorsolateral prefrontal BOLD responses in unipolar depression: related and independent features. *Biol Psychiatry, 61,* 198–209.

Steffens, D. C., McQuoid, D. R., Welsh-Bohmer, K. A., and Krishnan, K. R. (2003). Left orbital frontal cortex volume and performance on the Benton visual retention test in older depressives and controls. *Neuropsychopharmacology, 28,* 2179–2183.

Steptoe, A. (2006). *Depression and Physical Illness.* Cambridge, MA: Cambridge University Press.

Strigo, I. A., Simmons, A. N., Matthews, S. C., Craig, A. D., and Paulus, M. P. (2008a). Increased affective bias revealed using experimental graded heat stimuli in young depressed adults: evidence of "emotional allodynia". *Psychosom Med, 70,* 338–344.

Strigo, I. A., Simmons, A. N., Matthews, S. C., Craig, A. D., and Paulus, M. P. (2008b). Major depressive disorder is associated with altered functional brain response during anticipation and processing of heat pain. *Arch Gen Psychiatry, 65,* 1275–1284.

Surguladze, S. A., Young, A. W., Senior, C., Brebion, G., Travis, M. J. et al (2004). Recognition accuracy and response bias to happy and sad facial expressions in patients with major depression. *Neuropsychology, 18,* 212–218.

Taylor, W. D., Kuchibhatla, M., Payne, M. E., Macfall, J. R., Sheline, Y. I. et al (2008). Frontal white matter anisotropy and antidepressant remission in late-life depression. *PLoS ONE, 3,* e3267.

Taylor, W. D., Steffens, D. C., McQuoid, D. R., Payne, M. E., Lee, S. H. et al (2003). Smaller orbital frontal cortex volumes associated with functional disability in depressed elders. *Biol Psychiatry, 53,* 144–149.

Taylor. W. D., Steffens, D. C., Payne, M. E., MacFall, J. R., Marchuk, D. A. et al (2005). Influence of serotonin transporter promoter region polymorphisms on hippocampal volumes in late-life depression. *Arch Gen Psychiatry, 62,* 537–544.

Tremblay, L. K., Naranjo, C. A., Graham, S. J., Herrmann, N., Mayberg, H. S. et al (2005). Functional neuroanatomical substrates of altered reward processing in major depressive disorder revealed by a dopaminergic probe. *Arch Gen Psychiatry, 62,* 1228–36.

Urry, H. L., van Reekum, C. M., Johnstone, T., Kalin, N. H., Thurow, M. E. et al (2006). Amygdala and ventromedial prefrontal cortex are inversely coupled during regulation of negative affect and predict the diurnal pattern of cortisol secretion among older adults. *J Neurosci, 26,* 4415–4425.

Vakili, K., Pillay, S. S., Lafer, B., Fava, M., Renshaw, P. F. et al (2000). Hippocampal volume in primary unipolar major depression: a magnetic resonance imaging study. *Biol Psychiatry, 47,* 1087–1090.

van der Veen, F. M., Evers, E. A., Deutz, N. E., and Schmitt, J. A. (2007). Effects of acute tryptophan depletion on mood and facial emotion perception related brain activation and performance in healthy women with and without a family history of depression. *Neuropsychopharmacology, 32,* 216–224.

Vogt, B. A. (Ed.). (2009). *Cingulate Neurobiology and Disease.* New York: Oxford University Press.

Wacker, J., Dillon, D. G., and Pizzagalli, D. A. (2009). The role of the nucleus accumbens and rostral anterior cingulate cortex in anhedonia: integration of resting EEG, fMRI, and volumetric techniques. *Neuroimage, 46,* 327–37.

Wang, L., LaBar, K. S., Smoski, M., Rosenthal, M. Z., Dolcos, F. et al (2008). Prefrontal mechanisms for executive control over emotional distraction are altered in major depression. *Psychiatry Res, 163,* 143–155.

Wenzlaff, R. M., and Bates, D. E. (1998). Unmasking a cognitive vulnerability to depression: how lapses in mental control reveal depressive thinking. *J Pers Soc Psychol, 75,* 1559–1571.

Zald, D. H. (2003). The human amygdala and the emotional evaluation of sensory stimuli. *Brain Res, 41,* 88–123.

Zald, D. H., and Rauch, S. L. (Eds.). (2006). *The Orbitofrontal Cortex.* New York: Oxford University Press, 2006.

Chapter 53

The Electric Brain and Behavioral Medicine

J. Richard Jennings, Ydwine Zanstra, and Victoria Egizio

1 Introduction

Electrophysiological measures of brain function were developed well before the advent of brain imaging techniques. Electrophysiological measures assess the summated electrical activity generated by neural membrane potentials that is detectible most frequently from the scalp, but occasionally by either depth electrodes or electrodes on the brain surface. Relative to magnetic resonance and positron emission tomography imaging, electrophysiological measures are known to directly assess neural activity as opposed to vascular support for that activity. Electrophysiological measures occupy an important area in the space/time topology of brain indices. Electrical activity occurs over a millisecond time frame in synchrony with summated neural membrane changes. Transient neural events thus can be readily detected in the recorded electrical potentials. In contrast magnetic resonance imaging and positron emission tomography depend on relatively sustained neural activation that stimulates a cerebral blood flow response (see Chapter 50). Electrophysiological measures thus have relatively greater and excellent temporal sensitivity. Their drawback is spatial sensitivity. When assessments are made from the scalp or even brain surface, the source of summated measures assessed is only approximately known. The brain is largely a conductive medium so electrical changes travel readily through this medium away from their source. Analytic techniques can accurately determine how a signal from a particular source is expressed at the brain surface, but determining the source(s) of the electrical changes from surface changes is a complex problem (termed the "inverse problem"). Approximations to this "inverse problem" can be made, and with large electrode arrays and sophisticated software some spatial localization is possible with electrophysiological measures. As with any scientific problem, a clear analysis of the problem should permit the investigator to decide whether his question is well answered by a temporally sensitive measure – such as electrophysiology – or a measure with clearer spatial resolution – such as magnetic resonance imaging. A promising approach, but one with many technical and practical challenges, is multi-modal imaging of the brain. The combination of techniques such as electroencephalography and magnetic resonance imaging ultimately has the promise of enhanced assessment of both temporal and spatial properties of the brain as it processes information of interest.

A brief introduction to electrophysiological measures is appropriate, but the interested reader is encouraged to refer as well to any of a number of excellent reviews for a thorough coverage of the topic (Andreassi, 2007; Niedermeyer and Lopes da Silva, 2004; Rugg and Coles, 1995). The electroencephalogram (EEG) is the most common electrophysiological

J.R. Jennings (✉)
Department of Psychiatry, University of Pittsburgh,
Western Psychiatric Institute and Clinic, 3811 O'Hara
St, Pittsburgh, PA 15213, USA
e-mail: jenningsjr@upmc.edu

A. Steptoe (ed.), *Handbook of Behavioral Medicine*, DOI 10.1007/978-0-387-09488-5_53,
© Springer Science+Business Media, LLC 2010

measure in human studies. This measure is typically taken from scalp electrodes. These electrodes assess naturally occurring changes in voltage (in the microvolt range) arising from the brain. Localization is assisted by standardized placement of electrodes, often following the 10–20 system (Niedermeyer and Lopes da Silva, 2004). Although information can be gained from only a few electrodes, recent attempts to better localize the source of electrophysiological changes have led to expanded numbers of electrodes, e.g., 128 over the scalp. Electrical signals at the scalp are thought to primarily arise from summated pre- and postsynaptic potentials. Electrical activity is continuously detectible and the resting EEG signal is a complex of changing waveforms that can be analyzed into components with different wavelengths. Early work identified subjective state with the degree to which the complex waveform was made up of a particular wavelength. Quiet peaceful resting was, for example, associated with a preponderance of alpha waves (8–12 Hz); while active thought was found to be associated with higher frequency beta (12–30 Hz) and gamma (30 Hz and higher) waves. Extending this frequency analysis approach into sleep resulted in the classification of stages of sleep based in part on the frequency characteristics of the EEG (see Chapter 49). Stage 4 sleep, for example, is characterized by slow, delta waves (up to 4 Hz). The EEG can thus used to monitor subjective state related to a disease or risk factor.

The same electrodes and measure apparatus are used to assess brain reactions as well. Initial work examined cortical evoked potentials. These were "evoked" by a known and carefully controlled physical stimulus, e.g., a light flash or tone. Reliable waveforms were elicited with components unfolding over time that could be roughly associated with processing in particular brain areas. Event-related, as opposed to evoked, potentials are often of greater interest to the psychologist. These are neural responses to mental events, e.g., attending to an upcoming stimulus, recalling a word. The initiating "stimulus" is a mental event whose timing should be known, but an event that is less readily identified than

an environmental stimulus. With either event-related (ERPs) or evoked potentials (EPs) the signal occurs in the context of the ongoing complex EEG waveform. Typically the stimulus or event must be repeated numerous times so an average across these presentations can be computed. The segments of EEG surrounding the stimulus or event are aligned by the event/stimulus time and an average is computed across this ensemble. The transient changes in brain activity elicited by the event are synchronized with the event but these changes are small and often masked by ongoing variability in the EEG. Aligning the data with the onset of the event and averaging across occurrences of the event eliminates the non-synchronized activity and leaves the "event-related potential" or "evoked response." Components of these average waves are labeled (roughly) by their polarity and timing, e.g., P300, a positive wave occurring about 300 ms after the event. These components are then typically examined to see if they are related to, for example, enhanced attention to an event or recollection of a word. A typical and frequently used experimental paradigm is the "oddball." Tones of a particular frequency and amplitude are presented to a participant repetitively with reasonably close spacing. An occasional tone of a different frequency (or amplitude), the oddball, is presented in the midst of the repetitive tones (often termed the standard). The oddball is known to elicit a large P300 ERP.

A very limited amount of human work uses the exposed brain and can assess field or single unit potentials that are much more spatially specific. These techniques are very relevant for animal model work, but we will not review them here.

The use of EEG in behavioral medicine research is relatively low compared to the use in areas such as cognitive and affective psychology. Among the papers that we reviewed only 24% were published in journals commonly viewed as relevant to behavioral medicine. At some variance is the use of electrophysiological measures in clinical medicine. Electrophysiological measures of the brain are routinely applied in the assessment of epilepsy, level of consciousness after head injury, central conduction times, and in sleep disorders. These clinical applications are extended to research issues occasionally and we shall review some such studies. Often, a neurological perspective is taken in these papers, using EEG as a marker of brain state or EPs as measures of conduction times. We have attempted to exhaustively review the use of brain electrophysiology in behavioral medicine studies that directly concern a disease state, disease etiology, or disease risk factor. The review spans the years from 1950 (Ovid Medline) and 1967 (Psych Info) to March 2009 as represented in online data bases. Appendix 1 gives the search criteria used to identify articles. Next, final selection of articles based on their relevance for this review was made by two independent reviewers followed by a conference to achieve an agreed upon set of articles to review. This approach leads naturally to an organization of the review by disease entity and within that an organization by type of electrophysiology (EEG, event-related potential, or other technique). Of note, we have followed the convention (a rather odd one) of excluding psychiatric and neurologic disease from our coverage of diseases of relevance to behavioral medicine. Certain topics of relevance to behavioral medicine were missed by the search strategy, most notably the placebo effect (Colloca et al, 2008; Wager and Nitschke, 2005). Fortunately, a recent review of this literature provides a comprehensive overview detailing the role of electrophysiology in placebo analgesia research (Ng et al, 2004). Electrophysiological measures are very widely used in psychiatric research. Again this application has been reviewed elsewhere (Allen and Kline, 2004; Bagic and Sato, 2007; Davidson et al, 2000). We briefly consider the application of electrophysiology to health behaviors, smoking, alcohol use, eating, and exercise. The literature directed solely at understanding these risk factors (as opposed to their pathogenic or health effects) is quite large and thereby beyond the scope of the current review. We would, for example, be overwhelmed by examining the EEG/ERP studies of acute alcohol or tobacco intake. Finally, we confined our review to the

articles identified through the electronic search criteria. Review of the articles clearly suggested that the electronic criteria had failed to identify all the articles using electrophysiological measures in an area. Thus, the current review should not be considered exhaustive within any particular disease/health behavior category.

Our review led us to four conclusions concerning electrophysiological measures in behavioral medicine. (1) As noted above, electrophysiological measures are employed rather rarely in behavioral medicine research, (2) Existing applications focus more on cognitive function despite the sensitivity of these measures to affective and motivational states, (3) The sensitivity of EEG and ERP measures to both biological insults and psychological states forces the investigators to adopt an integrated biopsychological approach to disease/patient health, and (4) EEG/ERP measures to date have been used primarily as markers of disease state or pharmacological effect as opposed to examining processes influenced by or inherent to the disease.

2 Cardiovascular Disease

Electrophysiological measures have been applied in cardiovascular disease in various different ways; an initial example examines pharmacological effects. Denolle and colleagues (2002) examined cognitive effects of treatment with antihypertensive drugs in hypertensive patients. They examined the possible neuroprotective effects of a specific type of antihypertensive drug (nicardipine, a calcium-channel blocker) on the EEG, in comparison to an antihypertensive drug that is known to have sedative side effects (clonidine, an alpha-receptor agonist). After 2 weeks of treatment, results suggested that nicardipine effects were mainly excitatory: a decrease of slow delta waves and increase in alpha power. Clonidine showed a sedative EEG profile. Psychometric tests did not show any changes in attention, vigilance, and memory in the nicardipine group, but in the clonidine group these parameters decreased. Antihypertensive effects of clonidine and nicardipine were similar. This study shows how EEG can be applied to examine differential cognitive effects of medication. The added value of EEG is that in this particular study it detected cognitive changes in the nicardipine group that were not detected up by the psychometric tests.

In an interesting application of ERP, Gray et al (2007) examined the relationship between myocardial function and brain potentials, to examine the role of the brain in arrhythmias. Stress was assumed to trigger enhanced sympathetic drive to the heart. They further assumed that the heart evoked potential (HEP), detected at frontal and central scalp sites, assesses cortical responsivity to cardiac afferent information and its subsequent control of myocardial changes, as measured using electrocardiogram. Indeed the HEP in the left temporal and lateral prefrontal surface electrodes was found to be associated with changes in myocardial indices during stress. This study shows a novel way to examine the role of stress in cardiovascular disease in that it uses ERP as a central measure of stress-related cardiac activation to examine abnormal afferent feedback mechanisms that may be involved in arrhythmiogenesis (Gray et al, 2007).

Several studies examined the relationship between sleep and cardiovascular disease, using polysomnography (Guilleminault et al, 1996; Lee et al, 2008; Taheri et al, 2007; von Kanel et al, 2007; Zaregarizi et al, 2007). The polysomnogram was used to measure factors relating to respiration during sleep, sleep-disordered breathing (snoring, apneas, hypopneas) (Taheri et al, 2007; Lee et al, 2008), and upper airway resistance syndrome (Guilleminault et al, 1996). The polysomnogram involves the simultaneous measurement of some or all of the following parameters: 2-lead EEG, EOG (electrooculogram), ECG (electrocardiogram), EMG (electromyogram), oxygen saturation, and a respiration belt. Apnea is a complete cessation of breathing for at least 10 s, whereas hypopnea is a partial cessation of breathing as derived from the polysomnogram. A number of studies focused on respiratory components of the polysomnogram and factors

relevant to cardiovascular disease. Taheri and colleagues (2007) found no association between sleep duration or sleep-disordered breathing and C-reactive protein (CRP). The authors suggest body mass index may mediate the association between sleep-disordered breathing and CRP, but do not report any mediation analyses. Lee and colleagues (Lee et al, 2008) examined snoring as an aspect of the obstructive sleep apnea/hypopnea syndrome (OSAHS), which has been found to be associated with cerebrovascular disease. Although carotid atherosclerosis was related to snoring, polysomnography measures could not be shown to mediate the relationship. Guilleminault and colleagues (1996) found a suggestive association between transient blood pressure increases and acute instances of the upper airway resistance syndrome (heightened inspiratory effort without significant hypoxemia). These studies involve EEG only as a component on the polysomnogram while emphasizing the potential importance of respiration during sleep as related to cardiovascular risk.

In other studies examining the role of EEG in the association between sleep and heart disease, polysomnography was applied to examine factors relating to sleep quality and disruption (von Kanel et al, 2007) and napping (Zaregarizi et al, 2007). Von Kanel and colleagues (2007) looked at the role of sleep disturbances and prothrombotic changes. Polysomnography measures of sleep disruption were associated with prothrombotic parameters such as those that are associated with endothelial damage (von Willebrandt factor, soluble tissue factor; sTF), hypercoagulability (d-dimer), and fibrinolysis (PAI enzyme). In contrast to the majority of the studies reviewed, a substantial sample was employed; patients were 153 hypertensive, predominantly overweight individuals. Sleep disruption parameters were found to be predictive of both increased VWF and sTF. Furthermore, sleep apnea was associated with higher levels of fibrinolytic factors.

Napping is a protective factor; having a siesta regularly is associated with a 37% decrease in risk for myocardial infarction. Zaregarizi and colleagues (2007) examined whether this reduction in risk is due to the daytime nap itself, a supine posture, or the expectancy of a nap. The nap, particularly one with short sleep-onset time, seemed to relate most strongly to blood pressure.

In summary, EEG and ERP appear useful in examining psychologically mediated risk for arrhythmia and for evaluating medication side effects. Sleep has been examined with polysomnography both because of its impact on heart disease and as an etiologic factor. Results show the promise of objective polysomnography but the papers reviewed did not relate these to self-reports of sleep quality. Self-reported sleep has previously been related to heart disease in epidemiologic work (Ayas et al, 2003).

3 Diabetes and Neuroendocrine Disorder

Research using EEG/ERP directed at diabetes has been characterized by use of both EEG as a measure of state and EP's/ERP's as a probe of cognitive or sensory function. Both measures are largely directed at the impact of glucose dysregulation on neural function. Hypoglycemia is a fall in blood glucose levels that can occur as a complication of insulin treatment in diabetes mellitus. Hypoglycemia, if uncontrolled, can spiral through autonomic, cognitive, and affective disruption down to coma. Early awareness of hypoglycemia is important, as is the long-term effect of glucose dysregulation in general.

3.1 Hypoglycemia

Hypoglycemia's impact on neural processing has been documented reasonably well using EEG, EP, and ERP. The application of these measures to this aspect of diabetes was among the most thorough in the literature.

Lingenfelser et al (1993) examined auditory EP's. Diabetic patients were exposed to three hypoglycemic episodes whereas in patients

in the control group, glucose levels were strictly controlled around a set point. As glucose levels fell in the experimental group, the expected increased awareness of hypoglycemia was observed as well as expected counter regulatory blunting of adrenaline and cortisol responses. Mid latency components of the auditory EP were delayed, reflecting slowed auditory processing.

Auditory ERPs, e.g., the P300, during hypoglycemia were examined to document cognitive and neural processing deficits (Strachan et al, 2003). Diabetic patients were exposed to euglycemic (a control condition during which glucose levels were normal) or induced hypoglycemia states. Significant effects of hypoglycemia on performance on two neuropsychological tests, the digit symbol test and the trail-making B test, were found, but no significant effects were found for early negative and late positive, especially P300, components of the auditory ERP. Psychometric tests were generally more sensitive to the effects of hypoglycemia on cognitive function than EEG measures. Lobmann and colleagues (2000) did a similar study, however, and found effects of hypoglycemia on ERP components interpreted as reflecting stimulus selection (selection negativity) and response selection (lateralized readiness potential) in both diabetics and controls. Performance in the selective attention task was affected by hypoglycemia too. After restoration of euglycemia, performance and selection negativity recovered in diabetics but not in controls. Diabetes patients appeared to cope with the effects of hypoglycemia better than the controls, presumably due to enhanced cerebral glucose uptake in diabetics. This enhancement of cerebral glucose uptake may, however, contribute to reduced glucose awareness among diabetics (Lobmann et al, 2000).

Howorka and colleagues (2000) examined EEG parameters interpreted as reflecting vigilance to the hypoglycemic state in Type 1 diabetes patients who had a history of hypoglycemia. The EEG was obtained during relaxation, while participants were in a non-hypoglycemic state. In comparison to non-diabetic controls those with a history of hypoglycemia showed a reduction of power in the beta band, whereas those without recurrent hypoglycemia showed a small reduction in delta power in comparison to a healthy control group. No direct comparisons between the diabetes patient groups (with or without recurrent hypoglycemia) were reported. These results were interpreted as showing less internalized vigilance in those with a history of hypoglycemia. No differences were found on self-report measures examining motivational state, arousal, and well-being.

Jauch-Chara and colleagues (2007) examined the effects of hypoglycemia during and after sleep. Nocturnal hypoglycemia was expected to affect vigilance, cognition, and mood on the next day, an effect that might be less pronounced in diabetics compared to healthy controls, presumably due to habituation. On one night participants were exposed to hypoglycemia whereas during the other night, participants' plasma glucose concentration levels were normal (euglycemia condition). In addition to polysomnographic measures during the euglycemic and hypoglycemic nights, on the following day, mood, performance, and auditory ERPs were measured. In both patients and controls, hypoglycemia increased tiredness, depression, and restlessness. Nevertheless, no effects of hypoglycemia could be demonstrated on the auditory ERPs. Group differences in sleep parameters were found using the polysomographic measures; hypoglycemia increased time spent awake during the first part of the night and this effect was worse in healthy controls.

An interesting issue is whether glycemic state and insulin induce separable influences. Kern and colleagues (2001) examined the effects of insulin on mood, bodily symptoms, and cognitive function in healthy individuals. Participants were exposed to a euglycemic clamp procedure where glucose levels were kept constant while participants were infused with insulin. In this way, the effects of insulin were examined, independent of glucose. Participants performed an oddball task. The P300 latency and amplitude were enhanced in a high insulin condition

as compared to a low insulin condition (Kern et al, 2001). Furthermore, insulin was found to improve performance on a working memory task. These positive results argue for further study within diabetic as well as normal participants.

3.2 Hypoglycemic Awareness

Awareness of hypoglycemic changes has been examined using the EEG state measures (Howorka et al, 1996; Tribl et al, 1996). Patients with impaired hypoglycemic awareness may be more likely to progress into severe hypoglycemia because their inability to detect a state in which blood glucose is low will prevent them from taking appropriate measures. Furthermore, recurrent neuroglycopenia may result in reduced hypoglycemic awareness (Frier, 2001). Tribl and colleagues (1996) used a hypoglycemia protocol to examine patients varying in reported awareness. EEG was recorded as a function of decreasing glucose levels (normoglycemia, mild hypoglycemia, moderate hypoglycemia, and severe hypoglycemia). During the normoglycemic stage, those with poor hypoglycemia awareness showed less theta power and more alpha power. During mild hypoglycemia, these effects were the reversed, however; higher theta power and lower alpha power in those with poor hypoglycemia awareness. In the lowest hypoglycemic levels, no differences were found between those with and those without hypoglycemia awareness. Howorka and colleagues (1996) similarly examined the hypoglycemic state in patients classified as "unaware" or "aware." During hypoglycemia, participants performed a mental arithmetic task during which the EEG was recorded. Unaware patients had significantly higher alpha power, but lower power in delta and theta frequency bands. The authors interpret this EEG pattern as suggesting lower vigilance in unaware patients and suggest that this may, at least partly, be responsible for impaired hypoglycemia perception. These two papers both support a relationship of brain state and hypoglycemia awareness, though both experimental conditions and results differed somewhat between studies.

A wide range of applications of EEG technique has been used to examine the effects of hypoglycemia and hypoglycemia awareness in diabetes. Both glycemic state and individual differences in awareness were found to impact EEG measures. The number of studies available and relatively small samples prevent definitive interpretation. Level of hypoglycemia and whether or not the study involved mental task performance appeared to influence the results and these parameters were not typically consistent across studies.

3.3 Long-Term Effects of Diabetes

Longer term effects of diabetes on the central nervous system have been implicated by observed cognitive performance deficits among diabetes patients relative to controls on a range of tasks (learning, problem solving, mental and motor speed) (Dey et al, 1997; Pozzessere et al, 1991).

Two studies examined the P300 in insulin-dependent diabetes mellitus patients. Pozzessere and colleagues (1991) examined sixteen patients and sixteen (age- and sex-) matched healthy controls during performance of an oddball task. P300 latencies were lengthened in patients as compared to controls. Furthermore, diabetes patients performed significantly worse on a memory test (digit span backward). P300 latency and digit span task performance, however, were not significantly correlated in either the diabetes or the control group. The authors suggest that memory task performance and the P300 examine different aspects of cognitive functioning in diabetes and should be combined to evaluate the effects of diabetes on the brain. Dey and colleagues (1997) examined effects of long-standing diabetes in 28 patients in comparison to 28 healthy controls. P300 latencies in diabetes patients were significantly longer than in controls. Dey and colleagues (1997)

obtained a significant correlation between blood glucose levels and P300 latencies; as blood glucose levels increased, P300 latencies were less delayed – an effect not examined by Pozzessere et al (1991). This particular finding suggests that hypoglycemia plays a role in the obtained differences between patients and controls. In order to examine the long-term detrimental effects of diabetes the alternative explanation needs to be ruled out that the observed differences between patients and healthy controls could be due to the short-term effects of hypoglycemia.

Catterall and colleagues (1984) examined the potential role of diabetic neuropathy, hypothesizing that this may result in sleep apnea, which could explain sudden death in diabetes patients. Polysomnography-derived measures did not differ between the groups and therefore it was concluded that neuropathy-induced sleep apneas are not responsible for sudden unexplained deaths in diabetic neuropathy patients. This conclusion may, however, be deemed premature due to the limited sample size (eight patients and eight controls).

The promise of understanding influences on the brain of diabetes and treatment maintenance remains, but the studies reviewed were typically rather small and the measurement approach limited the interpretations that could be made.

4 EEG and the Effects of Hormone Treatment

The administration of hormone replacement therapy (HRT) offers the promise of normalization of function, but EEG/ERP has been used to determine whether general brain state or cognitive function indeed improved with treatment. Schneider and colleagues (2005) examined the effects of growth hormone (GH) replacement deficiency on the sleep EEG, using polysomnography in growth hormone-deficient patients. Results showed that the values for the obtained sleep parameters were similar to those for healthy individuals as reported in the literature and therefore, the authors conclude that 6 months of GH replacement therapy did not adversely affect night sleep or daytime sleep propensity (Schneider et al, 2005).

Golgeli and colleagues (2004) examined the effects of growth hormone (GH) replacement therapy on cognitive function in women with Sheehan's syndrome. Sheehan's syndrome is also known as postpartum hypopituitarism, a pituitary hormone deficiency as a result of life-threatening blood loss during or after childbirth. At baseline, amplitude and latencies of auditory oddball ERPs of patients showed longer latencies than those of controls. After 6 months of hormone replacement therapy, patients showed decreased P300 latencies compared to pre-treatment levels. The authors conclude that Sheehan's syndrome is associated with cognitive impairment as demonstrated by prolonged P300 latencies and the improvement with GH replacement. The conclusions of this study could have been strengthened if the paper had reported EEG measures in the control group as well, after a 6-month period.

In a similar study on the effects of thyroxine treatment in congenital hypothyroidism, Oerbeck and colleagues (2007), in a cross-sectional paradigm, used an auditory oddball paradigm to examine P300 and earlier cognitive (P1, N1, P2) ERP components. Significant group differences in amplitude and latency were found on early ERP components (P1, N1). P300 latency and amplitude in the congenital hypothyroidism group were negatively correlated with duration of treatment. The authors interpret these findings as suggesting that early treatment may have helped to normalize the P300 component.

These studies demonstrate the potential added value of EEG to examine treatment effects; principally the ability to register subtle changes in brain processing that may not be evident on performance tests. Most of the studies reviewed above examine the effects of treatment on the P300. Some of the paradigms above involve before and after measurements of the P300, assuming that changes in the P300 will reflect changes in treatment, an assumption which may be questionable in the absence of control group comparisons. The P300 component is strongly affected by state, and control of this factor is essential for interpretation of treatment effects.

5 Stress

Hall and colleagues (2000) examined the association between quantitative sleep measures using the EEG (spectral analysis), subjective sleep complaints, stress, and depression. Participants were fourteen individuals who were diagnosed with primary insomnia. It was hypothesized that self-reports of stress and depression would be positively correlated with measures of hyper-arousal during sleep. Hyperarousal during sleep was operationalized as subjective sleep quality as well as an increase in alpha and beta power in the EEG and a decrease in delta power. Results showed that subjective stress burden was negatively correlated with delta power and depression was associated with increased alpha power in the EEG. Intrusion tendency was positively correlated with beta power and negatively associated with subjective sleep quality. The authors point out that these results are in contradiction of previous findings suggesting a discrepancy between subjective measures of sleep and indices of sleep quality/duration derived from visual scoring of the EEG. It is suggested that traditional visual sleep stage scoring may be overestimating sleep quality and duration. The authors argue that spectral measures of EEG may be a more valid measure (Hall et al, 2000).

Frey and colleagues (2002) examined the effects of sleep deprivation and long shifts in physicians on their sleep quality and quantity, cognitive performance, perceived stress, and EEG power spectra. EEG data were collected while the participants relaxed. Data were collected twice (morning and evening) during a 24-h shift. There were two conditions: a no-rest condition and a rest condition. During the rest condition, physicians were allowed to sleep for 4 h in the afternoon. In the no-rest condition, delta power was increased from morning to evening in comparison to the rest condition, suggesting increased fatigue. No differences were found on cognitive performance tests, however (e.g., Pauli test, RT tasks). It would have been interesting to see how the self-report measures were associated with the EEG data, however, this was not reported.

These two studies show how EEG (polysomnography) can be applied to examine the relationship between sleep and stress.

6 Cancer

Electrophysiological measures have been employed in the study of various forms of cancer. The most common use of electrophysiological recording is in the assessment of patients' cognitive functioning. While some studies explicitly examine neuropsychological processing in the context of certain types of potentially neurotoxic medical treatments, others examine neuropsychological processing as a function of diagnosis alone.

Multiple studies have examined neuropsychological processing in individuals who are long-term survivors of leukemia or solid tumor malignancy. In a study comparing adolescent survivors of acute leukemias or solid tumor malignancy to control participants, both patient groups showed longer P300 latencies in response to an oddball task (Lahteenmaki et al, 2001). For the most part, there were no differences in P300 latency between patient groups or based on patient irradiation history. However, P300 latency did vary in association with time since diagnosis, age at diagnosis, and across various forms of chemotherapy treatment. These results are similar to those reported in previous research also comparing young adult survivors of leukemia and solid tumor malignancies to a control group (Heukrodt et al, 1988). In that study, both patient groups also had longer P300 latencies in an oddball task than control participants. Moreover, participants in both patient groups who experienced learning problems had longer P300 latencies than patients without learning

problems. Among leukemia patients, chemotherapy treatment and radiation effects may account for some of the variation in P300 latency. Another study explored electroencephalogram recordings of young adult survivors of childhood acute lymphoblastic leukemia (Ueberall et al, 1997). Participants who were between the ages of 2 and 5 years at diagnosis showed more electroencephalogram abnormalities than children diagnosed within other age ranges. Nonsignificant trends indicated that participants with abnormal electroencephalogram recordings may have more deficits in cognitive functioning as assessed by a neuropsychological test battery that examined the domains of attention and memory. Differences in electroencephalogram activity did not vary as a function of disease or treatment characteristics. Also, participants with abnormal electroencephalogram recordings did not appear to have morphological abnormalities as captured via magnetic resonance imaging scans. Thus, it appears that increased P300 latencies have been documented among long-term survivors of leukemia and solid tumor malignancies. Moreover, this electrophysiological index has been shown to share some association with learning problems and lesser cognitive problems.

Complementing this literature, electrophysiological recording has been used in a variety of applications. For example, in a study of women undergoing chemotherapy to treat breast cancer, asymmetry of the alpha rhythm of the electroencephalogram was found primarily in women receiving high-dose chemotherapy in comparison to women receiving low-dose chemotherapy or control participants (Schagen et al, 2001). Asymmetry refers to a difference in the preponderance of alpha waves between the right and left hemispheres of the brain. Negative affect has been associated with right-hemisphere dominance (Henriques and Davidson, 1990). Although increased P300 latency assessed via an oddball task was associated with poorer performance on a variety of neuropsychological assessments, it did not differ as a function of patient or non-patient status. Increased P300 latencies were, however, reported in a sample of adults with solid tumor malignancies (Siddiqui et al, 1992). Polysomnography research in adults with solid tumor malignancy showed decreased quantity and quality of nocturnal sleep, increased latency to the onset of rapid eye movement sleep and a decreased percentage in this stage of sleep, decreased sleep efficiency, and low levels of slow-wave sleep (Parker et al, 2008).

In sum, these studies identify electrophysiological differences in different forms of cancer with the most common finding being an increased P300 latency. This is typically seen as a cognitive deficit although concurrent cognitive assessment has often not been done. The variety of cancers, treatments, and types of patients has clearly not been fully explored. Rather these studies only support the potential utility of electrophysiological measures.

7 Immunological Disorders

The most commonly studied immunological conditions that are examined using electrophysiological methodology are hepatitis B and C and human immunodeficiency virus. However, some research has investigated the autoimmune disorder lupus (Langosch et al, 2008).

7.1 Hepatitis B and C

Electrophysiological measures have mainly been used to assess the side effects of interferon treatment on cognitive and psychological function in patients with hepatitis B and C (Tanaka et al, 2004). In one of the earliest reports of this kind, hepatitis C patients who were treated with interferon-alpha had higher delta, theta-1, and theta-2 power values, and lower alpha-2 and beta power values as measured by EEG (Kamei et al, 2002). These changes were recorded when comparing baseline values to those obtained during the course of treatment. Another study compared baseline EEG recordings and psychological functioning to that assessed at various time points during interferon treatment in hepatitis B

and C patients, abnormal EEG activity (e.g., general slowing of the basic rhythm and of the alpha wave) was associated with increased incidence of various psychological symptoms including mania, depression, and sleep disorders (Tanaka et al, 2004). This association appeared to be independent of multiple medical or treatment factors. Amodio et al (2005) confirmed the general slowing of the mean dominant frequency in hepatitis C patients and also observed increases in frontal alpha power and parietal theta power. These results, unlike those of Tanaka et al (2004), were unrelated to cognitive or other psychological factors.

This group of studies largely supports the contention that interferon treatment given to hepatitis patients influences EEG activity; however, it remains unclear what effects, if any, these changes may have on cognitive and psychological function. Variation in the precise brain indices related to treatment limit inference, but likely relate to variation in measurement, differences in instruments used, and participant differences (which were often not well described).

7.2 Human Immunodeficiency Virus and Lupus

Deficits in cognitive functioning have been the focus of EEG/ERP work on acquired immunodeficiency syndrome (AIDS) and human immunodeficiency virus (HIV). This is based on the observation of deficits on neuropsychological test performance associated with AIDS/HIV (Bungener et al, 1996). In some cases, the spectral content of the EEG is interpreted as reflecting cognitive state. In a study examining EEG activity in HIV-positive homosexual men, CD-8 cell count showed a significant positive correlation with theta, alpha, and beta wave power (Gruzelier et al, 1996). These authors also reported a trend toward decreased CD-4 cell count and increased activity in theta, alpha, and beta power. Subsequent EEG research indicates that HIV-positive patients who are symptomatic, in comparison to HIV-positive non-symptomatic patients or control participants, show increased power in the alpha and theta wave bands; after controlling for the effects of antiretroviral medication, this association appeared to persist mainly among untreated patients (Baldeweg and Gruzelier, 1997). Furthermore, while increased alpha wave amplitude in HIV-positive symptomatic patients was associated with increased rates of depressive symptoms, decreased alpha wave amplitude in HIV-positive asymptomatic patients was associated with increased rates of depressive symptoms. These results show a sensitivity of EEG waves to the disease and treatment but the authors offer little interpretation of shifts in both lower and higher frequency bands.

Other work has inferred cognitive state from ERP observed in the oddball paradigm. Chao and colleagues (Chao et al, 2004) found that HIV-positive individuals had decreased P200 and 300 amplitudes and longer P300 latencies than controls. Moreover, among HIV-positive patients, depressive symptoms were positively correlated with N1 latency. Similar slowing of components was observed by Jabbari et al (1993). Among HIV-positive patients relative to controls, they suggest that diffuse EEG slowing may be associated with increased reaction time, there may be lower amplitude of visual evoked potentials and brain-stem evoked potentials, and there may be prolonged P300 and N2 latency (Jabbari et al, 1993). The increased latency of N100 and N200 waves in the oddball task was confirmed in a sample with HIV-positive homosexual males and control participants (Bungener et al, 1996). An association was also found between decreased P300 amplitude and emotional blunting. Similarly, in a study of the chronic multisystem autoimmune disease systematic lupus erythematosus, which we will not review in great detail, results showed that patients who scored higher on a measure of emotional lability had reduced response latencies to ERP indices of pre-attentive and early orienting responses to auditory stimuli (Langosch et al, 2008). In summary, this research suggests that activation of the immune system in HIV patients may be associated with higher amplitude of slow-wave frequencies typically associated with drowsiness/inattention. This seems combined with a slowing of early ERP components in the oddball task as well as a reduction in amplitude of these and later components. The absence of performance testing, as well as some correlations with depressive symptoms, questions whether these changes are best characterized as cognitive. An impact of the disease on the brain is clearly implied, but results to date are rather non-specific and minimally interpreted.

8 Chronic Pain

A variety of chronic pain conditions including rheumatoid arthritis, low back pain, fibromyalgia, and chronic fatigue syndrome have been studied using electrophysiological measures.

8.1 Fibromyalgia

Electrophysiological research on fibromyalgia has examined sleep, pain processing, general health, and cognitive function. The diagnosis of fibromyalgia is based on diffuse pain in four body quadrants with tenderness upon palpation at certain musculoskeletal points (Landis et al, 2004). Patients often complain of sleep problems such as experiencing non-restorative, restless sleep. A small literature suggests that alpha wave sleep enduring throughout the sleep cycle may characterize chronic pain conditions, particularly fibromyalgia (Rains and Penzien, 2003). Instead of falling into a deep sleep, fibromyalgia patients may remain in a stage predominated by alpha waves, a waveform typically associated with drowsy wakefulness. Recent research has not strongly supported this observation. In a study of patients undergoing polysomnography to diagnose probable sleep disorders, a subset of patients who had abnormal alpha wave activity were identified (Rains and Penzien, 2003). Less than 40% of these patients with abnormal alpha wave activity suffered from a chronic pain condition, including fibromyalgia. Another study examined alpha wave activity in female fibromyalgia patients who were allowed to sleep undisturbed for 60 min and then were awoken throughout the night to complete a battery of memory tests (Perlis et al, 1997). Patients were categorized as high or low alpha generators based on levels of alpha wave activity recorded during the period of undisturbed sleep. High alpha fibromyalgia patients did characterize their sleep as shallow, but their alpha did not mediate memory differences among the patients. Women with fibromyalgia also appear to have less spindles per minute during non-rapid eye movement sleep than controls (Landis et al, 2004). Spindles, an indicant of transition to a deeper sleep stage, also have a slightly shorter duration among fibromyalgia patients. These results were influenced by patients' experience of pain intensity. Thus, while alpha wave activity may not be a defining feature of fibromyalgia, sleep spindles appear to show promise warranting future research.

ERP studies have asked whether pain stimuli are processed differently by fibromyalgia patients. Fibromyalgia patients, compared to control participants, have been shown to have reduced P200 wave and late positive slow-wave amplitudes during a task requiring them to categorize words as unpleasant and pain related or neutral (Montoya et al, 2005). Another study with a similar word categorization protocol failed to separate fibromyalgia and control patients despite a sensitivity to pain stimuli found in patients with recent injuries (Fossey et al, 2004). These two studies illustrate an interesting methodology, but their conflicting findings raise issues of sample size and co-occurring group differences, which were not investigated.

In addition to these studies of sleep and pain processing, electrophysiological research incorporating measures of general health has been conducted. The only study in this area found that, in comparison to control participants, fibromyalgia patients had greater latency and lower amplitude P300 recordings during an oddball task (Alanoglu et al, 2005). However, these electrophysiological findings were not related to

a measure of general health, the length of time since fibromyalgia diagnosis, or tenderness upon palpation at various musculoskeletal points.

Research regarding cognition has relied on measures of ERPs in response to oddball tasks as a marker of cognitive function (Yoldas et al, 2003). This work showed that fibromyalgia patients' N2 to P3 wave amplitudes were lower than those of control participants and their P300 latency was negatively correlated with levels of pain elicited by palpation. The authors included measures of pain perception and psychiatric function with their electrophysiological indices, providing an interesting integration of psychological and physiological variables. However, as the authors claim their results have relevance for cognitive functioning, the inclusion of a neuropsychological battery would have been particularly effective.

Potentially important differences in sleep and cognitively elicited ERP's have thus been reported for fibromyalgia patients relative to controls. Interpretation must be made very cautiously though as sample sizes were small and validity is also potentially threatened by the failure in most cases to thoroughly assess group characteristics, such as age and concomitant psychopathology, that might be as important as fibromyalgia for the results reported. Finally, while Yoldas and colleagues included measures of pain perception and psychiatric function in conjunction with electrophysiological assessment, other researchers often do not. The inclusion of psychological assessments such as these provides a richer, more integrated framework in which to interpret electrophysiological findings. As such, future research would do well to include such additional measures.

8.2 Chronic Fatigue Syndrome

Chronic fatigue syndrome is a diagnosis whose etiology remains unknown but symptoms include severe chronic fatigue, impaired short-term memory, difficulty concentrating, sore throat, tender lymph nodes, muscle pain, joint pain, headaches, un-restorative sleep, and malaise. Very little research has been conducted in this area. One study examined polysomnography recordings in this population (Scheffers et al, 1992). When comparing chronic fatigue patients, individuals with narcolepsy, and control participants, chronic fatigue patients had the highest prevalence of sleep disorders, as diagnosed via polysomnography. One study examined cognitive function in chronic fatigue syndrome patients and control participants (Yoldas et al, 2003). No group differences in the P300 and N2 components of the ERP were observed during an attention and an oddball task. Although both of these studies collected data on cognitive and psychological factors, neither examined how these measures interacted with electrophysiological findings or sample characteristics.

8.3 Rheumatoid Arthritis and Low Back Pain

A small literature has examined electrophysiological activity in the context of rheumatoid arthritis and low back pain. Regarding rheumatoid arthritis, research suggests that patients, in comparison to healthy control participants, show larger amplitude N1 and P2 responses following repetitive, painful stimulation (Hummel et al, 2000). While patients' neural responses to stimuli were significantly different from controls, patients and control participants showed similar responses as measured by a peripheral index of pain sensitivity. This was taken to indicate that central influences may play a primary role in the experience of pain in rheumatoid arthritis patients. Finally, continuous EEG recordings measured in patients with low back pain who received heat therapy showed decreased power in the beta-1 and beta-2 frequency bands in comparison to low back pain patients who received analgesic treatment (Kettenmann et al, 2007).

9 Respiratory Diseases

A small number of respiratory-related conditions have been examined with electrophysiological measures ranging from respiratory-related allergies to chemical intolerance. Major pulmonary diseases such as chronic obstructive pulmonary disease and asthma appear though to be minimally investigated. An exception to this is a study directed at using ERP to evaluate cognitive function in chronic obstructive pulmonary disease patients. Kirkil et al (2007) examined hypoxic but stable patients during an attack and when recovered, as well as controls. The P300 to the oddball in this paradigm was delayed in its onset in the constrictive pulmonary obstruction group (regardless of within or beyond an attack phase) relative to control participants. The latency of the P300 was negatively correlated with oxygen saturation and forced expiratory volume measures. The P300 results are interpreted as a cognitive effect although no performance tests were administered to validate this interpretation.

Allergic rhinitis is highly prevalent and one identified study examined how relevant medications may affect neurophysiological functioning, particularly sleepiness and alertness. Ng and colleagues (2004) failed to find any differences between first and second generation antihistamines in a study of children using a cross-over design that also included a placebo condition. The latency of the P300 in an oddball task was increased by both antihistamines relative to placebo although sleepiness/alertness ratings were unaltered. The authors suggest that the electrophysiology measures were more sensitive than ratings and should be used to determine the effects on alertness of antihistamines.

Chemical odor intolerance remains a controversial, but increasingly important clinical condition. Electrophysiological studies have provided biological assessment of differences between those reporting this intolerance relative to those that do not. Staudenmayer and Selner (1990) compared patients referred for odor intolerance, for various forms of psychopathology, or controls referred for an unrelated disease, e.g., asthma, lactose intolerance. Resting EEG was classified into patterns related to the predominance of certain frequencies of the alpha rhythm and the co-occurrence of these rhythms with the slightly slower theta rhythm. Classifications were based on EEG observed at the parietal, P4, electrode site. Classification frequencies were then compared between the three groups. These frequencies were interpreted as showing that the control group differed from both the psychologic and odor intolerant groups, but that the latter two did not differ from each other. The exact basis for the classification of the EEG patterns was unclear, as was the claim for similarity of the psychologic and odor intolerant groups (as opposed to lack of significant difference). The further controversial interpretation was made that odor intolerant patients might project psychologic problems upon environmental stimuli.

Bell et al (1998) examined the question of electrophysiological signs of chemical odor intolerance in college samples selected via questionnaire to show particularly strong or minimal intolerance. This sample was then cross-classified by the presence or absence of depressive symptoms. Spectral power in the different resting EEG bands was assessed during a pre-task period and during rest periods separating odor and cognitive stimulation. Differences in theta and beta waves were reported between groups replicating the general finding of Staudenmayer and Selner, but not using their category technique. Importantly depressive symptoms did not appear related to EEG patterns. Based on the literature and their somewhat scattered pattern of results, Bell and colleagues (1998) argue that psychological symptoms cannot explain odor intolerance and that the theta findings may indicate increased drowsiness among odor intolerant patients.

A subsequent paper by this group (Bell et al, 1999) examined community volunteers who reported chemical sensitivity either with or without associated avoidance behaviors. A similar design assessing EEG during exposure to odors and during interposed rest periods was used, but with a repeated session approximately 2 weeks after the first session. The authors note, but do not report directly, a replication of their prior resting EEG findings. The main result from this paper was a sensitization of slow wave. Delta power increased after exposure to odors, but only during the second session and only among participants with chemical sensitivity and no reported associated avoidant behavior. They also suggest that the increased delta power reflects an induction of "spaciness" in those affected.

The design of these studies of odor intolerance seems based on the assumption that the obtained EEG pattern is a biological trait that could be related to the odor intolerance of the participants. The EEG frequencies collected under resting conditions are interpreted as reflecting an arousal continuum. Arousability as witnessed by shifts in EEG power in response to either a psychologic or an odor manipulation was measured in one study (Bell et al, 1999), but the results were complex and difficult to interpret. An issue has been the psychological characteristics of these patients. Interested readers may wish to consult a review that mentions EEG but considers chemical intolerance more generally (Bell et al, 1999).

10 Kidney/Blood Diseases

Electroencephalographic measures have been used primarily in the study of the effectiveness of dialysis in the treatment of kidney failure. Frequency analysis of resting EEG as well as evoked potentials has been examined, generally with a neurological perspective, i.e., looking for general changes in frequency characteristics or changes in neural conduction times. The studies discussed later do, however, often include assessment of cognitive function and quality of life as well in part due to the dementia associated with late-stage kidney disease. EEG/ERP measures have, by and large, not correlated highly with these psychological/behavioral assessments. The studies we identified were largely clinical in scope and used relatively small patient samples. An early study by Tennyson and colleagues (1985) is illustrative.

Ten patients with chronic renal failure were assessed pre- and post- dialysis and with similarly timed tests on a non-dialysis day. A cognitive test (a digit symbol test) and an auditory oddball test using ERP's were administered on each occasion. The oddball task intermixed low probability (.2) "odd" tones with more probable (.8) standard tones with a fixed frequency and loudness. The amplitude of the P300 increased post-dialysis, but no shift in the latency of this component was demonstrated. Presumably, this was the P300 to the "odd" stimuli, but this is not clear. The latency of a number of ERP components related to changes in serum chemistry (chloride, sodium, potassium, and blood urea nitrogen) even though no pre–post changes in latency were evident. Cognitive performance did not change significantly with dialysis. Prior to treatment cognitive performance was related to individual difference in P300 latency, but changes in ERP latency and amplitude after dialysis were unrelated to changes in performance. Later work continued to examine the same question though varying the precise timing of assessments. Gallai and colleagues (1994), for example, examined the P300 and cognitive tests at the onset and offset of dialysis in a slightly larger group of patients. In their work, the P300 latency shortened, effects on amplitude were minimal, and cognitive performance improved significantly. Much more recently, Vos et al (2006) performed a quite similar study but assessed whether doubling the frequency of home dialysis for a 6-month period would yield changes in cognitive function, quality of life, and EEG (rather than ERP) characteristics. Differences between the effects of two dialysis regimens were, however, minimal – a transient change in quality of life ratings and the frequency of the EEG alpha rhythm. A similar conclusion was drawn from a study of children with two frequencies of dialysis which closely examined conduction times in a somatosensory evoked potential study (Hurkx et al, 1995). Although latency of very early EP components was delayed in these patients relative to normative data, the two dialysis regimens did not yield significant differences in conduction time or component amplitudes.

Iron deficiency anemia is another disease that is addressed by improving blood constituents. A similar scientific approach to the dialysis studies was taken in a treatment trial of oral iron therapy with both EEG and ERP (p300 measures) as outcome variables (Kececi and Degmirmenci, 2008). Pre-post measures were taken circumscribing 3 months of successful oral iron therapy in 51 patients. Over most scalp sites and for most ERP components, shortened latencies and enhanced amplitudes were observed after treatment relative to pre-treatment values. The power in EEG frequency bands all shifted toward lower frequencies except for the highest frequency (gamma) band. A subanalysis suggested that the improvements were more closely related to changes in hemoglobin rather than the changes in iron concentrations.

In sum, applications of electrophysiological measures to kidney disease have focused on the response to dialysis treatment, examining the possible remediating effects of this treatment on the dementia related to late-stage kidney disease. A neurological approach was taken, but changes were typically not striking and often more evident in later ERP components. This and the report in some studies of cognitive improvement suggest effects of dialysis on processing in cortical areas rather than on conduction pathways. A study of anemia suggested that improvement might be related to hemoglobin and the oxygen carrying capacity of the blood. Studies comparing different blood cleansing/improving treatments have not, however, convincingly demonstrated an active constituent that leads to the changes observed rather consistently in ERP components and somewhat variably in EEG spectra. Studies in this area were generally characterized by a neurological approach with standardized techniques and less attention to patient state and functional/cognitive status.

11 Health Behaviors

In contrast to disease-related studies, health-related studies using EEG were rare using our search terms. The reason for this may be that the terms were constrained to identify articles linking health behaviors and disease, while most articles in areas such as human exercise/sport, eating, alcohol, or tobacco use examine these areas without drawing inferences to disease. EEG measures appear underutilized in health behavior areas. For example, a review of studies of exercise/sport makes this point and suggests the utility of the measures (Thompson et al, 2008).

We can only illustrate the nature of the literature briefly here using smoking as an example. Early as well as later reviews have emphasized the sensitivity of electrophysiological measures both to the biological factors, such as nicotine, and to the psychological and environmental context within which smoking occurs (Hasenfratz and Baettig, 1993; Knott, 1991; Knott et al, 2008; O'Connor and Langlois, 1993). Other work examines factors related to smoking cessation, such as the surprisingly long-lasting brain changes that follow cessation in chronic smokers (Gilbert et al, 2004). A current interest is in the use of these indices as genetic endophenotypes that are suitable for understanding genetic factors in the initiation maintenance and cessation of smoking (Lerman et al, 2009; see Chapter 32).

12 Biofeedback

The field of behavioral medicine was initiated in part because of the scientific and public interest in the reported success of biofeedback as a treatment modality. Biofeedback of EEG contributed to this initial enthusiasm and continued to be an important modality for biofeedback treatment. Our search terms yielded a relatively small number of applications of EEG biofeedback to physical disease. EEG biofeedback often is offered as a relaxation technique. Indeed our review suggests that EEG biofeedback assists patients with coping with their disease, although specific changes in the EEG do not seem to mediate this.

Biofeedback has application to cardiovascular disease, but feedback of cardiovascular rather than EEG measures is more common. EEG biofeedback studies typically focus on patient stress rather than on cardiovascular outcomes. A case study by Norris and colleagues (2001) seems to typify the area and it also cites a number of excellent early reviews of EEG biofeedback. In their study a hypertensive patient is taught to increase alpha wave power in the EEG over 26 sessions. Ability to maintain appropriate blood pressure without medication as well as changes in performance and well-being were reported although these changes were not related to the EEG change over the sessions. A much larger study was directed at altering cardiac patient anxiety through enhancing beta wave (16–40 Hz) power (Michael et al, 2005). Training of the beta waves was not uniformly successful, but substantial improvements in anxiety were observed.

Biofeedback for conditions thought to relate more closely to brain function would be expected to more directly alter the disease state if successful. Our search terms again seemed to only sample this area. Siniatchkin et al (2000) provided feedback on a slow cortical potential related to attention/preparation (contingent negative variation) in a group of children with migraine and a comparison group of healthy children. Training in control of the brain wave was used, i.e., both increasing and decreasing its amplitude. Children with migraine learned more slowly than control children but were able to achieve control. The frequency and duration of migraine episodes also decreased across training, but, as with the prior studies reviewed, change in the ERP was not clearly related to the clinical outcome. A similar result was obtained with biofeedback for fibromyalgia patients. Biofeedback was successful in altering frequency/amplitude of EEG bands (Mueller et al, 2001), but the authors did not relate changes in EEG activity to reported changes in pain or psychiatric symptomatology. One study of pain was identified that did link outcomes. Miltner and colleagues (1988) used biofeedback of relatively early components of the somatosensory-evoked potential to modify pain sensations. Feedback was given to both increase and decrease the size of the peak to peak difference between negativity and positivity in the 150–260 ms time frame after the mild electrical stimulus. Control of this difference was generally achieved after a single session with decreasing of the amplitude more successful than increasing. Pain perception was also decreased during decrease training. These effects were promising, but not large and not immediately applicable to clinical issues.

In sum, biofeedback appears to have clinical utility, but this often appears to be due to non-specific effects of the treatment. Studies typically have quite small number of patients with a subset of these patients obtaining clearer benefit than the others. Given the intensive nature of biofeedback this is understandable, but it does limit interpretation. Overall, biofeedback of EEG/ERP in medical samples cannot be said to have the specific positive effects that have been reported for neurologic/psychiatric conditions, such as headache (Nestoriuc et al, 2008). An exciting use of biofeedback that may become increasing relevant is for bionics. EEG and ERP's of persons with disabilities can be used to guide external devices permitting the patients to regain functions, such as mobility and communication. Typically, patients are trained to show a particular EEG pattern that can then be used to control a "robot" executing the action associated with that brain pattern. Significant progress with this technology has been made. Our search identified one illustrative article (Cincotti et al, 2008).

13 Conclusion

Electrophysiological measures provide relatively inexpensive, sensitive indices of brain state and responsivity. As such, they could be useful additions to many behavioral medicine studies. Our review led us to suggest that the current, rather sparse literature could usefully be expanded through use of electrophysiological measures to assess affective and motivational as well as cognitive states. Such measures should be used to infer disease/health-related processes, likely in conjunction with other measures of brain processes. With some exceptions, current studies were characterized by small samples and a limited measurement/assessment approach. Future work would certainly benefit from enhanced sample size, thorough assessment of patient characteristics, well-matched controls, and careful designs. Beyond these basic concerns, more creative and conceptual application of EEG/ERP would likely be productive. Theoretical and methodological developments in the EEG/ERP field, such as dopamine models of the lateralized readiness potential, or the use of 128 electrode arrays, were largely not represented in the literature reviewed. Conceivably, these measures will be increasingly used as brain measures, such as magnetic resonance imaging, which reveal important central components of disease. These central components may then be defined more clearly using the temporal resolution and specificity of electrophysiological techniques. Research focused on affect and psychological conditions (work excluded from this chapter) has productively used advanced electrophysiological techniques and related these to imaging results. Richard Davidson and colleagues' work on positive and negative affect is illustrative of such approaches (Davidson, 2003; Davidson et al, 2007; Urry et al, 2006). Substantial progress can be anticipated from studies using such approaches and focused on processes specifically altered by a health behavior, a disease state or influenced by a therapeutic intervention.

Acknowledgments We thank Ester Saghafi, Med, MLS, for performing the literature search. We also acknowledge support provided by Pittsburgh Mind-Body Center (HL 076852 / 076858) and Training Grant HL07560.

Appendix

Below the keywords used in Ovid Medline are listed. A similar list of search terms was used in Psych Info, but due to the structure of the databases, the search terms used in Ovid Medline differed from those in Psych Info.

Electrophysiology terms:

- Electroencephalography
- Alpha rhythm
- Beta rhythm
- Cortical synchronization
- Delta rhythm
- Theta rhythm
- Polysomnography
- Evoked potentials

Disease terms:

- Disease syndrome
- Chronic disease
- Neoplasms (neoplasms or cancer)
- Musculoskeletal diseases
- Digestive system diseases
- Stomatognathic diseases
- Respiratory tract diseases
- Otorhinolaryngologic diseases
- Nervous system diseases
- Eye diseases
- Male urogenital diseases
- Cardiovascular system
- Heart (cardiology or cardiac or heart disease or cardiovascular)
- Cardiovascular diseases
- Congenital, hereditary, and neonatal diseases and abnormalities
- Endocrine system diseases
- Diabetes mellitus or diabetes
- Immune system diseases
- Female urogenital diseases
- Pregnancy complications
- Hematologic diseases
- Lymphatic diseases
- Connective tissue diseases
- Skin diseases
- Metabolic diseases
- Nutrition disorders
- Occupational diseases
- Wounds and injuries
- Surgical procedures, operative postoperative period
- Pain Surgery

Health psychology terms:

- Behavior therapy
- Behavior control
- Behavior modification
- Health behavior
- Patient compliance
- Medication adherence
- Self-examination
- Treatment refusal
- Pain management
- Exercise
- Muscle stretching exercises
- Resistance training
- Life style
- Health promotion
- Health education
- Consumer health information
- Patient education as topic
- Sex education
- Tobacco use cessation
- Smoking cessation
- Community networks
- Social support
- Social isolation
- Social problems
- Socialization
- Internal–external control
- Interpersonal relations
- Life style
- Morale
- Psychosocial deprivation
- Personality
- Assertiveness
- Authoritarianism
- Character
- Creativeness
- Dependency (psychology)
- Empathy
- Individuality
- Intelligence
- Leadership
- Machiavellianism
- Negativism
- Personality development
- Ego
- Introversion
- Self-concept

- Type a personality
- Temperament
- Emotions
- Attitude
- Attitude to death
- Attitude to health
- Adaptation, psychological
- Behavior
- Motivation
- Quality of Life
- Human activities
- Activities of daily living
- Feedback, psychological
- Orientation
- Personal autonomy
- Sleep
- Placebo effect
- Placebos

Exclusion terms:

- Substance-related disorders
- Alcohol-related disorders
- Psychotic disorders
- Schizophrenia
- Schizotypal personality disorder
- Attention deficit and disruptive behavior disorders
- Attention deficit disorder with hyperactivity
- Conversion disorder
- Brain injuries
- Traumatic brain hemorrhage
- Parkinsonian disorders
- Dementia
- Alzheimer disease
- Epilepsy
- Seizures
- Affective disorders, psychotic
- Bipolar disorder
- Depressive disorder

References

Alanoglu, E., Ulas, U. H., Ozdag, F., Odabasi, Z., Cakci, A. et al (2005). Auditory event-related brain potentials in fibromyalgia syndrome. *Rheumatol Int, 25,* 345–349.

Allen, J. J., and Kline, J. P. (2004). Frontal EEG asymmetry, emotion, and psychopathology: The first, and the next 25 years. *Biol Psychol, 67,* 1–5.

Amodio, P., Valenti, P., Del Piccolo, F., Pellegrini, A., Schiff, S. et al (2005). P300 latency for the diagnosis of minimal hepatic encephalopathy: evidence that spectral EEG analysis and psychometric tests are enough. *Dig Liver Dis, 37,* 861–868.

Andreassi, J. L. (2007). *Psychophysiology: Human Behavior and Physiological Response, 5th Ed.* Mahwah, NJ: Lawrence Erlbaum Associates Publishers.

Ayas, N. T., White, D. P., Manson, J. E., Stampfer, M. J., Speizer, F. E. et al (2003). A prospective study of sleep duration and coronary heart disease in women. *Arch Intern Med, 163,* 205–209.

Bagic, A., and Sato, S. (2007). Principles of electroencephalography and magnetoencephalography. In *Functional Neuroimaging in Clinical Populations* (pp. 71--96). New York, NY: Guilford Press.

Baldeweg, T., and Gruzelier, J. H. (1997). Alpha EEG activity and subcortical pathology in HIV infection. *Int J Psychophysiol, 26,* 431–442.

Bell, I. R., Baldwin, C. M., Fernandez, M., and Schwartz, G. E. (1999). Neural sensitization model for multiple chemical sensitivity: overview of theory and empirical evidence. *Toxicol Ind Health, 15,* 295–304.

Bell, I. R., Kline, J. P., Schwartz, G. E., and Peterson, J. M. (1998). Quantitative EEG patterns during nose versus mouth inhalation of filtered room air in young adults with and without self-reported chemical odor intolerances. *Int J Psychophysiol, 28,* 23–35.

Bungener, C., Le Houezec, J. L., Pierson, A., and Jouvent, R. (1996). Cognitive and emotional deficits in early stages of HIV infection: an event-related potentials study. *Prog Neuropsychopharmacol Biol Psychiatry, 20,* 1303–314.

Catterall, J. R., Calverley, P. M., Ewing, D. J., Shapiro, C. M., Clarke, B. F. et al (1984). Breathing, sleep, and diabetic autonomic neuropathy. *Diabetes, 33,* 1025–1027.

Chao, L. L., Lindgren, J. A., Flenniken, D. L., and Weiner, M. W. (2004). ERP evidence of impaired central nervous system function in virally suppressed HIV patients on antiretroviral therapy. *Clin Neurophysiol, 115,* 1583–1591.

Cincotti, F., Mattia, D., Aloise, F., Bufalari, S., Schalk, G. et al (2008). Non-invasive brain-computer interface system: towards its application as assistive technology. *Brain Res Bull, 75,* 796–803.

Colloca, L., Benedetti, F., and Porro, C. A. (2008). Experimental designs and brain mapping approaches for studying the placebo analgesic effect. *Eur J Appl Physiol, 102,* 371–380.

Davidson, R. J., Jackson, D. C., and Larson, C. L. (2000). Human electroencephalography. In *Handbook of Psychophysiology, 2nd Ed* (pp. 27–52). New York, NY: Cambridge University Press.

Davidson, R. J. (2003). Affective neuroscience and psychophysiology: toward a synthesis. *Psychophysiology, 40*, 655–665.

Davidson, R. J., Fox, A., and Kalin, N. H. (Eds.). (2007). *Neural Bases of Emotion Regulation in Nonhuman Primates and Humans.* New York, NY: Guilford Press.

Denolle, T., Sassano, P., Allain, H., Bentue-Ferrer, D., Breton, S. et al (2002). Effects of nicardipine and clonidine on cognitive functions and electroencephalography in hypertensive patients. *Fundam Clin Pharmacol, 16*, 527–535.

Dey, J., Misra, A., Desai, N. G., Mahapatra, A. K., and Padma, M. V. (1997). Cognitive function in younger type II diabetes. *Diabetes Care, 20*, 32–35.

Fossey, M., Libman, E., Bailes, S., Baltzan, M., Schondorf, R. et al (2004). Sleep quality and psychological adjustment in chronic fatigue syndrome. *J Behav Med, 27*, 581–605.

Frey, R., Decker, K., Reinfried, L., Klosch, G., Saletu, B. et al (2002). Effect of rest on physicians' performance in an emergency department, objectified by electroencephalographic analyses and psychometric tests. *Crit Care Med, 30*, 2322–2329.

Frier, B. M. (2001). Hypoglycaemia and cognitive function in diabetes. *Intl J Clin Pract Suppl, 123*, 30–37.

Gallai, V., Alberti, A., Buoncristiani, U., Firenze, C., and Mazzotta, G. (1994). Changes in auditory P3 event-related potentials in uremic patients undergoing haemodialysis. *Electromyogr Clin Neurophysiol, 34*, 397–402.

Gilbert, D. G., McClernon, F., Rabinovich, N. E., Sugai, C., Plath, L. C. et al (2004). Effects of quitting smoking on EEG activation and attention last for more than 31 days and are more severe with stress, dependence, DRD2 Al allele, and depressive traits. *Nicotine Tob Res, 6*, 249–267.

Golgeli, A., Tanriverdi, F., Suer, C., Gokce, C., Ozesmi, C. et al (2004). Utility of P300 auditory event related potential latency in detecting cognitive dysfunction in growth hormone (GH) deficient patients with Sheehan's syndrome and effects of GH replacement therapy. *Eur J Endocrinol, 150*, 153–159.

Gray, M. A., Taggart, P., Sutton, P. M., Groves, D., Holdright, D. R. et al (2007). A cortical potential reflecting cardiac function. *Proc Natl Acad Sci U S A, 104*, 6818–6823.

Gruzelier, J., Burgess, A., Baldeweg, T., Riccio, M., Hawkins, D. et al (1996). Prospective associations between lateralized brain function and immune status in HIV infection: analysis of EEG, cognition and mood over 30 months. *Int J Psychophysiol, 23*, 215–224.

Guilleminault, C., Stoohs, R., Shiomi, T., Kushida, C., and Schnittger, I. (1996). Upper airway resistance syndrome, nocturnal blood pressure monitoring, and borderline hypertension. *Chest, 109*, 901–908.

Hall, M., Buysse, D. J., Nowell, P. D., Nofzinger, E. A., Houck, P. et al (2000). Symptoms of stress and depression as correlates of sleep in primary insomnia. *Psychosom Med, 62*, 227–230.

Hasenfratz, M., and Baettig, K. (1993). Psychophysiological interactions between smoking and stress coping? *Psychopharmacology, 113*, 37–44.

Henriques, J. B., and Davidson, R. J. (1990). Regional brain electrical asymmetries discriminate between previously depressed and healthy control subjects. *J Abnorm Psychol, 99*, 22–31.

Heukrodt, C., Powazek, M., Brown, W. S., Kennelly, D., Imbus, C. et al (1988). Electrophysiological signs of neurocognitive deficits in long-term leukemia survivors. *J Pediatr Psychol, 13*, 223–236.

Howorka, K., Heger, G., Schabmann, A., Anderer, P., Tribl, G. et al (1996). Severe hypoglycaemia unawareness is associated with an early decrease in vigilance during hypoglycaemia. *Psychoneuroendocrinology, 21*, 295–312.

Howorka, K., Pumpria, J., Saletu, B., Anderer, P., Krieger, M. et al (2000). Decrease of vigilance assessed by EEG-mapping in type 1 diabetic patients with history of recurrent severe hypoglycaemia. *Psychoneuroendocrinology, 1*, 85–105.

Hummel, T., Schiessl, C., Wendler, J., and Kobal, G. (2000). Peripheral and central nervous changes in patients with rheumatoid arthritis in response to repetitive painful stimulation. *Int J Psychophysiol, 37*, 177–183.

Hurkx, W., Hulstijn-Dirkmaat, I., Pasman, J., Rotteveel, J., Visco, Y. et al (1995). Evoked potentials in children with chronic renal failure, treated conservatively or by continuous ambulatory peritoneal dialysis. *Pediatr Nephrol, 9*, 325–328.

Jabbari, B., Coats, M., Salazar, A., Martin, A., Scherokman, B. et al (1993). Longitudinal study of EEG and evoked potentials in neurologically asymptomatic HIV infected subjects. *Electroencephalogr Clin Neurophysiol, 86*, 145–151.

Jauch-Chara, K., Hallschmid, M., Gals, S., Schmid, S. M., Oltmanns, K. M. et al (2007). Hypoglycemia during sleep impairs consolidation of declarative memory in type 1 diabetic and healthy humans. *Diabetes Care, 30*, 2040–2045.

Kamei, S., Sakai, T., Matsuura, M., Tanaka, N., Kojima, T. et al (2002). Alterations of quantitative EEG and mini-mental state examination in interferon-alpha-treated hepatitis C. *Eur Neurol, 48*, 102–107.

Kececi, H., and Degmirmenci, Y. (2008). Quantitative EEG and congnitive evoked potentials in anemia. *Clin Neurophysiol, 38*, 137–143.

Kern, W., Peters, A., Fruehwald-Schultes, B., Deininger, E., Born, J. et al (2001). Improving influence of insulin on cognitive functions in humans. *Neuroendocrinology, 74*, 270–280.

Kettenmann, B., Wille, C., Lurie-Luke, E., Walter, D., and Kobal, G. (2007). Impact of continuous low level heatwrap therapy in acute low back pain patients:

subjective and objective measurements. *Clin J Pain, 23*, 663–668.

Kirkil, G., Tug, T., Ozel, E., Bulut, S., Tekatas, A. et al (2007). The evaluation of cognitive functions with P300 test for chronic obstructive pulmonary disease patients in attack and stable period. *Clin Neurol Neurosurg, 109*, 553–560.

Knott, V., Cosgrove, M., Villeneuve, C., Fisher, D., Millar, A. et al (2008). EEG correlates of imagery-induced cigarette craving in male and female smokers. *Addict Behav, 33*, 616–621.

Knott, V. J. (1991). Neurophysiological aspects of smoking behaviour: a neuroelectric perspective. *Br J Addict, 86*, 511–515.

Lahteenmaki, P. M., Holopainen, I., Krause, C. M., Helenius, H., Salmi, T. T. et al (2001). Cognitive functions of adolescent childhood cancer survivors assessed by event-related potentials. *Med Pediatr Oncol, 36*, 442–450.

Landis, C. A., Lentz, M. J., Rothermel, J., Buchwald, D., and Shaver, J. L. (2004). Decreased sleep spindles and spindle activity in midlife women with fibromyalgia and pain. *Sleep, 27*, 741–750.

Langosch, J., Rand, S., Ghosh, B., Sharma, S., Tench, C. et al (2008). A clinical electrophysiological study of emotional lability in patients with systemic lupus erythematosus. *J Neuropsychiatr Clin Neurosci, 20*, 201–209.

Lee, S. A., Amis, T. C., Byth, K., Larcos, G., Kairaitis, K. et al (2008). Heavy snoring as a cause of carotid artery atherosclerosis. *Sleep, 31*, 1207–1213.

Lerman, C., Perkins, K. A., and Gould, T. (2009). Nicotine dependence endophenotypes in chronic smokers. Chapter 9 in National Cancer Institute Tobacco Control Monograph No. 20, *Phenotypes and Endophenotypes: Foundations for Genetic Studies of Nicotine use and Dependence* (pp. 403–484). Bethesda, MD: U.S. Department of Health and Human Services, National Institutes of Health, National Cancer Institute. NIH Publication No. 08-6366.

Lingenfelser, T., Pickert, A., Pfohl, M., Renn, W., Radjaipour, M. et al (1993). Hypothalamic-pituitary activation does not differ during human and porcine insulin-induced hypoglycemia in insulin-dependent diabetes mellitus. *Clin Investigat, 72*, 56–59.

Lobmann, R., Smid, H., Pottag, G., Wagner, K., Heinze, H. J. et al (2000). Impairment and recovery of elementary cognitive function induced by hypoglycemia in type-1 diabetic patients and healthy controls. *J Clin Endocrinol Metab, 85*, 2758–2766.

Michael, A. J., Krishnaswamy, S., and Mohamed, J. (2005). An open label study of the use of EEG biofeedback using beta training to reduce anxiety for patients with cardiac events. *Neuropsychiatr Dis Treat, 1*, 357–363.

Miltner, W., Larbig, W., and Braun, C. (1988). Biofeedback of somatosensory event-related potentials: can individual pain sensations be modified

by biofeedback-induced self-control of event-related potentials? *Pain, 35*, 205–213.

Montoya, P., Pauli, P., Batra, A., and Wiedemann, G. (2005). Altered processing of pain-related information in patients with fibromyalgia. *Eur J Pain, 9*, 293–303.

Mueller, H. H., Donaldson, C. C., Nelson, D. V., and Layman, M. (2001). Treatment of fibromyalgia incorporating EEG-driven stimulation: a clinical outcomes study. *J Clin Psychol, 57*, 933–952.

Nestoriuc, Y., Martin, A., Rief, W., and Andrasik, F. (2008). Biofeedback treatment for headache disorders: a comprehensive efficacy review. *App Psychophysiol Biofeedback, 33*, 125–140.

Ng, K. H., Chong, D., Wong, C. K., Ong, H. T., Lee, C. Y. et al (2004). Central nervous system side effects of first-and second- generation antihistamines in school children with perennial allergic rhinitis: a randomized, double-blind, placebo-controlled comparative study. *Pediatrics, 113*, e116-e121.

Niedermeyer, E., and Lopes da Silva, F. (2004). *Electroencephalography: Basic Principles, Clinical Applications, and Related Fields* NewYork, NY: Lippincott Williams and Wilkins.

Norris, S., Lee, C. -T., Burshteyn, D., and Cea-Aravena, J. (2001). The effects of performance enhancement training on hypertension, human attention, stress, and brain wave patterns: a case study. *J Neurother, 4*, 29–44.

O'Connor, K., and Langlois, R. (1993). Situational typing and graded smoking reduction. *Psychol Rep, 72*, 747–751.

Oerbeck, B., Reinvang, I., Sundet, K., and Heyerdahl, S. (2007). Young adults with severe congenital hypothyroidism: cognitive event related potentials (ERPs) and the significance of an early start of thyroxine treatment. *Scand J Psychol, 48*, 61–67.

Parker, K. P., Bliwise, D. L., Ribeiro, M., Jain, S. R., Vena, C. I. et al (2008). Sleep/wake patterns of individuals with advanced cancer measured by ambulatory polysomnography. *J Clin Oncol, 26*, 2464–2472.

Perlis, M. L., Giles, D. E., Bootzin, R. R., Dikman, Z. V., Fleming, G. M. et al (1997). Alpha sleep and information processing, perception of sleep, pain, and arousability in fibromyalgia. *Int J Neurosci, 89*, 265–280.

Pozzessere, G., Valle, E., Decrignis, S., Cordischi, V. M., Fattaposta, F. et al (1991). Abnormalites of cognitive functions in IDDM revealed by P300 event-related potential analysis – comparison with short-latency evoked-potentials and psychometric tests. *Diabetes, 40*, 952–958.

Rains, J. C., and Penzien, D. B. (2003). Sleep and chronic pain: challenges to the alpha-EEG sleep pattern as a pain specific sleep anomaly. *J Psychosom Res, 54*, 77–83.

Rugg, M. D., and Coles, M. G. H. (1995). *Electrophysiology of Mind: Event-Related Brain Potentials and Cognition*. New York, NY: Oxford University Press.

Schagen, S. B., Hamburger, H. L., Muller, M. J., Boogerd, W., and van Dam, F. S. (2001). Neurophysiological evaluation of late effects of adjuvant high-dose chemotherapy on cognitive function. *J Neurooncol, 51*, 159–165.

Scheffers, M. K., Johnson, R., Jr., Grafman, J., Dale, J. K., and Straus, S. E. (1992). Attention and short-term memory in chronic fatigue syndrome patients: an event-related potential analysis. *Neurology, 42*, 1667–1675.

Schneider, H. J., Oertel, H., Murck, H., Pollmacher, T., Stalla, G. K. et al (2005). Night steep EEG and daytime steep propensity in adult hypopituitary patients with growth hormone deficiency before and after six months of growth hormone replacement. *Psychoneuroendocrinology, 30*, 29–37.

Siddiqui, T., Deshmukh, V. D., and Karimjee, N. (1992). Subclinical cognitive deficits in cancer patients: a preliminary P300 study. *Clin Electroencephalography, 23*, 132–136.

Siniatchkin, M., Hierundar, A., Kropp, P., Kuhnert, R., Gerber, W. D. et al (2000). Self-regulation of slow cortical potentials in children with migraine: an exploratory study. *Appl Psychophysiol Biofeedback, 25*, 13–32.

Staudenmayer, H., and Selner, J. C. (1990). Neuropsycholophysiology during relaxation in generalized, universal 'allergic' reactivity to the environment: a comparison study. *J Psychosom Res, 34*, 259–270.

Strachan, M. W. J., Ewing, F. M. E., Frier, B. M., McCrimmon, R. J., and Deary, I. J. (2003). Effects of acute hypoglycaemia on auditory information processing in adults with Type I diabetes. *Diabetologia, 46*, 97–105.

Taheri, S., Austin, D., Lin, L., Nieto, F. J., Young, T. et al (2007). Correlates of serum C-reactive protein (CRP) – no association with sleep duration or sleep disordered breathing. *Sleep, 30*, 991–996.

Tanaka, Y., Nagaki, M., Tomita, E., Murase, M., Enya, M. et al (2004). Psychoneurological symptoms during interferon therapy in patients with chronic hepatitis: prospective study on predictive use of Cornell Medical Index and electroencephalogram. *Liver Int, 24*, 407–412.

Tennyson, T. E., Brown, W. S., Vaziri, N. D., and Jennison, J. H. (1985). Event-related potential changes during hemodialysis. *Intl J Artific Organs, 8*, 269–276.

Thompson, T., Steffert, T., Ros, T., Leach, J., and Gruzelier, J. (2008). EEG applications for sport and performance. *Methods (Duluth), 45*, 279–288.

Tribl, G., Howorka, K., Heger, G., Anderer, P., Thoma, H. et al (1996). EEG topography during insulin-induced hypoglycemia in patients with insulin-dependent diabetes mellitus. *Eur Neurol, 36*, 303–309.

Ueberall, M. A., Wenzel, D., Hertzberg, H., Langer, T., Meier, W. et al (1997). CNS late effects after ALL therapy in childhood. Part II: conventional EEG recordings in asymptomatic long-term survivors of childhood ALL--an evaluation of the interferences between neurophysiology, neurology, psychology, and CNS morphology. *Med Pediatr Oncol, 29*, 121–131.

Urry, H. L., van Reekum, C. M., Johnstone, T., Kalin, N. H., Thurow, M. E. et al (2006). Amygdala and ventromedial prefrontal cortex are inversely coupled during regulation of negative affect and predict the diurnal pattern of cortisol secretion among older adults. *J Neurosci, 26*, 4415–4425.

von Kanel, R., Loredo, J. S., Ancoli-Israel, S., Mills, P. J., Natarajan, L. et al (2007). Association between polysomnographic measures of disrupted sleep and prothrombotic factors. *Chest, 131*, 733–739.

Vos, P. F., Zilch, O., Jennekens-Schinkel, A., Salden, M., Nuyen, J. et al (2006). Effect of short daily home haemoldialysis on quality of life, cognitive functioning and the electroencephalogram. *Nephrol Dial Transplant, 21*, 2529–2535.

Wager, T. D., and Nitschke, J. B. (2005). Placebo effects in the brain: linking mental and physiological processes. *Brain Behav Immun, 19*, 281–282.

Yoldas, T., Ozgocmen, S., Yildizhan, H., Yigiter, R., Ulvi, H. et al (2003). Auditory p300 event-related potentials in fibromyalgia patients. *Yonsei Med J, 44*, 89–93.

Zaregarizi, M., Edwards, B., George, K., Harrison, Y., Jones, H. et al (2007). Acute changes in cardiovascular function during the onset period of daytime sleep: comparison to lying awake and standing. *J Appl Physiol, 103*, 1332–1338.

Part IX
Statistical Methods

Chapter 54

Reporting Results in Behavioral Medicine

Michael A. Babyak

1 Introduction

The landscape of statistical analysis is evolving at an unprecedented rate. Modern computational power, channels of instant communication and dissemination, and, ultimately, dissatisfaction with conventional statistical methods have fomented a new era in terms of data analysis and methodology. Powerful new analytic approaches, important innovations in methodological standards, and even new thinking in fundamental philosophy are upon us with a breathtaking pace. These developments are quite welcome but also sobering – we (behavioral medicine and related fields) remain in many ways far behind even the older waves of innovation that preceded this newer deluge. Consequently, although the primary aim of this chapter is to discuss how to present research data, I take the opportunity to consider a number of issues dealing with data analysis per se. After all, the quality of the analysis is immutably linked to the quality of the report. My choices as to which data analysis topics to address here are admittedly idiosyncratic and obviously quite incomplete, but are based on my experience as a reviewer for many years for a wide variety of journals in psychology and medicine and also as a statistical editor for the journal *Psychosomatic*

Medicine, where a relatively large volume of manuscripts came across my desk. Although many submissions were excellent from an analytic perspective, there also were far too many with substantial problems and misconceptions, often clearly reflecting a failure to keep up with modern practice. I chose to focus my aim in the present chapter on the issues that I felt could be readily remediated without a monumental amount of retraining.

The chapter is organized to correspond roughly with the order of sections in a typical research manuscript, from background and rationale through the discussion and interpretation. Within each section I introduce what I believe are most relevant, immediately accessible topics. I do take a bit of extra time with multivariable modeling, as this technique now constitutes the vast majority of our analytic practice.

This chapter, of course, can only touch upon a limited number of topics and even then only briefly. The excellent book by Lang and Secic (2006) provides a detailed treatment of a much wider variety of topics in reporting statistics and would serve as a valued reference for anyone interested in learning more. In addition, there are several useful papers that provide an overview of common reporting problems from the perspective of journal editors and reviewers, including Harris et al (2009) and Byrne (2000). In terms of modern statistical ideas, while there are many outstanding texts on modern statistical practice, the primary influences on my own work and in terms of the present chapter is undoubtedly Harrell's regression book (Harrell, 2001). In addition to texts, there are now a

M.A. Babyak (✉)
Department of Psychiatry and Behavioral Sciences,
Duke University Medical Center, Box 3119 DUMC,
Durham, NC 27707, USA
e-mail: babya001@mc.duke.edu

A. Steptoe (ed.), *Handbook of Behavioral Medicine*, DOI 10.1007/978-0-387-09488-5_54,
© Springer Science+Business Media, LLC 2010

number of relatively widely accepted consensus guidelines for reporting the results of studies of various designs. These include, among others, CONSORT (Altman et al, 2001) for clinical trials, STROBE (Noah, 2008) for observational studies, QUOROM (Moher et al, 1999) and MOOSE (Stroup et al, 2000) for meta-analysis. The International Conference on Harmonisation of Technical Requirements for Registration of Pharmaceuticals for Human Use (ICH) (ICH, 2009), although focused on pharmaceutical trials, provides every information that behavioral medicine researchers might find helpful. In addition, the Equator Network (http://www.equator-network.org/) provides an excellent overview of reporting guidelines for health-related data. Many peer-reviewed journals now require as a matter of policy that these guidelines be followed. Further, a number of journals also have begun to implement specific "statistical guidelines" in the hope of improving and standardizing the analytic practice and reporting that they publish (Cooper et al, 2003; Freedland et al, 2005).

Finally, as you read this chapter, or any of the aforementioned texts and guidelines, I encourage the reader to be constantly mindful of the startling rate of change in these ideas. With any luck, much of what I present here, especially pertaining to the current fashion of relying almost solely on null hypothesis testing and p-values to draw conclusions about what was observed in a study, will be obsolete within the next two decades.

2 Some General Principles

Although there are far too many specific data analytic and reporting scenarios to address in a single chapter, there are some general principles that apply to virtually all that we might do analytically. They are as follows:

– State the aims of the study as explicitly as possible, including if applicable, specific hypotheses.

– Explain how the analyses address the study aims.
– Identify where the study falls along the confirmatory/exploratory continuum.
– Preserve the original measurement properties of the instrument: this includes avoiding artificial categorization of continuous variables in the analysis stage.
– Provide enough information for replication.
– Show as much of the raw data as is practical.
– Emphasize point estimates and intervals of effect size: p-values should be only a part of evaluating the scientific merit of a study finding.
– Avoid selective reporting and discussion. Many philosophers of science argue that disconfirmatory (null or those opposite of expectation) results are more important for the growth of scientific knowledge than "positive" results. If you did the test, report it. If you report it, discuss it.

Some of the above points may seem obvious or elementary, while others may be more opaque. Hopefully, in the coming pages we will reinforce the elementary points and illuminate the less obvious or familiar areas.

3 The Introduction and Background Section

Perhaps an odd place to begin a chapter on presenting results but the opening section of a research report prepares the reader for all that follows – the methods, analysis, results, and interpretation. The styles and length of this section differ considerably across disciplines and individual journals; many medical journals insist on very brief background sections, often only a very short paragraph, while journals in other disciplines, for example, psychology, tend to prefer longer introductions with an emphasis on theoretical material. Regardless of the style and length, the introductory section at a minimum should review the most relevant prior work in the area and how the present study fits with what is already known. Here the hypotheses are stated as explicitly as possible, indicating the direction and, if possible, the expected magnitudes of the hypothesized relations between the critical study variables. A simple example might be, "We hypothesize that at the end of the treatment period the Active Treatment group will score, on average, at least 4 points (0.5 standard deviations) lower than the Usual Care group on the Beck Depression Inventory." Even though our current fashion of null hypothesis testing does not easily allow for a formal test of the magnitude of difference, it is still very helpful to compare the prediction to the result by "eyeballing."

It is also useful to try and locate the study on the continuum of exploratory versus confirmatory at this point. If much is already known about a question, and the study has a strong explicit hypothesis or hypotheses with a focused set of variables under study, the study is more likely on the confirmatory side of the spectrum. On the other hand, there are times we may have only a vague intuition about what we might find and perhaps no hypotheses at all. In this case, the study is labeled as exploratory or hypotheses generating. Science needs studies across the full range of this spectrum to make progress.

The introduction section also can be used to describe briefly the implications of the range of possible findings. If positive, to what extent does this confirm or support the hypothesis given the design and previous literature? Although some authors are reluctant to do so, the introduction should also briefly entertain what a negative or "reversal" finding might mean. Making these explicit statements at the beginning provides the reader with a coherent thread that can be followed through the design, analysis, results, and interpretation.

4 The Methods Section

4.1 Design Considerations

The methods section typically begins with a section that includes a description of recruitment and, if the study compares randomized groups,

the details of the randomization procedures. Randomization procedures not only are critical to the validity and generalizability of a trial but also determine how the data should be analyzed. Randomization of study participants should be carried out using concealment, or what is often referred to as blind allocation, that is, no one involved in the decision to enroll a patient should have foreknowledge of the next treatment assignment. In fact, the randomization procedure should be designed such that the staff cannot even guess as to what the next assignment would be. Studies have shown that when study staff members are aware of the impending treatment assignment, subtle (and at times not so subtle) biases can be introduced (Schulz and Grimes, 2002). Imagine, for example, that a potential participant in relative fragile health arrives to be evaluated for inclusion in a trial. If the evaluator is aware that the next assignment is to the active treatment arm, they may be subtly or unconsciously inclined to reject the candidate. In addition to blind allocation, assessment at all phases of the study also should be blind to treatment condition if at all possible for obvious reasons. Remaining blind to treatment assignment during assessment is often challenging in behavioral treatment studies because some assessments may naturally elicit responses that reveal the treatment assignment to the evaluator. Of course, in behavioral treatment studies, it is impossible for study participants to be blind to their treatment condition.

If the study is sufficiently large, randomization usually manages to create reasonable baseline balance on background characteristics across treatment arms, thus minimizing concerns about confounding. When the study is relatively small, however, around $N < 200$, random imbalances may occur across treatment arms (Lachin, 2000), which in turn may bias the estimate of the treatment effect. If the imbalances are not large, covariate adjustment at the analytic stage is sufficient to produce unbiased treatment effect estimates. Some researchers choose to avoid risking the possibility of large baseline imbalances by adopting stratified sampling. In stratified sampling, the researcher identifies a small set of background characteristics that may be of particular concern in terms of confounding, for example, gender and age. The potential sample is divided into a set of subgroups based on the characteristics of interest. For example, if age and gender are the stratification variables, four subgroups might be identified: younger women, younger men, older women, and older men (age must be artificially categorized here). A separate randomization list is then created for each subgroup, ensuring that the number of participants assigned to each treatment arm is equivalent within each subgroup.

In practice, because the number of subgroups increases exponentially as the number of stratification factors increase, more than a few factors can quickly become unwieldy and often impractical. In addition, imbalances may still arise on other variables not in the stratification scheme. Pocock and Simon (1975) offer an alternative procedure called minimization. Briefly, minimization evaluates imbalance "on the fly," estimating the imbalance that would result from assignment of a new participant to a given treatment arm. Minimization has the advantage of being able to manage a relatively large number of background variables.

A final thought with respect to design concerns clustered observations. Clustered observations occur when there is a natural correlation among members within a subgroup, such as within a family or treatment site. Studies that include clustered observations, sometimes even randomizing at the cluster level, have become increasingly common (Bland, 2004). Failure to account for the clustering, even in the case of relatively weak within cluster correlations, can distort the standard errors used for testing and interval estimation. The correct standard errors can be generated using modern techniques available in mixed models (for example, Littell et al, 2006) or using special procedure such as the Huber–White sandwich (robust variance) estimator (Williams, 2000).

4.2 Describing Measures

It is not possible to fully evaluate the results of statistical analyses without knowing the measurement properties of the variables involved. For one, the reliability of a measure can have a direct influence on the effect size estimate, with lower reliability attenuating the estimate (Cohen et al, 2002). Measures should be described in terms of content and measurement properties. Describe exactly what the instrument is presumed to measure and include precedents showing that it has been used in similar settings. This latter issue is a special challenge in behavioral medicine, where some measurement instruments may not have been used extensively in the special populations that we often study. For example, a self-report measure of anxiety may have been used frequently in clinical psychiatric samples, but perhaps only rarely, if ever, used for patients with pulmonary disease. The psychometric properties established for the instrument in the psychiatric population may be less desirable in the pulmonary population, which would have important implications in interpreting the results of analyses based on that instrument. Further, the measurement properties for an instrument may be quite different across ethnic or cultural groups (Whitfield et al, 2008).

Report the potential range of each measure and how to interpret the scores, for example, "scores can range from 1 to 40, with higher scores indicating poorer neuropsychological performance." If available, indexes of reliability and validity should be presented. For self-report instruments, internal consistency (alpha) and test–retest reliability are the most commonly used reliability coefficients. A common error in reporting reliability is to confuse an internal consistency index, such as Cronbach's alpha, with a measure of unidimensionality. Alpha, in fact, has very little to do with how many dimensions underlie a psychometric scale. It is easy to show that a scale with many underlying dimensions can still have a high alpha coefficient (Green et al, 1977). Factor analytic techniques are the more appropriate choice for assessing dimensionality. For diagnostic tests, inter-rater reliability and sensitivity/specificity should be reported. Indicate clinically or theoretically meaningful values for the scale. For examples, "scores of 14 or greater on the depression scale are typically interpreted as indicating clinically significant levels of symptoms." I emphasize here, however, that although clinical cutpoints are necessary in the clinic, and potentially important in interpreting the analyses, they have virtually no useful place in the data analysis phase of a study. Statisticians have been pleading with scientists for decades to avoid cutting up continuous variables (Cohen, 1983; Peters and van Voorhis, 1940), yet the practice persists. The problems created by making artificial categories are manifold and well-documented, including loss of power in univariate analyses, increased type I error in multivariable models, loss of ability to detect nonlinearity, vulnerability to residual confounding (see for example, MacCallum et al, 2002; Maxwell and Delaney, 1993; Royston et al, 2006). Cutpoints can be useful for descriptive purposes, for example, to show how the sample data compare with widely accepted clinical groupings (or with prior studies that commit the categorization error), but they are a potential source of serious distortion in the analytic phase of a study. The argument is often made that cutpoints were used in the analysis because they are used in clinical decision-making or that they are based on published clinical practice guidelines (for example, definitions of hypertension or obesity). This position, however, puts the cart far before the horse. Clinical cutpoints can be made with far greater reliability based on data that have been analyzed using the full, continuous form of a measure. It is literally impossible to evaluate the tenability or usefulness of cutpoints if the cuts are made before the analysis.

4.3 The Analytic Plan

The trend for journals to reduce the space allocated to the analytic plan or to put it in smaller font type is contrary to the spirit of good scientific reporting. The analysis section, like the methods section of any good scientific report, is meant not only to describe what was done but also to supply enough detail to allow the methods to be replicated entirely by a competent independent party. Fortunately, with the advent of widespread access to the Internet, many technical details can now be made available in an online appendix. The movement toward increased transparency of research practice and sharing of technology, especially for publically funded research, has also resulted in increased sharing of annotated programming code for all analyses in such appendices (Rossini and Leisch, 2003). By providing this code with annotation, the interested reader can fully evaluate what assumptions were made about the analysis and how they were (or were not) dealt with. In addition, posting code allows an extra layer of quality control over scientific results.

In the data analysis section, the full analytic approach is laid out in the context of the study questions. The statistical models should be completely spelled out, preferably in equation form, accompanied by an explanation of how each model relates to the hypotheses. A simple example might be, "the primary hypothesis that weight loss, adjusted for age, would be associated with a clinically meaningful reduction in systolic blood pressure will be tested using a general linear model, with the form blood pressure $= a + b_1 \times$ weight loss $+ b_2 \times$ age, where a is the intercept, b_1 and b_2 are the regression weights." If there are many analyses or models, things can get quite tangled in a reader's mind pretty quickly. In these cases, it may be helpful to include a table, flowchart, or list to display how the analyses were organized.

Include the software and specific procedure within the software package used for each analysis. For example, "Cox proportional hazards models were estimated using the survreg package available in R (http://cran-r.org)." If any special algorithms were developed for the analyses that were not part of the standard software, the algorithm should be made available in an appendix. If intellectual property rights to the algorithm are not clear, provide at least a general description of the function. Finally, describe how the assumptions of the model were tested and what was done if the assumptions were not met. For example, "We examined model assumptions, including linearity, influential observations, additivity, and homoscedastic residuals using the techniques outlined by Harrell. When an assumption was violated, we modified our analyses accordingly, as described in the results section."

The description of the analytic plan also includes any special preprocessing of measures, such as collapsing of sparse cells, rescaling or transformation, and how outliers were evaluated and managed. A common misconception in preprocessing is that all variables must be normally distributed. Very few modern analytic procedures assume or require a variable to be normally distributed. In fact, for a variable on the predictor side of a regression model there is no distributional assumption at all (of course, we hope the predictor has sufficient range and variability, or prevalence). In Gaussian-based models, such as multiple regression or the general linear model, the critical assumption is that the *residuals* of the model are normal. Often, when the response variable (the criterion or dependent variable) in the regression is not normally distributed, the residuals also will not be normally distributed, but this is not always the case. Conversely, a normally distributed response variable does not guarantee that the residuals will be normally distributed. The best approach, therefore, is to examine the residuals carefully regardless of the distribution of the response variable. Of course, there are also now many modern modeling approaches that can accommodate a number of non-normal error distributions, such as the generalized linear model (McCullagh and Nelder, 1989).

A special case of preprocessing data occurs when data are missing. If the proportion of missing cases is very small (<5%) or the reason for missingness is completely random, it is possible to delete the case with the missing value or to use simple mean or median substitution without introducing much bias (Harrell, 2001). It is more often the case, however, that data are missing in some systematic way. For example, participants who are more depressed, sicker, older, or more hostile might be more prone to having missing data points. In cases where the missing data mechanism is systematic, modern practice almost uniformly discourages deleting

cases with missing data; instead we now prefer to use the special methods available for preserving cases with missing data. These methods usually involve a modeling or resampling technique to impute several possible values for the missing data point (or points). A series of new data sets are generated, each containing a different set of plausible guesses at what the missing data points might be. A separate analysis is then performed on each data set, and the results of the analyses are averaged to yield a single final result (Little and Rubin, 2002). In addition to allowing cases with missing data to be used in the analysis, multiple imputation also incorporates information about the fact that the missing data point was only estimated and not observed. Simpler methods, such as substituting the mean or median for a missing value, fail to take this uncertainty into account and can lead to standard errors that are too small (and hence p-values that are too small). Intuitively, it may seem that imputation of missing data is "making data up." There is ample evidence, however, that compared to the conventional approach of deleting cases with missing data from the analysis, imputation produces less biased estimates of the effect of interest (Little and Rubin, 2002). The methods section should include a description of the specific method for dealing with missing data. Later, in the results section or in an appendix, the frequency and patterns of missing data should be described. For a very accessible and practical introduction to missing data methods, see McKnight and colleagues (2007).

The proper management of missing data is especially important in clinical trials, where the intent-to-treat (ITT) principle (Lachin, 2000) has become the standard. ITT requires that the primary analysis of the treatment effect includes all study participants who were randomized, regardless of their actual level of participation in the trial after randomization. An ITT includes even those participants who dropped out of the study immediately after randomization. Thus, ITT requires that we must somehow find a way to include in the analysis participants with missing data on outcomes. Lachin (2000) notes that unless data are missing completely at random (that is, there is no systematic reason for missingness, such as age, illness severity), simple approaches such as last-observation-carried forward and even some of the more sophisticated modern methods for handling missing data, such as random effects models and generalized estimating equations, may not remove bias created by missing data. When there are systematic mechanisms underlying missingness, the aforementioned multiple imputation (Little and Rubin, 2002) or special applications of finite maximum likelihood (Enders, 2006) are preferred.

In contrast to ITT is the so-called per-protocol or efficacy subset analysis, in which the analysis includes only participants who are deemed adherent to the treatment. ITT analysis answers the broad policy question, "What is the estimated benefit for anyone walking into the clinic room and being prescribed a given treatment, irrespective of adherence?" In contrast, per-protocol answers the question, "If the participant did complete the protocol as desired, what is the treatment effect?" Although the per-protocol question seems perfectly reasonable, there are a number of reasons for preferring ITT to per-protocol. Foremost among these reasons is that ITT minimizes bias due to differential dropout. Consider, for example, a two-group trial comparing an active treatment group to a placebo. Imagine that the experimental treatment creates untoward side effects in a particularly vulnerable group of participants, such as those who were more severely ill at study entry. Those side effects could cause those sicker participants in the active treatment arm to drop out before completing the study. Participants in the control group with comparable levels of illness severity, however, would not have experienced those side effects and would be more likely to stay in the study. Thus, at the end of the study, the participants in the treatment arm would be, on average, healthier than those in the control arm solely due to differential dropout. The estimate of the treatment effect would therefore be too optimistic. More broadly, dropout has the effect of spoiling the randomization, which of course would render any analysis suspect. Interestingly, contrary

to popular belief, ITT is not always more conservative than per-protocol in terms of identifying a treatment effect (Lachin, 2000). One potential means of better answering the question that naïve per-protocol analysis attempts is Rubin's complier average causal effect (CACE) model (Little and Rubin, 2000). The technical details of the CACE model are beyond the scope of this chapter, but the broader concept is to identify the background characteristics of the subset of study participants who adhered to the protocol and then find participants in the control group who are similar on those background characteristics and then perform the comparison on the two subsets. Borman and Dowling (2006) have recently published a study that provides an accessible example of how the CACE model might be applied.

4.4 The Confirmatory Versus Exploratory Continuum

Returning to the more general topic of inference and design, a study may contain a combination of both confirmatory and exploratory analyses. There should be a clear statement distinguishing any exploratory analysis from those planned before the data were collected. Exploratory analyses can take a variety of forms, including those planned before data collection, but whose rationale is somewhat speculative, and also those decided upon after examining the data. If exploratory analyses were carried out, describe them in as much detail as possible, particularly why those particular analyses were selected. A typical exploratory analysis might take the form of repeating an analysis on particular subgroups of the original sample. See below for a discussion of "subgroup analyses."

Exploratory analyses play an important part of the scientific process, but do not represent the same strength of evidence in terms of inference compared to confirmatory analyses. Unfortunately, we have developed a scientific culture in which investigators are reluctant to label a finding as preliminary or to report a result with a non-significant *p*-value. This norm must change if we are to gain all we can from our data. All data provide information. Our role as scientists is to ensure that we interpret it in the context of what we know about the strength of the inference.

4.5 Statistical Power

Particularly in the present era when conventional *p*-values are still used to evaluate the success or failure of a hypothesis test, provide a full description of how the sample size and power were determined. The description should include the level of alpha, power, sample size, effect size, and any other assumptions about the data, such as attrition, drop-in (such as when a patient in a control or usual care group decides to find additional treatment), missing data, and the inclusion of adjustment covariates. Effect size estimates from pilot studies are rarely sufficiently stable to use in a power analysis (Kraemer et al, 2006). In addition, depending on the statistical methodology, even effect sizes reported in larger studies are often overly optimistic (see Steyerberg, 2009) and should not necessarily be used as a firm guide as to what a desirable effect size might be. Instead, a power analysis should be based on what a clinically or theoretically meaningful effect would be for the outcome variable. In other words, design the study with enough power to detect an effect of the size you would not want to miss.

The power section is also a natural place for presenting how multiplicity (control of type I error due to multiple hypothesis testing) will be addressed. If no correction is made for multiplicity, we must justify this choice. Power analyses also should be reported for observational studies, including secondary analyses of existing data sets (Noah, 2008). In this latter case, although the sample size is already fixed, it is important to know whether that sample size would afford the power to detect a meaningful effect size. If the sample size is not large enough, there may be a

need to revisit the analytic plan or the design, or even to abandon the study.

5 The Results Section

5.1 Describing the Sample

For clinical trials, the CONSORT guidelines suggest presenting a flowchart of the number of participants throughout the various phases of data collection, from the earliest screening and recruitment to the final analysis. Indicate the number of patients who remained in the study at each phase of the study, along with the number who were no longer included and the reasons for exclusion or dropout. The flowchart should include the number of study participants who had complete data and also the number who were included in the final analysis. Good examples of the CONSORT flowchart can be found in any issue of *JAMA*, which requires them for all clinical trial reports.

After the flowchart and narrative description of the participant flow, the conventional "Table 1" can be presented. This table should include the demographic characteristics of the sample and any other baseline variables that will aid the reader in judging the generalizability of the study to other populations. For some studies, where there are clearly defined groups, such as treatment arms in a clinical trial, or comparison of men and women, or individuals with and without a diagnosis, the descriptive table can be broken out by those groups, along with a final column summarizing the entire cohort. For categorical variables, present the number of participants in a given category along with the percentage that the number represents with respect to the group. For quantitative variables with reasonably normal distributions, present the mean and standard deviation; if the distribution is skewed or asymmetric, present instead the median and interquartile range. When comparing randomized groups, the CONSORT statement discourages the use of hypothesis tests for baseline balance across the groups (Senn, 2008, p. 98), although there are some who dissent from this view (Berger, 2005). The use of hypothesis tests to compare groups in observational studies is less controversial, but one must be mindful that if those variables are used together later in a multivariable model, they may behave quite differently in that model compared to how they behaved in a so-called univariate analysis. As we will discuss a bit later, we should avoid the temptation to use the p-values from the table as a criterion of inclusion in a subsequent multivariable model (Harrell, 2001).

Finally, as a general rule, not just for the first table but throughout the report, round, round, and round some more (Wainer, 1992). Rounded values can convey their meaning far more immediately than values carried to many decimal places. It also may make no scientific sense to report, for example, blood pressure to the third decimal place when the margin of error in the measurement is at least several whole millimeters of mercury. Lang and Secic (2006) suggest that there is rarely an instance where more than three decimal places are necessary in medical studies. Lang and Secic are also quick to point out, however, that the rounding should take place only in presentation, not in the statistical analysis.

There is some disagreement about the level of precision of p-values. Some authorities suggest reporting p-values to the second decimal place. Others, however, suggest using three places in order to allow meta-analysts to recover effect sizes more easily. There is agreement that p-values that are below 0.001 should be reported as <0.001. Many researchers seem to believe that small p-values somehow make the result "extra significant." This, of course, is not true, as the magnitude of a p-value is influenced not only by the observed effect size but also by the sample size of the study and the variability and reliability of the measures under consideration. In all other cases, regardless of whether the p-value is considered "significant," p-values should be reported exactly and not as a comparison to a critical value. For example, report $p = 0.030$ rather than $p < 0.05$.

5.2 Primary Results

Virtually all authoritative sources suggest that the first result reported should be the primary hypothesis tests, followed by supportive or secondary analyses (Lang and Secic, 2006). Presenting the most impressive result first based on significance or effect size regardless of the original analytic plan may give the false impression that these handsome results were tests of the primary hypotheses, which, of course, may or may not be true. It is well known that the sampling distribution, and hence the type I error rate, is very different for a large number of tests compared to a few prespecified tests (Maxwell and Delaney, 2004). Reporting effects based on their impressiveness rather than on the prespecified analytic plan is a form of selective reporting. In order to address the problem of selective reporting, some journals now require that the original analysis plan, for example, the funding application, be submitted or made available along with the manuscript.

5.3 Secondary Outcomes and Analyses

After the tests of the primary hypotheses are presented, additional analyses can be included. These latter analyses should be clearly labeled as secondary or exploratory. Secondary analyses may be prespecified or post hoc. Prespecified secondary analyses may, for example, include analyses of the primary outcome using a less well-known measure or experimental assessment device or additional measures that build a more comprehensive picture of the effects of a treatment. These latter types of analyses are sometimes referred to as "supportive" analyses. For example, in a clinical trial of hypertension, blood pressure may be the primary outcome, but the treatment effect on other measures of cardiovascular health or cardiovascular risk factors would be of interest and help flesh out the full impact of the treatment. These analyses might even include formal tests of prespecified mediators that explain the mechanism underlying the treatment effect. Secondary analyses also might include more exploratory post hoc information. One typical kind of exploratory analysis is examining subgroups after a primary analysis has been conducted. Subgroup tests are highly controversial and generally discouraged by statisticians, and for a number of good reasons (Assmann et al, 2000). Among these reasons, the two most important are the inflated error rate and the differential power of the tests. Conducting many tests of any kind inflates the type I error rate. Correction for multiple testing in these cases can be of some help, but unless the study was designed specifically for the subgroup test, the power can and usually will be quite different for different subgroups. Hence, some subgroup tests will have more power than others, making it virtually impossible to manage the error rate coherently. If subgroup tests are of interest, the sampling plan must take them into account before the study is carried out to ensure adequate and consistent power across them. The inferences from pre-planned subgroup analyses are, of course, more robust than those which arose from post hoc analyses. If the design did not take these tests into account, subgroup analyses should either not be conducted at all or should be interpreted as highly preliminary.

Finally, if we do choose to carry out subgroup analyses, the preferred approach is to test the corresponding interaction term rather than to examine subgroups separately (Altman and Bland, 2003; Altman and Matthews, 1996; Matthews and Altman, 1996a, b). (There are also Bayesian methods, which may overcome some of the problems with conventional subgroup analyses [see Dixon and Simon, 1992; Simon, 2002].) For example, if one is interested in whether a treatment is more effective in one ethnic group than another, the proper test is a treatment group by ethnicity interaction term. Conducting separate within-group analyses for each group is prone again to the problem of differential power and also does not exploit the information from the entire sample when

estimating standard errors (and hence p-values and confidence intervals are incorrect). In a multivariable model setting, when more than one interaction term is of interest, the error rate can be minimized by entering all the interaction terms of interest in the model as a block simultaneously and testing the change in model fit associated with the block (Cohen et al, 2002; Harrell, 2001). If the test of the entire block is not significant, then the individual interaction terms are interpreted as inconclusive or noise. I add a reminder here that in most statistical models nowadays all lower order component terms must be included in the model with a higher order term such as interaction. For example, if we are testing a treatment group by ethnicity interaction, we also must include the treatment group and ethnicity main effects – otherwise the interaction term is not really interpretable as an interaction in the conventional sense of the concept.

Finally, for all results, include measures of effect size and not just p-values. For group differences, effect sizes can be reported in the form of standardized differences, such as "Cohen's δ," which is simply the group difference divided by the pooled standard deviation[1] (Cohen et al, 2002). For regression-type models, partial r^2 values or properly scaled regression coefficients, odds ratios, and hazard ratios provide immediately meaningful indexes of effect size.

5.4 Some Specific Cases

In the sections below, I will present suggestions for reporting in some of the most frequently encountered situations. These include the reporting of group means as is often encountered in a clinical trial and also reporting the results of multivariable models, including multiple regression, logistic regression, and survival

[1] There are many variations of this type of effect size. See, for example, Johnson and Eagly (2000).

analysis. In the section on modeling I also include a brief discussion of predictor scaling, sample size, and the distinction between a confounder and a mediator.

5.4.1 Group Means or Frequencies

Some studies are designed to compare groups on a measure of central tendency, such as a mean or a median. One question immediately arises: a table or a figure? There are proponents of each approach. My own view is decidedly noncommittal: it depends. I tend to generate both and decide which conveys the result in the clearest, most intuitive, and *most memorable* fashion. I will discuss tables and figures more generally in a separate section that follows. If a table is presented to display group means, present the means along with a measure of variability for each group. The table should include the number of participants that were used for a given analysis. If space permits, both raw means and model-based means should be shown. Showing the raw means provides the reader with some sense of what the raw data looked like; presenting model-generated values is important because these are the values upon which the actual hypothesis tests and confidence intervals are based. For unadjusted means, the standard deviation is a suitable index of variability. Despite its use in many medical journals, the use of "+/–" for the standard deviation is inappropriate, as the standard deviation is not an interval, but a single estimate of variability. Instead enclose the standard deviation value in parentheses. For adjusted or fitted means, present the 95% confidence interval rather that the standard error of the mean, the latter having no immediate intuitive interpretation. Since the central aim of comparing groups is to show differences between groups, why make the reader do the mental calculation? Report the differences directly in the table, along with 95% CI of the difference in the same table. If *p*-values are required, include them along with the degrees of freedom for the test. Annotate the table, explaining how the means were generated,

for example, "fitted means were generated from a general linear model using multiple imputation and are adjusted for covariates, *x*, *y*, *z*." The text should summarize what is in the table, not repeat it. Of course, the arithmetic mean is not always the best measure of central tendency and may in fact not represent at all what is really "happening" with the data. With variables whose distributions are skewed, the median, or one of several special types of means (Wilcox, 1998), or even ranks (LaVange and Koch, 2006) might be preferred. If the values to be reported are counts (frequencies), report the raw values along with the proportion or percentage that the value represents and, critically, tell the reader explicitly what the denominator was for calculating the value. Table 54.1 was created using Harrell's summary function in the R software package (http://biostat.mc.vanderbilt.edu/twiki/pub/Main/StatReport/summary.pdf) and displays one way in which group data can be displayed. In this case, the values for continuous measures are the median (in bold) surrounded by the 25th and 75th percentile, while the values for count data are displayed as group percentages, including the fraction used to calculate the percentage.

5.4.2 Multivariable Models: Some General Considerations

In this section I discuss a few ideas regarding several types of multivariable models that are very frequently encountered in behavioral medicine research, including multiple regression, logistic regression, and time-to-event models. I do not, however, address the relatively vast topics of structural equation models and mixed or hierarchical linear models, under which are subsumed a very large array of approaches, including confirmatory factor analysis, path analysis, partial least squares, growth curve modeling. For further information on these latter models, see Chapters 56, 57, and 58).

Multivariable models are now among the most frequently reported analyses in behavioral medicine and we will thus spend a bit more time with them than other types of analyses.

Table 54.1 Descriptive statistics by mental stress ischemia

	N	No ischemia N = 112	Ischemia N = 26	Combined N = 138	Test statistic
Age, years	138	56 **62** 71	51 **60** 69	55 **62** 70	$F_{1,136}=0.5, p=0.5^1$
Gender	138				$\chi^2_1=0.3, p=0.6^2$
Men		71% $\frac{79}{112}$	65% $\frac{17}{26}$	70% $\frac{96}{138}$	
Ethnicity	138				$\chi^2_2=7, p=0.03^2$
African American		15% $\frac{17}{112}$	31% $\frac{8}{26}$	18% $\frac{25}{138}$	
Caucasian		81% $\frac{91}{112}$	58% $\frac{15}{26}$	77% $\frac{106}{138}$	
Other ethnicity		4% $\frac{4}{112}$	12% $\frac{3}{26}$	5% $\frac{7}{138}$	
Education	138				$\chi^2_2=2, p=0.4^2$
High school or less		29% $\frac{32}{112}$	27% $\frac{7}{26}$	28% $\frac{39}{138}$	
Some college		35% $\frac{39}{112}$	23% $\frac{6}{26}$	33% $\frac{45}{138}$	
College or more		37% $\frac{41}{112}$	50% $\frac{13}{26}$	39% $\frac{54}{138}$	
Hypertension	138	54% $\frac{60}{112}$	58% $\frac{15}{26}$	54% $\frac{75}{138}$	$\chi^2_1=0.1, p=0.7^2$
Diabetes	138	19% $\frac{21}{112}$	38% $\frac{10}{26}$	22% $\frac{31}{138}$	$\chi^2_1=5, p=0.03^2$
Current smoking	138	12% $\frac{14}{112}$	12% $\frac{3}{26}$	12% $\frac{17}{138}$	$\chi^2_1=0.02, p=0.9^2$
Quit smoking	138	64% $\frac{72}{112}$	58% $\frac{15}{26}$	63% $\frac{87}{138}$	$\chi^2_1=0.4, p=0.5^2$
Past myocardial infarction	138	56% $\frac{63}{112}$	58% $\frac{15}{26}$	57% $\frac{78}{138}$	$\chi^2_1=0.02, p=0.9^2$
Past revascularization	138	45% $\frac{50}{112}$	46% $\frac{12}{26}$	45% $\frac{62}{138}$	$\chi^2_1=0.02, p=0.9^2$
Total cholesterol, mg/dL	136	160 **180** 205	166 **183** 197	161 **180** 201	$F_{1,134}=0.05, p=0.8^1$
LDL, mg/dL	136	87 **97** 124	88 **114** 125	87 **98** 125	$F_{1,134}=0.4, p=0.5^1$
HDL, mg/DL	136	39 **45** 54	35 **40** 47	38 **44** 52	$F_{1,134}=6, p=0.02^1$
Triglycerides, mg/dL	136	102 **141** 211	100 **138** 166	102 **140** 210	$F_{1,134}=0.02, p=0.9^1$
LVEF at rest, %	138	51 **58** 66	51 **56** 63	51 **57** 65	$F_{1,136}=0.1, p=0.7^1$

a represents the lower quartile, b the median, and c the upper quartile for continuous

N is the number of non-missing values

Tests used: [1]Wilcoxon test; [2]Pearson test

A few general words about multivariable models to start, starting with a little tidying up of nomenclature. The term "multi*variate*" is often used incorrectly to describe regression models with more than one predictor. "Multi*variate*" really refers to a class of models that have more than one response, or dependent variable. "Multi*variable*" is a more precise term for models with one response variable and several predictors.

One important aim of multivariable models is to generate predictions for clinical or theoretical use. In this application, the notion of overfitting (Babyak, 2004) is particularly important. Broadly speaking, overfitting is the problem of trying to squeeze more predictors in a model than the data will really support. As you increase the number of predictors, the role of chance increases – some variables will look like good predictors owing merely to random sampling error, thus leading to what looks like a good prediction. The more predictors you enter, the more likely the model will include some of these spuriously good-looking predictors. Overfitting and the larger related problem of variable selection are topics worthy of an entire book. Indeed, large portions of the texts by Harrell (2001) and Steyerberg (2009) are devoted to this topic. As a general rule of thumb, one should not use p-values, especially the conventional $p < 0.05$ criterion, to determine which variable to include in a multivariable model. Thus, if one wants to avoid an overfitted and hence unreliable "final" model, it is probably best to avoid univariate pre-screening and certainly the so-called automated selection techniques, unless special steps are taken to validate the procedures and to correct the estimates to account for all of the variables that were screened for inclusion (Greenland, 2000; Moons et al, 2004; Tibshirani, 1997; Ye, 1998). Unless the sample size is extremely large, we are almost always better off developing a multivariable model by selecting predictors based on prior knowledge.

As noted above, power and sample size estimates are typically generated to allow a false null hypothesis to be rejected at a given rate or to ensure that confidence intervals are sufficiently narrow for a reasonable scientific conclusion to be drawn. Sample size also plays an important role in ensuring that multivariable models produce reproducible results. Again, this issue is discussed in great detail in the Harrell (2001) and Steyerberg (2009) texts. The sample size requirements in this regard differ depending on the type of model. Generally speaking, the rule of 10–15 cases per predictor under study seems to be supported by several simulation studies (Concato et al, 1995; Peduzzi et al, 1996). However, what is often not understood is that what counts as a "case" differs depending on the model (Harrell, 2001). In a multiple regression model, which assumes a continuous outcome and normally distributed errors, each individual observation may be counted as a case. In other words, if there are 200 individuals with data on the measures under study, it is safe to study about 13–20 variables in the model. (In more precise terminology, we can use about 13–20 degrees of freedom in the model.) For logistic regression models, in which the outcome is a binary variable, the effective sample size is the count of events or nonevents, whichever is the smaller number of the two. For example, if there are 200 individuals in the sample, and 20 had an event, the effective sample size is 20, not 200, and at best 2 variables can be studied with reasonable confidence. If there were 180 events rather than 20, the effective sample size would still be 20. In more technical parlance, the number of cases in a logistic regression model with a binary response is $min(q, n - q)$, where min represents "the minimum of the following quantities," q is the number of events, and n is the total sample size. For survival models, where time-to-event is the outcome, the effective sample size is the number of events. Again, if there are 1000 cases, but only 10 events, the effective sample size is 10. As is true of all rules of thumb, these are only general guidelines, and in certain circumstances, such as models where the primary focus is on a predictor that is expected to have a very large effect size or that has been studied fairly extensively already, the sample size requirements may be smaller (Vittinghoff and McCulloch, 2007).

Nevertheless, unless data are very expensive to collect or process, more is always better.

As already discussed in the measures section, we generally want to avoid making artificial categories out of continuous variables. Some scientists prefer making categories because the resulting regression coefficients are easily interpreted as the expected value of the response variable for one category compared to another. However, as described earlier, the distortions introduced by categorizations may not be worth easier interpretation. It is something like the intoxicated man crawling on his hands and knees in the alley under the streetlight looking for his lost car keys. A friend comes by to ask the hapless man where he thinks he might have dropped the keys, the intoxicated man points further down the alley. Puzzled, the friend asks why he is not looking there, and the man responds, "Because the light is so much better over here." The problem of making meaningful regression coefficients for continuous predictors is actually quite easily addressed. The unstandardized regression coefficient represents the change in the response for every one unit change in the predictor; it is useful to consider the magnitude of that unit. If the unit is inherently meaningful and represents a theoretically important distance on the predictor's scale, no rescaling needs to be done. However, when units are quite small and not necessarily clinically or theoretically meaningful, rescaling can be very useful. Consider the example of a regression model in which the predictor is total cholesterol, measured in units of mg/dL. The resulting unstandardized regression weight would represent the change in the response variable for every 1 mg/dL change in cholesterol. A 1 mg/dL change in cholesterol may simply not be large enough to be biologically interesting. It would instead be preferable to select a range across the predictor that had some biological meaning or that at least was beyond the range of measurement error, say 10 mg/dL. The rescaling can be accomplished in several ways. In a linear model, the unstandardized coefficient can simply be multiplied by the scaling constant. If the regression weight was 0.2 for a 1-unit increase in the predictor, then a 10-unit increase

in the predictor would be associated with a $0.2 \times 10 = 2$ in the response variable. For coefficients derived from nonlinear models, such as the hazard or odds ratio, the idea is the same but the mathematics must accommodate the underlying model. If the hazard ratio from a time-to-event model is 1.1 for a 1-unit increase in the predictor, the hazard ratio for a 10-unit increase will be $1.1^{10} = 2.6$. Alternatively, the rescaling can be done prior to the analysis by simply dividing the value of the original predictor by the newly desired range, a scaling constant. Thus, the new regression coefficient for cholesterol would represent the change in the response for every 10 mg/dL change in cholesterol (for a more complete discussion of rescaling, see Babyak, 2009).

Finally, be clear about how categories were coded. If dummy or contrast variables were included, show the coding, and if applicable, state which category was used as the reference. Beware that in some coding schemes, the tests of the individual coefficients are dependent on one another and it may be safer to test those coefficients as a block before interpreting the individual coefficients (Cohen et al, 2002).

5.4.3 Results from Regression Models

Regardless of the type of model being estimated, the critical information to report about the model are the parameter estimates (usually in the form of regression weights, odds ratios, or hazard ratios, depending on the type of model) and the fit of the model. For linear regression, many software packages produce unstandardized and standardized parameter estimates[2] as part of the default output. The unstandardized weight should always be reported. The conventional standardized coefficient (where the predictor and

---

[2] Typically, the unstandardized coefficient is referred to with Roman letter 'b' while the standardized coefficient is referred to with Greek beta, β. However, this usage is not consistent across all texts, as some use the Greek β to refer to any type of regression coefficient.

response variables are scaled to one standard deviation units), however, has fallen out of favor to some extent. This is because the standard deviations of the study variables will necessarily vary across samples, making comparison impossible. Instead of the conventional standardized weight, a coefficient scaled to some meaningful distance on the predictor, as described earlier, can be reported in addition to the unstandardized weight. In addition to the weights for each predictor, report the 95% confidence limits for each coefficient, the *p*-value, and the degrees of freedom expended for the test. If one predictor is of critical importance to the hypothesis, also report some estimate of effect size. In linear regression, the partial correlation or partial r^2 can serve as an effect size estimate. The fit of a linear regression model is typically reported in the form of multiple R^2, along with the adjusted R^2. The adjusted R^2 is usually a more realistic estimate of the likely fit of the model outside of the sample. The results enumerated above can easily be presented in a table format. However, graphical representation of regression models also can be effective. If one predictor is of particular interest,

the fitted regression line for the primary predictor of interest can be presented, along with confidence bands, after adjustment for other variables in the model. If more than one predictor in the model is of interest, a figure showing the point estimates and confidence intervals can be presented. The section below on logistic regression includes an example of this type of figure.

For logistic regression and time-to-event models, the above recommendations hold with a few exceptions. The relation between a predictor and outcome in a logistic regression model can be displayed with the values of the predictor on the *x*-axis against the predicted probability and confidence bands of the binary outcome on the *y*-axis. Figure 54.1 is an example of a multivariable logistic regression model that might be presented graphically. The model was constructed to show associations of a variety of background variables with whether a patient had been prescribed an antidepressant (Waldman et al, 2009). Note that since odds ratios are being plotted, a logarithmic scale was used for the *x*-axis.

For the time-to-event model, the raw survival curves using the Kaplan–Meier method

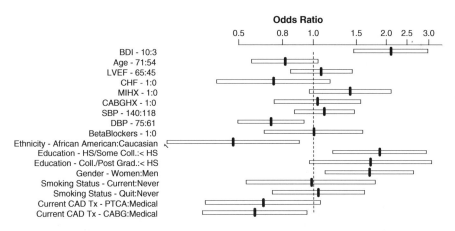

Fig. 54.1 Presentation of multivariable logistic regression model results predicting antidepressant use. The *bold* vertical bars represent the point estimates, while the *empty bars* represent the 95% confidence limits of the estimate. The predictor variable names are listed on the left-hand side, along with the comparison that was made to generate the estimate. For example, the odds ratio for the ethnicity variable is the ratio of the odds of antidepressant use for African Americans compared to the odds

for Caucasians. Similarly, for continuous variables, the values next to the predictor names represent the scaling. For example, for the BDI (Beck Depression Inventory) the odds ratio compares the odds of antidepressant use for a person with a BDI score of 10 (75th percentile) with the odds for a person with a score of 3 (25th percentile). In other words, the estimate compares a person in the middle of the upper half of the distribution to a person in the middle of the lower half are typically reported and provide the reader with a good sense of how the raw data looked. Including the number at risk at reasonable intervals is also informative. Figure 54.2 is adapted from Martinu and colleagues (2008) and shows a typical Kaplan–Meier curve, plotting the survival curves for three groups of lung transplant recipient grouped by values of their pretransplant 6 min walk test. The values at the bottom of the figure are the number at risk for each year of the study. If more sophisticated modeling is used, such as Cox proportional hazards modeling, one very useful way to display the relation between an important continuous predictor and survival is to plot the values of the predictor against predicted probability of survival at some selected point during the follow-up time. Figure 54.3, again adapted from Martinu et al, displays the association between the 6 min walk distance, modeled as a continuous variable, and the probability of survival 30 months after being listed for a lung transplant. The hatch marks across the top of the plot represent individual values for the 6 min walk test, giving the reader an indication of the distribution of the test values.

5.4.4 Confounding and Mediation

In many cases, the aim of including additional adjustment variables in an analysis is to rule out that the effect of the predictor of interest is not confounded, that is, mixed with the effect of one more of those other variables. I often use the following conceptual example of confounding with my students. Imagine that you are near the bottom of a long, deep ravine and are able to see in the distance a train trestle that crosses the ravine. Because of your location, you can see only the trestle itself and not anything beyond the trestle on either side of the ravine. Suddenly you see a small boy frantically running across the trestle, followed closely by a much larger boy. You conclude that the larger boy is chasing the smaller boy, or in other words, the large boy is *causing* the small boy to run. A few

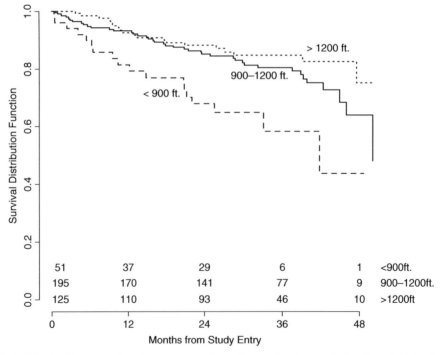

Fig. 54.2 Kaplan–Meier curves for three groups of 6 min walk test distance for patients listed for lung transplant. The *curves* are labeled directly in the figure rather than from a legend. The values at the bottom of the table are the number at risk for each of the three groups at each year of follow-up. Although categorizing the continuous 6 min walk distance would not be recommended for developing the best regression estimate, it is a serviceable means of describing the raw data in this case

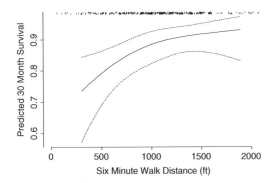

Fig. 54.3 Predicted probability of 30-month survival in transplant patients as a function of the 6 min walk test distance. The *solid line* is derived from a model in which 6 min walk distance is modeled as a continuous variable. The *dotted lines* are the 95% confidence limits. In this particular instance, the relation was clearly linear (the conversion of the relation from log hazard to a probability introduced a slight nonlinearity). Had there been a nonlinear or threshold effect, this plot would have clearly demonstrated the presence of inflections, which might be important for clinical decision-making. The *tick marks* at the top of the plot represent the individual values for the 6 min walk distance, giving the reader a sense of the distribution of distances

seconds later, however, you see a large steam engine barreling down the tracks not far behind both boys. Only now do you realize that both boys were running from the train – the apparent cause of the small boy running was not the larger boy, but the train. The larger boy just happened to be running from the train, too. Thus, you had initially confused one possible causal agent for another. Had you turned and looked away, you might not have seen the train, and perhaps even gone on to write an editorial in a scientific journal warning of the dangers that large boys pose to smaller boys! A more data-based example of confounding is presented by Rubin (1997), in which pipe and cigar smokers were compared with cigarette smokers on the incidence of cancer mortality. In an unadjusted analysis, cigar and pipe smokers were shown to have higher rates of cancer mortality than cigarette smokers. Cigar and pipe smokers, however, also were considerably older on average than cigarette smokers. Therefore, the difference in mortality rates may have been a function not of the type of tobacco taken, but merely by age. When the mortality rates were adjusted for age,

in fact, the cigarette group had the higher mortality rate. The criteria for confounding are as follows: (1) the predictor must be related to the outcome; (2) the potential confounder must be related to the outcome; (3) the predictor of interest and the potential confounder must be related to one another; (4) the confounder cannot be a causal consequence of the predictor. Stated more simply, all three variables, the predictor, potential confounder, and outcome, must be related, but the confounder cannot be caused by the predictor. Confounding is usually then tested by adjusting for the potential confounder. If the relation between the predictor and the outcome is eliminated or substantially diminished, there is strong evidence that confounding is present.[3]

Confounding is often confused with mediation, and for good reason. Mediation is identical mathematically to confounding – no statistical technique can distinguish the two. The criteria are precisely the same as the first three listed above for confounding. The difference is that while the confounder cannot be part of the causal sequence between the predictor and the outcome, the mediator is presumed to be a causal consequence of the predictor (see Chapter 55, and also Cole and Hernan, 2002; MacKinnon, 1994; MacKinnon and Dwyer, 1993; Pearl, 2005 for further details).

6 Tables

Tables in a results section provide a way to organize findings in a way that (1) directly addresses the research question and (2) is readily meaningful to the reader. Wainer (1992) provides an excellent guide to making effective tables. First, as previously discussed, round wherever possible. Similarly, if the scale of a measure requires many places beyond the decimal, for example, 0.0023 kg, convert the value to, say, 2.3 g. The

---

[3] We discuss only 'positive' confounding here. It is also possible for confounding to be negative, in which case adjusting for a confounder would actually increase the estimated effect of the predictor.

Table 54.2 Possible organization of tables reporting means measured before and after a treatment in a two group experiment. Table 54.2a requires the reader to make an awkward skip in order to compare the post treatment means, which are of primary interest. Table 54.2b is an improvement, but the reader must make a mental or hand calculation to obtain the actual group difference. Table 54.2c reports the group differences directly, while Table 54.2d adds the within group change, which, although generally secondary to the aim of the design, may be of clinical interest. In an actual report, confidence intervals for each estimate also would be included

		Active treatment		Control	
(a)	Before treatment	After treatment		Before treatment	After treatment
	30.2	25.0		31.0	22.0
		Active treatment	Control		
(b)	Before treatment	30.2	31.0		
	After treatment (unadjusted)	25.0	22.0		
		Active treatment	Control	Difference (active treatment – control)	
(c)	Before treatment	30.2	31.0	–0.8	
	After treatment (unadjusted)	25.0	22.0	3.0	
		Active treatment	Control	Difference (active treatment – control)	
(d)	Before treatment	30.2	31.0	–0.8	
	After treatment	25.0	22.0	3.0	
	Change from before to after treatment	–4.8	–9.0		

table itself can be organized so that values are in some natural order, such as by time, and also in a way that invites immediate inspection or comparison of the most salient data points. For example, in comparing the means before and after treatment, it is more effective to put the values being compared side by side, rather than a few columns or rows apart. Compare the following tables (I do not include p-values or 95% CIs for the sake of illustration):

In Table 54.2a, the reader must skip over a column to compare the group means before and after treatment; in the second table the values are much more easily compared because they are side by side. Table 54.2b also orders the rows more naturally by time. We can do even better than Table 54.2b, however. When differences are of interest (which is almost always the case), why not directly display the differences, in addition to the means? Table 54.2c presents not only the values before and after treatment, but also arguably the value of most scientific interest, the difference between the groups. We could even

add a direct display to the within-group change over time, as in Table 54.2d. (I should note that in actual application, these tables also would include at least the 95% confidence intervals for each value.)

Wainer also points out that there is nothing wrong with highlighting important data points. Highlighting might be accomplished, for example, by simply using a different font for the important data points. When there is no a priori logical order to the values being presented (for example, no time order or no hierarchy of hypotheses), one also can reorder the data in order to bring out the more important or interesting data points.

7 Graphics

A good deal of excellent literature now exists with regard to the graphical display of data and these sources should be consulted for further detail than space allows here. Cleveland (1993), Tufte (2001), and Wainer (2005) are well worth studying. The central aim of a figure is to convey information about a pattern that might not otherwise be obvious from merely looking at numeric values. For example, a trend over time is often much easier to interpret when arranged in a plot than in a table, especially if several series of data are being compared. Relative differences between more than two data points are also more interpretable as physical distance on a plot than in a table.

A general principle to live by in presenting graphics is the keep the "ink-to-information ratio" as low as possible. Despite their popularity, bar charts are an excellent example of violating the principle of low ink-to-information ratio, as the ink wasted on the bars below the values conveys absolutely no information (Harrell, 2008). Moreover, we tend to perceive bar charts in terms of length rather than location, leading to distortions in interpretation. This is especially true when the zero point is not included on the y-axis. The problem is made even worse when the bars are shaded with geometric patterns, such as oblique hatching. For similar reasons, pie charts are of very dubious use in a scientific publication. In addition, although perhaps aesthetically

pleasing and again apparently very popular, using a 3-dimensional plot to plot 2-dimensional data provides no useful information and should be avoided. Instead, unless the data are truly 3-dimensional, use a 2-dimensional plot with characters that show the upper and lower dimensions of the response variable.

So what, then, instead of bar/dynamite plots? There are a number of alternatives, depending on how many data points there are and the intent of the display. When there are not too many data points, the raw data should be displayed. There are at least two important reasons for displaying the data with small samples. First, it is simply better to see the raw data whenever feasible. Second, analyses conducted with small data sets are particularly vulnerable to being influenced by just a few data points. Even with larger samples, summary calculations such as regression lines or fitted means can hide a passel of sins. In the left panel of Fig. 54.4, for example, one outlying data point in the upper right corner, where $x = 11$ and $y = 20$, is apparently responsible for the entire "finding" – when that data point is removed (right panel), the regression line is far less exciting. The issue of hidden data holds true for plots of group means or medians, too, of course. Figure 54.5 is adapted

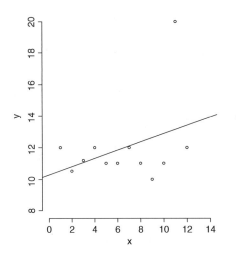
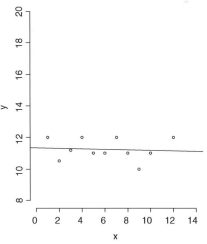

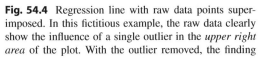

Fig. 54.4 Regression line with raw data points superimposed. In this fictitious example, the raw data clearly show the influence of a single outlier in the *upper right area* of the plot. With the outlier removed, the finding

is far less exciting. Although I purposely constructed an extreme example for illustrative purposes, failing to show the data whenever feasible obscures anomalies obvious or subtle. Adapted from Harrell and Slaughter (2009)

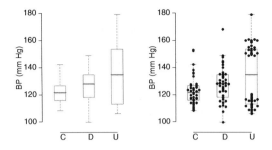

Fig. 54.5 Plots of mean and 95% confidence limits comparing fictional blood pressure response across three treatments. As in the prior example, failure to display the data hides the "real story"

from course material provided by Harrell and Slaughter (2009). The boxplot in the left panel suggests that the median for the third condition on the far right is higher than that of the other two groups. We see that the variability around the median is also larger in the third group but the plot gives us no indication of why. By displaying the raw data points over the boxplots, as in the right panel, we immediately see what is happening – there is a bimodal response in the third group, which renders the use of the mean or median for that group inappropriate.

When there are too many data points to display without overwhelming the plot, one alternative is to plot a random sample of the data points. If plotting a random sample is not feasible, box-and-whiskers (BW) plots provide the reader with a good deal of information about the distributional properties of the data. There are a number of variants of the BW plot that emphasize different aspects of the data. A selection of these plots can be seen at the online R graphics gallery: http://addictedtor.free. fr/graphiques/RGraphGallery.php?graph=102. Generally speaking, BW plots show not only one or more indexes of central tendency (such as mean and median) but the shape of the distribution, including outlying values.

The choice of axis scale is also important in portraying data accurately. When a zero point is possible on a measure, the zero point should be included in the plot. If zero is not a likely value for a variable (for example, blood pressure), the choice of axis scale becomes a bit more complex. When plotting means for example, it may be tempting to magnify an axis so that the differences look large. However, if the axis is magnified such that only a small range of the possible values for the variable are shown, the plot may give a misleading sense that size of the effect is very large. One approach is to construct the axis so that it covers at least the 25th to 75th percentiles of a variable's range. In conjunction with the direct display of the variability of the variable (standard deviation or 95% CI), distances between point estimates can be interpreted in the context of the variability of the data. An additional consideration is whether the values of the scale reside along equal intervals. Odds ratios and hazard ratios, for example, are best plotted on a logarithmic scale so that the distances can be compared accurately.

As noted earlier in the tables section, it can be useful to present not only the values of a given variable but also the result of a comparison of interest. In the case of comparing means across groups, for example, one can plot not only the means but also the difference between means. Figure 54.6 is again based on R code developed by Harrell (2004) and displays both the mean

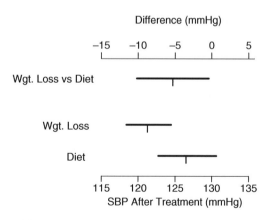

Fig. 54.6 Fictional blood pressure data across two treatment groups. The *bottom two lines* represent the mean and 95% blood pressure in each group. Since the difference between the two groups is of primary interest, the plot also displays this directly on the top axis, relieving the reader of the need to do the calculation. Adapted from Harrell (2004)

blood pressure for groups and also the pair-wise differences between the groups.

8 Interpretation

We close this chapter with a brief discussion on how results are interpreted. Although the primary purpose of the discussion or conclusions section is to place the findings in the context of theory and prior findings, there are at least a few statistical issues that bear on this process. I mentioned at the outset that we are currently experiencing substantial and widespread changes in how data are analyzed and interpreted. The vast majority of us currently conduct our hypothesis tests using what statisticians call the *frequentist* approach, which includes the conventional null hypothesis testing and *p*-values. Among the biggest changes likely to come in the next decade will be the growing influence, if not total adoption, of Bayesian methods over our current frequentist approach. Several journals, including, for example, *Annals of Emergency Medicine* (Cooper et al, 2003), have made it a policy to de-emphasize *p*-values and focus instead on point estimates, confidence intervals, with a preference for Bayesian methods. I will not address Bayesian methods here in any detail – a satisfactory treatment would require considerably more space, but it is clear that Bayesian methods are gaining a substantial following. The *British Medical Journal* has published several very accessible articles on Bayes techniques in a medical setting in the past decade or so (Freedman, 1996; Lilford and Braunholtz, 1996; Spiegelhalter et al, 1999). As pertains to our discussion here, the Bayesians offer a form of inference that yields what we seem to want the most intuitively – an estimate of the probability that our hypotheses are true. Whether the Bayesian influence is ultimately a good thing is a matter of persistent debate (see, for example, Skrepnek and Skrepnek, 2007). Regardless of the debate, there is little doubt that we will be seeing a good deal more from the Bayesians

in the near future, and the implications for this change may be quite profound.

While most of us are still tarry here in the frequentist world we can still avoid at least some of the pitfalls associated with frequentist testing methods. First, we can interpret the null hypothesis tests correctly. A typical error is to confuse the failure to reject null with accepting the null. A related error is to believe that the *p*-value offers information about the extent to which our hypothesis might be true, a mistake often compounded by the false belief that the smaller the *p*-value, the more likely it is that the observed effect is "real." Of course, this is not true. A *p*-value in the frequentist world does not have any bearing on the probability of the alternative hypothesis being true. Null hypothesis testing can only tell us how "odd" an observed result is if the null hypothesis is true in the population. In a clinical trial comparing two groups, for example, if the outcome is "significantly different," we can say that the result we observed would be very unusual if the null hypothesis were actually true. The *p*-value itself cannot tell us how important that difference is or how likely it is that the difference we see is the difference that exists in the population. A "non-significant" *p*-value can only tell us that there is not enough evidence to conclude that the effect being tested is a function of sampling error or not (for excellent discussion of this issue, see Thompson, 1998; Vickers, 2006).

Second, we can emphasize the effect size, not the *p*-value. A *p*-value provides only one piece of information about the finding, that is, how unusual it would be for one to see the observed effect if the null hypothesis were true. Although many journal editors and reviewers are still entirely wed to the idea that if *p* is not less than 0.05, the finding cannot be published, there are some signs that this convention is beginning to fade, albeit slowly. The critical issues to address with effect sizes in the discussion are, "Are these effects something we should care about and why?" There are a variety of approaches to these questions. We could, for example, compare our effect size to those seen in other studies. If the outcome is an event, such as an illness or death, we can calculate the number of excess events associated with the variable under study. We also could compare the effect to the effect of another variable that is well known. For example, the relation between depressive symptoms and cardiac disease might be compared to the relation of cigarette smoking and heart disease – for example, does a high score on a depression symptom inventory compare to, say, smoking a half of a pack of cigarettes everyday? Such a comparison, of course, cannot be very precise and rests heavily on the choice of scaling (how many points on the depression inventory versus how many cigarettes, and at what rate?). But with careful selection of scaling and cautious language, the reader can get a sense of the importance of the association.

Finally, consistent with the principle of reporting all results, be sure to discuss all results, irrespective of the extent to which they support your favorite position. We seem to have a natural tendency to spend a lot of time explaining the positive findings, digging deep into precedents and possible mechanisms, but less time on results that do not fit our expectations. The imbalance may exist in part because we simply know much more about the positive finding. Nevertheless, a contrary or null finding should be entertained as fully as possible, both in substantive and in statistical terms (for example, power, effect size). Again, using the effect size rather than statistical significance can be beneficial in helping us sort out what the data are really telling us.

References

Altman, D. G., and Bland, J. M. (2003). Statistics Notes: Interaction revisited: the difference between two estimates. *BMJ*, *326*, 219.

Altman, D. G., and Matthews, J. N. S. (1996). Statistics Notes: Interaction 1: heterogeneity of effects. *BMJ*, *313*, 486.

Altman, D. G., Schulz, K. F., Moher, D., Egger, M., Davidoff, F., Elbourne, D. et al (2001). The revised CONSORT statement for reporting randomized trials: explanation and elaboration. *Ann Intern Med*, *134*, 663–694.

Assmann, S. F., Pocock, S. J., Enos, L. E., and Kasten, L. E. (2000). Subgroup analysis and other (mis)uses of baseline data in clinical trials. *Lancet*, *355*, 1064–1069.

Babyak, M. A. (2004). What you see may not be what you get: a brief, nontechnical introduction to overfitting in regression-type models. *Psychosom Med*, *66*, 411–421.

Babyak, M. A. (2009). Rescaling predictors in regression models. Retrieved Oct. 13, 2009, from http://stattips.blogspot.com/

Berger, V. (2005). *Selection Bias and Covariate Imbalances in Randomized Clinical Trials*. Hoboken, NJ: Wiley.

Bland, M. J. (2004). Cluster randomised trials in the medical literature: two bibliometric surveys. *BMC Med Res Methodol*, *4*, 21.

Borman, G. D., and Dowling, N. M. (2006). Longitudinal achievement effects of multiyear summer school: evidence from the Teach Baltimore Randomized Field Trial. *Educ Eval Pol Ans*, *28*, 25–48.

Byrne, W. D. (2000). Common reasons for rejecting manuscripts at medical journals: a survey of editors and peer reviewers. *Sci Edit*, *23*, 39–44.

Cleveland, W. S. (1993). *Visualizing Data*. Summit, NJ: Hobart.

Cohen, J. (1983). The cost of dichotomization. *Appl Psychol Meas*, *7*, 249–253.

Cohen, J., West, S. G., Aiken, L., and Cohen, P. (2002). *Applied Multiple Regression/Correlation Analysis for the Behavioral Sciences, 3rd Ed*. London: Taylor & Francis.

Cole, S. R., and Hernan, M. A. (2002). Fallibility in estimating direct effects. *Int J Epidemiol*, *31*, 163–165.

Concato, J., Peduzzi, P., Holford, T. R., and Feinstein, A. R. (1995). Importance of events per independent variable in proportional hazards analysis I. Background, goals, and general strategy. *J Clin Epidemiol*, *48*, 1495–1501.

Cooper, R. J., Wears, R. L., and Schriger, D. L. (2003). Reporting research results: recommendations for improving communication. *Ann Emerg Med*, *41*, 561–564.

Dixon, D. O., and Simon, R. (1992). Bayesian subset analysis in a colorectal cancer clinical trial. *Stat Med*, *11*, 13–22.

Enders, C. K. (2006). A primer on the use of modern missing-data methods in psychosomatic medicine research. *Psychosom Med*, *68*, 427–436.

Freedland, K. E., Babyak, M. A., McMahon, R. J., Jennings, J. R., Golden, R. N. et al (2005). Statistical guidelines for psychosomatic medicine. *Psychosom Med*, *67*, 167.

Freedman, L. (1996). Bayesian statistical methods. *BMJ*, *313*, 569–570.

Green, S. B., Lissitz, R., and Mulaik, S. (1977). Limitations of coefficient alpha as an index of test unidimensionality. *Educ Psychol Meas*, *37*, 827–838.

Greenland, S. (2000). When should epidemiologic regressions use random coefficients? *Biometrics, 56,* 915–921.

Harrell, F. E. (2001). *Regression Modeling Strategies: With Applications to Linear Modeling, Logistic Regression, and Survival Analysis.* New York: Springer.

Harrell, F. E. (2004). S for statistical data analysis and graphics. Retrieved Oct 8, 2009, from http://biostat.mc.vanderbilt.edu/wiki/pub/Main/StatCompCourse/sCompGraph.pdf

Harrell, F. E. (2008). Dynamite plots. Retrieved Oct 13, 2009, from http://biostat.mc.vanderbilt.edu/twiki/bin/view/Main/DynamitePlots

Harrell, F. E., and Slaughter, J. C. (2009). Introduction to biostatistics for biomedical research (class material). Retrieved Oct 8, 2009, from https://data.vanderbilt.edu/biosproj/CI2/handouts.pdf

Harris, A. H. S., Reeder, R., and Hyun, J. K. (2009). Common statistical and research design problems in manuscripts submitted to high-impact psychiatry journals: what editors and reviewers want authors to know. *J Psychiatr Res, 43,* 1231–1234.

ICH (2009). The international conference on harmonisation of technical requirements for registration of pharmaceuticals for human use (ICH). Retrieved Oct 9, 2009, from http://www.ich.org/

Johnson, B. T., and Eagly, A. H. (2000). Quantitative synthesis of social psychological research. In H. T. Reis & C. M. Judd (Eds.), *Handbook of Research Methods in Social and Personality Psychology* (pp. 496–528). New York: Cambridge University Press.

Kraemer, H. C., Mintz, J., Noda, A., Tinklenberg, J., and Yesavage, J. A. (2006). Caution regarding the use of pilot studies to guide power calculations for study proposals. *Arch Gen Psychiatry, 63,* 484–489.

Lachin, J. M. (2000). Statistical considerations in the intent-to-treat principle. *Control Clin Trials, 21,* 167–189.

Lang, T. A., and Secic, M. (2006). *How to Report Statistics in Medicine: Annotated Guidelines for Authors, Editors, and Reviewers.* Philadelphia: American College of Physicians.

LaVange, L. M., and Koch, G. G. (2006). Rank score tests. *Circulation, 114,* 2528–2533.

Lilford, R. J., and Braunholtz, D. (1996). For debate: the statistical basis of public policy: a paradigm shift is overdue. *BMJ, 313,* 603–607.

Littell, R. C., Milliken, G. A., Stroup, W. W., Wolfinger, R. D., and Schabenberger, O. (2006). *SAS for Mixed Models, 2nd Ed.* Cary, NC: SAS Institute.

Little, R. J., and Rubin, D. B. (2000). Causal effects in clinical and epidemiological studies via potential outcomes: concepts and analytical approaches. *Annu Rev Public Health, 21,* 121–145.

Little, R. J. A., and Rubin, D. B. (2002). *Statistical Analysis with Missing Data, 2nd Ed.* New York: Wiley.

MacCallum, R. C., Zhang, S., Preacher, K., and Rucker, D. (2002). On the practice of dichotomization of quantitative variables. *Psychol Methods, 7,* 19–40.

MacKinnon, D. P. (1994). Analysis of mediating variables in prevention intervention studies. In A. Cazares & L. A. Beatty (Eds.), *Scientific Methods for Prevention Intervention Research* (pp. 127–153). Washington, DC: DHHS Pub.

MacKinnon, D. P., and Dwyer, J. H. (1993). Estimating mediated effects in prevention studies. *Eval Rev, 17,* 158.

Martinu, T., Babyak, M. A., O'Connell, C. F., Carney, R. M., Trulock, E. P. et al (2008). Baseline 6-min walk distance predicts survival in lung transplant candidates. *Am J Transplant, 8,* 1498–1505.

Matthews, J. N. S., and Altman, D. G. (1996a). Statistics Notes: Interaction 2: compare effect sizes not P values. *BMJ, 313,* 808.

Matthews, J. N. S., and Altman, D. G. (1996b). Statistics Notes: Interaction 3: how to examine heterogeneity. *BMJ, 313,* 862.

Maxwell, S. E., and Delaney, H. D. (1993). Bivariate median splits and spurious statistical significance. *Psychol Bull, 113,* 20.

Maxwell, S. E., and Delaney, H. D. (2004). *Designing Experiments and Analyzing Data: A Model Comparison Approach, 2nd Ed.* Mahwah, NJ: Lawrence Erlbaum.

McCullagh, P., and Nelder, J. (1989). *Generalized Linear Models.* London: Chapman and Hall.

McKnight, P. E., McKnight, K. M., Sidani, S., and Figueredo, A. J. (2007). *Missing Data: A Gentle Introduction.* NY: Guilford Press.

Moher, D., Cook, D. J., Eastwood, S., Olkin, I., Rennie, D. et al (1999). Improving the quality of reports of meta-analyses of randomised controlled trials: the QUOROM statement. Quality of Reporting of Meta-analyses. *Lancet, 354,* 1896–1900.

Moons, K. G. M., Donders, A. R. T., Steyerberg, E. W., and Harrell, F. E. (2004). Penalized maximum likelihood estimation to directly adjust diagnostic and prognostic prediction models for overoptimism: a clinical example. *J Clin Epidemiol, 57,* 1262–1270.

Noah, N. (2008). The STROBE initiative: STrengthening the Reporting of OBservational studies in Epidemiology (STROBE). *Epidemiol Infect, 136,* 865.

Pearl, J. (2005). *Direct and Indirect Effects: Technical Report R-273.* Paper presented at the Proceedings of the American Statistical Association, Minneapolis, MN.

Peduzzi, P., Concato, J., Kemper, E., Holford, T. R., and Feinstein, A. R. (1996). A simulation study of the number of events per variable in logistic regression analysis. *J Clin Epidemiol, 49,* 1373–1379.

Peters, C. C., and van Voorhis, W. R. (1940). *Statistical Procedures and Their Mathematical Bases.* New York: McGraw-Hill.

Pocock, S. J., and Simon, R. (1975). Sequential treatment assignment with balancing for prognostic factors in the controlled clinical trial. *Biometrics*, *31*, 102–115.

Rossini, A., and Leisch, F. (2003). Literate statistical practice. Working Paper 194. *UW Biostatistics Working Paper Series*. Retrieved from http://www.bepress.com/uwbiostat/paper194

Royston, P., Altman, D. G., and Sauerbrei, W. (2006). Dichotomizing continuous predictors in multiple regression: a bad idea. *Stat Med*, *25*, 127–141.

Rubin, D. B. (1997). Estimating causal effects from large data sets using propensity scores. *Ann Intern Med*, *127*, 757–763.

Schulz, K. F., and Grimes, D. A. (2002). Allocation concealment in randomised trials: defending against deciphering. *Lancet*, *359*, 614–618.

Senn, S. (2008). *Statistical Issues in Drug Development*. Hoboken, NJ: Wiley.

Simon, R. (2002). Bayesian subset analysis: application to studying treatment-by-gender interactions. *Stat Med*, *21*, 2909–2916.

Skrepnek, G. H., and Skrepnek, G. H. (2007). The contrast and convergence of Bayesian and frequentist statistical approaches in pharmacoeconomic analysis. *Pharmacoeconomics*, *25*, 649–664.

Spiegelhalter, D. J., Myles, J. P., Jones, D. R., and Abrams, K. R. (1999). Methods in health service research: an introduction to Bayesian methods in health technology assessment. *BMJ*, *319*, 508–512.

Steyerberg, E. W. (2009). *Clinical Prediction Models*. New York: Springer.

Stroup, D. F., Berlin, J. A., Morton, S. C., Olkin, I., Williamson, G. D. et al (2000). Meta-analysis of observational studies in epidemiology: a proposal for reporting. Meta-analysis Of Observational Studies in Epidemiology (MOOSE) group. *JAMA*, *283*, 2008–2012.

Thompson, B. (1998). Statistical significance and effect size reporting: portrait of a possible future. *Res Schools*, *5*, 33–38.

Tibshirani, R. (1997). The lasso method for variable selection in the Cox model. *Stat Med*, *16*, 385–395.

Tufte, E. R. (2001). *The Visual Display of Quantitative Information*, *2nd Ed*. Cheshire, CT: Graphics Press.

Vickers, A. (2006). Michael Jordan won't accept the null hypothesis: notes on interpreting high p-values. *Medscape Business of Medicine*, May 3, 2009, from http://www.medscape.com/viewarticle/531928

Vittinghoff, E., and McCulloch, C. E. (2007). Relaxing the rule of ten events per variable in logistic and Cox regression. *Am J Epidemiol*, *165*, 710–718.

Wainer, H. (1992). Understanding graphs and tables. *Educ Res*, *21*, 14–23.

Wainer, H. (2005). *Graphic Discovery: A Trout in the Milk and Other Visual Adventures*. Princeton, NJ: Princeton University Press.

Waldman, S. V., Blumenthal, J. A., Babyak, M. A., Sherwood, A., Sketch, M. et al (2009). Ethnic differences in the treatment of depression in patients with ischemic heart disease. *Am Heart J*, *157*, 77–83.

Whitfield, K. E., Allaire, J. C., Belue, R., and Edwards, C. L. (2008). Are comparisons the answer to understanding behavioral aspects of aging in racial and ethnic groups? *J Gerontol B Psychol Sci Soc Sci*, *63*, P301-P308.

Wilcox, R. R. (1998). How many discoveries have been lost by ignoring modern statistical methods? *Am Psychol*, *53*, 300–314.

Williams, R. L. (2000). A note on robust variance estimation for cluster-correlated data. *Biometrics*, *56*, 645–646.

Ye, J. (1998). On measuring and correcting the effects of data mining and model selection. *J Am Stat Assoc*, *93*, 120–131.

Chapter 55

Moderators and Mediators: The MacArthur Updated View

Helena Chmura Kraemer

1 Introduction

The terms "moderators" and "mediators" have been used in both behavioral and medical research for at least the last half century. Early on, however, the terms were typically used idiosyncratically, meaning whatever seemed to be implied from the context of the statement in which they were used. Terminology so loosely defined carries little impact in scientific research, whatever the scientific field (Finney, 1994). This situation changed with the publication of a seminal paper by Baron and Kenny in 1986, that presented both conceptual definitions for the two terms and proposed statistical methods to determine which term applied in specific situations.

Baron and Kenny (B&K) proposed that "moderation" and "mediation" described a relationship connecting three variables in a population: the target variable, T, the moderator or mediator, M, and the outcome, O. They suggested that

- M moderates the effect of T on O if M suggests on whom or under what conditions T is associated with O.
- M mediates the effect of T on O if M suggests how or why T is associated with O.

These conceptual definitions not only defined the concepts of moderation and mediation and distinguished between them but also clearly indicated why such concepts might be very important to full understanding of biobehavioral processes.

Unfortunately, the statistical methods proposed to implement these conceptual definitions did not, for a variety of reasons, resolve the problem. The methods proposed were based on a linear model and on "statistical significance," an emphasis consistent with the methodology of the time. In the years since, it has been better recognized that to declare than "$p < 0.05$" usually only means that the study design was adequate to detect a non-random association. Many such "statistically significant" results (no matter the actual value of p) were of no clinical significance. More recently, both the American Psychological Association in its Publication Manual (2001) and the American Medical Association with the CONSORT guidelines (Altman et al, 2001; Begg et al, 1999; Piaggio et al, 2006; Rennie, 1996) have emphasized the importance of presenting an interpretable effect size with every "p value." When the result is statistically significant, such an effect size guides consideration of its clinical significance; when the result is not statistically significant, the effect size provides a clue as to whether this is because the effect is of no potential clinical significance or because the study was inadequately powered to detect a clinically significant result (Kraemer and Kupfer, 2006).

While the linear model proposed does not well fit all situations in which moderation or

H.C. Kraemer (✉)
Department of Psychiatry and Behavioral Sciences, Stanford University, 1116 Forest Avenue, Palo Alto, CA 94301, USA
e-mail: hckhome@pacbell.net

A. Steptoe (ed.), *Handbook of Behavioral Medicine*, DOI 10.1007/978-0-387-09488-5_55,
© Springer Science+Business Media, LLC 2010

mediation might be important, it continues to be the most commonly used. However, when the emphasis shifted from "*p* values" to effect sizes, several problems emerged.

First of all, B&K suggested that the interaction of *M* and *T* on *O* be included in the linear model for moderation, but be assumed to be absent for mediation. If there is an interaction in the population that is not included in the linear model, the results of fitting the model are biased, and the power both to detect the association and to precisely estimate the effect sizes are reduced. Moreover, conceptually, *T* may not only affect the level of *M* but also affect the way *M* influences *O*, and both may contribute to the effect size of *T* on *O*. For example, in a randomized clinical trial comparing two treatments (*T*1 versus *T*2), there may be a difference between the two treatments in compliance, which may explain part of the differential effect of treatments on the outcome. However, it may also be that compliance with *T*1 has a much greater influence on *O* than does compliance with *T*2 and that too may contribute to understanding the differential effect of treatments on the outcome (The MTA Cooperative Group, 1999). Thus, for both mathematical and conceptual reasons, the interaction should not simply be assumed to be zero in documenting a mediation effect.

To show that *M* moderates the effect of *T* on *O* in the linear model, B&K required that the interaction be shown to be "statistically significant." Two problems then arise. If the existence of an interaction may indicate mediation, then the distinction between the moderator and mediator is no longer clear. Moreover, basing the definition on "statistical significance" in a sample instead of on the population relationship among *M*, *T*, and *O*, means that, with very large sample sizes, moderation or mediation may exist, whereas in the same situation, with small sample sizes, it does not. "Moderation" and "mediation" must be defined in terms of the population and then demonstrated to exist by statistical analyses of samples from that population.

Further problems arose, not from the definitions "per se," but from how they were later used. "Moderation" was often used as a synonym of

"interaction," and "mediation" as a synonym of "cause." The definition of moderation/mediation became inextricably confounded with general applications of the linear model, with multiple "mediators," and assuming all interactions to be zero. With increasing confusion between moderation and mediation, inevitably discussion of variables that were "moderator-mediators" and "mediator-moderators" resulted. In fact, it became increasingly clear that by the B&K criteria, with three correlated random variables, any one of these variables could be shown to both moderate and mediate, to be moderated by or to be mediated by, any other of these variables on the remaining variable, provided only that the sample size was large enough! The B&K conceptual definitions seemed valid and strong, but the criteria suggested had not completely resolved the existing problems.

In the 1990s, the MacArthur Network on Developmental Psychopathology, seeking to develop interventions to prevent preteen psychopathology, became increasingly aware of the fact that virtually all risk factors for early onset behavioral problems had very small effect sizes (Kraemer et al, 1999). Clearly no one risk factor, and no linear combination of risk factors, would accomplish their goal. To prevent such onset they needed to understand on whom or under what conditions certain risk factors influenced onset in order to "target" appropriate prevention efforts (moderators) and how and why certain risk factors influenced onset (mediators) to "tailor" the appropriate prevention efforts (King et al, 2008). This motivated reconsideration of the B&K approach, retaining the conceptual definitions, but identifying where the problems in implementing those definitions lay, modifying them appropriately, and beginning to develop methods to implement those modifications.

In the following discussion we will present the resulting MacArthur approach to moderators and mediators (Kraemer et al, 2001, 2002, 2005, 2006). A full discussion as to what modifications were made to the B&K approach and why is discussed in Kraemer et al (2008). The linear model proposed by B&K will here continue to be used to describe the population, although a non-parametric approach to the problem has been developed and may be useful in some circumstances (Kraemer, 2008), and other approaches are possible.

2 *M* Moderates the Effect of *T* on *O*

To show that M moderates the effect of T on O, it must be shown that

- M precedes T which precedes O in time;
- M is not correlated with T;
- The effect of T on O depends on what the value of M is.

The linear model posits that in the population:

$$O = \beta_0 + \beta_1 T + \beta_2 M + \beta_3 TM + \varepsilon,$$

where ε, the error term, has a distribution that is independent of T and M. As is true in all linear models, with inclusion of an interaction, the meaning of the regression coefficients depends on how each of the variables is coded (Kraemer and Blasey, 2004).

For example, if T were choice of treatment in a randomized controlled trial (RCT) comparing two treatments ($T1$ and $T2$) for Alzheimer's disease and M were age of onset, it may be that age of onset moderates the effect of treatment on outcome. If, in this situation, T were coded 1 for $T1$ and 0 for $T2$ and M were coded as age at time of onset in years (as is often done), β_1 would indicate the $T1$ versus $T2$ difference in outcome O for those with Alzheimer's disease at birth (age=0), which is, of course, ludicrous. Here β_2 is the slope of O on M for $T2$ only, which is easily misinterpreted.

For this reason, when interactions are included in any linear model, care must be taken to code the predictors in such a way that the regression coefficients to be estimated and tested are meaningful in context (Kraemer and Blasey, 2004). For the purpose of moderation analysis, a binary variable (whether T or M) is coded $+1/2$ and $-1/2$, an ordinal variable (whether T

or M) is coded as deviations from the population mean. Thus in the above illustration, had treatment choice been coded $+1/2$ and $-1/2$ and age of onset as deviations from the mean age of onset, β_1 would be the effect of treatment on the patient at the mean age of onset, β_2 would be the average slope in the two groups of O on age of onset, and β_3 would be the difference in those slopes in the two groups.

Then, if $\beta_3=0$, the effect of T on O is the same for any value of M, namely β_1. If not, the effect of T on O differs depending on what M is, i.e., M indicates on whom or under what conditions T affects O (hence a moderator). In an RCT, any baseline variable is uncorrelated with T because of randomization. Any baseline variable, then, that interacts with T in its effect on O is a moderator of T. In an observational study, it would have to be shown that M precedes T, that M is uncorrelated with T (at least that the correlation was of trivial size) and that there is a non-zero interactive effect of M and T on O.

Perhaps the most intriguing potential moderators are genetic moderators of environmental risk factors on outcome. For example, it has been suggested that a certain genotype (fixed at birth) moderates the effect of childhood abuse on adult violent behavior (Jaffee et al, 2005). There are very few medical outcomes (e.g., heart disease, cancer, and all psychiatric disorders) for which strong genetic predictors have yet been shown, despite the fact that the financial investment in finding such predictors has been both longstanding and enormous. If, however, some genes influence outcome by moderating the effect of environmental factors, that might totally change our understanding and would make nonsense of the nature-nurture arguments. Similarly in RCTs, genes may moderate the effect of treatment on outcome (Murphy et al, 2004), the basis of the emerging field of pharmacogenetics.

3 *M* Mediates the Effect of *T* on *O*

To show that M mediates the effect of T on O, it must be shown that

- *T* precedes *M* which precedes *O*.
- *T* and *M* are correlated.
- The effect of *T* on *O* depends completely (total mediation) or in part (partial mediation) on the effect of *T* on *M*.

Here, the same linear model is used. However, the situation differs. For *T* to precede *M* does not simply mean that *T* is measured at one time and *M* at a later time; it means that *M* is an event or change that follows *T*. In mediation analysis when *M* is binary, it is coded 1 if it occurs and 0 if it does not; if *M* is ordinal, it is coded as deviations from 0, i.e., from the situation that pertains at the time of *T*.

The effect size of *T* on *O* can be computed from this population model (Kraemer et al, 2008). From that effect size, it is apparent that *either* a non-zero β_2 or β_3 will indicate mediation, for either an effect of *T* on *M* changing its level (β_2), or an effect of *T* on *M* changing how *M* relates to *O* (β_3) may explain some or all of how *T* affects *O*.

From these definitions, it is immediately apparent that no one variable can both moderate and mediate a *T* on an outcome *O*, for a moderator must precede and be uncorrelated with the *T* it moderates and a mediator must follow and be correlated with the *T* it mediates.

4 Issues Raised in the Consideration of the MacArthur Approach

4.1 Cross-Sectional and Longitudinal Studies

It is immediately apparent that moderation and mediation cannot be studied in cross-sectional studies: there must be at least two time points in a longitudinal design. In an RCT, this is automatic, for any baseline variable is eligible as a moderator of choice of treatment (*T*) on outcome (*O*) and any change that takes place between the baseline and the determination of treatment outcome is eligible to be considered as a possible

mediator of *T* on *O*. In observational studies, determining the time line is more difficult (e.g., Essex et al, 2006). This is troublesome, for many existing studies of moderators and mediators in the research literature are based on cross-sectional samples, with conclusions questionable under the MacArthur approach (Jacobi et al, 2004).

4.2 Variable Definition

But surely, some would say, the notion that no variable can be both a moderator and a mediator of *T* on *O* must be wrong! For example, in an RCT comparing *T*1 and *T*2, surely social support may both moderate and mediate a treatment choice on an outcome.

This query reflects a degree of imprecision sometimes seen in defining variables. Social support prior to choice of treatment may indeed moderate the effect of treatment on outcome. Change in social support during treatment may indeed mediate the effect of treatment on outcome, with the same treatment and the same outcome. However, social support prior to treatment and change in social support during treatment are *not* the same variable and may not even be highly correlated to each other. Care must be taken to define precisely what is being measured and when.

4.3 First Moderation, then Mediation

Another issue relates to the relationship between moderation and mediation. No variable can be both a moderator and a mediator of the effect of *T* on *O*, but there is a strong and important connection between the moderators and the mediators of *T* on *O*. If *M* moderates the effect of *T* on *O*, that means the effect of *T* on *O* differs depending on what *M* is. This in turn raises the possibility that the mediators of the effect of *T* on *O* may also be different in the subgroups defined by the moderator.

For example, if, in an RCT, gender moderated the effect of $T1$ versus $T2$ on the outcome O, not only does it mean that the $T1$ versus $T2$ effect size is different for men and women but also it raises the possibility that the process by which $T1$ affects O and that by which $T2$ affects O may also be different for men and women. Thus the mediators of T on O may be different for men and women. Consequently, once a moderator of T on O is identified, the search for mediators should focus separately on moderator-defined subgroups.

4.4 The Problem of Causal Inferences

All causal factors leading from T to O are, by the MacArthur definition, mediators of T on O. However, not all factors that are mediators of T on O are causal. It takes a great deal more than showing an association between M, T, and O to infer a causal effect: one cannot infer causation simply from correlation.

To some extent, the problem here relates to different standards for claiming causality in social psychology (B&K) and in medicine (MacArthur). In observational studies in social psychology, a causal association is assumed to exist and if the data do not refute that assumption, the causal assumption remains viable. In medicine inferences of causality usually require RCTs. To understand why this is so, consider the inference drawn from the observational study in 1985 that use of hormone replacement therapy (HRT) protects against heart disease (Stampfer et al, 1985), later refuted by an RCT that showed that the use of HRT increased the risk of heart disease, as well as that of breast cancer. (Writing Group for the Women's Health Initiative Investigators, 2002). After the 1985 study, many women began and continued HRT with the hope of avoiding the most common cause of death in women: heart disease. Following the 2002 study and the subsequent sudden decrease in use of HRT, cancer rates also dramatically decreased, suggesting (but not proving) the harm done by the earlier premature

inference of causality (Jemal et al, 2007). After publication of the 2002 study, the 1986 data were reexamined. It was then suggested that age moderated the effect of HRT on heart disease and thus that the original causal inference was overly inclusive as to the relevant population. Since the 2002 RCT sampled women largely beyond the age window now suggested, it could neither confirm nor deny this new hypothesis. As a result, there is still confusion among clinicians and patients as to the value or danger of use of HRT. From experiences such as this, claims of causality are viewed more suspiciously in medicine than in other fields.

In an RCT in which subjects in a population are randomly assigned to $T1$ and $T2$, it is appropriate to infer that any differential effect of $T1$ versus $T2$ on outcome O is *caused* by the choice of T, and even that the differential effect of $T1$ versus $T2$ on a mediator M is *caused* by the choice of T. It is not, however, appropriate to infer that any association between M and O is causal. To show this causal effect, the most direct way would be to do an RCT in which M is experimentally manipulated within $T1$ and within $T2$ and the effect of that manipulation on O assessed.

Finally, there is the issue of "backward" causation or "reciprocal" causation. Suppose that the stress level at time 1 ($S1$) was measured, followed by the change in cortisol level in the next time interval ($C2$), followed by the change in stress in the next time interval ($S3$), followed by the change in cortisol level in the next time interval ($C4$), etc. Then if $S1$ and $C2$ were correlated, it may be that $C2$ mediates the effect of $S1$ on $S3$. The same could be said for $C2$ being mediated by the effect of $S3$ on $C4$, etc. If these were all mediating relationships, one would have established a mediator chain across time. According to the MacArthur model, none of these mediators are necessarily causal, but they certainly may be. If they were, it must be noted that $S1$, $S3$, $S5$, etc., *neither* are the same variables nor are $C2$, $C4$, $C6$, etc. Thus each causal factor would temporally precede its outcome. There is no backward causation or reciprocal causation in the MacArthur approach. In fact, this type of situation would constitute a "feedback loop," one likely both common and important to consider in biobehavioral processes.

4.5 When Treatment Choice Moderates Event/Change on Outcome

Suppose in an RCT, an event or change (M) that occurs between choice of treatment (T) onset and outcome (O) (hence not a moderator of T) is not correlated with choice of treatment (hence not a mediator of T) but has an interactive effect with T on O. What then? The answer is simple: The fact that M follows T, is uncorrelated with T, and has an interactive effect with T on O means that T moderates the effect of M on O. What is confusing here is only that in RCTs, the focus is generally on moderators and mediators of treatment choice, where in this case, the direction of moderation is reversed. It is convenient to label the three variables M, T, and O, but what we choose to label a variable does not determine its role.

For example, in an RCT comparing two treatments of major depressive disorder, it may be that some patients during treatment experience the death of a loved one or another such traumatic life event. Random treatment assignment is unlikely to affect the occurrence of such a traumatic life event. However, it may be that one of the treatments fosters better coping with that life event, resulting in a much better outcome for those affected in that treatment group. This would result in an interaction between treatment choice and the life event on outcome. Since the effect of the life event on outcome depends on the earlier treatment choice, here treatment choice moderates the effect of the life event on outcome, not vice versa.

4.6 How Distinct Must M, T, O Be?

In comparing a drug treatment with group psychotherapy, neither drug level in the blood nor degree of participation in therapy group interactions can logically be considered as possible mediators of treatment, since each is completely tied only to one of the two treatments. Similarly, in comparing two strategies to induce smoking cessation, the decrease in the number of cigarettes per day at 11 months from baseline should not be considered as a possible mediator when the outcome measure is the decrease in the number of cigarettes per day at 12 months, since these measure substantially the same outcome. To obtain useful results, there must be a certain conceptual distinction among M, T, and O. Otherwise, while the MacArthur approach continues to "work," the logic would falter.

There are many more such questions that arise, but at least to date, most seem to yield to application of the MacArthur criteria. Inevitably, problems will sooner or later be found with this approach that do not so yield, and as was the case with the B&K approach, modifications or extensions will be eventually be required.

5 Extensions to Other Relationships

What was clear from the outset in developing the MacArthur approach was that moderation and mediation do not cover all the possible important associations connecting two variables (M and T) with an outcome (O).

5.1 M Is Proxy to T with Respect to O

To demonstrate that M is proxy to T with respect to O, it must be shown that

- Either T precedes M or there is no time precedence between M and T, but both precede O;
- M and T are correlated;
- When M and T are jointly considered, only M is related to O.

For example, gender is said to be associated with teenage onset of depression, with girls more likely to have onset than boys. Also, girls tend not to throw a ball as hard and straight as do boys in the preteen years. Consequently, if ball-throwing ability were to be correlated with teenage onset of depression, it would not be surprising to see some association. However, if both gender and ball-throwing ability were entered into the linear model, the influence of ball-throwing ability on later onset of depression would likely disappear, and it probably makes little sense to teach girls how to throw a ball better in order to prevent depression. This is a case, one of many, in which a factor (here ball-throwing ability) serves as a proxy for another factor (here gender) when that second factor is not considered. Non-causal mediators, for example, are often proxy to causal mediators. In trying to understand the factors that lead to a particular outcome, factors recognized as proxy factors should be set aside. Including proxy factors along with the factors they are proxy to increases the problems associated both with increased dimensionality and multicollinearity problems. T.S. Eliot is quoted as asking: "Where is the knowledge we have lost in information?" This is one case where too much information may impede the search for knowledge.

5.2 M *and* T *Are Overlapping Risk Factors with Respect to* O

To demonstrate that M and T are overlapping risk factors with respect to O, it must be shown that

- There is no temporal precedence between M and T, and both precede O.
- M and T are correlated;
- When jointly considered in prediction of O, both M and T matter.

It often happens that there are valid multiple measures related to the same underlying construct (hence no temporal precedence). If one of these measures is much more reliable than the others, the other measures are likely to be

identified as proxy to the more reliable one and discarded. However, if they are all more or less of equal but not very high reliability, it may be that combining such measures (as is done with the linear model) might serve to disattenuate the effects of unreliability, in which case none will be identified as proxy to another. This is the case with "overlapping" risk factors. When this happens, it would be preferable to identify all such overlapping risk factors and either to select one to represent them all or, better yet, to combine them into one measure more reliable and more valid a measure of their common construct than any single one of the measures. To do so would facilitate the identification of the underlying common construct as a moderator or mediator of T on O. To do otherwise, once again, would risk having too much information impede the search for knowledge.

For example, in the United States, ethnicity is typically correlated with education, income, and other factors related to socio-economic status. It is not surprising that these are often overlapping risk factors in risk studies. The redundancy should somehow be removed.

5.3 M *and* T *Are Independent Risk Factors for* O

If none of the above sets of conditions are satisfied, M and T are independent risk factors for O. This is the case when M and T are not correlated, but neither moderates the effect of the other on O. In short they are independent factors that have independent effects on O. Gender and ethnicity in many risk studies prove to be independent factors for outcomes related to both.

6 Implementation Questions

6.1 *Population Specificity*

The criteria of the MacArthur approach all refer to a specified population. It is quite possible that

M moderates/mediates the effect of *T* on *O* in one population and not in another (e.g., a clinical population and not a community population or vice versa). Sampling the appropriate population is important.

6.2 Studies to Detect and to Confirm Moderation or Mediation

To demonstrate that the criteria are satisfied, one needs to draw a sample from the population of interest, measure whatever variables are of interest, and (for example) estimate and test the effects. To have power to get precise estimates of the effects, the sample size must be large enough to detect effects of clinical significance. With a specific "a priori" hypothesis of a moderator–mediator relationship and an empirical rationale and justification for such an "a priori" hypothesis, the problem of designing a study to estimate and test the effects is a familiar one. The more difficult practical problem is not how to test an "a priori" hypothesis, but where one would find the empirical rationale and justification for such a hypothesis, and the background information necessary to create a powerful enough design.

Such information is obtained in exploratory data analysis (hypothesis-generating studies), easiest done as secondary data analysis on studies done to test other "a priori" hypotheses (whether RCTs or longitudinal observational studies). In many areas of clinical research data sharing is uncommon and thus secondary data analysis is often quite limited. In a cutting-edge area, where few previous hypothesis-testing studies are available, it would be appropriate to propose a large study specifically for the purpose of hypothesis generation. However, such proposals are often given short shrift in the current funding review process, as well as in the publication review process, often pejoratively described as "mere fishing expeditions." Yet the success of any hypothesis-testing study depends on having a strong hypothesis and a powerful design, which requires the kind of information only obtainable

in such exploratory studies. Consequently, until the culture shifts to put appropriate emphasis on hypothesis-generating studies along with hypothesis-testing studies, the primary source of preliminary information will be secondary data analysis on the researchers' own existing hypothesis-testing studies, to generate hypotheses of moderators and mediators to be tested in subsequent hypothesis-testing studies designed for that purpose.

6.3 "Proving" Lack of Correlation

Other implementation questions also have no comfortable solutions as yet. For example, how does one "prove" that two variables are uncorrelated? To date, to show correlation, a double criterion is used: the association must be statistically significant (e.g., $p < 0.01$) and the magnitude of the correlation above a certain cutpoint (e.g., $|r| > .2$). Otherwise, the correlation is treated as absent. Clearly this is not optimal, but a better criterion has yet to be proposed.

6.4 The Clinical Significance of Moderation/Mediation?

Perhaps the most important and interesting of the unresolved implementation questions is how to describe the effect size due to moderation or mediation in a way that would facilitate consideration of its clinical significance. To see the complexity of the problem, consider the illustrations in Fig. 55.1. Here we have a hypothetical RCT comparing two treatments *T*1 and *T*2, with a binary moderator (say gender, coded $\pm 1/2$ in the analysis but 0 and 1 in the figure) or with a binary mediator (say adequate compliance: 1 coded for yes, 0 for no). Shown are the two lines indicating the regression of outcome *O* on *M* (here exactly the same in both graphs).

Since in an RCT, gender is uncorrelated with treatment choice, the mean of *M* is the same

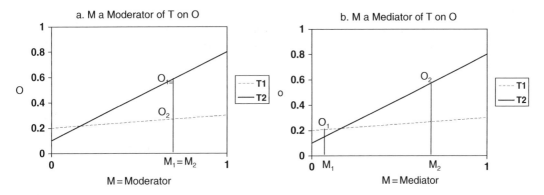

Fig. 55.1 Illustration of a binary moderator (gender) and of a binary mediator (compliance) of choice of treatment (*T*1 versus *T*2) on outcome (*O*) in a hypothetical randomized controlled trial (RCT)

in both groups (e.g., the percentage of men in each group). The average response, O, in each of the two treatment groups is the value of O on the regression line corresponding to that common mean M. The difference between these two average responses is the observed mean difference in O for the two groups. If the O response lines were parallel ($\beta_3 = 0$), this mean difference in O would be the same as the mean difference in O for males as well as for females. However, the lines are not parallel ($\beta_3 \neq 0$), and thus the observed mean difference in O underestimates the treatment effect size for one gender and overestimates it for the other (in fact suggests the wrong treatment as preferred for that gender). Simply reporting β_3 (or standardized β_3) does not convey the information in Fig. 55.1a necessary to allow clinicians to decide whether to make the same choice between $T1$ and $T2$ for men and women, i.e., to consider the clinical significance of this moderator.

In Fig. 55.1b, if M (compliance) is a mediator of treatment choice on outcome, the average M is different in $T1$ (say $M1$) from that in $T2$ (say $M2$). The points on the corresponding lines above those two means are the observed outcomes in the two groups, and the observed treatment effect is indicated by the difference in height of those two points (here with $T2$ having higher outcome than $T1$). This observed treatment effect reflects three impacts of the treatment choice: (1) how much difference in O is induced in M between

the two groups ($M1$ versus $M2$), (2) how much difference is induced by the fact that both lines are not flat (β_2), and (3) how much difference is induced by the fact that the two lines are not parallel (β_3). Is it here worthwhile to consider adding components to $T1$ that would increase compliance and possibly make it more effective against $T1$? Again no single effect size seems to convey the information in the graphic necessary to guide this decision.

6.5 Will Methods Developed for the B&K Model Still "Work" with the MacArthur Model? Will Conclusions Change?

Clearly the Baron and Kenny approach has been used in multiple research studies since its introduction in 1986 and it is natural to ask whether the testing procedures that have been developed for the B&K approach will also be applicable using the MacArthur approach and whether conclusions based on the B&K approach remain valid under the updated approach. Unfortunately, each such test or inference will have to be reevaluated. Some will be validated, some not. Let us take as an example the Sobel mediation test (Sobel, 1982).

The B&K approach is based on two standard linear regression models:

$M = \alpha_0 + \alpha_1 T + \varepsilon_1$, where ε_1 is assumed to be independent of T and normally distributed with variance σ_1^2, and $O = \beta_0 + \beta_1 T + \beta_2 M + \varepsilon_2$, where ε_2 is assumed to be independent of T and M and normally distributed with variance σ_2^2. The Sobel test for mediation proposed the null hypothesis that $\alpha_1\beta_2=0$.

First, suppose X_1, X_2, and X_3 were three variables having a trivariate normal distribution with the correlation between any pair of them $\rho > 0$. If we then evaluated whether X_2 mediated the effect of X_1 on X_3 using the Sobel test, $\alpha_1 = \rho$ and $\beta_2 = \rho/(1 + \rho)$ and thus, since $\rho > 0$, $\alpha_1\beta_2 > 0$. A large enough sample size with a valid test would document that fact.

However, the very same proof shows that X_1 mediates the effect of X_2 on X_3, or that X_3 mediates the effect of X_1 on X_2, or any other of the six permutations of these three variables to the roles of T, M, and O. In fact, with any three correlated variables, even when the three pair-wise correlations are not equal, one can often use the Sobel test to document that any one mediates the effect of any other on the remaining third. It is to prevent this kind of ambiguity that the MacArthur approach explicitly requires that, before considering the possibility of mediation, it is clear from the design that T precedes M that precedes O in time.

However, this is probably a minor problem. The Baron and Kenny model is often described using a diagram in which T is connected to M which is connected to O using single-pointed arrows in that order, strongly suggesting that the time precedence required explicitly in the MacArthur model is tacitly assumed in the Baron and Kenny model. The problem is only with users who have applied the moderator and mediator analyses using the B&K model with cross-sectional data or other types of data in which temporal precedence is indeterminate.

But now suppose that the temporal order condition is satisfied. Then the Sobel mediation test and other related tests (MacKinnon et al, 2002) require that one perform a linear regression analysis relating M to T, resulting in an estimate a of α_1 and its standard error $s(a)$, then a linear regression analysis relating O to M and T,

resulting in an estimate b of β_2 and its standard error $s(b)$. The test then computes a z-statistic, where, for example, the Sobel equation:

$$z\text{ - value} = ab/(b^2 s(a)^2 + a^2 s(b)^2)^{1/2}.$$

The statistical problem is that $s(a)$ computed from a standard linear regression is not the true standard error of a but the standard error conditional on the T sample, as $s(b)$ is the standard error of b conditional on the (T,M) sample. Their true standard errors are much larger and determined by the unknown joint distribution of (T,M). Conditional on the (T,M) sample, the distributions of a and b are normal, but the unconditional distributions are mixtures of normal distributions, not themselves normal distributions. The distribution of ab, the product of two variables, with unknown unconditional distributions is unlikely to be normal. All these problems have been realized in the poor performance of the Sobel test, resulting in the current recommendations to use bootstrap methods to obtain a confidence interval for $\alpha_1\beta_2$ and to reject the null hypothesis of absence of mediation if the value zero is not within that confidence interval.

But then the problem is whether $\alpha_1\beta_2$ is an unambiguous indicator of mediation in the MacArthur Model. Figure 55.2 is an example, with binary T ($T1$ versus $T2$), ordinal O (with means $O1$ and $O2$ in the two groups), ordinal M (with means $M1$ and $M2$ in the two groups), in which all the βs equal 5 and α_1 equals 6. (Such results are general, but negative distances are hard to visualize.) Then β_0 is the value of the intercept of the $T1$ line at $M=0$. β_1 is the distance from that intercept to the intercept of the $T1$ line at $M=0$. Then α_1 is the distance between $M1$ and $M2$. Three auxiliary lines are drawn: two horizontal lines, one through the lower intercept at $(0,\beta_0)$ and one through the point showing the response to $T1$ at $(M1, O1)$, and a line through the upper intercept at $(0, \beta_0+\beta_1)$ parallel to the lower line (showing what the response would have been if the two lines were parallel). Then components of the difference between $O2$ and $O1$ can then be seen:

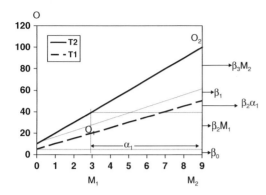

Fig. 55.2 Graphical display of the mediator effect. The two *heavy lines* represent the regression of O on M in groups $T1$ and $T2$. The means of M for $T1$ and $T2$ are $M1$ and $M2$; the difference between them is α_1. The means of O in $T1$ and $T2$ are $O1$ and $O2$, and the difference is graphically dissected into its three components: the main effect β_1, the Sobel mediation effect of $\alpha_1\beta_2$, and the portion due to an interaction effect ($\beta_2 M2$)

- β_1, the main effect of treatment, here equal to the difference in response had no post-treatment change or event occurred;
- $\alpha_1\beta_2$, the effect size used in the Sobel and other related tests;
- $\beta_3 M2$, which in this illustration is the major portion of that difference, is due to the interaction effect that is assumed to be zero in the Baron and Kenny model.

A remarkable fact now evident is that Sobel mediator effect size can be determined without knowing where the response line for $T2$ is located, a consequence of assuming that the response lines are parallel. That is not true for the MacArthur approach.

If an interaction exists in the population but is assumed zero in the model, the two lines shown in Fig. 55.2 would be fitted by two different lines still going through the points ($M1, O1$) and ($M2, O2$), but with a common slope that is a weighted average of the two different actual slopes. Which weighted average depends on the size of the population interactions, the relative sizes of the $T1$ and $T2$ groups, and the size of the correlation between M and T. Then because the Sobel mediator effect is determined by that slope, what it actually means is uninterpretable.

In summary the Sobel test, using bootstrap estimation, is a clear indicator of mediation if and only if the linear model holds and there is no interaction in the population, in which case the MacArthur approach will give the same answer. However, the MacArthur approach gives the correct answer under the linear model whether or not the lines are parallel and can be used when the linear model is not appropriate. A similar comment probably to other tests and inferences derived under the B&K model – sometimes the two approaches will concur and sometimes not.

7 Conclusions

The MacArthur approach is more than a redefinition of moderators and mediators, although that is essentially its core, but represents a way of thinking essential to understanding complex biobehavioral processes. As such, it remains very much a "work in progress."

References

Altman, D. G., Schulz, K. F., Hoher, D., Egger, M., Davidoff, F. et al (2001). The revised CONSORT statement for reporting randomized trials: explanation and elaboration. *Ann Intern Med, 134*, 663–694.

Baron, R. M., and Kenny, D. A. (1986). The moderator-mediator variable distinction in social psychological research: conceptual, strategic, and statistical considerations. *J Pers Soc Psychol, 51*, 1173–1182.

Begg, C., Cho, M., Eastwood, S., Horton, R., Moher, D. et al (1999). Improving the quality of reporting of randomized controlled trials: the CONSORT statement. *JAMA, 276*, 637–639.

Essex, M. J., Kraemer, H. C., Armstong, J. M., Boyce, W. T., Goldsmith, H. H. et al (2006). Exploring risk factors for the emergence of children's mental health problems. *Arch Gen Psychiatry, 63*, 1246–1256.

Finney, D. J. (1994). On biometric language and its abuses. *Biometric Bull*, 11, 2–4.

Jacobi, C., Hayward, C., deZwaan, M., Kraemer, H. C., and Agras, W. S. (2004). Coming to terms with risk factors for eating disorders: application of risk terminology and suggestions for a general taxonomy. *Psychol Bull, 130*, 19–65.

Jaffee, S. R., Caspi, A., Moffitt, T. E., Dodge, K. A., Rutter, M. et al (2005). Nature X nurture: genetic vulnerabilities interact with physical maltreatment to promote conduct problems. *Devel Psychopathol, 17,* 67–84.

Jemal, A., Ward, E., and Thun, M. J. (2007). Recent trends in breast cancer incidence rates by age and tumor characteristics among U.S. women. *Breast Cancer Res, 9,* R28.

King, A. C., Ahn, D. F., Atienza, A. A., and Kraemer, H. C. (2008). Exploring refinements in targeted behavioral medical intervention to advance public health. *Ann Behav Med, 35,* 251–260.

Kraemer, H. C. (2008). Toward non-parametric and clinically meaningful moderators and mediators. *Stat Med, 27,* 1679–1692.

Kraemer, H. C., and Blasey, C. (2004). Centring in regression analysis: a strategy to prevent errors in statistical inference. *Int J Method Psychiat Res, 13,* 141–151.

Kraemer, H. C., Frank, E., and Kupfer, D. J. (2006). Moderators of treatment outcomes: clinical, research, and policy importance. *JAMA, 296,* 1286–1289.

Kraemer, H. C., Kazdin, A. E., Offord, D. R., Kessler, R. C., Jensen, P. S. et al (1999). Measuring the potency of a risk factor for clinical or policy significance. *Psychol Methods,* 4, 257–271.

Kraemer, H. C., Kiernan, M., Essex, M. J., and Kupfer, D. J. (2008). How and why criteria defining moderators and mediators differ between the Baron and Kenny and MacArthur Approaches. *Health Psychol, 27,* S101–S108.

Kraemer, H. C., and Kupfer, D. J. (2006). Size of treatment effects and their importance to clinical research and practice. *Biol Psychiatry, 59,* 990–996.

Kraemer, H. C., Lowe, K. K., and Kupfer, D. J. (2005). *To Your Health: How to Understand What Research Tells us About Risk.* Oxford: Oxford University Press.

Kraemer, H. C., Stice, E., Kazdin, A., and Kupfer, D. (2001). How do risk factors work together to produce an outcome? Mediators, moderators, independent, overlapping and proxy risk factors. *Am J Psychiatry, 158,* 848–856.

Kraemer, H. C., Wilson, G. T., Fairburn, C. G., and Agras, W. S. (2002). Mediators and moderators of treatment effects in randomized clinical trials. *Arch Gen Psychiatry, 59,* 877–883.

MacKinnon, D. P., Lockwood, C. M., Hoffman, J. M., West, S. G., and Sheets, V. (2002). A comparison of methods to test mediation and other intervening variable effects. *Psychol Methods, 7,* 83–104.

Murphy, G. M. J., Hollander, S. B., Rodrigues, Kremer, C., and Schatzberg, A. F. (2004). Effects of the serotonic transporter gene promoter polymorphism on Mirtazapine and Paroxetine efficacy and adverse events in geriatric major depression. *Arch Gen Psychiatry, 61,* 1163–1169.

Piaggio, G., Elbourne, D. R., Altman, D. G., Pocock, S. J., and Evans, S. J. W. (2006). Reporting of noninferiority and equivalence randomized trials: an extension of the CONSORT statement. *JAMA, 295,* 1152–1160.

American Psychological Association (2001). *Publication Manual of the American Psychological Association, 5th Ed.* Washington, DC: American Psychological Association.

Rennie, D. (1996). How to report randomized controlled trials: The CONSORT Statement. *JAMA, 276,* 649.

Sobel, M. E. (Ed.). (1982). *Asymptotic Intervals for Indirect Effects in Structural Equations Models.* San Francisco, CA: Jossey-Bass.

Stampfer, M. J., Willett, W. C., Colditz, G. A., Rosner, B., Speizer, F. E. et al (1985). A prospective study of postmenopausal estrogen therapy and coronary heart disease. *New Engl J Med,* 313, 1044–1049.

The MTA Cooperative Group. (1999). Moderators and mediators of treatment response for children with attention-deficit/hyperactivity disorder. *Arch Gen Psychiatry, 56,* 1088–1096.

Writing Group for the Women's Health Initiative Investigators. (2002). Principal results from the Women's Health Initiative randomized controlled trial. *JAMA, 288,* 321–333.

Chapter 56

Multilevel Modeling

1 Introduction

The term "multilevel" refers to the distinct levels or units of analysis, which usually, but not always, consist of individuals (at lower level) who are nested within contextual/aggregate units (at higher level). Indeed, individuals are organized within a nearly infinite number of levels of organization, from the individual up (for example, families, neighborhoods, counties, and states), from the individual down (for example, body organs, cellular matrices, and DNA), and for overlapping units (for example, area of residence and work environment). It is, therefore, necessary that links should be made between these different levels of analysis. Multilevel methods consist of statistical procedures that are pertinent when (i) the observations that are being analyzed are correlated or clustered or (ii) the causal processes are thought to operate simultaneously at more than one level and/or (iii) there is an intrinsic interest in describing the variability and heterogeneity in the phenomenon, over and above the focus on average (Diez Roux, 2002; Subramanian, 2004; Subramanian et al, 2003).

Multilevel methods are specifically geared toward the statistical analysis of data that have a nested structure. The nesting, typically, but not always, is hierarchical. For instance, a two-level structure would have many level-1 units nested within a smaller number of level-2 units. In educational research, the field that provided the impetus for multilevel methods, level-1 usually, consists of pupils who are nested within schools at level-2. Such structures arise routinely in health and social sciences, such that level-1 and level-2 units could be workers in organizations, patients in hospitals, and individuals in neighborhoods, respectively. In this chapter, for exemplification, we will consider the structure of individuals nested within neighborhoods (used to reflect one practical realization of place) (see Chapter 24).

The existence of nested data structures is neither random nor ignorable; for instance, individuals differ but so do the neighborhoods. Differences among neighborhoods could either be directly due to the differences among individuals who live in them or groupings based on neighborhoods may arise for reasons less strongly associated with the characteristics of the individuals who live in them. Regardless, once such groupings are established, even if their establishment is random, they will tend to become differentiated. This would imply that the group (for example, neighborhoods) and its members (for example, individual residents) can exert influence on each other suggesting different sources of variation (for example, individual induced and neighborhood induced) in the outcome of interest and thus compelling analysts to consider covariates at the individual and at the neighborhood level. Ignoring this multilevel

S.V. Subramanian (✉)
Department of Society, Human Development and Health, Harvard School of Public Health, 677 Huntington Avenue, Kresge Building, 7th Floor, Boston MA 02115, USA
e-mail: svsubram@hsph.harvard.edu

A. Steptoe (ed.), *Handbook of Behavioral Medicine*, DOI 10.1007/978-0-387-09488-5_56,
© Springer Science+Business Media, LLC 2010

structure of variations not simply risks over-looking the importance of neighborhood effects, but has implications for statistical validity (Goldstein, 2003; Raudenbush and Bryk, 2002).

Clustered data also arise as a result of sampling strategies. For instance, while planning large-scale survey data collection, for reasons of cost and efficiency, it is usual to adopt a multistage sampling design. A national population survey, for example, might involve a three-stage design, with regions sampled first, then neighborhoods, and then individuals. A design of this kind generates a three-level hierarchically clustered structure of individuals at level-1 nested within neighborhoods at level-2, which in turn are nested in regions at level-3. Individuals living in the same neighborhood can be expected to be more alike than they would be if the sample were truly random. Similar correlation can be expected for neighborhoods within a region. Much documentation exists on measuring this "design effect" and correcting for it. Indeed, clustered designs (for example, individuals at level-1 nested in neighborhoods at level-2 nested in regions at level-3) are often a nuisance in traditional analysis. However, individuals, neighborhoods, and regions can be seen as distinct structures that exist in the population that should be measured and modeled.

2 Multilevel Framework: A Necessity for Understanding Ecologic Effects

Figure 56.1 identifies a typology of designs for data collection and analyses (Blakely and Woodward, 2000; Kawachi and Subramanian, 2006; Subramanian et al, 2007; Subramanian et al, 2009), where the rows indicate the level or the unit at which the outcome variable is being measured (that is, at the individual level (y) or at the ecological level (Y)) and the columns indicate whether the exposure is being measured at the individual level (x) or at the ecological

		Exposure	
		Individual (x) (measured at individual level)	Ecologic (X) (measured at ecological level)
Outcome	Individual (y)	(y,x) Traditional risk factor study	(y,X) Multilevel study
	Ecologic (Y)	(Y,x)[(A)]	(Y,X) Ecological study

Fig. 56.1 Typology of studies (Subramanian et al, 2007) Note: [(A)]This type of study is impossible to specify as it stands. Practically speaking, it will either take the form of (y,x), that is, ecological study, where X will now simply be central tendency of x. Or, if dis-aggregation of Y is possible, so that we can observe y, then it will be equivalent to (y,x)

level (X). The ecological level, in this illustration, relates to the neighborhood level. Study type (y,x) is most commonly encountered when the researcher aims to link exposure to outcomes, with both being measured at the individual level. Study type (y,x) typically ignores ecological effects (either implicitly or explicitly).

Conversely, study type (Y,X) – referred to as an "ecological study" – may seem intuitively appropriate for research where higher levels (for instance, neighborhoods, regions, states, and schools) are the targets of interest. However, study type (Y,X) conflates the genuinely ecological and the aggregate or "compositional" (Moon et al, 2005) and precludes the possibility of testing heterogeneous contextual effects on different types of individuals. Ecological effects reflect predictors and associated mechanisms operating primarily at the contextual level. The search for such measures and their scientific validation and assessment is an area of active research (Raudenbush, 2003). Aggregate effects, in contrast, equate the effect of a neighborhood with the sum of the individual effects associated with the people living within the neighborhood. In this situation the interpretative question becomes particularly relevant. If common membership of a neighborhood by a set of individuals brings about an effect that is over and above those resulting from individual characteristics, then there may indeed be an ecological effect.

Study type (y,X) provides a multilevel approach, that is, in which an ecological exposure is linked to an individual outcome. A more complete representation would be type (y,x,X) whereby we have an individual outcome (y), individual confounders (x), and neighborhood exposure (X) reflecting a multilevel structure of individuals nested within neighborhoods. A fundamental motivation for study type (y,x,X) is to distinguish "neighborhood differences" from "the difference a neighborhood makes" (Moon et al, 2005). Stated differently, ecological effects on the individual outcome should be ascertained after individual factors that reflect the composition of the places (and may be potential confounders) have been controlled. Indeed, compositional explanations for ecological variations in health are common. It nonetheless makes intuitive sense to test for the possibility of ecological effects. Besides anticipating their impact on individual outcomes, compositional factors may vary by context. Thus, unless contextual variables are considered, their direct effects and any indirect mediation through compositional variables remain unidentified. Moreover, composition itself has an intrinsic ecologic dimension; the very fact that individual (compositional) factors may "explain" ecologic variations serves as a reminder that the real understanding of ecologic effects is likely to be complex.

The multilevel framework with its simultaneous examination of the characteristics of the individuals at one level and the context or ecologies in which they are located at another level accordingly offers a comprehensive framework for understanding the ways in which places can affect people (contextual) and/or people can affect places (composition). It likewise allows for a more precise distinction between aggregative fallacy (which is the invalid transfer of results observed at an aggregate level to the individual level) and ecologic effects (which is the effect of aggregate ecologies on individual outcomes) (Subramanian et al, 2009).

3 A Typology of Multilevel Data Structures

The idea of multilevel structure can be recast, with great advantage, to address a range of circumstances where one may anticipate clustering.

Outcomes as well as their causal mechanisms are rarely stable and invariant over time, producing data structures that involve repeated measures, which can be considered a special case of multilevel clustered data structures. Consider the "repeated cross-sectional design" that can be structured in multilevel terms with neighborhoods at level-3, year/time at level-2, and individuals at level-1. In this example, level-2 represents repeated measurements on the neighborhoods (level-3) over time. Such a structure can be used to investigate what sorts of individuals and what sorts of neighborhoods have changed with respect to the outcome. Alternatively, there is the classic "longitudinal or panel design" in which the level-1 is the measurement occasion, level-2 is the individual, and level-3 is the neighborhood. This time, the individuals are repeatedly measured at different time intervals so that it becomes possible to model changing individual behaviors within a contextual setting of, say, neighborhoods.

When different responses/outcomes are correlated, it could be seen as generating a "multivariate" multilevel data structure in which level-1 are sets of response variables measured on individuals at level-2 nested in neighborhoods at level-3. The "multivariate responses" could be, for instance, different aspects of, say, health behavior (for example, smoking and drinking). In addition, such responses could be a mixture of "quality" (do you smoke/do you drink) and "quantity" (how many/how much) producing "mixed multivariate responses." The substantive benefit of this approach is that it is possible to assess whether different types of behavior and whether the qualitative and quantitative aspects of each behavior are related to individual characteristics in the same or different ways. Additionally, we can also ascertain whether neighborhoods that are high for one behavior are also high for another and whether neighborhoods with high prevalence of smoking, for instance, are also high in terms of the number of cigarettes smoked.

While the previous examples are strictly hierarchical, in that all level-1 units that form a level-2 grouping are always in the same group at any higher level, data structures could be non-hierarchical. For example, a model of health behavior (for instance, smoking) could be formulated with individuals at level-1 and both residential neighborhoods and workplaces at level-2 not nested but crossed and are also called as the "cross-classified structures." Individuals are then seen as occupying more than one set of contexts, each of which may have an important influence. For instance, individuals in a particular workplace may come from different neighborhoods and individuals in a neighborhood may go to several worksites.

A related structure occurs when an individual can be considered to belong simultaneously to several neighborhoods with the contributions of each neighborhood being weighted in relation to its distance (if the interest is spatial) from the individual. This generates a structure that is referred to as "multiple membership" data structures which are non-hierarchical in design. In summary, between some combinations of hierarchical structures, cross-classified nesting, and multiple memberships, a great deal of complexity that is imprinted either explicitly or implicitly in data can be incorporated via multilevel models.

4 The Distinction Between Levels and Variables

Each of the levels that were discussed in the previous section (for example, neighborhoods) can be considered as variables in a regression equation with an indicator variable specified for each neighborhood. Conversely, why are many categorical variables such as gender, ethnicity/race, and social class not a level? Critical to treating neighborhoods, for example, as a level is

because neighborhoods are treated as a population of units from which we have observed one random sample. This enables us to draw generalizations for a particular level (for example, neighborhoods) based on an observed sample of neighborhoods. Further, it is more efficient to model neighborhoods as a random variable given the (likely) large number of neighborhoods. On the other hand, gender, for instance, is not a level because it is not a sample out of all possible gender categories. Rather, it is an attribute of individuals. Thus, male or female in our gender example is a "fixed" discrete category of a variable with the specific categories only contributing to their respective means. They are not a random sample of gender categories from a population of gender groupings. Further, we would usually wish to ascribe a fixed effect to each gender, but not each neighborhood. Rather, we wish to model an ecologic attribute at the neighborhood level. It is possible to consider "levels" as "variables". Thus, when neighborhoods are considered as a variable, they are typically reflective of a fixed classification. While this may be useful in certain circumstances, doing so robs the researcher of the ability to generalize to all neighborhoods and inferences are only possible for the specific neighborhoods observed in the sample.

5 Multilevel Analysis

There are three constitutive components of multilevel analysis which are now discussed.

5.1 Evaluating Sources of Variation: Compositional and/or Contextual

A fundamental application of multilevel methods is disentangling the different sources of variations in the outcome. Evidence for variations in poor health, for instance, between different neighborhoods can be due to factors that are intrinsic to, and are measured at, the neighborhood level. In other words, the variation is due to what can be described as *contextual* or *neighborhood effects*. Alternatively, variations between neighborhoods may be *compositional*, that is, certain types of people who are more likely to be in poor health due to their individual characteristics happen to be clustered in certain neighborhoods. The issue, therefore, is not whether variations between different neighborhoods exist (they usually do), but what is the primary source of these variations. Put simply, are there significant contextual differences in health between neighborhoods, after taking into account the individual compositional characteristics of the neighborhood? The notions of contextual and compositional sources of variation have general relevance and they are applicable whether the context is administrative (for example, political boundaries), temporal (for example, different time periods), or institutional (for example, schools or hospitals).

5.2 Describing Contextual Heterogeneity

Contextual differences may be complex such that they may not be the same for all types of people. Describing such contextual heterogeneity is another aspect of multilevel analysis and can have two interpretative dimensions. First, there may be a different amount of neighborhood variation, such that, for example, for high social class individuals it may not matter in which neighborhoods they live (thus a lower between-neighborhood variation) but it matters a great deal for the low social class and as such show a large between-neighborhood variation. Second, there may be a differential ordering: neighborhoods that are high for one group are low for the other and vice versa. Stated simply, the multilevel analytical question is whether the contextual neighborhood differences in poor health, after taking into account the individual

composition of the neighborhood, are different for different types of population groups.

5.3 Characterizing and Explaining the Contextual Variations

Contextual differences, in addition to people's characteristics, may also be influenced by the different characteristics of neighborhoods. Stated differently, individual differences may interact with context, and ascertaining the relative importance of individual and neighborhood covariates is another key aspect of a multilevel analysis. For example, over and above social class (individual characteristic), health may depend upon the poverty levels of the neighborhoods (neighborhood characteristic). The contextual effect of poverty can either be the same for both the high and the low social class suggesting that while neighborhood poverty explains the prevalence of poor health, it does not influence the social class inequalities in health. On the other hand, the contextual effects of poverty may be different for different groups, such that neighborhood poverty adversely affects the low social class, but does the opposite for the high social class. Thus, neighborhood level poverty may not only be related to average health achievements but also shapes social inequalities in health. The analytical question of interest is whether the effect of neighborhood level socioeconomic characteristics on health is different for different types of people?

Presence of a multilevel data structure along with an interest in understanding contextual effects provides substantive as well as technical motivation to use multilevel statistical models (Goldstein, 2003; Raudenbush and Bryk, 2002). We shall not review the basic principles of multilevel modeling here as they have been described elsewhere in the context of health research (Blakely and Subramanian, 2006; Moon et al, 2005; Subramanian et al, 2003), but instead provide a brief overview of the type of models invoked for identifying ecological effects.

6 Specifying Multilevel Models

Like all statistical regression equations, multi-level models have the same underlying function, which can be expressed as

Response = Fixed/Average Parameters
+(Random/Variance Parameters).

While in a conventional regression model the random part of the model is usually restricted to a single term (that are called as "error terms" or "residuals"), in the multilevel regression model the focus or innovation is on expanding the random part of a statistical model.

In order to exemplify multilevel models we consider the following example. Suppose we are interested in studying the variation in body mass index (BMI), as a function of certain individual and neighborhood predictors. Let us assume that the researcher collected data on a sample of 50 neighborhoods and, for each of these neighborhoods, a random sample of individuals. We then have a two-level structure where the outcome is BMI y, for individual i in neighborhood j. We will restrict this exemplification to one individual-level predictor, poverty, x_{1ij}, coded as 0 if not poor and 1 if poor, for every individual i in neighborhood j, and one neighborhood predictor, w_{1j}, a socioeconomic deprivation index in neighborhood j.

7 Variance Component or Random Intercepts Model

Multilevel models operate by developing regression equations at each level of analysis. In the illustration considered here, models would have to be specified at two levels, level-1 and level-2. The model at level-1 can be formally expressed as

$$y_{ij} = \beta_{0j} + \beta_1 x_{1ij} + e_{0ij}. \qquad (56.1)$$

In this level-1 model, β_{0j} (associated with a constant, x_{0ij}, which is a set of 1s, and therefore, not written) is the mean BMI for the *jth*

neighborhood for the non-poor group; β_1 is the average differential in BMI associated with individual poverty status (x_{1ij}) across all neighborhoods. Meanwhile, e_{0ij} is the individual or the level-1 residual term. To make this a genuine two-level model we let β_{0j} become a random variable as

$$\beta_{0j} = \beta_0 + u_{0j}, \qquad (56.2)$$

where u_{0j} is the random neighborhood-specific displacement associated with mean BMI (β_0) for the non-poor group. Since we do not allow, at this stage, the average BMI differential for the poor group (β_1) to vary across neighborhoods, u_{0j} is assumed to be same for both groups. Eq. (56.2) is then the level-2 between-neighborhood model.

It is worth emphasizing that the "neighborhood effect", u_{0j}, can be treated in one of two ways. One can estimate each neighborhood separately as a fixed effect (that is, treat them as a variable; with 50 neighborhoods there will be 49 additional parameters to be estimated). Such a strategy may be appropriate if the interest is in making inferences about just those sampled neighborhoods. On the other hand, if neighborhoods are treated as a (random) sample from a population of neighborhoods (which might include neighborhoods in future studies if one has complete population data), the target of inference is the variation between neighborhoods in general. Adopting this multilevel statistical approach makes u_{0j} a random variable at level-2 in a two-level statistical model.

Substituting the level-2 model (Eq. 56.2) into level-1 model (Eq. 56.1) and grouping them into fixed and random part components (the latter shown in brackets) yields the following combined, also referred to as *random intercepts* or *variance components*, model:

$$y_{ij} = \beta_0 + \beta_1 x_{1ij} + (u_{0j} + e_{0ij}). \qquad (56.3)$$

We have now expressed the response y_{ij} as the sum of a fixed part and a random part. Assuming a normal distribution with a 0 mean, we can estimate a variance at level-1 (σ_{e0}^2: the between-individual within-neighborhood variation) and level-2 (σ_{u0}^2: the between-neighborhood variation), both conditional on fixed poverty differences in BMI. It is the presence of more than one residual term (or the structure of the random part more generally) that distinguishes the multilevel model from the standard linear regression models or analysis of variance type analysis. The underlying random structure (variance–covariance) of the model specified in Eq. (56.3) is $\text{Var}[u_{0j}] \sim N(0, \sigma_{u0}^2)$; $\text{Var}[e_{0ij}] \sim N(0, \sigma_{e0}^2)$; and $\text{Cov}[u_{0j}, e_{0ij}] = 0$. It is this aspect of the regression model that requires special estimation procedures in order to obtain satisfactory parameter estimates (Goldstein, 2003).

The model specified in Eq. (56.3) with the above random structure is typically used to partition variation according to the different levels, with the variance in y_{ij} being the sum of σ_{u0}^2 and σ_{e0}^2. This leads to a statistic known as *intraclass correlation*, or *intra-unit correlation*, or more generally *variance partitioning coefficient* (Goldstein et al, 2002), representing the degree of similarity between two randomly chosen individuals within a neighborhood. This can be expressed as

$$\rho = \frac{\sigma_{u0}^2}{\sigma_{u0}^2 + \sigma_{e0}^2}. \qquad (56.4)$$

Note that Eq. (56.3) estimates a variance based on the observed sample of neighborhoods. While this is important to establish the overall importance of neighborhoods as a unit or level, another quantity of interest may pertain to estimating whether living in neighborhood j_1, as compared to neighborhood j_3, for example, predicts a different BMI conditional on compositional influences of covariates. Given Eq. (56.3), we can estimate for each level-2 a unit:

$$\hat{u}_{0j} = E(u_{0j}|Y, \hat{\beta}, \hat{\Omega}) \qquad (56.5)$$

The quantity $\hat{u}_{0j}$ is referred to as "estimated" or "predicted" residuals, or using Bayesian ter-

minology, as "posterior" residual estimates, and is calculated as

$$\hat{u}_{0j} = r_j \times \frac{\sigma_{u0}^2}{\sigma_{u0}^2 + \sigma_{e0}^2/n_j}, \qquad (56.6)$$

where σ_{u0}^2 and σ_{e0}^2 are as defined above, r_j is the mean of the individual-level raw residuals for neighborhood j, and n_j is the number of individuals within each neighborhood j. This formula for $\hat{u}_{0j}$ uses the level-1 and level-2 variances and the number of people observed in neighborhood j to scale the observed level-2 residual (r_j). As the level-1 variance declines or the sample size increases, the scale factor approaches 1 and thus estimated $\hat{u}_{0j}$ approaches r_j.

These neighborhood-level residuals are random variables that are seen to be coming from a distribution and whose parameter values quantify the variation among the higher level or neighborhood units (Goldstein, 2003). Another interpretation is that each $\hat{u}_{0j}$ estimates neighborhood j's departure from the expected mean outcome. This interpretation is premised on the assumption that each neighborhood belongs to a population of neighborhoods, and the distribution of the population provides information about plausible values for neighborhood j (Goldstein, 2003). For a neighborhood with only a few individuals, we can obtain more precise estimates by combining the population and neighborhood-specific observations than if we were to ignore the population membership assumption and use only the information from that neighborhood. When the estimated residuals at higher level units are of interest in their own right, we need to provide standard errors, interval estimates, and significance tests as well as point estimates for them (Goldstein, 2003).

8 Modeling Places: Fixed or Random?

It is worth drawing parallels between the multilevel or a random-effects model Eq. (56.3) and the conventional ordinary least squares or fixed-effects regression model. Consider the fixed-effects model, whereby the neighborhood effect is estimated by including a dummy for each neighborhood, as shown below:

$$y_{ij} = \beta_0 + \beta x_{ij} + \beta N_j + (e_{0ij}), \qquad (56.7)$$

where N_j is a vector of dummy variables for $N - 1$ neighborhoods. The key conceptual difference between the fixed and the random-effects approach to modeling neighborhoods is that while the fixed part coefficients are estimated separately, the random part differentials (u_{0j}) are conceptualized as coming from a distribution (Goldstein, 2003). This conceptualization results in three practical benefits (Jones and Bullen, 1994):

(i) *pooling information* between neighborhoods, with all the information in the data being used in the combined estimation of the fixed and random part; in particular, the overall regression terms are based on the information for all neighborhoods;

(ii) *borrowing strength*, whereby neighborhood-specific relations that are imprecisely estimated benefit from the information for other neighborhoods; and

(iii) *precision-weighted estimation*, whereby unreliable neighborhood-specific fixed estimates are differentially down-weighted or shrunk toward the overall city-wide estimate. A reliably estimated within-neighborhood relation will be largely immune to this shrinkage.

The random-effects and the fixed-effects estimates for each neighborhood, meanwhile, are related (Jones and Bullen, 1994). The neighborhood-specific random intercept (β_{0j}) in a multilevel model is a weighted combination of the specific neighborhood coefficient in a fixed-effects model (β_{0j}^*) and the overall multilevel intercept (β_0), in the following way:

$$\beta_{0j} = w_j \beta_{0j}^* + (1 - w)\beta_0, \qquad (56.8)$$

with the overall multilevel intercept being a weighted average of all the fixed intercepts:

$$\beta_0 \left(\sum w_j \beta_{0j}^* \right) \Big/ \sum w_j. \qquad (56.9)$$

Each neighborhood weight is the ratio of the true between-neighborhood parameter variance to the total variance, which additionally includes sampling variance resulting from observing a sample from the neighborhood. Consequently, the weights represent the reliability or precision of the fixed terms:

$$w_j = \frac{\sigma_{uo}^2}{v_j^2 + \sigma_{uo}^2}, \qquad (56.10)$$

where the random sampling variance of the fixed parameter is

$$v_j^2 = \frac{\sigma_e^2}{n_j}, \qquad (56.11)$$

with n_j being the number of observations within each neighborhood. When there are genuine differences between the neighborhoods and the sample sizes within a neighborhood are large, the sampling variance will be small in comparison to the total variance. As a result, the associated weight will be close to 1, with the fixed neighborhood effect being reliably estimated, and the random effect neighborhood estimate will be close to the fixed neighborhood effect. As the sampling variance increases, however, the weight will be less than 1 and the multilevel estimate will increasingly be influenced by the overall intercept based on pooling across neighborhoods. Shrinkage estimates allow the data to determine an appropriate compromise between specific estimates for different neighborhoods and the overall fixed estimate that pools information across places over the entire sample (Jones and Bullen, 1994).

Importantly, the fixed-effects approach to modeling neighborhood differences using cross-sectional data is not a choice for a typical multilevel research question, where there is an intrinsic interest in an exposure measured at the

level of neighborhood such as the one specified in Eq. (56.3); in such instances, a multilevel
modeling approach is a necessity. This is because
the dummy variables associated with the neighborhoods (measuring the fixed effects of each
neighborhood) and the neighborhood exposure
is perfectly confounded and, as such, the latter is
not identifiable (Fielding, 2004). Thus, the fixed-
effects specification to understand neighborhood
differences is unsuitable for the sort of complex questions which multilevel modeling can
address.

9 Random Coefficient or Random Slopes Model

We can expand the random structure in Eq.
(56.3) by allowing the fixed effect of individual
poverty (β_1) to randomly vary across neighborhoods in the following manner:

$$y_{ij} = \beta_{0j} + \beta_{1j}x_{1ij} + e_{0ij}. \qquad (56.12)$$

At level-2, there will now be two models:

$$\beta_{0j} = \beta_0 + u_{0j}, \qquad (56.13)$$

$$\beta_{1j} = \beta_1 + u_{1j}. \qquad (56.14)$$

Substituting the level-2 models in Eqs.
(56.13) and 56.14 into the level-1 model in Eq.
(56.12) gives

$$y_{ij} = \beta_0 + \beta_1 x_{1ij} + (u_{0j} + u_{1j}x_{1ij} + e_{0ij}). \qquad (56.15)$$

Across neighborhoods, the mean BMI for
non-poor is β_0, the mean BMI for the poor is
$\beta_0 + \beta_1$, and the mean "poverty-differential" is
β_1. The poverty differential is no longer constant across neighborhoods, but varies by the
amount u_{1j} around the mean β_1. Such models
are also referred to as *random slopes* or *random coefficient models*. These models have a

much more complex variance–covariance structure than before:

$$\mathrm{Var}\begin{bmatrix} u_{0j} \\ u_{1j} \end{bmatrix} \sim N\left(0, \begin{bmatrix} \sigma_{u0}^2 & \\ \sigma_{u0u1} & \sigma_{u1}^2 \end{bmatrix}\right) \qquad (56.16)$$

and

$$\mathrm{Var}[e_{0ij}] \sim N(0, \sigma_{e0}^2). \qquad (56.17)$$

With this formulation, it is no longer straightforward to think in terms of a summary intraclass
correlation statistic ρ as the level-2 variation is
now a function of a individual predictor variable
x_{1ij}. In our exemplification when x_{1ij} is a dummy
variable, we will have two variances estimated at
level-2: one for non-poor which is

$$\sigma_{u0}^2 \qquad (56.18)$$

and one for poor which is

$$\sigma_{u0}^2 + 2\sigma_{u0u1}x_{1ij} + \sigma_{u1}^2 x_{1ij}^2. \qquad (56.19)$$

That is, level-2 variation will be a "quadratic"
function of the individual predictor variable
when x_{1ij} is a continuous predictor. Thus the
notion of "random intercepts and slopes", while
intuitive, is not entirely appropriate. Rather, what
these models are really doing is modeling variance as some function (constant, quadratic, or
linear) of a predictor variable (Subramanian et al,
2003).

Building on the above perspective of modeling the variance–covariance function (as
opposed to "random intercepts and slopes"), we
can extend the concept to modeling variance
function at level-1. It is extremely common to
assume that the variance is "homoskedastic" in
the random part at level-1 (σ_{e0}^2; Eq. (56.15)),
and indeed, researchers seldom report whether
this assumption was tested or not. One strategy
would be to model the different variances for
poor and non-poor of the following form:

$$\begin{aligned} y_{ij} = \beta_0 + \beta_1 x_{1ij} &+ (u_{0j} + u_{1j}x_{1ij} \\ &+ e_{1ij}x_{1ij} + e_{2ij}x_{2ij}), \end{aligned} \qquad (56.20)$$

where, $x_{1ij} = 0$ for non-poor, 1 for poor, and the new variable $x_{2ij} = 1$ for non-poor, 0 for poor, with σ_{e1}^2 giving the variance for poor and σ_{e2}^2 giving the variance for non-poor, and $Cov[e_{1ij}, e_{2ij}] = 0$. There are other parsimonious ways to model level-1 variation in the presence of a number of predictor variables (Goldstein, 2003; Subramanian et al, 2003). With this specification, we do not have an interpretation of the random level-1 coefficients as "random slopes" as we did at level-2. The level-1 parameters, σ_{e1}^2 and σ_{e1}^2, describe the complexity of level-1 variation, which is no longer homoskedastic (Goldstein, 2003). Anticipating and modeling heteroskedasticity or heterogeneity at the individual level may be important in multilevel analysis as there may be cross-level confounding – what may appear to be neighborhood heterogeneity (level-2) to be explained by some ecological variable could be due to a failure to take account of the between-individual (within-neighborhood) heterogeneity (level-1).

10 Modeling the Fixed Effect of a Neighborhood Predictor

An attractive feature of multilevel models – one that is perhaps most commonly used in health and social science research – is their utility in modeling neighborhood *and* individual characteristics, and any interaction between them, simultaneously. We will consider the underlying level-2 model related to Eq. (56.20), which is exactly the same as specified in Eqs. (56.13) and (56.14), but now including a level-2 predictor: w_{1j}, the deprivation index for neighborhood j:

$$\beta_{0j} = \beta_0 + \alpha_1 w_{1j} + u_{0j}, \qquad (56.21)$$

$$\beta_{1j} = \beta_1 + \alpha_2 w_{1j} + u_{1j}. \qquad (56.22)$$

Note that the separate specification of micro and macro models correctly recognizes that the contextual variables (w_{1j}) are predictors of between-neighborhood differences. The extension of Eq. (56.20) will now be

$$y_{ij} = \beta_0 + \beta_1 x_{1ij} + \alpha_1 w_{1j} + \alpha_2 w_{1j} x_{1ij}$$
$$+ (u_{0j} + u_{1j} x_{1ij} + e_{1ij} x_{1ij} + e_{2ij} x_{2ij}). \qquad (56.23)$$

The combined formulation in Eq. (56.23) highlights an important feature, the presence of an interaction between a level-2 and level-1 predictor ($w_{1j} \cdot x_{1ij}$), represented by the fixed parameter α_2. Now, α_1 estimates the marginal change in BMI for a unit change in the neighborhood deprivation index for the non-poor and α_2 estimates the extent to which the marginal change in BMI for unit change in the neighborhood deprivation index is different for the poor. This multilevel statistical formulation allows cross-level effect modification or interaction between individual and neighborhood characteristics to be robustly specified and estimated.

In summary, multilevel models are concerned with modeling both the average and the variation around the average, at different levels. To accomplish this they consist of two sets of parameters: those summarizing the average relationships(s) and those summarizing the variation around the average at both the level of individuals and neighborhoods. Models presented in the preceding section can be easily adapted to other structures with nesting of level-1 units within level-2 units. Additionally, these models can be extended to three or more levels. While the preceding discussion considered a single normally distributed response variable for illustration, multilevel models are capable of handling a wide range of responses. These include binary outcomes, proportions (as logit, log–log, and probit models), multiple categories (as ordered and unordered multinomial models), and counts (as Poisson and negative binomial distribution models). In essence, these models work by assuming a specific, "non-Gaussian" distribution for the random part at level-1, while maintaining the normality assumptions for random parts at higher levels. Consequently, the discussion presented in this entry focusing at the neighborhood level would continue to hold regardless of the nature of the response variable, with some exceptions. For instance, determining intraclass correlation or partitioning variances across individual and neighborhood levels in complex non-linear multilevel logistic models is not straightforward (see elsewhere for details: (Browne et al, 2005; Goldstein et al, 2002)).

11 Exploiting the Flexibility of Multilevel Models to Incorporating "Realistic" Complexity

Current implementations of multilevel models have generally failed to exploit the full capabilities of the analytical framework (Leyland, 2005; Moon et al, 2005; Subramanian, 2004). Much, if not all, of the current research linking neighborhoods and health is cross-sectional and assumes a hierarchical structure of individuals nested within neighborhoods. This simplistic scenario ignores, for instance, the possibility that an individual might move several times and as such reflect neighborhood effects drawn from several contexts or that other competing contexts (for example, schools, workplaces, and hospital settings) may simultaneously contribute to contextual effects. Figure 56.2 provides a visual illustration of one complex, but realistic multilevel structure for neighborhoods and health research, where time measurements (level-1)

are nested within individuals (level-2) who are in turn nested within neighborhoods (level-3). Importantly, individuals are assigned different weights for the time spent in each neighborhood. For example, individual 25 moved from neighborhood 1 to neighborhood 25 during the time period t1–t2, spending 20% of her time in neighborhood 1 and 80% in her new neighborhood. This multiple membership design would allow control of changing context as well as changing composition. Such designs could be extended to incorporate memberships to additional contexts, such as workplaces or schools. It can also be extended to enable consideration of weighted effects of proximate contexts (Langford et al, 1998). So, for example, the geographic distribution of disease can be seen not only as a matter of composition and the immediate context in which an outcome occurs but also as a consequence of the impact of nearby contexts with nearer areas being more influential than more distant ones. This is also called *spatial autocorrelation* and forms an important area of spatial statistical research (Lawson, 2001). While such analyses require high-quality longitudinal and context-referenced data, models that incorporate such "realistic complexity" (Best et al, 1996) are likely to improve our understanding of true neighborhood effects. While the foregoing discussion provides a sound rationale to adopt a multilevel analytic approach for modeling ecologic effects, they obviously do not overcome the limitations intrinsic to any observational study design, single-level or multilevel.

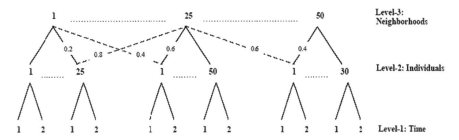

Fig. 56.2 Multilevel structure of repeated measurements of individuals over time across neighborhoods with individuals having multiple membership to different neighborhoods across the time span
Source: Subramanian (2004)

12 Summary

The multilevel statistical approach – an approach that explicitly models the correlated nature of the data arising either due to sampling design or because populations are clustered – has a number of substantive and technical advantages.

From a substantive perspective, it circumvents the problems associated with ecological fallacy (the invalid transfer of results observed at the ecological level to the individual level); individualistic fallacy (occurs by failing to take into account the ecology or context within which individual relationships happen); and atomistic fallacy (arises when associations between individual variables are used to make inferences on the association between the analogous variables at the group/ecological level). The issue common to the above fallacies is the failure to recognize the existence of unique relationships being observable at multiple levels and each being important in its own right. Specifically, one can think of an individual relationship (for example, individuals who are poor are more likely to have poor health); an ecological–contextual relationship (for example, places with a high proportion of poor individuals are more likely to have higher rates of poor health); and an individual–contextual relationship (for example, the greatest likelihood of being in poor health is found for poor individuals in places with a high proportion of poor people). Multilevel models explicitly recognize the level-contingent nature of relationships.

From a technical perspective, the multilevel approach enables researchers to obtain statistically efficient estimates of fixed regression coefficients. Specifically, using the clustering information, multilevel models provide correct standard errors and thereby robust confidence intervals and significance tests. These generally will be more conservative than the traditional ones that are obtained simply by ignoring the presence of clustering. More broadly, multilevel models allow a more appropriate and realistic specification of complex variance structures at each level. Multilevel models are also precision weighted and capitalize on the advantages that accrue as a result of "pooling" information from all the neighborhoods to make inferences about specific neighborhoods.

While the advances in statistical research and computing have shown the potential of multilevel methods for health and social behavioral research there are issues to be considered while developing and interpreting multilevel applications. First, it is important to clearly motivate and conceptualize the choice of higher levels in a multilevel analysis. Second, establishing the relative importance of context and composition is probably more apparent than real and necessary caution must be exercised while conceptualizing and interpreting the compositional and contextual sources of variation. Third, it is important that the sample of neighborhoods belong to well-defined population of neighborhoods such that the sample shares exchangeable properties that are essential for robust inferences. Fourth, it is important to ensure adequate sample size at all levels of analysis. In general, if the research focus is essentially on neighborhoods then clearly the analysis requires more neighborhoods (as compared to more individuals within a neighborhood). Lastly, like all quantitative procedures, the ability of multilevel models to make causal inferences is limited and innovative strategies including randomized neighborhood-level research designs (via trials or natural experiments) in combination with multilevel analytical strategy may be required to convincingly demonstrate causal effects of social contexts such as neighborhoods.

Acknowledgment S. V. Subramanian is supported by the National Institutes of Health Career Development Award (NHLBI 1 K25 HL081275).

References

Best, N. G., Spiegelhalter, D. J., Thomas, A., and Brayne, C. E. G. (1996). Bayesian analysis of realistically complex models. *J Roy Stat Soc A, 159,* 232–342.

Blakely, T., and Subramanian, S. V. (2006). Multilevel studies. In M. Oakes & J. Kaufman (Eds.),

Methods for Social Epidemiology (pp. 316–340). San Francisco: Jossey Bass.

Blakely, T. A., and Woodward, A. J. (2000). Ecological effects in multi-level studies. *J Epidemiol Commun Health, 54*, 367–74.

Browne, W. J., Subramanian, S. V., Jones, K., and Goldstein, H. (2005). Variance partitioning in multilevel logistic models that exhibit overdispersion. *J Royal Stat Soc A, 168*, 599–613.

Diez Roux, A. V. (2002). A glossary for multilevel analysis. *J Epidemiol Commun Health, 56*, 588–594.

Fielding, A. (2004). The role of the Hausman test and whether higher level effects should be treated as random or fixed. *Multilevel Modeling Newsletter, 16*, 3–9.

Goldstein, H. (2003). *Multilevel Statistical Models, 3rd Ed.* London: Arnold.

Goldstein, H., Browne, W. J., and Rasbash, J. (2002). Partitioning variation in multilevel models. *Understanding Stat, 1*, 223–232.

Jones, K., and Bullen, N. (1994). Contextual models of urban house prices: a comparison of fixed- and random-coefficient models developed by expansion. *Econ Geogr, 70*, 252–272.

Kawachi, I., and Subramanian, S. V. (2006). Measuring and modeling the social and geographic context of trauma: a multilevel modeling approach. *J Trauma Stress, 19*, 195–203.

Langford, I. H., Bentham, G., and McDonald, A. L. (1998). Multilevel modelling of geographically aggregated health data: a case study on malignant melanoma mortality and UV exposure in the European Community. *Stat Med, 17*, 41–57.

Lawson, A. B. (2001). *Statistical Methods in Spatial Epidemiology, 2nd Ed.* Chichester, UK: Wiley.

Leyland, A. H. (2005). Assessing the impact of mobility on health: implications for life course epidemiology. *J Epidemiol Commun Health, 59*, 90–91.

Moon, G., Subramanian, S. V., Jones, K., Duncan, C., and Twigg, L. (2005). Area-based studies and the evalua-tion of multilevel influences on health outcomes. In A. Bowling & S. Ebrahim (Eds.), *Handbook of Health Research Methods: Investigation, Measurement and Analysis* (pp. 266–292). Berkshire, England: Open University Press.

Raudenbush, S., and Bryk, A. (2002). *Hierarchical Linear Models: Applications and Data Analysis Methods.* Thousand Oaks: Sage Publications.

Raudenbush, S. W. (2003). The quantitative assessment of neighborhood social environment. In I. Kawachi & L. F. Berkman (Eds.), *Neighborhoods and Health.* New York: Oxford University Press.

Subramanian, S. V. (2004). Multilevel methods, theory and analysis. In N. Anderson (Ed.), *Encyclopedia of Health and Behavior* (pp. 602–608). Thousand Oaks, CA: Sage Publications.

Subramanian, S. V., Jones, K., and Duncan, C. (2003). Multilevel methods for public health research. In I. Kawachi & L. Berkman (Eds.), *Neighborhoods and Health* (pp. 65–111). New York: Oxford Press.

Subramanian, S. V. (2004). The relevance of multilevel statistical methods for identifying causal neighbor-hood effects. *Soc Sci Med, 58*, 1961–1967.

Subramanian, S. V. (2004). The relevance of multilevel statistical models for identifying causal neighborhood effects. *Soc Sci Med, 58*, 1961–1967.

Subramanian, S. V., Glymour, M. M., and Kawachi, I. (2007). Identifying causal ecologic effects on health: a methodologic assessment. In S. Galea (Ed.), *Macrosocial Determinants of Population Health* (pp. 301–331). New York: Springer Media.

Subramanian, S. V., Jones, K., and Duncan, C. (2003). Multilevel methods for public health research. In I. Kawachi & L. F. Berkman (Eds.), *Neighborhoods and Health* (pp. 65–111). New York: Oxford University Press.

Subramanian, S. V., Jones, K., Kaddour, A., and Krieger, N. (2009). Revisiting Robinson: the perils of individualistic and ecologic fallacy. *Int J Epidemiol, 38*, 342–360.

Chapter 57

Structural Equation Modeling in Behavioral Medicine Research

Maria Magdalena Llabre

1 Introduction

Structural equation modeling (SEM) is a broad data analytic framework that can subsume most of the analyses performed within the behavioral medicine research field. Over the past 30 years SEM has gone from a novel methodology to mainstream statistical analysis, expanding beyond general linear models to address nonlinear models, categorical outcomes, and multilevel models, to name a few. While SEM was initially considered to be most useful for testing causal models, the heuristic aspects of the framework go beyond causal hypothesis testing. In fact, the specification of the models, a necessary step in SEM, is a valuable tool in itself, helping researchers better understand their research questions and their data. Models are specified either through a system of structural equations or through a path diagram. The path diagram is a valuable way to visually describe how variables are expected to relate to one another within a specified research context, forcing the researcher to think critically about every variable relevant to the phenomenon under study.

This chapter is designed to provide a brief overview of principles and current topics in SEM. The chapter strives for breadth rather than depth, but will give readable references

for those interested in delving deeper into any one topic. I begin with an introduction to the framework and provide a general overview of relevant aspects of SEM. I present some hypothetical examples and also provide a few references to published examples. Readers interested in a more technical introduction may want to read Bollen (1989) or the more recent work by Kaplan (2000). Those who want a very readable conceptual introduction are referred to Kline (2010). New developments have been described in many places, including some edited books such as Marcoulides and Schumaker (2001) and Hancock and Mueller (2006).

2 Model Specification

SEM is most useful when the data analysis is based on theory. That is partly because a necessary first step in any SEM analysis is the specification of the model to be tested. A model includes the observed variables to be analyzed, the constructs to be inferred, the unobserved but ever present errors or disturbances, and the ways in which these observed and unobserved variables are related to one another. All statistical analyses are based on some model. For example, when conducting an independent t-test we imply a simple linear model, which we do not bother to specify but which is

$$Y = \alpha + \beta X + e,$$

M.M. Llabre (✉)
Department of Psychology, University of Miami,
P.O. Box 24-8185, Coral Gables, FL 33124, USA
e-mail: mllabre@miami.edu

A. Steptoe (ed.), *Handbook of Behavioral Medicine*, DOI 10.1007/978-0-387-09488-5_57,
© Springer Science+Business Media, LLC 2010

where X is a 0, 1 dummy coded variable. The parameters in this model include α and β, the structural parameters, as well as the variances of X and e. α is the mean of the group coded 0 and β is the difference between the means of the two groups. The t-test is the test of the β, obtained by dividing its sample estimate by its standard error. Multiple regression analysis is based on a more general linear model which we sometimes present. As we move toward more complex models, there is a greater need to describe them. Because of the multivariate nature of SEM, the models can have multiple equations, and each must be specified.

2.1 Notation

While this chapter will keep formulas and notation to a minimum, some basic definitions are necessary. We will use X or Y to indicate observed variables, also called indicators. X will be used for exogenous variables, those variables whose causes are not part of our model, and Y for endogenous variables, the variables whose causes are posited by our model. These are the variables we measure, the operational definitions of our constructs. In SEM we can go beyond observed variables and work with latent variables, the constructs of interest to us. A latent variable, like a construct, cannot be observed directly, but is inferred from the covariances among its indicators. For example, we cannot observe depression directly, but diagnose it from responses to a structured interview that cover affective, cognitive, behavioral, and somatic reported symptoms (APA, 1994). We will use F to denote a latent variable, also referred to as a factor. Errors will be identified with the symbols E or D. The distinction lies in the use of D, a disturbance, to indicate the residuals associated with unmeasured variables in a prediction equation not part of a measurement model, while E will be restricted to those equations that relate latent variables to their indicators in a measurement model.

Many find it easier to specify the model with a path diagram rather than with a system of equations. But for many computer programs (AMOS is an exception; Arbuckle, 2003), the diagram must be converted to model equations. We will first consider model specification with a diagram which we will then convert to a set of equations.

2.2 Path Diagram

Let us consider an example of a hypothetical overly simplistic model in behavioral medicine research. Many of us believe that stress influences health because stress activates the sympathetic nervous system (SNS) as well as the immune system, two important pathways linking the mind and the body. Suppose we have collected a measure of perceived stress from a sample of participants on three separate occasions during a 1-month period, as well as physiological measures of stress reactivity in the form of blood pressure reactivity and C-reactive protein (CRP) levels assayed from blood. In this population the relevant indicators of health might be a rating of fatigue, the number of visits to the doctor, and a general rating of health, all in reference to the previous month. At this point we will focus on a few key features in the example to describe the elements of a path diagram. These elements are ovals, rectangles, and arrows. The arrows are either single headed or double headed. Single-headed arrows indicate direct effects called path coefficients (β's). Double-headed arrows indicate covariance which, when both arrows point to the same variable, is a variance. In Fig. 57.1 we see that stress and health are shown in ovals because they are latent variables, not directly observed. The observed variables are shown in rectangles. Errors and disturbances are also shown in ovals because they, also, cannot be directly observed. The direct effects of errors and disturbances on the variables are always fixed to equal 1. This is necessary to be able to identify the models. Stress is the underlying latent variable manifested in the observed measures of perceived stress. This relationship is depicted by

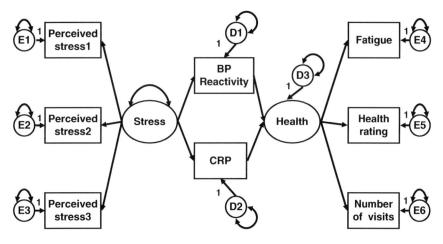

Fig. 57.1 Path diagram of mediators of stress and health with latent variables

an arrow stemming from the stress latent variable and pointing to each of the three observed measures of perceived stress.

Similarly, health is an underlying construct that determines the observed measures of fatigue, number of doctor's visits, and general rating of health. These relationships between the latent variable and its indicators represent the *measurement model* aspect of the SEM. Each of the indicators is measured with some error; they are not perfectly valid and/or reliable. The measurement error in each indicator is captured by the ovals with the E labels in each. These measurement errors contain other influences on the measures of either stress or health that may be specific to how or when the measures were taken. The path diagram also indicates the relation between stress and health is not direct, but rather mediated (see Chapter 55) by two different pathways: blood pressure reactivity and CRP. This part of the model represents the structural aspect of SEM. The mediator variables are measured with a single indicator each, which is a weakness in this model. The assumption is that they have been measured with perfect reliability (an assumption we generally make in all analyses that do not incorporate a measurement model). Reactivity, CRP, and the latent variable of health are all endogenous. In other words, the model specifies its predictors, but this prediction is not perfect; thus a disturbance term is specified for each. The arrows in the path diagram are model parameters to be estimated.

We can now translate our diagram into a set of structural equations. We begin with the equations for the measurement model with one equation for each indicator as shown below. For simplicity, we initially work with centered variables and the equations will have intercepts of zero:

$$
\begin{aligned}
X1 &= \lambda1F1 + E1, \\
X2 &= \lambda2F1 + E2, \\
X3 &= \lambda3F1 + E3, \\
X4 &= \lambda4F2 + E4, \\
X5 &= \lambda5F2 + E5, \\
X6 &= \lambda6F2 + E6.
\end{aligned}
\tag{57.1}
$$

In terms of the structural aspect of the model we have three equations corresponding to the three endogenous variables:

$$
\begin{aligned}
Y1 &= \beta1F1 + D1, \\
Y2 &= \beta2F1 + D2, \\
F2 &= \beta3Y1 + \beta4Y2 + D3.
\end{aligned}
$$

Note that the path diagram does not specify double-headed curved arrows among residuals or between residuals and other predictors, thus assuming independence of errors.

The purpose of the analysis of this model will be twofold. First, we wish to test whether the specified model fits the data well. And simultaneously, we want to estimate the parameters and test them for significance. In particular we wish to estimate the direct effects from stress to the indicators of SNS and CRP and, in turn, the extent to which those indicators predict health. Once we have estimated direct effects, we will also want to quantify the indirect effect for a test of mediation.

3 Parameter Estimation and Model Fit

The popularity of SEM results from advances in methods of estimation of the structural equation parameters. Karl Joreskog (see Cudeck et al, 2001, for references to his work and new areas of development) and the LISREL program (Joreskog and Sorbom, 1996) made this framework accessible to applied researchers. In addition to LISREL other software programs currently available to conduct these analyses include EQS (Bentler, 1995), AMOS (Arbuckle, 2003), Mx (Neal et al, 2002), and Mplus (Muthen and Muthen, 1998–2004). For a description of these and other programs, see Kline (2010).

The most common method of estimation used in these programs is maximum likelihood (ML), performed iteratively to arrive at an admissible solution. The idea is as follows: Once a model is specified, such as that in Fig. 57.1, one can make initial guesses at the values of the parameter estimates. In fact, if we had superpowers and knew the population values for those parameters, given our model, we could work backward and tell the values of the variances and covariances of our variables. These would form the model-implied variance–covariance matrix which we will label $\Sigma(\Theta)$. For our data with eight indicators it would be an 8×8 variance–covariance matrix with variances along the diagonal and covariances in the off-diagonals. For illustration, let us take the

third structural equation (1): $Y3 = \beta3F1 + D3$. If we know the values of $\beta3$, the variance of $F1$, and the variance of $D3$, we could calculate the variance of $Y3$, as implied by the equation because $\text{Var}(Y3) = \beta3^2 \times \text{Var}(F1) + \text{Var}(D3)$, using covariance algebra. This will hold for other variances and covariances as well. We can then compare the model-implied variance–covariance matrix to the one generated from the data, which we will call Σ, to test the hypothesis that the model fits the data:

$$H_0 : \Sigma = \Sigma(\Theta).$$

One minor problem is that we do not know the values of the population parameters, but have to estimate them from the data. The algorithms used by the computer programs perform the parameter estimation and test of model fit simultaneously and iteratively. They begin with starting values, guesses about the values of these parameters, which are used to generate a model-implied matrix. The model-implied matrix is compared to the data-based matrix for a calculation of a residual matrix. If the residuals are large, model parameters are modified in an attempt at minimizing the residuals. In ML estimation a fit function is used such that the parameter values estimated have the greatest likelihood of having given rise to the sample values obtained, assuming a multivariate normal distribution. For more detailed explanations of this and other methods of estimation, see Bollen (1989).

The typical output from a computer analysis will have indices of model fit, as well as the parameter estimates, their standard errors, and z-values used to test them for statistical significance. The primary statistic used in testing the hypothesis of perfect fit is a χ^2 obtained by multiplying $N–1$ times the minimum value of the ML fit function. A nonsignificant χ^2 is indicative of good model fit, but may be difficult to obtain with large samples because of its direct dependence on sample size. With large samples, even small differences between the two matrices may be picked up as indicative of lack of fit. Several other indices have been developed and proposed as either alternatives or companions to the χ^2. The ones that have been recommended and are included in current versions of computer programs are the comparative fit index (CFI; Bentler, 1990), the root mean squared error of approximation (RMSEA; Steiger, 1990), and the standardized root mean residual (SRMR). As the name indicates, CFI compares the fit of the specified model to a null model which posits no relationships among the variables. Models with values of CFI greater than 0.95 are desirable (Hu and Bentler, 1999). The RMSEA is based on a non-central χ^2 distribution, the distribution of the test statistic under the alternative hypothesis, and measures the degree of lack of fit of the model per degree of freedom. Values less than 0.06 are considered indicative of models with close fit to the data. A value of 0.08 for any given standardized residual is considered acceptable and so when the average value across all residuals (SRMR) is less than 0.10, the model is considered acceptable.

Beyond overall measures of fit, it is important to make sure that parameter estimates make sense in relation to the problem being investigated. For example, variances should all be positive and the signs of effects in the expected direction.

Examples of SEM are not as common in the behavioral medicine literature as they are in the social sciences. One recent example is work by Bleil et al (2008) who tested a model of cardiac autonomic function, measured by high frequency heart rate variability, predicted by negative emotions. Another example is the work by Weaver et al (2005) who tested a stress and coping model of medication adherence and its relation to viral load in HIV-positive individuals, including a test of an alternative model. Testing of alternative models is uncommon but necessary to strengthen the causal inferences often associated with SEM. Sometimes researchers improperly assume that models that fit the data represent reality, without recognizing there are always multiple alternative models that fit just as well. Models can be rejected but not proven. This is not to suggest that causal inference can never be entertained, but rather to remind readers

of the importance of considering design features such as the use of longitudinal data, instrumental variables, randomization, experimentation, or inclusion of other variables that help dissect confounded relations.

Alternative models that are nested can be compared statistically. Nested models are models that have the same variables but where the parameters estimated in one model represent a subset of the parameters estimated in the more general model. When models are nested, the difference between their χ^2 is also a χ^2 and, therefore, the difference can be tested for statistical significance, with degrees of freedom calculated from the difference in degrees of freedom between the two models. When the result of the difference test is statistically significant, the more general model with more parameters estimated should be retained. On the other hand, when the result is not significant, the more parsimonious model should be retained. Often, alternative models are not nested and the χ^2 difference test cannot be used. In that case, there are alternative descriptive indices, such as the Akaike Information Criterion (Akaike, 1974) or the Bayesian Information Criterion (Schwarz, 1978), that take both fit and parsimony into consideration. For both lower indices are associated with preferred models.

3.1 Path Analysis

If instead of latent variables for measuring stress and health in the path diagram of Fig. 57.1 we had a single indicator for each one, the resulting model would be a path analysis model shown in Fig. 57.2. Path analysis is a special case of SEM where all variables are observed (except for the errors) and assumed to be perfectly reliable. To the extent the reliability assumption is true, the path coefficients from the path model versus the structural model should be the same. But when reliability is not perfect, and the indicators contain measurement error, the path coefficients from the path model will be biased, typically underestimated.

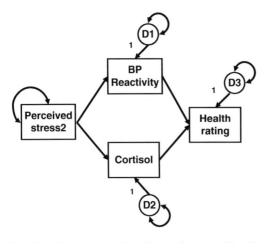

Fig. 57.2 Path diagram of mediators of stress and health with single indicators

Path analysis models have the direction of effects going one way only. These are called recursive models. Recursive models are all identified, meaning solutions may be obtained for all of the parameters in the model. When effects go both ways, say X to Y and also Y to X, the models are no longer path analysis models. These models are called nonrecursive. Under certain conditions nonrecursive models can be identified and analyzed in SEM. While the issue of identification will not be covered in this chapter, it is worth pointing out that a necessary condition for identification of any model is that the number of parameters to be estimated be less than or equal to the number of variances and covariances in the data. This will always be true for path analysis models. If our model has, for example, $p = 4$ variables, there will be $p \times (p + 1)/2$ or $4 \times (4 + 1)/2 = 10$ unique variances and covariances. This is the information used for model estimation. In our model in Fig. 57.2 there are $q = 8$ parameters to be estimated. The difference between p and q is the degrees of freedom (df). When df is 0, the model is just identified and cannot be tested for model fit because it fits the data perfectly, meaning the model-implied variance–covariance matrix perfectly matches the one obtained from the data. These models are also called saturated models. In this case the focus is not on model fit but

rather on estimation of model parameters, their test of significance, and the explanatory power of the model. When df is greater than 0, as is the case in our example, the model is overidentified and model fit can be tested. The 2 df $(10 - 8)$ imply that there are two different ways in which our model could be incorrect. In our example, they come from the fact that we specified complete mediation between stress and health, i.e., there is no direct effect linking those two variables (1 df). Also, the two mediators are not specified to be correlated in this model beyond what results from sharing the common predictor of stress (1 df). There is neither a single-headed nor a double-headed arrow linking those two. If either one of those conditions is true our model will be rejected.

3.2 Model Parameters

It is worth taking time to consider model parameters in the structural aspect of SEM. The parameters of primary interest are the path coefficients, the direct effects among the variables. Also counted as parameters are the variances of the disturbances and any covariances they may share. These covariances represent shared variance among endogenous variables that are external to the model. If converted to correlations, these would be partial correlations, controlling for the explanatory variables in the model. The variances and covariances among the exogenous variables are also counted as model parameters.

4 Measurement Model

One of the key features of SEM that distinguishes it from other general linear models is the ability to incorporate a measurement model for the constructs of interest while simultaneously analyzing their interrelations. Often when we work with observed variables we forget they are frequently measured with some amount of error. Classical test theory (Crocker and Algina,

1986) reminds us that an observed score is made up of two components, a true score and an error score as depicted below:

$$X = T + E.$$

When we assess the reliability of a measurement procedure, we are estimating the proportion of variance in an observed score that is true score or that is not error. This can be accomplished in several ways, most of which assume parallel measurement. Parallel measures are measures of the same construct with the same metric (units of measurement) and equal error variances. I purposely chose to include the same measure of perceived stress taken at three different times to assess the stress construct in Fig. 57.1 to make this point. These three measures are parallel if the path coefficients (λ, factor loadings) from the stress latent variable to the three indicators all equal 1, and if the three error variances are equal to each other. In that case the retest reliability of the stress measure may be estimated by taking the variance of the stress latent variable and dividing it by the variance of the stress latent variable plus the error variance. This proportion of variance in the total that is explained by the latent variable is reported in most SEM programs:

$$\text{Reliability} = \text{Var}(F1)/[\text{Var}(F1) + \text{Var}(E)].$$

The stress latent variable is defined by the shared variance among the three parallel measures and does not contain random measurement error. The error variance is separate because under the assumption of independence, it does not contribute to the shared variance. Thus, when we estimate the effect of stress on, say blood pressure reactivity, the stress latent variable does not introduce random noise to that estimation. It follows that anytime a researcher can work with a latent variable based on multiple indicators, she/he has the advantage of eliminating a source of error and bias. One way to improve upon our model in Fig. 57.1 would be to add multiple measures of blood pressure reactivity as well as multiple measures of CRP.

In SEM this measurement model is not restricted to multiple parallel measures. The SEM measurement model is more general. It is called a congeneric model. In a congeneric model the indicators are assumed to reflect a unidimensional latent variable. But they do not need to have the same metric nor equal error variances. The measurement model of health represents this type of congeneric model. Its three indicators reflect different aspects of health (or lack thereof) quantified in different ways with varying amounts of measurement error. The health latent variable still represents the shared variance among the three indicators. Because this latent variable is not an observed quantity it does not have a metric of its own. Unlike the situation with parallel measurement where the metric is constant across the indicators and is applied to the latent variable, in a congeneric model the researcher decides which of the indicators will contribute its metric in order to identify the latent variable. In the absence of either a gold standard or a most reliable indicator, this decision is arbitrary. But although it will influence the parameter estimates that are metric based, in most situations it does not influence model fit. This metric assignment is done by fixing the loading for the selected indicator to a value of 1, instead of estimating it. As is the interpretation of a regression coefficient, the value 1 implies a change of 1 unit in $X4$ for every change of 1 unit in $F2$, a one-to-one correspondence:

$$X4 = 1F2 + E4.$$

The loadings for the other indicators are freely estimated. An alternative way to assign a metric to a latent variable is to standardize it by giving the latent variable a variance of 1.

SEM measurement models are also more common in psychology than in behavioral medicine. Shen and colleagues (2006) used a second-order model to examine the structure of the metabolic syndrome. My colleagues and I (Llabre et al, 2006) also used a second-order model to separate estimates of reliability and validity in measures of medication adherence.

These examples show that measurement models are relevant to behavioral medicine.

4.1 Measurement Model Parameters

In strictly measurement models, the parameters to be estimated are the factor loadings (except for the indicator which sets the metric), the measurement error variances, the variances of the latent variables, and the covariances among latent variables when there are more than one. Sometimes, some error covariances are also estimated. This happens when some of the measures used to reflect a latent variable share method variance.

4.2 Formative Indicators

The measurement model previously described assumes that the latent variable is responsible for the indicators; thus the arrows flow from the latent variable to its indicators. In this case the indicators are "reflective" because they represent a reflection of the underlying latent variable. In this type of model one expects for the correlations among the indicators to be moderate to high, as they share an underlying cause. What is important is their commonality and not their uniqueness. In fact, their uniqueness is separated into the error term. The loss of any one indicator, when there are many, is not catastrophic, as they are considered interchangeable.

This type of measurement model does not fit all situations encountered in behavioral medicine research. For example, there has been emerging interest in quantifying childhood socioeconomic status (SES), as it has been shown to find its way "under the skin" (Miller et al, 2009). SES is commonly defined in terms of measures of parent education, income, and occupation, but each of these is considered a critical piece of the construct. They in combination define SES. Similarly, checklists of life events are used to define what is considered life stress. These items are not interchangeable, and they are not always correlated. Individuals who experienced the death of a parent are not necessarily those who recently change jobs or whose spouse was incarcerated. In this case there is no underlying latent variable that generates the indicators; instead, the indicators define the latent variable. This type of measurement model is depicted by arrows pointing from the indicators to the latent variable and is called formative measurement. Formative measurement models are more difficult to work with because they can only be estimated when the latent variable is used to predict some subsequent outcome, and different outcomes can alter the meaning of the latent variable (see Bollen and Lennox, 1991; Howell et al, 2007).

5 Mean Structures

So far we have been concerned with models that focus on relationships among variables and have made the assumption that our variables were centered, meaning we have subtracted the mean from the original variable to simplify our equations and eliminate the intercept. This is appropriate when analyzing covariances or correlations which are invariant when adding or subtracting constants. However, centering can be limiting because there are many important research questions in behavioral medicine that require retaining information about the means. For instance, in randomized clinical trials the focus is often a comparison of two group means. Questions related to health disparities often require testing hypotheses about group means. Longitudinal studies of health outcomes also often focus on changes in mean levels over time. Therefore, if the SEM latent variable framework is to be useful in those situations, we need to consider means.

When we work with mean structures, our equations include intercepts. You may recall when learning about regression that the intercept was associated with a vector of 1's in the data. This is because when we regress a variable, say Y, on the constant 1, the regression coefficient is the mean of Y. Also, if we regress a variable Y on a constant 1 and another predictor, say X, the regression coefficient for the constant is the intercept. These concepts apply in SEM. In a path diagram we indicate the inclusion of means and/or intercepts by specifying a triangle with the number 1 in it. This triangle represents a constant which will be useful in estimating means and intercepts. The arrows going from the triangle to a variable represent either a mean or an intercept, depending on whether there are other predictors also going to the variable.

As I mentioned earlier, mean structures are useful when comparing multiple groups or examining change in a group over time. In a subsequent section, I will introduce latent growth models, which are relevant for studying change over time.

6 Multiple Groups

SEM can be applied to a single group or multiple groups. When analyzing multiple groups all parameters in a model (i.e., means, variances, and path coefficients) may be compared between groups. The general approach is to compare two models: one where the parameter or parameters of interest are specified to be equal between groups, we say constrained equal, and another model which allows the parameters to vary between groups. Each model is associated with a χ^2 test of model fit. Importantly, these models are nested; the model with constrained parameters is nested within the more general model. In this fashion, groups can be compared on many different dimensions without restrictive assumptions. For instance, recall how in the analysis of variance when we compare group means we assume their variances are equal. With multiple group SEM we can compare means in the presence of unequal variances.

7 Latent Growth Model

Latent growth models (LGMs) are special cases of SEM applied to longitudinal data where the interest is in the estimation of parameters of change over time (Duncan et al, 1999). They are closely related to mixed models or multilevel models of longitudinal data (see Chou et al, 1998; MacCallum et al, 1996, for a comparison of approaches). The idea is that there is an underlying latent process of change responsible for the data, and the goal is to capture the parameters of the change process. Requirements for LGM are data from at least three time points with interval scale measurement using the same metric at all time points. The researcher specifies a general functional form for the growth over time. This function could be linear or nonlinear, but the form is limited by the number of time points available. With three time points we are restricted to a linear function with an intercept and a slope, a common form in many studies. Parameters of interest are the average intercept and slope, as well as the variability in individuals' intercepts and slopes. LGM has been applied to the investigation of cardiovascular reactivity and recovery from stress (Llabre et al, 2001) where a piecewise function was used to model both reactivity and recovery separately, but simultaneously. Reactivity was modeled with a linear function, while the recovery curve was quadratic. In another application (Llabre et al, 2004), we illustrated how LGM could be used to compare cardiovascular recovery across stressors and across groups. For a brief example, let us examine a path diagram of an LGM from a hypothetical model of change in Beck Depression Inventory scores over a 6-month interval in cancer patients starting right after a diagnosis (Time 0) and repeated 3 (Time 3) and 6 months (Time 6) later, as shown in Fig. 57.3 with solid lines. The latent variables in this model are the characteristics of the hypothesized linear change process for the given time interval. Any line is characterized by an intercept, labeled Baseline, and a slope, labeled Change. What makes this measurement model an LGM is that the loadings linking the latent variables to the indicators are not estimated, but rather are used to specify the time structure of the data in months. This is conveyed also in the equations shown below

Fig. 57.3 Latent growth
model path diagram of linear
change

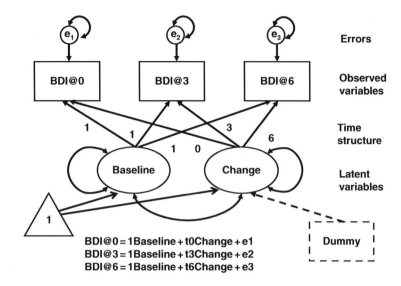

BDI@0 = 1Baseline + t0Change + e1
BDI@3 = 1Baseline + t3Change + e2
BDI@6 = 1Baseline + t6Change + e3

the figure. The parameters of interest are the
means of the Baseline and Change latent variables, indicated by the paths from the constant
1; the variances of the latent variables, quantifying individual differences in the trajectory of
change; the covariance between the Baseline and
Change; and the error variances which are often
assumed to be equal across time. If we wanted to
compare the change in depression between participants randomized to an intervention designed
to reduce symptoms of depression and control
participants, we could add a dummy coded (0,
1) indicator for this group classification with an
arrow pointing to the Change latent variable (see
dashed lines). The estimate of this added parameter represents the difference between the means
of the two groups on the Change latent variable.
In this revised model, the path from the constant
to the Change latent variable is now the mean
slope for the control group.

LGM is very flexible and can be embedded in
more complex SEM models. With a little imagi-
nation, you can envision that LGM variables can
be used, not only as outcome variables but also
as predictors of other outcomes. So, for example, one can investigate whether the change in
depression might be associated with changes in
inflammation or with other markers of disease.
These models are ideally suited to test the types
of mechanism hypotheses generated in many
behavioral medicine laboratories.

7.1 Latent Difference Scores

A related set of models to examine change that
is free of measurement error comes from work
by McArdle and colleagues (Hamagami and
McArdle, 2000; McArdle and Hamagami, 2000)
and generally referred to as latent difference
scores. In their framework, the change process
is segmented into change scores, which take
advantage of multiple repeated measurements
in order to be able to separate it from the error.
These latent difference scores can be influenced by an overall change process (Constant
change), as assumed in LGM, and also by the
preceding level of the variable (Proportional
change). These models are particularly useful
for studying reciprocal influences in multiple
change processes. King and colleagues (2006)
have made this methodology quite accessible to
readers in their application to trauma recovery
(King et al, 2006).

8 Missing Data

When working in the SEM framework with ML
it is possible to take advantage of its full information capabilities to include all of the available data. Often referred to as full information
maximum likelihood (FIML), this approach has

been shown to yield unbiased estimates of group parameters when missingness (whether data are missing or not) is related to variables that are accessible for analysis (Little and Rubin, 2002; Schafer and Graham, 2002). This condition or assumption, sometimes confusing because it is called missing at random (MAR), implies that once the variables that predict missingness are controlled in the analysis, the remaining mechanism responsible for the missingness is a random process. This approach is superior to older deletion or imputation approaches such as listwise or pairwise deletion, or mean, regression or hotdeck imputation, and comparable to multiple imputation (Collins et al, 2001). The older methods are less powerful and produce biased parameter estimates unless the missingness is the result of a completely random process, referred to as missing completely at random (MCAR). MCAR is a stricter assumption than MAR, particularly in longitudinal studies when attrition can often be predicted from variables collected at baseline, such as disease severity. For a clear explanation of this and other modern methods, see Enders (2006).

9 Sample Size and Power

The appropriate sample size in an SEM analysis must be considered keeping in mind several issues including model complexity, estimation method, and statistical power. With samples of less than 100 participants, the models must be simple and the variables normally distributed, otherwise the researcher will likely find problems with convergence. As a general rule, more complex models or non-normal data will require more participants because more parameters will have to be estimated. Kline (2010) provides some rules for classifying studies into small ($n<100$), medium ($100< n < 200$), and large (>200). But given all of the factors that bear on the question of sample size, these general rules may not be relevant for a given study.

There are two power considerations in SEM: the power associated with the test of the overall

model and the power associated with the test of each parameter or set of parameters in the model. Power analyses can be performed in the design phase of a study to determine the appropriate sample size or after the analyses to determine whether the study was sufficiently powered for a given effect size. MacCallum et al (1996) provided a useful approach to power determination for the overall model based on the RMSEA. Hancock (2006) shows how to calculate power for individual parameters or sets of parameters. Muthén and Muthén (2002) illustrate the use of Monte Carlo simulation in power estimation in SEM.

10 Categorical Outcomes

As stated earlier, ML estimation assumes continuous variables and multivariate normality. Often in behavioral medicine, variables of interest are dichotomous (have a disease or not), represent count variables, or have a preponderance of zeros. Various strategies are available for working with categorical data and non-normal distributions (Finney and DiStefano, 2006). These include various types of adjustments to the χ^2 test and the standard errors of the parameters, using robust weighted least squares methods, including mean and/or variance adjusted weighted least squares (WLSMV; Muthén, 1984), or bootstrapping the standard errors. An important consideration in determining the appropriate method is whether the underlying variable is truly continuous, but the measures available cannot make fine discriminations, as opposed to variables that are truly categorical. One available program, Mplus, is particularly useful for these situations. Using the Mplus framework, researchers can incorporate non-normal and/or categorical outcomes within more comprehensive SEM models and conduct discrete time survival analyses (Muthen and Masyn, 2005) while accounting for measurement error (Masyn, 2008). Advances in this area will make SEM more relevant to current problems in behavioral medicine.

11 Latent Class and Mixture and Multilevel Models

Up to now we have been considering models that apply to single populations. However, it is possible to consider situations where our participants come from different subpopulations not previously identified and to use the SEM to identify these mixtures of populations. In this context the mixtures or subpopulations represent latent classes, identified with a categorical latent variable. In latent class analysis the latent classes are determined on the basis of the associations among categorical outcomes. But the latent classes could be subgroups that, for example, have different trajectories in LGM or have different factor structures in measurement models or have different path models (Muthén, 2001). When these subpopulations are known ahead of time, their models may be compared with multiple group SEM as described earlier. But it is when the classes are unknown that the researcher can employ these more exploratory methods and determine the number of classes (Nylund et al, 2007), the probability associated with belonging to a given class, and estimate the parameters within classes. Jung and Wickrama (2008) present a step-by-step illustration on a growth mixture model analysis; Lubke et al (2007) also provides an instructive application of this methodology.

Given that the factors that affect health occur at multiple levels (for example, the cell, the person, the family, and the community) some of the models of health or disease will benefit from a multilevel data structure. Multilevel models are considered in a separate chapter. However, it is worth mentioning that multilevel models can be specified within an SEM framework (Heck, 2001; Mehta and Neale, 2005), with different influences specified at different levels.

12 Concluding Comments

In this chapter I have attempted to provide an overview of the principles involved in using an SEM framework, as well as some introductory comments on more advanced topics. Adopting this framework when designing and analyzing data has several advantages, including control for measurement error, the examination and testing of mechanisms, and the quantification of change. SEM allows the researcher to match the analyses to the complex questions of interest in behavioral medicine research.

References

Akaike, H. (1974). A new look at the statistical model identification. *IEEE Trans Automat Contr, 19,* 716–723.

American Psychiatric Association (1994). *Diagnostic and statistical manual of mental disorders, 4th Ed (DSM-IV).* Washington, DC: Author.

Arbuckle, J. L. (2003). *Amos 5.* Chicago: SmallWaters.

Schwarz, G. E. (1978). Estimating the dimension of a model. *Ann. Statist, 6,* 461–464.

Bentler, P. M. (1990). Comparative fit indexes in structural models. *Psychol Bull, 107,* 238–246.

Bentler, P. M. (1995) *EQS Structural Equations Program Manual.* Encino, CA: Multivariate Software.

Bleil, M. E., Gianaros, P. J., Jennings, J. R., Flory, J. D., and Manuck, S. B. (2008). Trait negative affect: toward an integrated model of understanding psychological risk for impairment in cardiac autonomic function. *Psychosom Med, 70,* 328–337.

Bollen, K. (1989). *Structural Equations with Latent Variables.* New York: Wiley and sons.

Bollen, K., and Lennox, R. (1991). Conventional wisdom on measurement: a structural equation perspective. *Psychol Bull, 110,* 305–314.

Chou, C., Bentler, P. M., and Pentz, M. A. (1998). Comparisons of two statistical approaches to study growth curves: the multilevel model and the latent curve analysis. *Struct Equation Model, 5,* 247–266.

Collins, L. M., Schafer, J. L., and Kam, C. M. (2001). A comparison of inclusive and restrictive strategies in modern missing data procedures. *Psychol Methods, 6,* 330–351.

Crocker, L., and Algina, J. (1986). *Introduction to Classical and Modern Test Theory.* New York: Holt, Rinehart and Winston.

Cudeck, R., Du Toit, S., and Sorbom, D. (Eds.). (2001). *Structural Equation Modeling: Present and Future.* Chicago: Scientific Software International.

Duncan, T. E., Duncan, S. C., Strycker, A. L., Li, F., and Alpert, A. (1999). *An Introduction to Latent Variable Growth Curve Modeling: Concepts, Issues, and Applications.* Mahwah, NJ: Erlbaum.

Enders, C. K. (2006). Analyzing structural equation models with missing data. In G. R. Hancock & R. O. Mueller (Eds.), *Structural Equation Modeling:*

A Second Course (pp. 313–344). Greenwich, CT: Information Age Publishing.

Finney, S. J., and DiStefano, C. (2006). Nonnormal and categorical data in structural equation modeling. In G. R. Hancock & R. O. Mueller (Eds.), *Structural Equation Modeling: A Second Course* (pp. 269–312). Greenwich, CT: Information Age Publishing.

Hamagami, F., and McArdle, J. J. (2000). Advanced studies of individual differences linear dynamic models for longitudinal data analysis. In G. Marcoulides & R. Schumaker (Eds.), *New Developments and Techniques in Structural Equations Modeling* (pp. 203–246). Mahwah, NJ: Erlbaum.

Hancock, G. R. (2006). Power analysis in covariance structure modeling. In G. R. Hancock & R. O. Mueller (Eds.), *Structural Equation Modeling: A Second Course* (pp. 69–118). Greenwich, CT: Information Age Publishing.

Howell, R. D., Breivik, E., and Wilcox, J. B. (2007). Reconsidering formative measurement. *Psychol Methods, 12*, 205–218. Plus comments and reply.

Hancock, G. R., and Mueller, R. O. (2006) *Structural Equation Modeling: A Second Course*. Greenwich, CT: Information Age Publishing.

Heck, R. H. (2001) Multilevel modeling with SEM. In G. A. Marcoulides & R. E. Schumaker (Eds.), *New Developments and Techniques in Structural Equation Modeling* (pp. 89–128). Mahwah, NJ: Erlbaum.

Hu, L., and Bentler, P. M. (1999). Cutoff criteria for fit indices in covariance structure analysis: conventional criteria vs new alternatives. *Struct Equ Modeling, 6*, 1–55.

Joreskog, K. G., and Sorbom, D. (1996). *LISREL 8: User's Reference Guide*. Chicago: Scientific Software International.

Jung, T., and Wickrama, K. A. S. (2008). An introduction to latent class growth analysis and growth mixture modeling. *Soc Personal Psychol Compass, 2*, 302–317.

Kaplan, D. (2000). *Structural Equation Modeling: Foundations And Extensions*. Thousand Oaks: Sage.

King, L. A., King, D. W., McArdle, J. J., Doron-LaMarca, S., and Orazem, R. J. (2006). Latent difference score approach to longitudinal trauma research. *J Traumatic Stress, 19*, 771–785.

Kline, R. (2010). *Principles and Practice of Structural Equation Modeling, 2nd Ed.* New York: Guilford Press.

Little, R. J., and Rubin, D. B. (2002). *Statistical Analysis with Missing Data, 2nd Ed.* Hoboken, NJ: Wiley.

Llabre, M. M., Spitzer, S. B., Saab, P. G., and Schneiderman, N. (2001). Piecewise latent growth curve modeling of systolic blood pressure reactivity and recovery from the cold pressor test. *Psychophysiology, 38*, 951–960.

Llabre, M. M., Spitzer, S., Siegel, S., Saab, P. G., and Schneiderman, N. (2004). Applying latent growth curve modeling to the investigation of individual differences in cardiovascular recovery from stress. *Psychosom Med, 66*, 29–41.

Llabre, M. M., Weaver, K., Duran, R., Antoni, M., McPhearson-Baker, S., and Schneiderman, N. (2006). A measurement model of medication adherence to highly active antiretroviral therapy and its relation to viral load in HIV+ adults. *AIDS Patient Care STDS, 20*, 701–711

Lubke, G., Muthen, B., Moilanen, I. K. et al (2007). Subtypes versus severity differences in attention-deficit/ hyperactivity disorder in the Northern Finnish birth cohort. *J Acad Child Adolesc Psychiat, 46*, 1584–1593.

MacCallum, R. C., Browne, M. W., and Sugawara, H. M. (1996). Power analysis and determination of sample size for covariance structure modeling. *Psychol Methods, 1*, 130–149.

Marcoulides, G. A., and Schumaker, R. E. (2001). *New Developments and Techniques in Structural Equation Modeling*. Mahwah, NJ: LEA.

Masyn, K. E. (2008). Modeling measurement error in event occurrence for single, non-recurring events in discrete-time survival analysis. In G. R. Hancock & K. M. Samuelsen (Eds.), *Advances in Latent Variable Mixture Models* (pp. 105–145). Charlotte, NC: Information Age Publishing, Inc.

McArdle, J. J., and Hamagami, F. (2000). Linear dynamic analysis of incomplete longitudinal data. In L. Collins & A. Sayer (Eds.), *New Methods for the Analysis of Change* (pp. 139–175). Wash DC: APA.

Mehta, P., and Neale, M. (2005). People are variables too: Multilevel structural equations modeling. *Psychol Methods, 10*, 259–284.

Miller, G. E., Chen, E., Fok, A. K., Walker, H., Lim, A. et al (2009). Low early-life social class leaves a biological residue manifested by decreased glucocorticoid and increased proinflammatory signaling. *Proc Natl Acad Sci USA, 106*, 14716–14721.

Muthén, B. (1984). A general structural equation model with dichotomous, ordered categorical, and continuous latent variable indicators. *Psychometrika, 49*, 115–132.

Muthén, B. (2001). Second-generation structural equation modeling with a combination of categorical and continuous latent variables: new opportunities for latent class/latent growth modeling. In L. M. Collins & A. Sayer (Eds.), *New Methods for the Analysis of Change* (pp. 291–322). Washington, DC: APA.

Muthen, B., and Masyn, K. (2005). Discrete time survival mixture analysis. *J Educ Behav Stats, 30*, 27–28.

Muthen, L., and Muthen, B. (1998-2004). *Mplus (version 5.1)*. Los Angeles: Muthen and Muthen.

Muthén, L. K. and Muthén, B. O. (2002). How to use a Monte Carlo study to decide on sample size and determine power. *Struct Equ Modeling, 4*, 599–620.

Neal, M. C., Boker, S. M., Xie, G., and Maes, H. H. (2002). *Mx: Statistical Modeling, 6th Ed.* Richmond: Virginia Commonwealth University.

Nylund, K. L., Asparouhov, T., and Muthen, B. (2007). Deciding on the number of classes in latent class analysis and growth mixture modeling. A Monte Carlo simulation study. *Struct Equ Modeling, 14*, 535–569.

Schafer, J. L., and Graham, J. W. (2002). Missing data: our view of the state of the art. *Psychol Methods, 7*, 147–177.

Shen, B. J., Goldberg, R. B., Llabre, M. M., and Schneiderman, N. (2006). Is the factor structure of the metabolic syndrome comparable between men and women and across three ethnic groups: The Miami Community Health Study. *Ann Epidemiol, 16*, 131–137.

Steiger, J. H. (1990). Structural model evaluation and modification: an interval estimation approach. *Multivar Behav Res, 25*, 173–180.

Weaver, K. E.., Llabre, M. M., Durán, R. E., Antoni, M. H., Ironson, G. et al (2005) A stress and coping model of medication adherence and viral load in HIV+ men and women on highly active antiretroviral therapy (HAART). *Health Psychol, 24*, 385–392.

Chapter 58

Meta-analysis

Larry V. Hedges and Elizabeth Tipton

1 Introduction

The research literature in behavioral medicine, like that in other areas of medicine, is experiencing dramatic growth. This expansion has made it essential that systematic reviews of research be conducted that can organize and synthesize findings. The fundamental statistical tool in systematic reviews of research is meta-analysis, which represents the results of research studies (such as clinical trials) by numerical indices of effect sizes and then summarizes these results across studies by using statistical procedures. There are many non-statistical aspects of carrying out systematic reviews in any area (see Cooper et al, 2009; Counsell, 1997; Meade and Richardson, 1997). However, this chapter provides an introduction to meta-analysis for clinical trials in behavioral medicine. For a more complete introduction to meta-analysis we recommend Borenstein et al (2009) and Cooper et al (2009).

2 Effect Sizes

Effect sizes are numerical indices of study results. They are selected to represent the results of a study in a manner that will be comparable across studies. Depending on the design of the study, different effect sizes may be more natural,

and often more than one effect size index might be chosen. In this chapter we will focus on studies that will compare a treated group with a control group (as in most randomized controlled trials). When the outcome is measured as a discrete variable (e.g., alive or not), the natural effect sizes are the risk ratio or the odds ratio (although the risk difference is sometimes used as well). When the outcome is measured as a continuous variable (such as a cognitive test score or a subjective rating of pain), but not measured on exactly the same scale in every study, a natural measure of effect size is the standardized mean difference (sometimes called Cohen's d). Finally, when both the independent variables and the outcome are continuous variables, a natural measure of the effect size is the Pearson correlation coefficient ρ.

The effect sizes usually used in meta-analysis have the property that they are approximately normally distributed with standard errors that are largely a function of the sample size in the study and can be computed from analytical formulas. In this section we describe several effect size indices and show how to compute their sampling variances (the square of their standard errors). The (sample) effect size (estimates) and their variances are the basic inputs required from each study in the meta-analysis.

All of the effect size estimates that we describe in this section have approximately normal sampling distributions. For each of these, we can therefore construct 95% confidence intervals of the following form:

$$T - 1.96\sqrt{v} \leq \theta \leq T + 1.96\sqrt{v},$$

L.V. Hedges (✉)
Department of Statistics, Northwestern University, 2046
Sheridan Road, Evanston, IL 60208, USA
e-mail: l-hedges@northwestern.edu

A. Steptoe (ed.), *Handbook of Behavioral Medicine*, DOI 10.1007/978-0-387-09488-5_58,
© Springer Science+Business Media, LLC 2010

where θ is the parameter of interest, T the sample estimate, and $\sqrt{v}$ the standard error or the estimate.

2.1 Studies Measuring Outcomes on a Binary Scale

Suppose that each study measures the outcome on a binary scale (such as survived to 6 months or not), with one of those two outcomes selected as a target outcome. Let π^T and π^C be the underlying parameters describing the proportion of individuals in the treatment and control groups, respectively, that experience the target outcome. One might describe these proportions as the "risks" of the target outcome in the treatment and control groups. A treatment effect (and therefore effect size indices) can be defined in one of three ways. The simplest but least statistically satisfactory is the risk difference:

$$\Delta = \pi^T - \pi^C.$$

Although it is simple, the risk difference has the undesirable property that its range is limited by the baseline risk (the risk in the control group); for example, if $\pi^C = 0.05$, the risk difference can be no smaller than –0.05, even if the treatment reduces the risk to 0. There are also technical shortcomings that suggest that the risk difference may not be the ideal index to use in summarizing effects across studies.

An alternative representation of a treatment effect is the risk ratio:

$$\Delta = \pi^T / \pi^C.$$

The risk ratio is an intuitive index that is frequently used in epidemiological studies, which has advantages over the risk difference for summarizing estimates across studies.

A third representation of a treatment effect is the odds ratio:

$$\omega = \frac{\pi^T / \left(1 - \pi^T\right)}{\pi^C / \left(1 - \pi^C\right)} = \frac{\pi^T \left(1 - \pi^C\right)}{\pi^C \left(1 - \pi^T\right)}.$$

Note that the odds (in the sense of betting on a horserace) of the target outcome in the treatment group are $\pi^T/(1 - \pi^T)$ and the odds of the target outcome in the control group are $\pi^C/(1 - \pi^C)$, so the odds ratio ω is literally the ratio of the odds in the treatment group to that in the control group. When the prevalence π^C (and therefore usually π^T) are small, then $(1 - \pi^C)/(1 - \pi^T)$ will be close to unity and the odds ratio will be close to the risk ratio.

Of these three measures, the odds ratio is generally preferable for the statistical analysis. In addition to having superior mathematical properties, the odds ratio can be computed in both retrospective and prospective studies, while the risk ratio and risk difference can only be calculated in prospective studies. Additionally, some empirical investigations have found that the odds ratio is the more consistent estimate across studies. However, an important disadvantage of the odds ratio is that it is less intuitive and harder to interpret than the risk difference and the risk ratio. Consequently, it is sometimes useful to carry out a meta-analysis in the metric of odds ratios, and then convert the resulting measure back into a risk ratio or risk difference for interpretation. Such a conversion requires that a value of the prevalence (π^C) be assumed, which is often selected as a typical value that might be expected.

The data from a study with binary outcomes can be summarized in a 2×2 table such as Table 58.1.

In a prospective study such as randomized trial, any of the three effect sizes can be estimated from the data given in Table 58.1. The simplest estimates arise by substituting the sample proportions for the corresponding population parameters in the definitions of the effect size (that is substituting $p^T = a/(a + b)$ for π^T and $p^C = c/(c + d)$ for π^C.

Table 58.1 Generic data summary table from a study with binary outcome

	Outcome		
	Target	Non-target	Total
Treatment	a	b	n^T
Control	c	d	n^C
Total	$a + c$	$b + d$	N

The estimate of the risk difference is

$$D = p^T - p^C = \frac{a}{a+b} - \frac{c}{c+d},$$

and the variance of D is estimated by

$$v = \frac{p^T(1-p^T)}{n^T} + \frac{p^C(1-p^C)}{n^C}$$

$$= \frac{ab}{(a+b)^3} + \frac{cd}{(c+d)^3}.$$

The estimate of the risk ratio is

$$r = \frac{p^T}{p^C} = \frac{a(c+d)}{c(a+b)}.$$

Statistical analyses involving risk ratios (including meta-analyses) typically use the (natural) logarithm of the risk ratio, not the raw risk ratio. The variance of $\ln(r)$ is estimated by

$$v = \frac{1-p^T}{n^T p^T} + \frac{1-p^C}{n^C p^C} = \frac{b}{a(a+b)} + \frac{d}{c(c+d)}.$$

Note that if either $p^C = 0$ or $p^T = 0$ (that is if $c = 0$ or $a = 0$ in Table 58.1), neither the estimate $\ln(r)$ of the log-risk ratio nor its variance can be calculated. In this case, we usually add $\frac{1}{2}$ to each cell of Table 58.1, so that the estimate of the risk ratio becomes $[(a + \frac{1}{2})(c + d + 1)]/[(c + \frac{1}{2})(a + b + 1)]$ and the estimate of the variance of $\ln(r)$ becomes

$$v = \frac{b + \frac{1}{2}}{(a + \frac{1}{2})(a + b + 1)} + \frac{d + \frac{1}{2}}{(c + \frac{1}{2})(c + d + 1)}.$$

The estimate of the odds ratio is

$$o = \frac{p^T(1 - p^C)}{p^C(1 - p^T)} = \frac{ad}{bc}.$$

As in the case of the risk ratio, statistical analyses involving odds ratios (including meta-analyses) typically use the (natural) logarithm of the odds ratio, not the raw odds ratio. The estimated variance of $\ln(o)$ is

$$v = \frac{1}{n^T p^T} + \frac{1}{n^T(1-p^T)} + \frac{1}{n^C p^C} + \frac{1}{n^C(1-p^C)}$$

$$= \frac{1}{a} + \frac{1}{b} + \frac{1}{c} + \frac{1}{d}.$$

Note that if either p^C or p^T is 0 or 1 (that is if any of a, b, c or d in Table 58.1 is 0), neither the estimate $\ln(o)$ of the log-odds ratio nor its variance can be calculated. In this case, we usually add $\frac{1}{2}$ to each cell of Table 58.1, so that the estimate of the odds ratio becomes $[(a + \frac{1}{2})(d + \frac{1}{2})]/[(b + \frac{1}{2})(c + \frac{1}{2})]$ and the variance becomes

$$v = \frac{1}{(a + \frac{1}{2})} + \frac{1}{(b + \frac{1}{2})} + \frac{1}{(c + \frac{1}{2})} + \frac{1}{(d + \frac{1}{2})}.$$

2.2 Studies Measuring Outcomes on a Continuous Scale

Suppose that each study evaluates the effect of a treatment by comparing the mean of a group of treated individuals with the mean of a group of control individuals. If the outcome measurements are normally distributed within the treatment groups with equal variances, the natural analysis would involve a t-test or an analysis of variance. The natural effect size parameter in this case is the standardized mean difference (sometimes called Cohen's d):

$$\delta = \frac{\mu^T - \mu^C}{\sigma},$$

where the parameters μ^T and μ^C are the treatment and control group means and the parameter σ is the within-group standard deviation. The quantity δ represents the treatment effect in standard deviation units. However because δ is a population parameter, it is not observed. In fact we carry out the study to estimate or draw inferences about δ. The natural estimate of δ is the sample standardized mean difference:

$$d = \frac{\overline{Y}^T - \overline{Y}^C}{S}.$$

where $\overline{Y}^T$ and $\overline{Y}^C$ are the treatment and control group sample means and S is the pooled within-group standard deviation. This estimate is often modified slightly to adjust for small sample bias to produce an unbiased estimate of δ (sometimes called Hedges' g):

$$g = d \left(1 - \frac{3}{4\left(n^T + n^C\right) - 9}\right)$$

where n^{T} and n^{C} are the sample sizes in the treatment and control groups of the study.

The variance of g is determined (mostly) by the sample sizes and (slightly) by the magnitude of g. Specifically, the variance, v, of g can be computed as

$$v = \frac{n^{\mathrm{T}} + n^{\mathrm{C}}}{n^{\mathrm{T}} n^{\mathrm{C}}} + \frac{g^2}{2\left(n^{\mathrm{T}} + n^{\mathrm{C}}\right)}.$$

The effect size g is approximately normally distributed with a mean of δ and a variance of v.

Finally, suppose that both the outcome and independent variables are continuous measures as in the case when the studies are correlational. In this case, the natural effect size parameter is ρ, the Pearson correlation coefficient. Its sample estimate is r, where

$$r = \frac{\sum\limits_{i=1}^{n} (x_i - \bar{x})(y_i - \bar{y})}{\sqrt{\sum\limits_{i=1}^{n} (x_i - \bar{x})^2 \sum\limits_{i=1}^{n} (y_i - \bar{y})^2}}.$$

In order to apply normal theory, we must use a transformation of r, the Fisher z transformation, where

$$z = \frac{1}{2} \ln\left(\frac{1+r}{1-r}\right).$$

The result, z, is unbiased, with mean

$$\zeta = \frac{1}{2} \ln\left(\frac{1+\rho}{1-\rho}\right)$$

and variance $v = 1/(n-3)$. Here n is the total sample size in the correlational study.

Finally, note that it is possible to compute confidence intervals for both δ and ζ from single values of g or z, so that we can compute the confidence interval for the effect size from each study in the meta-analysis.

3 Combining Estimates of Effect Size Across Studies

Methods for combining estimates of effect size across studies are generally the same, regardless of the effect size index used. The one exception is when studies being combined have binary outcomes and very small sample sizes, a case in which special methods (so-called Mantel-Haenszel methods) are needed. Therefore, we will present the methods for meta-analysis using a general effect size parameter which will be denoted by θ, and a general effect size estimate denoted by T, and its variance denoted by v. Thus the raw data for the meta-analysis of k studies are the effect size estimates $T_1, \ldots, T_k$ and their variances $v_1, \ldots, v_k$. The estimate from the ith study T_i estimates the unknown effect size parameter θ_i.

The summary of a collection of effect sizes via meta-analysis addresses two basic questions. The first concerns the typical or average value of the effect sizes. The second concerns the consistency of effect sizes across studies. The typical effect size in meta-analyses is estimated by averaging estimates across studies. However, because some studies produce more precise estimates (that is, they have smaller variances) than others, it makes sense to give more weight to some (the more precise) estimates than others. Two major statistical approaches to meta-analysis differ in how they compute these weights. Fixed effects methods do not include between-study differences in computing weights, while random effects methods include between-study variations in computing weights. We will describe each one of them below.

3.1 Fixed Effects Methods Combining Estimates

If the effect size parameters are identical across studies so that $\theta_1 = \cdots = \theta_k = \theta$, then the most precise estimate of θ is given by the weighted mean effect size

$$\bar{T}_\bullet = \frac{\sum\limits_{i=1}^{k} w_i T_i}{\sum\limits_{i=1}^{k} w_i},$$

where $w_i = 1/v_i$, so that the weight given to a particular effect size is the inverse of its variance. Because each of the effect size estimates is normally distributed, the weighted mean $\overline{T}_\bullet$ is also normally distributed and the variance $v_\bullet$ of $\overline{T}_\bullet$ is the reciprocal of the sum of the weights:

$$v_\bullet = \left(\sum_{i=1}^{k} w_i \right)^{-1}.$$

A 95% confidence interval for θ is given by

$$\overline{T}_\bullet - 1.96\sqrt{v_\bullet} \le \theta \le \overline{T}_\bullet + 1.96\sqrt{v_\bullet}.$$

In cases such as the risk ratio or the odds ratio where the statistical analysis is carried out in the log metric, the confidence interval is first computed in that transformed metric, then the confidence limits are transformed back to the metric of the effect size by using the exponential function $\exp(x) = e^x$. For example, the 95% confidence interval in the log metric (e.g., for the log-risk ratio or log-odds ratio) is transformed back to the unlogged metric (e.g., the risk ratio or odds ratio) as

$$\exp\left(\overline{T}_\bullet - 1.96\sqrt{v_\bullet}\right) \le \theta \le \exp\left(\overline{T}_\bullet + 1.96\sqrt{v_\bullet}\right).$$

A test of the hypothesis that $\theta = 0$ uses the test statistic

$$Z = \frac{\overline{T}_\bullet}{\sqrt{v_\bullet}}.$$

The level α two-tailed test rejects the null hypothesis when $|Z|$ exceeds the 100α percent critical value of the standard normal distribution (e.g., 1.96 for $\alpha = 0.05$). When the statistical analysis is performed in the log metric (e.g., for risk ratios or odds ratios), the significance test is conducted in the metric of the log-transformed effects. The reason is that the null hypothesis that $\rho = 1$ is equivalent to the null hypothesis that $\ln(\rho) = 0$ and similarly the null hypothesis that $\omega = 1$ is equivalent to the null hypothesis that $\ln(\omega) = 0$.

The weighted mean provides a summary of the common effect size estimates if they are reasonably homogeneous, but it is important to understand whether the hypothesis that $\theta_1 = \cdots = \theta_k$ is reasonably consistent with the evidence. To test the hypothesis that the effect sizes are the same across studies, we usually use the statistic

$$Q = \sum_{i=1}^{k} w_i \left(T_i - \overline{T}_\bullet\right)^2.$$

When the effect size parameters are identical, Q has a chi-square distribution with $(k - 1)$ degrees of freedom. Therefore a test of the hypothesis that effect sizes are identical across studies at significance level α consists of comparing the obtained value of Q with the upper α critical value of the chi-square distribution with $(k - 1)$ degrees of freedom, and rejecting the hypothesis of identical effect sizes if Q exceeds this critical value.

Note, however, that this test need not be very powerful if the number of studies is small or if the variances of the effect sizes are large (e.g., if the sample sizes in most studies are small) (see Hedges and Pigott, 2001). Thus one should not routinely conclude that effect size parameters are identical (or essentially identical) across studies unless the number of studies is large and they also have large sample sizes (and thus v_i are small).

3.1.1 Example

A systematic review and meta-analysis of $k = 10$ studies of interventions for smoking cessation for pregnant women was reported by Naughton and colleagues (2008). The data reported in Table 58.2 are from ten of their studies that used assignment of individuals (as opposed to clusters of individuals) to treatment. The number of individuals assigned to treatment who ceased smoking, the number who did not, and the total number assigned to treatment, the number assigned to the control condition who ceased smoking, the number who did not, and the total number assigned to control (a, b, n^T, c, d, and n^C from Table 58.1) are given in the columns two to seven of Table 58.2. The next three columns

Table 58.2 Example data for computing fixed and random effects meta-analyses by combining log-odds ratios

Study	Treatment			Control			o	$\ln(o)=T$	v	w	w^2	wT	wT^2	w^*	w^*T
	a	b	n^T	c	d	n^C									
1	14	88	102	2	102	104	8.114	2.094	0.593	1.687	2.848	3.533	7.396	1.427	2.988
2	29	97	126	12	104	116	2.591	0.952	0.138	7.260	52.708	6.912	6.581	4.069	3.874
3	56	388	444	18	191	209	1.532	0.426	0.081	12.311	151.570	5.248	2.237	5.285	2.253
4	4	42	46	1	23	24	2.190	0.784	1.317	0.759	0.576	0.595	0.467	0.702	0.550
5	9	34	43	11	36	47	0.866	−0.144	0.259	3.858	14.883	−0.554	0.079	2.723	−0.391
6	57	343	400	35	379	414	1.800	0.588	0.052	19.354	374.572	11.371	6.680	6.263	3.680
7	12	86	98	3	98	101	4.558	1.517	0.438	2.281	5.201	3.459	5.248	1.830	2.776
8	12	181	193	11	187	198	1.127	0.120	0.185	5.402	29.182	0.646	0.077	3.412	0.408
9	5	21	26	0	30	30	15.605	2.748	2.261	0.442	0.196	1.215	3.339	0.422	1.160
10	4	46	50	0	47	47	9.194	2.219	2.265	0.442	0.195	0.980	2.173	0.421	0.935
Totals										53.796	631.931	33.405	34.277	26.554	18.233

give the odds ratio, the log-odds ratio, and the variance of the log-odds ratio. Note that studies 9 and 10 have 0 individuals in the control group who experienced smoking cessation; therefore, we added $\frac{1}{2}$ to each of the a, b, c, and d values for those two studies in order to compute the odds ratio and its variance.

Using the summaries in Table 58.2 we see that the weighted mean of the log-odds ratios is

$$\bar{T}_{\bullet} = 33.405/53.796 = 0.621$$

with a variance of

$$v_{\bullet} = 1/53.796 = 0.019,$$

which leads to a confidence interval for the log-odds ratio $\ln(\omega)$ of

$$0.354 = 0.621 - 1.96\sqrt{0.019} \leq \ln(\omega) \leq 0.621$$
$$+1.96\sqrt{0.019} = 0.888.$$

Converting these into the metric of (unlogged) odds ratio ω yields the estimate $o = \exp(0.621) = 1.86$ and the 95% confidence interval

$$1.42 = \exp(0.354) \leq \omega \leq \exp(0.888) = 2.43$$

The test for the homogeneity of effect sizes is computed as

$$Q = 34.227 - (33.405)^2/53.796 = 13.534$$

Comparing $Q = 13.534$ with the critical values of the chi-square distribution with $(10 - 1) = 9$ degrees of freedom, we see that a large Q value could occur between 10 and 15% of the time by chance if the odds ratios were identical across studies.

3.2 Mantel-Haenszel Methods

A special problem arises in the meta-analysis of studies with binary outcomes when the individual studies are very small. When only one or a few have 2×2 data tables with empty cells (a, b, c, or d from Table 58.1 are zero), the methods described above may be used after adding $\frac{1}{2}$ to the numbers in each cell. However when individual studies are very small, a large proportion of studies may have empty cells. In this case, special methods, known as Mantel-Haenszel methods, may be more appropriate. There is no hard and fast rule as to when Mantel-Haenszel methods are needed, but it might be wise to use these methods whenever more than a small proportion of studies (say 5%) have empty cells. We describe Mantel-Haenszel methods for estimating the odds ratio, but there are analogous methods for the risk ratio and the risk difference (see Greenland, 1982; Tarone, 1981).

The Mantel-Haenszel method of combining odds ratios uses the statistic:

$$o_{MH} = \frac{\sum_{i=1}^{k} \frac{a_i d_i}{N_i}}{\sum_{i=1}^{k} \frac{b_i c_i}{N_i}},$$

where a_i, b_i, c_i, and d_i are the quantities in Table 58.1 for the ith study, and $N_i = a_i + b_i + c_i + d_i$ is the total sample size for the ith study. Note that the Mantel-Haenszel statistic computes the summary directly from the cell counts and dispenses with the intermediate computation of odds ratios from each study. As long as none of the N_i are zero, it is unnecessary (and it would be incorrect) to add $\frac{1}{2}$ to the cell counts in order to compute the Mantel-Haenszel statistic, even if some of the a_i, b_i, c_i, and d_i are zero.

An (somewhat complex) expression for the variance of $\ln(o_{MH})$ is

$$v_{MH} = \frac{\sum_{i=1}^{k} P_i R_i}{2\left(\sum_{i=1}^{k} R_i\right)^2} + \frac{\sum_{i=1}^{k} (P_i S_i + Q_i R_i)}{2\left(\sum_{i=1}^{k} R_i\right)\left(\sum_{i=1}^{k} S_i\right)}$$
$$+ \frac{\sum_{i=1}^{k} Q_i S_i}{2\left(\sum_{i=1}^{k} S_i\right)^2},$$

where

$$P_i = \frac{a_i + d_i}{N_i},$$

$$Q_i = \frac{c_i + b_i}{N_i},$$

$$R_i = \frac{a_i d_i}{N_i},$$

and

$$S_i = \frac{b_i c_i}{N_i}.$$

To compute confidence intervals for the odds ratio ω, we first compute a confidence interval for the $\ln(\omega)$ and then use the exponential function $\exp(x) = e^x$ to convert the confidence limits for the log-odds into confidence limits for the (unlogged) odds ratio. For example, a 95% confidence interval for ω is given by

$$\exp\left(\ln(o_{\mathrm{MH}}) - 1.96\sqrt{v_{\mathrm{MH}}}\right) \leq \omega$$
$$\leq \exp\left(\ln(o_{\mathrm{MH}}) + 1.96\sqrt{v_{\mathrm{MH}}}\right).$$

The Mantel-Haenszel method is basically a fixed effects procedure. There is no entirely satisfactory way to extend this method to random effects analysis. There are methods with the same motivation, such as those based on generalized mixed model procedures (see, e.g., Schall, 1991; or Breslow and Clayton, 1993).

3.2.1 Example

Return to our example of $k = 10$ studies of interventions to promote smoking cessation among pregnant women. Table 58.3 illustrates the calculation of the quantities necessary for computing the Mantel-Haenszel estimate o_{MH} of the odds ratio and the variance of $\ln(o_{\mathrm{MH}})$ directly. The estimate of the odds ratio is

$$o_{\mathrm{MH}} = 83.494/45.252 = 1.98,$$

which is very similar to the odds ratio estimate of 1.86 computed by averaging the log-odds ratios.

The variance of $\ln(o_{\mathrm{MH}})$ is computed as

$$v_{\mathrm{MH}} = \frac{42.351}{2(83.494)^2} + \frac{20.687 + 41.142}{2(83.292)(42.252)}$$
$$+ \frac{21.565}{2(42.252)^2} = 0.018,$$

which is quite similar to the variance of the log-odds ratio of 0.019 computed by averaging the log-odds. Note that neither estimate required adding $\frac{1}{2}$ to compensate for the zero cell counts in studies 9 and 10. A 95% confidence interval for ω based on the Mantel-Haenszel estimate is given by

$$1.52 = \exp\left(\ln(1.98) - 1.96\sqrt{0.018}\right) \leq \omega$$
$$\leq \exp\left(\ln(1.98) + 1.96\sqrt{0.018}\right) = 2.57.$$

This confidence interval is quite similar to the interval of 1.42–2.43 computed in connection with the analysis that averaged the log-odds ratios.

3.3 Random Effects Methods

If the effect size parameters are not identical (or almost so) across studies, an alternative method for combining estimates across studies is the random effects model. In this model, studies are considered as a sample of possible studies and their effect size parameters are considered as a sample from a universe of possible effect size estimates. In this model the object is to estimate the mean μ and variance τ^2 of the population of effect sizes (the population of θ values) from which the observed study effect sizes are sampled.

If the effect size parameters corresponding to the studies in our sample of studies $(\theta_1, \ldots, \theta_k)$ were observed, we could simply compute their variance as a sample estimate of τ^2. Because they are not observed we must estimate their variance indirectly by noting that the variance of the observed effect size estimates $(T_1, \ldots, T_k)$ depends partly on v_i, which represent estimation

Table 58.3 Example data for computing fixed effects meta-analyses using the Mantel-Haenszel method

	Control		Treatment											
Study	a	b	c	d	N	P	Q	R	S	PR	PS	QR	QS
1	14	88	2	102	206	0.563	0.437	6.932	0.854	3.903	0.481	3.029	0.373
2	29	97	12	104	242	0.550	0.450	12.463	4.810	6.849	2.643	5.613	2.166
3	56	388	18	191	653	0.378	0.622	16.380	10.695	6.196	4.046	10.184	6.650
4	4	42	1	23	70	0.386	0.614	1.314	0.600	0.507	0.231	0.807	0.369
5	9	34	11	36	90	0.500	0.500	3.600	4.156	1.800	2.078	1.800	2.078
6	57	343	35	379	814	0.536	0.464	26.539	14.748	14.215	7.900	12.324	6.849
7	12	86	3	98	199	0.553	0.447	5.910	1.296	3.267	0.717	2.643	0.580
8	12	181	11	187	391	0.509	0.491	5.739	5.092	2.921	2.592	2.818	2.500
9	5	21	0	30	56	0.625	0.375	2.679	0.000	1.674	0.000	1.004	0.000
10	4	46	0	47	97	0.526	0.474	1.938	0.000	1.019	0.000	0.919	0.000
Totals						5.125	4.875	83.494	42.252	42.351	20.687	41.142	21.565

Note: There are no columns for ad/N or bc/N because $ad/N = R$ and $bc/N = S$

errors and partly on τ^2, which represents true heterogeneity among θ_i. The Q-statistic used to test heterogeneity is a weighted sample variance that can be used to obtain an indirect estimate of τ^2. In particular,

$$\hat{\tau}^2 = \frac{Q - (k - 1)}{c},$$

if the quantity on the right-hand side of the equation is positive, and zero otherwise, where c is a normalizing constant given by

$$c = \sum_{i=1}^{k} w_i - \frac{\sum_{i=1}^{k} w_i^2}{\sum_{i=1}^{k} w_i}.$$

Random effects methods compute the weighted mean effect size as

$$\overline{T}_\bullet{}^* = \frac{\sum_{i=1}^{k} w_i^* T_i}{\sum_{i=1}^{k} w_i^*},$$

where $w_i^* = 1/v_i^* = 1/(v_i + \hat{\tau}^2)$. This corresponds to weighting each effect size by the inverse of a new variance, $v_i^* = v_i + \hat{\tau}^2$, which includes a component of between-study variation. As in the fixed effect case, the weighted mean $\overline{T}_\bullet{}^*$ is also normally distributed, the variance $v_\bullet^*$ of $\overline{T}_\bullet{}^*$ is the reciprocal of the sum of the weights

$$v_\bullet{}^* = \left(\sum_{i=1}^{k} w_i^*\right)^{-1},$$

and a 95% confidence interval for the average effect size μ is given by

$$\overline{T}_\bullet{}^* - 1.96\sqrt{v_\bullet^*} \le \theta \le \overline{T}_\bullet{}^* + 1.96\sqrt{v_\bullet^*}.$$

A test of the hypothesis that $\theta = 0$ uses the test statistic

$$Z* = \frac{\overline{T}_\bullet^*}{\sqrt{v_\bullet^*}}.$$

The level α two-tailed test rejects the null hypothesis when $|Z|$ exceeds the 100α percent critical value of the standard normal distribution (e.g., 1.96 for $\alpha = 0.05$).

The fixed and random effects weighted means are similar in form and differ only in the weights used to compute them. When $\hat{\tau}^2 > 0$, the w_i^* are more similar to one another than the w_i. This means that studies receive more equal weights in the random effects weighted mean than in the fixed effects weighted mean, where one study can dominate (receive very large weight) if it has a very small variance (usually because it has a very large sample size). By contrast, in the random effects weighted mean, where the weight given to each study is more similar, no single study can completely dominate. Similarly, when $\hat{\tau}^2 > 0$, each w_i^* is larger than the corresponding w_i. Because the variance of the weighted mean is the inverse of the sum of the weights, this means that the variance $v_\bullet^*$ of the random effects weighted mean $\overline{T}_\bullet{}^*$ is larger than the variance $v_\bullet$ of the fixed effects weighted mean $\overline{T}_\bullet$. One implication of this is that confidence intervals for the random effects weighted mean are longer than those of the fixed effects weighted mean.

Note that the test of the hypothesis that $\tau^2 = 0$ in the random effects analysis is exactly the test of the hypothesis that $\theta_1 = \cdots = \theta_k$ based on the Q-statistics described in connection with the fixed effects analysis, since if $\tau^2 = 0$, the effect size parameters will be identical.

A quantitative description of the amount of heterogeneity can be provided in either one of two ways. The estimate of τ^2 provides one such estimate. The square root of this estimate, $\hat{\tau}$, is an estimate of the standard deviation of the distribution of the effect size parameters across studies. An alternative way to characterize heterogeneity is to describe the proportion of variation in the observed effect size estimates that is due to τ^2. The estimate

$$I^2 = \left(\frac{Q - (k - 1)}{Q}\right) \times 100\%$$

does just this. Because $\hat{\tau}$ describes the *absolute* amount of variation in θ_s and I^2 describes the amount of variation *relative* to the total variation of estimates (including the amount of variation due to both variation of θ_s and errors of estimation), both are complementary ways to describe variation in effect size parameters.

3.3.1 Example

Returning to our example of $k = 10$ studies of interventions to promote smoking cessation among pregnant women, we use the quantities in Table 58.2 to compute and give an estimate of the between-studies variance component (τ^2), the random effects weight w^*, w^*T, and their sums. First compute the normalizing constant c as

$$c = 53.796 - 631.931/53.796 = 42.05,$$

then use this quantity along with the Q-statistic computed in the fixed effects analysis ($Q = 13.534$) to compute the estimate of τ^2 as

$$\hat{\tau}^2 = \frac{13.534 - (10 - 1)}{42.05} = 0.108.$$

This value is used to compute the w^* values and the w^*T values in Table 58.2, for example, the random effects weight in study 1 is $w_1^* = 1/(0.593 + 0.108) = 1.427$. Using these random effects weights, the random effects weighted mean of the log-odds ratios is

$$\bar{T}_\bullet = 18.233/26.554 = 0.687$$

with a variance of

$$v_\bullet = 1/26.554 = 0.038,$$

which leads to the 95% confidence interval for the log-odds ratio $\ln(\omega)$ of

$$0.306 = 0.687 - 1.96\sqrt{0.038} \leq \ln(\omega) \leq 0.687 + 1.96\sqrt{0.038} = 1.067.$$

Converting these into the metric of (unlogged) odds ration ω yields the estimate $o = \exp(0.687)$ = 1.99 and the 95% confidence interval

$$1.36 = \exp(0.306) \leq \omega \leq \exp(1.067) = 2.91.$$

Note that the point estimate of the odds ratio is slightly larger than that computed using the fixed effects model, and the variance of the log-odds ratio computed using the random effects model is twice as large as the value of 0.019 computed using the fixed effects model. Similarly the confidence interval for ω computed using the random effects model is wider (1.36–2.91) than that computed using the fixed effects model (1.42–2.43).

Using the value of the Q statistic of $Q = 13.534$ computed in the example for the fixed effects analysis, the value of I^2, representing the proportion of variance in the estimates that is due to variation in effect size parameters across studies is

$$I^2 = 100\% \times [13.534 - (10 - 1)]/13.534$$
$$= 33.5\%$$

4 Methods for Testing for Differences Between Groups of Studies

There are also meta-analytic methods for modeling variation across studies as a function of study level covariates. Perhaps the most common such analyses are designed to determine whether the average effect sizes of subgroups of studies differ from one another, a meta-analytic generalization of analysis of variance. Another type of analysis examines the relation between continuously measured covariates and effect size, a meta-analytic generalization of regression analysis (sometimes called meta-regression). For more information about the fixed effects versions of these techniques, see Konstantopoulos and Hedges (2009), and for information about the random effects versions of these techniques, see Raudenbush (2009).

5 Forest Plots

Note that for all the effect size indices we have considered (and a great many more as well) that it is possible to compute a confidence interval for the effect size parameter from a single value of the effect size estimate, so that we can compute a confidence interval for the effect size parameter associated with each study in the meta-analysis. A plot depicting all the confidence intervals from all of the studies in a meta-analysis is called a forest plot (as in seeing the forest and the trees). A forest plot provides an overview of all the effect size estimates in a meta-analysis along with their uncertainties (depicted by the error bars in the confidence intervals).

An example of a forest plot arising from the data used in Naughton and colleagues (2008) example is given below (Fig. 58.1). Particularly note two things about this forest plot. First the error bars are of much different lengths, denoting that the sampling uncertainties of different studies are quite different. Second, note that the centers of these error bars (denoting the point estimates of effect sizes from different studies) are somewhat different from one another, indicating that there is variation in the effect size estimates across studies.

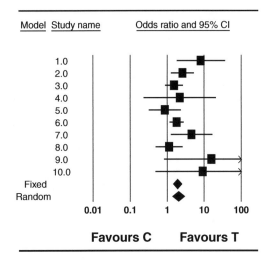

Fig. 58.1 Forest plot of odds ratios found in Table 58.2

6 Publication Bias

Publication selection is the tendency of studies that are published, reported, or otherwise available for review to be a non-random sample of the studies that were actually conducted. If studies producing effect size estimates that tend to be smaller are less likely to be available (e.g., if effects that are too small to be statistically significant are less likely to be published) then publication selection may lead to biases in the effect size estimates computed from observed studies. Such biases can be severe when selection is severe. There is a substantial literature on the detection and possible correction of publication bias which is beyond the scope of this chapter (see Rothstein et al, 2005; Sutton, 2009).

7 Conclusion

Meta-analysis can be a valuable tool for summarizing research findings across studies. It permits reviewers to describe the results of each study on a common effect size metric, combine information from many studies in an optimal fashion, and understand the degree to which the findings from different studies agree with one another.

References

Borenstein, M., Hedges, L. V., Higgins, J. P. T., and Rothstein, H. (2009). *Introduction to Meta-analysis*. London: Wiley.

Breslow, N. E., and Clayton, D. G. (1993). Approximate inference in generalized linear mixed models. *J Am Stat Assoc, 88*, 9–25.

Cooper, H., Hedges, L. V., and Valentine, J. (2009). *The Handbook of Research Synthesis and Meta-analysis, 2nd Ed.* New York: Russell Sage Foundation.

Counsell, C. (1997). Formulating questions and locating primary studies for inclusion in systematic reviews. *Ann Intern Med, 127*, 380–387.

Greenland, S. (1982). Interpretation and estimation of summary ratios under heterogeneity. *Stat Med, 1,* 217–227.

Hedges, L. V., and Pigott, T. D. (2001). The power of statistical tests in meta-analysis. *Psychol Methods, 6,* 203–217.

Konstantopoulos, S., and Hedges, L. V. (2009). Fixed effects models. In H. Cooper, L. V. Hedges, & J. Valentine (Eds.), *The Handbook of Research Synthesis and Meta-analysis, 2nd Ed* (pp. 279–294). New York: Russell Sage Foundation.

Meade, M. O., and Richardson, W. S. (1997). Selecting and appraising studies for a systematic review. *Ann Intern Med, 127,* 531–537.

Naughton, F., Prevost, A. T., and Sutton, S. (2008). Self-help smoking cessation interventions in pregnancy: a systematic review and meta-analysis. *Addiction, 103,* 566–579.

Raudenbush, S. W. (2009). Random effects models. In H. Cooper, L. V. Hedges, & J. Valentine (Eds.), *The Handbook of Research Synthesis and Meta-analysis, 2nd Ed* (pp. 295–316). New York: Russell Sage Foundation.

Rothstein, H., Sutton, A., and Borenstein, M. (Eds.) (2005). *Publication Bias in Meta-analysis.* New York: Wiley.

Schall, R. (1991). Estimation in generalized linear models with random effects. *Biometrika, 78,* 719 727.

Sutton, A. (2009). Publication bias. In H. Cooper, L. V. Hedges, & J. Valentine (Eds). *The Handbook of Research Synthesis and Meta-analysis, 2nd Ed* (pp. 435–451). New York: Russell Sage Foundation.

Tarone, R. E. (1981). On summary estimators of relative risk. *J Chron Dis, 34,* 463–468.

Part X
Behavioral and Psychosocial Interventions

Chapter 59

Trial Design in Behavioral Medicine

Kenneth E. Freedland, Robert M. Carney, and Patrick J. Lustman

1 Introduction

The design of a clinical trial depends on the purpose of the study. Most behavioral medicine trials test the efficacy of an intervention under carefully controlled conditions or its effectiveness in clinical practice. However, some trials are conducted for other purposes, and they may not be designed the same way as standard efficacy or effectiveness trials. Also, many efficacy trials can be designed in more than one way. Design decisions frequently involve difficult tradeoffs and they can be controversial. Investigators, grant reviewers, institutional review boards, and other interested parties often disagree about these decisions. Differences of opinion about control groups drive many of these disagreements.

These differences can widen when the decision makers represent multiple disciplines or fields of research with different methodological traditions. Researchers who only conduct drug trials may be unfamiliar with the distinctive challenges involved in designing and conducting randomized trials of nonpharmacological interventions. Social and behavioral scientists who only conduct trials involving healthy subjects may be unaware of the complex design and logistical challenges involved in studies of medically ill patients. These crosswinds often buffet trialists who work at the nexus of behavioral and biomedical research.

This chapter is not intended to be a comprehensive guide to clinical trial design. Instead, it focuses on design issues that are particularly relevant to contemporary behavioral medicine research. It may not resolve the controversies that often surround trial design decisions, but it should at least help to clarify some of the reasons why they are controversial.

2 Control Conditions

2.1 Control vs. Comparison

In a randomized controlled trial (RCT), there is at least one experimental group and at least one control group. The latter is so named because its primary purpose is to "control" for threats to internal validity, i.e., the validity of conclusions about the causal relationship between the intervention and the outcome (Campbell and Stanley, 1966). However, some control groups have other purposes, in addition to controlling for threats to internal validity. In some trials, participants are randomly assigned to a new, experimental intervention or to an existing, standard treatment. The aim is to determine whether the new treatment is superior, or at least equivalent, to the standard treatment. Thus, the principal reason for including the standard treatment arm is to

K.E. Freedland (✉)
Behavioral Medicine Center, Department of Psychiatry,
Washington University School of Medicine, 4320 Forest
Park Avenue, Suite 301, St. Louis, MI 63108, USA
e-mail: freedlak@bmc.wustl.edu

A. Steptoe (ed.), *Handbook of Behavioral Medicine*, DOI 10.1007/978-0-387-09488-5_59,
© Springer Science+Business Media, LLC 2010

compare it to the experimental treatment. This design does control for most of the standard threats to internal validity, but if that were the only consideration, a different control condition such as a placebo might be a better choice. When designing a trial, both the control and the comparison functions of the control group(s) must be considered (Kazdin, 2003b).

In a randomized comparison of two active treatments, the positive outcomes of both interventions could be due to factors such as the placebo effect rather than to their putative active ingredients. On the other hand, both treatments could actually be *less* effective than a mere placebo if their side effects were too aversive. Neither possibility would be apparent unless a placebo control group was included in the trial design. However, adding a placebo arm would increase costs and could raise ethical concerns. Given these constraints, it is necessary to consider whether comparison of the active interventions would be sufficiently informative to justify the trial, even without a placebo arm. An RCT of two interventions may be worth conducting even if some threats to internal validity cannot be completely ruled out.

2.2 The Standard Hierarchy of Control Conditions

Control conditions differ with respect to the amount of manipulation or intervention they deliver. The minimal condition is a no-treatment control arm. It can only be used when it is possible to ensure that (1) Group A is given the experimental treatment and Group B is not, (2) Group B cannot obtain it any other way, and (3) Group B cannot obtain any other treatment for the same indication. A recent trial (Wolfe et al, 2003) compared a community-based dating violence prevention program for at-risk youth to a no-treatment control condition. The program was not available from any other source, and no other treatment for this problem was available in the community. Consequently, the

investigators could be confident that the control group would not receive any dating violence prevention services during the trial.

If it is possible to employ a true, no-treatment control condition, then it is also possible to construct a hierarchy of control conditions that range from less to more intervention: (1) no treatment; (2) wait list; (3) nonspecific intervention or placebo; (4) isolated component(s) of an active treatment; (5) a complete, active treatment. Wait lists provide more intervention than no-treatment conditions in the sense that the participants are expecting to receive the experimental treatment. Nonspecific and placebo control conditions do not provide the putative active ingredients of the experimental intervention, but they do provide an intervention that can affect outcomes via therapist contact, expectations for improvement, or other mechanisms. Treatment component conditions are active interventions, albeit missing one or more ingredients of the full experimental intervention. Active treatment control arms generally provide as much intervention as the experimental treatment(s) to which they are compared; they simply represent different forms of treatment. Both treatment component and active treatment control conditions also have nonspecific or placebo effects.

This hierarchy, or something similar, is presented in many research methodology textbooks (e.g., Kazdin, 2003b). It assumes that it is possible to withhold treatment altogether from untreated controls. This is possible in many experimental environments, but most clinical research in behavioral medicine is conducted in settings wherein pristine, no-treatment control conditions are *not* possible. If the target problem or disorder involves physical and/or mental health and if the participants have access to health-care services, then a true, no-treatment control condition is usually not an option. If the participants are randomly assigned to a nominal "no-treatment" condition, they may still receive some form of usual care (UC) or treatment as usual (TAU). They have access to non-study clinical services, whether or not they utilize them. Thus, in many trials, one cannot guarantee that the participants will refrain from non-study treatment.

2.3 Usual Care, Treatment as Usual, and Standard of Care Controls

"Usual care" and "treatment as usual" are often used interchangeably, but they have different connotations. UC is the preferred term in medical research (e.g., Minneci et al, 2008). It implies that the non-study care extends beyond the specific treatment or disorder being studied. For example, cancer patients enrolled in a psychosocial intervention trial might be receiving non-study treatment not only for cancer and its complications but also for other medical and psychiatric problems, whether related or unrelated to cancer. TAU terminology is used more often in mental health services research and psychosocial intervention studies than in medical research (Street and Luoma, 2002). It implies that an identifiable treatment of some sort is routinely provided for the target problem or disorder. It does not imply that other forms of care are being provided in the trial setting, although it does not preclude this either.

UC might be very narrowly construed as including only the non-study psychiatric, psychological, social work, or primary care services that are available to the participants for the same psychosocial problem that is the target of the experimental intervention. It could be viewed more broadly as including services for any mental health problem, whether or not targeted in the trial, or even more broadly as comprising all of the health services the participants are receiving for all of their medical and psychiatric problems. This last definition not only is the most comprehensive but also captures more threats to internal validity. For example, care received for other medical problems can affect psychosocial adjustment. Also, UC often refers not only to health services that are actually utilized but also to services that *could* be utilized. Assignment to a UC control group does not necessarily mean that all participants will actually receive treatment for the disorder in question. Some might not pursue, be offered, or accept treatment.

UC typically includes whatever health services a patient would routinely receive, regardless of clinical trial participation. In contrast, *enhanced* usual care (EUC) conditions provide something other than purely naturalistic usual care. There are several circumstances in which an EUC control might be employed instead of a naturalistic UC condition. One of the most common occurs when the patient's health-care provider(s) must be informed, for ethical and/or clinical reasons, about the results of assessments performed for the study. Doing so enhances usual care and might trigger additional non-study tests or treatments that would not have occurred if the patient were not participating in the trial. Even minimal enhancement of usual care can have substantial effects on the patient's care and medical outcomes.

Another reason to use an EUC control is to ensure that all participants receive the current, guideline-adherent standard of care. Even if a novel treatment is found to be superior to UC, it will not necessarily be seen as representing a significant advance in medical care unless the UC was state-of-the-art. An EUC control condition may be needed to provide this level of care.

This can create a dilemma for behavioral trialists working at tertiary or quaternary care medical centers. Consider a trial that would compare a behavioral intervention to improve glycemic control in outpatients with Type 2 diabetes, to UC for diabetes. The behavioral intervention would be added on to UC for diabetes. Thus, the design can be depicted as comparing UC plus behavioral intervention to UC alone. If the researcher casts a broad net in recruiting for the trial, some of the participants might be receiving their diabetes care from the medical center's renowned, state-of-the-art diabetes specialty clinic, while others might be receiving it from their own primary care physician, a community health center, or some other provider. The quality of UC for diabetes is likely to differ markedly across these settings. If it does, the researcher will not be able to claim that the behavioral intervention improves outcomes above and beyond state-of-the-art medical care for diabetes, even if the trial's results are positive. One alternative would be to restrict recruitment to the diabetes specialty clinic, where UC is uniformly state-of-the-art. The disadvantages of this approach are that it would limit recruitment and jeopardize the feasibility and generalizability of the trial. Another alternative would be to stratify by site. This approach would permit a comparison with state-of-the-art care within the specialty clinic sample, but it would only be possible to do this if the trial were fairly large. Yet another approach would be to ensure that all participants receive the best possible care, even if some of them would otherwise receive care that falls short of the state-of-the-art. This would change the trial design to EUC + behavioral intervention vs. EUC alone.

This sort of enhancement is also easier said than done. The trialist would either have to arrange for all participants to be seen at the diabetes specialty clinic, and thereby increasing the cost of the trial and possibly alienating the participants' primary care physicians, or else find a way to ensure that the all of the primary care physicians provide state-of-the-art diabetes care. Neither possibility would be a realistic option for some behavioral medicine research centers.

Another reason to employ an EUC control is to standardize the non-study care received by all participants, in order to reduce extraneous variability in exposure to relevant treatments. A trial of a behavioral treatment for insomnia might compare the experimental treatment to UC. In this design, some participants in both arms might receive medications for insomnia from their own physicians, while others might not receive any medication, so UC would not consist of the same sort of medical treatment for insomnia from one patient to the next. In an EUC alternative, these physicians might be asked to prescribe the same medication, at the same dosage, to every patient. Of course, trialists usually cannot dictate non-study care or guarantee that every physician will comply with their requests to standardize care.

The more the UC is enhanced, the more it resembles an experimental intervention in its own right and the more it diverges from actual clinical practice. Thus, a trial comparing a novel experimental intervention to extensively enhanced UC is, essentially, a comparison of two active interventions. For these reasons, UC or minimally enhanced UC controls are more common than substantially enhanced or standardized EUC controls in behavioral medicine research.

Evidence-based clinical guidelines exist for many different conditions and treatments. Treatments that are of the highest quality and that adhere closely to state-of-the-art clinical guidelines or to well-established best practices are often labeled standard of care (SoC). SoC should not be confused with standard care (SC), which is usually synonymous with usual or routine care. There are many reasons why the usual care in a particular setting or community might not always conform to established standards of care. There are unfortunate reasons, such as disparities in the quality of health care that fall along socioeconomic, demographic, or geographic lines (Werner et al, 2008). Entire health-care systems can differ with respect to their institutional commitment to, or ability to, provide state-of-the-art care. There is also a good reason for variability in UC: expert clinicians often depart from guidelines when doing so is clinically indicated. A basic example is a physician's decision to withhold a guideline-recommended medication if the patient is allergic to it. Another is a therapist's effort to tailor an evidence-based intervention to the idiosyncratic needs of an individual patient. Thus, appropriately individualized care (IC) accounts for some of the variability in usual care.

In some circumstances, individualized care might yield better outcomes than rigid adherence to a specific SoC, but in others, the best way to achieve optimal outcomes might be to uniformly follow the SoC. Thus, the most rigorous comparator in some RCTs might be IC rather than SoC, and in some trials, it might be the reverse. It might even be desirable in some cases to compare a novel intervention to both an SoC and an IC control condition (Thompson and Schoenfeld, 2007). Like other three-arm designs, however, this type of trial may be prohibitively expensive in many instances, and it may be necessary to choose just one of these control conditions even if it would be informative to include both.

UC, SoC, and other conditions that are not entirely (or not at all) determined by the investigator's research protocol can change over time. The chances that consequential change will occur increase over time. This pertains both to the length of the intervention phase of the trial and to the overall duration of the trial itself. The longer the patients remain in the intervention phase of a trial, the greater the chance that their non-study care will evolve. For example, non-study cardiac treatment regimens are unlikely to change over the course of a 4-week intervention phase in a group of patients with stable coronary disease, but they could very well change if the trial's intervention phase lasts 6 months or a year. Similarly, the longer the trial as a whole takes to complete, the greater is the chance that there will be changes in the ways that the study population will be treated. New drugs can enter the market, existing ones can fall abruptly into disfavor, and new or revised clinical guidelines can be issued, to state just a few examples. Thus, temporal variability in usual care can be problematic in trials that involve long intervention phases and in ones that take years to complete.

Clearly, UC, EUC, SoC, and IC can be rather complex control conditions. Failure to give due consideration to the characteristics of these control conditions can have unfortunate consequences for clinical trials, and even for entire lines of research (Burns, 2009). The composition of UC in any given trial depends upon the problem or disorder in question, the other problems that are present, the state-of-the-art of treatment for the target problem, the availability of treatment services, the patient population being studied, and the settings from which the participants are recruited. In multicenter studies, usual care may differ from one center to the next or from one recruitment venue to the next within a single center. It can differ from one patient to the next within the same setting, and it can change in the middle of the study. Given its heterogeneity, it is essential to document key elements of UC. For example, it is important to systematically document any non-study medications that participants were taking during the trial.

Data on non-study treatments can be very useful for analyses of the roles of *differential treatment intensification* and *differential adherence* in study outcomes, particularly in behavioral RCTs that cannot be double blinded and that involve some form of usual care. Differential treatment intensification occurs when one group tends to receive more intensive non-study care than another group, and differential adherence occurs when the patients in one group tend to adhere more closely to their non-study treatment regimens than those in another group.

For example, patients with arthritis might be randomly assigned to a coping skills intervention plus usual care for arthritis or to usual care alone. The intervention might, either inadvertently or by design, encourage the participants to contact their physician more frequently or to be more assertive in requesting medications or other non-study treatments. Consequently, they may receive more frequent or intensive non-study medical care than the UC participants. Depending upon the aims of the intervention, this form of differential intensification could be viewed either as a rival explanation for better outcomes in the intervention arm or as a mechanism of action through which the intervention produced better outcomes. Conversely, the UC participants in such a trial might seek more non-study treatment than their counterparts in the intervention arm, because they are not receiving any special intervention for their arthritis and may have more difficulty coping with it. This might turn out to be a potential explanation for why there was *no* significant difference between the groups in the primary study outcome. Differential adherence can have the same causes and effects as differential intensification. The coping intervention might, for example, induce closer patient adherence to non-study treatments for arthritis in the intervention than in the usual care arm.

Treatment intensification measurement methods have only recently started to gain attention. So far, most of the emphasis has been on the intensification of medication regimens, as indicated by increases in the number of drug classes, increased dosages within a drug class, or switches to different drug classes (Schmittdiel et al, 2008; Selby et al, 2009). Other dimensions of treatment intensification, such as whether there is an increased frequency of non-study outpatient clinic visits, may also be useful to measure in some behavioral RCTs. Measurement of patient adherence is addressed in Chapter 7.

2.4 Usual Care and Its Variants in the Hierarchy of Control Conditions

UC does not fit into the standard hierarchy of control conditions. In fact, if non-study clinical care is available to the participants of a trial, the standard hierarchy disintegrates. In the presence of UC, there is often no way to guarantee that participants randomly assigned to no-treatment control conditions will abstain from non-study treatment for the target problem or disorder (Kazdin, 2003a). For example, in a trial of a psychotherapeutic intervention for depression, some "no-treatment" participants might obtain antidepressants from their own physicians, as might some in the treatment arm. In addition, the presence of UC in the background of a trial often precludes pure controls for placebo or nonspecific treatment effects, as well as pure comparisons with treatment components or active interventions. If the depression trial were designed to compare the full experimental psychotherapeutic intervention against a treatment component condition, for example, the design would ordinarily be described simply as a comparison of the component in question vs. that component + the remaining ingredients. However, a more complete description would be UC + treatment component vs. UC + treatment component + the remaining ingredients, given that UC is present in the background of the trial.

The UCs do not necessarily cancel each other out in this type of design because UC may interact differentially with the two conditions. For example, if the remaining ingredients in our example included educational materials about treatments for depression, the participants in the full intervention arm might be more likely than those in the component-only arm to seek non-study antidepressants. This potential source of differential intensification of non-study care should be addressed whenever an RCT is conducted with a UC control group or even when UC is merely present in the trial's milieu. This also holds for EUC, SoC, and IC controls.

Clinical trials targeting problems that are not routinely (or ever) addressed in the setting of interest or for the population of interest might be regarded as an exception to this rule, but even these types of trials can be affected by UC. For example, self-forgiveness has been shown to predict better psychosocial adjustment and quality of life among women being treated for breast cancer (Romero et al, 2006). If a research team were to propose a clinical trial of self-forgiveness therapy, they would probably find that UC for breast cancer at their medical center does not include formal self-forgiveness therapy. If they were to dig a little deeper, however, they might find that the center's pastoral care or support groups encourage self-forgiveness. Even if the medical center were bereft of self-forgiveness services, the participants would still be receiving interventions (e.g., visits with their physician or social worker) that could influence some of the outcomes of the self-forgiveness trial, such as quality of life. Thus, even if the experimental intervention is only available to trial participants, UC is still non-ignorable.

3 Design Issues in Behavioral Medicine Research

3.1 Efficacy and Effectiveness Trials

In addition to obliterating the standard hierarchy of control conditions, the presence of UC blurs the distinction between efficacy and effectiveness. In principle, the efficacy of an intervention should be tested under tightly controlled conditions, and its generalizability and effectiveness should subsequently be tested in the "real world" of clinical practice. However, when efficacy studies are conducted in clinical settings, the presence of UC constrains the investigator's control over the conditions to which the participants are exposed (Kazdin, 2003a). Also, many behavioral medicine RCTs are designed to adapt or extend to medically ill patients, interventions that have already proven to be efficacious in medically well subjects. Consequently, many of our "efficacy" trials are actually efficacy–effectiveness hybrids.

In effectiveness trials, interventions with known efficacy are tested as replacements for current practices or as ways to augment them. The control arm is either UC or EUC. The basic replacement effectiveness design compares a translational intervention to UC or EUC. The basic augmentation effectiveness design is similar except that the new intervention is added to existing practice: UC or EUC + translational intervention vs. UC or EUC alone.

Some efficacy trials in behavioral medicine are analogous to augmentation effectiveness studies, except that the efficacy of the intervention has not yet been established, at least not in the setting of interest or for the population of interest. They compare UC or EUC + an experimental intervention to UC or EUC alone. For example, we recently compared two experimental interventions for depression in patients with a recent history of coronary artery bypass graft (CABG) surgery to UC (Freedland et al, 2009). For simplicity, the present discussion focuses on just one of the interventions, cognitive behavior therapy (CBT). We chose CBT because it had well-established efficacy for depression in psychiatric patients and could be adapted to address the needs and problems of post-CABG patients, but its efficacy had not yet been established in this population. We compared CBT to EUC for depression which, in this patient population, sometimes includes antidepressants but rarely includes psychotherapy. About half of

the participants were already taking an antidepressant but were still depressed at enrollment in the trial. They were permitted to continue their antidepressants regardless of group assignment. Consequently, about half of the patients in the experimental arm received a combination of CBT plus non-study antidepressants, and the other half received only CBT for depression. Similarly, half of the control group received non-study antidepressants, and the other half received no treatment for depression at all. The participants and their physicians were informed of the patient's depression status at baseline. Thus, this trial provides an example of minimally enhanced usual care and the following design: EUC + CBT vs. EUC alone.

Criticism of the UC or EUC control condition is common in this type of trial, particularly by reviewers who are uncomfortable with departures from more familiar efficacy designs. A frequent concern is that this design does not control for attention or placebo effects. It is true that the participants in the EUC arm are unlikely to receive as much clinical attention as their intervention arm counterparts, since CBT provides ample clinical attention. However, researchers may disagree about whether it is necessary or even desirable to control for attention in this type of study. Because the presence of UC in the background of a trial generally precludes pure placebo or attention controls, controlling for attention implies this design: EUC + attention vs. EUC + attention + other ingredients of CBT. A serious drawback of this design is that it is uninformative as to whether CBT yields better depression outcomes than UC alone after CABG surgery. That may seem like an effectiveness rather than an efficacy question, but as discussed above, the presence of UC blurs the distinction between efficacy and effectiveness. Unless CBT is first shown to be superior to UC for depression in this patient population, there is little reason for researchers, clinicians, patients, administrators, or policymakers to care whether its apparent effects are due to attention rather than to the other ingredients of CBT.

One way to overcome this limitation would be to add an EUC-only group to the design. This three-arm trial would require a larger sample and it would cost more than a two-arm trial. Would it be worth the additional expense? That depends on how important it is to determine the extent to which clinical attention explains the effects of CBT and that is not a simple question. Unlike the standard threats to internal validity (e.g., history, maturation, or regression to the mean), attention is not a rival explanation for the effects of CBT. Attention is an integral *part* of CBT, so the attention control design is analogous to the treatment component design, and its principal function is comparison rather than control. In other words, this design does not truly "control" for attention, since attention is not a threat to internal validity; instead it permits a comparison of the full intervention (CBT) to one of its key ingredients (clinical attention).

However, clinical attention cannot be extracted from the therapy in which it is embedded and delivered in a pure, active ingredient-free form. Attention group therapists cannot simply sit and stare at their patients for the same number of hours that the experimental group therapists interact with theirs. They have to provide some sort of intervention in order to have a vehicle within which to deliver clinical attention. Furthermore, CBT provides a distinctive form of clinical attention known as a collaborative therapeutic relationship, in which the patient and therapist collaborate on cognitive-behavioral treatment goals and strategies (Beck, 1995). This special relationship cannot be extracted from CBT without changing it. At best, an attention condition might approximate CBT's collaborative relationship, but there would still have to be some sort of non-CBT therapeutic content for the collaboration to form around.

Assuming that a credible UC or EUC + attention condition can be implemented, what is gained from comparing it to the full intervention? In basic psychotherapy research, it is important to determine whether the particular form of therapy under investigation provides benefits above and beyond clinical attention. In applied behavioral medicine research, determining whether particular therapies have specific

active ingredients is usually less important than ascertaining whether the therapies are beneficial. Nonspecific therapies, the kind of interventions that may be used as attention control conditions for established interventions such as CBT, may require less training and experience, may be less expensive to deliver, and may or may not be as efficacious as the experimental intervention. These are important but secondary questions. The more pressing goal for behavioral medicine RCTs is to develop highly efficacious interventions for clinically significant problems.

However, the behavioral medicine research community is increasingly aware of the need for behavioral and psychosocial interventions that are not only highly efficacious but effective and practical to implement in clinical practice (Glasgow and Emmons, 2007). Practical clinical trials (Glasgow et al, 2006; Tunis et al, 2003) are expected to play an increasingly important role in testing interventions in clinical practice settings. In some instances, two or more evidence-based interventions for a given problem may already be available to practitioners, but whether, for whom, and under which circumstances one intervention is superior to another, is unknown. A comparative effectiveness trial can address such questions. In other instances, practical clinical trials are needed for further evaluation of innovative behavioral interventions that have been found to be superior to other therapies, medications, and/or control conditions in tightly controlled efficacy studies. In these cases, the new intervention should be compared with the current standard of care, if one exists. If there is no evidence-based standard of care, or if current clinical practices in the settings of interest do not adhere to whatever evidence-based guidelines may be available, then comparison to some form of usual care would be appropriate (Glasgow et al, 2006).

3.2 Factorial Designs in Efficacy Research

Factorial trial designs are uncommon in most areas of medical research, including behavioral medicine, but they can be very useful. The Canadian Cardiac Randomized Evaluation of Antidepressant and Psychotherapy Efficacy (CREATE) trial (Frasure-Smith et al, 2006; Lesperance et al, 2007) is a good example. Patients with stable coronary disease and major depression were randomly assigned to either clinical management (CM) or interpersonal psychotherapy (IPT) + CM. Within each group, the participants were then randomized to citalopram or to a pill placebo. This yielded four groups: IPT + CM + pill placebo, IPT + CM + citalopram, CM + pill placebo, and CM + citalopram, and it permitted independent comparisons of citalopram vs. placebo and IPT vs. CM. Because the participants were medical patients, UC was present in the background of all four groups; this will be ignored here, for simplicity.

The key advantage of this design is that it requires fewer subjects to test the two hypotheses (i.e., drug vs. placebo and IPT vs. CM) than if two separate trials were conducted instead. A critical assumption is that there is no interaction between the two interventions (Frasure-Smith et al, 2006; Friedman et al, 1998). If there is an interaction, the effects of each intervention depend upon whether the other is co-administered. This is more likely to occur when the two interventions have similar mechanisms of action than when they operate through different pathways. Consequently, it is an appropriate design for simultaneously testing the efficacy of a drug and a behavioral or psychotherapeutic intervention. It might not be a good design for simultaneously testing two similar drugs or two forms of psychotherapy.

A factorial design can also be used to test interaction hypotheses (Piantadosi, 2005). For example, a trial might be designed to determine whether the combination of a drug plus a behavioral intervention produces greater weight loss in obese subjects than either the drug or the behavioral intervention alone. The control group receives neither treatment, but like all of the other participants, they may, depending on the setting and population, receive some form of UC. Double randomization is not required for this type of study. Instead, the participants would be randomly assigned just once, to the drug alone, to the behavioral intervention alone, to combination therapy, or to neither treatment. A larger sample is required for this type of trial than for the double-randomization factorial RCT design discussed above (Friedman et al, 1998).

3.3 Safety Trials

The ultimate goals of medical care are to save lives, prevent or decrease disability, and maintain or improve quality of life. Unfortunately, many medical and surgical therapies have been found to increase the risk of death or disability, or to diminish quality of life, despite being efficacious for a target condition of some sort. The Cardiac Arrhythmia Suppression Trial (CAST) is a classic example. CAST showed that certain medications decrease cardiac arrhythmias but do so at the expense of increasing the risk of mortality (CAST Investigators, 1989). Such findings have generated widespread skepticism about claims of treatment efficacy that are based on improvements in surrogate end points such as arrhythmias without concomitant evidence of improved functioning, survival, or quality of life (Fleming and DeMets, 1996).

In behavioral medicine, many trials target outcomes that could be considered surrogate end points, and do so without being designed or powered to evaluate survival or other ultimate end points. There are often good reasons for this. Depression, for example, is a risk factor for morbidity and mortality in patients with heart disease, but it is also a disorder in its own right. In the post-CABG depression trial discussed earlier, the goal was to test the efficacy of an intervention for depression in a patient population that had been excluded from almost every other depression trial ever conducted. It is possible, but unlikely, that exposure to CBT during the year after CABG surgery increases the risk of mortality. To determine whether it indeed poses this risk would have required a much larger trial. Conducting a large, expensive trial simply to confirm that CBT is not lethal would have been hard to justify. It is essential to monitor serious adverse events (SAEs) in any RCT, but few medical or behavioral trials are adequately powered to analyze group differences in SAEs (Tsang et al, 2009).

Safety is a more serious consideration when antidepressants are used to treat depression in patients who also have heart disease or other serious medical conditions. The sertraline antidepressant heart attack randomized trial (SADHART) evaluated the safety and efficacy of sertraline for major depression in patients with a recent acute myocardial infarction (MI). Left ventricular ejection fraction (LVEF) was the primary indicator of the drug's safety, and other cardiac variables (e.g., angina) were secondary indicators. The trial was not adequately powered to study mortality, but deaths were analyzed in an exploratory analysis.

SADHART was a double-blind, placebo-controlled trial. All of the participants received UC for heart disease and other medical problems, but they were not permitted to take non-study antidepressants while participating in the trial. In this sense, something was subtracted from the participants' usual care, and replaced with either sertraline or a pill placebo. So, instead of receiving *enhanced* UC for depression, they received *restricted* usual care (RUC). In this type of design, it may be necessary to enhance some aspects of UC while restricting others. The SADHART team notified the participant's cardiologist if significant cardiac abnormalities were found. Thus, although SADHART is usually described simply as a placebo-controlled trial, a complete description of the design compares EUC for heart disease, etc., + RUC for depression + sertraline to EUC for heart disease, etc., + RUC for depression + pill placebo.

3.4 Mediation Trials

Successful mediation trials are the "holy grail" in many areas of behavioral medicine research.

They are designed to show that medical outcomes can be improved by treating behavioral problems. They are pragmatic trials in that they aim to yield new approaches to preventing or treating medical conditions, but they are also explanatory studies in that they are designed to determine whether the behavioral problem is a causal risk factor rather than a non-causal risk marker. They are referred to herein as mediation trials, because they target putative mediators of medical outcomes, rather than the medical outcomes themselves.

For example, considerable evidence has accumulated that both depression and low perceived social support (LPSS) increase the risk of morbidity and mortality after acute MI. It is not known, however, whether these variables are causal risk factors or whether modifying them can reduce the incidence of recurrent infarction and death. The enhancing recovery in coronary heart disease (ENRICHD) clinical trial was designed to address these questions. Patients with a recent MI plus depression and/or LPSS were randomly assigned to an intervention that included CBT and, in some cases, sertraline, or to minimally enhanced UC for depression. The intervention had modest effects on depression and LPSS, but no effect on the combined primary end point of reinfarction-free survival (Berkman et al, 2003). The findings provided a reasonably clear answer to the pragmatic question of whether post-MI depression and LPSS are treatable: they are, but the best available treatments have relatively weak effects on these problems. They yielded an ambiguous answer to the pragmatic question of whether post-MI medical outcomes can be improved by treating depression and LPSS. The medical outcomes did not differ between the groups, but they might have differed if the intervention had stronger effects on depression and LPSS. The findings also left open the explanatory issue of whether depression and LPSS are causal risk factors: they may be, but ENRICHD neither proved nor disproved this.

ENRICHD illustrates some of the challenges involved in conducting behavioral mediation trials. The intervention targeted two behavioral risk markers which, assuming that they are even part of a causal process that leads to reinfarction or cardiac death after an MI, are distal mediators. The processes that are involved in blood clot formation are, in contrast, proximal mediators of recurrent infarction. All else being equal, it would be much easier to demonstrate that aspirin and clopidogrel prevent reinfarction, because they target proximal mediators. Establishing that a behavioral problem predicts adverse medical outcomes is a precondition for conducting a trial such as ENRICHD. The trial tests the mediation hypothesis by demonstrating that (1) the intervention improves medical outcomes, (2) it improves the behavioral risk factor, and (3) the improvement in medical outcomes is due, at least partially, to improvement in the behavioral risk factor. Whether the hypothesis will be supported depends on (1) the strength of the association between the behavioral risk factor and the medical outcome, (2) the efficacy of the intervention in relation to the behavioral risk factor, and (3) whether the intervention affects the medical outcome via other pathways. The strength of the association between the risk factor and the medical outcome is not something that the investigator can control, but it is an important consideration in deciding whether the trial should be conducted in the first place. If the intervention is not very efficacious for the behavioral risk factor, then there is little hope that it will affect the medical outcome even if the risk factor is a strong determinant of it. This was problematic in ENRICHD; the differences in depression and social support between the intervention and EUC groups were too small to affect the medical outcomes. If the intervention operates through multiple pathways, then it may be challenging to demonstrate behavioral mediation even if the medical outcomes improve. For example, sertraline is an antidepressant but it also interferes with blood clotting by binding with platelet receptors. If sertraline helps to prevent MIs (a potential benefit which has not yet been proven), it might do so by improving depression, inhibiting platelet activation, or both.

These issues make it difficult to demonstrate that behavioral interventions can improve medical outcomes and even more difficult to test

causal hypotheses. It is often said that unlike observational studies, clinical trials are experiments and therefore provide stronger tests of causal hypotheses about risk factors (Elwood, 2007). They are indeed experiments, but they are less tightly controlled than most laboratory experiments. Also unlike laboratory research, the experimental manipulation in a behavioral trial does not necessarily produce distinct groups. In SADHART, for example, depression was neither totally abolished in the sertraline arm nor uniformly persistent in the placebo arm. No known treatment is efficacious enough to turn a depressed sample into a 100% fully remitted sample, and the placebo effect and spontaneous improvement conspire to ensure that some control subjects will partially or fully remit. In general, mediation trials should only be conducted if highly efficacious treatments for the behavioral risk factor exist. However, many behavioral problems are difficult to treat. Treatment development and efficacy studies are needed to pave the way for multicenter mediation trials.

In any RCT, the efficacy of an experimental intervention is judged in relation to the control condition. The effect size has as much to do with the control condition as it does with the experimental treatment (Mohr et al, 2009). For example, antidepressant medications are more efficacious in relation to no-treatment controls than to pill placebos. This is especially important in mediation trials, which require highly efficacious treatments for behavioral targets in order to affect medical outcomes and to provide strong tests of the mediation hypotheses.

For clinical problems like depression in medical patients, no-treatment control groups are not an option because of the presence of UC. Among the designs that are feasible in this circumstance, UC or minimally enhanced UC control designs are the most powerful. To employ a UC + attention control instead of UC or EUC could defeat the purpose of a mediation trial. If sufficient resources are available, it might be possible to add a third arm in order to "control" for attention, but doing so might not serve the primary aims of the trial. It could serve a secondary aim, but whether this is a wise use of limited resources in an explanatory mediation trial should be questioned. It might be better to wait until more pragmatic questions come to the fore; in other words, after it has been shown that treating the behavioral risk factor can improve medical outcomes. Once this has been accomplished, it is then time to address such questions as whether the risk factor can be treated more rapidly, less expensively, and in a broader range of settings.

On the other hand, if an applicable intervention has a powerful effect on a behavioral risk factor that is known to have a strong relationship with a medical outcome, it may be preferable to move directly to a more stringent mediation trial design. The Diabetes Prevention Program (DPP; Knowler et al, 2002) is an example. The DPP randomly assigned individuals at risk for Type 2 diabetes to an intensive lifestyle intervention, metformin, or placebo. The lifestyle intervention was designed to reduce obesity and increase physical activity. UC was enhanced by a brief lifestyle education intervention and by assisting the patients' non-study health-care providers in following treatment guidelines for concomitant conditions such as hypertension. UC was also restricted in that treatments that could have affected study outcomes were discouraged if alternate treatments were available. The intensive lifestyle group lost more weight and engaged in more physical activity than the other groups. The incidence of diabetes was reduced by 58% in the lifestyle group and by 31% in the metformin group, as compared with the placebo group. The lifestyle intervention was also more efficacious than metformin. Thus, the DPP showed that the intensive lifestyle intervention is an efficacious treatment for obesity and physical inactivity in individuals at risk for Type 2 diabetes, and that it also helps to prevent the onset of diabetes in this population. It did so even though stringent control conditions were employed.

3.5 Statistical Power and Trial Design

As noted previously, the effect size of an intervention depends not only on the intervention itself but also on the condition to which it is compared (Mohr et al, 2009). A corollary of this fact is that trial design also affects statistical power. For example, if an RCT is designed to test the efficacy of an intervention in which positive outcome expectations are likely to be associated with better outcomes (as is the case with many psychosocial interventions), then for any given sample size, the statistical power of the primary hypothesis test will be lower if the RCT includes a placebo control group than if the control group receives no treatment.

Comparative efficacy and effectiveness trials tend to require relatively large samples because they are usually designed to compare two active interventions to one another. In some trials, however, two different active interventions are compared to a control condition such as a placebo or usual care. In the DPP trial, both of the active treatments reduced the incidence of diabetes, in comparison to the placebo. Furthermore, the trial was large enough to compare the two active interventions to one another, and the results showed that the lifestyle intervention was superior to metformin (Knowler et al, 2002).

Smaller trials with similar designs may have sufficient power to compare both active interventions to the control condition, but not to compare the active treatments to each other. This was the case, for example, in our recent trial of treatments for depression in patients with a recent history of CABG surgery. There was adequate power to compare the cognitive-behavioral and stress management interventions to the EUC control condition, but not enough to compare the interventions to each other (Freedland et al, 2009).

In such a trial, even if Treatment A has a bigger effect than Treatment B vis-à-vis the control condition, it is not clear whether Treatment A is superior to Treatment B. Consequently, there will be some uncertainty about the clinical implications of the results. It could be argued that Treatment A is the more efficacious intervention, yet one cannot say with certainty that Treatment A is more efficacious than Treatment B. Thus, whenever possible, these sorts of trials should be powered to support comparisons among all of the groups, not just between the active intervention and control arms.

3.6 Falsification Research

The philosopher of science Karl Popper argued that a hypothesis is scientific only if it is falsifiable (Popper, 1972). Much of the research that is conducted in our field is designed to determine whether behavioral variables are risk factors for adverse medical outcomes. Much less research aims to falsify these hypotheses. For example, there is a strong association between depression and Type 2 diabetes (Anderson et al, 2001). This raises the question of whether treatment of depression can prevent diabetes. If so, that would lend support to the hypothesis that depression is a causal risk factor for diabetes. It is also possible that diabetes and depression are associated because diabetes causes depression. An RCT targeting glycemic control in diabetes, with depression as the primary outcome, would test this hypothesis. However, reciprocal causality is also possible. Consequently, even if diabetes treatment were shown to decrease depression, this would not literally falsify the hypothesis that depression causes diabetes. Nevertheless, if diabetes treatment was shown to prevent or improve depression, but depression treatment could not be shown to prevent or improve diabetes, then the "depression causes diabetes" hypothesis would essentially have been falsified. It would be almost impossible to design a clinical trial that could completely falsify any of behavioral medicine's major hypotheses in one fell swoop. Falsification can emerge from a line of research, but it is unlikely to result from a single trial.

3.7 Mechanistic Research

Long after behavioral variables such as mental stress, anger, or anxiety have been established as risk factors for a disease or an adverse medical outcome, questions tend to remain about the underlying mechanism(s). Observational studies and laboratory experiments comprise most of the mechanistic studies in behavioral medicine, but clinical trials also provide opportunities to test mechanistic hypotheses. If a candidate mechanism has been associated in cross-sectional research both with a behavioral risk factor and with an adverse medical outcome that the risk factor predicts, one of the next questions to ask is whether change in the risk factor is associated with change in the candidate mechanism. This can be accomplished by correlating the change scores derived from an observational study, but not if the risk factor tends to remain stable. By intervening in the risk factor, an investigator can induce change, or promote more rapid change than would otherwise occur, and thereby create the variability needed to correlate the risk factor and candidate mechanism change scores.

This strategy utilizes an intervention to perturb a behavioral risk factor. The purpose of the study is not to test the efficacy of the intervention, but rather to use an intervention with established efficacy to manipulate the risk factor. There is no need to control for threats to any conclusions that might be drawn about the efficacy of the treatment, so an uncontrolled, "open label" trial is a satisfactory way to test this type of hypothesis. Including a control group would waste resources and needlessly expose additional subjects to experimentation. For example, Carney et al (2000) used CBT to treat a group of patients with stable coronary disease and comorbid depression in an uncontrolled trial. The aim was to induce change in depression, in order to correlate it with change in various indicators of cardiovascular autonomic dysregulation, including heart rate and heart rate variability. CBT was chosen because it was an efficacious, nonpharmacological treatment for depression. It was considered to be less likely than antidepressant medications to have direct, physiological effects on the cardiovascular variables of interest, i.e., effects that are not mediated by change in depression.

Since CBT and antidepressants improve depression via different pathways, it might have been informative to conduct a randomized comparison of CBT vs. an antidepressant. The primary aim would still have been to correlate change in depression with change in cardiovascular variables, but this design would make it possible to determine whether the type of treatment explained any of the variance in the cardiovascular change scores. This might have provided some new insights into the cardiovascular effects of antidepressants, but it would not have provided better data than the uncontrolled trial with regard to whether cardiovascular autonomic dysregulation is a plausible mechanism linking depression to cardiac events. It would also have been more expensive and expose more subjects to experimentation. Here again, a trial design may seem appear at first glance to be rigorous by familiar methodological standards, yet not serve the purpose of the study as well as a seemingly less rigorous design.

Mechanistic questions can also be investigated as ancillary studies within standard efficacy RCTs. These trials need control groups, unlike in the kinds of studies discussed above. The controls are justified by the primary (efficacy) aims of the trial, not by the mechanistic aims. If the control group data are useful for ancillary mechanistic studies, all the better, but that is not why the control groups are included in these studies.

Although there are not many examples in the behavioral medicine literature to draw upon, RCTs can also be used to falsify mechanistic hypotheses. For example, depression is known to increase the risk of Type 2 diabetes, but the mechanisms underlying this risk have not been firmly established. Glucose dysregulation is one of the leading candidates. However, it is also possible that glucose dysregulation causes depression. If the causal arrow runs in this direction, then glucose dysregulation may be a "third variable" cause of both depression and diabetes. One way to study this question would be to randomly assign a sample of depressed, pre-diabetic individuals to treatment with either a metformin or a selective serotonin reuptake inhibitor. If the antidepressant failed to improve glucose control despite improving depression, and if the metformin improved depression by

improving glucose control, this would help to falsify the hypothesis that depression causes diabetes by causing glucose dysregulation. This would be a two-arm comparison of two active treatments, with no placebo control arm. A placebo could have mild effects on both depression and on glycemic control, so the inclusion of a placebo control arm would probably not be very informative.

4 Summary

Clinical trial designs that are suitable for a given purpose, population, or setting may not be suitable for others. The design of a trial should match its purpose, even if this means challenging some common assumptions about what a rigorous trial should look like. For example, a trial whose primary purpose is to test a mechanistic hypothesis should not necessarily resemble a treatment efficacy trial.

Many behavioral medicine researchers conduct their trials in medical care settings and enroll participants who either already have or are at risk for developing medical illnesses. The pervasive influence of usual care in these settings is a salient consideration for trial designers. It is especially important to take usual care into account when choosing control groups.

Careful consideration of these issues could help to resolve many of the controversies that surround the design of clinical trials in behavioral medicine, including disagreements about control conditions. Greater agreement about trial design issues among all interested parties (including investigators, grant reviewers, and institutional review boards) would help to foster the growth of clinical trials in behavioral medicine.

References

Anderson, R. J., Freedland, K. E., Clouse, R. E., and Lustman, P. J. (2001). The prevalence of comorbid depression in adults with diabetes: a meta-analysis. *Diabetes Care, 24*, 1069–1078.

Beck, J. S. (1995). *Cognitive Therapy: Basics and Beyond*. New York: Guilford.

Berkman, L. F., Blumenthal, J., Burg, M., Carney, R. M., Catellier, D. et al (2003). Effects of treating depression and low perceived social support on clinical events after myocardial infarction: the Enhancing Recovery in Coronary Heart Disease Patients (ENRICHD) Randomized Trial. *JAMA, 289*, 3106–3116.

Burns, T. (2009). End of the road for treatment-as-usual studies? *Br J Psychiatry, 195*, 5–6.

Campbell, D. T., and Stanley, J. C. (1966). *Experimental and Quasi-experimental Designs for Research*. Chicago: R. McNally.

Carney, R. M., Freedland, K. E., Stein, P. K., Skala, J. A., Hoffman, P. et al (2000). Change in heart rate and heart rate variability during treatment for depression in patients with coronary heart disease. *Psychosom Med, 62*, 639–647.

CAST Investigators (1989). Preliminary report: effect of encainide and flecainide on mortality in a randomized trial of arrhythmia suppression after myocardial infarction. The Cardiac Arrhythmia Suppression Trial (CAST) Investigators. *New Engl J Med, 321*, 406–412.

Elwood, J. M. (2007). *Critical Appraisal of Epidemiological Studies and Clinical Trials, 3rd Ed*. Oxford: Oxford University Press.

Fleming, T. R., and DeMets, D. L. (1996). Surrogate end points in clinical trials: are we being misled? *Ann Intern Med, 125*, 605–613.

Frasure-Smith, N., Koszycki, D., Swenson, J. R., Baker, B., van Zyl, L. T. et al (2006). Design and rationale for a randomized, controlled trial of interpersonal psychotherapy and citalopram for depression in coronary artery disease (CREATE). *Psychosom Med, 68*, 87–93.

Freedland, K. E., Skala, J. A., Carney, R. M., Rubin, E. H., Lustman, P. J. et al (2009). Treatment of depression after coronary bypass surgery: a randomized, controlled trial. *Arch Gen Psychiatry, 66*(4), 387–396.

Friedman, L. M., Furberg, C., and DeMets, D. L. (1998). *Fundamentals of Clinical Trials, 3rd Ed*. New York: Springer.

Glasgow, R. E., Davidson, K. W., Dobkin, P. L., Ockene, J., and Spring, B. (2006). Practical behavioral trials to advance evidence-based behavioral medicine. *Ann Behav Med, 31*, 5–13.

Glasgow, R. E., and Emmons, K. M. (2007). How can we increase translation of research into practice? Types of evidence needed. *Ann Rev Public Health, 28*, 413–433.

Kazdin, A. E. (2003a). *Methodological Issues and Strategies in Clinical Research, 3rd Ed*. Washington, DC: American Psychological Association.

Kazdin, A. E. (2003b). *Research Design in Clinical Psychology, 4th Ed*. Boston: Allyn and Bacon.

Knowler, W. C., Barrett-Connor, E., Fowler, S. E., Hamman, R. F., Lachin, J. M. et al (2002). Reduction in the incidence of type 2 diabetes with lifestyle intervention or metformin. *New Engl J Med, 346*, 393–403.

Lesperance, F., Frasure-Smith, N., Koszycki, D., Laliberte, M. A., van Zyl, L. T. et al (2007). Effects of citalopram and interpersonal psychotherapy on depression in patients with coronary artery disease: the Canadian Cardiac Randomized Evaluation of Antidepressant and Psychotherapy Efficacy (CREATE) trial. *JAMA, 297*, 367–379.

Minneci, P. C., Eichacker, P. Q., Danner, R. L., Banks, S. M., Natanson, C. et al (2008). The importance of usual care control groups for safety monitoring and validity during critical care research. *Int Care Med, 34*, 942–947.

Mohr, D. C., Spring, B., Freedland, K. E., Beckner, V., Arean, P. et al (2009). The selection and design of control conditions for randomized controlled trials of psychological interventions. *Psychother Psychosom, 78*, 275–284.

Piantadosi, S. (2005). *Clinical Trials: A Methodologic Perspective, 2nd Ed*. Hoboken, NJ: Wiley-Interscience.

Popper, K. R. (1972). *The Logic of Scientific Discovery, 6th impression revised Ed*. London: Hutchinson.

Romero, C., Friedman, L. C., Kalidas, M., Elledge, R., Chang, J. et al (2006). Self-forgiveness, spirituality, and psychological adjustment in women with breast cancer. *J Behav Med, 29*, 29–36.

Schmittdiel, J. A., Uratsu, C. S., Karter, A. J., Heisler, M., Subramanian, U. et al (2008). Why don't diabetes patients achieve recommended risk factor targets? Poor adherence versus lack of treatment intensification. *J Gen Intern Med, 23*, 588–594.

Selby, J. V., Uratsu, C. S., Fireman, B., Schmittdiel, J. A., Peng, T. et al (2009). Treatment intensification and risk factor control: toward more clinically relevant quality measures. *Med Care, 47*, 395–402.

Street, L. L. and Luoma, J. B. (2002). Control groups in psychosocial intervention research: ethical and methodological issues. *Ethics Behav, 12*, 1–30.

Thompson, B. T., and Schoenfeld, D. (2007). Usual care as the control group in clinical trials of nonpharmacologic interventions. *Proc Am Thorac Soc, 4*, 577–582.

Tsang, R., Colley, L., and Lynd, L. D. (2009). Inadequate statistical power to detect clinically significant differences in adverse event rates in randomized controlled trials. *J Clin Epidemiol, 62*, 609–616.

Tunis, S. R., Stryer, D. B., and Clancy, C. M. (2003). Practical clinical trials: increasing the value of clinical research for decision making in clinical and health policy. *JAMA, 290*, 1624–1632.

Werner, R. M., Goldman, L. E., and Dudley, R. A. (2008). Comparison of change in quality of care between safety-net and non-safety-net hospitals. *JAMA, 299*, 2180–2187.

Wolfe, D. A., Wekerle, C., Scott, K., Straatman, A. L., Grasley, C. et al (2003). Dating violence prevention with at-risk youth: a controlled outcome evaluation. *J Consult Clin Psychol, 71*, 279–291.

Chapter 60

Methodological Issues in Randomized Controlled Trials for the Treatment of Psychiatric Comorbidity in Medical Illness

David C. Mohr, Sarah W. Kinsinger, and Jenna Duffecy

1 Why Do We Need RCTs for Treatments for Psychiatric Disorders in Medical Patients?

An enormous literature has validated the use of a variety of psychological and behavioral treatments for many common psychiatric disorders, including the mood and anxiety disorders (Cuijpers et al, 2008) that commonly afflict people with medical illnesses. Presumably many of these trials enroll participants who are reasonably representative of the general public, which includes many people with many medical illnesses. So why do we need randomized controlled trials (RCTs) of psychological and behavioral treatments for psychiatric disorders in patients with medical illness? Why not accept the findings of RCTs conducted in the general public?

There are at least three broad answers to that question: First, RCTs of psychological and behavioral treatments are needed when there are questions of whether a validated treatment generalizes from one population to another. Second, treatments are sometimes altered to meet the specific needs of a patient population. For example, treatments may include components to manage symptoms of the medical illness, such as pain or fatigue, or may be delivered differently to accommodate disabilities. These alterations may change the efficacy of the treatment. Finally, we will propose that trials are needed in part because our ability to accurately diagnose psychiatric disorders is diminished by medical illness. We will argue that when outcomes in RCTs of validated psychological and behavioral treatments are substantially smaller in medical populations than in non-medical populations, the problem may lie in our ability to accurately identify the psychiatric disorder in that population, rather than in the intervention. We will discuss the implications of this for RCT design.

2 The Influences of Medical Illness on Psychological Functioning

2.1 Occurrence of Psychiatric Disorders in Medical Populations

The literature on the relationship between medical illness and psychiatric disorders is mixed. By far the largest literature on comorbid psychiatric problems and medical illness has focused on depressive symptoms and disorders. Chronic medical conditions have generally been associated with increased prevalence of depression and anxiety (Scott et al, 2007). Rates of depression have been shown to be higher among patients with coronary artery disease, particularly following myocardial infarction and stroke (Connerney et al, 2001; Hackett et al, 2005), chronic obstructive pulmonary disease (COPD)

D.C. Mohr (✉)
Department of Preventive Medicine, Northwestern University, Feinberg School of Medicine, 680 N. Lakeshore Drive, Suite 1220, Chicago, IL 60611, USA
e-mail: d-mohr@northwestern.edu

A. Steptoe (ed.), *Handbook of Behavioral Medicine*, DOI 10.1007/978-0-387-09488-5_60,
© Springer Science+Business Media, LLC 2010

(Yohannes et al, 2000), autoimmune diseases such as multiple sclerosis (Patten et al, 2003) and inflammatory bowel disease (IBD) (Graff et al, 2009), rheumatoid arthritis (Dickens et al, 2002), hepatitis C (Carta et al, 2007), and sickle cell disease (Levenson et al, 2008), just to name a few.

However, not all medical conditions are consistently associated with increased psychiatric distress. For example, while depression and anxiety are high among patients with traumatic conditions such as limb amputations or spinal cord injuries up to 2 years post-amputation, these rates fall to general population levels once the condition stabilizes (Horgan and MacLachlan, 2004). Among illnesses that are not necessarily stable, the prevalence of psychiatric disorders may vary with the amount of disease activity. For example, patients whose epilepsy is uncontrolled are at greater risk for depression, while prevalence among patients with controlled epilepsy is similar to the general population (Kanner, 2003). However, even when the prevalence of diagnosable psychiatric disorders is not elevated, this does not mean that there is no distress. For example, among diabetes patients, rates of diagnosable depression have been shown to be similar to the general population, however, subthreshold depressive symptoms remain elevated (Fisher et al, 2007).

These patterns of variable relationships between psychiatric illness, severity of psychiatric symptoms, and medical illness are also seen within disease groups. There are fairly consistent findings that rates of depression are higher among cancer patients generally. However, rates are particularly high among some cancer populations (oropharyngeal, pancreatic, breast, lung) and lower in others (colon, gynecological, lymphoma) (Massie, 2004). Psychiatric disorders are also more prevalent in the first year or two after diagnosis, but become equivalent to the general population thereafter (Stanton, 2006). Although rates of diagnosable psychiatric problems decline, patients may nevertheless continue to experience adjustment difficulties. There is a substantial literature indicating that many cancer patients experience long-term psychosocial difficulties, including impaired quality of life and disease-specific concerns (e.g., fears of recurrence, body image concerns, sexual dysfunction) (Stanton, 2006).

The increased rates of psychiatric disorders among medical populations may be attributable to either psychosocial or biological factors. Arguments for the role of psychosocial factors in producing psychiatric symptoms generally fit into a diathesis-stress model (Banks and Kerns, 1996), in which stress triggers a psychiatric disorder among a subset of the population with a specific illness who also carry specific genetic, biological, psychological, or social vulnerabilities. Perceived threats or losses in health, well-being, and social functioning coupled with the belief that these threats or losses cannot be effectively managed or controlled can increase risk of psychological distress in vulnerable individuals. The decline in prevalence of psychiatric disorders following initial adjustment to a medical problem may be related to patients' capacities to adjust to adverse events and circumstances such as disability or threat of recurrence (Burgess et al, 2005; Horgan and MacLachlan, 2004; Kanner, 2003). On the other hand, other disease-related symptoms, most notably pain, are more difficult to adjust to and may constitute an ongoing stressor that triggers increased psychological distress (Banks and Kerns, 1996).

Psychiatric symptoms may also be directly related to the disease processes. This can occur in at least two ways. Increased psychiatric symptoms can result from anatomical pathology related to the medical disorder. For example, illnesses that result in the destruction of brain tissue, such as cerebrovascular disease or multiple sclerosis, can produce lesions in regions of the brain that regulate emotion and behavior, resulting in increased risk of psychological and behavioral symptoms (Fang and Cheng, 2009; Feinstein et al, 2004). To the degree that the anatomical pathology is chronic, the vulnerability to psychological and behavioral symptoms may also be permanent. Alternatively, disease processes or the pathogenesis of medical illness may produce psychiatric symptoms. For example, inflammation-associated injury, such as spinal cord injury, can produce psychological and behavioral symptoms of depression and anxiety that subside as inflammation decreases (Riegger et al, 2009). Alternatively, inflammatory diseases such as multiple sclerosis (MS) and IBD are characterized by periodic increases in inflammation that may result in symptoms of depression and anxiety (Gold and Irwin, 2006; Rosenkranz, 2007). Likewise, neuroendocrine dysregulation associated with medical diseases such as cardiovascular disease could produce depressive symptoms (Joynt et al, 2003). In many cases these pathogenic causes may exert episodic and time-limited influences on psychiatric symptoms.

Admittedly, the conceptual distinctions between psychosocial and biological or between anatomical pathology and pathogenesis may be somewhat blurred in reality. That is, inflammation may also increase pain, which in turn may contribute to psychological distress. Damage to central nervous system tissue may produce both permanent damage and inflammation that varies over time. Also, as noted in Chapters 44 and 45, psychiatric symptoms can cause changes in neuroendocrine and immune function. Despite the overlapping and recursive nature of these relationships, it is useful to consider these sources independently when considering the effects of medical illness on RCTs for psychiatric disorders.

2.2 Identifying Psychiatric Disorders in Medical Populations

A critical component of an RCT is selecting a sample of patients with the disorder or problem that the intervention is intended to treat. A sample that is well defined with respect to the target problem will support a good test of the experimental treatment. A sample that is poorly defined, containing misdiagnoses or false positives, is less likely to provide an accurate test of the intervention. Much of medicine has improved diagnostic validity and reliability through the use of laboratory tests, imaging, and other technologies. In contrast, psychiatric diagnosis continues to rely on clusters of symptoms that are often relatively non-specific and

which, even among patients without medical illness, produce groups that are likely heterogeneous in terms of the underlying etiology of the symptoms used in diagnosis. This heterogeneity can decrease power in RCTs, since those who are false positives may be less likely to respond to the treatments (Cipriani et al, 2009). The degree to which medical illness creates symptoms that mimic, but are unrelated to psychiatric disorders, the problem of heterogeneity is only aggravated. An example of this are symptoms used to diagnose post-stroke depression, which can have a variety of etiologies including brain tissue damage, inflammation, and psychosocial stress-related reactions (Fang and Cheng, 2009). The heterogeneity of etiological factors underlying symptoms of post-stroke depression is further evidenced by the frequent lack of responsiveness to antidepressant medications (Hackett et al, 2008). Thus, among patients with medical illness and presumed comorbid psychiatric diagnoses, the symptoms used to diagnose psychiatric illness may be caused by the medical illness rather than the psychiatric disorder.

Complicating the matter, there is no reason why any individual symptom must have a single etiology. For example, fatigue is a common symptom in MS experienced by 65–97% of all patients (Bakshi, 2003). Depression is also common, with 15–26% of patients experiencing a major depressive episode in a 12-month period (Patten et al, 2003) and nearly 50% experiencing significant symptoms of depression (Chwastiak et al, 2002). Thus, for many patients with MS, fatigue may be multiply determined. Simply understanding whether or not the symptom is caused by the medical illness may not necessarily be of assistance in determining whether or not it should be counted as a symptom for a psychiatric assessment.

2.3 Measurement Issues Specific to Medical Populations

The potential complications of confounded symptoms emerge in RCTs in the assessment of the psychiatric disorder. Numerous symptoms of psychiatric disorders may be confounded with medical illness, such as fatigue, changes in sleep and appetite, agitation and/or tremors, sweating, gastrointestinal symptoms, and neuropsychological changes (Koenig et al, 1997; Mohr et al, 1997). Thus, assessments of psychiatric disorders in populations or samples with medical illnesses may produce false positives, both on symptoms and diagnoses, and may result in elevated levels of symptom severity.

Several methods have been proposed to handle the problem of confounded symptoms (Cohen-Cole and Harpe, 1987). The *etiologic* approach requires the evaluator to determine the etiology of the symptom. This can be effective, but requires a high level of expertise from the evaluators (Koenig et al, 1995). The *exclusive* approach simply excludes those symptoms that are confounded. This is reliable, as the decision can be made a priori and not on a case-by-case basis, but it requires making a diagnostic determination based on a smaller number of symptoms, which may reduce validity. The *substitutive* approach substitutes non-confounded symptoms for confounded ones. For example, social withdrawal might be substituted for fatigue in the diagnosis of major depressive episode. This can also be reliable, but it is unclear if modified diagnostic criteria will identify the same patients as the original categories. Finally, the *inclusive* approach includes any symptom, without consideration of its potential etiology. While these different approaches likely identify different groups of people as meeting diagnostic criteria, no method is necessarily superior to any other (Koenig et al, 1997). Not surprisingly, inclusive approaches are among the most reliable, since there is no determination, either by the evaluator or a priori by the investigator, as to whether a psychiatric symptom is confounded with a medical symptom or not. However, inclusive approaches produce high false-positive rates. Exclusive approaches, on the other hand, may increase false negatives. When following patients longitudinally, as in an RCT, an approach that excludes symptoms based on etiology has been shown to be the most sensitive to change, although it likely produces false negatives (Koenig et al, 1997). Etiologic approaches are a middle road. However, etiologic approaches require a high level of skill on the part of evaluating clinicians in making such determinations (Koenig et al, 1995), and thus may be beyond the budgets of many RCTs.

The relationship between medical illness and psychiatric symptoms is complex and has important implications for RCTs. Psychiatric and medical symptoms often overlap and symptom etiology is not always clear. These comorbidities can interfere with accurate detection of psychiatric disorders, thereby increasing heterogeneity and false-positive rates in an RCT sample. We encourage researchers to consider the ways in which these overlapping symptoms can influence recruitment and assessment when designing RCTs of psychological and behavioral treatments.

3 Effects of Medical Illness and Environmental Factors on Psychiatric Symptoms Longitudinally: Implications for RCTs

Much of the discussion above has focused mainly on the impact of medical illness on psychiatric disorders at a single point in time. However, both medical illness and psychiatric comorbidities can change over time, as can the relationship between the two. The complexity of these relationships can make designing an RCT with medically ill populations particularly challenging. On the medical side of the equation, the pathological and pathogenic features of an illness can change over time or exert a consistent influence on psychiatric symptoms. Treatment of the medical illness can also change over time and influence psychiatric symptoms. On the psychiatric comorbidity side of the equation, the natural history of the disorder can change – indeed many psychiatric problems improve to some degree without treatment. A person's ability to adapt to the symptoms, problems, and sequelae of long-term medical illness can also change over time.

Environmental factors complicate the picture even further. Environmental factors specific to medical patients can influence psychiatric symptoms during the course of an RCT. For example, patients with chronic medical conditions are treated in medical centers where they are more likely to have their psychiatric symptoms may be identified and treated (Harman et al, 2005), which can produce effects that compete with the treatment effect under scrutiny in the trial. Thus, to understand the relationship between medical illness and psychiatric disorders in an RCT, one must conceptualize these variables as processes that occur and interact with each other over time, and not just as fixed, unchanging constructs.

3.1 Interactions Between Medical Illness and Psychiatric Symptoms Longitudinally

The interaction between medical illness and psychiatric disorder over the course of an RCT is displayed graphically in Fig. 60.1. The relationship between medical illness and psychiatric disorder at baseline is depicted as arrow (a). As described above, this relationship includes pathological and pathogenic processes related to the medical illness that produce symptoms that aggravate or mimic the symptoms of psychiatric illness, as well as psychological reactions related to symptoms and adjustment. Below we will describe many potential relationships between medical illness and psychiatric disorders that can occur over time. Each potential relationship is represented by an arrow.

As noted above, many medical illnesses produce symptoms of psychiatric disorders. In some cases these may be comparatively stable symptoms, at least over the course of a 2–4 month trial of a psychological or behavioral treatment. This is depicted in arrow (c). In other words, the medical illness might be expected to exert a fairly consistent effect on the

psychiatric disorder (and measured outcome) over the course of the trial. For example, among post-stroke patients, depression does not change appreciably in the first weeks and months following stroke, and response to psychological and behavioral treatment is very modest at best (Hackett et al, 2008). The persistence of depressive symptoms and their apparent resistance to treatments that are known to work in other populations suggests that these symptoms are in part driven by pathologic or pathogenic features of the medical disease. The relatively small effect produced by psychological and behavioral treatments indicates that very large samples would be required for trials that were adequately powered.

Trials sometimes select time points at which depression is likely to be most prevalent or most severe. This can occur inadvertently or by design. For example, selecting patients when the psychiatric disorder is at its worst often happens inadvertently, since people often seek treatment when symptoms have worsened. Randomization with an appropriate control arm should control for any improvement that occurs as part of the natural course of the illness (Mohr et al, 2009). A problem particular to trials in behavioral medicine occurs when the heightened psychiatric symptoms are due to medical illness, as illustrated by arrow (b). In this case, the baseline medical condition affects not only the baseline psychiatric symptoms (a), but also symptoms of depression later in the course of the RCT (b). An example of this is trials that examine interventions for depression following myocardial infarction (MI). There is considerable interest in post-MI depression, given the strong relationships between depression, and mortality and morbidity in this population (Carney et al, 2002). This has prompted numerous trials examining treatment for depression, most of which have generally produced small or even negligible effect sizes (Thombs et al, 2008). Part of the reason for the failure of these trials may lie in the effect of heart disease on depressive symptoms. While depression is very common immediately following MI, spontaneous remission occurs frequently, with nearly half of all depressions

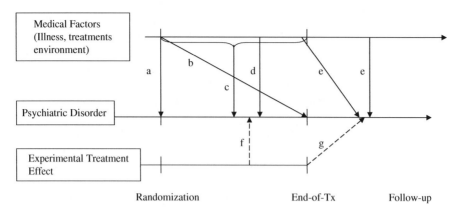

(a) Relationship between medical factors and psychiatric outcome at baseline

(b) Medical factors exert a relatively constant effect over time on psychiatric disorder over
the course of the RCT.

(c) Changes in the course of medical illness may affect the course of psychiatric disorder.

(d) Medical disease events (e.g. exacerbations, relapses, etc) can impact psychiatric
disorder.

(e) Medical factors can impact maintenance of gains in psychiatric symptoms during the
post-treatment follow-up period

(f) Experimental treatment is expected to have an effect on the psychiatric disorder during
the treatment period

(g) Experimental treatment is expected to have an effect on the psychiatric disorder after
treatment cessation

Fig. 60.1 Temporal relationship between medical
factors, psychiatric disorder, and experimental treatments (solid lines indicate effects increasing psychiatric
symptoms; dashed lines indicate effects decreasing
psychiatric symptoms)

remitting within a year following the MI (Hance
et al, 1996). This change in depressive symptoms
may be in part due to changes in pathogenic factors of cardiovascular disease such as neuroendocrine dysregulation or inflammation that may
cause symptoms similar to depression (Joynt
et al, 2003). Improvement in these factors in the
months following MI may lead to decreasing
depressive symptoms. If a substantial number
of patients in a trial experience improvement in
measures of psychiatric outcomes that are the
result of improvements in medical conditions
(e.g., reduced depression resulting from lower
inflammation), the trial will require a larger sample size to be powered to detect a difference.
Thus, the prognosis at baseline for the psychiatric symptoms, and for the medical factors
that may drive depression, should be taken into
account when designing clinical trials.

Medical illnesses also may have pathogenic
and clinical features that are episodic or

relapsing remitting. For many such illnesses,
including MS, IBD, sickle cell, and others, these
relapses are associated with significant increases
in psychiatric symptoms such as depression and
anxiety (Dalos et al, 1983; Graff et al, 2009;
Levenson et al, 2008), which can result in a
unique set of disease-related effects on psychiatric outcomes in an RCT (see arrow (d)). MS is
a good example of this phenomenon. Multiple
sclerosis is in part an autoimmune disease in
which many patients experience sudden exacerbations or increases in inflammation and symptoms that can last a period of weeks or months.
During disease exacerbation, distress may be
experienced by as many as 90% of patients
(Dalos et al, 1983). Depression in MS may be
due in part to the increased inflammation and
cytokine production that are part of the pathogenesis of multiple sclerosis (Gold and Irwin,
2006). Furthermore, these exacerbations are
most commonly treated with high-dose infusions

of corticosteroids, which are known to produce side effects that include euphoria, and less commonly depression and psychosis (Lyons et al, 1988). Typically trials of treatments for psychiatric disorders among illnesses like MS exclude patients from enrollment while exacerbations are occurring to reduce the likelihood of spontaneous improvement in psychiatric symptoms resulting from resolution of the exacerbation (Mohr et al, 2005). This avoids problems illustrated above with arrow (c), in which changes in illness-driven psychiatric symptoms result in high rates of spontaneous remission. However, given MS patients with relapsing forms of the disease may have an exacerbation every 1–2 years, 16.7–33.3% of all patients enrolled in a trial might be expected to experience an exacerbation during the course of a 16-week intervention, resulting in MS-related increases in psychiatric symptoms. Assuming that an exacerbation may last 2 months, 8.4–16.7% of the sample could be in exacerbation at the time of the outcome assessment. The process of randomization should remove any bias in analyses comparing treatment arms. However, the potential influence of increased psychiatric symptoms resulting from exacerbation and inflammation could increase error variance, reduce variance associated with time by treatment effects, and thereby reduce a study's power to detect treatment differences.

Because waxing and waning symptoms that are potentially linked to the primary outcome could have an impact on power, it is advisable to consider these potential effects during study design, and adjust the sample size accordingly. If one is solely interested in the question of whether or not a treatment is efficacious, it may be useful to include the occurrence of sudden increases in the disease exacerbations in the analytic model as a time-dependent covariate.

Maintenance of gains is an increasingly important question in RCTs of psychological and behavioral treatments (Hollon et al, 2005). The effects of medical illness on psychiatric outcomes may be different during post-treatment follow-up, compared to during treatment. For example, in MS, disease severity, level of

cognitive impairment (a common symptom of MS), and brain lesion volume are generally unrelated to the efficacy of treatments for depression (Mohr et al, 2003a). However, depression is significantly more likely to worsen during the first 6 months of post-treatment follow-up among patients with greater neuropsychological impairment and greater brain lesion volume. This suggests that treatment may buffer the negative effects that medical illness has on psychiatric symptoms while treatment is occurring, as illustrated by arrow (f). But once treatment is completed, the effects of the medical illness (arrow e) are no longer buffered by the treatments (arrow g), and the psychiatric symptoms can return. Including follow-up periods to examine maintenance of gains is particularly important in trials conducted with medically ill populations. It is also important to examine potential moderating effects of medical illness factors not only on treatment outcome, but also on maintenance of gains.

3.2 The Influence of Environmental Factors on Psychiatric Symptoms

The environments of medical patients, compared to the environments of non-medical populations, may contain factors that have unique influences on their psychiatric symptoms. For example, many medical patients have frequent contact with the medical providers. Given that most RCTs of psychological and behavioral treatments do not preclude pharmacotherapy for the target psychiatric problems, the increased potential for competing treatments may increase power requirements, compared to trials focused on populations that do not have frequent contact with medical clinics. On the other hand, many of the treatments for medical illness can produce psychiatric side effects. For example, medications such as interferon-alpha, beta blockers, or chemotherapies can increase the risk of depression (Ried et al, 2005; Russo and Fried, 2003; Wichers et al, 2006), while other medications such as levodopa and corticosteroids can produce symptoms of mania and psychosis (Black and Friedman, 2006; Lyons et al, 1988). Similar to how features of the medical illness can have variable effects on psychiatric symptoms, so can treatments of the illness. These treatments can exert continuous or episodic influences on psychiatric symptoms, potentially influencing RCT outcomes.

Changing patterns of contact with medical providers may also exert effects on psychological adjustment during an RCT. For example, the transition from active treatment to early survivorship (i.e., re-entry phase) can be a particularly distressing time for cancer patients (Stanton et al, 2005). This difficult adjustment period is thought to be in part due to the loss of a "safety net." Patients typically have less frequent contact with health-care providers following active treatment and they might receive less support from family and friends as they transition back to their "normal" lives. Continued side effects from treatment (e.g., fatigue, menopause, sexual dysfunction, lymphodema) are often unexpected and can also contribute to this difficult transition. There is some evidence that most patients do not experience significant psychiatric distress during the re-entry phase (Costanzo et al, 2007) and only a subset of patients experience adjustment difficulties. However, preliminary evidence suggests that psychological and behavioral treatments aimed at facilitating adjustment during this phase can be beneficial, particularly for patients at high risk for adjustment difficulties (e.g., younger women with breast cancer) (Scheier et al, 2005). Just as characteristics of the disease should be considered when designing RCTs of psychological and behavioral treatments for medical patients, so should these environmental factors.

4 The Effects of Medical Illness on Access and Adherence to Psychological and Behavioral Treatments

RCTs of psychological interventions in patients with medical illnesses are plagued by problems of generalizability resulting from who is enrolled and completes studies. RCTs of psychological and behavioral treatments often focus on samples drawn from narrow socioeconomic strata. For example, critiques of the oncology literature argue that ethnic minorities, men, patients with advanced cancer, and patients of lower socioeconomic status are underrepresented in RCTs of psychological and behavioral treatments in cancer (Helgeson, 2005). Samples may be further biased, as barriers to psychological and behavioral care can reduce access to treatments and treatment arms that require frequent clinic visits. Up to two-thirds of general primary care patients identify one or more barriers to attending psychological and behavioral treatments and that rate rises to 75% among patients with depression (Mohr et al, 2006). While cost is certainly a barrier, other barriers include transportation problems, time constraints, interference from medical symptoms, and living too far from specialized care. These barriers are even more pronounced among medical patients, given that aspects of the illness likely aggravate these factors. For example, approximately 40% of individuals screened for a recent RCT examining treatment for depression following coronary artery bypass graft surgery were excluded due to transportation issues (Freedland et al, 2009). This is not uncommon even in well executed trials such as this one. The resulting biases may reduce both the generalizability of findings to a broader population and limit the potential public health impact of such interventions.

Over the past 15–20 years there has been a growing effort to develop and to evaluate treatments that overcome barriers to access, primarily by bringing the treatment to the patient. Some studies have examined extending psychological and behavioral care by providing home visits, for example in treating post-partum depression (Dennis, 2005) and distress in terminal cancer patients (Mohr et al, 2003b). Increasingly, the telephone has been examined as a tool to deliver treatments to patients who have cancer, HIV, MS, are blind, are elderly, or are caregivers of disabled patients, just to name a few patient populations. A recent meta-analysis suggests that telephone-delivered treatment results in rates of attrition that are much lower than those seen in face-to-face delivery (Mohr et al, 2008). More recently there has been a remarkable increase in investigations into internet-delivered treatments, which hold promise as cost-effective methods of delivering treatments (Spek et al, 2007; see Chapter 64). Advances in telecommunication are greatly increasing the capacity to bring treatments to patients.

Evaluations of these trials have focused almost exclusively on efficacy, which may be appropriate for early-stage evaluations. However, many of these interventions are being developed for medical populations with the goal of overcoming barriers to care. Yet this goal remains largely untested. In the design of these trials, access to care remains an implicit rather than explicit goal that is not measured or analyzed. The use of different treatment delivery methods may decrease some barriers while creating entire classes of new barriers (Eysenbach, 2005). As these telemental health treatments begin to show initial efficacy, it will be important to make the goals of increasing reach and adherence explicit and to develop designs that can test these hypotheses directly.

5 Reconceptualizing RCTs of Psychological and Behavioral Treatments in Medical Populations to Include Prognosis

RCTs of psychological and behavioral Treatments in treating psychiatric disorders in patients with medical disorders often produce effect sizes that compare quite favorably to those seen in trials with medically healthy populations (Freedland et al, 2009). However, not uncommonly the outcomes are more mixed, less robust than seen in healthy populations, or the treatments are simply ineffective (Hackett et al, 2008; Sheard and Maguire, 1999). A common

response in the field is to attempt to alter the treatment by tailoring it more specifically to the needs of the population. We will argue here that a second approach is to refine our diagnostic capabilities and incorporate the evaluation of prognostic indicators into RCTs.

Much of the discussion in this chapter has involved problems that arise from difficulties in detecting and measuring symptoms of psychiatric disorders in medical populations. Diagnosis is used clinically to determine the utility of a treatment, and under good circumstances it provides some information about the differential prognoses associated with various treatment options. Hence, the oft-quoted notion in psychiatry that diagnosis is prognosis (Goodwin and Guze, 1974). However, if our diagnostic system is producing a highly heterogeneous group, with numerous false positives who either do not respond to treatment or improve even without treatment, then that diagnosis is no longer providing much prognostic value. The identification and validation of prognostic indicators that can differentiate patients who are likely to respond to treatment or who do not need treatment, would substantially improve our ability to provide effective and efficient care. Randomized trials (using control arms or comparative outcome designs) should supply the evidence upon which this prognostic information is based.

The RCT design has generally been conceptualized as a method of testing the efficacy or effectiveness of an intervention or therapy. However, when conducting an RCT of a validated intervention or therapy in a medical population, the conceptual clarity of the RCT methodology is muddied, largely due to the confounding factors discussed earlier. Therefore, when we conduct an RCT of a validated treatment in a medical population, we are really asking if that treatment, which is known to be effective in a psychiatric population without a single medical comorbidity, is *also* effective in the medical population. There are two reasons why a validated treatment may not be effective under these circumstances. One reason is that factors related to the medical illness could interfere with the efficacy of the treatment. As described earlier in the chapter, many features of medical illness and its treatment can threaten the validity of RCTs of psychological and behavioral treatments. That is, the patients in fact have the psychiatric disorder, but something is preventing the treatment from working properly. The other reason that a validated treatment might be less effective in a medical population is that the method of identifying patients is producing large numbers of false positives. In other words, when validated treatments fail to have results similar to those seen in a medically healthy population, the problem may not be the treatment – the treatment failure may reflect our inability to accurately diagnose the psychiatric disorder in that medical population.

From this perspective, an RCT is required not only to test the effectiveness of an experimental treatment for a psychiatric disorder, but also to *know if our diagnostic procedures are identifying the disorder for which the treatment is known to be effective*. If we explicitly recognize that part of the reason for conducting RCTs of otherwise validated treatments in medical populations is because we are unable to accurately identify psychiatric problems in these populations, this has substantial implications for the design of RCTs. In other words, an RCT under these circumstances, to be of maximum benefit, has two broad aims. One is the question of whether the treatment works. The other is to reduce unexplained heterogeneity in the targeted samples. To address this second aim, the focus of RCTs would have to include methodologies that identify symptoms, features, or characteristics of patients that can be used to provide prognostic information as to who is likely to improve and who is likely not to improve, and reduce unexplained heterogeneity in the sample, with respect to the target psychiatric disorder.

The design of such a *prognostic trial* would require careful consideration of which psychiatric symptoms may likely remain unaffected by the medical illness, which symptoms may be confounded, which measureable features of the medical illness predict non-response, and potentially even define the mechanisms by which the confounding may occur. Such a design would

essentially use the active treatment, validated in non-medical populations, as a method of identifying prognostically useful features in the patient population. Once identified, the prognostic model would have to be tested, using the treatment response as the predictive criterion validity for the diagnostic model. Validation could only occur if the prognostic strategy were identified a priori.

One argument against this thesis is that by identifying symptoms that are responsive to our treatments, we are confounding diagnosis and outcome in a way that could lead to a loss of diagnostic clarity. Traditionally, methodology in clinical research suggests that first a problem should be identified (diagnosis) and only afterwards can a solution to that problem (treatment) be developed. To identify symptoms that predict response to treatment is in effect developing a solution and then looking for a problem that it fixes.

The drawback of using a traditional linear approach to validate psychological and behavioral treatments with medical patients is that it limits our ability to develop effective care strategies for populations who experience significant psychological and psychiatric difficulties and it is out of keeping with practices and standards that are currently the norm among clinical investigators in medicine. We would counter this argument for a linear approach with three points. First, the process of problem identification and evaluation of solutions is not nearly so linear in practice. Certainly the development of pharmaceutical therapies usually begins with the identification of a specific problem and the attempt to manufacture a pharmacological therapy that is safe and effective. But it is not uncommon for the target of a promising compound to change as more is learned about the effects of the agent. And the development of off-label alternative uses, even for problems that are not clearly diagnosable under the International Classification of Diseases, is also common. Second, we are not suggesting developing a new diagnosis. Rather, we are suggesting identifying prognostic factors that can augment the diagnosis in medical populations, thereby providing information that could be very useful for clinicians and policymakers. Third, it is true that expecting a trial to validate a treatment, investigate predictors of response, and test a prognostic model would overburden any single RCT. But treatments are not validated by single trials; they are validated by programs of research and multiple trials. Likewise, no single study could validate both a diagnostic/prognostic strategy and a treatment. However, programs of research in which initial trials include methodological components that promote the identification of prognostic indicators, and later trials that validate those indicators, have the potential to move behavioral medicine forward in populations where validated treatments have been less effective than in medically healthy populations.

6 Summary

Given the prevalence of psychiatric disorders in medically ill populations, there is great interest in understanding whether traditional psychological and behavioral treatments of psychiatric disorders are effective for these patients. Unfortunately, there are numerous confounding features of a medical illness that can threaten validity and influence outcomes in a standard RCT. The illness itself, the treatment of the illness, and the environmental factors can all interact with psychiatric symptoms. Furthermore, in an RCT, medical illnesses and psychiatric disorders change over time, and the relationship between the two can change across all stages of a trial, from recruitment to post-treatment follow-up. Despite these challenges, RCTs of psychological and behavioral treatments in medical populations provide unique opportunities. We have proposed a modification in RCT conceptualization that makes explicit the challenges of diagnosis and the role of prognosis in RCTs of psychological and behavioral treatments in medical populations. By designing trials aimed at identifying prognostic features, behavioral medicine researchers have the opportunity to gain valuable information about the specific features that do or do not predict treatment response

among these patient groups and thereby improve our ability to provide effective targeted care.

References

Bakshi, R. (2003). Fatigue associated with multiple sclerosis: diagnosis, impact and management. *Multi Scler, 9*, 219–227.

Banks, S. M., and Kerns, R. D. (1996). Explaining high rates of depression in chronic pain: a diathesis-stress framework. *Psychol Bull, 119*, 95–110.

Black, K. J., and Friedman, J. H. (2006). Repetitive and impulsive behaviors in treated Parkinson disease. *Neurology, 67*, 1118–1119.

Burgess, C., Cornelius, V., Love, S., Graham, J., Richards, M. et al (2005). Depression and anxiety in women with early breast cancer: five year observational cohort study. *Brit Med J, 330*, 702–705.

Carney, R. M., Freedland, K. E., Miller, G. E., and Jaffe, A. S. (2002). Depression as a risk factor for cardiac mortality and morbidity: a review of potential mechanisms. *J Psychosom Res, 53*, 897–902.

Carta, M. G., Hardoy, M. C., Garofalo, A., Pisano, E., Nonnoi, V. et al (2007). Association of chronic hepatitis C with major depressive disorders: irrespective of interferon-alpha therapy. *Clin Pract Epidemiol Ment Health, 3*, 22.

Chwastiak, L., Ehde, D. M., Gibbons, L. E., Sullivan, M., Bowen, J. D. et al (2002). Depressive symptoms and severity of illness in multiple sclerosis: epidemiologic study of a large community sample. *Am J Psychiatry, 159*, 1862–1868.

Cipriani, A., Furukawa, T. A., Salanti, G., Geddes, J. R., Higgins, J. P. et al (2009). Comparative efficacy and acceptability of 12 new-generation antidepressants: a multiple-treatments meta-analysis. *Lancet, 373*, 746–758.

Cohen-Cole, S. A., and Harpe, C. (1987). Diagnostic assessment of depression in the medically ill. In A. Stoudemire & B. S. Fogel (Eds.), *Principles of Medical Psychiatry* (pp. 23–36). New York: Grune and Stratton.

Connerney, I., Shapiro, P. A., McLaughlin, J. S., Bagiella, E., Sloan, R. P. et al (2001). Relation between depression after coronary artery bypass surgery and 12-month outcome: a prospective study. *Lancet, 358*, 1766–1771.

Costanzo, E. S., Lutgendorf, S. K., Mattes, M. L., Trehan, S., Robinson, C. B. et al (2007). Adjusting to life after treatment: distress and quality of life following treatment for breast cancer. *Br J Cancer, 97*, 1625–1631.

Cuijpers, P., Brannmark, J. G., and van Straten, A. (2008). Psychological treatment of postpartum depression: a meta-analysis. *J Clin Psychol, 64*, 103–118.

Dalos, N. P., Rabins, P. V., Brooks, B. R., and O'Donnell, P. (1983). Disease activity and emotional state in multiple sclerosis. *Ann Neurol, 13*, 573–577.

Dennis, C. L. (2005). Psychosocial and psychological interventions for prevention of postnatal depression: systematic review. *Brit Med J, 331*, 15.

Dickens, C., McGowan, L., Clark-Carter, D., and Creed, F. (2002). Depression in rheumatoid arthritis: a systematic review of the literature with meta-analysis. *Psychosom Med, 64*, 52–60.

Eysenbach, G. (2005). The law of attrition. *J Med Internet Res, 7*, e11.

Fang, J., and Cheng, Q. (2009). Etiological mechanisms of post-stroke depression: a review. *Neurol Res, 31*, 905–909.

Feinstein, A., Roy, P., Lobaugh, N., Feinstein, K., O'Connor, P., and Black, S. (2004). Structural brain abnormalities in multiple sclerosis patients with major depression. *Neurology, 62*, 586–590.

Fisher, L., Skaff, M. M., Mullan, J. T., Arean, P., Mohr, D. et al (2007). Clinical depression versus distress among patients with type 2 diabetes: not just a question of semantics. *Diabetes Care, 30*, 542–548.

Freedland, K. E., Skala, J. A., Carney, R. M., Rubin, E. H., Lustman, P. J. et al (2009). Treatment of depression after coronary artery bypass surgery: a randomized controlled trial. *Arch Gen Psychiat, 66*, 387–396.

Gold, S. M., and Irwin, M. R. (2006). Depression and immunity: inflammation and depressive symptoms in multiple sclerosis. *Neurol Clin, 24*, 507–519.

Goodwin, D. W., and Guze, S. B. (1974). *Psychiatric Diagnosis*. New York: Oxford University Press.

Graff, L. A., Walker, J. R., and Bernstein, C. N. (2009). Depression and anxiety in inflammatory bowel disease: a review of comorbidity and management. *Inflamm Bowel Dis, 15*, 1105–1118.

Hackett, M. L., Anderson, C. S., House, A., and Halteh, C. (2008). Interventions for preventing depression after stroke. *Cochrane Database Syst Rev*, CD003689.

Hackett, M. L., Yapa, C., Parag, V., Anderson, C. S., Hackett, M. L. et al (2005). Frequency of depression after stroke: a systematic review of observational studies. *Stroke, 36*, 1330–1340.

Hance, M., Carney, R. M., Freedland, K. E., and Skala, J. (1996). Depression in patients with coronary heart disease: a 12-month follow-up. *Gen Hosp Psychiatry, 18*, 61–65.

Harman, J. S., Edlund, M. J., Fortney, J. C., and Kallas, H. (2005). The influence of comorbid chronic medical conditions on the adequacy of depression care for older Americans. *J Am Ger Soc, 53*, 2178–2183.

Helgeson, V. S. (2005). Recent advances in psychosocial oncology. *J Cons Clin Psychol, 73*, 268–271.

Hollon, S. D., DeRubeis, R. J., Shelton, R. C., Amsterdam, J. D., Salomon, R. M. et al (2005). Prevention of relapse following cognitive therapy vs medications in moderate to severe depression. *Arch Gen Psychiatry, 62*, 417–422.

Horgan, O., and MacLachlan, M. (2004). Psychosocial adjustment to lower-limb amputation: a review. *Disabil Rehabil, 26*, 837–850.

Joynt, K. E., Whellan, D. J., and O'Connor, C. M. (2003). Depression and cardiovascular disease: mechanisms of interaction. *Biol Psychiatry, 54*, 248–261.

Kanner, A. M. (2003). Depression in epilepsy: prevalence, clinical semiology, pathogenic mechanisms, and treatment. *Biol Psychiatry, 54*, 388–398.

Koenig, H. G., George, L. K., Peterson, B. L., and Pieper, C. F. (1997). Depression in medically ill hospitalized older adults: prevalence, characteristics, and course of symptoms according to six diagnostic schemes. *Am J Psychiatry, 154*, 1376–1383.

Koenig, H. G., Pappas, P., Holsinger, T., and Bachar, J. R. (1995). Assessing diagnostic approaches to depression in medically ill older adults: how reliably can mental health professionals make judgments about the cause of symptoms? *J Am Ger Soc, 43*, 472–478.

Levenson, J. L., McClish, D. K., Dahman, B. A., Bovbjerg, V. E., de A. Citero, V. et al (2008). Depression and anxiety in adults with sickle cell disease: The PiSCES project. *Psychosom Med, 70*, 192–196.

Lyons, P. R., Newman, P. K., and Saunders, M. (1988). Methylprednisolone therapy in multiple sclerosis: a profile of adverse effects. *J Neurol Neurosurg Psychiatry, 51*, 285–287.

Massie, M. J. (2004). Prevalence of depression in patients with cancer. *J Natl Cancer Inst Monogr, 32*, 57–71.

Mohr, D. C., Epstein, L., Luks, T. L., Goodkin, D., Cox, D. et al (2003a). Brain lesion volume and neuropsychological function predict efficacy of treatment for depression in multiple sclerosis. *J Cons Clin Psychol, 71*, 1017–1024.

Mohr, D. C., Goodkin, D. E., Likosky, W., Beutler, L., Gatto, N. et al (1997). Identification of Beck Depression Inventory items related to multiple sclerosis. *J Behav Med, 20*, 407–414.

Mohr, D. C., Hart, S. L., Howard, I., Julian, L., Vella, L. et al (2006). Barriers to psychotherapy among depressed and nondepressed primary care patients. *Ann Behav Med, 32*, 254–258.

Mohr, D. C., Hart, S. L., Julian, L., Catledge, C., Honos-Webb, L. et al (2005). Telephone-administered psychotherapy for depression. *Arch Gen Psychiatry, 62*, 1007–1014.

Mohr, D. C., Moran, P. J., Kohn, C., Hart, S., Armstrong, K. et al (2003b). Couples therapy at end of life. *Psychooncology, 12*, 620–627.

Mohr, D. C., Spring, B., Freedland, K. E., Beckner, V., Arean, P. H. et al (2009). The selection and design of control conditions for randomized controlled trials of psychological interventions. *Psychother Psychosom, 78*, 275–284.

Mohr, D. C., Vella, L., Hart, S., Heckman, T., and Simon, G. (2008). The effect of telephone-administered psychotherapy on symptoms of depression and attrition: a meta-analysis. *Clin Psychol Sci Pract, 15*, 243–253.

Patten, S. B., Beck, C. A., Williams, J. V., Barbui, C., and Metz, L. M. (2003). Major depression in multiple sclerosis: a population-based perspective. *Neurology, 61*, 1524–1527.

Ried, L. D., Tueth, M. J., Handberg, E., Kupfer, S., and Pepine, C. J. (2005). A study of antihypertensive drugs and depressive symptoms (SADD-Sx) in patients treated with a calcium antagonist versus an atenolol hypertension treatment strategy in the International Verapamil SR-Trandolapril Study (INVEST). *Psychosom Med, 67*, 398–406.

Riegger, T., Conrad, S., Schluesener, H. J., Kaps, H. P., Badke, A., Baron, C. et al (2009). Immune depression syndrome following human spinal cord injury (SCI): a pilot study. *Neuroscience, 158*, 1194–1199.

Rosenkranz, M. A. (2007). Substance p at the nexus of mind and body in chronic inflammation and affective disorders. *Psychol Bull, 133*, 1007–1037.

Russo, M. W., and Fried, M. W. (2003). Side effects of therapy for chronic hepatitis C. *Gastroenterology, 124*, 1711–1719.

Scheier, M. F., Helgeson, V. S., Schulz, R., Colvin, S., Berga, S. et al (2005). Interventions to enhance physical and psychological functioning among younger women who are ending nonhormonal adjuvant treatment for early-stage breast cancer. *J Clin Oncol, 23*, 4298–4311.

Scott, K. M., Bruffaerts, R., Tsang, A., Ormel, J., Alonso, J. et al (2007). Depression-anxiety relationships with chronic physical conditions: results from the World Mental Health Surveys. *J Affect Dis, 103*, 113–120.

Sheard, T., and Maguire, P. (1999). The effect of psychological interventions on anxiety and depression in cancer patients: results of two meta-analyses. *Br J Cancer, 80*, 1770–1780.

Spek, V., Cuijpers, P., Nyklicek, I., Riper, H., Keyzer, J. et al (2007). Internet-based cognitive behaviour therapy for symptoms of depression and anxiety: a meta-analysis. *Psychol Med, 37*, 319–328.

Stanton, A. L. (2006). Psychosocial concerns and interventions for cancer survivors. *J Clin Oncol, 24*, 5132–5137.

Stanton, A. L., Ganz, P. A., Rowland, J. H., Meyerowitz, B. E., Krupnick, J. L. et al (2005). Promoting adjustment after treatment for cancer. *Cancer, 104*, 2608–2613.

Thombs, B. D., de Jonge, P., Coyne, J. C., Whooley, M. A., Frasure-Smith, N. et al (2008). Depression screening and patient outcomes in cardiovascular care: a systematic review. *JAMA, 300*, 2161–2171.

Wichers, M. C., Kenis, G., Leue, C., Koek, G., Robaeys, G. et al (2006). Baseline immune activation as a risk factor for the onset of depression during interferon-alpha treatment. *Biol Psychiatry, 60*, 77–79.

Yohannes, A. M., Baldwin, R. C., and Connolly, M. J. (2000). Depression and anxiety in elderly outpatients with chronic obstructive pulmonary disease: prevalence, and validation of the BASDEC screening questionnaire. *Int J Ger Psychiatry, 15*, 1090–1096.

Chapter 61

Quality of Life in Light of Appraisal and Response Shift

Sara Ahmed and Carolyn Schwartz

The value of evaluating quality of life (QOL) has always resonated in the minds of patients, clinicians, and society at large. While the term has existed since the time of Pigou in 1920 (Pigou, 1920), it is only in the past two decades that QOL has been operationally defined and that standardized measures exist to allow us to attach a meaningful metric that can be considered for monitoring patient progress and clinical research.

The accumulation of such advances in the development of QOL measures and of other patient-reported outcomes (PRO) is reflected in two major changes that serve as the foundation for the practical application of PROs in research and clinical care. The first is the 2006 publication of the Food and Drug Administration (FDA) Guidance on the use of PROs in medical product development to support labeling claims (Guidance for Industry, 2006). This Guidance formalized the use of PROs in drug development and emphasized the use of symptom and function measures in such research (Puhan et al, 2004). The Guidance also provided a clear and unignorable link between PROs and commercial products aimed at improving health (see Chapter 8).

The second is that psychometric methods and theory have grown substantially. These methods have opened the door to a deeper and more nuanced approach to working with data as well as for thinking about change over time. They have also provided useful tools for characterizing clinically important change (Browne and Cudeck, 1993), of relevance, both for individual patient monitoring and for assessment of treatment value (Maltais et al, 2008).

Theoretical advances have focused on the impact of adaptation on the interpretation of QOL scores. For example, the meaning of change depends on where you start (Hays and Woolley, 2000). Such "response shifts" represent health-related changes in the meaning of measured concepts, due to changes in the individual's internal standards, values, and conceptualization of the concept(s) being measured. The growing evidence base for response shift suggests that it is of primary importance in rehabilitation research, since many interventions aimed at helping people with disability outcomes involve teaching response shifts. If they are not adequately measured, the intervention may appear to have no impact because relevant changes are obfuscated.

This chapter discusses the relevance of QOL to clinical care and research. We will also describe the evolution of the theoretical scope of QOL research, extending from theories in psychology and other social sciences. We also highlight methodological challenges with evaluating change in QOL and how these may be mitigated by incorporating appraisal and response shift assessments.

C. Schwartz (✉)
DeltaQuest Foundation Inc, 31 Mitchell Road, Concord, MA, USA; Research Professor of Medicine and Orthopaedic Surgery, Tufts University School of Medicine, Boston, MA, USA
e-mail: carolyn.schwartz@deltaquest.org

A. Steptoe (ed.), *Handbook of Behavioral Medicine*, DOI 10.1007/978-0-387-09488-5_61,
© Springer Science+Business Media, LLC 2010

1 Patient-Reported Outcomes of Quality of Life

PROs are measurements of any aspect of a patient's QOL or health status that comes directly from a patient. QOL is defined by the WHO as *an individual's perception of his/her position in life in the context of the culture and value systems in which he/she lives, and in relation to his/her goals, expectations, standards and concerns. It is a broad-ranging concept, incorporating in a complex way the person's physical health, psychological state, level of independence, social relationships, and their relationship to salient features of their environment* (World Health Organization, 1998). QOL can be thought of as a hierarchical concept, similar to Maslow's hierarchy of needs (Maslow, 1943; Smith, 1981) (Fig. 61.1). This hierarchy would have at its base physical aspects of functioning, including mobility, fatigue, and pain. At the next layer would be social functioning, participation, etc., followed by emotional functioning. At the top of the pyramid would be existential well-being, including such concepts as purpose in life and self-acceptance. All of the domains are best assessed by PROs because they are subjective by nature and thus require the unique perspective of the patient. QOL PROs

may provide finer-grained estimates of QOL by including standardized evaluations of pain, fatigue, disability, participation in life roles, and other domains related to physical, social, and emotional functions. Such measures are important for evaluating the impact of disease and for assessing the efficacy of treatments (Donaldson, 2006; Greenhalgh et al, 2005; Haywood, 2007; Lipscomb et al, 2007; Stull et al, 2007).

Health-related quality of life (HRQL) is a more restricted term in that it refers specifically to the impact of disease and treatment on the lives of patients and is defined as "the capacity to perform the usual daily activities for a person's age and major social role" (Guyatt et al, 1993). The concepts we describe in this chapter can be applied to any PRO, but from this point on we refer to QOL as it is all-encompassing of other PRO domains.

1.1 Generic and Disease-Specific Measures

Generic measures of QOL include broad domains and can be used across a wide range of healthy and chronic disease populations. The advantage of generic measures is that they

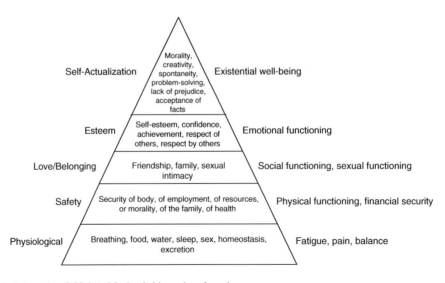

Fig. 61.1 Integrating QOL into Maslow's hierarchy of needs

allow for comparisons across groups and have often been used in population and health services delivery studies. Commonly used measures include the SF-36 (Ware Jr., 2000; Ware Jr. et al, 1994), the Sickness Impact Profile (SIP) (Bergner et al, 1976; Bergner et al, 1981), and the WHO-QOL (World Health Organization, 1998).

Clinical researchers recognized that generic measures were not specific enough to capture changes in clinical populations. Consequently, over the years, several disease-specific measures have emerged that capture particular domains of relevance to a specific patient population. Some examples for HIV include the MOS-HIV (Holmes and Shea, 1999; O'Leary et al, 1998), WHOQOL-HIV (WHOQOL HIV Group, 2004) and for cancer are the Functional Assessment of Cancer Therapy-General (FACT-G) (Cella et al, 2002b; Cormier et al, 2008) and the EORTC Core Quality of Life Questionnaire (EORTC QLQ-C30) (Groenvold et al, 1997). While disease-specific measures may be more sensitive to changes in a particular patient population, they do not allow for broad comparisons across populations. To benefit from both types of measures some developers have used a *modular approach* whereby a disease-specific component is built as an adjunct to a core generic measure that allows for greater generalisability.

1.2 The Value of Evaluating QOL

With advances in medical technology and drug therapy, individuals in developed countries are living longer with chronic illness (Bodenheimer et al, 2002). This has broadened the focus from only measuring outcome indicators, such as survival, to also evaluating the impact of disease and treatment on the QOL of individuals for the years gained (e.g., Quality-Adjusted Life Year (QALY)) (Donaldson, 2006).

QOL assessments have been used as an outcome, a predictor, or an intervention. As an outcome measure, QOL assessments have provided information about the benefits of an intervention in randomized controlled trials (Lim et al, 2003; Mayo et al, 2000) to attach a value to an increased length of survival (Siddiqui et al, 2008) and to evaluate the long-term impact of illness (Mayo et al, 2001).

The importance of QOL measures for capturing concepts beyond clinical indicators is reflected in the prognostic value of QOL scores (Sprangers, 2002). In cancer research there is evidence that HRQL is an independent predictor of survival (Siddiqui et al, 2008) and in some studies QOL was found to be even more predictive of survival than known biologic prognostic factors (Sprangers, 2002).

QOL assessments have also been used as an intervention in clinical care by providing a mechanism to improve patient–clinician communication (Chumbler et al, 2007; Jacobsen et al, 2002). This allows doctors to identify areas that may otherwise go unnoticed and that can be treated by the medical team if they are medically related problems, such as symptoms or activity limitations. If the problems are non-medical, they may lead to referrals to social workers or psychologists.

Therefore, QOL evaluations can play a central role in enhancing the richness of the patient–clinician encounter. In clinical care, the prognostic value of QOL assessments, supported by studies in cancer research, may allow QOL assessments to be used to tailor medical and psychosocial therapy for patients soon after diagnosis.

2 Methodological Advances in QOL Research

Methodological advances from educational testing using item response theory (IRT) (Embretson and Reise, 2000) have been applied to HRQL assessments, leading to a paradigm shift in patient-reported outcomes assessment (see Chapter 9). These methods allow the selection of items for short forms based on the range of the underlying trait that is of most interest. Thus, short forms can be created for different disease groupings or levels of disabilities, rather than having one short form for all.

These IRT methods have also led to the development of generic computerized adaptive tests, expanded and made widely available through the NIH-Roadmap initiative called Patient-Reported Outcome Measurement Information System (PROMIS). The PROMIS collaboration has yielded item banks for 11 different QOL domains for use across patient populations (Reeve et al, 2007). Static short forms and dynamic computerized adaptive tests were developed for the following domains: Emotional Distress (Anger, Anxiety, Depression); Fatigue; Pain (Behavior, Impact); Physical Function; Satisfaction (with Discretionary Social Roles, with Social Roles); Sleep Disturbance; and Wake Disturbance. Additionally, a static short form was developed for Global Health. It is unknown, however, how well these computerized adaptive tests function for disease-specific applications. A comparison of the responsiveness of generic computerized adaptive tests and disease-specific short forms is essential for determining the best tool battery for use in clinical research and patient monitoring.

3 The Influence of Adaptation and Appraisal Processes on QOL Evaluations

Clinicians have often noted that their clients are continually adapting to their illness and recognize that often patients who would be expected to feel despair given their physical health report being happier and more satisfied with life than expected. Over the past 10 years the QOL field has taken note of the possible influence of "response shift" on the QOL assessments. When individuals experience a health-state change, they may change their internal standards (i.e., recalibration), values (i.e., reprioritization), or meaning (i.e., reconceptualization) of the target

construct one is asking them to self-report, in this case QOL (Schwartz and Sprangers, 1999; Sprangers and Schwartz, 1999). For example, people with a substantial physical disability may experience a severity of fatigue that they did not know prior to the development of the disability. Consequently, they would *recalibrate* what "severe fatigue" means to them, making it difficult to compare their pre-disability and post-disability ratings of fatigue as it relates to physical health. They may also *reprioritize* life domains, such that sense of community and interpersonal intimacy become more important to their sense of well-being than career success or material gains. Finally, they may *reconceptualize* QOL to focus on those domains where they continue to have control and be effective when rating their QOL. These subtle and not-so-subtle response shifts are to be expected with evaluative constructs, which are assessed by idiosyncratic rather than objective criteria (Sprenkle et al, 2004). Evaluative ratings of participation are products of an appraisal process, where individuals must consider what QOL means to them, what experiences they have had that are relevant to QOL, how experiences compare to desired circumstances or outcomes, and the relative importance of different experiences (Rapkin and Schwartz, 2004). Although clinicians and philosophers have long noted response shift phenomena, with early references linked to Aristotle (Jette et al, 2008) and Heraclitus (Kahn, 1981), the challenge for researchers has been to operationalize the construct in ways that are measurable and robust.

3.1 History of Response Shift

Response shift was originally noticed and studied in educational intervention and management science research in the 1970s, where investigators noticed that students' internal standards of competency changed as a result of learning more about the subject (Armenakis and Zmud,

1979; Hoogstraten, 1982). For example, students rated their abilities or knowledge in a particular area as stronger or better until they learned more about it, and then, after learning more, rated their abilities as less or the same as before the educational intervention. Similarly, people with spinal disorders may rate themselves as more disabled after treatment than they did before treatment because the yardstick has changed.

In the 1990s, interest in response shift developed in studying QOL. Clinicians began to recognize that response shift could obfuscate important treatment-related changes and indeed might even be the subtext or the desired effect in rehabilitation and psychosocial interventions (Schwartz and Sprangers, 1990; Schwartz et al, 1999, 2007). Response shift has now been studied and recognized to affect adaptation to a wide degree of health conditions, including multiple sclerosis (Christensen et al, 1999; Brandtstadter and Renner, 1990; Helson, 1964; Schwartz and Sendor, 1999), cancer (Ahmed et al, 2009a; Bernhard et al, 1999, 2001; Boyd et al, 1990; Breetvelt and Van Dam, 1991; Cella et al, 2002a; Hagedoorn et al, 2002; Jansen et al, 2000; Kagawa-Singer, 1993; Oort et al, 2005; Schwartz et al, 1999; Sprangers et al, 1999), stroke (Ahmed et al, 2003, 2004, 2005), diabetes (Li and Rapkin, 2009; Postulart and Adang, 2000), geriatrics (Daltroy et al, 1999; Rapkin, 2009), palliative care (Schwartz et al, 2002, 2004a, 2005), dental disorders (Ring et al, 2005), and, most recently, orthopedics (Razmjou et al, 2006). A meta-analysis done on response shift reported that response shift findings ranged from moderate to small effect sizes (Schwartz et al, 2006). Although this may seem of minor clinical significance, Oort and colleagues demonstrated that adjusting for response shift in the data analytic phase of a study can boost effect sizes from moderate to large for clinical interventions for cancer patients (Oort et al, 2005). Other research has demonstrated that adjusting for response shift can even reverse putative null or deleterious findings (Schwartz et al, 2007), seemingly a Type II error can occur if response shift is not accounted for (Ring et al, 2005).

3.2 Theoretical Foundation of Response Shift

The motivation for research in response shift in relation to QOL outcomes began in the late 1990s with the development of the Sprangers and Schwartz (Sprangers and Schwartz, 1999) response shift theoretical model. Within this framework, response shift refers to health-related changes in the self-evaluation of a concept (e.g., health, quality of life, pain) due to (1) changes in internal standards (i.e., recalibration); (2) changes in values (i.e., reprioritization); or (3) changes in the conceptualization (i.e., reconceptualization) (Sprangers and Schwartz, 1999).

The model proposed that with a change in a person's health as a catalyst, antecedents (i.e., stable characteristics of the individual such as gender, personality, expectations, and spiritual identity) interact with mechanisms (i.e., behavioral, cognitive, and affective processes that accommodate the catalyst) that may initiate a response shift and result in an overestimation or underestimation of HRQL as measured by objective criteria (Sprangers and Schwartz, 1999).

Rapkin and Schwartz (Rapkin and Schwartz, 2004; Sprenkle et al, 2004) (Fig. 61.2) further expanded the model to distinguish mechanisms that are initial responses to catalysts from

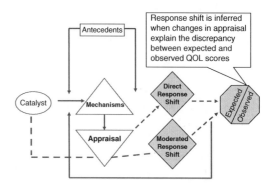

Fig. 61.2 Rapkin and Schwartz Model of appraisal and quality of life.
Adapted and reprinted with permission from BioMed Central (Rapkin and Schwartz, 2004)

response shifts that continue the process of adaptation. In an attempt to make these distinctions, the Rapkin and Schwartz model incorporates appraisal processes as a possible explanation for intra-individual variations in HRQL change scores.

Based on the Rapkin and Schwartz model (Rapkin and Schwartz, 2004) individual differences in longitudinal changes in appraisal will affect how people respond to HRQL items. Any response to a HRQL item is dependent on four distinct cognitive processes which correspond to psychological aspects of coping and adjustment. These include (1) induction of a frame of reference; (2) recall and sampling of salient experiences; (3) use of standards of comparison to appraise experiences; and (4) application of a subjective algorithm to prioritize and combine appraisals to arrive at a QOL rating (Rapkin and Schwartz, 2004). Within the appraisal framework, response shift is inferred when changes in appraisal explain discrepancies between expected and observed HRQL scores.

3.3 The Relationship Between QOL and Response Shift to Other Frameworks from Psychology and the Social Sciences

Empirically based research on adaptation increasingly highlights that the personal level of happiness is more flexible and thus changeable than was previously thought (Diener, 2006). The field of positive psychology has provided mounting evidence that sustainable increases in happiness levels are possible via interventions that teach ways of refocusing one's perspective and priorities, and that these increases are sustained over time (Lyubomirsky and Sheldon, 2005; Lyubomirsky et al, 2006; McCullough, 2000; Otake et al, 2006; Seligman et al, 2005). In contrast to this demonstrated flexibility is the increasingly documented genetic influence on HRQOL (Christensen et al, 1999; Kendler et al, 2000; Leinonen et al, 2005; Lykken and

Tellegen, 1996; Romeis et al, 2000, 2005; Roysamb, 2002; Roysamb et al, 2003; Stubbe et al, 2005; Svedberg et al, 2005, 2006). Although distinct, these areas of research have in common that they provide new insights into the changeability of quality of life (research on adaptation and positive psychology) versus its stability (genetic research). The convergence of these lines of investigation thus supports a state (i.e., situational) and trait (i.e., genetic) conceptualization of HRQOL (Schwartz and Sprangers, 2009).

This trait and state distinction has implications for methods and clinical applications of response shift. Measuring relevant personality characteristics may be needed to predict who will undergo response shifts, with what magnitude and in which direction. While personality is included under Antecedents in the original theoretical model proposed by Sprangers and Schwartz (1999), the work on the genetic predisposition for personality and well-being underscores the need to measure it. Further, it points to the need to take different personality characteristics into account that encompass "affective reserve." One may also want to measure targeted characteristics, such as resilience or emotional flexibility.

For healthcare professionals to help patients achieve a response shift, we should focus on those aspects that can change. For example, we can teach better affective, behavioral, and cognitive methods for dealing with health state changes but these may only work optimally for people who have an adequate "affective reserve" or emotional flexibility. This notion does not mean, however, that the constellation of personality characteristics underlying "affective reserve" is given and unchangeable. It is possible that this affective reserve is something that can be hidden or obfuscated by maladaptive traits that can be modified by affective, behavioral, or cognitive methods. For example, cognitive behavioral interventions that teach people how to modify negative appraisals or self-talk may also help people to uncover or enliven traits related to their response shift potential. Thus, interventions to teach response shifts may be able to heighten one's response shift proneness. We have to keep in mind that only 50% of a personality trait is estimated to be genetically determined; thus the remaining 50% is amenable to change.

4 Limitations of Current Measures of QOL in Light of Response Shift

4.1 Psychometric Properties of QOL Measures in Light of Response Shift

One of the most challenging aspects of response shift research is that it calls into question fundamental assumptions of questionnaires (e.g., measurement invariance) and psychometric criteria, such as reliability, validity, and responsiveness. Schwartz and Rapkin (2004) noted that every quantitative index of reliability, validity, and responsiveness may be distorted by reasonable and expected adaptation-related changes over time. For example, high internal consistency (reliability) and cross-measure correlations (validity) provide little psychometric information about what a measure is evaluating, but rather support the idea that people are answering a set of items in a similar way and that these items reflect a narrow "bandwidth" of a given construct. Similarly, for inter-observer agreement to be high (another aspect of reliability), observers must share a frame of reference, sample the same experiences, apply the same standards, and give experiences equal priority. It is likely, however, that observers may differ in many aspects of QOL appraisal, particularly if their health trajectory has been quite different (Schwartz and Rapkin, 2004).

Responsiveness, another key psychometric index that is an extension of validity (Hays and Hadorn, 1992), may also not reflect what is assumed. A measure that is not responsive, that is, it does not change in step with objective indices of health, may be reflecting a provisionally stable set point, to which an individual returns despite a constant level of stress (Carver and Scheier, 2000; Helson, 1964; Schwartz et al, 2004b). This unresponsiveness or stability may be due to habituation (Folkman et al, 1997) or active coping (Brandtstadter and Renner, 1990) and may follow a pattern described by engineers and economists as hysteresis (Mayergoyz, 1991). That is, stress may be added without inducing apparent change in a system (or a person), up to a certain level of tolerance, beyond which the system may undergo permanent and profound change that makes it impossible to returning to earlier tolerances.

The impact of these response shifts on psychometric characteristics such as reliability, validity, and responsiveness is not only conceptually important but also operationally important because they influence the interpretation of clinical research findings.

4.2 Implications of Response Shift for Evaluation of Psychosocial and Healthcare Interventions

As HRQL is increasingly becoming part of the evaluation profile for interventions, particularly for chronic disease and for those interventions involving health services delivery, developing an estimator of HRQL that differentiates between objective change and changes in standards, conceptualization, and values is essential for the interpretation of the results. The strength of randomized trials is that balance is achieved at the outset on measured and unmeasured variables, which would include conceptualization of HRQL and internal standards. However, in trials where the intervention involves a psychosocial component or support from a healthcare team, the intervention arm may receive information and support to help them cope and manage their illness. As a consequence, the intervention arm may induce a response shift leading to a differential response shift in the two groups.

This differential response shift effect may attenuate or exaggerate findings from clinical trials that use HRQL as an end-point (Schwartz and Sprangers, 1999). The implications are that the conclusions drawn from evaluations of the impact of disease or health interventions on HRQL may be incorrect and in turn may guide clinical-care decisions in the wrong direction. The dynamic nature of individuals' standpoint regarding their health may explain several paradoxical findings in health care. Even a small response shift effect can move an effect size from small to moderate or moderate to large (Oort et al, 2005). The impact of response shift on evaluations of change in HRQL has been reported in a number of studies including those that have evaluated the effects of support groups (Schwartz, 1999) and self-management programs (Ahmed et al, 2009b; Osborne et al, 2006).

5 Methodological Advances in Evaluating Changes in QOL and Response Shift Detection

In order to draw appropriate conclusions regarding treatment effects and to fully understand the impact of illness over time, methodological approaches that detect response shift are needed before scores are analyzed and interpreted as actual change. Diverse approaches for assessing response shift have been developed (Schwartz and Sprangers, 1999; Schwartz et al, 2006; Visser et al, 2005). Some of these stem from work initiated in the educational (Howard, 1979) and management sciences (Schmitt, 1982; Schmitt et al, 1984) (Golembiewski et al, 1976; Norman and Parker, 1996). The range and details of these approaches have been outlined in detail elsewhere (Ahmed et al, 2009b; Schwartz and Sprangers, 1999, 2000). This chapter highlights recent advances, mainly statistical approaches, which show promise in being able to monitor and provide estimates that distinguish response shift from changes in QOL for an individual patient.

Current methods for detecting response shifts are evolving from a predominant focus on the 'then-test' design approach to an emphasis on statistical or individualized methods. The then-test defines the magnitude of the response-shift as the difference between the pre-assessment and *then*-test, which is a retrospective rating of the pre-assessment (Howard and Bray, 1979; Sprangers et al, 1999). The then-test approach has the advantage of being easy to administer and analyze but the disadvantages of random error and/or confounding with recall bias as well as being difficult to interpret. For these reasons, we now briefly describe promising statistical or individualized methods that have evolved in the past few years.

There are three statistical methods that have been applied to response shift detection that hold promise: structural equation modeling, latent trajectory analysis with subject-centered residuals, and classification and regression tree analysis. All of these methods require substantial sample sizes, on the order of 10 subjects per variable and a minimum of 200. These methods vary in terms of how much they focus on aggregate analyses versus individual patient-focused, and thus how sensitive they are to individual response shifts.

Originally evolving from factor analytic methods, *structural equation modeling* (SEM) is a technique that combines factor analysis and regression analysis to solve multivariate research questions at a group level (Bollen, 1989; Hoyle, 1995) (see Chapter 57). By analyzing covariance matrices, these models test measurement and structural models to first test the assumption of measurement invariance and then to examine whether relationships among variables are similar over time (i.e., the structural model). Recent advances of this method were made by Oort and colleagues (Oort et al, 2005), to clarify how distinct changes detectable with SEM reflect different aspects of response shift. This work extended earlier work done by Schmitt (1982) and yielded more sensitive algorithms for detecting response shifts. Although this method has the advantage of allowing secondary analysis of existing data to test response shift hypotheses, it has the disadvantage of being sensitive to response shifts only when a majority of the sample does so (Ahmed et al, 2009a, b). Since preliminary estimates of the prevalence of response shift suggests that about one-half to one-third of respondents exhibit response shifts that are detectable by these methods (Finkelstein et al, 2009; Mayo et al, 2009), one would have to over-sample people prone to response shifts to be able to detect such change using SEM. Over-sampling will be feasible when we are better able to predict who experiences response shifts.

Latent trajectory analysis with subject-centered residuals is a method developed by Mayo and colleagues that focuses on the individual and seeks to develop a predictive model to examine patterns in discrepancies between expected and observed scores (Bryk and Raudenbush, 1992; Mayo et al, 2009). By obtaining and scaling model residuals, Mayo creates subject-centered residuals to categorize respondents as either (Cupples and McKnight, 1994) (1) exhibiting no response shift, i.e., the person's residuals are consistent over time, but there was some change in their perceived QOL; (2) exhibiting a positive response shift, i.e., the person's evaluation started low, and then shifted or reassessed upward; or (3) exhibiting a negative response shift, i.e., started higher than expected and then reassessed down over time. This method is of interest because it classifies response shift at the individual rather than group level, and because it distinguishes groups based on the timing as well as the direction of the response shift. It is useful for stratified analyses with existing data and thus does not impose additional demands on the respondent. Its primary weakness is that it cannot distinguish random error from response shift. Like other statistically sophisticated methods, it requires a substantial sample size measured over multiple time points to create a predictive model.

Classification and regression tree analysis (CART) (Breiman et al, 1993; Haykin, 2002) is a method applied by Li and Rapkin (Li and Rapkin, 2006; Li et al, 2007; Li and Rapkin, 2009) that combines qualitative and quantitative methods to yield a rich analysis of complex data. These investigators utilized the Appraisal Profile developed by Rapkin (Rapkin and Schwartz, 2004), which yields qualitative text data in response to open-ended questions

as well as quantitative data in response to multiple choice questions. The tool measures four distinct parameters of the appraisal process: (a) *Framing*, i.e., what does quality of life mean to the individual; (b) *Sampling*, i.e., What relevant experiences do I have; (c) *Evaluating*, i.e., How do experiences compare to relevant standards; (d) *Combining*, i.e., what is the relative importance of different experiences.

These data are then content analyzed to yield categories (Li and Rapkin, 2009) amenable to quantitative analysis, and "trees" are generated. The final product of this analysis is homogenous groupings of respondents who share patterns of appraisal. In this example, Li and Rapkin evaluated appraisal processes in 644 AIDS patients 6 months after enrollment into a study evaluating how appraisal patterns were related to reported general health. The method revealed substantial differences in level of reported general health as a function of distinct combinations of appraisal preferences (Li and Rapkin, 2006, 2009; Li et al, 2007).

All of the above-mentioned methods require large sample sizes, which can be a hindrance for researchers conducting small trials or observational studies. We would make two suggestions for response shift detection methods for such researchers. First, we would suggest collecting data using the Rapkin Appraisal Profile (Rapkin and Schwartz, 2004) and working with the data descriptively. For example, one could simply describe how patients answered the open-ended questions using qualitative methods or summarize the most frequent categories endorsed in the multiple choice questions.

A second suggestion would be to use another individualized method, the Schedule for the Evaluation of Individual Quality of Life (SEIQOL) (Joyce et al, 1999). This method explicitly allows the cues, levels, and weights to vary within and across individuals. This approach reduces the ambiguity of QOL scores by making this variation explicit and measurable, while retaining the option of comparing a global score over time. In contrast, current QOL measures such as the SF-36 (Ware Jr. et al, 1994) commonly compare overall scores

Table 61.1 Summary of strengths of response shift detection methods

Strength	Then-test	SEM	Latent	CART	SEIQOL
Easy to use	✓		✓	✓	
Easy to analyze	✓				
Meaningful interpretation		✓ if expert involved	TBD	✓ if expert involved	✓
Individual-level interpretation					✓
Low participant burden		✓	✓	✓	
RSP adjustment possible		✓		✓	
RSP stratification possible			✓		
Does not need large samples	✓				✓

but they do not query or contain information about the disparate domains, cues, or anchors being considered and combined in these overall scores.

All of the methods described above have strengths and weaknesses, as summarized in Table 61.1. Regardless of the response shift detection approach however, the investigator should adhere to the following guidelines: always have a comparison/control group to enable theory-driven hypothesis testing; have clearly stated hypotheses about when the response shift will occur (catalyst and change); use a combination of approaches to provide information about convergence among methods; and include an objective clinical criterion measure so that it is possible to distinguish between expected and observed change in quality of life over time.

6 Future Directions in QOL and Response Shift Research

The theoretical and methodological developments of QOL assessments have progressed over the past decade. As work using advanced psychometric approaches continues, the routine use of QOL in clinical care will become more feasible. Future developments based on methods that can generate a response shift parameter for each individual will provide stronger insight into our ability to evaluate and account for response shift when estimating change in QOL.

Our understanding of response shift will change as different disease trajectories are investigated using existing and novel approaches currently being developed, building on existing tools.

Evaluating the biopsychosocial determinants of QOL appraisal will also be critical in understanding whether individuals differ in their cognitive and affective capacities relevant to QOL appraisal, what factors influence different kinds of changes in QOL appraisal, and the timing of changes in appraisal. Not only will this help inform methodological developments for assessing response shift but it will also lead to a better understanding of when, how, and for whom to intervene to improve QOL (Rapkin, 2009).

Considering response shift and appraisal can enrich and increase the detected impact of illness and behavioral and psychosocial interventions on individuals' well-being and QOL. Further QOL research that integrates appraisal and response shift evaluations will ensure that scores are interpreted correctly and that the patient perspective is accurately reflected in the resulting change estimates.

References

Ahmed, S., Mayo, N., Hanley, J., And Wood-Dauphinee, S. (2003). Individualized health-related quality of life (Hrql) post stroke: revealing response shift. *Qual Life Res, 12*, 765.

Ahmed, S., Mayo, N. E., Wood-Dauphinee, S., Hanley, J. A., and Cohen, S. R. (2004). Response shift influenced estimates of change in health-related quality of life poststroke. *J Clin Epidemiol, 57*, 561–570.

Ahmed, S., Mayo, N. E., Wood-Dauphinee, S., Hanley, J. A., and Cohen, R. (2005). The structural equation modeling technique did not show a response shift, contrary to the results of the then test and the individualized approaches. *J Clin Epidemiol, 58*, 1125–1133.

Ahmed, S., Schwartz, C., Ring, L., and Sprangers, M. A. (2009a). Applications of health-related quality of life for guiding healthcare: advances in response shift research. *Ed J Clin Epidemiol, 62*(11), 1115–1117.

Ahmed, S., Bourbeau, J., Maltais, F., and Mansour, S. (2009b). The Oort structural equation modeling approach detected a response shift after a COPD self-management program not detected by the Schmitt technique. *J Clin Epidemiol, 62*, 1165–1172.

Armenakis, A. A., and Zmud, R. W. (1979). Interpreting the measurement of change in organizational research. *Person Psychol, 32*, 709–723.

Bergner, M., Bobbitt, R. A., Pollard, W. E., Martin, D. P., and Gilson, B. S. (1976). The sickness impact profile: validation of a health status measure. *Med Care, 14*, 57–67.

Bergner, M., Bobbitt, R. A., Carter, W. B., and Gilson, B. S. (1981). The sickness impact profile: development and final revision of a health status measure. *Med Care, 19*, 787–805.

Bernhard, J., Hurny, C., Maibach, R., Herrmann, R., and Laffer, U. (1999). Quality of life as subjective experience: reframing of perception in patients with colon cancer undergoing radical resection with or without adjuvant chemotherapy. *Ann Oncol, 10*, 775–782.

Bernhard, J., Lowy, A., Maibach, R., and Hurny, C. (2001). Response shift in the perception of health for utility evaluation. An explorative investigation. *Eur J Cancer, 37*, 1729–1735.

Bodenheimer, T., Lorig, K., Holman, H., and Grumbach, K. (2002). Patient self-management of chronic disease in primary care. *Jama, 288*, 2469–2475.

Bollen, K. A. (1989). *Structural Equations With Latent Variables*. New York, NY: Wiley And Sons.

Boyd, N. F., Sutherland, H. J., Heasman, K., Tritchler, D., and Cummings, B. (1990). Whose utilities for decision analysis? *Med Decis Making, 10*, 58–67.

Brandtstadter, J., and Renner, G. (1990). Tenacious goal pursuit and flexible goal adjustment: explication and age-related analysis of assimilative and accommodative strategies of coping. *Psychol Aging, 5*, 58–67.

Breetvelt, I. S., and Van Dam, F. S. (1991). Underreporting by cancer patients: the case of response-shift. *Soc Sci Med, 32*, 981–987.

Breiman, L., Friedman, J. H., Olshen, R. A., and Stone, C. J. (1993). *Classification and Regression Trees*. New York, NY: Chapman and Hall/Crc.

Browne, M., and Cudeck, R. (1993). Alternative ways of assessing model fit. In K. A. Bollen & J. S. Long (Eds.), *Testing Structural Equation Models* (pp. 136–162). London: Sage Publications.

Bryk, A. S., and Raudenbush, S. W. (1992). *Hierarchical Linear Models: Applications and Data Analysis Methods*. Thousand Oaks,CA: Sage Publications.

Carver, C. S., and Scheier, M. F. (2000). Scaling back goals and recalibration of the affect system are processes in normal adaptive self-regulation: understanding 'response shift' phenomena. *Soc Sci Med, 50*, 1715–1722.

Cella, D., Hahn, E. A., and Dineen, K. (2002a). Meaningful change in cancer-specific quality of life scores: differences between improvement and worsening. *Qual Life Res, 11*, 207–221.

Cella, D., Eton, D. T., Fairclough, D. L., Bonomi, P., Heyes, A. E. et al (2002b). What is a clinically meaningful change on the functional assessment of cancer therapy-lung (Fact-L) questionnaire? Results From Eastern Cooperative Oncology Group (Ecog) Study 5592. *J Clin Epidemiol, 55*, 285–295.

Christensen, K., Holm, N. V., Mcgue, M., Corder, L., and Vaupel, J. W. (1999). A Danish population-based twin study on general health in the elderly. *J Aging Health, 11*, 49–64.

Chumbler, N. R., Mkanta, W. N., Richardson, L. C., Harris, L., Darkins, A. et al (2007). Remote patient-provider communication and quality of life: empirical test of a dialogic model of cancer care. *J Telemed Telecare, 13*, 20–25.

Cormier, J. N., Ross, M. I., Gershenwald, J. E., Lee, J. E., Mansfield, P. F. et al (2008). Prospective assessment of the reliability, validity, and sensitivity to change of the functional assessment of cancer therapy-melanoma questionnaire. *Cancer, 112*, 2249–57.

Cupples, M. E., and Mcknight, A. (1994). Randomised controlled trial of health promotion in general practice for patients at high cardiovascular risk. *BMJ, 309*, 993–996.

Daltroy, L. H., Larson, M. G., Eaton, H. M., Phillips, C. B., and Liang, M. H. (1999). Discrepancies between self-reported and observed physical function in the elderly: the influence of response shift and other factors. *Soc Sci Med, 48*, 1549–1561.

Diener, E. (2006). Guidelines for national indicators of subjective well-being and illbeing. *J Happiness Stud, 7*, 397–404.

Donaldson, M. (2006). Using patient-reported outcomes in clinical oncology practice:benefits, challenges and next steps. *Expert Rev Pharmacoecon Outcomes Res, 6*, 87–95.

Embretson, S. E., and Reise, S. P. (2000). *Item Response Theory for Psychologists*. Mahwah, NJ: Lawrence Erlbaum Associates.

Finkelstein, J. A., Razmjou, H., and Schwartz, C. E. (2009). Response shift and outcome assessment in orthopedic surgery: is there is a difference between complete vs. partial treatment? *J Clin Epidemiol, 62*, 1189–1190.

Folkman, S., Moskowitz, J. T., Ozer, E. M., Park, C. L., and Gottlieb, B. H. (1997). positive meaningful events and coping in the context of HIV/AIDS. In B. H. Gottlieb (Ed,), *Coping with Chronic Stress* (pp. 293–315). New York, NY: Plenum Press.

Golembiewski, R. T., Billingsley, K., and Yeager, S. (1976). Measuring change and persistence in human affairs: types of change generated by Od designs. *J Appl Behav Sci, 12*, 133–157.

Greenhalgh, J., Long, A. F., and Flynn, R. (2005). The use of patient reported outcome measures in routine clinical practice: lack of impact or lack of theory? *Soc Sci Med, 60*, 833–843.

Groenvold, M., Klee, M. C., Sprangers, M. A., and Aaronson, N. K. (1997). Validation of the Eortc Qlq-C30 quality of life questionnaire through combined qualitative and quantitative assessment of patient-observer agreement. *J Clin Epidemiol, 50*, 441–450.

Guidance For Industry: Patient-Reported Outcome Measures: Use In Medical Product Development To Support Labeling Claims: Draft Guidance (2006). *Health Qual Life Outcomes, 4*, 79.

Guyatt, G. H., Feeny, D. H., and Patrick, D. L. (1993). Measuring health-related quality of life. *Ann Intern Med, 118*, 622–629.

Hagedoorn, M., Sneeuw, K. C. A., and Aaronson, N. K. (2002). changes in physical functioning and quality of life in patients with cancer - response shift and relative evaluation of one's condition. *J Clin Epidemiol, 55*, 176–183.

Haykin, S. (2002). *Neural Networks: A Comprehensive Foundation, 2nd Ed.* Delhi, India: Pearson Education (Singapore).

Hays, R. D., and Hadorn, D. (1992). Responsiveness to change: an aspect of validity, not a separate dimension. *Qual Life Res, 1*, 73–75.

Hays, R. D., and Woolley, J. M. (2000). The concept of clinically meaningful differnce in health-related quality-of-life research: how meaningful is it? *Pharmacoeconomics, 18*, 419–423.

Haywood, K. L. (2007). Patient-reported outcome ii: selecting appropriate measures for musculoskeletal care. *Muscoskel Care, 5*, 72–90.

Helson, H. (1964). *Adaptation Level Theory.* New York, NY: Harper and Row.

Holmes, W. C., and Shea, J. A. (1999). Two approaches to measuring quality of life in the HIV/AIDS population: Hat-Qol and Mos-HIV. *Qual Life Res, 8*, 515–527.

Hoogstraten, J. (1982). The retrospective pretest in an educational training context. *J Exp Educ, 50*, 200–204.

Howard, G. S. (1979). Response-Shift bias: a source of contamination of self-report measures. *J Appl Psychol, 64*, 144–150.

Howard, G. S., and Bray, J. H. (1979). Internal invalidity in studies employing self-report instruments: a suggested remedy. *J Educ Meas, 16*, 129–135.

Hoyle, R. H. (1995). *Structural Equation Modeling: Concepts, Issues, And Application.* Thousand Oaks: Sage Publications, C1995.

Jacobsen, P. B., Davis, K., and Cella, D. (2002). Assessing quality of life in research and clinical practice. *Oncology (Williston Park) 16(9 Suppl 10): 133–9.*

Jansen, S. J., Stiggelbout, A. M., Nooij, M. A., Noordijk, E. M., and Kievit, J. (2000). Response shift in quality of life measurement in early-stage breast cancer patients undergoing radiotherapy. *Qual Life Res, 9*, 603–615.

Jette, A. M., Haley, S. M., Ni, P., Olarsch, S., and Moed, R. (2008). Creating a computer adaptive test version of the late-life function and disability instrument. *J Gerontol A Biol Sci Med Sci, 63*, 1246–1256.

Joyce, C. R. B., O'boyle, C. A., and Mcgee, H. (1999). Individualising qestionnaires. In C. R. B. Joyce, C. A. O'boyle, & H. Mcgee (Eds.), *Individual Quality of Life. Approaches to Conceptualization and Assessment* (pp. 87–104). Amsterdam: Harwood.

Kagawa-Singer, M. (1993). Redefining health: living with cancer. *Soc Sci Med, 37*, 295–304.

Kahn, C. H. (1981). *The Art and Thought of Heraclitus: An Edition of the Fragments with Translation and Commentary.* London: Cambridge University Press.

Kendler, K. S., Myers, J. M., and Neale, M. C. (2000). A multidimensional twin study of mental health in women. *Am J Psychiatry, 157*, 506–513.

Leinonen, R., Kaprio, J., Jylha, M., Tolvanen, A., Koskenvuo, M. et al (2005). Genetic influences underlying self-rated health in older female twins. *J Am Geriatr Soc, 53*, 1002–1007.

Li, Y., and Rapkin, B. (2006). HIV/AIDS patients' quality of life appraisal depends on their personal meaning of quality of life and frame of reference. *Qual Life Res, E-Suppl 15*, A–36.

Li, Y., and Rapkin, B. (2009). Classification and regression tree uncovered hierarchy of psychosocial determinants underlying quality-of-life response shift in HIV/AIDS. *J Clin Epidemiol, 62*, 1138–1147.

Li, Y., Rapkin, B., and Patel, S. (2007). Attainment of goals in HIV/AIDS patients in New York City. *Qual Life Res Suppl, A-39.*

Lim, W. K., Lambert, S. F., and Gray, L. C. (2003). Effectiveness of case management and post-scute services in older people after hospital discharge. *Med J Aust, 178*, 262–266.

Lipscomb, J., Gotay, C. C., and Snyder, C. F. (2007). Patient-reported outcomes in cancer: a review of recent research and policy initiatives. *Ca Cancer J Clin, 57*, 278–300.

Lykken, D. T., and Tellegen, A. (1996). Happiness is a stochastic phenomenon. *Psychol Sci, 7*, 186–189.

Lyubomirsky, S., and Sheldon, K. M. (2005). Pursuing happiness: the architecture of sustainable change. *Rev Gen Psychol, 9*, 111–131.

Lyubomirsky, S., Sousa, L., and Dickerhoof, R. (2006). The costs and benefits of writing, talking, and thinking about life's triumphs and defeats. *J Pers Soc Psychol, 90*, 692–708.

Maltais, F., Bourbeau, J., Shapiro, S., Lacasse, Y., Perrault, H. et al (2008). Effects of home-based pulmonary rehabilitation in patients with chronic obstructive pulmonary disease: a randomized trial. *Ann Intern Med, 149*, 869–878.

Maslow, A. H. (1943). A theory of human motivation. *Psychol Rev, 50*, 370–396.

Mayergoyz, I. D. (1991). *Mathematical Models of Hysteresis.* New York, NY: Springer-Verlag.

Mayo, N., Scott, C., and Ahmed, S. (2009). Case management post-stroke did not induce response shift: the value of residuals. *J Clin Epidemiol, 62*, 1148–1156.

Mayo, N. E., Wood-Dauphinee, S., Cote, R., Gayton, D., Carlton, J. et al (2000). There's no place like home : an evaluation of early supported discharge for stroke. *Stroke, 31*, 1016–1023.

Mayo, N. E., Wood-Dauphinee, S., Cote, R., Durcan, L., and Carlton, J. (2001). Activity, participation, and quality of life six months post-stroke. *Arch Phys Med Rehabil, 83*, 1035–1042.

Mccullough, M. E. (2000). *Forgiveness : Theory,Research, And Practice.* New York, NY: Guilford Press.

Norman, P., and Parker, S. (1996). The interpretation of change in verbal reports: implications for health psychology. *Psychol Health, 11*, 301–314.

O'Leary, J. F., Ganz, P. A., Wu, A. W., Coscarelli, A., and Petersen, L. (1998). Toward a better understanding of health-related quality of life: a comparison of the medical outcomes study hiv health survey (MOS-HIV) and the HIV overview of problems-evaluation system (Hopes). *J Acquir Immune Defic Syndr Hum Retrovirol, 17*, 433–441.

Oort, F. J., Visser, M. R., and Sprangers, M. A. (2005). An application of structural equation modeling to detect response shifts and true change in quality of life data from cancer patients undergoing invasive surgery. *Qual Life Res, 14*, 599–609.

Osborne, R. H., Hawkins, M., and Sprangers, M. A. (2006). Change of perspective: a measurable and desired outcome of chronic disease self-management intervention programs that violates the premise of preintervention/postintervention assessment. *Arthritis Rheum, 55*, 458–465.

Otake, K., Shimai, S., Tanaka-Matsumi, J., Otsui, K., and Fredrickson, B. L. (2006). Happy people become happier through kindness: a counting kindnesses intervention. *J Happiness Stud, 7*, 361–375.

Pigou, A. C. (1920). *The Economics of Welfare.* London: Mac Millan.

Postulart, D., and Adang, E. M. (2000). response shift and adaptation in chronically ill patients. *Med Decis Making, 20*, 186–193.

Puhan, M. A., Behnke, M., Laschke, M., Lichtenschopf, A., Brandli, O. et al (2004). Self-administration and standardisation of the chronic respiratory questionnaire: a randomised trial in three German-speaking countries. *Respir Med, 98*, 342–350.

Rapkin, B. (2009). Considering the application of the trait/state distinction for response shift research: continuing the conversation. *J Clin Epidemiol, 62*, 1124–1125.

Rapkin, B. D., and Schwartz, C. E. (2004). Toward a theoretical model of quality-of-life appraisal: implications of findings from studies of response shift. *Health Qual Life Outcomes, 2*, 14.

Razmjou, H., Yee, A., Ford, M., and Finkelstein, J. A. (2006). Response shift in outcome assessment in patients undergoing total knee arthroplasty. *J Bone Joint Surg, 88*, 2590–2595.

Reeve, B. B., Burke, L. B., Chiang, Y. P., Clauser, S. B., Colpe, L. J. et al (2007). Enhancing measurement in health outcomes research supported by agencies within the US Department of Health and Human Services. *Qual Life Res, 16 Suppl*, 175–186.

Ring, L., Hofer, S., Heuston, F., Harris, D., and O'boyle, C. A. (2005). Response Shift masks the treatment impact on patient reported outcomes (Pros): the example of individual quality of life in edentulous patients. *Health Qual Life Outcomes, 3*, 55.

Romeis, J. C., Scherrer, J. F., Xian, H., Eisen, S. A., Bucholz, K. et al (2000). Heritability of self-reported health. *Health Serv Res, 35*, 995–1010.

Romeis, J. C., Heath, A. C., Xian, H., Eisen, S. A., Scherrer, J. F. et al (2005). Heritability of Sf-36 among middle-age, middle-class, male-male twins. *Med Care, 43*, 1147–1154.

Roysamb, E. H. (2002). Subjective well being. sex specific effects of genetic and environmental factors. *Pers Indiv Differ, 32*, 211–223.

Roysamb, E., Tambs, K., Reichborn-Kjennerud, T., Neale, M. C., and Harris, J. R. (2003). Happiness and health: environmental and genetic contributions to the relationship between subjective well-being, perceived health, and somatic illness. *J Pers Soc Psychol, 85*, 1136–1146.

Schmitt, N. (1982). The use of analysis of covariance structures to assess beta and gamma change. *Multivariate Behav Res, 17*, 343–358.

Schmitt, N., Pulakos, E., and Lieblein, A. (1984). Comparison of three techniques to assess group-level beta and gamma change. *Appl Psychol Meas, 8*, 249–260.

Schwartz, C. E. (1999). Teaching coping skills enhances quality of life more than peer support: results of a randomized trial with multiple sclerosis patients. *Health Psychol, 18*, 211–220.

Schwartz, C. E., and Rapkin, B. D. (2004). Reconsidering the psychometrics of quality of life assessment in light of response shift and appraisal. *Health Qual Life Outcomes, 2*, 16.

Schwartz, C. E., and Sendor, M. (1999). Helping others helps oneself: response shift effects in peer support. *Soc Sci Med, 48*, 1563–1575.

Schwartz, C. E., and Sprangers, M. A. G. (1990). Introduction to symposium on the challenge of response shift in social science and medicine. *Soc Sci Med, 48,* 1505–1506.

Schwartz, C. E., and Sprangers, M. A. (1999). Methodological approaches for assessing response shift in longitudinal health-related quality-of-life research. *Soc Sci Med, 48,* 1531–1548.

Schwartz, C. E., and Sprangers, M. A. G. (2000). *Adaptation to Changing Health Response Shift in Quality-of-Life Research, 1st Ed.* Washington, DC: American Psychological Association.

Schwartz, C. E., and Sprangers, M. A. G. (2009). Reflections on genes and sustainable change: toward a trait and state conceptualization of response shift. *J Clin Epidemiol, 62,* 1118–1123.

Schwartz, C. E., Feinberg, R. G., Jilinskaia, E., and Applegate, J. C. (1999). An evaluation of a psychosocial intervention for survivors of childhood cancer: paradoxical effects of response shift over time. *Psycho-Oncology, 8,* 344–354.

Schwartz, C. E., Wheeler, H. B., Hammes, B., Basque, N., Edmunds, J. et al (2002). Early intervention in planning end-of-life care with ambulatory geriatric patients: results of a pilot trial. *Arch Intern Med, 162,* 1611–1618.

Schwartz, C. E., Merriman, M. P., Reed, G. W., and Hammes, B. J. (2004a). Measuring patient treatment preferences in end-of-life care research: applications for advance care planning interventions and response shift research. *J Palliat Med, 7,* 233–245.

Schwartz, C. E., Sprangers, M. A. G., Carey, A., and Reed, G. (2004b). Exploring response shift in longitudinal data. *Psychol Health, 19,* 51–69.

Schwartz, C. E., Merriman, M. P., Reed, G., and Byock, I. (2005). Evaluation of the Missoula-Vitas quality of life index--revised: research tool or clinical tool? *J Palliat Med, 8,* 121–135.

Schwartz, C. E., Bode, R., Repucci, N., Becker, J., Sprangers, M. A. et al (2006). The clinical significance of adaptation to changing health: a meta-analysis of response shift. *Qual Life Res, 15,* 1533–50.

Schwartz, C. E., Andresen, E. M., Nosek, M. A., Krahn, G. L., And Rrtc Expert Panel On Health Status Measurement (2007). Response shift theory: important implications for measuring quality of life in people with disability. *Arch Phys Med Rehabil, 88,* 529–36.

Seligman, M. E., Steen, T. A., Park, N., and Peterson, C. (2005). Positive psychology progress: empirical validation of interventions. *Am Psychol, 60,* 410–421.

Siddiqui, F., Pajak, T. F., Watkins-Bruner, D., Konski, A. A., Coyne, J. C. et al (2008). Pretreatment quality of life predicts for locoregional control in head and neck cancer patients: a radiation therapy oncology group analysis. *Int J Radiat Oncol Biol Phys, 70,* 353–60.

Smith, J. A. (1981). The idea of health: a philosophical inquiry. *Ans Adv Nurs Sci, 3,* 43–50.

Sprangers, M. A. (2002). Quality-of-life assessment in oncology. Achievements and challenges. *Acta Oncol, 41,* 229–237.

Sprangers, M. A., and Schwartz, C. E. (1999). Integrating response shift into health-related quality of life research: a theoretical model. *Soc Sci Med, 48,* 1507–1515.

Sprangers, M. A., Van Dam, F. S., Broersen, J., Lodder, L., Wever, L. et al (1999). Revealing response shift in longitudinal research on fatigue--the use of the thentest approach. *Acta Oncol, 38,* 709–718.

Sprenkle, M. D., Niewoehner, D. E., Nelson, D. B., and Nichol, K. L. (2004). The veterans short form 36 questionnaire is predictive of mortality and healthcare utilization in a population of veterans with a self-reported diagnosis of asthma Or Copd. *Chest, 126,* 81–89.

Stubbe, J. H., Posthuma, D., Boomsma, D. I., and De Geus, E. J. (2005). Heritability of life satisfaction in adults: a twin-family study. *Psychol Med, 35,* 1581–1588.

Stull, D. E., Leidy, N. K., Jones, P. W., and Stahl, E. (2007). Measuring functional performance in patients with Copd: a discussion of patient-reported outcome measures. *Curr Med Res Opin, 23,* 2655–65.

Svedberg, P., Gatz, M., Lichtenstein, P., Sandin, S., and Pedersen, N. L. (2005). Self-rated health in a longitudinal perspective: a 9-year follow-up twin study. *J Gerontol B Psychol Sci Soc Sci, 60,* S331–S340.

Svedberg, P., Bardage, C., Sandin, S., and Pedersen, N. L. (2006). A prospective study of health, life-style and psychosocial predictors of self-rated health. *Eur J Epidemiol, 21,* 767–776.

Visser, M. R., Oort, F. J., and Sprangers, M. A. (2005). Methods to detect response shift in quality of life data: a convergent validity study. *Qual Life Res, 14,* 629–39.

Ware, J. E. Jr. (2000). Sf-36 health survey update. *Spine, 25,* 3130–3139.

Ware, J. E., Jr.. Kosinski, M., and Keller S.D. (1994). *Sf-36 Physical and Mental Scales: A User's Manual.* Boston, MA: The Health Institute, New England Medical Center.

Whoqol HIV Group (2004). Whoqol-HIV for quality of life assessment among people living with HIV and AIDS: results from the field test. *Aids Care, 16,* 882–9.

World Health Organization Quality Of Life Assessment (Whoqol): Development And General Psychometric Properties (1998). *Soc Sci Med, 46,* 1569–1585.

Chapter 62

Behavioral Interventions for Prevention and Management of Chronic Disease

Brian Oldenburg, Pilvikki Absetz, and Carina K.Y. Chan

1 Background

Many different factors influence changing patterns of morbidity, mortality, and the spread of diseases, both globally and within and between countries. Global economic forces influence health trends around the world, as do demographic changes related to population growth, ageing, and social patterns. More locally, changes in people's living and working environments and other settings, where individuals' health is more directly affected, also play a crucial role. An impressive amount of epidemiological evidence collected over the past 50 years has identified the influence of a number of key behavioral determinants and lifestyle risk factors on social, physical, and mental health.

A small subset of these health behaviors are particularly critical lifestyle risk factors for noncommunicable chronic diseases, their management and progression (WHO, 2005). Physical inactivity, unhealthy eating, alcohol consumption, and tobacco use are the primary behavioral risk factors for cardiovascular and respiratory disease. These potentially modifiable behavioral risk factors are contributing to an ever increasing global burden of disease and rising health-care costs in most countries (WHO, 2005). Indeed, tobacco use is a risk factor for

six of the eight leading causes of death in the world and is the single most preventable cause of death today (WHO, 2008). Sedentary lifestyle and poor nutrition are major risk factors for overweight and obesity which lead to adverse metabolic changes including increases in blood pressure, unfavorable cholesterol levels, and increased resistance to insulin, which then lead to an increased risk of coronary heart disease (CHD), stroke, diabetes mellitus, and several forms of cancer (WHO, 2002). The World Health Organization's 2002 World Health Report indicated that physical inactivity alone now causes about 15% of the disease burden associated with diabetes, heart disease, and some cancers (WHO, 2002). Additionally, poor nutrition, including low intake of fruit and vegetables and high intake of (saturated) fat, sugar, and salt, is responsible for almost 3 million deaths a year due to the resulting development of cardiovascular disease (CVD) and cancer (WHO, 2002).

Ischemic heart disease and cerebrovascular disease were identified as the global leading causes of mortality, accounting for 42.4% of all deaths across the world in 2000 (WHO, 2001). It has been estimated that without action to address the underlying lifestyle risk factors, noncommunicable chronic diseases will account for a further 17% of deaths globally by 2015 (WHO, 2005). Of even greater concern is the fact that while unhealthy lifestyle behaviors and their associated diseases are already at high levels in developed countries, they are now also becoming increasingly prevalent in developing countries as well (WHO, 2002).

B. Oldenburg (✉)
Department of Epidemiology and Preventive Medicine,
Monash University, 89 Commercial Rd, Melbourne,
VIC 3004, Australia
e-mail: brian.oldenburg@med.monash.edu.au

A. Steptoe (ed.), *Handbook of Behavioral Medicine*, DOI 10.1007/978-0-387-09488-5_62,   969
© Springer Science+Business Media, LLC 2010

In summary, the established links between behavior and health are now very considerable. Research in a number of different chronic diseases has now clearly established the complex interplay that occurs between behavioral, psychological, social, and environmental factors and how collectively all of these factors can have an important bearing on disease progression, quality of life, and health outcomes (WHO, 2002). Addressing key lifestyle risk factors can lead to improved health (primary prevention), reduced risk of disease (secondary prevention), and improved health outcomes (tertiary prevention). While a substantial evidence base has established the effectiveness of lifestyle change approaches as an important component of smoking cessation (Barth et al, 2008; DiClemente et al, 1991), chronic disease prevention and management through lifestyle changes related to diet and physical activity are not nearly as well developed (Yach et al, 2005). For example, the first *US Surgeon General's Report on Smoking and Health* was published in 1964 (US Department of Health and Human Services, 1964), but the first *US Surgeon General's Reports* on *Nutrition* (US Department of Health and Human Services, 1988, 1996) and on *Physical Activity* (US Department of Health and Human Services, 1988, 1996) were not published until over 20 years later, in 1988 and 1996, respectively. Furthermore, a number of self-care behaviors such as regular blood glucose monitoring and adherence to treatment regimens that involve the taking of multiple medications and also complex clinical care are also often required for management of chronic diseases such as heart disease and diabetes. Therefore, it is important to establish the effectiveness of approaches targeting self-care behaviors either alone or in combination with other lifestyle behaviors.

This chapter reviews the existing evidence base for behavioral interventions in relation to the prevention and management of chronic disease. Our focus is on key lifestyle and self-care behaviors – dietary behaviors, exercise, smoking, and disease management behaviors – that are causally linked to circulatory and commonly related conditions, including CVD, diabetes, and respiratory conditions. The review is conducted in three steps. First, we consider the evidence for the effectiveness for behavioral interventions by considering the systematic reviews in this field. Next, we supplement these findings with issues and findings from relevant narrative reviews. Finally, we discuss the implications of these findings for future research and practice in the field.

2 Overview of Systematic Reviews of Behavioral Change Interventions

2.1 Search Strategy and Selection Criteria

We identified and conducted a review of systematic reviews of behavioral intervention trials targeting lifestyle risk factors related to the prevention and/or management of circulatory and related conditions. Suitable reviews were identified by conducting an electronic search with the Database of Systematic Reviews of the *Cochrane Library* (Issue 3, 2009) and by crossing the keywords 'diet,' 'eating,' 'physical activity,' 'exercise,' 'smoking,' 'nutrition,' 'lifestyle,' 'behavior,' 'change,' 'smoking,' 'obesity,' 'overweight,' and 'adiposity.' These were crossed separately with 'cardiovascular,' 'heart disease,' 'coronary,' 'metabolic syndrome,' 'type 2 diabetes,' 'pre-diabetes,' and 'chronic disease.' Last, the search was combined with 'intervention' or 'trial.' We identified 165 reviews published between 1997 and 2009. We selected only reviews that were published in English and related to adults aged 18 or above. Reviews were excluded if they were: (1) related to medical conditions other than circulatory and associated conditions (e.g., psychiatric disorders, pregnancy, HIV/AIDS, cancer); (2) pharmacological interventions and did not incorporate any explicit lifestyle or behavioral change strategies; (3) primarily focused on interventions to treat biological mechanisms; (4) focused primarily on determinants of health behaviors rather than health behavior change per se; and (5) primarily narrative or qualitative reviews. We identified 27 reviews that met these inclusion criteria and these reviews form the basis of our evaluation of the effectiveness of lifestyle interventions for this chapter. Additionally, we conducted a search that also included other databases (PSYCINFO, MEDLINE) in order to identify non-systematic and narrative reviews that considered other relevant issues that are not usually well addressed by systematic reviews. These other issues are discussed in more detail in the final section of this chapter.

Among the 27 systematic reviews included from the Cochrane Library, there were six on nutrition and diet (Table 62.1, SR1–6), four on exercise (SR7–10), three on both diet and exercise (SR11–13), five on smoking (SR14–18), and one on multiple risk factors (SR19). Another eight reviews evaluated interventions targeting different aspects of disease management (SR20–27).

2.2 Characteristics of the Intervention Trials in the Systematic Reviews

2.2.1 Target Population

The reviews considered lifestyle interventions that target adult populations on a continuum from healthy people to people with elevated disease risk through to people with established disease.

2.2.2 Intervention Setting

Diet and physical activity interventions were predominantly conducted in health-care settings, although some worksite and other community interventions were also represented in the reviews. Smoking intervention settings were more varied and included other community settings and delivery systems, including the use of mass media. Disease management interventions were most often delivered via health-care or related settings.

2.2.3 Mode of Delivery

Channels of delivery were varied and diverse, although face-to-face delivery – either individually or in groups – was the most common approach utilized. Other approaches included delivery via telephone, internet, mail, and mass media. Most interventions were delivered by health professionals. Many different kinds of professionals were involved in delivery of smoking interventions including counselors, psychotherapists, teachers, and pharmacists, in addition to nurses and physicians. There were two systematic reviews of intervention delivery by peers.

2.2.4 Purpose of Systematic Reviews

The primary objective for all reviews was to establish the efficacy of the interventions in terms of clinical, behavioral, and/or other outcomes. Typically, a number of comparisons were included, with the main one being a comparison between a single intervention condition and some kind of usual or routine care. A number of reviews also assessed the relative efficacy of different types of interventions (e.g., diet only vs. diet and exercise); different modes of delivery (e.g., physicians vs. nurses; individuals vs. groups); or different intensities or duration of interventions. Often, however, when these latter comparisons were a secondary objective of the review, the data available and sample sizes were insufficient for drawing any definitive conclusions. Except for a few exceptions, the reviews did not evaluate the influence of setting or delivery on outcomes.

Table 62.1 Summary of systematic reviews

Authors	Brief titles	Outcomes Behavior	Physiological and anthropometric outcomes	Disease outcomes	Quality of life/ cost-effectiveness	Mortality
SR1 (Hooper et al, 2004)	Dietary salt reduction for preventing CVD	N/A	Urinary sodium excretion: −35.5 mmol/l Systolic RR: −1.1 mmHg Diastolic RR: −0.6 mmHg	Cardiovascular events inconsistently defined/reported	N/A	Deaths inconsistently defined/reported
SR2 (Hooper et al, 2000)	Dietary fat reduction for preventing CVD	N/A	N/A	Cardiovascular events: −16% for all studies; −24% for studies with follow-up > 2 years	N/A	Cardiovascular mortality: non-significant trend Total mortality: no effect
SR3 (Brunner et al, 2007)	Dietary advice for reducing cardiovascular risk	Fruit/vegetable intake: +1.25 servings/day Fiber intake: + 6 g/day Total fat intake: −4.5% E Saturated fat intake: −2.4% E	Urinary sodium excretion: −44.2 mmol/l Systolic RR: −2.1 mmHg Diastolic RR: −1.1 mmHg Total cholesterol: −0.16 mmol/l LDL cholesterol: −0.18 mmol/l	N/A	N/A	N/A
SR4 (Nield et al, 2008)	Dietary advice for the prevention of T2DM in adults	N/A	Significant (p<0.05) reductions in BMI, risk ratio, triglycerides, and improvements in HDL cholesterol, insulin resistance, and glucose tolerance in one study	Incidence of type 2 diabetes: −33% (6 years) in one study	N/A	N/A
SR5 (Nield et al, 2007)	Dietary advice for treatment of T2DM in adults	N/A because of heterogeneity/poor quality of data	N/A because of heterogeneity/poor quality of data	N/A because of heterogeneity/poor quality of data	N/A	N/A because of heterogeneity/poor quality of data
SR6 (Thompson et al, 2003)	Dietary advice for cholesterol reduction	N/A	Total cholesterol: −0.25 mmol/l dietitian versus doctor; ns. dietitian versus self-help; N/A dietitian versus nurse	N/A	N/A	N/A
SR7 (Rees et al, 2004b)	Exercise-based rehabilitation for heart failure	Exercise duration: +2.38 min Distance on 6-min walk: +40.9 m	VO₂max: +2.16 ml/kg/min Work capacity: +15.1 Watts		HRQoL: 7/9 studies found improvements	

Table 62.1 (Continued)

Authors	Brief titles	Outcomes Behavior	Physiological and anthropometric outcomes	Disease outcomes	Quality of life/cost-effectiveness	Mortality
SR8 (Jolliffe et al, 2001)	Exercise-based rehabilitation for coronary heart disease	Smoking: comprehensive rehabilitation no effect	All findings from comprehensive rehabilitation: Total cholesterol: −0.57 mmol/l LDL cholesterol: −0.51 mmol/l Triglycerides: −0.29 mmol/l	Non-fatal myocardial infarction: no effect	HRQoL: small improvements or no effect in 11 studies	Total cardiac mortality/all cause mortality: exercise only −31%/−27%; comprehensive rehabilitation −26%/−13%
SR9 (Thomas et al, 2006)	Exercise for T2DM	N/A	VO_2max: no effect in two studies HbA_{1c}: −0.6% BMI: no effect Visceral adipose tissue: −45.4 cm^2 Total cholesterol: no effect Triglycerides: −0.25 mmol/l Systolic and diastolic RR: no effect	N/A	QoL: no effect in one study	N/A
SR10 (Ashworth et al, 2005)	Home versus center-based physical activity programs in older adults	1-year adherence to exercise program: 75–79% home based/53% center based in two studies Peak walking time: center-based improved significantly more Smoking: no effect in one study	VO_2max: significant improvement in home- and center-based exercise groups at 6 months Lipids: no significant changes at 1 year, no difference between home- versus center-based exercise groups BMI: no effect	N/A	HRQoL: no change or small improvement in three studies; no differences between home versus center-based exercise groups	N/A
SR11 (Orozco et al, 2008)	Exercise or exercise and diet for preventing T2DM	N/A	Weight, BMI, waist circumference: improvement in exercise plus diet versus control compromised by high statistical heterogeneity Systolic RR: −4 mmHg Diastolic RR: −2 mmHg Fasting plasma glucose: −0.59 exercise plus diet versus control 2-h GTT: improvement in exercise plus diet	Incidence of type 2 diabetes: −37% in exercise plus diet interventions; no difference between diet only/exercise only and control or with each other	Cost-effectiveness: two studies concluded to be cost-effective	N/A

Table 62.1 (Continued)

Authors	Brief titles	Outcomes Behavior	Physiological and anthropometric outcomes	Disease outcomes	Quality of life/ cost-effectiveness	Mortality
			Total, LDL, and HDL cholesterol: no effect Triglycerides: −0.14 mmol/l in exercise plus diet versus control			
SR12 (Norris et al, 2005b)	Long-term non-pharmacological weight loss interventions for pre-diabetes adults	N/A	Weight: −2.8 kg at one year. BMI: −1.3 kg/m^2 HbA$_{1c}$: −0.3 to 0.0%. Systolic and diastolic RR: small decrease in most studies Lipids: minor improvements	Incidence of type 2 diabetes: significant reduction in 3/5 studies.	N/A	N/A
SR13 (Norris et al, 2005a)	Long-term non-pharmacological weight loss interventions for adults with T2DM	N/A	Weight: −1.7 kg or 3.1% for any intervention versus control with 1–2 year f-u HbA$_{1c}$: −2.6 to 1.0% in different types of interventions	N/A	N/A	N/A
SR14 (Rice and Stead, 2008)	Nursing interventions for smoking cessation	Risk ratio for quitting: overall 1.28; weak evidence for lower intensity interventions; weak evidence for additional telephone support	N/A	N/A	N/A	N/A
SR15 (Stead et al, 2008)	Physician advice for smoking cessation	Risk ratio for quitting: overall 1.66; intensive versus minimal 1.37; follow-up versus no follow-up 1.52	N/A	Lung cancer: no effect at 20 years in one study	NNT = 35–120	Total mortality and coronary disease mortality: no effect at 20 years in one study
SR16 (Barth et al, 2008)	Psychosocial interventions for smoking cessation in CHD patients	Odds ratio (OR) for quitting: overall 1.66; intensive versus brief 1.98; behavioral therapies versus usual care 1.69; telephone support versus usual care 1.58; self-help versus usual care 1.48	N/A	N/A	NNT = 10	N/A

Table 62.1 (Continued)

Authors	Brief titles	Outcomes Behavior	Physiological and anthropometric outcomes	Disease outcomes	Quality of life/cost-effectiveness	Mortality
SR17 (Carr and Ebbert, 2006)	Interventions for tobacco cessation in dental setting	OR for tobacco abstinence rate: 1.44; no difference between those actively seeking versus not seeking treatment	N/A	N/A	NNT = 33	N/A
SR18 (Sowden et al, 2003)	Community interventions for preventing smoking in young people	Smoking prevalence: 2/13 studies reported differences between community intervention versus control	N/A	N/A	N/A	N/A
SR19 (Ebrahim et al, 2006)	Multiple risk factor interventions for primary prevention of CHD	OR for reduction in smoking prevalence: 0.80.	Systolic RR: −3.6 mmHg. Diastolic RR: −2.8 mmHg Total cholesterol: −0.07 mmol/l	N/A	N/A	CHD mortality: no effect Total mortality: no effect
SR20 (Schedlbauer et al, 2004)	Interventions to improve adherence to lipid lowering medication	Adherence: significant effect in 3/8 studies	Total cholesterol: 1/4 studies reported significant improvement	N/A	N/A	N/A
SR21 (Welschen et al, 2005)	Self-monitoring of blood glucose in patients with T2DM who are not using insulin	N/A	HbA$_{1c}$: small but significant improvement in 2/6 studies	N/A	HRQoL: no effect in one study	N/A
SR22 (Vermeire et al, 2005)	Interventions for improving adherence to treatment recommendations in people with T2DM	Smoking cessation incidence: −15% higher in intervention versus comparison in one study	HbA$_{1c}$: small but significant improvement in 10/13 studies with different types of interventions	N/A	HRQoL: no effect in one study	N/A

Table 62.1 (Continued)

Authors	Brief titles	Outcomes Behavior	Physiological and anthropometric outcomes	Disease outcomes	Quality of life/ cost-effectiveness	Mortality
SR23 (Deakin et al, 2005)	Group-based training for self-management strategies in people with T2DM	Heterogeneous measures for self-management, exercise, diet, foot care, self-monitoring: modest findings in support of intervention in 5/6 studies	Weight: −1.6 kg Systolic blood pressure: −5 mmHg Total cholesterol: no effect Triglycerides: no effect HbA_{1c}: −1.4% at 4–6 months; −0.8% at 12–14 months; −1.0% at 2 years Fasting blood glucose: −1.2 mmol/l	N/A	QoL: no significant effect OR for reduced need for diabetes medication: 11.8 (NNT = 5) Cost-effectiveness: $2.12 per point gained in QoL in one study	N/A
SR24 (Duke et al, 2009)	Individual patient education for people with T2DM	Smoking cessation: weak evidence from two studies	BMI: no effect (individual vs. usual care/group) Systolic/diastolic RR: no effect (individual vs. usual care/group) Total cholesterol: no effect (individual vs. usual care/group) HbA_{1c}: no overall effect for individual versus usual care; −0.3% among participants with baseline HbA_{1c} > 8%; no difference individual versus group	N/A	HRQoL: mixed findings from two studies	N/A
SR25 (Rees et al, 2004a)	Psychological interventions for CHD	Smoking: mixed findings in eight studies	Total cholesterol: −0.27 mmol/l LDL, HDL cholesterol: no effect Triglycerides: no effect	OR for reduction in non-fatal reinfarction: 0.78	Anxiety: SMD−0.08 Depression: SMD−0.3 Composite measure for mental health: SMD−0.22	Cardiac mortality: no effect Total mortality: no effect
SR26 (Dale et al, 2008)	Peer support telephone calls for improving health	Smoking : no effect in 1/3 studies Recovery behaviors: no effect in 1/3 studies	BMI, cholesterol, HbA_{1c}: no effect in 1/3 studies	N/A	HRQoL: no effect in 2/3 studies	N/A
SR27 (Foster et al, 2007)	Self-management education programs by lay leaders for people with chronic conditions	Exercise: SMD 0.20	N/A	N/A	HRQoL: no effect	N/A

QOL= quality of life; HRQOL= health-related quality of life; HbA_{1}c= glycated hemoglobin; OR = odds ratio; SMD=standardized mean difference

2.3 Intervention Outcomes

2.3.1 Dietary Interventions

Evaluation of dietary advice to reduce disease risk factors or to treat an existing disease is based on six reviews with approximately 44,000 participants. Outcomes of these reviews are listed in Table 62.1 (SR1–6). Usually, they were physiological or anthropometric risk factors. While behavior was reported in some trials as an indicator of intervention compliance, it was rarely measured as an outcome. Quality of life and cost-effectiveness were not reported. Overall, small but statistically significant improvements were found in physiological and anthropometric outcomes (Table 62.1, SR1–6). Only one review (Brunner et al, 2007) reported on behavioral outcomes: in comprehensive dietary interventions for reducing CVD risk, modest beneficial changes in behavior were translated into statistically significant improvements in physiological and anthropometric outcomes. Beneficial disease outcomes included reduction of cardiovascular events, but this effect could only be established for interventions to reduce fat (Hooper et al, 2000). Another disease outcome was reduction of type 2 diabetes incidence (Nield et al, 2008), but the finding was based on just one trial and therefore provided only weak evidence. Outcome evaluation of diet only interventions in treatment of type 2 diabetes (Nield et al, 2007) was rendered impossible by the heterogeneity and poor quality of the studies. The only review on dietary interventions capable of reporting on mortality (Hooper et al, 2000) found no statistically significant effects on either cardiovascular or total mortality.

Effects of intervention delivery and duration were evaluated in two of the dietary intervention reviews. While dietary advice from a dietitian was more effective than advice from a doctor, it was no more effective than fairly simple self-help material. Comparison between dietitians versus nurses was not possible because of limited data (Thompson et al, 2003). The beneficial effect of fat reduction to cardiovascular

events was limited to trials with intervention extending over 2 years (Hooper et al, 2000). Although one review (Hooper et al, 2000), p. 18) specifically referred to the potential benefits of applying a behavioral theory for improving intervention outcomes, none actually discussed the interventions within any sort of theoretical framework.

2.3.2 Exercise Only Interventions

Evaluation of exercise interventions covers over 10,000 participants but it is mainly based on reviews among patient populations. The intervention programs were heterogeneous (e.g., exercise alone or as part of comprehensive rehabilitation program including educational or psychological interventions) – often meaning that the independent effect of exercise could not be separated. A range of outcome measures was covered but typically the focus was on physiological measures and as a secondary outcome, quality of life. Morbidity and mortality were rarely studied, and no review reported on cost-effectiveness. Behavior was regarded as a compliance factor rather than a primary intervention outcome. None of the reviews discussed behavioral theories used in the interventions although the comprehensive rehabilitation programs often included an educational or psychosocial component.

Overall, exercise training was found to improve several of the measured physiological or anthropometric factors (Table 62.1, SR7–10), such as glycated hemoglobin (HbA_{1c}) among patients with type 2 diabetes (Thomas et al, 2006) and lipid profile among patients in comprehensive cardiac rehabilitation (Jolliffe et al, 2001). No reduction was found in body mass index (BMI), but body composition changed significantly, with adipose tissue decreasing and fat-free mass increasing. In most cases only short-term effects on risk factors could be established due to lack of long-term follow-ups. However, the one review with a longer follow-up was able to show reduction in both all cause and cardiac mortality (Jolliffe et al, 2001). Findings on quality of life were mixed, although most studies tended to have found small improvements.

Duration of the interventions ranged widely, and one review evaluated its effect on outcomes. Among patients with type 2 diabetes, decrease in HbA_{1c} was greater for briefer (< 6 months) interventions than for longer interventions (6–12 months) (Thomas et al, 2006). One review also evaluated the effects of intervention delivery on outcomes (Ashworth et al, 2005). Assessment of home- versus center-based physical activity programs in older adults showed that on the short term, center-based training produced better outcomes. However, two studies in the review were able to evaluate longer-term adherence (1–2 years) which was shown to be better in the home-based program.

2.3.3 Combined Diet and Exercise/Weight Reduction Interventions

Altogether 15,000 patients are included in the assessment of the efficacy of combined diet and exercise or weight reduction interventions on prevention (Norris et al, 2005b; Orozco et al, 2008) and treatment (Norris et al, 2005a) of type 2 diabetes. Prevention interventions included participants with elevated risk for type 2 diabetes, who typically (but not necessarily) had an impaired glucose tolerance. Behavior was not reported as a specific outcome measure although one review included physical activity and diet as indicators of compliance (Orozco et al, 2008). Typically, outcomes included incidence of type 2 diabetes and physiological and anthropometric risk factors (Table 62.1, SR11–13). None of the reviews were able to report on behavior or mortality. No aggregated data was provided for cost-effectiveness although two trials in one review provided support for cost-effectiveness (Orozco et al, 2008). Length of follow-up ranged from 12 months to 10 years (Norris et al, 2005b). Although most of the reviews mentioned the use of behavioral theories and/or specific intervention strategies (including goal setting, self-monitoring and feedback, and

stress management and coping), these were not systematically evaluated.

Small improvements were found in weight, BMI, and waist circumference (Table 62.1, SR11–13), although statistical heterogeneity for these outcomes was high and effects were minimized by significant weight loss in the comparison groups (Norris et al, 2005a). Modest, but statistically significant improvements were shown on many physiological and anthropometric outcomes. Both reviews on prevention of type 2 diabetes reported statistically significant reductions in the incidence of type 2 diabetes, but only one provided a pooled effect (Orozco et al, 2008).

Intervention duration per se was not shown to effect outcomes although the number of contacts correlated positively with weight loss among adults with pre-diabetes (Norris et al, 2005b). Furthermore, examination of different intervention arms suggested that multi-component interventions with low or very low calorie diets might help to achieve weight loss among patients with type 2 diabetes (Norris et al, 2005a).

2.3.4 Tobacco Control Interventions

Evaluation of tobacco control interventions is based on nearly 110,000 participants including mainly healthy adults. Without exception, the outcomes were always measured in terms of behavior. For interventions addressing cessation the outcome was abstinence, in prevention interventions it was smoking behavior (Table 62.1, SR14–18). None of the reviews reported on physiological or anthropometric outcomes or quality of life, and only one study reported on disease or mortality outcomes. Cost-effectiveness was not commonly reported although three reviews estimated the number required to treat one individual successfully (NNT). Unlike the dietary and exercise interventions, smoking interventions were commonly based on theoretical models, especially if they were delivered by professionals other than physicians or nurses. However, none of the reviews compared different theoretical approaches to behavior change.

Nursing interventions (Rice and Stead, 2008), physician advice (Stead et al, 2008), psychosocial interventions (Barth et al, 2008), and interventions delivered by oral health professionals in connection with oral examination (Carr and Ebbert, 2006) were all shown to be effective. The overall likelihood for quitting was 28–66% higher in these interventions in comparison to usual care. Heterogeneity of community interventions prevented pooling of those data, so overall quitting rates could not be established. However, only 2 out of the 13 community interventions were more effective than no treatment (Sowden et al, 2003). Estimated NNT ranged between 10 and 120, the lowest NNT being in CHD patients who tend to have high unassisted quit rates anyhow (30–50%) (Barth et al, 2008) and the highest NNT was in primary care patients, whose unassisted quit rate was estimated to be only 2–3% (Stead et al, 2008). The minimum follow-up time for all interventions was 6 months and the majority had 12 month or longer follow-up.

Higher intensity interventions increased the effectiveness of interventions. Psychosocial interventions including behavioral therapies outperformed usual care, as did those based on self-help or telephone support, but none of these were found superior to each other. Furthermore, a subgroup analysis among patients in the dental setting showed the interventions effective regardless of whether participants had actively sought treatment (Table 62.1).

2.3.5 Multiple Risk Factor Interventions

One extensive review with almost 150,000 participants evaluated the effects of multiple risk factor interventions among adults without clinical evidence of established CVD. All the trials compared an intervention comprising some form of education or counseling targeting combinations of diet, exercise, weight loss, smoking cessation, diabetes management, and use of medication with control groups receiving either usual care or no treatment. Behavioral theories underlying the interventions were rarely specified, with a few studies using the Transtheoretical Model of Stages of Change as an exception (DiClemente et al, 1991). Smoking was the most common behavioral outcome included, other reported outcomes included blood pressure, cholesterol, and mortality. Quality of life outcomes or cost-effectiveness were not reported.

Overall, the interventions had a small, positive effect on smoking prevalence (Table 62.1, SR19). Also, modest but statistically significant improvements were shown in blood pressure and cholesterol, but these were most likely related to pharmacological treatments rather than the lifestyle interventions used. Ten of the trials provided data on CHD mortality and total mortality, but overall, no effect could be established. Studies where participants had highest initial risk factor levels demonstrated larger improvements in these factors (Ebrahim et al, 2006).

2.3.6 Disease Management Interventions

Interventions for improving risk or disease management were assessed among almost 30,000 patients with vascular conditions. Included were interventions with a narrow focus to adherence to treatment recommendations (Table 62.1, SR20–21) as well as broader self-management education and support programs delivered by professionals (SR22–25) and peers (SR26–27). Reporting on outcomes focused on physiological and anthropometric risk factors but also behavior and quality of life were included. Only one review reported on disease outcomes and mortality.

The disease management interventions were probably even more heterogeneous in content, intensity, and duration than the other lifestyle interventions already described in this chapter. While some tackled only relatively simple behaviors (such as blood glucose monitoring or taking a lipid lowering medicine), others addressed very complex sets of behaviors (e.g., comprehensive disease management including lifestyle, self-care, and adherence to medical care). Rather surprisingly, the interventions targeting simpler behaviors were often more heterogeneous and more poorly described in the reviews. They also typically lacked any description of the behavioral component(s). The more comprehensive programs, however, were often theory based, well described, and they also allowed comparison of different modes of delivery.

Behavioral outcomes were rarely established in interventions targeting adherence (Table 62.1, SR20–21) and improvements in physiological outcomes tended to be small at best. None of the few studies including quality of life measures showed any significant effects on it. Morbidity and mortality outcomes were not reported for adherence interventions. The effect of intervention characteristics on the outcomes was not evaluated in any of the reviews.

The more comprehensive self-management programs delivered by professionals (Table 62.1, SR22–25) provided heterogeneous results in terms of behavior change. In terms of physiological or anthropometric outcomes among patients with type 2 diabetes, individual patient education was no better than usual care or group education (Duke et al, 2009). However, group training resulted in moderate improvement in most of these risk factors (Deakin et al, 2005). Disease and mortality outcomes were only measured among CHD patients. No effect was found on mortality, and the significant reduction in the number of non-fatal reinfarction was found to be influenced by publication bias (Rees et al, 2004a). Quality of life outcomes in interventions among type 2 diabetes patients were mixed, but CHD patients were shown to gain modest psychological benefit from the interventions in terms of reductions in anxiety and depression (Rees et al, 2004a).

Self-management programs by lay leaders had very little effect on behaviors, physiological and anthropometric outcomes, or quality of life (Table 62.1, SR26–27). None of the studies reported on morbidity or mortality (Dale et al, 2008; Foster et al, 2007).

3 Relevant Findings from Narrative Reviews

3.1 Intervention Settings

Some settings are likely to make recruitment, targeting, and tailoring of interventions easier than others. For example, schools and worksites are community settings where many people can easily be reached. However, findings from worksite diet and exercise programs (L. Anderson et al, 2009) only showed very modest reductions in weight and BMI. The worksite interventions were typically based on informational and behavioral strategies, with few having promoted changes to the work environment to support healthy behavioral choices. As with similar interventions in other settings, more intensive interventions (duration, number of components, structured vs. unstructured) were more effective (L. Anderson et al, 2009). It also seems that workplace interventions have tended to be quite focused compared to more generic lifestyle interventions. A recent meta-analysis (Abraham and Graham-Rower, 2009) showed more than three-fold effect sizes for physical activity interventions in comparison to general lifestyle change interventions.

3.2 Information and Communications Technology in Intervention Delivery

3.2.1 Web-Based Interventions

Information and communications technology (ICT) has become an increasingly popular channel for delivery of interventions. However, despite the exciting potential for ICT-delivered interventions, program reach and adherence are still a significant concern. Wantland et al reviewed web-based interventions with nearly 12,000 participants (Wantland et al, 2004). Compared with interventions utilizing more "traditional" means of delivery, web-based interventions report reaching an equal proportion of men and women. Although the average drop-out rate was relatively low (only 21%), this needs to be considered in relation to measures of program exposure and intensity. For example, participants showed significant variation in time spent per session (4.5–45 min). Some had only few logons while others entered the intervention site very frequently (from 2.6 over 32 weeks to 1008 logons/person over 36 weeks). The interventions included one-time studies, self-paced interventions, and longitudinal, repeated measures intervention studies (3–78 weeks). Despite wide variation in intensity, nearly all (16/17) studies revealed improved knowledge and/or behavioral outcomes (e.g., exercise duration, 18-month weight loss maintenance, participation in health care). Among users with chronic disease (Murray, 2006), interactive health communication applications have also been shown to improve knowledge, social support, self-efficacy, health behaviors, and clinical outcomes.

3.2.2 Interventions Delivered via Telephone

The telephone provides another channel with easy access for participants. Eakin et al reviewed 26 studies on diet and physical activity interventions, most delivered by different health professionals but some with automated telephone systems (that fully free the participants from both temporal and spatial restrictions) (Eakin et al, 2007). Recruitment methods influenced reach, with studies recruiting highly selected clinical samples and having stringent criteria reporting higher participation rates. However, few of the studies reported how representative their study populations were. Unlike many other interventions reviewed in this chapter, a majority of the telephone interventions were based on one or more specific theories, with Transtheoretical Model, Social Cognitive Theory, and/or Motivational Interviewing being the most commonly reported, however, the effect

of theory was not formally evaluated in the review.

The majority of the studies (20/26) reported significant behavioral improvements with a medium average effect size (0.60, [0.24–1.19]). Positive outcomes were reported for 69% of exercise studies, 83% of dietary behavior studies, and 75% of studies addressing both behaviors. Furthermore, the positive outcomes were associated with duration and intensity (number of calls) of the intervention (Eakin et al, 2007).

3.3 Effectiveness of Theory-Based Interventions

We found only a couple of reviews where the effectiveness of theory-based interventions was formally evaluated. Stage models propose that individuals can be distinguished by their behavior-related cognitions into discrete stages of action readiness, hence behavior change interventions are claimed to be most effective when tailored to match the needs of groups defined by the stages. van Sluijs et al reviewed effectiveness of stage-based lifestyle interventions in primary care with two kinds of outcomes: positive stage changes and behavior changes (van Sluijs et al, 2004). For physical activity and smoking, neither kind of change was achieved. For diet, limited evidence supported an effect on stage change and an effect on behavior change. Altogether, the findings do not lend much support for stage theories.

Motivational Interviewing (MI) (Miller and Rollnick, 2002) is a theory-based technique rather than a theory. It is based on the empowerment ideology (J. M. Anderson, 1996) and Self-Determination Theory (Deci and Ryan, 1980). It was first developed as a counseling method for working with patients with substance abuse, but it is increasingly frequently used also in other lifestyle interventions. Dunn et al reviewed 29 randomized trials using motivational interviewing interventions across different behaviors including diet and exercise (Dunn et al, 2001).

Although this method was found effective in substance abuse interventions, data were inadequate to judge the effects in other domains. However, increase in exercise was consistent in size and direction (although many of the studies were underpowered). A positive finding across domains was that the effects of MI did not diminish with longer follow-ups. Interactions between client attribute and treatment were understudied and "sparse and inconsistent findings revealed little about the mechanism by which MI works" (p. 1725). Furthermore, it remained unknown what levels of MI training, skill, and duration would be optimal.

Self-regulation theories emphasize the importance of goal setting, planning, and review in behavior change and maintenance. Reviewing worksite physical activity interventions, Abraham et al (Abraham and Graham-Rower, 2009) found that setting specific goals that defined the frequency and duration of physical activity, setting of graded tasks, and goal review techniques enhanced outcomes of the interventions in comparison to interventions without these techniques. Furthermore, interventions providing advice, even if it was individually tailored, were not effective (Abraham and Graham-Rower, 2009). Another review suggested that problem solving strategies – also a technique based on self-regulation theories – might be a critical intervention element in promoting long-term weight loss (Seo and Sa, 2008).

4 Lifestyle Change – Current Issues and Future Challenges

While systematic reviews are a good method for identifying and summarizing the effects of lifestyle change interventions on important behavioral, clinical, and disease outcomes, it is important to acknowledge that they do have some significant limitations. Importantly, information on many key issues can be very limited in systematic reviews and detailed information

cannot be reported from all the original studies on issues and topics that would be important for the research question being addressed in the review. The analysis of and reporting on sub-questions can also be problematic because of the small number of studies and/or sample sizes related to these. We have outlined some of the important unresolved issues and questions in relation to behavioral interventions in Table 62.2. The problems related to study designs and measurements have been adequately discussed in the original reviews and also in the previous section, so they will not be addressed further here. In this final section, we will discuss major findings from the reviews in light of the two other sets of issues, the intervention features and delivery, and sustainability and future uptake of the interventions.

4.1 Features of the Intervention and Its Delivery

Generally, it is impossible to say whether interventions targeted to one specific behavioral component or behavior are more effective in addressing it than a more comprehensive intervention might be. When targeting physical activity in the worksite, less comprehensive interventions were not necessarily more effective. When addressing disease management, more comprehensive interventions were reportedly more effective. Many interventions were shown to have a positive effect on some lifestyle behaviors or clinical risk factors, while not affecting others. This strongly suggests that a number of interventions and delivery components are likely needed to address all aspects of behavior change related to preventing and managing a specific chronic disease such as CVD or diabetes. This is certainly the case at a population level, however, it is also likely to be the case at a more individual level as well. This view is more strongly supported by the evidence from the field of tobacco control (WHO, 2008) with further support coming from community intervention trials over the past 30 years

Table 62.2 Important issues arising from systematicreviews of interventions targeting lifestyle factors

1. Study design and measurement
  o Small, underpowered studies
  o Heterogeneity and lack of specificity in relation to participants:
    – Socio-demographic characteristics
    – Clinical characteristics
  o Heterogeneity in measurement
    – Different outcomes
    – Lack of key outcomes in relation to behavior, morbidity, mortality, cost-effectiveness
    – Variability in the quality and type of measures used
  o Heterogeneity in length of follow-up
    – Lack of long-term follow-up
  o Lack of implementation and process measurement
  o Difficulty in disentangling the effects of other factors
    – Medication use
    – Mediating and moderating factors

2. Features of the intervention and its delivery
  o Heterogeneity and lack of specificity in relation to:
    – Content
    – Setting
    – Intensity
    – Duration
    – Delivery person/system
  o Intervention is a "black box," i.e., components are either undefined or impossible to separate
    from each other
  o Inadequate use and reporting of health behavior theory, including:
    – Theoretical model for expected behavior changes and determinants
    – Techniques to change behaviors
    – Compliance by program users with techniques to change behaviors
    – Systematic analysis of theory-based moderators and mediators

3. Intervention sustainability and future uptake
  o What were the necessary versus sufficient components?
  o Intensive interventions but small effects
  o Economic outcomes and costing data are lacking
  o Long-term outcomes are not established

(Sowden et al, 2003). It is further supported by more recent evidence in relation to interventions that focus on reducing absolute risk of a number of chronic diseases (Ebrahim et al, 2006; Goldstein et al, 2004; Pronk et al, 2004; WHO, 2002).

The fact that little particularly useful information was found in reviews in relation to settings for program delivery reflects the complexity of this issue as well. Clearly, some settings are likely to make recruitment, targeting, and tailoring of interventions easier than others. For example, schools and worksites are community settings where many people can easily be reached. When recruiting people for telephone interventions where no "natural" setting necessarily exists, recruitment was generally shown to be easier when conducted via a clinical setting (Eakin et al, 2007). Furthermore, as the review on exercise training among older adults showed (Ashworth et al, 2005), what works best setting wise might change over time as participants' needs change. Instead of thinking in terms of home-based versus center-based programs, maybe the ideal would be a program where the participant can choose from either or both and change back and forth between the options as their personal circumstances and needs change.

Intensity and duration are issues for which the reviews do provide some important findings. More intensive and longer interventions are generally more effective than less intensive and briefer interventions, and it is critically important that follow-up is included in an intervention in order to enhance maintenance and sustainability. However, there may be a trade-off between effectiveness and availability of resources, but this cannot be assessed without cost-effectiveness studies. Attrition can also be very problematic in long-lasting interventions. However, we do not know much about individual differences in relation to intervention intensity and duration. As the review on internet interventions showed (Strecher, 2007), if people get to choose for themselves, some will decide to be intensively involved for long periods of time while others only have very fleeting and brief contact with the intervention.

There is not much information in relation to which professionals are best able to delivery which kinds of lifestyle interventions. While physicians can deliver lifestyle advice and programs in an effective and durable fashion under certain circumstances, there are likely to be many other professionals who can do so much more cost-effectively. However, they do not necessarily have the same "window of opportunity" as physicians might have, particularly those in the primary care setting. There are also some interventions, such as dietary advice, which may be delivered quite effectively and efficiently through the use of information and communications technology. The delivery of such programs by lay leaders or peers (Dale et al, 2008; Foster et al, 2007) is another area that needs more investigation, particularly, when associated with management of a disease such as diabetes (Fisher et al, 2010).

Automated telephone programs and the internet also have great potential to supplement and support health-care settings and professionals as platforms for effective intervention delivery. The outcomes are by and large moderately positive on several measures (Dale et al, 2008; Eakin et al, 2007; Strecher, 2007). However, despite the burgeoning interest in internet-based interventions, the potential of the internet in interactivity – user navigation, collaborative filters, expert systems, and human-to-human interaction – is still poorly utilized and understood for the delivery of lifestyle change programs (Strecher, 2007). It is certainly the case that the internet provides tremendous opportunities for making use of the individual's characteristics as active ingredients for tailoring and delivery of programs. However, the ways these characteristics moderate the impact of interventions need to be explored first and then purposefully utilized. Furthermore, there are now tremendous opportunities to combine current knowledge with new interactive and mobile technologies, as well as with consumer and other (medical and public health) informatics systems (Strecher, 2007).

Probably more important than who or which system delivers an intervention per se is how well the intervention components and the system used to deliver these, properly address the participant's needs, and the extent to which these are related to their current knowledge, attitudes, skills or support, or most likely, a combination of all of these. The need for theory to inform more appropriately these issues as well as the development, implementation, and evaluation of lifestyle change programs is a really important issue which has received increasing attention in recent years and whole textbooks have been devoted to this issue (e.g. Bartholomew et al, 2006; Glanz et al, 2002). As already mentioned, few of the systematic reviews discussed in this chapter discuss in detail the importance of behavioral or other kinds of theories and only a couple of reviews actually analyzed the use of theory-based interventions. The Transtheoretical Model of Stages of Change (Prochaska and DiClemente, 1982) has been one of the most frequently cited theories in both smoking and telephone interventions in the reviews that have been considered in this chapter. Consequently, it is really the only theory with adequate data for recent evaluation. These data, however, only lend equivocal support to the theory. Abraham, among others, has critiqued stage models for oversimplifying "the cognitive architecture" by defining stage transitions by single determinants and for implying cognitive uniformity within stages (Abraham, 2008). Moreover, instead of stage-based interventions, he has suggested use of multi-determinant, multi-goal continuum approaches. Such an approach recognizes graded discontinuities throughout the development of action readiness from attitude formation to maintenance of behavior change as a process that is not linear and that includes movement in both directions (Abraham, 2008).

In addition to health behavior theories that help intervention designers to identify psychosocial determinants for behavior change and target and tailor interventions, the need for explicit use of theory-based health behavior techniques has also been acknowledged (Abraham and Michie, 2008). Reporting the use of these specific techniques in interventions would take the field forward and allow gathering of evidence for what works.

The approach advocated by Abraham is interesting, not just because of the perspective it provides on behavior change, but also because it provides a framework for conceptualizing a more menu-based approach to interventions. In other words, instead of providing one uniform or stage-specified intervention to all program participants, it is probably more appropriate to provide a menu of interventions from which potential program participants can then self-tailor a combination of interventions that best suit their personal needs and circumstances. Utilizing such an approach in relation to the interactive potential that different ICT and web-based systems can provide is likely to lead to a significant paradigm shift in the way in which lifestyle change interventions are provided to and accessed by the community over the next few years. This will lead to a shift away from the view of the individual/patient as an almost passive recipient of expert-driven interventions toward the individual becoming a much more active participant in deciding on their own needs and how to address these.

4.2 Intervention Sustainability in the "Real World" and Future Uptake of Interventions

With a few notable exceptions, most published lifestyle change intervention trials have only achieved at best, quite modest outcomes, even when evaluated under very controlled conditions. The further implementation and dissemination of such programs under more "real world" settings is often not evaluated very well (Glanz and Oldenburg, 2008), so we do not usually know whether even these modest effects are maintained. The Diabetes Initiative of the Robert Wood Johnson Foundation in the United States evaluated the resources and supports for self-management of diabetes in various community settings. The program identified six key supports for program success: individualized assessment and tailored measurement; collaborative goal setting; enhancement of key skills for disease management, health behaviors, and problem solving; continuity of high-quality, safe clinical care; ongoing follow-up and support; and a very important role for supportive community resources (Fisher et al, 2005). The authors conclude that the concept of "equifinality" is especially helpful for thinking about how such programs can work for individuals in community settings, that is, that different procedures, strategies, or programs can work in complementary ways to achieve similar ends or effects.

Generally speaking, intensive and costly lifestyle change interventions for people with minimal risk might not be very cost-effective, and therefore, more community-wide, population-based, or upstream social and economic interventions are likely to be more cost-effective. Given the increasing pressures on limited resources for health care and prevention in most countries and the increasing burden of chronic diseases, it is important that resources are prioritized for populations where the interventions will be most effective.

Although none of the systematic reviews we have described contained significant findings in relation to cost-effectiveness, a number of the authors raised the issue of interventions that were evaluated under very controlled conditions, being too resource intensive for broader uptake (Ebrahim et al, 2006). Further investigation of the cost-effectiveness of lifestyle interventions is essential in order to allow for priority setting and for governments and major donors to justify spending resources on modifying behavioral risk factors. The WHO has recognized the importance of reducing lifestyle risk factors in cost-effective ways, stating in their 2002 World Health Report that their ultimate goal is to help governments of all countries to raise the healthy life expectancy of their populations. However, the cost-effectiveness of lifestyle interventions to prevent mortality and morbidity from preventable chronic diseases should also be appropriately demonstrated in resource poor countries before recommending their "scaling up."

5 Summary

If properly developed, implemented and evaluated lifestyle change interventions have excellent potential to prevent disease, to improve the self-management of existing conditions, and to increase the quality of life of individuals in all countries. Some evidence also points to the cost-effectiveness of lifestyle change interventions, even when compared to more traditional medical interventions, but this is definitely a field that needs more research. Most importantly, however, it is clear that such approaches can not only have a beneficial impact on particular disease(s) or risk factor(s) in individuals, but they can also have significant effects and benefits for prevention in populations. Use of contemporary communication technologies is an especially exciting development, especially when combined with more traditional delivery approaches used by health professionals, peer leaders and others in health care and other community settings. Given the very rapid increase of disease burden attributable to chronic non-communicable disease as a result of lifestyle behaviors in developing regions of the world, these kinds of approaches also urgently need further development and adapting to the growing health needs and challenges of these part of the world as well (Beaglehole and Bonita, 2008).

Acknowledgment Thanks to Carla Renwick for so much invaluable assistance with the preparation and finalizing of the final manuscript.

References

Abraham, C. (2008). Beyond stages of change: multi-determinant continuum models of action readiness and menu-based interventions. *Applied Psychol, 57*, 30–41.

Abraham, C., and Graham-Rower, E. (2009). Are work-site interventions effective in increasing physical activity? A systematic review and meta-analysis. *Health Psychol Rev, 3*, 108–144.

Abraham, C., and Michie, S. (2008). A taxonomy of behavior change techniques used in interventions. *Health Psychol, 27*, 379–387.

Anderson, J. M. (1996). Empowering patients: issues and strategies. *Soc Sci Med, 43*, 697–705.

Anderson, L., Quinn, T., Glanz, K., Ramirez, G., Kahwati, L. et al (2009). The effectiveness of worksite nutrition and physical activity interventions for controlling employee overweight and obesity. *Am J Prev Med, 37*, 340–357.

Ashworth, N. L., Chad, K. E., Harrison, E. L., Reeder, B. A., and Marshall, S. C. (2005). Home versus center based physical activity programs in older adults. *Cochrane Database Syst* Rev, CD004017.

Barth, J., Critchley, J., and Bengel, J. (2008). Psychosocial interventions for smoking cessation in patients with coronary heart disease. *Cochrane Database Syst Rev*, CD006886.

Bartholomew, L. K., Parcel, G., Kok, G., and Gottlieb, N. (2006). *Planning Health Promotion Programs: An Intervention Mapping Approach, 2nd Ed.* San Francisco: Jossey-Bass.

Beaglehole, R., and Bonita, R. (2008). Global public health: a scorecard. *Lancet, 372*, 1988–1996.

Brunner, E. J., Rees, K., Ward, K., Burke, M., and Thorogood, M. (2007). Dietary advice for reducing cardiovascular risk.[update of Cochrane Database Syst Rev. 2005;(4)]. *Cochrane Database Syst Rev*CD002128.

Carr, A. B., and Ebbert, J. O. (2006). Interventions for tobacco cessation in the dental setting. *Cochrane Database Syst Rev*, CD005084.

Dale, J., Caramlau, I. O., Lindenmeyer, A., and Williams, S. M. (2008). Peer support telephone calls for improving health. *Cochrane Database Syst Rev*, CD006903.

Deakin, T., McShane, C. E., Cade, J. E., and Williams, R. D. (2005). Group based training for self-management strategies in people with type 2 diabetes mellitus. *Cochrane Database Syst* Rev, CD003417.

Deci, E. L., and Ryan, R. M. (1980). Self-determination theory – the iteration of psychophysiology and motivation. *Psychophysiology, 17*, 321.

DiClemente, C. C., Prochaska, J. O., Fairhurst, S. K., Velicer, W. F., Velasquez, M. M. et al (1991). The process of smoking cessation: an analysis of precontemplation, contemplation, and preparation stages of change. *J Consult Clin Psychol, 59*, 295–304.

Duke, S. A., Colagiuri, S., and Colagiuri, R. (2009). Individual patient education for people with type 2 diabetes mellitus. *Cochrane Database Syst Rev*, CD005268.

Dunn, C., Deroo, L., and Rivara, F. P. (2001). The use of brief interventions adapted from motivational interviewing across behavioral domains: a systematic review. *Addiction, 96*, 1725–1742.

Eakin, E. G., Lawler, S. P., Vandelanotte, C., and Owen, N. (2007). Telephone interventions for physical activity and dietary behavior change: a systematic review. *Am J Prev Med, 32*, 419–434.

Ebrahim, S., Beswick, A., Burke, M., and Davey Smith, G. (2006). Multiple risk factor interventions for primary prevention of coronary heart disease. *Cochrane Database Syst Rev*, CD001561.

Fisher, E. B., Brownson, C. A., O'Toole, M. L., Shetty, G., Anwuri, V. V. et al (2005). Ecological approaches to self-management: the case of diabetes. *Am J Public Health, 95*, 1523–1535.

Fisher, E. B., Earp, J. A., Maman, S., and Zolotor, A. (2010). Cross-cultural and international adaptation of peer support for diabetes management. *Fam Pract, 27*(1), i6–16. Epub 2009 Mar 10.

Foster, G., Taylor, S. J., Eldridge, S. E., Ramsay, J., and Griffiths, C. J. (2007). Self-management education programmes by lay leaders for people with chronic conditions. *Cochrane Database Syst Rev*, CD005108.

Glanz, K., Lewis, F. M., and Rimer, B. (Eds.). (2002). *Health Behavior and Health Education: Theory, Research and Practice*. San Francisco: Jossey-Bass.

Glanz, K., and Oldenburg, B. (2008). Diffusions of Innovation. In K. Glanz, B. Rimer, & K. Viswanath (Eds.), *Health Behavior and Health Education: Theory, Research, and Practice, 4th Ed*. San Francisco: Jossey-Bass Inc.

Goldstein, M. G., Whitlock, E. P., DePue, J., and Planning Committee of the Addressing Multiple Behavioral Risk Factors in Primary Care, P. (2004). Multiple behavioral risk factor interventions in primary care. Summary of research evidence. *Am J Prev Med, 27*, 61–79.

Hooper, L., Bartlett, C., Davey, S. G., and Ebrahim, S. (2004). Advice to reduce dietary salt for prevention of cardiovascular disease. *Cochrane Database Syst Rev*, CD003656.

Hooper, L., Summerbell, C. D., Higgins, J. P., Thompson, R. L., Clements, G. et al (2000). Reduced or modified dietary fat for prevention of cardiovascular disease. *Cochrane Database Syst Rev*, CD002137.

Jolliffe, J. A., Rees, K., Taylor, R. S., Thompson, D., Oldridge, N. et al (2001). Exercise-based rehabilitation for coronary heart disease. *Cochrane Database Syst Rev*, CD001800.

Miller, W. R., and Rollnick, S. (2002). *Motivational Interviewing: Preparing People for Change, 2nd Ed*. New York: Guilford Press.

Murray, S. (2006). Doubling the burden: chronic disease. *CMAJ, 174*, 771.

Nield, L., Moore, H. J., Hooper, L., Cruickshank, J. K., Vyas, A. et al (2007). Dietary advice for treatment of type 2 diabetes mellitus in adults. *Cochrane Database Syst Rev*, CD004097.

Nield, L., Summerbell, C. D., Hooper, L., Whittaker, V., and Moore, H. (2008). Dietary advice for the prevention of type 2 diabetes mellitus in adults. *Cochrane Database Syst Rev*, CD005102.

Norris, S. L., Zhang, X., Avenell, A., Gregg, E., Brown, T. J. et al (2005a). Long-term non-pharmacologic weight loss interventions for adults with type 2 diabetes. *Cochrane Database Syst Rev*, CD004095.

Norris, S. L., Zhang, X., Avenell, A., Gregg, E., Schmid, C. H. et al (2005b). Long-term non-pharmacological weight loss interventions for adults with prediabetes. *Cochrane Database Syst Rev*, CD005270.

Orozco, L. J., Buchleitner, A. M., Gimenez-Perez, G., Roque, I. F. M., Richter, B. et al (2008). Exercise or exercise and diet for preventing type 2 diabetes mellitus. *Cochrane Database Syst Rev*, CD003054.

Prochaska, J. O., and DiClemente, C. C. (1982). Transtheoretical therapy: toward a more integrative model of change. *Psychother Theory Res Pract, 19*(3), 276–288.

Pronk, N. P., Peek, C. J., and Goldstein, M. G. (2004). Addressing multiple behavioral risk factors in primary care. A synthesis of current knowledge and stakeholder dialogue sessions. *Am J Prev Med, 27*, 4–17.

Rees, K., Bennett, P., West, R., Davey, S. G., and Ebrahim, S. (2004a). Psychological interventions for coronary heart disease. *Cochrane Database Syst Rev*, CD002902.

Rees, K., Taylor, R. S., Singh, S., Coats, A. J., and Ebrahim, S. (2004b). Exercise based rehabilitation for heart failure. *Cochrane Database Syst Rev*, CD003331.

Rice, V. H., and Stead, L. F. (2008). Nursing interventions for smoking cessation. *Cochrane Database Syst Rev*, CD001188.

Schedlbauer, A., Schroeder, K., Peters, T. J., and Fahey, T. (2004). Interventions to improve adherence to lipid lowering medication. *Cochrane Database Syst Rev*, CD004371.

Seo, D. C., and Sa, J. (2008). A meta-analysis of psycho-behavioral obesity interventions among US multiethnic and minority adults. *Prev Med, 47*, 573–582.

Sowden, A., Arblaster, L., and Stead, L. (2003). Community interventions for preventing smoking in young people. *Cochrane Database Syst Rev*, CD001291.

Stead, L. F., Bergson, G., and Lancaster, T. (2008). Physician advice for smoking cessation. *Cochrane Database Syst Rev*, CD000165.

Strecher, V. (2007). Internet methods for delivering behavioral and health-related interventions (eHealth). *Annu Rev Clin Psychol, 3*, 53–76.

Thomas, D. E., Elliott, E. J., and Naughton, G. A. (2006). Exercise for type 2 diabetes mellitus. *Cochrane Database Syst Rev, 3*, CD002968.

Thompson, R. L., Summerbell, C. D., Hooper, L., Higgins, J. P., Little, P. S. et al (2003). Dietary advice given by a dietitian versus other health professional or self-help resources to reduce blood cholesterol. *Cochrane Database Syst Rev*, CD001366.

US Department of Health and Human Services (1964). *Smoking and Health: A Report of the Surgeon General*. Washington.

US Department of Health and Human Services (1988). *The Surgeon General's Report on Nutrition and Health*. Washington.

US Department of Health and Human Services (1996). *Physical Activity and Health: A Report of the Surgeon General*. Washington.

van Sluijs, E., van Poppel, M., and van Mechelen, W. (2004). Stage-based lifestyle interventions in primary care – Are they effective? *Am J Prev Med, 26*, 330–343.

Vermeire, E., Wens, J., Van Royen, P., Biot, Y., Hearnshaw, H. et al (2005). Interventions for improving adherence to treatment recommendations in people with type 2 diabetes mellitus. *Cochrane Database Syst Rev*, CD003638.

Wantland, D. J., Portillo, C. J., Holzemer, W. L., Slaughter, R., and McGhee, E. M. (2004). The effectiveness of web-based vs. non-web-based interventions: a meta-analysis of behavioral change outcomes. *J Med Internet Res, 6*, e40.

Welschen, L. M., Bloemendal, E., Nijpels, G., Dekker, J. M., Heine, R. J. et al (2005). Self-monitoring of blood glucose in patients with type 2 diabetes who are not using insulin. *Cochrane Database Syst Rev*, CD005060.

WHO (2001). *World Health Report- Mental Health: New Understanding, New Hope*. Geneva: World Health Organization.

WHO (2002). *The World Health Report 2002. Reducing Risks, Promoting Health Life*. Geneva: World Health Organization.

WHO (2005). *Chronic Disease Risk Factors*. Geneva: World Health Organization.

WHO (2008). *WHO Report on the Global Tobacco Epidemic: The MPOWER Package*. Geneva: World Health Organization.

Yach, D., McKee, M., Lopez, A. D., and Novotny, T. (2005). Improving diet and physical activity: 12 lessons from controlling tobacco smoking. *BMJ, 330*, 898–900.

Chapter 63

Psychosocial–Behavioral Interventions and Chronic Disease

Neil Schneiderman, Michael H. Antoni, Frank J. Penedo, and Gail H. Ironson

1 Introduction

According to the World Health Organization (WHO, 2008) the leading causes of death worldwide are coronary heart disease (CHD), stroke, chronic obstructive pulmonary diseases, diarrhea, and HIV/AIDS. Using a slightly different metric that aggregates cancers, it is observed that cancer is either the first or second leading cause of mortality (WHO, 2009). As McGinnis and Foege (2004) have pointed out, however, reporting of deaths, diseases, and disabilities using traditional diagnostic categories obscures the importance of antecedent factors that are responsible for disease outcomes. Mokdad and colleagues (2004), for instance, have reported that about half of all deaths in the United States could be attributable to a very limited number of largely preventable behaviors and exposures. Furthermore, the INTERHEART Study has provided evidence that nine potentially modifiable risk factors associated with myocardial infarction (MI) account for more than 90% of population attributable MI risk worldwide (Yusuf et al, 2004). According to INTERHEART, smoking, abdominal obesity, hypertension, diabetes, and psychosocial stressors are associated with increased risk, whereas daily consumption of fruits or vegetables, moderate exercise, and alcohol consumption are protective. The population attributable risk associated with psychosocial stressors is 32.5% (Rosengren et al, 2004).

Most of the risk factors identified in INTERHEART, particularly smoking, abdominal obesity and psychosocial stressors have also been associated with the mortality risk for cancer (Duffy et al, 2009) and other diseases. Of further interest to behavioral scientists is that for the most part the risk factors identified in INTERHEART are amenable to behavior modification. Even when patients reach the stage where they are in need of medication, behavioral skills can help to improve adherence. During the past several decades behavioral scientists have developed a number of psychosocial–behavioral interventions based upon research showing how psychosocial and biobehavioral factors influence quality of life and disease-related outcomes. Whereas early studies adhered to a strict dichotomy between psychosocial and behavioral interventions, it has become increasingly apparent that efficacious interventions for patients with chronic disease require behavioral skill interventions that address psychosocial, lifestyle, and medical adherence issues. This chapter describes some of the psychosocial and biobehavioral factors that moderate and/or mediate the outcomes of chronic disease prevention and management programs with particular reference to CHD, HIV/AIDS, and cancer.

N. Schneiderman (✉)
Department of Psychology, University of Miami, P.O. Box 248185, Coral Gables, FL 33124-0751, USA
e-mail: nschneid@miami.edu

A. Steptoe (ed.), *Handbook of Behavioral Medicine*, DOI 10.1007/978-0-387-09488-5_63,

2 Coronary Heart Disease

2.1 Risk Factors

The leading cause of death worldwide is CHD (WHO, 2008). Although atherosclerosis, the preclinical antecedent of CHD, begins in childhood, the clinical manifestations of CHD occur in adulthood and include angina pectoris, MI, heart failure, and sudden death. Major cardiovascular risk factors are those that independently influence the development of atherosclerosis and CHD. More than a half century ago the Framingham Heart Study identified cigarette smoking, elevated serum cholesterol, hypertension, and advancing age as major risk factors (Dawber et al, 1951). Since then, conventional wisdom has come to accept that four modifiable traditional cardiovascular risk factors (i.e., smoking, hypertension, hypercholesterolemia, type 2 diabetes mellitus) account for "only 50%" of the risk for CHD (Braunwald, 1997; Hennekens, 1998). However, some investigators have contended that the 50% figure is a myth and that traditional risk factors account for far more than half the prevalence of CHD (Canto and Iskandrian, 2003). In fact, given what we now know about modifiable risk factors, it appears that they account for almost all CHD mortality. INTERHEART was a standardized case-control study of acute MI in 52 countries representing every inhabited continent (Yusuf et al, 2004). As might be expected in a study whose age distribution is determined by MI, the median age in years for men was in the 50 s and for women in the 60 s although there was a variation related to geographic region and ethnic origin. The 15,152 cases and 14,820 controls were compared in terms of self-reported smoking, history of hypertension, history of diabetes, dietary patterns, physical activity, consumption of alcohol, and psychosocial factors as well as by tape measurements for adiposity and blood measurement for apolipoproteins (Apo). Abnormal lipids, smoking, hypertension, diabetes, abdominal obesity, and psychosocial stressors were found to be associated with increased risk, whereas daily consumption of fruits or vegetables, moderate or strenuous exercise, and consumption of alcohol were protective. INTERHEART found that the major risk factors having odds ratios (OR) of 2 or greater in univariate analyses included smoking, abnormal lipids, psychosocial factors, hypertension, diabetes, and abdominal obesity. They were qualitatively similar and consistently adverse in all regions of the world and in all ethnic groups.

INTERHEART (Yusuf et al, 2004) made an important contribution to our knowledge of cardiovascular risk by documenting the generalizability of modifiable risk factors across diverse regions and ethnicities. In order to accomplish this monumental task, the investigators made a number of important compromises. Thus, rather than using fasting blood to evaluate triglycerides, HDL-, and LDL-cholesterol, they used the ratio of ApoB/ApoA1 from non-fasting blood as an index of abnormal lipids. Neither blood pressure, blood glucose nor plasma insulin were assessed directly. Similarly, psychosocial stress was examined by four simple questions about stress at work and at home, financial stress, and major life events in the past year (Rosengren et al, 2004). Depression was evaluated by a modified version of the short form of the composite international diagnostic interview questionnaire (Patten, 1997). Interestingly, all of these psychosocial variables were associated with increased risk of MI. For severe global stress, the size of the effect appeared to be less than that for smoking, but comparable with that for hypertension and abdominal obesity.

The measurement deficiencies in INTERHEART, essential as they may have been in order to meet study objectives, suggest that some of the methods used may have led to variations in estimated risk that could be improved by more sensitive measurement (e.g., blood pressure, fasting lipids, impaired glucose tolerance, psychosocial distress). This would be particularly important for planning secondary prevention in CHD patients who, although usually offered pharmacological treatment for traditional risk factors, may have 5–7 times the relative risk of recurrent MI when compared with the general population of same age adults (National Cholesterol Education Program, 1994). Thus, in such patients it is important that both psychosocial behavioral and pharmacological treatment should be guided by an understanding of the variables likely to be mediating the associations between traditional risk factors and cardiovascular mortality including inflammation, insulin resistance, oxidative stress, and platelet coagulation. The design of such rehabilitation programs for post-MI patients should consider behavioral variables including medication adherence and lifestyle modification, reduction of sympathetic nervous system arousal and glucocorticoid dysregulation, and the bidirectional interaction between behavior and stress. There is also need to assess the role of moderating variables such as low socioeconomic status (e.g., Marmot et al, 1984) (see Chapter 22), whose adverse effects upon cardiovascular mortality may operate through behavioral, biological, psychosocial, and environmental (including access to health care, fresh fruits and vegetables, and safe neighborhoods) risk factors (Albert et al, 2006; Steptoe and Marmot, 2002).

2.2 Psychosocial–Behavioral Interventions with Acute Coronary Syndrome Patients

Several meta-analyses have examined randomized psychosocial–behavioral interventions in patients with CHD (Clark et al, 2005; Dusseldorp et al, 1999; Linden et al, 1996, 2007). Most of the studies that were analyzed compared a psychosocial–behavioral intervention with usual care. The meta-analysis by Dusseldorp and colleagues examined the effects of health education and stress management in 37 studies and found a 34% reduction in cardiovascular mortality, a 29% reduction in MI recurrence and significant positive effects for blood pressure, cholesterol, body weight, smoking, physical exercise, and eating habits.

Cardiac rehabilitation programs that were successful in improving traditional risk factor profiles were also more effective in decreasing cardiovascular mortality and MI recurrence than those that were not successful in risk factor reduction.

Linden et al (1996) conducted a meta-analysis on 3,180 CHD patients in 23 randomized controlled trials (RCTs) and found that patients who did not receive psychosocial–behavioral treatment showed greater mortality (OR=1.70; 95% confidence interval [CI], 1.09–2.64) and MI recurrence (OR=1.84; CI, 1.12–2.99) than those who did. Similarly, Clark et al (2005) conducted a meta-analysis on 21,295 CHD patients in 63 RCTs and reported an OR=0.85; CI, 0.77–0.94 for all-cause mortality and OR=0.83; CI, 0.74–0.94 for recurrent MI. More recently in a meta-analysis conducted on 9,856 CHD patients in 43 RCTs, Linden et al (2007) found that trials initiating treatment at least 2 months after a cardiovascular event revealed greater mortality savings than those beginning treatment sooner (OR=0.28; CI, 0.11–0.70 vs OR=0.87, CI, 0.86–1.15, respectively). Moreover the mortality benefits applied only to men (OR=0.73; CI, 0.57–1.00) but not to women (OR=1.01, CI, 0.87–1.72). In general then, meta-analyses have confirmed that psychosocial–behavioral interventions in MI patients can improve cardiovascular risk factor profiles, decrease mortality, and reduce recurrent MI. Beneficial effects appear to be more likely if the intervention begins at least 2 months after the MI and are more likely in men than in women. Although meta-analyses are useful in providing a broad overview of outcomes in a research area, it is important to examine key RCT in order to assess the quality of the data and to begin to understand differences and similarities in outcomes.

Among the psychosocial–behavioral RCTs that have been conducted upon post-MI patients, there have been exceptionally few large-scale trials that meet the reporting criteria of the Consolidated Standards of Reporting Trials (CONSORT) statement (Moher et al, 2001). The few trials that have approximated these standards have yielded both positive and null results. Because of the heterogeneity of the procedures employed, the exact reasons for the discrepancies in results have not been entirely obvious.

The Recurrent Coronary Prevention Project (RCPP) randomized 862 post-MI patients (90% men; 98% white) into either a control condition receiving group-based traditional risk factor counseling (diet, exercise, medication adherence) or an intervention condition receiving group-based risk factor counseling plus cognitive behavior therapy (CBT) to reduce type A behaviors (i.e., hostility, impatience, time urgency) and relaxation training to decrease behavioral arousal (Friedman et al, 1986). Patients were enrolled at least 6 months after their MI. The average control participant attended 25 (76% of total available) sessions and the average intervention participant attended 38 (61% of total available) sessions over 4.5 years. Rate of combined fatal and nonfatal recurrence was significantly lower in the intervention than in the control group. Participants in the intervention group also showed significant decreases in hostility, time urgency, impatience, and depressed mood as well as reliable gains in perceived self-efficacy (Mendes de Leon et al, 1991).

In a subsequent RCT, Jones and West (1996) randomized 2,328 post-MI patients into either an intervention condition receiving seven weekly psychological counseling and therapy, relaxation, and stress management sessions (some in a group format) or a usual care condition. Other components of rehabilitation dealing with smoking, diet, weight control, or exercise were not included in the program. Patients were enrolled within 28 days after their MI. Data on the age, sex distribution, or racial/ethnicity of participants are not described in the published article. The investigators found no significant differences within or between groups in reported anxiety and depression between baseline and 6 months and no differences between conditions in clinical complications, clinical sequaelae, or mortality after 1 year.

The Montreal Heart Attack Readjustment Trial (M-HART) was an RCT carried out in 1,376 post-MI patients assigned to an intervention or control condition (Frasure-Smith et al, 1997). Intervention participants were telephoned by a research assistant 1 week after discharge, then monthly for a year. They responded to the 20-item general health questionnaire (Goldberg, 1972), which assesses psychological distress from anxiety, depressed mood, and activity impairment. Participants scoring 5 or higher on the questionnaire or were readmitted to the hospital were then contacted by a cardiology nurse who made a home visit and provided reassurance, education, practical advice, and when necessary referral to a health-care provider. Nurses were not given specific training for implementing the protocol beyond their cardiology nursing training. About 75% of patients in the intervention condition received on average 5–6 1-h nursing visits. In general, the program had no overall impact upon either cardiac or all-cause mortality or on psychological outcomes (depressive symptoms, anxiety, anger, or perceived social support) between intervention and control groups. However, treated women did reveal marginally greater all-cause mortality than control women (OR=1.99; CI, 0.99–4.00) suggesting that the intervention may actually have been harmful to women. The OR for cardiac mortality was 1.96 (CI, 0.95–4.06).

Subsequently, the enhancing Recovery in Coronary Heart Disease (ENRICHD) trial randomized 2,481 post-MI patients (44% women; 34% ethnic minority), selected because they were depressed and/or had low social support, into a CBT-based psychosocial–behavioral intervention or to usual medical care (Berkman et al, 2003). The intervention was initiated at a median of 17 days after MI for a median of 11 individual sessions throughout 6 months. During this 6-month period 30% of participants also received group-based CBT and relaxation training and were placed on a selective serotonin reuptake inhibitor if they had severe depression or less than 50% reduction in Beck's depression inventory scores after 5 weeks of intervention.

By 6 months after randomization ENRICHD modestly decreased depression and increased social support in the intervention compared with the control group. However, after an average follow-up of 29 months, there was no significant difference in event-free survival between the usual care and the psychosocial intervention conditions. Because ENRICHD was designed to enroll large numbers of women and minorities, it was possible to conduct a secondary analysis examining the outcome of sex by ethnicity subgroups (Schneiderman et al, 2004). This secondary analysis indicated that the intervention decreased the incidence of both cardiac death (OR=0.63; CI, 0.40–0.99) and nonfatal MI (or=0.61; CI, 0.40–0.92) in white men but not in the other subgroups.

Most recently, the Stockholm Women's Intervention Trial for Coronary Heart Disease (SWITCHD) randomized 237 patients with severe CHD incidents into a group-based psychosocial–behavioral intervention program or usual medical care (Orth-Gomér et al, 2009). Initiated 4 months after hospitalization, intervention groups of 4–8 women met for a total of 20 sessions over the course of an entire year. The intervention program, in which 75% of the women attended 15–20 sessions, included education about risk factors, self-care, and adherence to medical advice, as well as skills training in relaxation and coping with stress exposure from family and work. The nurses who delivered the intervention were pre-trained and certified in the behavior modification techniques used in the trial. From randomization until the end of follow-up (mean duration 7.1 years), the intervention yielded an almost threefold protective effect on mortality rate (OR=0.33; CI, 0.1–0.74).

The meta-analyses that have been conducted on psychosocial–behavioral interventions in patients with severe CHD-related events indicate that such treatments can reduce the incidence of nonfatal and/or fatal events. Examination of major studies carried out on such patients reveals that the studies reporting positive results were initiated several months after the index event, used a group-based format, conducted the intervention for a relatively long temporal duration, and followed the patients for a number of years (Friedman et al, 1986; Orth-Gomér et al, 2009). These trials addressed a broad range of modifiable traditional and psychosocial risk factors, medication adherence, and lifestyle adjustment as well as provided training in behavior change methods by group leaders who themselves were certified in such procedures. Some of the conclusions drawn from these trials are based on post hoc analyses and reviews of trial data, so prospective replication studies are needed.

3 HIV/AIDS

3.1 Disease Processes in HIV/AIDS

Human immunodeficiency virus infection and acquired immune deficiency syndrome (HIV/AIDS) are caused by the HIV retrovirus, which is transmitted most commonly through unprotected sexual intercourse or intravenous drug use. HIV selectively targets a subset of lymphocytes expressing a surface T4 glycoprotein, most commonly found in a subpopulation of lymphocytes referred to as CD4+ T helper cells. These CD4+ T cells serve as the host cells for the transcription of HIV RNA and protein synthesis, which begins the process of creating new HIV virions that target other host cells. The infected person undergoes a progressive loss of CD4+ T cells while HIV virus concentration in the circulation (i.e., viral load) is increasing (Pantaleo et al, 1993). The rapid replication and mutation rate of HIV thwarts the effectiveness of immune mechanisms in controlling the infection. Later individuals may develop full-blown AIDS defined as a decline in the number of CD4+ cells to critically low levels (<200 cell/mm^3) or AIDS-defining opportunistic infections such as pneumonia or neoplasias such as Kaposi's Sarcoma, Burkitt's lymphoma, and invasive cervical cancer.

There is substantial individual variability in the rate at which immunologic status declines (CD4+T-cell counts), viral load increases, and clinical symptoms manifest over a given time period in persons with HIV. These individual differences may be due to negative health behaviors such as substance use or poor medication adherence as well as differences in the ability to preserve an immune repertoire that is vital for responding to pathogens and neoplastic processes. The variability in some of these immune parameters has been related to negative mood and stress-related processes in persons with HIV (Antoni and Carrico, in press).

3.2 Factors Influencing HIV Disease Progression

3.2.1 Mood and Affect

One of the most widely studied mental health challenges in HIV/AIDS is the elevated risk of affective and anxiety disorders (Cielsa and Roberts, 2001). Depression and other mental health challenges may impact disease course in HIV via difficulties with health behaviors (increased substance use and poorer HIV medication adherence) and/or via psychoneuroimmunologic (PNI) processes (Antoni and Carrico, in press). Longitudinal investigations in men and women with HIV reveal that depressive symptoms are associated with more rapid CD4+ cell count decline (Burack et al, 1993), greater HIV viral load (Ironson et al, 2005), faster progression to AIDS (Leserman et al, 1999; Page-Shafer et al, 1996), heightened risk of developing an AIDS-defining clinical condition (Leserman et al, 2002), and hastened mortality (Ickovics et al, 2001; Mayne et al, 1996). Other mood states, including anger and anxiety, have been associated with faster progression to AIDS (Leserman et al, 2002) and greater HIV viral load (Evans et al, 2002). Conversely, positive psychological states predict less rapid CD4+ cell decline and greater longevity in men and women

with HIV (Ickovics et al, 2006; Moskowitz, 2003).

3.2.2 Medication Adherence

Due to the substantial reductions in morbidity and mortality associated with the advent of antiretroviral therapy (ART) medication regimens, HIV infection is now commonly conceptualized as a chronic illness (Bangsberg et al, 2001). However, not all HIV-positive patients treated with ART display adequate viral suppression, which may largely be due to suboptimal levels of adherence as well as the emergence of medication-resistant strains of the virus. A substantial number of individuals with advanced HIV disease experience significant structural, social, and psychological barriers to initiating treatment (Morin et al, 2002). These barriers may directly contribute to late presentation for HIV medical care and failure to initiate ART (Keruly and Moore, 2007), which can substantially increase risk for hastened AIDS-related mortality.

ART is a demanding treatment regimen that requires high levels of patient adherence up to 95% to maximize the clinical benefits (Friedland and Williams, 1999). Further complicating adherence to ART are the special indications (e.g., taking medications with food) that accompany many medications in order to attenuate the severity of side effects, maximize bioavailability, and ensure a constant therapeutic dose. In fact, medication intolerance is the most commonly cited reason among patients for terminating ART (Park et al, 2002); greater number and severity of medication side effects is also associated with poorer self-reported adherence among those who continue to take ART. Specific side effects such as nausea, vomiting, skin problems, and memory impairment have been independently associated with reporting less than 90% adherence to ART (Johnson et al, 2005).

There is evidence that depressive symptoms and other forms of negative affect can influence ART non-adherence (Weaver et al, 2005). Since affect can adversely influence ART adherence, it is possible that medication non-adherence may mediate the previously shown association between depression and poorer health outcomes in persons with HIV.

3.2.3 Stressors and Stress-Related Processes

Cumulative negative life events have been associated with reduced natural killer (NK) and cytotoxic/suppressor (CD8+) T-cell counts over a 2-year period in HIV-positive gay men (Leserman et al, 1997), faster disease progression over 5- to 9-year follow-up (Leserman et al, 1999; Leserman et al, 2002), and increases in HIV viral load (Ironson et al, 2005). Other work indicates that stressor appraisals (fatalism, optimism, benefit finding) and coping strategies (active coping, denial) may moderate the impact of stressors and distress states on disease progression and related physiological processes in persons with HIV. Social relationships may improve patients' psychological adjustment to HIV and its physical course by way of multiple pathways, including as a stress buffer (Cohen and Wills, 1985), source of personal disclosure (Fekete et al, 2009), decreased HIV stigma (Galvan et al, 2008), and enhanced medication adherence (Gonzalez et al, 2004). Processes proposed to explain the effects of affective disorders and stress-related processes on HIV disease progression include health behaviors, such as substance use and poor medication adherence, and PNI pathways tied to sympathetic nervous system (SNS) and hypothalamic pituitary adrenal (HPA) neuroendocrine regulation (Carrico et al, 2008). There is emerging evidence that neuroendocrine factors may mediate stress effects on HIV disease progression through direct effects on dysregulation of Th1 cytokines, chemokines, and HIV transcription factors that favor increased HIV replication rate, which predates increased viral load in the circulation and ultimately clinical disease progression (Cole, 2008).

3.3 Psychosocial–Behavioral Intervention in HIV/AIDS

The research on psychosocial interventions in the context of HIV/AIDS generally focus on one of the three major aims: (1) primary prevention to reduce viral transmission risk behaviors via injection drug use or unprotected sex (Kalichman, 2008); (2) secondary prevention to enhance medication adherence (Safren et al, 2006); and (3) secondary prevention to decrease depression and stress, promote optimal coping in order to optimize QOL, and possibly enhance health outcomes via PNI mechanisms (Antoni et al, 2007).

3.3.1 Primary Prevention Interventions

Recent reviews of sexual risk reduction interventions have summarized the efficacy for such programs and their likely cognitive and social mediators, especially in adolescent populations (DiClemente et al, 2008). These interventions, mostly based on Social Learning Theory and Social Cognitive Theory, incorporate modeling, behavioral rehearsal, and communication skills training to increase knowledge, change attitudes, and provide behavioral skills to enact safer sex behaviors (e.g., DiClemente et al, 2004). These programs have been shown to increase the use of condoms, delay the initiation of intercourse in adolescents, and reduce the number of sexual partners (e.g., Metzler et al, 2000). Future work in this field is moving in the direction of utilizing the family in the change process and building strategies for long-term maintenance (DiClemente et al, 2008). There is also evidence that among persons infected with HIV, poorer medication adherence often covaries with HIV transmission risk behaviors, which may increase the risk for transmitting resistant strains of HIV (Kalichman, 2008). Since substance use and depression are associated with both HIV transmission behaviors and non-adherence to ART, Kalichman has suggested that interventions that are able to address multiple targets simultaneously may improve effectiveness. In terms of interventions targeting substance use, behavioral programs targeting injection drug users have had an important impact on primary prevention of HIV. Most of these programs combine education about injection practices with access to sterile equipment, condoms, and treatment for drug abuse and addiction.

3.3.2 Secondary Prevention to Improve Antiretroviral Medication Adherence

Interventions designed to improve ART adherence have focused on modulating different psychological processes including cognitive appraisals and affect regulation. Simoni and colleagues (2006) conducted a meta-analytic review of 19 randomized controlled trials that examined the efficacy of innovative adherence interventions. The majority of these interventions employed CBT principles and results indicated that participants randomized to the intervention arm were significantly more likely to achieve 95% adherence. The use of CBT has also led to increases in adherence associated with decreases in depression (Safren et al, 2009). Thus, depressed men and women with HIV receiving 12-week individual CBT for adherence and depression showed significant reductions in depressive symptoms and concurrent increases in electronically monitored ART adherence compared to those who received a single-session adherence intervention.

3.3.3 Secondary Prevention to Reduce Depression and Stress-Related Processes

Recently published reviews have summarized the effects of CBT on anxiety and depressed mood (Crepaz et al, 2008). Crepaz et al (2008) conducted a meta-analytic review of 15 RCTs of CBT effects in persons with HIV which were published from 1988 to 2005. Most studies used interventions delivered over 3–17 sessions

(median = 10), in a group format, and used cognitive re-appraisal/cognitive restructuring (N = 15), coping skills training (N = 14), stress management skills training (N = 11), or social support (N = 7). Reported effect sizes ranged from 0.30 to 1.00 for anxiety and depression. Findings varied as a function of the techniques used in the interventions, with significant effects on depression and anxiety found only in studies providing stress management and in those having at least 10 intervention sessions.

A second recent review focused exclusively on the effects of psychological interventions on stress/affect, neuroendocrine regulation, and immune status in persons with HIV (Carrico and Antoni, 2008). This review was based on 14 RCTs published from 1987 to 2007 involving mostly group-based interventions and with a mode of 10-weeks duration. The majority of the studies that showed effects on psychological states (anxiety and depressed mood), neuroendocrine hormones (cortisol and catecholamines), and immune and viral parameters (lymphocyte proliferation, herpesvirus antibody titers, HIV viral load) involved at least 10 weeks of group-based CBT intervention. Those interventions that were most successful in improving psychological adjustment (reducing depressed mood, anxiety, distress) were more likely to have beneficial effects on neuroendocrine regulation and immune status. Much of the work covered in these reviews took place in the period prior to the adoption of highly active antiretroviral therapy (HAART) into clinical practice (prior to 1997).

The HAART era, beginning in the late 1990s, presented new opportunities. First, this period was marked by the explosion of new therapeutic approaches to HIV that incorporated cocktails of drugs including protease inhibitors that were shown to decrease viral load to undetectable levels. Second, the development of an ultrasensitive polymerase chain reaction assay capable of detecting very low concentrations (down to 50 RNA copies/ml) of HIV RNA in peripheral blood samples provided a sensitive assessment of viral load in a reasonably inexpensive manner. Third, longitudinal investigations revealed that avoidant coping, lower social support, and negative mood all predicted poorer HAART adherence, which in turn predicted greater viral load over time (Weaver et al, 2005). It was reasoned that if psychosocial interventions could improve negative mood by modifying coping and social support, then these interventions might help improve HAART adherence and/or HIV viral load. In fact CBT had been shown to decrease negative mood by enhancing adaptive coping and social support in men with HIV (Lutgendorf et al, 1998) and these decreases in negative mood paralleled decreases in 24-h urinary cortisol output (Antoni et al, 2000), improved immunologic control of herpes viruses (Lutgendorf et al, 1997) during the intervention, and preserved naïve T cells up to 1 year (Antoni et al, 2005). It seems likely that CBT may influence HIV disease progression (HIV viral load) by improving adherence and/or by modulating mood.

Since medication adherence training (MAT) programs had been shown to be effective in improving adherence (e.g., Safren et al, 2006) we examined whether combining CBT with relaxation training (Cognitive behavior stress management: CBSM) would provide added value to pharmacist-delivered MAT. In a trial with HIV-positive men who have sex with men comparing the combination of CBSM + MAT to MAT alone, an analysis utilizing all participants showed no intervention-related changes in viral load (Antoni et al, 2006). However, in the analysis only of men who had a detectable HIV viral load at baseline, the CBSM + MAT condition produced a $0.56 \log_{10}$ reduction in HIV viral load over the 15-month investigation period, an effect that held even after controlling for ART adherence over this entire period (Antoni et al, 2006). Men in CBSM + MAT also showed significant reductions in depressed mood over the intervention period and a structural equation model demonstrated that decreases in depressed mood during the CBSM + MAT intervention mediated its effects on viral load decreases over the 15-month follow-up period (Antoni et al, 2006). In addition, greater attendance to CBSM sessions was associated with lower HIV viral load at follow-up.

It is noteworthy that persons with uncontrolled viral load (but not those with undetectable viral load) who participated in a combined stress management and medication adherence intervention showed decreased viral load through 15 months of follow-up. This suggests that CBSM used in combination with MAT may be useful for disease management in those persons having difficulty in achieving viral suppression. For those whose viral load is under control (undetectable), the use of psychosocial interventions to modulate disease progression is not empirically supported. At least one explanation for the decreased viral load in men receiving CBSM and MAT appears to relate to decreased depressed mood. Future work examining putative neuroendocrine (urinary cortisol and catecholamines) and health behavior changes (substance use, sleep) that may co-vary with depressed mood changes may serve to explain these provocative effects. It is also important to determine, why some studies that produce improvements in mental health variables do not lead to improvements in disease status such as HIV viral load (Berger et al, 2008).

Much of what we know about the effects of psychosocial–behavioral interventions in persons with HIV has come from studies of middle class men who have sex with men. A small collection of studies, however, has begun to show that CBSM may reduce stress and improve emotional well-being among lower income minority women with HIV (Antoni et al, 2008), though little is known about their longer-term effects on disease course. Research aiming to modify psychosocial–behavioral processes in ethnic minority populations calls for careful targeting of the intervention material so as to be culturally sensitive as well as relevant to the nature of stressors that each population must deal with and use community-based participatory research methods. While group-based formats can be an efficient and effective means for delivering psychosocial intervention in clinic and community settings, more work needs to focus these interventions at the level of the romantic dyad (Fife et al, 2008) and the family system (Szapocznik et al, 2004) to ensure optimal carryover to the social milieu where longer-term coping skills will be enacted. Studies of processes that might mediate the effects of interventions on stress, depression, and disease progression in persons with HIV should include measures of psychosocial processes and neuroimmune changes on the one hand and changes in health behaviors such as medication adherence, sexual risk behaviors, and substance use on the other. There is a growing body of research in HIV-infected and at-risk populations demonstrating the effects of health behavior change interventions targeting these inter-related behaviors that have implications for primary and secondary prevention (Kalichman, 2008; Safren et al, 2006). For instance, the regular use of cocaine, crack, and methamphetamine has been associated with increased rates of HIV transmission risk behavior, acquisition of strains of HIV that are resistant to some classes of antiretroviral medications, impaired adherence to ART, and elevated HIV viral load (Johnson et al, 2008). There is also evidence that affective states can influence viral load through decreased stimulant use and better ART adherence (Carrico et al, 2007). Taken together with the work showing that CBSM can decrease viral load by way of decreases in negative mood (Antoni et al, 2006), there is converging evidence suggesting that such interventions used in combination with strategies targeting specific health behaviors may produce beneficial results in specific subpopulations of persons living with HIV.

been implicated in cancer risk. Similarly, factors such as radiation and chemical (e.g., smoking) exposure, viruses, and bacteria are some of the extrinsic risk factors associated with this disease. Other known risk factors include age, alcohol use, poor diet, obesity, and lack of physical activity. While having one or more risk factors increases the probability of developing cancer over the life course, most individuals who have these risk factors do not develop cancer.

Cancer is the second leading cause of death in the United States and is only exceeded by heart disease (ACS, 2009). Although there has been a considerable reduction in deaths associated with other major diseases such as heart disease, cerebrovascular disease, and pneumonia/influenza, cancer deaths have shown no significant decline over the past 50 years (Heron et al, 2009). However, the 5-year relative cancer survival rate (i.e., percent of patients who are alive after diagnosis/treatment) in the United States has increased from 50% in 1975–1977 to 66% between 1996 and 2004 although significant ethnic, social-economic status, and geographic disparities exist (ACS, 2009). Survival statistics also show that industrialized and economically developed societies report higher survival rates across multiple cancers relative to non-industrialized and low-income countries. Recent studies suggest that international variation in survival rates may be attributed to differential availability of screening and treatment services (Coleman et al, 2008).

4 Cancer

4.1 Risk Factors for Initiation, Promotion, and Recurrence

The reason why some individuals develop cancer and others do not is unknown, but a number of risk factors for cancer initiation have been identified (Abraham et al, 2005). Both intrinsic and extrinsic factors have been implicated in cancer development. For example, intrinsic factors such as heredity, diet, and endocrine processes have

4.2 Psychosocial Factors and Disease Progression

Although most patients adjust relatively well, a significant number of cancer survivors experience psychological responses ranging from common and normal feelings of vulnerability, sadness and fear, to clinical levels of depression and anxiety leading to significant disruptions in interpersonal functioning which require psychological intervention (Holland et al, 1998). Approximately 30% of oncology patients show significant levels of distress that warrant psychological treatment (e.g., Zabora et al, 2001). Such responses vary according to cancer site and stage. Patients experiencing advanced cancer in sites that show poor treatment response outcomes, such as lung, brain, and pancreas, report the greatest levels of psychological distress and need for treatment. Studying psychological responses to cancer diagnosis and treatment has received significant attention, because a growing number of studies have suggested that there is a significant association between psychosocial processes and health outcome in cancer. For example, in a recent review of 165 studies examining the contribution of psychosocial factors to cancer incidence and survival, Chida and colleagues (2008) showed that factors such as stressful life experiences, maladaptive coping styles, and depression are associated with greater cancer incidence and poorer prognosis and survival.

The term "cancer survivor" is used to describe any individual who has been diagnosed with cancer and is living, whereas "survivorship" is used to describe the experience of living with a diagnosis of cancer and its related treatments. Currently, there are about 10 million cancer survivors in the United States with breast (22%), prostate (17%), and colorectal (11%) cancers constituting the majority of diagnosed cases. About 61% of all cancer survivors are age 65 or older and one out of every six individuals over the age of 65 is a cancer survivor (Hewitt et al, 2006). Coping with a cancer diagnosis and its treatment can present individuals with a series of psychosocial challenges that may compromise both quality of life (QOL) and health outcomes. Cancer, even if treated successfully, is a chronic condition that involves ongoing status monitoring for possible disease recurrence (Abraham et al, 2005). Patients must cope with long-term and late effects of cancer treatment such as fatigue and cognitive difficulties. Interpersonal disruption and sexual dysfunction are not uncommon and may affect both intimate relationships and overall social functioning. Some cancer treatments such as those available for some head and neck cancers can lead to disfigurement and difficulty in eating and speaking, thus significantly compromising QOL and overall functional status (Harrison et al, 2009). In addition to these treatment-related side effects, several cancers associated with health risk behaviors such as smoking and alcohol use continue to carry a significant stigma that may compromise a patient's emotional well-being. Overall, these experiences require ongoing long-term adjustment to cancer treatment while continuing to monitor disease status or recurrence.

There is growing evidence suggesting that among cancer patients, psychosocial (e.g., appraisals, coping, social support, depression) and physiological (e.g., neuroendocrine function, immunologic status) factors may mediate relations among distress, QOL, and physical health status following a cancer diagnosis. These psychosocial factors have also been related to adjustment and disease management. For example, greater optimism, active coping styles (e.g., "fighting spirit", planning, positive reframing), accurate stressor appraisals, positive growth, and efficacious social networks have been significantly associated with positive adjustment at various stages of the disease (i.e., diagnosis, treatment, and survivorship) in various cancers (e.g., Cruess et al, 2000). In prostate cancer, for example, greater social support from a spouse and family or friends has been associated with higher general and disease-specific QOL (e.g., urinary function), while greater self-efficacy has been related to better sexual function and QOL. In contrast, social constraints have been associated with poorer general and emotional functioning (Eton et al, 2001). It is not surprising that some studies show that up to 30% of prostate cancer survivors report a need for psychological support (e.g., Steginga et al, 2001).

4.3 Psychosocial Interventions, Optimizing Health/Survival and Improving Quality of Life

A large number of studies indicate that group-based interventions in cancer reduce psychological distress (e.g., Gustafsson et al, 1979), including anxiety and depression (e.g., Fawzy et al, 1997); improve coping (e.g., Lieberman, 1988); and reduce physical symptoms such as pain, nausea, and vomiting (e.g., Meyer and Mark, 1995). Psychosocial interventions tailored to meet the needs of cancer patients include supportive-expressive group therapy (Luebbert et al, 2001), psychoeducational interventions (e.g., Lieberman, 1988), and multimodal intervention approaches. Research shows that effective components include (e.g., Gregoire et al, 1997): strategies, such as relaxation training (e.g., guided imagery) to lower arousal, disease information and management; an emotionally supportive environment where participants can address fears and anxieties; behavioral and cognitive coping strategies; and social support. In a meta-analysis of relaxation interventions targeting patients undergoing cancer treatments, relaxation significantly reduced treatment-related symptoms such as nausea and pain (Lepore and Helgeson, 1998). Similar effect sizes were found for the impact of relaxation training in reducing negative mood (i.e., depression, tension, anxiety, hostility, fatigue, and confusion).

Several interventions have been specifically developed to target smoking cessation among cancer survivors (de Moor et al, 2008). The successful smoking prevention programs included such features as high intensity delivery and long-term intervention, ongoing reinforcement of the benefits of smoking cessation, and training participants to make overall healthy lifestyle choices. However, a number of smoking cessation trials reviewed by de Moor and colleagues did not show significant effects. The authors suggest that these studies were limited by various factors including small sample sizes and overmatched control conditions that involved best practices for smoking cessation.

Currently, a considerable amount of work is focusing on the efficacy of physical activity interventions among cancer survivors. Multiple mental and physical health benefits are associated with physical activity including better health outcomes, better general and health-related QOL, better functional capacity, and better mood (Penedo and Dahn, 2005). Physical activity interventions may be particularly beneficial in reducing the risk and disease burden conveyed by co-morbid conditions (e.g. obesity, CHD) among cancer patients by reducing fatigue, elevating mood, improving physical functioning and reducing physical-role limitations (Schmitz et al, 2005). Among colorectal and prostate cancer survivors those engaged in physical activity levels recommended by the American Cancer Society (2009) (i.e., 30 min of moderately intense exercise at least 5 or more days per week) reported significantly greater HRQOL (Blanchard et al, 2004). In metastatic breast cancer, women randomized to a seated exercise program using a home video showed a slower decline in general QOL, less increase in fatigue, and less decline in physical well-being (Headley et al, 2004).

4.3.1 Improving Psychosocial Adjustment and QOL

The vast majority of psychosocial interventions in cancer populations aimed at facilitating post-diagnosis and -treatment adjustment have been delivered to breast cancer survivors and findings support efficacy of such interventions in reducing distress, and improving QOL. In a study involving a heterogeneous sample of breast cancer survivors, women participating in a 7-week mindfulness meditation intervention showed significant decreases in mood disturbance and stress symptoms immediately after intervention and at 6-month follow-up (Carlson et al, 2001). Among women with metastatic breast cancer, participants randomized to a supportive-expressive group therapy intervention showed significantly decreased trauma symptoms (i.e., intrusive and avoidant symptoms in response to having cancer) relative to patients assigned to a control condition. Notably, women who were most distressed at baseline showed most improvement (Classen et al, 2001) suggesting that those at greatest need may derive the most benefits.

Several studies have suggested the efficacy of group-based psychosocial interventions in improving general and disease-specific QOL in prostate cancer survivors. Gregoire et al (1997) reported that men who participated in a supportive group had a better understanding of their illness, perceived themselves as more involved in their treatment, felt reassured sharing their experiences with others, and had less anxiety and a more positive outlook. Lepore and Helgeson (1998) tested the extent to which patients participating in a support group developed self-efficacy through direct education or social sharing, and lowered cancer-related distress by targeting intrusive thoughts with the support of peers. Men in the intervention condition had greater improvements in mental health, fewer interpersonal conflicts, larger increases in perceived control over health, and lower distress associated with cancer. The intervention was especially beneficial to men with inadequate social resources and low social support from family and friends (Eton et al, 2001).

In work targeting prostate cancer survivors about 1-year post-treatment, Penedo and colleagues (2006) adapted a CBSM intervention to be delivered among men who had been treated with radical prostatectomy or radiation therapy for localized disease. Men were randomized either into a group-based 10-week CBSM intervention that targeted areas such as coping and communication skills, social support and relaxation training, and provided health information related to prostate cancer and sexual functioning or a 1-day stress management seminar where the techniques covered in the intervention were provided in a classroom format with no group process. Findings showed that relative to men randomized to the 1-day seminar, patients in the

CBSM condition showed significant improvements in QOL and benefit finding. Additionally, the acquisition of stress management skills (e.g., mobilizing social networks, ability to cognitively reframe negative stressor appraisals or engage in relaxation training) mediated the relationship between the group assignment and the study outcomes. Further analyses showed that for men who entered the study with higher levels of interpersonal anxiety and perceived stress, randomization into the CBSM condition was associated with significant improvements in sexual functioning and emotional well-being (Molton et al, 2008).

4.3.2 Psychosocial–Behavioral Intervention and Survival

Few psychosocial–behavioral intervention studies conducted in cancer patients have examined survival as an outcome. Although these trials appear to have reported at least as many null as positive results, an examination of these studies is informative.

Fawzy et al (1993) randomized 80 patients with early stage malignant melanoma into a six-session psychoeducation (health education, medical adherence, cancer prevention behaviors, stress management) or a control condition. The intervention condition revealed decreasing psychological distress, improved adaptive coping, and significant increases in natural killer (NK) cells and NK cytotoxicity relative to control participants. At 10-year follow-up, intervention participants showed a 1.9 times greater likelihood of survival (Fawzy et al, 2003). This study has been criticized because it did not follow an intent-to-treat principle and the dropout rate in the control condition was 25% (Coyne and Palmer, 2007). An attempt to replicate the study in Denmark with a larger sample was unsuccessful (Boesen et al, 2007).

Another pioneering study conducted by Spiegel et al (1989) randomized 86 women with metastasizing breast cancer into a 1 year, weekly supportive-expressive group therapy and self-hypnosis condition versus a control condition. Self-hypnosis was used to help control pain. After 10 years, participants in the intervention group were found to have lived an average of 18 months longer than participants in the control condition. Several attempts to replicate these findings have been unsuccessful (Goodwin et al, 2001; Kissane et al, 2007; Spiegel et al, 2007).

More recently Andersen et al (2008) randomized 227 women who were surgically treated for regional breast cancer into a psychosocial–behavioral intervention condition or an assessment only control condition. The group-based intervention consisted of 26 sessions conducted over a 1-year period and included strategies to reduce stress, improve mood, alter health behaviors, and maintain adherence to cancer treatment and care. After a median of 11 years of follow-up, intervention patients as compared to controls were found to have a reduced risk of death from breast cancer (OR=0.44; CI, 0.22–0.86) or breast cancer recurrence (OR=0.55; CI, 0.32–0.96). Previously, in the same cohort Andersen et al (2004) found that compared to the control condition, participants in the intervention condition showed significant decreases in anxiety and smoking as well as improvement in perceived social support, dietary habits, and T-cell proliferative responses to plant mitogens.

In view of the criticisms that have been leveled against other psychosocial–behavioral intervention studies that have examined survival from cancer as an outcome, it should be noted that the study by Andersen et al (2008) did a reasonable job of satisfying the reporting requirements of the CONSORT statement (Moher et al, 2001). Participants in each arm of the study were well-matched in terms of disease, prognostic factors, type of surgery received, adjuvant treatments planned and received, sociodemographic factors, age, and participant accrual sites.

5 Conclusions

Psychosocial–behavioral interventions have been shown to be efficacious in health-care situations ranging from the prevention of HIV/AIDS, enhancing QOL in cancer patients, improving medication adherence, decreasing HIV viral load, and reducing disease recurrence and mortality rate in CHD and cancer. Not all intervention attempts have been successful and the mediators in trials that have reported significant decreases in disease event recurrence or mortality rate still remain unknown. Almost invariably RCTs, even when reporting positive results with regards to clinical medical endpoints, have studied too few patients to allow adequate examination of potential mediators or to present confidence in treatment generalizability. Hence, even when positive, informative results have been obtained, the exact causal pathways between intervention components and outcomes are obscure.

On a more optimistic note, both the major cardiovascular (Friedman et al, 1986; Orth-Gomér et al, 2009) and cancer (Andersen et al, 2008) RCTs showing intervention-based improvement in clinical medical endpoints have shared several important attributes. First, they each used a group-based CBSM format. Second, they each used coping and behavioral skills learning in relation to relaxation, reframing, social support, improving self-efficacy, making lifestyle changes, and optimizing medication adherence. Third, the duration of the psychosocial–behavioral intervention was at least a year (approximately 25 sessions). Fourth, patients were followed on average from 4.5 to 11 years.

Until recently there has been insufficient data on which to conduct a cost-benefit analysis of psychosocial–behavioral intervention compared to other components of medical treatment with regard to medical endpoints. If 20–25 group-based CBSM sessions can indeed be shown to provide substantial medical benefits for up to 10 years in high-risk patients, the cost per patient is likely to compare favorably with other medical intervention components. Furthermore, the trials recently completed by Andersen's group and by Orth-Gomér and colleagues suggest that psychosocial–behavioral treatments can be well accepted by both severe CHD and breast cancer patients.

In conclusion, an examination of the literature regarding the relationship between psychosocial–behavioral interventions and the management of chronic diseases suggests that such interventions are useful in enhancing QOL and improving adherence to medical treatments. Recent RCTs indicate that psychosocial–behavioral interventions can also reduce disease recurrence and mortality rate in CHD and regional breast cancer. It would appear, however, that large multi-center RCTs are now warranted to confirm promising recent findings, determine the mediators of positive outcomes, and establish treatment generalizability. The need for a large number of participants to find important mediators appears likely, because some patients may benefit from improved medication adherence, whereas others may benefit from stress reduction, lifestyle changes, or improvement in self-efficacy in dealing with the many problems encountered in daily life. Underlying these adjustments are also likely to be changes that occur in inflammation, oxidative stress, fibrinolysis, neuroendocrine regulation, and other biological processes. These too need to be investigated as part of the causal pathway between psychosocial–behavioral intervention and clinical medical outcomes.

References

Abraham, J., Allegra, C., and Gulley, J. (2005). *Bethesda Handbook of Clinical Oncology, 2nd Ed.* Philadelphia: Lippincott Williams & Wilkins.

Albert, M. A., Glynn, R. J., Buring, J., and Ridker, P. M. (2006). Impact of traditional and novel risk factors on the relationship between socioeconomic status and incident cardiovascular events. *Circulation, 114*, 2619–2626.

American Cancer Society. (2009). *Cancer Facts and Figures 2009*. Atlanta, GA: American Cancer Society.

Andersen, B. L., Farrar, W. B., Golden-Kreutz, D. M., Glaser, R., Emery, C. F. et al (2004). Psychological, behavioral, and immune changes after a psychological intervention: a clinical trial. *J Clin Oncol, 22*, 3570–3580.

Andersen, B. L., Yang, H. C., Farrar, W. B., Golden-Kreutz, D. M., Emery, C. F. et al (2008). Psychologic intervention improves survival for breast cancer patients: a randomized clinical trial. *Cancer, 113*, 3450–3458.

Antoni, M. H., and Carrico, A. (in press). Psychological and bio-behavioral processes in HIV disease. In A. Baum & T. Revenson (Eds), *Handbook of Clinical Health Psychology*.

Antoni, M. H., Schneiderman, N. and Penedo, F. (2007) Behavioral interventions: immunologic mediators and disease outcomes. In R. Ader, R. Glaser, N. Cohen, & M. Irwin (Eds), *Psychoneuroimmunology, 4th Ed* (pp. 675–703). New York: Academic.

Antoni, M. H., Wagner, S., Cruess, D., Kumar, M., Lutgendorf, S. et al (2000) Cognitive behavioral stress management reduces distress and 24-hour urinary free cortisol among symptomatic HIV-infected gay men. *Ann Behav Med, 22*, 29–37.

Antoni, M. H., Cruess, D., Klimas, N., Carrico, A. W., Maher, K. et al (2005). Increases in a marker of immune system reconstitution are predated by decreases in 24-hour urinary cortisol output and depressed mood during a 10-week stress management intervention in symptomatic HIV-infected gay men. *J Psychosom Res, 58*, 3–13.

Antoni, M. H., Carrico, A. W., Durán, R. E., Spitzer, S., Penedo, F. et al (2006). Randomized clinical trial of cognitive behavioral stress management on human immunodeficiency virus viral load in gay men treated with highly active antiretroviral therapy. *Psychosom Med, 68*, 143–151.

Antoni, M. H., Pereira, D. B., Buscher, I., Ennis, N., Peake-Andrasik, M. Rose, R. et al (2008). Stress management effects on perceived stress and cervical intraepithelial neoplasia in low-income HIV infected women. *J Psychosom Res, 65*, 389–401.

Bangsberg, D. R., Perry, S., Charlebois, E. D., Clark, R. A., Roberston, M., et al (2001). Non-adherence to highly active antiretroviral therapy predicts progression to AIDS. *AIDS, 15(9)*, 1181–1183.

Berger, S., Schad, T., VonWyl, V., Ehlert, U., Zellweger, C. et al (2008). Effects of cognitive behavioral stress management on HIV-1 RNA, CD4 cell counts and psychosocial parameters of HIV-infected persons. *AIDS, 22*, 767–775.

Berkman, L. F., Blumenthal, J., Burg, M., Carney, R. M., Catellier, D. et al (2003). Effects of treating depression and low perceived social support on clinical events after myocardial infarction: the Enhancing Recovery in Coronary Heart Disease Patients (ENRICHD) Randomized Trial. *JAMA, 289*, 3106–3116.

Blanchard, C., Stein, K., Baker, F., Dent, M., Denniston, M. et al (2004). Association between current lifestyle behaviors and health-related quality of life in breast, colorectal and prostate cancer survivors. *Psychol Health, 19*, 1–13.

Boesen, E. H., Boesen, S. H., Frederiksen, K., Ross, L., Dahlstrom, K. et al (2007). Survival after a psychoeducational intervention for patients with cutaneous malignant melanoma: a replication study. *J Clin Oncol, 25*, 5698–5703.

Braunwald, E. (1997). Shattuck lecture – cardiovascular medicine at the turn of the millennium: triumphs, concerns and opportunities. *N Engl J Med, 337*, 1360–1369.

Burack, J. H., Barrett, D. C., Stall, R. D., Chesney, M. A., Ekstrand, M. L., and Coates, T. J. (1993). Depressive symptoms and CD4 lymphocyte decline among HIV-infected men. *JAMA, 270*, 2568–2573.

Canto, J. G., and Iskandrian, A. E. (2003). Major risk factors for cardiovascular disease: debunking the "only 50%" myth. *JAMA, 290*, 947–949.

Carlson, L. E., Ursuliak, Z., Goodey, E., Angen, M., and Speca, M. (2001). The effects of a mindfulness meditation-based stress reduction program on mood and symptoms of stress in cancer outpatients: 6-month follow-up. *Support Care Cancer, 9*, 112–123.

Carrico, A. W., and Antoni, M. H. (2008). The effects of psychological interventions on neuroendocrine hormone regulation and immune status in HIV-positive persons: a review of randomized controlled trials. *Psychosom Med, 70*, 575–584.

Carrico, A. W., Johnson, M. O., Moskowitz, J. T., Neilands, T. B., Morin, S. F. et al (2007). Affect regulation, stimulant use, and viral load among HIV-positive persons on anti-retroviral therapy. *Psychosom Med, 69*, 785–792.

Carrico, A. W., Johnson, M. O., Morin, S. F., Remien, R. H. Riley, E. D. et al (2008). Stimulant use is associated with immune activation and depleted tryptophan among HIV-positive persons on anti-retroviral therapy. *Brain Behav Immunity, 22*, 1257–1262.

Chida, Y., Hamer, M., Wardle, J., and Steptoe, A. (2008). Do stress-related psychosocial factors contribute to cancer incidence and survival? *Nat Clin Pract Oncol, 5*, 466–475.

Cielsa, J. A., and Roberts, J. E. (2001). Meta-analysis of the relationship between HIV infection and the risk for depressive disorders. *Am J Psychiatry, 158*, 725–730.

Clark, A. M., Hartling, L., Vandermeer, B., and McAlister, F. A. (2005). Secondary prevention program for patients with coronary artery disease: a meta-analysis of randomized control trials. *Ann Intern Med, 143*, 659–672.

Classen, C., Butler, L. D., Koopman, C., Miller, E., DiMiceli, S. et al (2001). Supportive-expressive group therapy and distress in patients with metastatic breast cancer: a randomized clinical intervention trial. *Arch Gen Psychiatry, 58*, 494–501.

Cohen, S., and Wills, T. A. (1985). Stress social support, and the buffering hypothesis. *Psychol Bull, 98*, 310-357.

Cole, S. W. (2008). Psychosocial influences on HIV-1 disease progression: neural, endocrine, and virologic mechanisms. *Psychosom Med, 70*, 562–568.

Coleman, M. P., Quaresma, M., Berrino, F., Lutz, J., De Angelis, R. et al (2008). Cancer survival in five continents: a worldwide population-based study (CONCORD). *Lancet Oncol, 9*, 730–756.

Coyne, J. C., and Palmer, S. C. (2007). Does psychotherapy extend survival? Some methodological problems overlooked. *J Clin Oncol, 25*, 4852–4853.

Crepaz, N., Passin, W., Herbst, J., Rama, S, Malow, R. et al (2008). Meta-analysis of cognitive behavioral interventions on HIV-positive person's mental health and immune functioning. *Health Psychol, 27*, 4–14.

Cruess, D. G., Antoni, M. H., McGregor, B. A., Kilbourn, K. M., Boyers, A. E. et al (2000). Cognitive-behavioral stress management reduces serum cortisol by enhancing benefit finding among women being treated for early stage breast cancer. *Psychosom Med, 62*, 304–308.

Dawber, T. R., Meadors, C. F., and Moore, F. E. (1951). Epidemiological approaches to heart disease: the Framingham Study. *Am J Public Health, 41*, 279–290.

de Moor, J. S., Elder, K., and Emmons, K. M. (2008). Smoking prevention and cessation interventions for cancer survivors. *Semin Oncol Nurs, 24*, 180–192.

DiClemente, R. J., Wingood, G., Harrington, K., Lang, D., Davies, S. L. et al (2004). Efficacy of an HIV prevention intervention for African American adolescent girls: a randomized controlled trial. *JAMA, 292*, 171–179.

DiClemente, R. J., Crittenden, C., Rose, E., Sales, J. M., Wingood, G. M. et al (2008). Psychosocial predictors of HIV-associated sexual behaviors and the efficacy of prevention interventions in adolescents at risk for HIV infection: what works and what doesn't work? *Psychosom Med, 70*, 598–605.

Duffy, S. A., Ronis, D. L., McLean, S., Fowler, K. E., Gruber, S. B. et al (2009). Pretreatment health behaviors predict survival among patients with head and neck squamous cell carcinoma. *J Clin Oncol, 27*, 1969–1975.

Dusseldorp, E., vanElderen, T., Maes, S., Meulman, J., and Kraaij, V. (1999). A meta-analysis of psychoeducational programs for coronary heart disease patients. *Health Psychol, 18*, 506–519.

Eton, D. T., Lepore, S. J., and Helgeson, V. S. (2001). Early quality of life in patients with localized prostate carcinoma: an examination of treatment-related, demographic, and psychosocial factors. *Cancer, 92*, 1451–1459.

Evans, D. L., Ten Have, T. R., Douglas, S. D., Gettes, D., Morrison, C. H. et al (2002). Association of depression with viral load, CD8 T lymphocytes, and natural killer cells in women with HIV infection. *Am J Psychiatry, 159*, 1752–1759.

Fawzy, F., Fawzy, N., and Hyun, C. (1993). Malignant melanoma: effects of an early structured psychiatric intervention, coping and affective state on recurrence and survival 6 years later. *Arch Gen Psychiatry, 50*, 681–689.

Fawzy, F. I., Fawzy, N. W., Hyun, C. S., and Weeler, J. F. (1997). Brief coping-oriented therapy for patients with malignant melanoma. In J. L. Spira (Ed.), *Group Therapy for Medically Ill Patients* (pp. 133–164). New York: Guilford Press.

Fawzy, F. I., Canada, A. L., and Fawzy, N. W. (2003). Malignant melanoma: effects of a brief, structured psychiatric intervention on survival and recurrence at 10-year follow-up. *Arch Gen Psychiatry, 60*, 100–103.

Fekete, E., Antoni, M. H., Lopez, C., Duran, R., Penendo, F. et al (2009). Men's serostatus disclosure to parents: associations among social support, ethnicity, and disease status in men living with HIV. *Brain Behav Immunity, 23*(5), 693–696.

Fife, B., Scott, L., Fineberg, N. and Zwickil, B. (2008). Promoting adaptive coping by persons with HIV disease: evaluation of a patient/partner intervention model. *J Assoc Nurse AIDS Care, 19*, 75–84.

Frasure-Smith, N., Lesperance, F., Prince, R., Verrier, P., Garber, R. A. et al (1997). Randomized trial of home-based psychosocial nursing intervention for patients recovering from myocardial infarction. *Lancet, 350*, 473–479.

Friedland, G. H., and Williams, A. (1999). Attaining higher goals in HIV treatment: the central importance of adherence. *AIDS, 13*, S61–S72.

Friedman, M., Thoresen, C. E., Gill, J., Ulmer, D., Powell, L. H. et al (1986). Alteration of Type A behavior and its effect on cardiac recurrences in post-myocardial infarction patients: summary results of the Recurrent Coronary Prevention Project. *Am Heart J, 112*, 653–665.

Galvan, F., Davis, E., Banks, D., and Bing, E. (2008). HIV stigma and social support among African Americans. *AIDS Patient Care STDs, 22*, 423–436.

Goldberg, D. P. (1972). *The Assessment of Psychiatric Illness by Questionnaire*. London: Oxford University Press.

Gonzalez, J. S., Penedo, F. J., Antoni, M. H., Duran, R. E., McPherson-Baker, S. et al (2004). Social support, positive states of mind, and HIV treatment adherence in men and women living with HIV/AIDS. *Health Psychol, 23*, 413–418.

Goodwin, P. J., Leszcz, M., Ennis, M., Koopmans, J., Vincent, L. et al (2001). The effect of group psychosocial support on survival in metastatic breast cancer. *N Engl J Med, 345*, 1719–1726.

Gregoire, I., Kalogeropoulos, D., and Corcos, J. (1997). The effectiveness of a professionally let support group for men with prostate cancer. *Urol Nursing, 17*, 58–66.

Gustafsson, H. H., Whitman, J. P., and Coleman, F. W. (1979). Group approaches for cancer patients: leaders and members. *AJN, 79*, 910–913.

Harrison, L. B., Sessions, R. B., and Hong, W. K. (Eds.). (2009). *Head and Neck Cancer: A Multidisciplinary Approach*, 3rd Ed (pp. 114–131). Philadelphia: Lippincott Williams & Wilkins.

Headley, J., Ownby, K., and John, L. (2004). The effect of seated exercise on fatigue and quality of life in women with advanced breast cancer. *Oncol Nurs Forum, 31*, 977–983.

Hennekens, C. H. (1998). Increasing burden of cardiovascular disease: current knowledge and future directions for research on risk factors. *Circulation, 97*, 1095–1102.

Heron, M., Hoyert, D. L., Murphy, S. L., Xu, J., Kochanek, J. D. et al (2009). National Vital Statistic Report-Deaths: Final Data for 2006. http://www.cdc.gov/nchs/data/nvsr57/nvsr57_14.pdf.

Hewitt, M., Greenfield, S., and Stovall, E. (Eds.). (2006). *From Cancer Patient to Cancer Survivor Lost in Translation* (pp. 17–26). Washington DC: The National Academies Press.

Holland, J. C., Breitbart, W., Jacobsen, P. B., Lederberg, M. S., Loscalzo, M. et al (Eds.). (1998). *Psycho-Oncology*. New York: Oxford University Press, Inc.

Ickovics, J. R., Hamburger, M. E., Vlahov, D., Schoenbaum, E. E., Schuman, P. et al (2001). Mortality, CD4 cell count decline, and depressive symptoms among HIV-seropositive women: longitudinal analysis from the HIV Epidemiology Research Study. *JAMA, 285*, 1460–1465.

Ickovics, J. R., Milan, S., Boland, R., Schoenbaum, E., Schuman, P. et al (2006). Psychological resources protect health: 5-year survival and immune function among HIV-infected women from four U.S. cities. *AIDS, 20*, 1851–1860.

Ironson, G., O'Cleirigh, C., Fletcher, M. A., Laurenceau, J. P., Balbin, E. et al (2005). Psychosocial factors predict CD4 and viral load change in men and women with human immunodeficiency virus in the era of highly active antiretroviral therapy. *Psychosom Med, 67*, 1013–1021.

Johnson, M. O., Charlebois, E., Morin, S. F., Catz, S. L., Goldstein, R. B. et al (2005). Perceived adverse effects of antiretroviral therapy. *J Pain Sympt Manage, 29*, 193–205.

Johnson, M. O., Carrico, A. W., Chesney, M. A., and Morin, S. F. (2008). Internalized heterosexism among HIV-positive gay-identified men: implications for HIV prevention and care. *J Consult Clin Psychol, 76*, 829–839.

Jones, D. A., and West, R. R. (1996). Psychological rehabilitation after myocardial infarction: multicentre randomized controlled trial. *Br Med J, 313*, 1517–1521.

Kalichman, S. (2008). Co-occurrence of treatment nonadherence and continued HIV transmission risk behaviors: implications for positive prevention interventions. *Psychosom Med, 5*, 70, 593–597.

Keruly, J. C. and Moore, R. D. (2007). Immune status at presentation to care did not improve among antiretroviral-naïve persons from 1990 to 2006. *Clin Infect Dis, 45*, 1369–1374.

Kissane, D. W., Grabsch, B., Clarke, D. M., Smith, G. C., Love, A. W. et al (2007). Supportive-expressive group therapy for women with metastatic breast cancer: survival and psychosocial outcome from a randomized controlled trial. *Psychooncology, 16*, 277–286.

Lepore, S., and Helgeson, V. S. (1998). Social constraints, intrusive thoughts and mental health after prostate cancer. *J Soc Clin Psychol, 17*, 89–106.

Leserman, J., Petitto, J. M., Perkins, D. O., Folds, J. D., Golden, R. N. et al (1997). Severe stress and depressive symptoms, and changes in lymphocyte subsets in human immunodeficiency virus infected men. *Arch Gen Psychiatry, 54*, 279–285.

Leserman, J., Jackson, E. D., Petitto, J. M., Golden, R. N., Silva, S. G. et al (1999). Progression to AIDS: the effects of stress, depressive symptoms and social support. *Psychosom Med, 61*, 397–406.

Leserman, J., Petitto, J. M., Gu, H., Gaynes, B. N., Barroso, J. et al (2002). Progression to AIDS, a clinical AIDS condition and mortality: psychosocial and physiological predictors. *Psychol Med, 32*, 1059–1073.

Lieberman, M. A. (1988). The role of self-help groups in helping patients and families cope with cancer. *Cancer, 38*, 162–168.

Linden, W., Stossel, C., and Maurice, J. (1996). Psychosocial interventions for patients with coronary artery disease. *Arch Intern Med, 156*, 745–752.

Linden, W., Phillips, M. J., and Leclerc, J. (2007). Psychological treatment of cardiac patients; a meta-analysis. *Euro Heart J, 28*, 2972–2984.

Luebbert, K., Dahme, B., and Hasenbring, M. (2001). The effectiveness of relaxation training in reducing treatment-related symptoms and improving emotional adjustment in acute non-surgical cancer treatment: a meta-analytical review. *Psycho-Oncology, 10*, 490–502.

Lutgendorf, S. K., Antoni, M. H., Ironson, G., Klimas, N., Kumar, M. et al (1997). Cognitive behavioral stress management intervention decreases dysphoria and herpes simplex virus-type 2 titers in symptomatic HIV-seropositive gay men. *J Consult Clin Psychol, 65*, 23–31.

Lutgendorf, S., Antoni, M. H., Ironson, G., Starr, K., Costello, N. et al (1998) Changes in cognitive coping skills and social support mediate distress outcomes in symptomatic HIV-seropositive gay men during a cognitive behavioral stress management intervention. *Psychosom Med, 60*, 204–214.

Marmot, M. G., Shipley, M. J., and Rose, G. (1984). Inequalities in death: specific explanations of a general pattern? *Lancet, 1*, 1003–1006.

Mayne, T. J., Vittinghoff, E., Chesney, M. A., Barrett, D. C., and Coates, T. J. (1996). Depressive affect and survival among gay and bisexual men infected with HIV. *Arch Intern Med, 156*, 2233–2238.

McGinnis, J. M., and Foege, W. H. (2004). Editorial: the immediate vs the important. *JAMA, 291*, 1263–1264.

Mendes de Leon, C. F., Powell, L. H. and Kaplan, B. (1991). Changes in coronary-prone behaviors in the recurrent coronary prevention project. *Psychosom Med, 53*, 407–419.

Metzler, C. W., Bigaln, A., Noell, J., Ary, D. V., and Ochs, L. (2000). A randomized controlled trial of behavioral intervention to reduce high-risk behaviors among adolescents in STD clinics. *Behav Ther, 31*, 27–54.

Meyer, T. J., and Mark, M. M. (1995). Effects of psychosocial interventions with adult cancer patients: a meta-analysis of randomized experiments. *Health Psychol, 14*, 101–108.

Mokdad, A. H., Marks, J. S., Stroup, D. F., and Gerberding, J. I. (2004). Actual causes of death in the United States, 2000. *JAMA, 291*, 1238–1245.

Moher, D., Schulz, K. F., and Altman, D. (2001). The CONSORT statement: revised recommendations for improving the quality of reports of parallel-group randomized trials. *JAMA, 286*, 1987–1991.

Molton, I. R., Siegel, S. D., Penedo, F. J., Dahn, J. R., Kinsinger, D. et al (2008). Promoting recovery of sexual functioning after radical prostatectomy with group-based stress management: the role of interpersonal sensitivity. *J Psychosom Res, 64*, 527–536.

Morin, S. F., Sengupta, S., Cozen, M., Richards, T. A., Shriver, M. D. et al (2002). Responding to racial and ethnic disparities in the use of HIV drugs: Analysis of state policies. *Public Health Rep, 117*, 263–272.

Moskowitz, J. T. (2003). Positive affect predicts lower risk of AIDS mortality. *Psychosom Med, 65*, 620–626.

National Cholesterol Education Program (1994). Second report of the expert panel on detection, evaluation, and treatment of high blood cholesterol in adults (Adult Treatment Panel II). *Circulation*; *89*, 1333–1445.

Orth-Gomér, K., Schneiderman, N., Wang, H., Walldin, C., Bloom, M., and Jernberg, T. (2009). Stress reduction prolongs life in women with coronary disease: The Stockholm Women's Intervention Trial for Coronary Heart Disease (SWITCHD). *Circulation: Cardiovasc Qual Outcomes, 2*, 25–32.

Page-Shafer, K., Delorenze, G. N., Satariano, W., and Winkelstein, W. (1996). Comorbidity and survival in HIV-infected men in the San Francisco Men's Health Survey. *Ann Epidemiol, 6*, 420–430.

Pantaleo, G., Graziosi, C., and Fauci, A. S. (1993). The immunopathogenesis of human immunodeficiency virus infection. *N Eng J Med, 328*, 327–335.

Park, W., Laura, Y., Scalera, A., Tseng, A., and Rourke, S. (2002). High rate of discontinuations of highly active antiretroviral therapy as a result of antiretroviral intolerance in clinical practice: missed opportunities for support? *AIDS, 16*, 1084–1086.

Patten, S. B. (1997). Performance of the composite international diagnostic interview short form for major depression in community and clinical samples. *Chronic Dis Can, 18*, 109–112.

Penedo, F. J., and Dahn, J. R. (2005). Exercise and well-being: a review of mental and physical health benefits associated with physical activity. *Curr Opin Psychiatry, 18*, 189–193.

Penedo, F. J., Molton, I., Dahn, J. R., Shen, B. J., Kinsinger, D. et al (2006). A randomized clinical trial of group-based cognitive-behavioral stress management in localized prostate cancer: development of stress management skills improves quality of life and benefit finding. *Ann Behav Med, 31,* 261–270.

Rosengren, A. Hawken, S., Ounpuu, S., Silwa, K., Zubaid, M. et al (2004). Association of psychosocial risk factors with risk of acute myocardial infarction in 11119 cases and 13648 controls from 52 countries (the INTERHEART study): case-control study. *Lancet, 364,* 953–962.

Safren, S., Knauz, R. O., O'Cleirigh, C., Lerner, J., Greer, J. et al (2006). CBT for HIV medication adherence and depression: process and outcome at post-treatment and three-month cross over. *Ann Behav Med, 31,* S006.

Safren, S., O'Cleirigh, C., Tan, J., Raminani, S., Reilly, L. et al (2009). Cognitive behavioral therapy for adherence and depression (CBT-AD) in HIV-infected individuals. *Health Psychol, 28,* 1–10.

Schmitz, K. H., Holtzman, J., Courneya, K. S., Mâsse, L. C., Duval, S. et al (2005). Controlled physical activity trials in cancer survivors: a systematic review and meta-analysis. *Cancer Epidemiol Biomarkers Prev, 14,* 1588–1595.

Schneiderman, N., Saab, P. G., Catellier, D., Powell, L. H., DeBusk, L. F. et al (2004). Psychosocial treatment within sex by ethnicity subgroups in the Enhancing Recovery in Coronary Heart Disease clinical trial. *Psychosom Med, 66,* 475–483.

Simoni, J. M., Pearson, C. R., Pantalone, D. W., Marks, G., and Crepaz, N. (2006). Efficacy of interventions in improving highly active antiretroviral therapy adherence and HIV-1 RNA viral load. A meta-analytic review of randomized controlled trials. *J AIDS, 43 Suppl 1,* S23–S35.

Spiegel, D., Bloom, J. R., Kraemer, H. C., and Gottheil, E. (1989). Effect of psychosocial treatment on survival of patients with metastatic breast cancer. *Lancet, 14,* 888–891.

Spiegel, D., Butler, L. D., Giese-Davis, J., Koopman, C., Miller, E. et al (2007). Effects of supportive-expressive group therapy on survival of patients with metastatic breast cancer: a randomized prospective trial. *Cancer, 110,* 1130–1138.

Steginga, S. K., Occhipinti, S., Dunn, J., Gardiner, R. A., Heathcote, P. et al (2001). The supportive care needs of men with prostate cancer. *Psychooncology, 10,* 66–75.

Steptoe, A., and Marmot, M. G. (2002). The role of psychobiological pathways in socio-economic inequalities in cardiovascular disease risk. *Eur Heart J, 23,* 13–25.

Szapocznik, J., Feaster, D. J., Mitrani, V. B., Prado, G., Smith, L. et al (2004). Structural ecosystems therapy for HIV-seropositive African American women: effects on psychological distress, family hassles, and family support. *J Consult Clin Psychol, 72,* 288–303.

Weaver, K. E., Llabre, M. M., Duran, R. E., Antoni, M. H., Ironson, G. et al (2005). A stress and coping model of medication adherence and viral load in HIV-positive men and women on highly active antiretroviral therapy (HAART). *Health Psychol, 24,* 385–392.

World Health Organization (2009). Cancer. Fact sheet Number 297, http://www.who.int/mediacentre/factsheets/fS297/en/print.html

World Health Organization (2008). The top 10 causes of death. Fact sheet Number 310, http://www.who.int/mediacentre/factsheets/f5310/en/index.html

Yusuf, S., Hawken, S., Ounpuu, S., Dans, T., Avezum, A. et al (2004). Effect of potentially modifiable risk factors associated with myocardial infarction in 52 countries (the INTERHEART study): case-control study. *Lancet, 364,* 937–952.

Zabora, J., BrintzenhofeSzoc, K., Jacobsen, P., Curbow, B., Piantadosi, S. et al (2001). A new psychosocial screening instrument for use with cancer patients. *Psychosomatics, 42,* 241–246.

Chapter 64

The Role of Interactive Communication Technologies in Behavioral Medicine

Victor J. Strecher

1 Introduction

Over the past 10 years, interactive communication technologies have extended to nearly all parts of the world, changing how we work, play, and learn. Interactive health communications, here given the broad term "eHealth," has paralleled these changes. Our implementation of robust eHealth applications, however, continues to lag well behind other interactive communication endeavors. Far more sophisticated uses of these strategies go into the online purchase of a pair of shoes than into assistance provided to a depressed patient. Most research examining the impact and potential uses of eHealth applications is stunted and likely to be outdated by the time it reaches publication. Even high-quality eHealth research is largely ignored in commercial eHealth applications, which continue to compete in a Wild West snake-oil environment. This situation is unfortunate since eHealth applications offer the potential for achieving tremendous impact on the public's health.

To date, most behavioral medicine intervention strategies fall into two categories: (1) those that have high efficacy but, when using population-based criteria of need, have low rates of participation or reach, such as group or individual therapy approaches; or (2) those strategies that have high reach but low efficacy, such as pamphlets, brochures, videos, and other mass communications (Bendryen and Kraft, 2008). Both strategies can be criticized for lacking significant population health impact. Programs developed using interactive communication technologies have the potential to reach large populations with content tailored to specific needs and interests of the individual user.

This chapter examines current and future *reach* and *efficacy* of eHealth applications relevant to behavioral medicine. These applications will first be discussed in terms of their access and use. This chapter then discusses efficacy of eHealth applications, examining different uses of this flexible communications strategy. Finally, future directions of eHealth field are examined, considering new technologies and the integration of informatics fields for behavioral medicine interventions.

2 The Reach of eHealth Applications

The reach of eHealth applications defined here as access to, and participation in, the intervention out of the total population in need will vary by the interactive communication technology employed and the organizations through which the applications are delivered.

V.J. Strecher (✉)
Department of Health Behavior and Health Education,
Center for Health Communications Research, School of
Public Health, University of Michigan, 300 N. Ingalls –
Room 5D-04 (0471), Ann Arbor, MI 48109-0471, USA
e-mail: stretcher@umich.edu

A. Steptoe (ed.), *Handbook of Behavioral Medicine*, DOI 10.1007/978-0-387-09488-5_64,
© Springer Science+Business Media, LLC 2010

2.1 Technology Channels

Today the most common delivery channel for eHealth applications is the Internet, a channel allowing detailed data collection and tailored feedback at a fraction of the cost of other intervention formats. The proportion of adults in the United States with access to the Internet now exceeds 78% (Center for the Digital Future, 2005). The largest increases in Internet access are among low-income and older Americans. The University of Southern California Annenberg School's Center for the Digital Future (2005) reported that 61% of respondents with incomes of less than $30,000 and 75% of respondents aged 56–65 were using the Internet in 2005.

While the Internet is likely to remain for years a dominant delivery channel for eHealth applications, a large portion of the world, particularly younger individuals and the developing world, utilize mobile phones for communication, entertainment, and education (ITU, 2009). As Fig. 64.1 indicates, the rate of mobile technology penetration has far exceeded that of the Internet.

The Internet, however, is also used as a source of information for mobile technologies. For example, in 2007, 32% of Americans reported downloading information to an iPod, cell phone, or personal digital assistant (PDA) (HINTS, 2009). As will be discussed later in this chapter,

mobile technology allows the collection of ecological momentary assessment (EMA) data while also providing interactive health coaching at any time of the day. It is likely that mobile phone devices will increasingly incorporate other features, including pedometry and biometric assessment. A current example of multiple resources incorporated into mobile phone technology is Apple's iPhone.

As Fig. 64.2 indicates, in the United States, a large portion of individuals (roughly 100 million) first go to the Internet to look for information about health or medical topics, nearly five times the number who seek a health-care provider or books and pamphlets, and nearly ten times the number who report going to a telephone information service (HINTS, 2009). Similar findings have been reported in European countries, where use of the Internet for health purposes exceeds 50% and continues to increase while the importance of traditional health information channels has decreased or remained the same (Kummervold et al, 2008).

The use of the Internet for the prevention of morbidity and mortality is lower than for treatment issues but is nonetheless significant: 51% of Americans with Internet access report using the Internet for information about diet, nutrition, vitamins, or nutritional supplements; 42% for information about exercise or fitness; and 7% for information about how to quit smoking (Fox, 2005). While 7% of all adult Internet users may

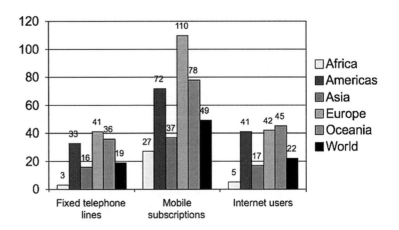

Fig. 64.1 International communication technologies rates per 100 inhabitants, 2007

Source: International Telecommunication Union, 2009

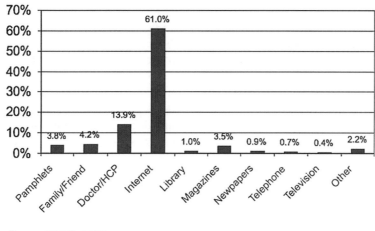

Source: HINTS, 2009

Fig. 64.2 First source for health or medical information, 2007

seem to be a small proportion, this amounts to more than 10 million individuals and compares favorably with the estimate that 800,000 smokers in the United States call quitlines each year for cessation advice (Ossip-Klein and McIntosh, 2003). In all of these areas, more females than males sought Web-based information. Seekers of Internet-based health information were more likely than non-seekers to be better educated, to have higher incomes, and to be younger.

Individuals are now taking advantage of the Internet in ways that transcend simple information transmission. In 2007, 34% of American Internet users were using social networking sites such as MySpace and Second Life and 10% were writing online diaries or blogs (web-logs) (HINTS, 2009). However, the use of online support groups remains small (5% of Internet users) despite persistent offerings of these programs over the past decade (HINTS, 2009). Low use of online support groups for somatic disease issues has also been found in Europe (van Uden-Kraan et al, 2009a, b).

2.2 Organizational Channels

At least as important as the specific technology channels for delivering eHealth applications

for behavioral medicine, the intermediary organizations delivering these applications can significantly influence reach. Current organizational channels include health plans (e.g., KPOnline of Kaiser Permanente), voluntary health organizations (e.g., American Cancer Society), employers, pharmaceutical companies, governments, schools, and universities. These organizational channels have different long-term goals for behavior change and decision-making programs. All of these organizations will be interested in improved health-related behaviors and better-informed decision-making. However, a health plan will be interested in Healthcare Effectiveness Data and Information Set (HEDIS) scores related to member satisfaction scores and utilization. An employer will be particularly interested in productivity and employee retention. A pharmaceutical company will be interested in medication adherence and persistence. A school will be interested in absenteeism and test scores. These pragmatic outcomes will be the criteria for sustaining the intervention within a particular channel and are therefore highly relevant to the eHealth application developer.

eHealth applications will increasingly be delivered with, or aligned with, medical and consumer products. The pharmaceutical industry has developed eHealth applications integrated with prescription and over-the-counter products for over 15 years. A good example of this type of application is the Internet-based smoking cessation programming offered with pharmacological smoking cessation products. These eHealth applications have demonstrated a benefit in smoking cessation as well as medication adherence (Strecher et al, 2005). Both outcomes are extremely important to the pharmaceutical sponsor and assure continued sustainability of the eHealth application. eHealth programming that is aligned, but not directly associated with, a particular product is likely to grow as well. Such programs have been developed for the management of chronic conditions, including diabetes and cardiovascular disease.

Reach is likely to vary by the type of organization through which the eHealth application is delivered. Anecdotally, employers appear to generate higher use of eHealth applications when offered than do health plans or governments. The specific factors underlying participation rates are not well understood and very few randomized trials have tested different methods for enhancing participation. Since efficacy of an intervention means little if no one uses it, the consideration of reach deserves far more attention that it has received to date. Given the high rates of Internet use for health-related reasons, research in this area is likely to result in important public health outcomes.

3 The Efficacy of eHealth Applications

The efficacy of eHealth applications is difficult to quantify due to the highly varied nature of these applications. Asking "Is eHealth effective?" is like asking: "Do movies entertain?" Clearly, some movies do and some do not. Our challenge is to determine the optimal fit of eHealth applications to individual needs and preferences. Three common strategies for eHealth programming reflect how individuals normally seek help: (1) they might go to a

library, bookstore, pamphlet rack, or other information source for self-navigated help-seeking; (2) they might seek an expert who will assess, diagnose, and then prescribe a treatment tailored to the needs of the individual; or (3) they might seek other individuals with a similar condition, either through a support group or as an individual. These three options are examined below.

3.1 Self-Navigated Help Seeking

The Internet, and increasingly mobile technology, resembles a vast library that requires the user to select applications that best apply to his or her needs. Similar to a library, the Internet has methods of searching for a large amount of available health information. Also like a library, however, the Internet does not necessarily make available the most relevant information or advice that an individual needs at a particular time. Moreover, the individual needs to work, and sometimes work hard, to get the right information.

An expectation that users will create their own educational experiences is common on the Internet, but just as in a library, users might not know precisely what to search for or may fail to search in the right places (Eveland and Dunwoody, 2002). This is particularly likely among individuals new to a subject or those who have little confidence or ability in a particular area (Gay, 1986; Ross and Morrison, 1989; Steinberg, 1977). As Ross and Morrison (1989) state, "In general, while high achievers seem capable of using most forms of learner control effectively, low achievers seem much less able to benefit from forms that require them to make decisions about instructional properties of a lesson (i.e., what, how and how much information is being taught)..." (p. 29). Bhavnani and colleagues (2002) found that domain expertise is a critical factor in the effective use of the Internet. Experienced Internet shoppers were far less efficient or accurate in obtaining medical information than were medical librarians when both groups were asked to find the criteria for individuals who should and should not get the flu vaccine. Medical librarians, on the other hand, were far less efficient in finding a low-priced digital camera on the Internet.

Once an individual identifies a specific Internet site or mobile application, he or she often finds that it offers little more than an electronic pamphlet rack. This experience is found on most Internet health portals, whether commercial or through voluntary health organizations. These sites are rarely evaluated and are likely to offer no better solution to health-related behavior change and decision-making problems than an actual pamphlet rack. As Cline and Haynes (2001) state in their appraisal of the field, "Much of the literature reviewed here focuses on the Internet as a high-tech conveyor in the rapid diffusion of information or health lessons. However, to do so is to ignore the very nature of the Internet."

3.2 Tailored Expert Systems

The general strategy of a tailored expert system is to: (1) collect, from the individual user, data relevant to the targeted behavior; (2) apply an algorithm to the data that generates messages tailored to the specific needs of the user; and (3) generate feedback that combines these messages in a clear, vivid manner. Data collected can be biometric, behavioral, medical, psychosocial, or genetic. The inferences made from the data are an attempt to reflect standards of a human expert (Velicer et al, 1993). Selection of factors on which to tailor feedback is one of the most important steps in the development of an expert system. Participants in a traditional tailored media application may answer questions related to personal and family health history, behavior triggers, barriers to change, and motivation to change (among others), and a high proportion of expert systems utilize some form of cognitive-behavioral programming (e.g., Cavanagh and Shapiro, 2004; Clarke et al, 2005; Hawkins et al, 2008; Lustria

et al, 2009; Noar et al, 2007; Proudfoot et al, 2004; Rothert et al, 2006; Strecher et al, 2005; Wagner et al, 2006).

A rapidly growing number of research studies have demonstrated that tailored expert system interventions are more effective than generic health behavior change materials, even among underserved populations. These studies cover a range of topics, including smoking cessation, weight management, dietary fat reduction, fruit and vegetable intake, and cancer screening (Brug et al, 1999; Kroeze et al, 2006; Lancaster and Stead, 2000; Lemmens et al, 2008; Neville et al, 2009; Noar et al, 2007; Skinner et al, 1999; Strecher, 1999) with somewhat less evidence of efficacy in the area of physical activity (Kroeze et al, 2006; Vandelanotte et al, 2007; van den Berg et al, 2007). Tailored mobile applications using short-message service (SMS) feedback has demonstrated positive short-term results in health-related behavior change and self-management (Fjeldsoe et al, 2009).

Current research in this area is focusing on: (1) mechanisms underlying the efficacy of tailored eHealth applications and (2) innovative measures and strategies for making the tailored feedback more relevant to the user. Tailored eHealth messages appear to work, at least in part, through greater cognitive elaboration of messages perceived to be relevant to the user (Dijkstra, 2005; Hawkins et al, 2008). A number of studies have demonstrated that tailored materials are perceived as being more relevant than untailored materials (Brug et al, 1999; Strecher, 1999), and that perceived relevance moderates the impact of tailored materials on behavior change (Strecher et al, 2008a, 2008b). Neuroimaging research exposing cigarette smokers to high- versus low-depth tailored cessation materials found greater activation of the prefrontal cortex and the precuneous portions of the brain related to self-relevance and long-term episodic memory (Chua et al, 2009).

Innovative tailored message studies have moved beyond the "usual suspects" measures examining the impact of tailoring to self-relevant and learning style factors. Tailoring to ethnic identity (Resnicow et al, 2009) and intrinsic motives and values (Resnicow et al, 2009) have both resulted in positive changes in fruit and vegetable consumption. Williams-Piehota and colleagues (2003) found that tailoring mammography screening messages to the user's need for cognition (degree to which a person likes to think, solve problems, consider issues) produced a positive effect on mammography screening behavior at 6-month follow-up. Similarly, Bakker (1999) found that an HIV prevention message in comic format best influenced the attitudes of subjects with a low need for cognition, whereas a text format of the message best influenced subjects with a high need for cognition.

Interpersonal relation characteristics such as empathy can also be integrated into expert system interfaces. Bickmore and colleagues (2005) found that the inclusion of relational characteristics in an automated longitudinal health behavior change intervention produced significant improvements in perceived trust, understanding, liking, respect, concern, and caring after roughly 1 month of use. Moreover, the inclusion of relational behaviors enhanced the desire to continue working with the program.

To date, most expert systems for health behavior change have used survey data collected at a single point in time to tailor information. Ecological momentary assessment or EMA typically uses portable monitoring devices to collect multiple data points in the relevant environment in real time (Stone and Shiffman, 1994). Sampling strategies can vary according to the type of information collected (Wheeler and Reis, 1991). For example, event-contingent recording can track the details of specific behavioral events, smoking or dietary behavior, episodes of nausea, or precipitants of pain. Other assessments might require information collected at specific intervals or at random, for example, when assessing cigarette or food cravings during particular times of the day or night.

An important new direction for behavioral medicine research and practice is the statistical examination of EMA patterns which, along with characteristics of the user (e.g., motives, self-efficacy), could predict subsequent behaviors of the user and identify potential interventions tailored to the specific behavioral trajectories of the user (Shiyko et al, 2008). An automated "health coach" on your mobile phone, for example, could monitor psychosocial and behavioral measures, resetting goals and continually identifying behavioral triggers. Ongoing assessment could also determine appropriate subsequent treatment strength and dosing (Collins et al, 2005). Richardson and colleagues (2007), for example, found that an automated goal setting program combined with a pedometer that connects to the automated system enhanced walking behavior among elderly diabetics by roughly 1 mile after 6 months.

3.3 Online Support Groups and Virtual Communities

As stated previously, only a small proportion of Internet users report using online support groups or virtual communities (HINTS, 2009; Stoddard et al, 2008; van Uden-Kraan et al, 2009). Yet, online support groups allow patients a convenient way to provide and receive informational and emotional support (Brennan et al, 1997; Shaw et al, 2000; Tate and Zabinski, 2004; van Uden-Kraan et al, 2009). The 24/7 accessibility to online support is considered a significant advantage to patients who, because of stress, pain, or the treatment itself, have irregular sleeping habits. Patients report frequent use of discussion groups late at night (Shaw et al, 2000). Again, anonymity is a frequently cited benefit of computer-mediated groups. As one person in the latter study states: "It's a gift to be able to tell people as much or as little as you want about yourself."

Most evaluative studies have found minimal or no effects of online support groups and virtual communities (Eysenbach et al, 2004). Reviews, however, have found most studies in this area lacking controlled experiental designs (Eysenbach et al, 2004; Klemm et al, 2003).

A large, well-designed, trial of a peer-to-peer virtual community for smoking cessation randomized smokers interested in quitting to an online smoking cessation program (smokefree.gov) with or without a virtual community (Stoddard et al, 2008). As found in the recent national survey (HINTS, 2009), only a small proportion (12%) of smokers offered the virtual community actually used it. There were no differences in cessation as a result of the virtual community.

4 The Future of eHealth

In 2007, director of the National Institutes of Health Elias Zerhouni stated: "We are in a revolutionary period of medicine that I call the four Ps: predictive, personalized, preemptive and participatory... As opposed to the doctor-centric, curative model of the past, the future is going to be patient-centric and proactive. It must be based on education and communication." (NIH/MedlinePlus, 2007). The eHealth field clearly dovetails with Dr. Zerhouni's vision of personalized medicine: the use of data to predict relevant outcomes; tailored feedback designed to improve health-related behaviors, thereby pre-empting negative outcomes; and the emphasis on self-management.

Emerging mobile technologies will likely allow greater accuracy and timeliness in assessments, thereby allowing more relevant, timely feedback to the user. A particularly interesting direction for EMA is the involvement of microelectromechanical systems technologies. Microsystem "labs on chips" (larger than nanoscale technologies) are currently being developed to regularly assess blood glucose, cholesterol, and other physiological data. Larger-scale physiological data collection devices (e.g., glucometers, instrumented inhalers, ambulatory blood pressure monitors) already collect parallel streams of psychological and physiological data (e.g., Guyll and Contrada 1998; Kamarck et al, 2005). These technologies will continue to become more portable and nearly invisible

to the user, embedded in mobile phones, clothing, shoes, product containers (e.g., soft drink cans, sunscreen bottles), and many other objects of daily use. Still other tools allowing genomic assessment will offer interesting and doubtless controversial intervention strategies.

4.1 Integration of Consumer and Medical Informatics Systems

Interactions will also emerge between the types of eHealth applications discussed in this chapter, often termed "consumer health informatics," and other informatics systems of clinical medicine, biology, and public health. With organizations such as the Veterans Administration taking a lead in demonstrating the effectiveness and efficiency of electronic medical records (EMR) systems (Murphy 2002), large managed care systems – including Kaiser Permanente and Group Health Cooperative – are beginning to integrate EMR and expert system applications to prompt, intervene on, and record cancer-related screening, counseling, and decision support activities.

Online communication between clinicians and patients would seem, on the face of it, to be another logical extension of the medical-consumer informatics integration. A trial evaluating the impact of increased access to physicians through a patient portal found increased satisfaction with communication and overall care (Lin et al, 2005). Roughly half of the subjects in the intervention condition were willing to pay an average of $2 (USD) for online correspondence with their physician. Katz and colleagues (2003) found both physicians and patients expressing preferences for some types of email interactions (e.g., simpler clinical issues and requests for normal lab results) over others (e.g., complex or sensitive issues such as mental health or pain management).

Current embodiments of medical/consumer health informatics integration continue to focus on patient-held medical records combined with a library of health information (so-called personal health records), with little attention paid to evidence-based tailored behavior-change applications. This may reflect a locus of power residing among the EMR developers, many of whom are clinicians with traditional views of health behavior change and decision-making. For nearly four decades, researchers have found that knowledge is generally unrelated to health behavior and that simple information transmission fails to change health-related behaviors. Yet the concept of the pamphlet rack outside of the doctor's office, even in electronic form, endures. Successful integration of these fields of informatics can probably yield outcomes greater than the sums of their parts, but a scientific, theoretically grounded understanding of both fields will be required to achieve success.

4.2 Integration of Consumer and Public Health Informatics Systems

Epidemiological data are increasingly being collected by major search engines through an analysis of aggregated search queries (Ratzan, 2009). Innovative approaches to alerting and monitoring the spread of disease outbreaks (e.g., SARS, influenza) and health-related behaviors (e.g., searches for bootleg cigarettes) could provide ongoing, inexpensive sources of important population-based health information (Eysenbach, 2009; Ratzan, 2009). The application of information technologies to public health research and practice will increasingly allow us to link geographically specific disease patterns with environmental, behavioral, demographic, and eventually, genetic data (Kopp et al, 2002). Data sources can include reportable diseases, diagnostic information for inpatients and outpatients, intensive care unit admissions, Medicare or Medicaid claims, poison information calls, Internet hits for medical information, road and transit usage, weather records, and school and

work absenteeism records (Pavlin, 2003). The rewards of this multilevel integration will be deeper understanding of the incidence, prevalence, distribution, and multifactor etiologies of disease (Ratzan, 2009; Eysenbach, 2009).

4.3 Integration of Consumer and Bioinformatics Systems

The application of statistical and computational methods to understanding the human genome should yield tremendous benefits in our understanding of disease susceptibility, responsiveness to prevention efforts, chronic disease management, and long-term survivorship. To date, estimates of an individual's health risk are calculated from population-based data (Beery et al, 1986). Health Risk Assessment, for example, uses population-based mortality data to calculate a "risk age" on the basis of an individual's demographic characteristics and health habits (Beery et al, 1986). Feedback from such health risk assessments can provide only averaged, usually bland, feedback regarding risk and generally has very little impact on behavior change (Kreuter and Strecher, 1996; Strecher and Kreuter, 1995).

Assessing and predicting an individual's risk using genotypic, environmental, medical, and behavioral data will ultimately allow more accurate, detailed, and personalized feedback to that individual. Once this feedback is provided, genetic information could be used in combination with behavioral, psychosocial, and environmental data to create a far more tailored intervention plan. For example, genetic data could inform the type and dosing of pharmacotherapy for smoking cessation in combination with a tailored behavioral treatment plan (Lerman and Berrettini, 2003).

Large-scale, population-based genetic testing will generate a need for eHealth-based genetic counseling applications. Genetic counselors are trained to convey the risks and benefits of a genetic screening decision in an unbiased manner. With the advent of rapid, easier tests for genetic conditions, however, our traditional genetic counseling facilities will soon be rapidly overwhelmed (Wang et al, 2005). Interactive health communication technologies may have a role in addressing this issue, but must demonstrate the capability of conveying genetic screening information with the same unbiased, highly informed qualities of genetic counselors. Initial trials of CD-ROM-based and tailored print-based eHealth applications for genetic counseling have been promising and warrant further research of risk communication and informed decision-making outcomes using interactive health communication technologies (Skinner et al, 2002; Wang et al, 2005).

5 Conclusion

Interactive communication technologies are changing our lives in significant ways. The use of these technologies to reach a greater proportion of the public, with more effective interventions, at a lower cost, is a reasonable goal of eHealth. Controlled trials comparing the impact of different interactivity approaches, media, content, and message frequency, among other factors, with characteristics of the individual would likely improve the quality and understanding of eHealth applications. A common mistake has been to generalize eHealth programs into one class of intervention.

We should also recognize that these applications are still in their infancy. Technology, access to this technology, data collection, and content will continue to improve. Linkages between consumer health informatics, medical informatics, bioinformatics, and public health informatices will create a new generation of more finely tuned and systematic behavioral health applications. Researchers will be challenged to remain abreast of these advances while developing and evaluating new eHealth applications.

References

Bakker, A. B. (1999). Persuasive communication about AIDS prevention: need for cognition determines the impact of message format. *AIDS Educ Prev, 11,* 150c162.

Beery, W. L., Schoenbach, V. J., Wagner, E. H., Graham, R., Karon, J. et al (1986). Health risk appraisal: methods and programs with annotated bibliography. *Department of Health and Human Services Publication No. (PHS),* 86–3396. Washington, DC: Natl. Cent. Health Serv. Res. Health Care Technol.

Bhavnani, S. K., Bichakjian, C. K., Schwartz, J. L., Strecher, V. J., Dunn, R. L. et al (2002). Getting patients to the right healthcare sources: from real-world questions to Strategy Hubs. Proc. *AMIA Symp,* 51–55.

Bendryen, H., and Kraft, P. (2008). Happy ending: a randomized controlled trial of a digital multi-media smoking cessation intervention. *Addiction, 103,* 478–484.

Bickmore, T., Gruber, A., and Picard, R. (2005). Establishing the computer-patient working alliance in automated health behavior change interventions. *Patient Educ Couns, 59*(1), 21–30.

Brennan, P., Fink, S., Street, R., Gold, W., and Manning, T. (Eds.). (1997). *Health Promotion, Social Support, and Computer Networks. In Health Promotion and Interactive Technology* (pp. 157–170). Mahwah, NJ: Erlbaum.

Brug, J., Campbell, M., and van Assema, P. (1999). The application and impact of computer-generated personalized nutrition education: a review of the literature. *Pat Educ Couns, 36,* 145–156.

Cavanagh, K., and Shapiro, D. A. (2004). Computer treatment for common mental health problems. *J Clin Psychol, 60,* 239–251.

Center for the Digital Future Project. (2005). Digital Future Report. http://www.digitalcenter.org.

Chua, H. F., Liberzon, I., Welsh, R. C., and Strecher, V. J. (2009). Neural correlates of message tailoring and self-relatedness in smoking cessation programming. *Biol Psychiatry, 65,* 165–168.

Clarke, G., Eubanks, D., Reid, E., Kelleher, C., O'Connor, E. et al (2005). Overcoming Depression on the Internet (ODIN) (2): a randomized trial of a self-help depression skills program with reminders. *J Med Internet Res, 7,* e16.

Cline, R. J., and Haynes, K. M. (2001). Consumer health information seeking on the Internet: the state of the art. *Health Educ Res, 16,* 671–692.

Collins, L. M., Murphy, S. A., Nair, V., and Strecher, V. S. (2005). A strategy for optimizing and evaluating behavioral interventions. *Ann Behav Med, 30,* 65–73.

Dijkstra, A. (2005). Working mechanisms of computer-tailored health education: evidence from smoking cessation. *Health Educ Res, 20,* 527–539.

Eveland, W. P., and Dunwoody, S. (2002). An investigation of elaboration and selective scanning as mediators of learning from the Web versus print. *J Broadcast Electron Media, 46*, 34–53.

Eysenbach, G. (2009). Infodemiology and infoveillance: framework for an emerging set of public health informatics methods to analyze search, communication and publication behavior on the Internet. *J Med Internet Res, 11*, e11.

Eysenbach, G., Powell, J., Englesakis, M., Rizo, C., and Stern, A. (2004). Health related virtual communities and electronic support groups: systematic review of the effects of online peer to peer interactions. *Brit Med J, 328*, 1166.

Fjeldsoe, B. S., Marshall, A. L., and Miller, Y. D. (2009). Behavior change interventions delivered by mobile telephone short-message service. *Am J Prev Med, 36*, 165–73.

Fox, S. (2005). Health information online. May 17. Pew Internet and American Life Project. http://www.pewinternet.org.

Gay, G. (1986). Interaction of learner control and prior understanding in computer-assisted video instruction. *J Educ Psychol, 78*, 225–227.

Guyll, M., and Contrada, R. J. (1998). Trait hostility and ambulatory cardiovascular activity: responses to social interaction. *Health Psychol, 17*, 30–39.

Hawkins, R. P., Kreuter, M., Resnicow, K., Fishbein, M., and Dijkstra, A. (2008). Understanding tailoring in communicating about health. *Health Educ Res, 23*, 454–466.

HINTS (Health Information National Trends Survey: How Americans find and use cancer information). (2009). National Cancer Institute. http://hints.cancer.gov.

International Telecommunication Union (2009). World Telecommunication/ ICT Indicators Database. Geneva. (available at: http://www.itu.int/ITU-D/ict/statistics/ict/index.html).

Kamarck, T. W., Schwartz, J. E., Shiffman, S., Muldoon, M. F., Sutton-Tyrrell, K. et al (2005). Psychosocial stress and cardiovascular risk: what is the role of daily experience? *J Personality, 73*, 1–26.

Katz, S. J., Moyer, C. A., Cox, D. T., and Stern, D. T. (2003). Effect of a triage-based E-mail system on clinic resource use and patient and physician satisfaction in primary care: a randomized controlled trial. *J Gen Intern Med, 18*, 736–44.

Klemm, P., Bunnell, D., Cullen, M., Soneji, R., Gibbons, P. et al (2003). Online cancer support groups: a review of the research literature. *Comput Inform Nurs, 21*, 136–142.

Kopp, S., Shuchman, R., Strecher, V., Gueye, M., Ledlow, J. et al (2002). Public health applications. *Telemed J e-Health 8*, 35–48.

Kreuter, M. W., and Strecher, V. J. (1996). Do tailored behavior change messages enhance the effectiveness of health risk appraisal? Results from a randomized trial. *Health Educ Res, 11*, 97–105.

Kroeze, W., Werkman, A., and Brug, J. (2006). A systematic review of randomized trials on the effectiveness of computer-tailored education on physicial; activity and dietary behaviors. *Ann Behav Med, 31*, 205–223.

Kummervold, P. E., Chronaki, C. E., Lausen, B., Prokosch, H. U., Rasmussen, J. et al (2008). eHealth trends in Europe 2005–2007: a population-based survey. *J Med Internet Res, 10*, e42.

Lancaster, T., and Stead, L. F. (2000). *Self-help interventions for smoking cessation.* Cochrane Database Syst. Rev. CD001118.

Lemmens, V., Oenema, A., Knut, I. K., and Brug, J. (2008). Effectiveness of smoking cessation interventions among adults: a systematic review of reviews. *Eur J Cancer Prev, 17*, 535–544.

Lerman, C., and Berrettini, W. (2003). Elucidating the role of genetic factors in smoking behavior and nicotine dependence. *Am J Med Genet B Neuropsychiatr Genet, 118*, 48–54.

Lin, C. T., Wittevrongel, L., Moore, L., Beaty, B. L., and Ross, S. E. (2005). An Internet-based patient-provider communication system: randomized controlled trial. *J Med Internet Res, 7*, e47.

Lustria, M. L., Cortese, J., Noar, S. M., and Glueckauf, R. L. (2009). Computer-tailored health interventions delivered over the web: review and analysis of key components. *Patient Educ Couns, 74*, 156–173.

Murphy, F. (2002). *Department of Veterans Affairs: Information Technology Can Improve Health Care Quality.* Health Legacy Conference and eHealth Initiative Annual Meeting. Washington, DC: Natl. Press Club.

Neville, L. M., O'Hara, B., and Milat, A. J. (2009). Computer-tailored dietary behaviour change interventions: a systematic review. *Health Educ Res, 24*(4), 699–720.

NIH/ Medline Plus. (2007). *The promise of personalized medicine.* Winter, *2*(1), 2–3.

Noar, S. M., Benac, C. N., and Harris, M. S. (2007). Does tailoring matter? Meta-analytic review of tailored print health behavior change interventions. *Psychol Bull, 113*, 673–693.

Ossip-Klein, D. J., and McIntosh, S. (2003). Quitlines in North America: evidence base and applications. *Am J Med Sci, 326*, 201–205.

Pavlin, J. A. (2003). Investigation of disease outbreaks detected by "syndromic" surveillance systems. *J Urban Health, 80*(2 Suppl. 1), i107–14.

Proudfoot, J., Ryden, C., Everitt, B., Shapiro, D. A., Goldberg, D. et al (2004). Clinical efficacy of computerised cognitive-behavioural therapy for anxiety and depression in primary care: randomised controlled trial. *Br J Psychiatry, 185*, 46–54.

Ratzan, S. (2009). 21st century opportunities in health: e-health and technology. *J Health Commun, 14*, 1–2.

Resnicow, K., Davis, R., Zhang, N., Tolsma, D., Alexander, G., et al (2009). Tailoring a fruit and vegetable intervention on ethnic identity: results of a randomized study. *Health Psychol, 28*(4), 394–403.

Richardson, C. R., Mehari, K. S., McIntyre, L. G., Janney, A. W., Fortlage, L. A. et al (2007). A randomized trial comparing structures and lifestyle goals in an internet-mediated walking program for people with type 2 diabetes. *Int J Behav Nutr Phys Act, 4,* 59.

Ross, S., and Morrison, G. (1989). In search of a happy medium in instructional technology research: issues concerning external validity, media replications, and learner control. *Educ Technol Res Dev, 37,* 19–33.

Rothert, K., Strecher, V. J., Doyl, L. A., Caplan, W. M., Joyce, J. S. et al (2006). Web-based weight management programs in an integrated health care setting: a randomized, controlled trial. *Obes Res, 14,* 266–272.

Shaw, B. R., McTavish, F., Hawkins, R., Gustafson, D. H., and Pingree, S. (2000). Experiences of women with breast cancer: exchanging social support over the CHESS computer network. *J Health Comm, 5,* 135–159.

Shiyko, M., Li, Y., Ostroff, J., and Burkhalter, J. E. (2008). *Predictors of Time-to-Non-Adherence in a Scheduled Reduced Smoking Cessation Treatment for Cancer Patients.* Presentation (poster) at the annual meeting of the Society of Behavioral Medicine, San Diego, CA.

Skinner, C. S., Campbell, M. K., Rimer, B. K., Curry, S., and Prochaska, J. O. (1999). How effective is tailored print communication. *Ann Behav Med, 21,* 290–298.

Skinner, C. S., Schildkraut, J. M., Berry, D., Calingaert, B., Marcom, P. K., et al (2002). Pre-counseling education materials for BRCA testing: does tailoring make a difference? *Genet Test, 6(2),* 93–105.

Steinberg, E. R. (1977). Review of student control in computer-assisted instruction. *J Comp Based Instr, 3,* 84–90.

Stoddard, J. L., Augustson, E. M., and Moser, R. P. (2008). Effect of adding a virtual community (bulletin board) to smokefree.gov: randomized controlled trial. *J Med Internet Res, 10,* e53.

Stone, A. A., and Shiffman, S. (1994). Ecological momentary assessment (EMA) in behavioral medicine. *Ann Behav Med, 16,* 199–202.

Strecher, V. J. (1999). Computer-tailored smoking cessation materials: a review and discussion. *Pat Educ Couns, 36,* 107–117.

Strecher, V. J., and Kreuter, M. W. (1995). The psychosocial and behavioral impact of health risk appraisals. In R. T. Croyle (Eds.) *Psychosocial Effects of Screening for Disease Prevention and Detection* (pp. 144–184). New York: Oxford University Press.

Strecher ,V. J., Shiffman, S., and West, R. (2005). Randomized controlled trial of a Web-based computer-tailored smoking cessation program as a supplement to nicotine patch therapy. *Addiction 100,* 682.

Strecher, V. J., McClure, J., Alexander, G., Chakraborty, B., Nair, V. et al (2008a). The role of engagement in a tailored web-based smoking cessation program: randomized controlled trial. *J Med Internet Res, 10,* e36.

Strecher, V. J., McClure, J., Alexander, G., Chakraborty, B., Nair, V. et al (2008b). Web-based smoking cessation program: results of a randomized yrial. *Am J Prev Med, 34,* 373–381.

Tate, D. F., and Zabinski, M. F. (2004). Computer and Internet applications for psychological treatment: update for clinicians. *J Consult Clin Psychol, 60(2),* 209–20.

Vandelanotte, C., Spathonis, K. M., Eakin, E. G., and Owen, N. (2007). Website-delivered physical activity interventions: A review of the literature. *Am J Prev Med, 33(1),* 54–64.

Van den Berg, M. H., Schoones, J. W., and Vliet Vlieland, T. P. (2007). Internet-based physical activity interventions: a systematic review of the literature. *J Med Internet Res, 9(3),* e26.

van Uden-Kraan, C. F., Drossaert, C. H., Taal, E., Seydel, E. R., and van de Laar, M. A. (2009a). Participation in online patient support groups endorses patients' empowerment. *Patient Educ Couns, 74(1),* 61–69.

van Uden-Kraan, C. F., Drossaert, C. H., Taal, E., Smit, W. M., Moens, H. B. et al (2009b). Health-related Internet use by patients with somatic diseases: frequency of use and characteristics of users. *Inform Health Soc Care, 34,* 18–29.

Velicer, W. F., Prochaska, J. O., Bellis, J. M., DiClemente, C. C., Rossi, J. S. et al (1993). An expert system intervention for smoking cessation. *Addict Behav, 18,* 269–290.

Wagner, B., Knaevelsrud, C., and Maercker, A. (2006). Internet-based cognitive-behavioral therapy for complicated grief: a randomized controlled trial. *Death Studies, 30,* 429–453.

Wang, C., Gonzalez, R., Milliron, K. J., Strecher, V. J., and Merajver, S. D. (2005). Genetic counseling for BRCA1/2: a randomized controlled trial of two strategies to facilitate the education and counseling process. *Am J Med Genet A, 134,* 66–73.

Wheeler, L., and Reis, H. T. (1991). Self-recording of everyday life events: origins, types, and uses. *J Personality, 59,* 339–354.

Williams-Piehota, P., Schneider, T. R., Pizarro, J., Mowad, L., and Salovey, P. (2003). Matching health messages to information processing styles: need for cognition and mammography utilization. *Health Commun, 15,* 375–392.

Chapter 65

Behavioral Medicine, Prevention, and Health Reform: Linking Evidence-Based Clinical and Public Health Strategies for Population Health Behavior Change

Judith K. Ockene and C. Tracy Orleans

1 Introduction

Tobacco use, unhealthy diet, physical inactivity, and risky alcohol use, the leading causes of chronic disease and premature death in the United States, impose a significant financial and social burden on our health-care system (Gordon et al, 2007; McGinnis and Foege, 1993; Mokdad et al, 2004; Oldridge et al, 2008). These behavioral health risks play a role in the development, treatment, and management of the nation's most costly and prevalent chronic diseases. They are most prevalent in populations with limited income and formal education, among ethnic/racial minority populations, and in under-resourced, low-income communities. Thus, health behavior change represents our single greatest hope for improving the health of the nation, reducing the nation's untenable burden, and reducing growing disparities in disease and health status. President Barack Obama made this clear in his June 15, 2009 address to the American Medical Association by noting that in addition to providing the best medical treatments to all Americans health reform efforts must increasingly focus on health behavior change for primary prevention of illness:

> Our federal government also has to step up its efforts to advance the cause of healthy living. Five

of the costliest illnesses and conditions – cancer, cardiovascular disease, diabetes, lung disease, and strokes – can be prevented. And yet only a fraction of every dollar goes to prevention or public health. That is starting to change with an investment we are making in prevention and wellness programs that can help us avoid diseases that harm our health and the health of our economy.

(Although we focus on the United States and its efforts addressing health-care reform, the principles noted could be applied to other countries that are addressing prevention in health care.) Population-wide health behavior change will require linking evidence-based individual-level clinical interventions with evidence-based population-level public health interventions. Awareness of this need is reflected in the Obama administration's definition of "health reform" which emphasizes that prevention and improving health and health care requires a two-pronged approach; that is, one that integrates clinical and public health prevention strategies. The importance of linkages also has been well articulated in the Summit on Linking Clinical Practice and the Community for Health Prevention (April 30–May 1) convened in 2008 by the United States Agency for Healthcare Research and Quality (AHRQ), the Association for State and Territorial Health Officers (ASTHO), and the American Medical Association (AMA) (Agency for Healthcare Research and Quality, Association for State and Territorial Health Officers, & Association, 2008). The focus of the Summit, as described by Dr. Steven Woolf, was to reduce the divide between health-care providers, institutions, and community resources, each of which frequently

J.K. Ockene (✉)
Division of Preventive and Behavioral Medicine, University of Massachusetts Medical School, 55, Lake Avenue North, Worcester, MA 01655-0214, USA
e-mail: judith.ockene@umassmed.edu

A. Steptoe (ed.), *Handbook of Behavioral Medicine*, DOI 10.1007/978-0-387-09488-5_65,
© Springer Science+Business Media, LLC 2010

works in silos, unaware of each other's activities because of a cultural divide. As the AHRQ Summit report put it: "Although these groups are working toward the same goal they are not working together." (Agency for Healthcare Research and Quality et al, 2008)

Linking clinical and community health behavior change interventions makes sense. As noted in the AHRQ Summit summary,

> Health care providers and institutions bring systematic identification of behaviors, brief advice, and goal setting, while community resources offer intensive assistance through skilled counselors and ongoing support. Collaborative systems offer a "win-win" arrangement: patients obtain intensive and convenient support; clinicians obtain relief from the demands of intensive counseling; and community resources receive more referrals/clients (Agency for Healthcare Research and Quality et al, 2008).

Unfortunately, the solid infrastructure of multiple components required for these linkages is often missing. However, with focused leadership, both funding and infrastructure for prevention and the linkage of clinical and public health approaches may get a boost under new health reform legislation.

In this chapter we briefly outline the growth of behavioral medicine from its origins in the mid-1980s – as a multi-disciplinary field focused on identifying the behavioral factors contributing to the prevention, treatment, and management of disease and developing individually focused clinical interventions to address them – to its current broader focus on combined clinical and public health strategies to influence health behaviors population-wide. Drawing from our experiences serving on the United States Preventive Services Task Force (USPSTF) and the Centers for Disease Control and Prevention Community Preventive Services Task Force (CTF), we describe the progress in behavioral medicine over the past 3 decades in developing and evaluating: (1) evidence-based clinical health-related lifestyle interventions and the related system changes and policies needed to assure their delivery as part of routine care and (2) effective community-based policies, programs, and environmental changes for fostering

and maintaining healthy lifestyles at the population level. In so doing, we outline the "paradigm shifts" that have taken place in understanding what the targets of effective interventions need to be to achieve meaningful and lasting changes in individual behavioral health practices, in provider and health plan delivery of recommended evidence-based clinical behavior change interventions, and in the health behaviors of populations and communities. We use examples from our experiences and the field to briefly illustrate progress in each of these spheres – clinical and public health – and in strategies to facilitate their linkage. We close with recommendations for future research and practice.

2 Behavioral Medicine and Health Behavior Change: History and Paradigms

Three Institute of Medicine (IOM) reports can be used to "bookend" critical stages in behavioral medicine's contributions to preventive health behavior change. These reports reflect the related "paradigm shifts" that have taken place in understanding what the targets of successful health behavior change programs and policies need to be – not just individual patients and individual providers, but the powerful public health contexts and health-care systems influencing their actions (Orleans and Cassidy, 2008). Each of these reports drew substantially on research and practice models developed by leaders in behavioral medicine research and practice.

Behavioral medicine's earliest approaches to health behavior change are described in the landmark 1982 United States IOM report *Health and Behavior: Frontiers of Research in the Biobehavioral Sciences* (Institute of Medicine, Hamburg et al, 1982). This seminal report was among the first to define the field of behavioral medicine and to establish the strong links between behavioral risk factors and disease. It charged behavioral medicine researchers to develop interventions that could help people change their unhealthy behaviors and improve their health outcomes. Early interventions relied heavily on individually oriented health risk education dispensed by primary care providers, emphasizing, for instance, the harms of smoking and the benefits of quitting and were based substantially on social learning models of health behavior (Bandura, 1977). The implicit underlying assumption was "if you tell them, they will change." However, the limited impact of these approaches and the growing dominance of social learning theories fueled the development of more effective multi-component techniques that combined educational, skill-based, and pharmacologic approaches.

Over the next 10 years, these effective treatments, initially delivered in multi-session face-to-face group or individual clinic sessions, were distilled into brief, lower-cost "minimal contact" primary care interventions that could be offered to all patients in a practice, health plan, or patient population (Lichtenstein and Glasgow, 1992). One major byproduct was the now famous "5-A" primary care model for health behavior change interventions – *Ask* about the health behavior; *Advise* specific changes; *Assess* readiness to quit; *Assist* with evidence-based skill-building counseling and/or medications; and *Arrange* for needed follow-up care (McGinnis and Foege, 1993). These brief office-based health behavior change counseling interventions have been recommended by the USPSTF as among the most effective and cost-effective of all clinical preventive services. But their limited reach and long-term effectiveness for tobacco use, physical activity, diet, and/or risky drinking indicated that they were not sufficient on their own to address the problem of unhealthy lifestyles and fueled a major "paradigm shift" in behavioral medicine's approach to prevention.

Almost 20 years after issuing *Health and Behavior*, the IOM published another groundbreaking report, *Promoting Health: Intervention Strategies from Social and Behavioral Research* (Institute of Medicine and Committee on Quality of Health Care in America, 2001). This report described a profound shift in understanding what the targets of successful health behavior change

interventions needed to be – not just individuals, but the powerful social contexts in which they lived, worked, and played. Drawing from a social ecological model of health behavior (Stokols, 1996), this report concluded that the field of behavioral medicine had met the challenge of developing effective clinical interventions, particularly individually oriented treatments, but it stressed the need to intervene on multiple levels – not just at the individual level – to achieve enduring population-level changes that would foster and support healthy behaviors.

The *Promoting Health* report underscored the need to modify important policies and environments at the organizational (e.g., school, worksite, health plan), community, and state and national policy levels. It emphasized that public health policies and environmental changes, such as tobacco tax increases, more stringent laws governing drinking and driving, or the creation of communities and neighborhoods with adequate sidewalks, bike paths, and healthy food access, were potentially much more powerful approaches to population-wide behavior change than those requiring active decision making by individuals. It concluded that far-reaching environmental and policy changes were required to strengthen the norms, supports, and incentives for healthy behaviors and that even the most effective individually focused and clinical interventions would continue to have limited impact without them (e.g., Orleans et al, 2003).

In the same year, the IOM's *Crossing the Quality Chasm report* (Institute of Medicine and Committee on Quality of Health Care in America, 2001) described a similar "paradigm shift" in understanding and changing the behavior of health-care providers. Until the 1990s, most clinician-focused behavior change efforts – including those aimed at boosting their delivery of evidence-based treatments – were educational, again reflecting an "if you tell them, they will change" assumption (Greco and Eisenberg, 1993). Many of these educational efforts sought to increase the proportion of primary care providers who routinely delivered evidence-based "5-A" health behavior change interventions (i.e., addressing tobacco use, diet, physical activity, alcohol use) (Coffield et al, 2001; Whitlock et al, 2002, 2004). But, few examined the critical role of office practice and wider systems. This changed in the late 1990s with the introduction of systems-based health-care quality improvement efforts.

Viewed as the charter for national health-care quality improvement in the United States, the *Quality Chasm* report shifted the focus of practice improvement interventions from educating providers to addressing the health-care system influences over provider behaviors. It concluded: "The current care system cannot do the job. Trying harder will not work. Changing systems of care will." (Institute of Medicine and Committee on Quality of Health Care in America, 2001). Coinciding with a "practice ecological model" (Crabtree et al, 1998), it stressed the need to identify and alter the powerful office practice and larger health-care system cues, prompts, supports, and incentives governing provider behavior.

The Quality Chasm report also introduced the Chronic Care Model (Fig. 65.1) as a practical model for understanding and aligning the multiple inter-locking office-level and broader health-care system supports and incentives needed to insure the consistent delivery of behaviorally focused chronic illness care and prevention (Wagner et al, 1996). Integrating "social" and "practice" ecological models, the Chronic Care Model specified the need to link practice-based provider and patient behavior change and self-management supports with community-based resources and public health policies to support and incentivize healthy behaviors at the population level.

The next three sections of this chapter briefly describe behavioral medicine's major contributions to the development of evidence-based clinical and public health interventions to foster healthy lifestyles. Reflecting the field's evolution and major paradigm shifts this review also highlights behavioral medicine's contributions to the integration of effective broad-spectrum clinical and public health models. It concludes with recommendations for the research and practice leadership needed to realize the full potential of evidence-based prevention particularly at a time when prevention is being positioned in the United States by the Obama administration as the backbone of health reform.

3 Evidence-Based Clinical and Public Health Behavior Change Interventions and Guidelines

The last 2-plus decades of rigorous behavioral medicine research have been systematically reviewed and synthesized by two national expert

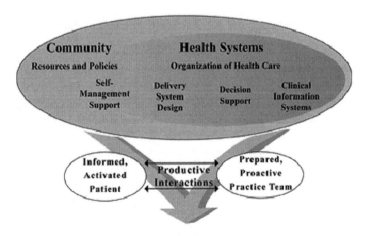

Fig. 65.1 The Chronic Care Model

Table 65.1 Clinical and community guides review of complementary interventions

Prevention strategy	Task force
Clinical screening, counseling, preventive medication	US Preventive Services Task Force
Health system change	
Community	Task Force on Community
Group education	Preventive Services
Policy change	
Environmental change	

panels, the USPSTF (Agency for Healthcare Research and Quality, 2005) and the CTF based at the Center for Disease Control and Prevention (CDC) (Institute of Medicine, 2009). These are the principal US agencies charged with the responsibility for developing national clinical and public health practice standards (Table 65.1). Their roles are to translate high-quality programmatic research into evidence-based guidelines and standards for national health care. The interventions they recommend are regarded as the kind of "top tier" evidence-based practices and programs that the White House Office of Management and Budget has identified as most worthy of federal funding (Orszag, 2009).

The USPSTF and CTF are convened and supported by the Agency for Healthcare Research and Quality (AHRQ) and the Centers for Disease Control and Prevention (CDC), respectively. Members of both task forces are nonfederal experts (including behavioral medicine specialists) drawn from academia, state and local governments, and the private sector, and both task forces work closely with a range of federal and nonfederal experts in science, program, and policy. Their recommendations are made on the basis of systematic reviews of a body of high-quality published research studies, and they provide essential information to providers, consumers, insurers, health plans, and government agencies for selecting and prioritizing effective preventive strategies. The reviews identify gaps in our information and suggest key areas for additional research (Ockene et al, 2007). At times like the present, when evidence-based interventions and comparative effectiveness evaluations are viewed as critical to guiding health reform and national health-care quality

improvement (Institute of Medicine, 2009), the strong behavioral medicine science base for health behavior change interventions is especially important.

The USPSTF focuses on clinical preventive services primarily delivered at the level of essentially healthy individual patients or patient cohorts seen in primary care settings, while the CTF focuses on preventive services targeted at entire communities and populations (Table 65.1) (Ockene et al, 2007). The problems of tobacco use and control, unhealthy diet, physical inactivity, risky drinking, and obesity prevention and treatment have been addressed by both task forces. Both task forces rely upon the tools of epidemiology to review the evidence and issue recommendations based on the quality of the evidence and the magnitude of intervention effects (Fielding and Teutsch, 2009). Their work is complementary and somewhat coordinated, though their recommendations and activities are independent, cover different domains, and are reported separately (Table 65.1).

3.1 The United States Preventive Services Task Force (USPSTF)

The USPSTF recommendations concern clinical preventive services focusing on preventive screening, medication, immunization, and health behavior change counseling in predominantly healthy patient populations. Each review is guided by an "analytic framework" or logic model to help determine whether a body of evidence indicates that a particular clinical service or intervention would improve health outcomes if implemented in a general patient population.

Well-designed randomized clinical trials are considered the "gold standard" for evaluating an intervention's effectiveness, though other controlled research designs also are included. The priority placed on the randomized clinical trial in the hierarchy of evidence driving national practice and policy is reinforced by the recent recommendations of the Coalition for Evidence-Based Policy (Coalition for Evidence-Based Policy, 2009). However, very few studies, even randomized clinical trials, provide direct evidence for determining that the intervention, such as breast cancer screening or counseling or pharmacotherapeutic treatments to promote tobacco use cessation or aspirin chemoprophylaxis to prevent acute myocardial infarction, improves ultimate health outcomes. Therefore, the task force also must consider indirect evidence, using an "analytic framework," to lay out a "chain of evidence" linking the clinical intervention to key intermediate and distal health outcomes. The quality of the individual studies used in this chain of evidence is assessed, and the overall strength of available evidence for each link is evaluated.

Evidence for benefits and possible harms of varied preventive interventions, including those aimed at health behavior change, are assessed and recommendations are made for services where evidence is sufficient to determine that benefits exceed harms. In cases where benefits are found to exceed harms, "A" or "B" recommendations are made (i.e., do it). The grade "C" is given when population benefits are smaller (i.e., do it selectively). When harms outweigh benefits a "D" recommendation is made (i.e., don't do it). The grade "I" denotes insufficient evidence to determine effectiveness (see Table 65.2). "I" statements tell researchers more work must be done in this area and identify critical gaps that new research must address. We will return to these statements and research needs later in this chapter. Current recommendations and clinical considerations are published annually in the *Guide to Clinical Preventive Services*. The current clinical guide and other clinical

preventive services products can be accessed at www.preventiveservices.ahrq.gov. (Agency for Healthcare Research and Quality, 2009)

As a result of decades of focused and rigorous behavioral medicine research, task force recommendations for primary care health behavior change interventions have been issued for most of the primary behavioral health risks. These recommendations and ratings have ranged from "A" for tobacco use and cessation counseling and medication, to "B" for dietary counseling, high-intensity obesity counseling, and counseling for risky drinking, to "I" for low-intensity and moderate-intensity treatment for obesity and physical activity counseling (www.preventiveservices.ahrq.gov) (Agency for Healthcare Research and Quality, 2009). The task force has not reviewed or made specific recommendations for interventions for multiple risk health behavior change other than for those used to prevent and treat obesity and diabetes and their broader complications (e.g., diet and physical activity).

3.2 The Community Preventive Services Task Force (CTF)

The CTF reviews the evidence for preventive interventions designed to improve health across a wide range of topics, including the leading behavioral risk factors for disease (e.g., tobacco and alcohol use, sedentary lifestyle, unhealthy diet, violence, motor vehicle injuries) at the level of a community or population (Teutsch and Briss, 2005); (Centers for Disease Control and Prevention, 2009). Interventions to promote health that are reviewed range from health-care policy and system changes and supports to improve the delivery of effective USPSTF-recommended clinical interventions (e.g., patient- and provider-oriented screening reminder systems, insurance coverage for effective clinical preventive services) to broader changes in public laws and policies that target schools, worksites, other organizations, or entire communities (e.g., smoke-free indoor air laws,

Table 65.2 United States Preventive Services Task Force Grades and Definitions (Agency for Healthcare Research and Quality, 2008)

Grade	Grade Definition	Suggestion for Practice
A	The USPSTF recommends the service. There is high certainty that the net benefit is substantial.	Offer or provide this service.
B	The USPSTF recommends the service. There is high certainty that the net benefit is moderate or there is moderate certainty that the net benefit is moderate to substantial.	Offer or provide this service.
C	The USPSTF recommends against routinely providing the service. There may be considerations that support providing the service in an individual patient. There is moderate or high certainty that the net benefit is small.	Offer or provide this service only if there are other considerations in support of the offering or providing the service in an individual patient.
D	The USPSTF recommends against the service. There is moderate or high certainty that the service has no net benefit or that the harms outweigh the benefits.	Discourage the use of this service.
I	The USPSTF concludes that the current evidence is insufficient to assess the balance of benefits and harms of the service. Evidence is lacking, of poor quality, or conflicting, and the balance of benefits and harms cannot be determined.	If offered the service, patients should understand the uncertainty about the balance of benefits and harms. Read "Clinical Considerations" section of USPSTF Recommendation Statement.

laws governing drinking and driving, school physical activity requirements, and school food standards).

Because RCTs are more difficult to conduct in studies of organizational, community, state, and national interventions, especially those involving policy and environmental changes, the CTF reviews studies with a greater range of designs than does the USPSTF (e.g., case control, quasi-experimental). Like the USPSTF, the CTF favors studies with adequate internal and external validity, especially those conducted in typical or "real world" health care or community settings. It also employs conceptual models and analytic frameworks to evaluate the evidence for hypothesized relationships between specific preventive interventions and their intermediate and distal health outcomes and to assess both benefits and harms (Teutsch and Briss, 2005).

Again, drawing on a large body of programmatic behavioral medicine-public health research, the CTF has issued evidence-based recommendations addressing all of the primary behavioral health risks (Centers for Disease Control and Prevention, 2009; Teutsch and Briss, 2005). For tobacco use, they include smoking bans and restrictions, increasing the unit price for tobacco products, mass media anti-tobacco campaigns combined with other interventions, restrictions on minors' access to tobacco products, use of health-care provider reminder systems, reductions in patient out-of-pocket costs for effective cessation therapies, and the use of multi-component cessation interventions that include telephone quitline support. For physical activity, they include informational approaches (community-wide campaigns, point of decision prompts), behavioral and social approaches to increasing physical activity (increasing the amount of moderate to vigorous physical activity in school physical education classes, individually adapted health behavior change programs, social support interventions in community settings), and environmental and policy approaches (creation of enhanced access to places for physical activity combined with informational outreach; and community- and street-scale urban design and land use policies). For alcohol, the CTF recommends a number of interventions limiting alcohol access to reduce and prevent risky drinking: regulating alcohol outlet density, increasing alcohol taxes, enacting and enforcing laws preventing sales to minors, and maintaining limits on days of sale. And while no evidence-based recommendations have yet been made for improving healthy eating or nutrition, two recommendations have been issued for multiple risk interventions found to reduce or prevent obesity: worksite programs to control overweight and obesity and behavioral interventions to reduce screen time (i.e., time watching TV, working on a computer screen, playing videogames, using the Internet) while simultaneously reducing sedentary activity (e.g., eating while watching TV).

3.3 Use of Evidence-Based Clinical and Public Health Behavior Change Strategies

The recommendations of both task forces for evidence-based clinical and community health behavior change interventions are regularly used by public health departments, state, local, and federal government agencies, health plans, employers, and community-based organizations to guide and support decisions about selecting and funding interventions and related research. The work of both task forces is also used as a core set of recommendations that can be tailored for particular audiences.

For example, recommendations made by the USPSTF for clinical preventive services have been prioritized by the National Commission on Prevention Priorities on the basis of their impact on clinically preventable burden and cost-effectiveness (Partnership for Prevention, 2008). The National Committee for Quality Assurance (NCQA) relied substantially on USPSTF recommendations in developing its health care effectiveness data and information set (HEDIS) measures introduced to provide

guidance and benchmarks for national health-care quality improvement efforts. The same is true for the *Employer's Guide to Health Improvement and Preventive* Services issued by the National Business Group on Health (www.businessgrouphealth.org) to provide practical advice to employers about structuring health benefits.

Similarly, the CFT's *Community Guide* is used by decision makers in a variety of clinical and public health settings to encourage use of, and funding for, effective interventions and for health-care and public health quality improvement (Teutsch and Briss, 2005). CTF recommendations have been used by the Institute of Medicine (IOM) to inform national health efforts and by public health programs (e.g., STEPS to a Healthier US, http://www.healthierus.gov/steps/) to inform ongoing public health activities. And they will be used increasingly as a guide to federal funding for evidence-based community interventions under the Obama administration. Peter Orszag, director of the White House Office of Management and Budget has made clear that it will be recommending more federal funding for "top tier" (recommended, evidence-based) community and public health programs found to "generate results" and "backed up by strong evidence." See: http://www.whitehouse.gov/omb/blog/09/06/08/BuildingRigorousEvidencetoDrivePolicy/.

An excellent example of how the work of both task forces now has been effectively linked can be found in state and national efforts that link clinical and community interventions to prevent and reduce tobacco use (M. Fiore et al, 2000). The CDC's 2007 "Best Practices for Comprehensive Tobacco Control Programs" recommends a set of integrated evidence-based clinical, community and state programs and policies, including mass media campaigns, cessation interventions, smoke-free air laws, and tobacco tax increases. Similarly, USPSTF clinical recommendations to reduce risky drinking on college campuses and the harms of alcohol use have been linked to CDC recommendations for policies limiting alcohol access on college campuses and surrounding communities. And USPSTF and CDC recommendations propose a range of clinical and community-oriented approaches that can be linked for maximum impact – from individually adapted behavioral interventions to creating more activity-friendly sidewalks, bike paths, parks, and playgrounds. In fact, these kinds of land use and community design changes are woven into proposed 2009 health reform legislation – legislation that explicitly seeks to link clinical health-care reforms with community public health reforms as part of broad new efforts to keep Americans healthy (Solomon, Standish, and Orleans, 2009).

While tremendous progress has been made in the development of evidence-based interventions at the clinical and community levels for behaviors such as tobacco use, problem alcohol use, and physical activity, there are gaps in evidence for these and other behaviorally related problems and in models that effectively link clinical and community-based services (Goldstein et al, 2004; Ockene et al, 2007). Perhaps the prime example is obesity prevention and control (Fielding and Teutsch, 2009). Finally, as Brownson and colleagues (Brownson et al, 2006; Glasgow et al, 2006; Klesges et al, 2007) point out, most of the well-controlled studies on which evidence-based recommendations are based have emphasized internal validity over external validity, contributing to difficulties translating from research to policy and practice, especially for assisting the underserved populations and communities in which behavioral health risks are most prevalent.

The remainder of this chapter presents examples of tested methods for linking comprehensive clinical and community-based services, with some conclusions about how far we have come and how far we still need to go to realize the full potential of combined or linked evidence-based clinical and public health strategies for health behavior change. Findings show that in addition to continued leadership and creativity, new funding and infrastructure for these innovations will be critical if we are to achieve the full benefit of the broader health reform vision now put forth in the new health care legislation

for the United States – a vision that links effective clinical *and* public health efforts to support healthy lifestyles and spreads health-promoting policies and environments. Clinical and public health leaders both must deliver this message to legislators and funding agencies.

4 Linking Evidence-Based Clinical and Community Strategies

In a growing number of reports, the IOM has recommended a multi-level perspective for health behavior change interventions, based on partnerships across health systems, communities, academia, business, and the media, in order to effectively improve the health of the population (Institute of Medicine, Committee on Immunization Finance Policies and Practices, and Division of Health Care Services and Division of Health Promotion and Disease, 2000; Institute of Medicine and Committee on Quality of Health Care in America, 2001). As noted earlier in this chapter, these recommendations are based on a cumulative body of behavioral medicine and related public health research showing that health behavior change interventions are most effective when they are broad-spectrum and cover multi-level determinants of healthy behavior and of provider practice patterns. Promising examples of linkage are described below.

4.1 Multiple Risk Health Behavior Change

Several informative "case studies" for effective linkages come from the Robert Wood Johnson Foundation (RWJF) *Prescription for Health* initiative, which was designed, implemented, and funded collaboration with the Agency for Healthcare Research and Quality. Informed by the Chronic Care Model (Glasgow et al, 2001; Wagner et al, 1996) *Prescription for Health* solicited and funded 27 studies developed by primary care practice-based research networks

(PBRNs) to discover and test innovative ways to help patients improve their health behaviors. Investigators working in "real world" practice-based research networks (PBRNs) developed and tested varied methods that would link practice-based clinical health behavior change counseling with community-based follow-up care to help their patients change two or more health behaviors: tobacco use, sedentary lifestyle, unhealthy diet, and/or risky drinking. Projects funded in Round 1 demonstrated that practices could identify at-risk patients and motivate them to make changes (Cifuentes et al, 2005; Woolf et al, 2005). In Round 2, grantees created linkages between clinical practices and community resources to help patients adopt and sustain healthier lifestyle behaviors. Each project required policy and environmental changes in the practice (e.g., reminder systems, patient registries, performance incentives) to facilitate provider delivery of evidence-based counseling and related treatments and to facilitate patient use of needed follow-up care and support from appropriate community services and resources.

One *Prescription for Health* project created a Community Health Educator Referral Liaison (CHERL) to link primary care patients receiving clinical treatments for multiple risk behaviors with diverse community resources for additional help with health behavior change (Holtrop et al, 2008). Patients with risky health behaviors were identified using routine screening questionnaires administered by the practice then subsequently referred to "CHERL" – a service that contacted them and provided patient-centered and motivational telephone-based behavior change support as well as referrals to other resources. With patient consent, *CHERL* provided confidential feedback about the patient to the practice's referring clinician. Patients who had access to a *CHERL* showed significant improvements in diet and physical activity (Holtrop et al, 2008).

A second *Prescription for Health* project, conducted by the Virginia Ambulatory Care Outcomes Research Network (ACORN), created "*eLinkS*" – an electronic linkage system designed to help physicians with the "assist" and "arrange" steps of the 5-As. A range of community organizations that were able to help offer behavior change assistance and follow-up support and interventions are identified. Automated electronic medical records (EMR) were used to link counselors and clinicians and to help counselors contact patients to provide proactive counseling via EMR prompts. Three options for health behavior change counseling were compared with usual care: access to a computer-based information library with e-counseling options, telephone counseling, and face-to-face group classes. Patients who enrolled in the program had lost significantly more weight at follow-up and were significantly more likely to quit smoking than usual care patients. Unfortunately, after funding ended, when patients were given an opportunity to continue using follow-up services for a fee, enrollment declined.

In both of the above examples, successful mechanisms for linking evidence-based primary care 5-A health behavior change counseling with follow-up community assistance and support were created and used, and in each case they led to significant improvements in the delivery of proven behavioral medicine interventions, and in at least some measures of health behavior change. Etz and colleagues (2008) analyzed eight Round 2 Prescription for Health projects and found that each team noted linkage design and implementation challenges that had to be repeatedly addressed, including the need for considerable assistance from outside the practice to initiate and maintain the program, for sustained good communication, and for financial resources. Similarly Orleans and colleagues (2006, p. 104) observed that "whether it is referring patients to quitlines or to other community services outside the practice, an effective system...could rarely be cobbled together by the practices themselves."

4.2 Tobacco Cessation and Control

A growing number of primary care practices, provider organizations, and health plans are using strategies guided by the Chronic

Care Model (Fig. 65.1) (Wagner et al, 1996) to integrate evidence-based clinical health behavior change interventions not only with community-based individual health behavior change resources, but also with efforts to implement health-promoting community policies and environments. Some of the most compelling examples come from the area of tobacco cessation and control (e.g., Institute of Medicine and Committee on Quality of Health Care in America, 2001; Smedley and Syme, 2001).

Nationally, rates of smoking have been significantly reduced over the last 40 years among adults through the combined effects of the individual-oriented clinical and community-focused public health interventions. Many successful examples have linked CTF-recommended health-care system and policy changes that facilitate and support provider adherence to USPSTF treatment guidelines with CTF-recommended community policy and environmental changes that facilitate and support patient adherence to recommended personal health practices (e.g. by banning smoking in bars, restaurants, and workplaces, and raising taxes on cigarettes). The examples that follow illustrate a variety of successful linkages at the practice, health plan, community, and state levels.

4.2.1 Practice-Level

The CTF, USPSTF, and USPHS tobacco treatment guidelines all recommend providing access to proactive telephone quitline counseling services as an evidence-based public health approach to tobacco use and addiction. Research and science-based advocacy by behavioral medicine experts led to the development and dissemination of proactive quitlines and to the federal policy implemented by US DHHS Secretary Tommy Thompson in 2004 mandating the creation of a network of state quitlines that would provide tobacco users in all 50 states, Puerto Rico, and the District of Columbia, with access to cost-free proactive quitline counseling (1-800-QUIT-NOW) (Fiore

et al, 2004). A 2005 survey of US state quitlines documented that 70% of state quitlines offered not just free counseling, but also (for eligible adults) free or low-cost cessation medication ((North American Quitline Consortium, 2006). Integrating evidence-based clinical services with evidence-based community public health resources, one of the projects in the RWJF *Prescription for Health* program used "faxed" telephone quitline referrals for the most time-consuming component, (i.e., assist), required by the "5-A" intervention model, cessation counseling essentially condensing it to "Ask-Advise-Refer" (Orleans et al, 2006). Similar models have become the norm for a variety of office practices and health plans across the country (Swartz et al, 2005). An and colleagues (2008) recently tested an innovative practice-based policy for increasing clinician quitline referral in a randomized trial comparing usual care ($n=25$ clinics) with matched clinics that offered a significant cash payment for 50 quitline referrals each ($n=24$ clinics). Providers in pay-for-performance clinics referred significantly more patients.

4.2.2 Health Plan Level

Successful combined clinical community approaches to screening and treatment for tobacco use and dependence, pioneered at Group Health Cooperative of Puget Sound, have been described using the Chronic Care Model (Glasgow et al, 2001). This staff-model Health Maintenance Organization (HMO) strategy employed each Chronic Care Model elements as follows:

- *Health-care organization* leaders made reducing tobacco use their top prevention priority, provided financial and other incentives to providers (including hiring dedicated clinic counselors), and eliminated patient co-pays for cessation counseling.
- *Clinical information systems* were used to create a registry of the tobacco users enrolled in the health plan, track their use of treatment

resources and programs, and generate proactive (i.e., outreach) telephone quitline calls for patients with feedback reports for providers.

- *Decision support tools* included extensive provider training, ongoing consultation, automated patient assessment and guideline algorithms, and reminder tools.
- *Practice re-design and self-management support* included self-help materials, face-to-face cessation clinics, and an HMO-based telephone quitline to deliver counseling and/or pharmacotherapy without burdening providers.
- *Community resources and policies* included referrals to community and local employer quit smoking clinics, worksite health promotion programs, and advocacy for increased state tobacco taxes and tax-based revenues for statewide tobacco control programs.

These integrated health plan, office, and community strategies dramatically reduced the prevalence of smoking among HMO enrollees from 25% in 1985 to 15.5% in 1993 with significant declines in smokers' use of inpatient and outpatient health-care services for tobacco-related diseases and conditions. Other health plans have achieved similar results using similar integrated clinical health-care system and public health community interventions, including Provident Health Systems in Portland, Oregon, Kaiser Permanente of Northern California and Health Partners in Minnesota (Amundson et al, 2005; Bentz, 2000; Schroeder, 2005).

4.2.3 Community Level

The CTF has recommended numerous evidence-based tobacco control policies as effective in increasing quitting and/or treatment use: tobacco tax increases, comprehensive clean indoor air laws, health-care benefits that reduce out-of-pocket treatment costs, and cessation media campaigns (Centers for Disease Control and Prevention, 2007). Capitalizing on these findings, in 2002, the New York City Department of Health combined a strong clean indoor air law with sizeable state and local tobacco tax increases, a primary care physician educational campaign, a citywide cessation media campaign that targeted low-income populations with higher smoking rates, and the promotion of free quitline services with a nicotine replacement therapy (patch) give-away program. The result was an 11% decline over 1 year in the city-wide smoking rate from 2002 to 2003 (the fastest drop in US smoking rates ever recorded) and a 15% decline over 2 years, from 2002 to 2004, producing 200,000 new ex-smokers and averting an estimated 60,000 premature deaths (Miller et al, 2005). By 2008, only 15.8% of adult New Yorkers smoked, down from 21.5% in 2002, representing a total drop of 350,000 smokers (Hartocollis, 2009)

4.2.4 State Level

An example of a statewide comprehensive coordinated tobacco treatment and control program is the statewide Massachusetts Tobacco Control Program (MTCP) (Robbins et al, 2002) funded by the 1992 Massachusetts Tobacco Tax Initiative that raised the state excise tax by 25 cents per pack and by the 1998 Master Settlement Agreement (Koh et al, 2005). Recognized by the Centers for Disease Control and Prevention (CDC) and others as a "best practice" program from its inception in 1993 through 2002, MTCP has incorporated clinical and community strategies, combining and connecting activities of clinical settings, the media, community agencies, academic institutions, and local and state policymakers. The MTCP included: (1) an innovative media campaign to change public opinion and community norms around tobacco use; (2) community mobilization to change local laws and health policies such as clean indoor air laws and restrictions on youth access; and (3) comprehensive tobacco treatment programs in clinics and community settings based on USPSTF, CTF, and USPHS guidelines to reduce tobacco use. A comparison of Massachusetts data to data for 40 states in the United States that had not had state programs in place through 1999

showed a more rapid decline in smoking prevalence in Massachusetts than in comparison states
during that time (Biener et al, 2000). Although
funding for the MTCP program was with-
drawn in 2002, a special tobacco treatment program, QuitWorks (Centers for Disease Control
and Prevention, 2004; Warner et al, 2002),
still exists. QuitWorks coordinates clinical and
community-based efforts by linking patients,
clinicians, and a proactive telephone counseling
quitline through the use of forms faxed to the
quitline. It is a collaboration of the MTCP and
major health plans in Massachusetts. Funding
is provided by the Massachusetts Department
of Public Health with funds allocated from the
legislature, the CDC, and the health plans.

5 Recommendations for the Future for Behavioral Medicine Research and Practice

Throughout this chapter we have discussed
the many contributions made to clinical and
community preventive services by behavioral
medicine researchers. We also have noted that
there remain gaps in evidence and in the linkage
and implementation of evidence-based clinical
and public health behavior change interventions. Each of the noted "gaps," i.e., limited
evidence for effective interventions for some
behaviors, limited evidence of effective linkages,
and weak external validity, represents important directions for behavioral medicine research
and practice. Addressing them will require new
behavioral medicine research and research funding paradigms and more visible and effective
behavioral medicine advocacy for the funding, resources, and infrastructure needed to
reap the full benefit of science-based interventions. As we go forward, we will need stronger
links between public health and behavioral
medicine practitioners, and more practice-based
research in "real world" settings like PBRNs and
Prescription for Health, especially in high-risk
underserved populations. Two-way relationships

will be needed between practitioners, policy
makers, and researchers, including those charged
with making decisions about health-care systems changes and policies, to assure that the
most policy-relevant questions are addressed,
including those about the costs and feasibility of
program implementation (Brownson et al, 2006).
Finally, as behavioral medicine researchers, we
must become more directly involved in translating gains in the science of clinical and community prevention to gains in public policy. We have
an unprecedented window of opportunity given
the growing recognition at all levels of health
care and government that clinical and community interventions that promote and support
healthy behaviors will be essential for success in
reducing the nation's most prevalent and costly
health problems and untenable health-care costs
and disparities. This is the kind of opportunity
that propelled the founders of our field 25 years
ago, and we are better prepared than ever in our
history to seize it.

Acknowledgments The views in this chapter do not
necessarily reflect those of the Robert Wood Johnson
Foundation or the University of Massachusetts Medical
School.

References

Agency for Healthcare Research and Quality.
  (2005). U.S. Preventive Services Task Force.
  Retrieved June 2, 2005, from http://www.ahrq.gov/
  clinic/uspstfix.htm
Agency for Healthcare Research and Quality.
  (2008). U.S. Preventive Services Task Force
  Grade Definitions. [Electronic Version] from
  http://www.ahrq.gov/clinic/uspstf/grades.htm.
Agency for Healthcare Research and Quality.
  (2009). Guide to Clinical Preventive Services.
  Retrieved September 28, 2009, from
  www.preventiveservices.ahrq.gov
Agency for Healthcare Research and Quality, Association
  for State and Territorial Health Officers, and
  Association, A. M. (2008). *Summit on Linking
  Clinical Practice and the Community for Health
  Promotion* (Meeting). Baltimore, MD.
Amundson, G., Gentilli, S., and Wehrle, D.
  (2005). Health Partners 2005 Clinical Indicators
  Report. 13. Retrieved October 6, 2009, from
  http://www.healthpartners.com/files/28455.pdf

An, L. C., Bluhm, J. H., Foldes, S. S., Alesci, N. L., Klatt, C. M. et al (2008). A randomized trial of a pay-for-performance program targeting clinician referral to a state tobacco quitline. *Arch Intern Med, 168,* 1993–1999.

Bandura, A. (1977). *Social Learning Theory.* Englewood Cliffs, NJ: Prentice-Hall.

Bentz, C. J. (2000). Implementing tobacco tracking codes in an individual practice association or a network model health maintenance organisation. *Tob Control, 9 Suppl 1,* I42-I45.

Biener, L., Harris, J., and Hamilton, W. (2000). Impact of the Massachusetts tobacco control programme: population based trend analysis. *Brit Med J, 321,* 351–354.

Brownson, R. C., Royer, C., Ewing, R., and McBride, T. D. (2006). Researchers and policymakers: travelers in parallel universes. *Am J Prev Med, 30,* 164–172.

Centers for Disease Control and Prevention. (2009). The Community Guide: Guide to Community Preventive Services. Retrieved September 28, 2009, from http://www.thecommunityguide.org/index.html

Centers for Disease Control and Prevention. (2004). *Telephone Quitlines: A Resource for Development, Implementation and Evaluation.* Atlanta: U.S. Department of Health and Human Services, National Center for Chronic Disease and Health Promotion, Office of Smoking and Health.

Centers for Disease Control and Prevention. (2007). Decline in Smoking Prevalence – New York City, 2002–2006. *MMWR, 56,* 604–608.

Cifuentes, M., Fernald, D. H., Green, L. A., Niebauer, L. J., Crabtree, B. F. et al (2005). Prescription for health: changing primary care practice to foster healthy behaviors. *Ann Fam Med, 3 Suppl 2,* S4–S11.

Coalition for Evidence-Based Policy. (2009). What Works and What Doesn't Work in Social Policy? Findings From Well-Designed Randomized Controlled Trials. Retrieved September 28, 2009, from http://www.evidencebasedprograms.org/static/

Coffield, A. B., Maciosek, M. V., McGinnis, J. M., Harris, J. R., Caldwell, M. B. et al (2001). Priorities among recommended clinical preventive services. *Am J Prev Med, 21,* 1–9.

Crabtree, B. F., Miller, W. L., Aita, V. A., Flocke, S. A., and Stange, K. C. (1998). Primary care practice organization and preventive services delivery: a qualitative analysis. *J Fam Pract, 46,* 403–409.

Etz, R. S., Cohen, D. J., Woolf, S. H., Holtrop, J. S., Donahue, K. E. et al (2008). Bridging primary care practices and communities to promote healthy behaviors. *Am J Prev Med, 35,* S390–S397.

Fielding, J. E., and Teutsch, S. M. (2009). Integrating clinical care and community health: delivering health. *JAMA, 302,* 317–319.

Fiore, M., Bailey, W., Cohen, S., Dorfman, S., Goldstein, M., Gritz, E. et al (2000). *Treating Tobacco Use and Dependence. Clinical Practice Guideline.* Rockville,

MD: US Department of Health and Human Services, Public Health Services.

Fiore, M. C., Croyle, R. T., Curry, S. J., Cutler, C. M., Davis, R. M. et al (2004). Preventing 3 million premature deaths, helping 5 million smokers quit: a national action plan for tobacco cessation. *Am J Public Health, 94,* 205–211.

Glasgow, R., Orleans, C., Wagner, E., Curry, S., and Solberg, L. (2001). Does the chronic care model serve also as a template for improving prevention? *Milbank Quart, 79,* 579–612.

Glasgow, R. E., Klesges, L. M., Dzewaltowski, D. A., Estabrooks, P. A., and Vogt, T. M. (2006). Evaluating the impact of health promotion programs: using the RE-AIM framework to form summary measures for decision making involving complex issues. *Health Educ Res, 21,* 688–694.

Glasgow, R. E., Orleans, C. T., and Wagner, E. H. (2001). Does the chronic care model serve also as a template for improving prevention? *Milbank Q, 79,* 579–612, iv–v.

Goldstein, M. G., Whitlock, E. P., and DePue, J. (2004). Multiple behavioral risk factor interventions in primary care. Summary of research evidence. *Am J Prev Med, 27 Suppl,* 61–79.

Gordon, L., Graves, N., Hawkes, A., and Eakin, E. (2007). A review of the cost-effectiveness of face-to-face behavioural interventions for smoking, physical activity, diet and alcohol. *Chronic Illn, 3,* 101–129.

Greco, P. J., and Eisenberg, J. M. (1993). Changing physicians' practices. *N Engl J Med, 329,* 1271–1273.

Hartocollis, A. (2009, September 14). Couch potatoes are next challenge for health chief. *New York Times,* p. 15.

Holtrop, J. S., Dosh, S. A., Torres, T., and Thum, Y. M. (2008). The community health educator referral liaison (CHERL): a primary care practice role for promoting healthy behaviors. *Am J Prev Med, 35 Suppl,* S365–S372.

Institute of Medicine (2009). *Initial National Priorities for Comparative Effectiveness Research.* Washington, DC.

Institute of Medicine, Committee on Immunization Finance Policies and Practices, and Division of Health Care Services and Division of Health Promotion and Disease. (2000). *Calling the Shots: Immunization Finance Policies and Practices.* Washington, DC: National Academy Press.

Institute of Medicine, and Committee on Quality of Health Care in America. (2001). *Crossing the Quality Chasm: A New Health System for the 21st Century.* Washington, DC: National Academy Press.

Institute of Medicine, Hamburg, D. A., Elliot, G. R., and Parron, D. L. (1982). *Health and Behavior: Frontiers of Research in the Biobehavioral Sciences.* Washington, DC: National Academy Press.

Klesges, R. C., Klesges, L. M., Vander Weg, M. W., DeBon, M., Poston, W. S. et al (2007). Characteristics of Air Force personnel who choose pharmacological aids for smoking cessation following an involuntary tobacco ban and tobacco control program. *Health Psychol, 26*, 588–597.

Koh, H. K., Judge, C. M., Robbins, H., Celebucki, C. C., Walker, D. K., and Connolly, G. N. (2005). The first decade of the Massachusetts Tobacco Control Program. *Public Health Rep, 120*, 482–495.

Lichtenstein, E., and Glasgow, R. (1992). Smoking cessation: what have we learned over the past decade? *J Consult Clin Psych, 60*, 518–527.

McGinnis, J. M., and Foege, W. H. (1993). Actual causes of death in the United States. *JAMA, 270*, 2207–2212.

Miller, N., Frieden, T. R., Liu, S. Y., Matte, T. D., Mostashari, F. et al (2005). Effectiveness of a large-scale distribution programme of free nicotine patches: a prospective evaluation. *Lancet, 365*, 1849–1854.

Mokdad, A. H., Marks, J. S., Stroup, D. F., and Gerberding, J. L. (2004). Actual causes of death in the United States, 2000. *JAMA, 291*, 1238–1245.

North American Quitline Consortium. (2006). Retrieved September 28, 2009, from http://www.naquitline.org/

Ockene, J. K., Edgerton, E. A., Teutsch, S. M., Marion, L. N., Miller, T. et al (2007). Integrating evidence-based clinical and community strategies to improve health. *Am J Prev Med, 32*, 244–252.

Oldridge, N., Furlong, W., Perkins, A., Feeny, D., and Torrance, G. W. (2008). Community or patient preferences for cost-effectiveness of cardiac rehabilitation: does it matter? *Eur J Cardiovasc Prev Rehabil, 15*, 608–615.

Orleans, C. T., and Cassidy, F. F. (2008). Health-Related Behavior. In A. P. Kovas & J. P. Knicknan (Eds.), *Health Care Delivery in the United States, 9th Ed* (pp. 267–297). New York, NY: Springer Publishing.

Orleans, C. T., Kraft, M. K., Marx, J. F., and McGinnis, J. M. (2003). Why are some neighborhoods active and others not? Charting a new course for research on the policy and environmental determinants of physical activity. *Ann Behav Med, 25*, 77–79.

Orleans, C. T., Woolf, S. H., Rothemich, S. F., Marks, J. S., and Isham, G. J. (2006). The top priority: building a better system for tobacco-cessation counseling. *Am J Prev Med, 31*, 103–106.

Orszag, P. R. (2009). Beyond economics 101: insights into healthcare reform from the Congressional Budget Office. *Healthc Financ Manage, 63*, 70–75.

Partnership for Prevention. (2008). Smoking Cessation Advice and Help To Quit. Retrieved September 28, 2009, from http://www.prevent.org/content/view/48/103/

Robbins, H., Krakow, M., and Warner, D. (2002). Adult smoking intervention programmes in Massachusetts:

a comprehensive approach with promising results. *Tob Control, 11 Suppl 2*, ii4–ii7.

Schroeder, S. A. (2005). What to do with a patient who smokes. *JAMA, 294*, 482–487.

Smedley, B. D., and Syme, S. L. (2001). Promoting health: intervention strategies from social and behavioral research. *Am J Health Promot, 15*, 149–166.

Solomon, L. S., Standish, M. B., and Orleans, C. T. (2009). Creating physical activity-promoting community environments: time for a breakthrough. *Prev Med, 36*(4), 351–357.

Stokols, D. (1996). Translating social ecological theory into guidelines for community health promotion. *Am J Health Promot, 10*, 282–298.

Swartz, S., Cowan, T., Klayman, J., Welton, M., and Leonard, B. (2005). Use and effectiveness of tobacco telephone counseling and nicotine therapy in Maine. *Am J Prev Med, 29*, 288–294.

Teutsch, S., and Briss, P. (2005). The Guide to Community Preventive Services: what works to promote health. Spanning the boundary between clinics and communities to address overweight and obesity in children. In S. Zaza, P. Briss, & K. Harris (Eds.), *Pediatrics*, Vol. 116 (pp. 240–241). New York, NY: Oxford University Press.

Wagner, E. H., Austin, B. T., and Von Korff, M. (1996). Organizing care for patients with chronic illness. *Milbank Q, 74*, 511–544.

Warner, D., Meneghetti, A., Pbert, L., Van Ness, J., DiPadova, P. et al (2002). *QuitWorks. A Department of Public Health collaboration with Eight Health Plans in Massachusetts Linking 12,000 Providers and Their Patients Who Smoke to Proactive Telephone Counseling*. Paper presented at the Proceedings of the 2002 National Conference on Tobacco or Health. p. 78 (Abstract #CESS–147), San Francisco, CA.

Whitlock, E. P., Orleans, C. T., Pender, N., and Allan, J. (2002). Evaluating primary care behavioral counseling interventions: an evidence-based approach. *Am J Prev Med, 22*, 267–284.

Whitlock, E. P., Polen, M. R., Green, C. A., Orleans, T., and Klein, J. (2004). Behavioral counseling interventions in primary care to reduce risky/harmful alcohol use by adults: a summary of the evidence for the U.S. Preventive Services Task Force. *Ann Intern Med, 140*, 557–568.

Woolf, S. H., Glasgow, R. E., Krist, A., Bartz, C., Flocke, S. A. et al (2005). Putting it together: finding success in behavior change through integration of services. *Ann Fam Med, 3 Suppl 2*, S20–S27.

Subject Index